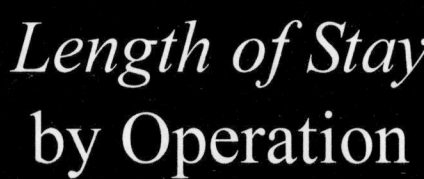

Length of Stay
by Operation
Western Region,
45th Edition

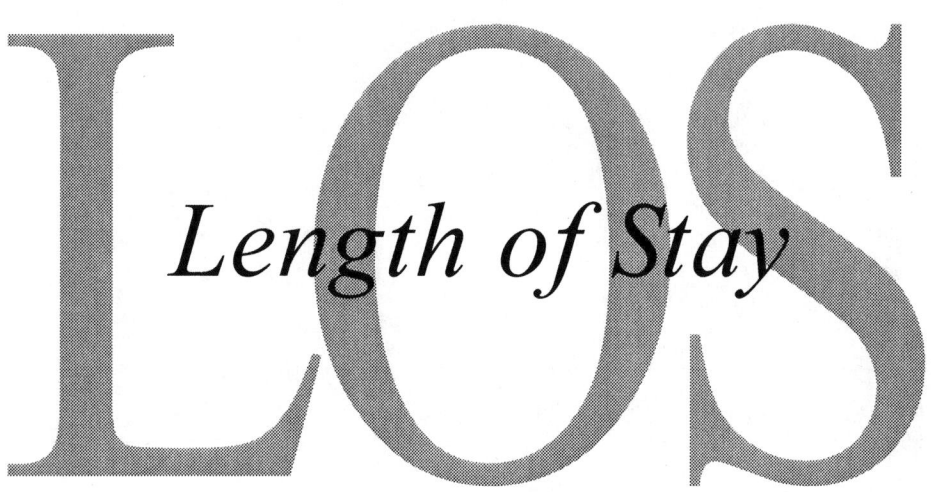

LOS

Length of Stay

ISBN   978-1-57372-427-2
ISSN   0895-9862

Statistics reported in the 45th edition are drawn from individual patient discharge records for the time period October 1, 2007, through September 30, 2008 (federal fiscal year 2008). This volume is one of the books in the *Length of Stay by Diagnosis and Operation* series

Length of Stay by Diagnosis and Operation, United States
ISSN 0895-9824

Length of Stay by Diagnosis and Operation, Northeastern Region
ISSN 0895-9838

Length of Stay by Diagnosis and Operation, North Central Region
ISSN 0895-9846

Length of Stay by Diagnosis and Operation, Southern Region
ISSN 0895-9854

Length of Stay by Diagnosis and Operation, Western Region
ISSN 0895-9862

Pediatric Length of Stay by Diagnosis and Operation, United States
ISSN 0891-1223

Thomson Reuters
777 E. Eisenhower Parkway
Ann Arbor, MI 48108
+1 800 366 7526

Length of Stay by Diagnosis and Operation, Western Region, 45th Edition

Printed and bound in the United States of America

Limitations of Thomson Reuters (The Publisher) Liability
It is understood by users of this publication that the information contained herein is intended to serve as a guide and basis for general comparisons and evaluations, but not as the sole basis upon which any specific material conduct is to be recommended or undertaken. All users of this publication agree to hold The Publisher harmless from any and all claims, losses, damages, obligations or liabilities, directly or indirectly relating to this publication, caused thereby or arising therefrom. In no event shall The Publisher have any liability for lost profits or for indirect, special, punitive, or consequential damages or any liability to any third party, even if The Publisher is advised of the possibility of such damages.

Publications Return Policy
Printed books may be returned, in good condition, for a full refund of the purchase price, within 21 days of shipment and must be pre-approved. All returns are subject to a 10% restocking fee unless otherwise approved. Shipping charges cannot be refunded. Electronic files (i.e. CDs, downloaded files (either PDF of Data Files)) are not refundable but are guaranteed against physical defects. Special order items and age-dated materials are final and cannot be returned for refund or credit. If your publication arrives damaged, or you need to return it for another reason, please call Customer Service immediately at (800) 568-3282.

ISSN 0895-9862
ISBN 978-1-57372-427-2

CONTENTS

INTRODUCTION

The *Length of Stay* Series: Real Patient Data for Powerful Decision Making

Today's health care professionals are challenged to reduce unnecessary stays and services without sacrificing quality of care. As a result, medical management continues to move toward a more aggressive style of managing inpatient care. This approach makes it essential to establish *Length of Stay* targets that are not only realistic, but based on real benchmark data that reflect the complexity of your patient population.

The *Length of Stay* (LOS) series is unique. It is the only resource based solely on objective, quantitative data that are consistent and complete across the United States. This methodology ensures that the focus is on statistical rather than anecdotal evidence. This series provides empirical data based on millions of discharges, enabling you to identify true utilization and achieve benchmark performance.

The *Length of Stay* series was created to help you provide quality care while reducing health care costs—by efficiently managing inpatient cases. With LOS percentiles and demographic breakdowns, this product is the industry's most powerful tool to determine stays by any sizable patient population—from the lowest realistic level to median stays, and stays at the highest outlier levels. While these percentiles are based on real data from actual inpatient records, other products' panel-determined goals are based on subjective analysis.

Each patient is unique, and the *Length of Stay* series allows you to factor in those differences. These LOS standards address the illness complexity and age of your patients by providing norms for both simple and more complex patients. Unlike some panel-determined goals, which address only the simple uncomplicated patient, our LOS provides figures for multiple diagnosis patients who have had a significant procedure performed and those who have not.

Designed for Easy Use

We designed the *Length of Stay by Diagnosis and Operation* series to be user-friendly. The front section of each book includes information on practical applications of the data, a step-by-step guide to using the tables, and a description of the data source. The LOS tables themselves include data organized by ICD-9-CM code and represent every diagnosis and procedure group. The tables examine average, median, and percentile length of stay for patients in five age groups, with single and multiple diagnoses or procedures, and according to whether the patient's stay included a significant procedure.

The appendices include counts of U.S. hospitals by bed size, region, census division, setting (rural or urban), and teaching intensity; a list of the states included in each LOS comparative region; and in the procedure volume, a table showing operative status of every procedure code included in the book. The glossary defines all of the terms used in the tables. An alphabetical index of diagnoses and procedures grouped according to classification categories can assist users who do not know the ICD-9-CM code for a particular diagnosis.

Length of Stay Data for a Variety of Needs

There are seven different editions of *Length of Stay*, making it easy to find the information you need. Each book in the series is updated annually.

Length of Stay by Diagnosis and Operation provides data representing every ICD-9-CM diagnosis and procedure group.

- National and regional (Northeastern, North Central, Southern, and Western) editions

- National Pediatric edition, with data for patients 19 years old and younger

Psychiatric Length of Stay by Diagnosis catalogs diagnoses unique to psychiatric and substance abuse treatment.

- National—available in electronic format only

Each title is available electronically for efficient analysis. The files load easily onto virtually any system, and give you the convenience to review, set LOS targets, and plan your utilization management quickly. With these files, you can generate custom reports and incorporate the data into your own decision support systems. Call at 800-568-3282 or send an email to healthcare.pubs@thomsonreuters.com for details.

About Thomson Reuters

Thomson Reuters is the world's leading source of intelligent information for businesses and professionals. We combine industry expertise with innovative technology to deliver critical information to leading decision makers in the financial, legal, tax and accounting, healthcare and science and media markets, powered by the world's most trusted news organization. With headquarters in New York and major operations in London and Eagan, Minnesota, Thomson Reuters employs more than 50,000 people and operates in over 100 countries. Thomson Reuters shares are listed on the Toronto Stock Exchange (TSX: TRI) and New York Stock Exchange (NYSE: TRI).

DESCRIPTION OF THE DATABASE

Thomson Reuters LOS standards are based on all-payer data gathered from more than 22 million actual inpatient records, representing more than 50 percent of discharges from U.S. hospitals annually. This detail-rich database is our Projected Inpatient Database (PIDB), which is the largest all-payer inpatient database available in the marketplace. The PIDB supports publications, products, and custom studies whose results are applicable to all short-term, general, nonfederal (STGNF) hospitals in the United States. This exclusive database combines data from both public and proprietary state data as well as individual and group hospital contracts. Updated quarterly, the PIDB is used to create the Length of Stay series and many other of our methodologies and products.

Methodology

The PIDB is created as an external, stable, consolidated database to enable users to make accurate evaluations about the entire universe of U.S. short-term, general, nonfederal (STGNF) hospitals. To make this possible, we project the data in the PIDB so that it accurately represents the universe. First, the data are standardized from all sources to create a consolidated patient record database. Then each discharge is assigned a projection factor (or weight) to indicate the number of discharges it represents. In this way, we project the data to represent the universe of all inpatient discharges.

To create the projection factors, we use the National Inpatient Sample (NIS) for creating the universe, and other sources such as the Medicare Provider Analysis and Review File (MedPAR) are used to validate the projections. NIS is a nationally representative sample produced and published by the Agency for Healthcare Research and Quality that describes the entire universe of non-federal, general (medical or surgical) or children's general, acute care hospitals in the United States. MedPAR, produced by the Centers for Medicare & Medicaid Services, contains a complete census of all Medicare inpatient discharges.

The universe of inpatients discharged from all acute care, general, non-federal U.S. hospitals is defined using NIS. The hospital characteristics are defined according to the American Hospital Association criteria:

Short-Term: The average length of stay for all patients at the facility is less than 30 days, or more than 50 percent of all patients are admitted to units in which the average length of stay is less than 30 days.

General: The primary function of the institution is to provide patient services, diagnostic and therapeutic, for a variety of medical conditions.

Nonfederal: The facility is controlled by a state, county, city, city-county, hospital district authority, or church.

U.S. hospitals include those in the 50 states and the District of Columbia. Data from long-term specialty institutions, e.g., long-term psychiatric or rehabilitation facilities, are also excluded. For the Length of Stay publications, several exclusions are applied to the average length of stay data to eliminate discharge records that do not represent a typical short-term inpatient stay. These exclusions include admission from other short-term hospitals, discharge to other short-term hospitals, discharge against medical advice, and death.

Data Quality and Validation

Data from all sources in the PIDB are standardized and run through a set of standard edit screens to ensure their quality. Examples of discrepancies detected by the audit include records with invalid diagnosis or procedure codes, invalid or unrecorded principal diagnosis, sex- or age-specific diagnosis or procedure inconsistencies, and incalculable age or length of stay. All records from hospitals with more than 5 percent of discharges failing any screen are deleted from the database.

The projection methodology ensures that the PIDB will be representative of the inpatient universe defined by NIS. Using data that were not used to create the projection factors, representativeness of the PIDB has been demonstrated at the ICD-9-CM diagnosis and procedure level as well as by MS-DRG.

To perform a comparison between PIDB data and NHDS, the weighted discharges in the PIDB were grouped within ICD-9-CM diagnosis and procedure chapters, as were the discharges in NIS. PIDB patients were compared to the NIS for the same age range. The diagnosis and procedure chapter distributions of the PIDB were found to be highly representative of NIS.

Concordance between MS-DRG-specific Medicare estimates from the PIDB and the actual Medicare counts as found in MedPAR were compared. The correlation between the PIDB and MedPAR counts is 99.9%. Because the PIDB projection methodology accounts for payer, the representativeness of the PIDB is not limited to the Medicare population, but rather is applicable across all payer types.

BENEFITS AND APPLICATIONS

The *Length of Stay* series is an invaluable standard reference for health care professionals who want to measure inpatient utilization. Using the hospital stay data found in this series, you can compare regional and national norms to an individual institution or a special population. Specifically, the *Length of Stay* series allows you to

- establish baselines (benchmarking);
- pre-authorize procedures;
- identify candidates for utilization review;
- project extended stay reviews;
- develop forecasts;
- and report lengths of stay versus benchmarks.

Patient severity, managed care market presence, and varying practice patterns all have significant impact on actual LOS statistics. As technological advances and financial pressures reduce inpatient days and increase outpatient volumes, only the most severely ill patients are left in the hospitals. Consequently, health care professionals must have detailed measurement criteria to make truly accurate, patient-focused assessments of appropriate lengths of stay.

Because the *Length of Stay* series is based on real patient data, you can tailor your LOS analyses to a particular patient age group, or compare the norms for patients with single or multiple diagnoses. You may also study regional variations, as well as specialized groups including pediatric and psychiatric patient populations. And the 10th, 25th, 50th, 75th, 95th, and 99th percentile groups enhance the average length of stay data by allowing you to pick a realistic goal for an individual patient. Our LOS data can help pinpoint whether patients are being cared for efficiently, targeting areas that may need further clinical analysis.

The proliferation of new laws regulating utilization management procedures—in part, by requiring the disclosure of criteria used—is fueling the demand for high quality data. To comply with these new legal stipulations and to track fluctuating LOS trends, utilization managers must have reliable, industry-accepted criteria sets. Because we update the *Length of Stay* series annually with millions of new patient records, it provides extremely useful trend information—including significant developments from one year to the next and over even longer periods of time. Compiled from our exclusive Projected Inpatient Database (PIDB), the largest all-payor inpatient database available in the marketplace, this series is the most comprehensive, current source for length of stay data available.

HOW TO USE THE TABLES

The data in each *Length of Stay* volume are organized numerically by the International Classification of Diseases, 9th Revision, Clinical Modification (ICD-9-CM) coding system. Each Diagnosis volume contains every diagnosis chapter (three-digit code), including both summary and valid detail codes, and the approximately 1,500 four- and five-digit codes highest in projected volume. Each Operation volume contains every procedure chapter (two-digit code) including both summary codes and valid detail codes, and the approximately 950 four-digit codes highest in projected volume.

Data are categorized by number of observed patients, average length of stay, variance, and distribution percentiles. In addition, two subtotals and a grand total are included. All data elements except the number of observed patients are calculated using the projection methodology described in the "Description of the Database" section.

Determining length of stay would be easy if all patients were identical, but they are not. Illness, complexity, age, and region of the country will cause some variation in the LOS of patients admitted with the same diagnosis or procedure. We recognize those differences and our data tables let you to do the same. The *Length of Stay* series gives you detailed length of stay breakdowns—by individual ICD-9-CM code—listed by age groups, single versus multiple diagnosis patient, and operated versus non-operated status. You can find specific length of stay norms by taking the following steps

Step 1 Find the desired ICD-9-CM code in the tables in one of the *Length of Stay* volumes. If you do not know a patient's ICD-9-CM code, refer to the index, which provides an alphabetical listing of the descriptive titles for all codes included in the book.

The **Observed Patients** column gives you the number of patients in the stratified group as reported in our projected inpatient database. "Observed" means that this data element, unlike the other elements in the LOS tables, is not projected. Patients with stays longer than 99 days (indicated as ">99") are not included.

Step 2 For each diagnosis code, patients are stratified by single or multiple diagnoses, operated or not operated status, and age. For each procedure code, patients are stratified by single or multiple diagnoses and age. Find the appropriate portion of the table for review by using the following patient information

- Number of diagnoses

- Operated status

- Age

Single or Multiple Diagnoses

More than 80 percent of all admissions are complicated (have more than one diagnosis). The data tables include rows for patients with single and multiple diagnoses. This enables you to identify stays that are realistic and on-target with the patient's unique characteristics.

Patients are classified in the multiple diagnoses category if they had at least one valid secondary diagnosis in addition to the principal one. The following codes are not considered valid secondary diagnoses for purposes of this classification

1. Manifestation codes (conditions that evolved from underlying diseases [etiology] and are in italics in ICD-9-CM, Volume 1)

2. Codes V27.0-V27.9 (outcome of delivery)

3. E Codes (external causes of injury and poisoning)

Operated or Not Operated

In the diagnosis tables, operated patients are those who had at least one procedure that is classified by CMS as an operating room procedure. CMS physician panels classify every ICD-9-CM procedure code according to whether the procedure would in most hospitals be performed in the operating room. This classification system differs slightly from that used in *Length of Stay* publications published before 1995, in which patients were categorized as "operated" if any of their procedures were labeled as Uniform Hospital Discharge Data Set (UHDDS) Class 1. Appendix C contains a list of procedure codes included in this series and their CMS-defined operative status.

Patient's Age

The data tables illustrate the impact of age by providing five age group breakouts. These ages are from the day of the patient's admission.

For diagnosis codes V30-V39, which pertain exclusively to newborns, age is replaced by birth weight in grams. Newborns with unrecorded birth weights with secondary diagnosis codes in the 764.01-764.99 and 765.01-765.19 ranges have been assigned to the appropriate birth weight category on the basis of the fifth digit of these codes. (Data for patients whose birth weights cannot be determined by using this method are included only in the Subtotal and Total rows of the table.)

Step 3 Choose from the average stay or the 10th, 25th, 50th, 75th, 95th, and 99th percentile columns to find the appropriate length of stay for your patient. Our LOS standards document the statistical range of stays for each patient group. These ranges are represented as percentiles, so that you can determine a more aggressive (benchmark) or less aggressive (norm) LOS for your patient, depending on individual variables, and are all backed by actual patient data.

Average Length of Stay

The average length of stay is calculated from the admission and discharge dates by counting the day of admission as the first day; the day of discharge is not included. The average is figured by adding the lengths of stay for each patient and then dividing by the total number of patients. Patients discharged on the day of admission are counted as staying one day. Patients with stays over 99 days (>99) are excluded from this calculation.

Median and Percentiles

A statistical range of stays are presented for each patient group. These ranges are represented as percentiles, so that you can determine a more aggressive or less aggressive LOS for your patient, depending on individual variables such as illness complications, age, etc. A length of stay percentile for a stratified group of patients is determined by arranging the individual patient stays from low to high. Counting up from the lowest stay to the point where one-half of the patients have been counted yields the value of the 50th percentile. Counting one-tenth of the total patients gives the 10th percentile, and so on.

The 10th, 25th, 50th, 75th, 90th, 95th, and 99th percentiles of stay are displayed in days. If, for example, the 10th percentile for a group of patients is four, then 10 percent of the patients stayed four days or fewer. The 50th percentile is the median. Any percentile with a value of 100 days or more is listed as >99. Patients who were hospitalized more than 99 days (>99) are not included in the total patients, average stay, and variance categories. The percentiles, however, do include these patients.

Step 4 Consult the total patient sample (**Observed Patients** column) and variance to consider the homogeneity of the data (i.e., to what extent length of stay averages are clustered or spread out within a particular patient group).

The **Total** row represents a subtotal for each of the patient age groups. The **Grand Total** row represents the total number of patients in the specified diagnosis or procedure category.

The **variance** is a measure of the spread of the data (from the lowest to the highest value) around the average. As such, it shows how much individual patient stays ranged around the average. The smallest variance is zero, indicating that all lengths of stay are equal. In tables in which there is a large variance and the patient group size is relatively small, the average stay may appear high. This sometimes occurs when one or two patients with long hospitalizations fall into the group.

FEATURES OF AN OPERATION TABLE

ICD-9-CM procedure code and title

01.1 SKULL/BRAIN DX PROCEDURE

Type of Patients	Observed Patients	Avg. Stay	Vari- ance	Percentiles						
				10th	25th	50th	75th	90th	95th	99th
1. SINGLE DX										
0–19 Years	78	4.4	20	1	1	3	6	11	11	28
20–34	62	2.6	8	1	1	1	3	5	7	14
35–49	82	4.1	21	1	1	4	4	7	10	18
50–64	92	3.5	17	1	1	2	4	7	9	26
65+	68	5.6	32	1	1	2	10	15	15	17
2. MULTIPLE DX										
0–19 Years	425	15.6	236	2	4	11	21	38	56	71
20–34	429	14.1	238	1	3	7	19	42	49	71
35–49	471	11.0	137	1	3	6	15	29	35	>99
50–64	471	8.5	77	1	3	5	9	21	31	37
65+	665	10.8	120	1	3	7	14	25	33	48
TOTAL SINGLE DX	**382**	**4.1**	**21**	**1**	**1**	**2**	**5**	**10**	**15**	**18**
TOTAL MULTIPLE DX	**2,337**	**11.7**	**159**	**1**	**3**	**7**	**16**	**29**	**40**	**62**
TOTAL										
0–19 Years	503	14.1	222	1	3	9	21	34	56	71
20–34	409	12.6	223	1	2	7	17	39	49	67
35–49	511	9.6	121	1	2	6	14	27	31	77
50–64	563	7.7	71	1	2	5	9	18	28	37
65+	733	10.4	115	1	3	7	14	25	30	48
GRAND TOTAL	**2,719**	**10.7**	**147**	**1**	**2**	**7**	**14**	**28**	**37**	**59**

Because each patient is unique, we stratify patients by single or multiple diagnoses and age.

Total number of patients

Length of stay (in days) by percentile document the statistical range of stays for each patient group, so you can determine the right length of stay for your patient.

Observed Patients is the actual number of patient discharges. We derive length of stay figures from real patient data projected to represent the inpatient universe. See "Description of the Database" for further explanation.

The variance shows how much individual patient lengths of stay ranged around the average.

Average length of stay, in days, calculated from the admission and discharge dates

LENGTH OF STAY TABLES
OPERATION CODES

SUMMARY OF ALL PATIENTS IN OPERATION CODES

Type of Patients	Observed Patients	Avg. Stay	Vari-ance	Percentiles							
				10th	25th	50th	75th	90th	95th	99th
1. SINGLE DX										
0–19 Years	116,802	2.1	2	1	1	2	2	4	5	8
20–34	203,223	2.0	2	1	1	2	2	3	4	5
35–49	36,491	2.1	4	1	1	2	2	4	5	8
50–64	22,416	2.3	5	1	1	2	3	4	5	9
65+	9,244	2.3	4	1	1	2	3	4	5	8
2. MULTIPLE DX										
0–19 Years	547,762	4.6	63	1	2	2	4	9	16	48
20–34	664,997	3.2	16	1	2	2	3	5	7	20
35–49	503,030	4.2	29	1	2	3	4	8	13	28
50–64	656,884	5.1	40	1	2	3	6	11	16	33
65+	999,706	5.5	32	1	2	4	7	11	16	28
TOTAL SINGLE DX	**388,176**	**2.1**	**2**	**1**	**1**	**2**	**2**	**3**	**4**	**7**
TOTAL MULTIPLE DX	**3,372,379**	**4.6**	**37**	**1**	**2**	**3**	**5**	**9**	**14**	**31**
TOTAL										
0–19 Years	664,564	4.1	53	1	2	2	4	7	14	43
20–34	868,220	2.9	13	1	2	2	3	4	6	18
35–49	539,521	4.1	28	1	2	3	4	8	12	27
50–64	679,300	5.0	39	1	2	3	6	10	15	32
65+	1,008,950	5.5	32	1	2	4	7	11	15	28
GRAND TOTAL	**3,760,555**	**4.4**	**34**	**1**	**2**	**3**	**5**	**9**	**13**	**30**

LOS by Diagnosis and Operation, Western Region, 45th Edition

Western Region, October 2007–September 2008 Data, by Operation

00.0: THERAPEUTIC ULTRASOUND

Type of Patients	Observed Patients	Avg. Stay	Vari-ance	Percentiles						
				10th	25th	50th	75th	90th	95th	99th
1. SINGLE DX										
0–19 Years	0									
20–34	0									
35–49	0									
50–64	1	1.0	0	1	1	1	1	1	1	1
65+	0									
2. MULTIPLE DX										
0–19 Years	0									
20–34	0									
35–49	0									
50–64	1	1.0	0	1	1	1	1	1	1	1
65+	1	2.0	0	2	2	2	2	2	2	2
TOTAL SINGLE DX	1	1.0	0	1	1	1	1	1	1	1
TOTAL MULTIPLE DX	2	1.5	<1	1	1	1	2	2	2	2
TOTAL										
0–19 Years	0									
20–34	0									
35–49	0									
50–64	2	1.0	0	1	1	1	1	1	1	1
65+	1	2.0	0	2	2	2	2	2	2	2
GRAND TOTAL	3	1.3	<1	1	1	1	2	2	2	2

00.1: PHARMACEUTICALS

Type of Patients	Observed Patients	Avg. Stay	Vari-ance	Percentiles						
				10th	25th	50th	75th	90th	95th	99th
1. SINGLE DX										
0–19 Years	8	1.0	0	1	1	1	1	1	1	1
20–34	0									
35–49	0									
50–64	2	2.0	2	1	1	1	3	3	3	3
65+	2	1.5	<1	1	1	2	2	2	2	2
2. MULTIPLE DX										
0–19 Years	75	9.8	232	2	3	5	9	26	40	90
20–34	197	5.4	41	2	3	4	5	9	11	38
35–49	474	4.8	11	2	3	4	6	8	11	16
50–64	848	5.7	26	2	4	4	6	10	15	25
65+	1,119	6.7	23	2	4	5	8	13	17	25
TOTAL SINGLE DX	12	1.2	<1	1	1	1	1	2	3	3
TOTAL MULTIPLE DX	2,713	6.1	33	2	3	5	7	11	15	27
TOTAL										
0–19 Years	83	9.0	217	1	2	4	8	18	40	90
20–34	197	5.4	41	2	3	4	5	9	11	38
35–49	474	4.8	11	2	3	4	6	8	11	16
50–64	850	5.7	26	2	3	4	6	10	15	25
65+	1,121	6.7	23	2	4	5	8	13	17	25
GRAND TOTAL	2,725	6.1	33	2	3	5	7	11	15	27

00.13: INJECT NESIRITIDE

Type of Patients	Observed Patients	Avg. Stay	Vari-ance	Percentiles						
				10th	25th	50th	75th	90th	95th	99th
1. SINGLE DX										
0–19 Years	0									
20–34	0									
35–49	0									
50–64	0									
65+	0									
2. MULTIPLE DX										
0–19 Years	0									
20–34	1	9.0	0	9	9	9	9	9	9	9
35–49	12	5.5	14	2	3	4	7	11	13	13
50–64	37	7.1	39	2	3	4	10	15	19	30
65+	164	6.0	15	2	4	5	7	11	13	19
TOTAL SINGLE DX	0									
TOTAL MULTIPLE DX	214	6.2	19	2	3	5	8	13	15	19
TOTAL										
0–19 Years	0									
20–34	1	9.0	0	9	9	9	9	9	9	9
35–49	12	5.5	14	2	3	4	7	11	13	13
50–64	37	7.1	39	2	3	4	10	15	19	30
65+	164	6.0	15	2	4	5	7	11	13	19
GRAND TOTAL	214	6.2	19	2	3	5	8	13	15	19

00.14: INJECT OXAZOL ANTIBIO

Type of Patients	Observed Patients	Avg. Stay	Vari-ance	Percentiles						
				10th	25th	50th	75th	90th	95th	99th
1. SINGLE DX										
0–19 Years	0									
20–34	0									
35–49	0									
50–64	0									
65+	0									
2. MULTIPLE DX										
0–19 Years	14	4.8	5	2	3	4	6	9	10	10
20–34	37	6.6	44	2	3	5	8	12	21	38
35–49	59	5.5	11	2	3	5	8	10	14	16
50–64	70	9.8	113	3	4	6	11	19	36	55
65+	131	7.4	27	3	4	6	9	14	17	24
TOTAL SINGLE DX	0									
TOTAL MULTIPLE DX	311	7.3	46	3	4	6	8	14	17	38
TOTAL										
0–19 Years	14	4.8	5	2	3	4	6	9	10	10
20–34	37	6.6	44	2	3	5	8	12	21	38
35–49	59	5.5	11	2	3	6	8	10	14	16
50–64	70	9.8	113	3	4	6	11	19	36	55
65+	131	7.4	27	3	4	6	9	14	17	24
GRAND TOTAL	311	7.3	46	3	4	6	8	14	17	38

Western Region, October 2007–September 2008 Data, by Operation

00.2: INTRAVASCULAR IMAGING

Type of Patients	Observed Patients	Avg. Stay	Vari-ance	Percentiles						
				10th	25th	50th	75th	90th	95th	99th
1. SINGLE DX										
0–19 Years	0									
20–34	0									
35–49	0									
50–64	0									
65+	0									
2. MULTIPLE DX										
0–19 Years	1	17.0	0	17	17	17	17	17	17	17
20–34	0									
35–49	1	3.0	0	3	3	3	3	3	3	3
50–64	8	2.4	3	1	1	1	4	6	6	6
65+	6	2.5	3	1	1	3	4	5	5	5
TOTAL SINGLE DX	**0**									
TOTAL MULTIPLE DX	**16**	**3.4**	**16**	**1**	**1**	**3**	**4**	**6**	**17**	**17**
TOTAL										
0–19 Years	1	17.0	0	17	17	17	17	17	17	17
20–34	0									
35–49	1	3.0	0	3	3	3	3	3	3	3
50–64	8	2.4	3	1	1	1	4	6	6	6
65+	6	2.5	3	1	1	3	4	5	5	5
GRAND TOTAL	**16**	**3.4**	**16**	**1**	**1**	**3**	**4**	**6**	**17**	**17**

00.3: COMPUTER ASSISTED SURG

Type of Patients	Observed Patients	Avg. Stay	Vari-ance	Percentiles						
				10th	25th	50th	75th	90th	95th	99th
1. SINGLE DX										
0–19 Years	0									
20–34	1	1.0	0	1	1	1	1	1	1	1
35–49	1	1.0	0	1	1	1	1	1	1	1
50–64	2	1.5	<1	1	1	1	2	2	2	2
65+	0									
2. MULTIPLE DX										
0–19 Years	1	7.0	0	7	7	7	7	7	7	7
20–34	0									
35–49	4	6.3	7	4	4	6	8	9	9	9
50–64	8	6.5	24	1	3	5	11	15	15	15
65+	5	5.0	12	2	3	4	5	11	11	11
TOTAL SINGLE DX	**4**	**1.3**	**<1**	**1**	**1**	**1**	**1**	**2**	**2**	**2**
TOTAL MULTIPLE DX	**18**	**6.1**	**15**	**2**	**3**	**5**	**9**	**11**	**15**	**15**
TOTAL										
0–19 Years	1	7.0	0	7	7	7	7	7	7	7
20–34	1	1.0	0	1	1	1	1	1	1	1
35–49	5	5.2	11	1	4	4	8	9	9	9
50–64	10	5.5	23	1	2	4	10	15	15	15
65+	5	5.0	12	2	3	4	5	11	11	11
GRAND TOTAL	**22**	**5.2**	**15**	**1**	**2**	**4**	**8**	**11**	**11**	**15**

00.15: HIGH-DOSE INTERLEUKIN-2

Type of Patients	Observed Patients	Avg. Stay	Vari-ance	Percentiles						
				10th	25th	50th	75th	90th	95th	99th
1. SINGLE DX										
0–19 Years	0									
20–34	0									
35–49	0									
50–64	0									
65+	0									
2. MULTIPLE DX										
0–19 Years	14	4.0	2	2	2	4	5	6	7	7
20–34	78	4.3	1	2	4	4	5	5	6	8
35–49	238	4.2	3	2	3	4	5	6	6	10
50–64	394	4.1	4	2	3	4	5	6	7	12
65+	53	4.2	4	2	4	4	5	6	6	14
TOTAL SINGLE DX	**0**									
TOTAL MULTIPLE DX	**777**	**4.2**	**3**	**2**	**3**	**4**	**5**	**6**	**6**	**10**
TOTAL										
0–19 Years	14	4.0	2	2	2	4	5	6	7	7
20–34	78	4.3	1	2	4	4	5	5	6	8
35–49	238	4.2	3	2	3	4	5	6	6	10
50–64	394	4.1	4	2	3	4	5	6	7	12
65+	53	4.2	4	2	4	4	5	6	6	14
GRAND TOTAL	**777**	**4.2**	**3**	**2**	**3**	**4**	**5**	**6**	**6**	**10**

00.17: INFUSE VASOPRESSOR AGENT

Type of Patients	Observed Patients	Avg. Stay	Vari-ance	Percentiles						
				10th	25th	50th	75th	90th	95th	99th
1. SINGLE DX										
0–19 Years	0									
20–34	0									
35–49	0									
50–64	1	1.0	0	1	1	1	1	1	1	1
65+	1	2.0	0	2	2	2	2	2	2	2
2. MULTIPLE DX										
0–19 Years	15	9.6	386	2	2	3	9	18	18	96
20–34	34	5.0	12	2	2	4	7	10	11	16
35–49	114	5.9	23	2	3	5	8	11	15	26
50–64	258	6.5	22	2	3	6	8	12	16	25
65+	707	6.8	22	2	4	6	9	13	17	25
TOTAL SINGLE DX	**2**	**1.5**	**<1**	**1**	**1**	**1**	**2**	**2**	**2**	**2**
TOTAL MULTIPLE DX	**1,128**	**6.7**	**29**	**2**	**3**	**5**	**8**	**12**	**16**	**25**
TOTAL										
0–19 Years	15	9.6	386	2	2	3	9	18	18	96
20–34	34	5.0	12	2	2	4	7	10	11	16
35–49	114	5.9	23	2	3	5	8	11	15	26
50–64	259	6.5	22	2	3	6	8	12	16	25
65+	708	6.8	22	2	4	6	9	13	17	25
GRAND TOTAL	**1,130**	**6.7**	**29**	**2**	**3**	**5**	**8**	**12**	**16**	**25**

LOS by Diagnosis and Operation, Western Region, 45th Edition

Western Region, October 2007–September 2008 Data, by Operation

00.4: ADJUNCT VASC SYST PX

Type of Patients	Observed Patients	Avg. Stay	Vari-ance	Percentiles						
				10th	25th	50th	75th	90th	95th	99th
1. SINGLE DX										
0–19 Years	0									
20–34	0									
35–49	0									
50–64	0									
65+	0									
2. MULTIPLE DX										
0–19 Years	0									
20–34	0									
35–49	2	2.0	0	2	2	2	2	2	2	2
50–64	10	3.1	13	1	1	2	3	4	13	13
65+	9	3.3	13	1	1	1	3	10	10	10
TOTAL SINGLE DX	**0**									
TOTAL MULTIPLE DX	**21**	**3.1**	**11**	**1**	**1**	**2**	**3**	**9**	**10**	**13**
TOTAL										
0–19 Years	0									
20–34	0									
35–49	2	2.0	0	2	2	2	2	2	2	2
50–64	10	3.1	13	1	1	2	3	4	13	13
65+	9	3.3	13	1	1	1	3	10	10	10
GRAND TOTAL	**21**	**3.1**	**11**	**1**	**1**	**2**	**3**	**9**	**10**	**13**

00.5: OTH CARDIOVASCULAR PX

Type of Patients	Observed Patients	Avg. Stay	Vari-ance	Percentiles						
				10th	25th	50th	75th	90th	95th	99th
1. SINGLE DX										
0–19 Years	0									
20–34	0									
35–49	6	1.8	3	1	1	1	2	5	5	5
50–64	6	1.0	0	1	1	1	1	1	1	1
65+	11	1.1	<1	1	1	1	1	1	2	2
2. MULTIPLE DX										
0–19 Years	12	5.3	103	1	1	2	5	5	10	49
20–34	59	4.9	73	1	1	2	7	10	14	61
35–49	258	4.3	25	1	1	2	6	9	13	28
50–64	1,328	4.3	30	1	1	2	6	10	16	25
65+	4,034	4.0	24	1	1	2	6	10	13	25
TOTAL SINGLE DX	**23**	**1.3**	**<1**	**1**	**1**	**1**	**1**	**2**	**2**	**5**
TOTAL MULTIPLE DX	**5,691**	**4.1**	**26**	**1**	**1**	**2**	**6**	**10**	**14**	**25**
TOTAL										
0–19 Years	12	5.3	103	1	1	2	5	5	10	49
20–34	59	4.9	73	1	1	2	7	10	14	61
35–49	264	4.2	25	1	1	2	6	9	12	28
50–64	1,334	4.3	29	1	1	2	6	10	16	25
65+	4,045	4.0	24	1	1	2	6	10	13	25
GRAND TOTAL	**5,714**	**4.1**	**26**	**1**	**1**	**2**	**6**	**10**	**14**	**25**

00.50: IMPL CRT-P TOTAL SYSTEM

Type of Patients	Observed Patients	Avg. Stay	Vari-ance	Percentiles						
				10th	25th	50th	75th	90th	95th	99th
1. SINGLE DX										
0–19 Years	0									
20–34	0									
35–49	0									
50–64	0									
65+	4	1.3	<1	1	1	1	2	2	2	2
2. MULTIPLE DX										
0–19 Years	7	2.4	2	1	1	2	4	5	5	5
20–34	8	11.2	409	1	1	4	6	61	61	61
35–49	13	4.3	15	1	1	3	7	10	13	13
50–64	86	3.4	13	1	1	2	5	8	9	22
65+	577	4.0	21	1	1	2	6	10	13	23
TOTAL SINGLE DX	**4**	**1.3**	**<1**	**1**	**1**	**1**	**2**	**2**	**2**	**2**
TOTAL MULTIPLE DX	**691**	**4.0**	**24**	**1**	**1**	**2**	**6**	**10**	**13**	**22**
TOTAL										
0–19 Years	7	2.4	2	1	1	2	4	5	5	5
20–34	8	11.2	409	1	1	4	6	61	61	61
35–49	13	4.3	15	1	1	3	7	10	13	13
50–64	86	3.4	13	1	1	2	5	8	9	22
65+	581	4.0	21	1	1	2	6	10	13	23
GRAND TOTAL	**695**	**4.0**	**24**	**1**	**1**	**2**	**6**	**10**	**13**	**22**

00.51: IMPL CRT-D TOTAL SYSTEM

Type of Patients	Observed Patients	Avg. Stay	Vari-ance	Percentiles						
				10th	25th	50th	75th	90th	95th	99th
1. SINGLE DX										
0–19 Years	0									
20–34	0									
35–49	6	1.8	3	1	1	1	2	5	5	5
50–64	5	1.0	0	1	1	1	1	1	1	1
65+	7	1.0	0	1	1	1	1	1	1	1
2. MULTIPLE DX										
0–19 Years	3	5.2	8	5	5	5	5	10	10	10
20–34	42	4.1	22	1	1	2	7	10	14	21
35–49	225	4.4	27	1	1	2	6	10	13	28
50–64	1,154	4.4	31	1	1	2	6	11	16	27
65+	3,188	4.1	25	1	1	2	6	10	13	25
TOTAL SINGLE DX	**18**	**1.3**	**<1**	**1**	**1**	**1**	**1**	**2**	**5**	**5**
TOTAL MULTIPLE DX	**4,612**	**4.2**	**27**	**1**	**1**	**2**	**6**	**10**	**14**	**25**
TOTAL										
0–19 Years	3	5.2	8	5	5	5	5	10	10	10
20–34	42	4.1	22	1	1	2	7	10	14	21
35–49	231	4.4	27	1	1	2	6	9	13	28
50–64	1,159	4.4	31	1	1	2	6	11	16	27
65+	3,195	4.1	25	1	1	2	6	10	13	25
GRAND TOTAL	**4,630**	**4.2**	**27**	**1**	**1**	**2**	**6**	**10**	**14**	**25**

LOS by Diagnosis and Operation, Western Region, 45th Edition

Western Region, October 2007–September 2008 Data, by Operation

00.52: IMPL LEAD COR VEN SYSTEM

Type of Patients	Observed Patients	Avg. Stay	Variance	Percentiles						
				10th	25th	50th	75th	90th	95th	99th
1. SINGLE DX										
0–19 Years	0									
20–34	0									
35–49	0									
50–64	0									
65+	0									
2. MULTIPLE DX										
0–19 Years	0									
20–34	5	3.6	14	1	1	3	3	10	10	10
35–49	6	2.0	2	1	1	1	4	4	4	4
50–64	30	3.2	9	1	1	2	4	7	11	13
65+	87	3.5	18	1	1	1	5	8	12	27
TOTAL SINGLE DX	0									
TOTAL MULTIPLE DX	128	3.4	15	1	1	2	4	7	11	17
TOTAL										
0–19 Years	0									
20–34	5	3.6	14	1	1	3	3	10	10	10
35–49	6	2.0	2	1	1	1	4	4	4	4
50–64	30	3.2	9	1	1	2	4	7	11	13
65+	87	3.5	18	1	1	1	5	8	12	27
GRAND TOTAL	128	3.4	15	1	1	2	4	7	11	17

00.54: IMPL CRT-D GENERATOR

Type of Patients	Observed Patients	Avg. Stay	Variance	Percentiles						
				10th	25th	50th	75th	90th	95th	99th
1. SINGLE DX										
0–19 Years	0									
20–34	0									
35–49	0									
50–64	1	1.0	0	1	1	1	1	1	1	1
65+	0									
2. MULTIPLE DX										
0–19 Years	0									
20–34	0									
35–49	12	2.8	4	1	1	2	4	5	7	7
50–64	46	3.6	47	1	1	1	3	7	13	44
65+	144	2.8	12	1	1	1	3	7	9	16
TOTAL SINGLE DX	1	1.0	0	1	1	1	1	1	1	1
TOTAL MULTIPLE DX	202	3.0	19	1	1	1	3	7	9	16
TOTAL										
0–19 Years	0									
20–34	0									
35–49	12	2.8	4	1	1	2	4	5	7	7
50–64	47	3.5	46	1	1	1	3	7	13	44
65+	144	2.8	12	1	1	1	3	7	9	16
GRAND TOTAL	203	3.0	19	1	1	1	3	7	9	16

00.6: BLOOD VESSEL PX

Type of Patients	Observed Patients	Avg. Stay	Variance	Percentiles						
				10th	25th	50th	75th	90th	95th	99th
1. SINGLE DX										
0–19 Years	7	1.4	<1	1	1	1	1	2	4	4
20–34	6	1.3	<1	1	1	1	2	2	2	2
35–49	60	1.3	<1	1	1	1	1	2	3	5
50–64	213	1.3	<1	1	1	1	1	2	2	4
65+	276	1.1	<1	1	1	1	1	1	2	3
2. MULTIPLE DX										
0–19 Years	43	3.6	18	1	1	2	4	9	12	21
20–34	337	3.2	9	1	2	2	3	6	8	17
35–49	7,532	2.6	7	1	1	2	3	4	6	12
50–64	29,557	2.5	8	1	1	2	3	5	6	14
65+	40,833	2.8	10	1	1	2	3	6	8	16
TOTAL SINGLE DX	562	1.2	<1	1	1	1	1	2	2	4
TOTAL MULTIPLE DX	78,302	2.7	9	1	1	2	3	5	8	15
TOTAL										
0–19 Years	50	3.3	16	1	1	1	4	9	9	21
20–34	343	3.1	9	1	2	2	3	6	8	17
35–49	7,592	2.6	7	1	1	2	3	4	6	12
50–64	29,770	2.5	8	1	1	2	3	5	6	14
65+	41,109	2.8	10	1	1	2	3	6	8	16
GRAND TOTAL	78,864	2.7	9	1	1	2	3	5	8	15

00.61: PERC ATHER PRECEREB VESS

Type of Patients	Observed Patients	Avg. Stay	Variance	Percentiles						
				10th	25th	50th	75th	90th	95th	99th
1. SINGLE DX										
0–19 Years	1	4.0	0	4	4	4	4	4	4	4
20–34	2	1.0	0	1	1	1	1	1	1	1
35–49	3	1.0	0	1	1	1	1	1	1	1
50–64	9	1.1	<1	1	1	1	1	2	2	2
65+	25	1.2	<1	1	1	1	1	2	2	3
2. MULTIPLE DX										
0–19 Years	5	1.1	<1	1	1	1	1	2	2	2
20–34	14	7.1	58	1	1	3	12	17	26	26
35–49	41	3.7	13	1	1	2	6	8	10	14
50–64	379	3.4	27	1	1	1	4	8	14	40
65+	1,211	2.6	11	1	1	1	3	6	9	16
TOTAL SINGLE DX	40	1.2	<1	1	1	1	1	2	2	4
TOTAL MULTIPLE DX	1,650	2.8	15	1	1	1	3	7	10	20
TOTAL										
0–19 Years	6	1.4	1	1	1	2	4	4	4	4
20–34	16	6.4	55	1	1	2	8	17	26	26
35–49	44	3.5	12	1	1	1	6	8	10	14
50–64	388	3.4	26	1	1	1	4	8	14	40
65+	1,236	2.5	11	1	1	1	3	6	9	16
GRAND TOTAL	1,690	2.8	15	1	1	1	3	7	10	20

LOS by Diagnosis and Operation, Western Region, 45th Edition

Western Region, October 2007–September 2008 Data, by Operation

00.62: PERC ATHER IC VESSEL

Type of Patients	Observed Patients	Avg. Stay	Vari-ance	Percentiles						
				10th	25th	50th	75th	90th	95th	99th
1. SINGLE DX										
0–19 Years	0									
20–34	1	1.0	0	1	1	1	1	1	1	1
35–49	0									
50–64	1	1.0	0	1	1	1	1	1	1	1
65+	0									
2. MULTIPLE DX										
0–19 Years	5	6.4	29	3	4	4	5	16	16	16
20–34	11	6.0	26	1	1	5	9	13	15	15
35–49	28	5.8	34	1	1	2	12	14	18	18
50–64	72	5.0	23	1	1	3	7	10	17	22
65+	74	6.1	25	1	2	5	9	12	15	27
TOTAL SINGLE DX	**2**	**1.0**	**0**	**1**	**1**	**1**	**1**	**1**	**1**	**1**
TOTAL MULTIPLE DX	**190**	**5.6**	**26**	**1**	**1**	**4**	**9**	**13**	**15**	**22**
TOTAL										
0–19 Years	5	6.4	29	3	4	4	5	16	16	16
20–34	12	5.6	26	1	1	5	9	13	15	15
35–49	28	5.8	34	1	1	2	12	14	18	18
50–64	73	5.0	23	1	1	3	7	10	17	22
65+	74	6.1	25	1	2	5	9	12	15	27
GRAND TOTAL	**192**	**5.6**	**26**	**1**	**1**	**4**	**9**	**12**	**15**	**22**

00.66: PTCA/ATHERECTOMY

Type of Patients	Observed Patients	Avg. Stay	Vari-ance	Percentiles						
				10th	25th	50th	75th	90th	95th	99th
1. SINGLE DX										
0–19 Years	6	1.1	<1	1	1	1	1	2	2	2
20–34	3	1.7	<1	1	1	2	2	2	2	2
35–49	57	1.3	<1	1	1	1	1	2	3	5
50–64	202	1.3	<1	1	1	1	1	2	2	4
65+	250	1.1	<1	1	1	1	1	1	2	3
2. MULTIPLE DX										
0–19 Years	33	3.7	19	1	1	2	5	9	12	21
20–34	309	2.9	6	1	2	2	3	5	7	12
35–49	7,460	2.6	7	1	1	2	4	6	6	12
50–64	29,093	2.5	8	1	1	2	5	5	6	13
65+	39,518	2.8	10	1	1	2	3	6	8	16
TOTAL SINGLE DX	**518**	**1.2**	**<1**	**1**	**1**	**1**	**1**	**2**	**2**	**4**
TOTAL MULTIPLE DX	**76,413**	**2.7**	**9**	**1**	**1**	**2**	**3**	**5**	**7**	**15**
TOTAL										
0–19 Years	39	3.3	17	1	1	1	3	9	9	21
20–34	312	2.9	6	1	2	2	3	5	7	12
35–49	7,517	2.6	6	1	1	2	4	6	6	12
50–64	29,295	2.5	8	1	1	2	5	5	6	13
65+	39,768	2.8	10	1	1	2	3	6	8	16
GRAND TOTAL	**76,931**	**2.7**	**9**	**1**	**1**	**2**	**3**	**5**	**7**	**15**

00.7: OTHER HIP PX

Type of Patients	Observed Patients	Avg. Stay	Vari-ance	Percentiles						
				10th	25th	50th	75th	90th	95th	99th
1. SINGLE DX										
0–19 Years	0									
20–34	2	3.5	<1	3	3	3	4	4	4	4
35–49	13	3.3	1	2	2	3	4	4	5	5
50–64	24	3.1	2	2	2	3	3	5	5	7
65+	14	3.3	<1	3	3	3	4	4	5	5
2. MULTIPLE DX										
0–19 Years	4	4.6	2	3	3	5	6	6	6	6
20–34	63	3.8	10	2	2	3	5	5	6	26
35–49	489	4.4	13	2	3	3	5	8	11	19
50–64	1,796	4.5	16	2	3	3	5	8	11	20
65+	3,758	5.1	17	3	3	4	6	9	12	22
TOTAL SINGLE DX	**53**	**3.2**	**1**	**2**	**3**	**3**	**4**	**4**	**5**	**7**
TOTAL MULTIPLE DX	**6,110**	**4.9**	**16**	**2**	**3**	**4**	**5**	**8**	**12**	**21**
TOTAL										
0–19 Years	4	4.6	2	3	3	5	6	6	6	6
20–34	65	3.8	9	2	3	3	4	5	6	26
35–49	502	4.4	12	2	3	3	5	7	11	18
50–64	1,820	4.5	16	2	3	3	5	7	10	20
65+	3,772	5.1	17	3	3	4	6	9	12	22
GRAND TOTAL	**6,163**	**4.9**	**16**	**2**	**3**	**4**	**5**	**8**	**11**	**21**

00.70: REV HIP REPL-BOTH COMP

Type of Patients	Observed Patients	Avg. Stay	Vari-ance	Percentiles						
				10th	25th	50th	75th	90th	95th	99th
1. SINGLE DX										
0–19 Years	0									
20–34	1	4.0	0	4	4	4	4	4	4	4
35–49	7	3.3	2	1	2	4	4	5	5	5
50–64	15	3.1	<1	2	3	3	4	4	5	5
65+	9	3.4	<1	3	3	3	4	5	5	5
2. MULTIPLE DX										
0–19 Years	1	4.0	0	4	4	4	4	4	4	4
20–34	37	3.4	1	2	3	3	4	5	6	6
35–49	257	4.6	13	2	3	3	5	8	13	19
50–64	957	4.5	15	2	3	3	7	7	11	22
65+	1,941	5.1	13	3	3	4	6	9	12	19
TOTAL SINGLE DX	**32**	**3.3**	**<1**	**2**	**3**	**3**	**4**	**4**	**5**	**5**
TOTAL MULTIPLE DX	**3,193**	**4.8**	**14**	**2**	**3**	**4**	**5**	**8**	**11**	**20**
TOTAL										
0–19 Years	1	4.0	0	4	4	4	4	4	4	4
20–34	38	3.4	1	2	3	3	4	5	6	6
35–49	264	4.5	13	2	3	3	5	8	12	19
50–64	972	4.5	14	2	3	3	6	7	11	22
65+	1,950	5.1	13	3	3	4	6	9	12	19
GRAND TOTAL	**3,225**	**4.8**	**13**	**2**	**3**	**4**	**5**	**8**	**11**	**20**

LOS by Diagnosis and Operation, Western Region, 45th Edition

Western Region, October 2007–September 2008 Data, by Operation

00.71: REV HIP REPL-ACETAB COMP

Type of Patients	Observed Patients	Avg. Stay	Vari-ance	Percentiles						
				10th	25th	50th	75th	90th	95th	99th
1. SINGLE DX										
0–19 Years	0									
20–34	1	3.0	0	3	3	3	3	3	3	3
35–49	3	4.0	0	4	4	4	4	4	4	4
50–64	4	2.5	<1	2	3	3	3	3	3	3
65+	1	3.0	0	3	3	3	3	3	3	3
2. MULTIPLE DX										
0–19 Years	1	6.0	0	6	6	6	6	6	6	6
20–34	11	3.9	1	3	3	4	5	5	6	6
35–49	96	4.0	5	2	3	3	5	7	8	17
50–64	290	4.0	7	2	3	3	4	7	9	16
65+	578	4.7	12	2	3	4	5	8	12	19
TOTAL SINGLE DX	9	3.1	<1	2	3	3	4	4	4	4
TOTAL MULTIPLE DX	976	4.4	10	2	3	3	5	7	10	18
TOTAL										
0–19 Years	1	6.0	0	6	6	6	6	6	6	6
20–34	12	3.8	1	3	3	4	5	5	6	6
35–49	99	4.0	5	2	3	3	5	7	8	17
50–64	294	4.0	7	2	3	3	4	6	9	16
65+	579	4.7	12	2	3	4	5	8	12	19
GRAND TOTAL	985	4.4	9	2	3	3	5	7	10	18

00.72: REV HIP REPL-FEM COMP

Type of Patients	Observed Patients	Avg. Stay	Vari-ance	Percentiles						
				10th	25th	50th	75th	90th	95th	99th
1. SINGLE DX										
0–19 Years	0									
20–34	0									
35–49	1	4.0	0	4	4	4	4	4	4	4
50–64	2	6.0	2	5	5	7	7	7	7	7
65+	4	3.0	<1	2	2	3	4	4	4	4
2. MULTIPLE DX										
0–19 Years	2	4.0	1	3	3	4	5	5	5	5
20–34	11	3.2	3	2	2	2	4	5	7	7
35–49	47	4.9	13	2	3	4	6	11	13	20
50–64	240	5.4	39	3	3	4	6	9	12	49
65+	628	6.3	29	3	3	5	7	11	15	26
TOTAL SINGLE DX	7	4.0	3	2	3	4	5	7	7	7
TOTAL MULTIPLE DX	928	6.0	31	3	3	4	7	10	14	26
TOTAL										
0–19 Years	2	4.0	1	3	3	4	5	5	5	5
20–34	11	3.2	3	2	2	2	4	5	7	7
35–49	48	4.9	13	2	3	4	6	11	13	20
50–64	242	5.4	39	3	3	4	6	9	12	49
65+	632	6.3	29	3	3	5	7	11	15	26
GRAND TOTAL	935	5.9	30	3	3	4	7	10	14	26

00.73: REV HIP REPL-LINER/HEAD

Type of Patients	Observed Patients	Avg. Stay	Vari-ance	Percentiles						
				10th	25th	50th	75th	90th	95th	99th
1. SINGLE DX										
0–19 Years	0									
20–34	0									
35–49	2	2.0	0	2	2	2	2	2	2	2
50–64	3	2.0	<1	1	1	2	3	3	3	3
65+	0									
2. MULTIPLE DX										
0–19 Years	0									
20–34	4	9.2	124	3	3	3	5	26	26	26
35–49	88	4.0	20	2	2	3	4	6	8	37
50–64	306	4.1	10	2	3	3	4	7	9	17
65+	607	4.6	19	2	3	3	5	7	11	22
TOTAL SINGLE DX	5	2.0	<1	1	2	2	2	3	3	3
TOTAL MULTIPLE DX	1,005	4.4	17	2	3	3	5	7	10	22
TOTAL										
0–19 Years	0									
20–34	4	9.2	124	3	3	3	5	26	26	26
35–49	90	4.0	19	2	3	3	4	6	8	37
50–64	309	4.0	10	2	3	3	4	7	9	17
65+	607	4.6	19	2	3	3	5	7	11	22
GRAND TOTAL	1,010	4.4	17	2	3	3	5	7	10	22

00.8: OTHER KNEE & HIP PX

Type of Patients	Observed Patients	Avg. Stay	Vari-ance	Percentiles						
				10th	25th	50th	75th	90th	95th	99th
1. SINGLE DX										
0–19 Years	2	2.0	0	2	2	2	2	2	2	2
20–34	6	2.7	<1	2	2	3	3	3	3	3
35–49	117	2.6	<1	2	2	3	3	3	4	5
50–64	150	2.7	<1	2	2	3	3	3	4	4
65+	24	2.8	1	2	2	3	3	4	5	5
2. MULTIPLE DX										
0–19 Years	18	3.2	8	1	1	2	3	8	11	11
20–34	65	3.6	5	2	2	3	4	7	8	12
35–49	800	3.3	6	2	2	3	4	5	6	11
50–64	3,021	3.6	6	2	3	3	4	5	7	13
65+	3,458	4.1	8	2	3	3	4	6	8	15
TOTAL SINGLE DX	299	2.6	<1	2	2	3	3	3	4	5
TOTAL MULTIPLE DX	7,362	3.8	7	2	3	3	4	6	7	14
TOTAL										
0–19 Years	20	3.1	7	1	2	2	3	8	11	11
20–34	71	3.5	5	2	2	3	3	6	8	12
35–49	917	3.2	5	2	2	3	3	5	6	9
50–64	3,171	3.5	6	2	3	3	4	6	7	12
65+	3,482	4.1	8	2	3	3	4	6	8	15
GRAND TOTAL	7,661	3.8	7	2	3	3	4	6	7	14

LOS by Diagnosis and Operation, Western Region, 45th Edition

Western Region, October 2007–September 2008 Data, by Operation

00.80: REV KNEE REPL-TOTAL

Type of Patients	Observed Patients	Avg. Stay	Variance	10th	25th	50th	75th	90th	95th	99th
1. SINGLE DX										
0–19 Years	0									
20–34	0									
35–49	4	2.8	<1	2	2	3	4	4	4	4
50–64	14	2.9	<1	2	3	3	3	4	4	4
65+	7	3.1	1	1	3	3	4	5	5	5
2. MULTIPLE DX										
0–19 Years	4	4.0	10	1	1	5	8	8	8	8
20–34	7	2.6	2	1	1	2	4	5	5	5
35–49	171	3.7	5	2	3	3	4	6	7	11
50–64	1,048	3.9	5	2	3	4	4	6	7	13
65+	1,618	4.2	8	3	3	4	5	6	8	15
TOTAL SINGLE DX	25	3.0	<1	2	3	3	3	4	4	5
TOTAL MULTIPLE DX	2,848	4.1	7	2	3	3	4	6	8	14
TOTAL										
0–19 Years	4	4.0	10	1	1	5	8	8	8	8
20–34	7	2.6	2	1	1	2	4	5	5	5
35–49	175	3.7	4	2	3	3	4	6	7	11
50–64	1,062	3.9	5	2	3	4	4	6	7	13
65+	1,625	4.2	8	3	3	4	5	6	8	15
GRAND TOTAL	2,873	4.1	6	3	3	3	4	6	8	14

00.81: REV KNEE REPL-TIB COMP

Type of Patients	Observed Patients	Avg. Stay	Variance	10th	25th	50th	75th	90th	95th	99th
1. SINGLE DX										
0–19 Years	0									
20–34	0									
35–49	1	2.0	0	2	2	2	2	2	2	2
50–64	6	2.5	1	1	2	2	3	4	4	4
65+	6	2.5	1	1	2	3	3	4	4	4
2. MULTIPLE DX										
0–19 Years	2	6.0	50	1	1	6	11	11	11	11
20–34	6	4.0	2	3	3	4	4	7	7	7
35–49	66	3.6	7	2	3	3	4	6	6	8
50–64	380	3.7	7	2	3	3	4	5	7	13
65+	555	3.8	5	2	3	3	4	6	7	14
TOTAL SINGLE DX	13	2.5	<1	1	2	2	3	4	4	4
TOTAL MULTIPLE DX	1,009	3.7	6	2	3	3	4	6	7	12
TOTAL										
0–19 Years	2	6.0	50	1	1	6	11	11	11	11
20–34	6	4.0	2	3	3	4	4	7	7	7
35–49	67	3.6	7	2	3	3	4	6	6	8
50–64	386	3.7	7	2	3	3	4	5	7	13
65+	561	3.8	5	2	3	3	4	6	7	14
GRAND TOTAL	1,022	3.7	6	3	3	3	4	6	7	12

00.82: REV KNEE REPL-FEM COMP

Type of Patients	Observed Patients	Avg. Stay	Variance	10th	25th	50th	75th	90th	95th	99th
1. SINGLE DX										
0–19 Years	0									
20–34	0									
35–49	3	2.3	<1	2	2	2	3	3	3	3
50–64	1	3.0	0	3	3	3	3	3	3	3
65+	1	3.0	0	3	3	3	3	3	3	3
2. MULTIPLE DX										
0–19 Years	4	3.4	14	1	1	1	5	11	11	11
20–34	13	4.4	7	2	4	4	6	8	9	9
35–49	64	3.9	7	2	3	3	4	6	8	17
50–64	322	3.8	8	2	3	3	4	6	7	13
65+	466	4.2	5	3	3	4	5	6	8	13
TOTAL SINGLE DX	5	2.6	<1	2	2	3	3	3	3	3
TOTAL MULTIPLE DX	869	4.0	6	2	3	3	4	6	8	13
TOTAL										
0–19 Years	4	3.4	14	1	1	1	5	11	11	11
20–34	13	4.4	7	2	4	4	6	8	9	9
35–49	67	3.9	7	2	3	3	4	6	8	17
50–64	323	3.8	8	2	3	3	4	6	7	13
65+	467	4.2	5	3	3	4	5	6	8	13
GRAND TOTAL	874	4.0	6	2	3	3	4	6	8	13

00.83: REV KNEE REPL-PAT COMP

Type of Patients	Observed Patients	Avg. Stay	Variance	10th	25th	50th	75th	90th	95th	99th
1. SINGLE DX										
0–19 Years	0									
20–34	0									
35–49	4	2.5	2	1	2	3	4	4	4	4
50–64	1	3.0	0	3	3	3	3	3	3	3
65+	1	2.0	0	2	2	2	2	2	2	2
2. MULTIPLE DX										
0–19 Years	0									
20–34	1	1.0	0	1	1	1	1	1	1	1
35–49	26	3.5	8	2	2	3	3	6	7	16
50–64	146	3.1	4	1	2	3	4	5	7	10
65+	219	3.2	3	2	2	3	4	5	6	11
TOTAL SINGLE DX	6	2.5	1	1	2	2	3	4	4	4
TOTAL MULTIPLE DX	392	3.2	4	1	2	3	4	5	6	12
TOTAL										
0–19 Years	0									
20–34	1	1.0	0	1	1	1	1	1	1	1
35–49	30	3.3	7	2	2	3	3	6	7	16
50–64	147	3.1	4	1	2	3	4	5	7	10
65+	220	3.2	3	2	2	3	4	5	6	11
GRAND TOTAL	398	3.1	4	1	2	3	4	5	6	11

LOS by Diagnosis and Operation, Western Region, 45th Edition

Western Region, October 2007–September 2008 Data, by Operation

00.84: REV KNEE REPL-TIB INSERT

Type of Patients	Observed Patients	Avg. Stay	Vari-ance	10th	25th	50th	75th	90th	95th	99th
1. SINGLE DX										
0–19 Years	0									
20–34	0									
35–49	2	2.0	2	1	1	3	3	3	3	3
50–64	2	4.0	8	2	2	5	6	6	6	6
65+	1	5.0	0	5	5	5	5	5	5	5
2. MULTIPLE DX										
0–19 Years	0									
20–34	5	7.8	14	3	6	7	11	12	12	12
35–49	57	3.2	3	1	2	3	4	5	5	12
50–64	361	4.1	16	2	2	3	5	7	10	22
65+	535	4.7	18	2	3	3	5	9	10	18
TOTAL SINGLE DX	5	3.4	4	1	2	3	5	6	6	6
TOTAL MULTIPLE DX	958	4.4	17	2	3	3	5	8	10	19
TOTAL										
0–19 Years	0									
20–34	5	7.8	14	3	6	7	11	12	12	12
35–49	59	3.2	3	1	2	3	4	5	5	12
50–64	363	4.1	16	2	2	3	5	7	10	22
65+	536	4.7	18	2	3	3	5	9	10	18
GRAND TOTAL	963	4.4	17	2	3	3	5	8	10	19

00.85: HIP RESURFACING-TOTAL

Type of Patients	Observed Patients	Avg. Stay	Vari-ance	10th	25th	50th	75th	90th	95th	99th
1. SINGLE DX										
0–19 Years	1	2.0	0	2	2	2	2	2	2	2
20–34	4	2.5	<1	2	2	2	3	3	3	3
35–49	94	2.6	<1	2	2	3	3	3	4	5
50–64	118	2.6	<1	2	2	3	3	3	4	4
65+	7	2.3	<1	2	2	2	3	3	3	3
2. MULTIPLE DX										
0–19 Years	6	2.3	<1	1	2	3	3	3	3	3
20–34	26	2.9	<1	2	2	3	3	4	5	5
35–49	378	2.9	<1	2	2	3	3	4	4	6
50–64	716	2.9	<1	2	2	3	3	4	4	6
65+	62	2.9	<1	2	2	3	3	4	5	6
TOTAL SINGLE DX	224	2.6	<1	2	2	3	3	3	4	4
TOTAL MULTIPLE DX	1,188	2.9	<1	2	2	3	3	4	4	6
TOTAL										
0–19 Years	7	2.3	<1	1	2	2	3	3	3	3
20–34	30	2.9	<1	2	2	3	3	4	4	5
35–49	472	2.9	<1	2	2	3	3	4	4	6
50–64	834	2.9	<1	2	2	3	3	4	4	6
65+	69	2.9	<1	2	2	3	3	4	5	6
GRAND TOTAL	1,412	2.9	<1	2	2	3	3	4	4	6

00.86: HIP RESURFACING-FEM HEAD

Type of Patients	Observed Patients	Avg. Stay	Vari-ance	10th	25th	50th	75th	90th	95th	99th
1. SINGLE DX										
0–19 Years	1	2.0	0	2	2	2	2	2	2	2
20–34	2	3.0	0	3	3	3	3	3	3	3
35–49	8	2.4	<1	1	2	3	3	3	3	3
50–64	7	3.1	<1	3	3	3	3	4	4	4
65+	0									
2. MULTIPLE DX										
0–19 Years	0									
20–34	6	2.7	<1	2	2	3	3	3	3	3
35–49	27	3.3	2	2	3	3	3	4	5	9
50–64	36	3.1	<1	2	3	3	3	4	4	5
65+	3	2.7	<1	2	2	3	3	3	3	3
TOTAL SINGLE DX	18	2.7	<1	2	2	3	3	3	4	4
TOTAL MULTIPLE DX	72	3.1	<1	2	3	3	3	4	4	9
TOTAL										
0–19 Years	1	2.0	0	2	2	2	2	2	2	2
20–34	8	2.8	<1	2	2	3	3	3	3	3
35–49	35	3.1	2	2	3	3	3	4	5	9
50–64	43	3.1	<1	2	3	3	3	4	4	5
65+	3	2.7	<1	2	2	3	3	3	3	3
GRAND TOTAL	90	3.0	<1	2	3	3	3	4	4	9

00.9: PX & INTERVENTION NEC

Type of Patients	Observed Patients	Avg. Stay	Vari-ance	10th	25th	50th	75th	90th	95th	99th
1. SINGLE DX										
0–19 Years	0									
20–34	0									
35–49	0									
50–64	0									
65+	0									
2. MULTIPLE DX										
0–19 Years	0									
20–34	0									
35–49	1	5.0	0	5	5	5	5	5	5	5
50–64	1	9.0	0	9	9	9	9	9	9	9
65+	0									
TOTAL SINGLE DX	0									
TOTAL MULTIPLE DX	2	7.0	8	5	5	9	9	9	9	9
TOTAL										
0–19 Years	0									
20–34	0									
35–49	1	5.0	0	5	5	5	5	5	5	5
50–64	1	9.0	0	9	9	9	9	9	9	9
65+	0									
GRAND TOTAL	2	7.0	8	5	5	9	9	9	9	9

LOS by Diagnosis and Operation, Western Region, 45th Edition

Western Region, October 2007–September 2008 Data, by Operation

01.0: CRANIAL PUNCTURE

Type of Patients	Observed Patients	Avg. Stay	Vari- ance	Percentiles						
				10th	25th	50th	75th	90th	95th	99th
1. SINGLE DX										
0–19 Years	4	4.2	1	3	4	4	4	6	6	6
20–34	2	1.5	<1	1	2	2	2	2	2	2
35–49	2	3.0	2	2	2	2	2	2	2	2
50–64	1	2.0	0	2	2	2	2	2	2	2
65+	2	1.5	<1	1	1	1	2	2	2	2
2. MULTIPLE DX										
0–19 Years	213	4.0	16	1	2	2	5	10	13	22
20–34	67	6.9	39	1	2	5	10	15	20	27
35–49	60	4.9	23	1	2	4	6	10	12	28
50–64	43	6.5	35	1	2	5	8	13	18	31
65+	79	6.9	28	2	3	5	10	16	19	25
TOTAL SINGLE DX	11	2.9	2	1	2	2	4	4	6	6
TOTAL MULTIPLE DX	462	4.7	22	1	2	3	6	11	15	23
TOTAL										
0–19 Years	217	4.0	16	1	2	2	5	10	13	22
20–34	69	6.7	38	1	2	5	9	15	20	27
35–49	62	4.9	23	1	2	4	6	9	12	28
50–64	44	6.4	35	1	2	5	8	13	18	31
65+	81	6.7	28	2	3	5	10	15	17	25
GRAND TOTAL	473	4.7	22	1	2	3	6	11	15	23

01.02: VENTRICULOPUNCT VIA CATH

Type of Patients	Observed Patients	Avg. Stay	Vari- ance	Percentiles						
				10th	25th	50th	75th	90th	95th	99th
1. SINGLE DX										
0–19 Years	1	4.0	0	4	4	4	4	4	4	4
20–34	0									
35–49	0									
50–64	0									
2. MULTIPLE DX										
0–19 Years	196	3.7	15	1	1	2	4	9	12	18
20–34	61	6.5	37	1	2	4	9	14	20	27
35–49	46	4.2	14	1	2	3	5	8	10	22
50–64	31	5.7	24	1	2	4	8	12	18	21
65+	45	6.8	27	2	3	5	10	16	19	21
TOTAL SINGLE DX	1	4.0	0	4	4	4	4	4	4	4
TOTAL MULTIPLE DX	379	4.3	19	1	2	3	5	10	13	22
TOTAL										
0–19 Years	197	3.7	14	1	1	2	4	9	12	18
20–34	61	6.5	37	1	2	4	9	14	20	27
35–49	46	4.2	14	1	2	3	5	8	10	22
50–64	31	5.7	24	1	2	4	8	12	18	21
65+	45	6.8	27	2	3	5	10	16	19	21
GRAND TOTAL	380	4.3	19	1	2	3	5	10	13	22

01.1: DXTIC PX ON SKULL/BRAIN

Type of Patients	Observed Patients	Avg. Stay	Vari- ance	Percentiles						
				10th	25th	50th	75th	90th	95th	99th
1. SINGLE DX										
0–19 Years	9	4.1	5	1	3	4	5	6	6	10
20–34	17	1.9	<1	1	1	2	2	3	4	4
35–49	25	2.2	4	1	1	1	3	6	7	7
50–64	22	1.9	2	1	1	1	3	3	3	6
65+	8	1.5	<1	1	1	1	2	3	3	3
2. MULTIPLE DX										
0–19 Years	136	10.5	223	1	2	5	13	29	38	88
20–34	154	10.9	202	1	2	5	14	30	48	71
35–49	230	9.7	133	1	2	6	12	26	35	58
50–64	415	7.4	90	1	1	4	10	17	27	46
65+	437	7.3	75	1	2	4	10	18	23	41
TOTAL SINGLE DX	81	2.4	3	1	1	2	3	5	6	10
TOTAL MULTIPLE DX	1,372	8.7	133	1	2	4	11	22	31	71
TOTAL										
0–19 Years	145	10.1	212	1	2	5	12	27	38	88
20–34	171	9.8	187	1	2	4	12	29	44	71
35–49	255	9.0	125	1	2	4	11	25	35	58
50–64	437	7.2	87	1	1	3	9	17	27	46
65+	445	7.2	74	1	2	4	10	17	22	41
GRAND TOTAL	1,453	8.4	128	1	2	4	10	21	30	61

01.10: IC PRESSURE MONITORING

Type of Patients	Observed Patients	Avg. Stay	Vari- ance	Percentiles						
				10th	25th	50th	75th	90th	95th	99th
1. SINGLE DX										
0–19 Years	1	6.0	0	6	6	6	6	6	6	6
20–34	2	2.0	2	1	1	1	3	3	3	3
35–49	1	3.0	0	3	3	3	3	3	3	3
50–64	0									
65+	0									
2. MULTIPLE DX										
0–19 Years	47	9.0	101	1	2	3	14	27	31	35
20–34	39	9.6	198	1	2	4	11	21	31	71
35–49	21	10.0	69	2	4	8	14	19	19	36
50–64	9	8.5	44	1	2	10	13	20	20	20
65+	9	10.3	112	2	4	6	13	33	33	33
TOTAL SINGLE DX	4	4.4	4	1	3	6	6	6	6	6
TOTAL MULTIPLE DX	125	9.3	115	1	2	4	14	23	31	55
TOTAL										
0–19 Years	48	8.9	98	1	2	4	14	27	31	35
20–34	41	9.2	192	1	2	4	10	21	31	71
35–49	22	9.7	68	2	3	8	14	19	19	36
50–64	9	8.5	44	2	3	10	13	20	20	20
65+	9	10.3	112	2	4	6	13	33	33	33
GRAND TOTAL	129	9.1	111	1	2	4	13	23	31	55

LOS by Diagnosis and Operation, Western Region, 45th Edition

Western Region, October 2007–September 2008 Data, by Operation

01.2: CRANIOTOMY & CRANIECTOMY

Type of Patients	Observed Patients	Avg. Stay	Vari-ance	Percentiles						
				10th	25th	50th	75th	90th	95th	99th
1. SINGLE DX										
0–19 Years	82	2.8	2	1	2	2	4	4	5	7
20–34	29	4.3	9	1	2	4	6	8	8	16
35–49	23	3.4	7	1	2	3	4	7	7	13
50–64	13	3.8	10	3	2	3	4	7	13	13
65+	3	4.3	5	3	3	3	7	7	7	7
2. MULTIPLE DX										
0–19 Years	358	9.3	163	2	3	4	8	23	45	60
20–34	333	9.9	140	2	3	6	11	23	39	84
35–49	368	11.6	187	2	4	7	14	29	43	85
50–64	397	11.1	190	2	4	6	12	27	41	84
65+	375	8.5	62	2	3	6	11	18	26	38
TOTAL SINGLE DX	**150**	**3.1**	**4**	**1**	**2**	**2**	**4**	**5**	**7**	**13**
TOTAL MULTIPLE DX	**1,831**	**10.0**	**152**	**2**	**3**	**5**	**11**	**23**	**39**	**68**
TOTAL										
0–19 Years	440	8.2	140	2	3	4	7	18	39	54
20–34	362	9.4	132	2	3	5	10	22	38	84
35–49	391	11.1	180	2	3	6	13	26	42	85
50–64	410	10.9	186	2	3	6	12	27	41	84
65+	378	8.5	62	2	3	6	11	18	26	38
GRAND TOTAL	**1,981**	**9.3**	**142**	**2**	**3**	**5**	**10**	**22**	**37**	**65**

01.23: REOPEN CRANIOTOMY SITE

Type of Patients	Observed Patients	Avg. Stay	Vari-ance	Percentiles						
				10th	25th	50th	75th	90th	95th	99th
1. SINGLE DX										
0–19 Years	0									
20–34	1	6.0	0	6	6	6	6	6	6	6
35–49	0									
50–64	0									
65+	1	3.0	0	3	3	3	3	3	3	3
2. MULTIPLE DX										
0–19 Years	8	32.4	641	10	14	24	65	65	65	65
20–34	21	8.9	90	3	4	6	8	21	43	>99
35–49	53	9.3	135	3	4	6	10	17	22	68
50–64	65	8.5	87	2	4	5	9	16	29	51
65+	33	9.9	90	2	4	7	14	17	29	49
TOTAL SINGLE DX	**2**	**4.5**	**4**	**3**	**3**	**6**	**6**	**6**	**6**	**6**
TOTAL MULTIPLE DX	**180**	**10.6**	**166**	**2**	**4**	**6**	**12**	**21**	**43**	**68**
TOTAL										
0–19 Years	8	32.4	641	10	14	24	65	65	65	65
20–34	22	8.7	86	3	4	6	8	21	43	>99
35–49	53	9.3	135	3	4	6	10	17	22	68
50–64	65	8.5	87	2	4	5	9	16	29	51
65+	34	9.7	89	2	3	7	14	17	29	49
GRAND TOTAL	**182**	**10.5**	**164**	**2**	**4**	**6**	**12**	**21**	**43**	**68**

01.13: CLOSED BRAIN BIOPSY

Type of Patients	Observed Patients	Avg. Stay	Vari-ance	Percentiles						
				10th	25th	50th	75th	90th	95th	99th
1. SINGLE DX										
0–19 Years	6	4.1	6	1	4	4	5	5	10	10
20–34	10	1.8	2	1	1	1	2	4	4	7
35–49	17	2.2	4	1	1	1	3	6	7	7
50–64	14	1.7	<1	1	1	1	3	3	3	3
65+	5	1.0	0	1	1	1	1	1	1	1
2. MULTIPLE DX										
0–19 Years	29	9.6	343	1	2	5	10	17	88	>99
20–34	55	7.1	132	1	1	3	7	16	32	61
35–49	100	6.4	61	1	1	3	9	18	25	31
50–64	243	5.5	63	1	1	3	7	13	17	32
65+	289	5.7	38	1	1	3	8	13	18	35
TOTAL SINGLE DX	**52**	**2.3**	**4**	**1**	**1**	**1**	**4**	**5**	**6**	**10**
TOTAL MULTIPLE DX	**716**	**6.2**	**89**	**1**	**1**	**3**	**8**	**14**	**20**	**52**
TOTAL										
0–19 Years	35	8.9	303	1	2	5	10	17	88	>99
20–34	65	6.3	115	1	1	2	7	15	22	61
35–49	117	5.8	55	1	1	2	8	17	25	31
50–64	257	5.3	60	1	1	2	7	13	17	32
65+	294	5.7	38	1	1	3	8	13	18	35
GRAND TOTAL	**768**	**6.0**	**84**	**1**	**1**	**3**	**7**	**13**	**18**	**40**

01.14: OPEN BIOPSY OF BRAIN

Type of Patients	Observed Patients	Avg. Stay	Vari-ance	Percentiles						
				10th	25th	50th	75th	90th	95th	99th
1. SINGLE DX										
0–19 Years	2	2.6	<1	1	3	3	3	3	3	3
20–34	5	1.9	<1	1	1	2	2	3	3	3
35–49	5	1.5	<1	1	1	2	2	2	2	2
50–64	6	2.5	3	1	1	2	3	6	6	6
65+	3	2.3	<1	2	2	2	3	3	3	3
2. MULTIPLE DX										
0–19 Years	39	12.5	276	1	2	7	17	29	72	>99
20–34	41	15.0	181	2	3	12	23	31	44	50
35–49	93	12.7	194	1	3	7	18	34	46	>99
50–64	135	11.0	133	2	3	7	15	27	38	51
65+	113	9.1	85	2	3	7	12	19	28	46
TOTAL SINGLE DX	**21**	**2.1**	**1**	**1**	**1**	**2**	**3**	**3**	**3**	**6**
TOTAL MULTIPLE DX	**421**	**11.5**	**167**	**1**	**3**	**7**	**15**	**29**	**41**	**72**
TOTAL										
0–19 Years	41	12.0	266	1	2	6	14	29	72	72
20–34	46	12.8	174	1	3	9	19	31	44	50
35–49	98	12.0	189	1	3	7	17	34	46	>99
50–64	141	10.6	130	1	3	6	14	27	36	51
65+	116	9.0	84	2	3	6	12	19	28	46
GRAND TOTAL	**442**	**11.0**	**162**	**1**	**2**	**7**	**15**	**29**	**41**	**72**

LOS by Diagnosis and Operation, Western Region, 45th Edition

Western Region, October 2007–September 2008 Data, by Operation

01.24: CRANIOTOMY NEC

Type of Patients	Observed Patients	Avg. Stay	Vari-ance	Percentiles 10th	25th	50th	75th	90th	95th	99th
1. SINGLE DX										
0–19 Years	61	2.9	2	1	2	2	4	5	5	7
20–34	20	3.4	3	1	2	2	4	6	8	8
35–49	15	4.1	9	2	2	3	5	7	13	13
50–64	8	4.3	14	1	3	4	4	13	13	13
65+	1	3.0	0	3	3	3	3	3	3	3
2. MULTIPLE DX										
0–19 Years	252	8.9	130	2	3	4	8	23	43	54
20–34	230	10.6	169	3	4	6	11	24	43	84
35–49	223	12.6	204	3	4	7	15	30	43	85
50–64	216	11.2	161	2	4	7	12	28	37	72
65+	252	8.4	56	2	4	6	10	17	24	35
TOTAL SINGLE DX	105	3.1	4	1	2	3	4	5	7	13
TOTAL MULTIPLE DX	1,173	10.0	141	2	3	6	11	24	39	60
TOTAL										
0–19 Years	313	7.8	111	2	3	4	7	18	34	53
20–34	250	10.0	159	3	3	6	11	23	40	84
35–49	238	12.1	196	2	4	7	15	29	43	85
50–64	224	10.9	157	2	4	7	12	27	37	72
65+	253	8.4	56	2	3	6	10	17	24	35
GRAND TOTAL	1,278	9.3	131	2	3	5	10	22	35	60

01.25: CRANIECTOMY NEC

Type of Patients	Observed Patients	Avg. Stay	Vari-ance	Percentiles 10th	25th	50th	75th	90th	95th	99th
1. SINGLE DX										
0–19 Years	21	2.6	<1	1	2	2	3	4	4	4
20–34	6	4.2	3	2	3	4	6	6	6	6
35–49	8	2.3	2	1	1	2	3	5	5	5
50–64	4	3.2	6	2	2	2	2	7	7	7
65+	0									
2. MULTIPLE DX										
0–19 Years	74	6.0	66	2	3	4	5	9	19	47
20–34	70	8.2	79	2	3	5	11	18	29	40
35–49	74	10.5	161	2	3	5	12	31	42	60
50–64	81	14.9	382	2	3	7	17	43	68	>99
65+	53	8.5	74	2	3	5	9	22	31	33
TOTAL SINGLE DX	39	2.7	2	1	2	2	4	4	6	7
TOTAL MULTIPLE DX	352	9.1	152	2	3	5	9	23	34	68
TOTAL										
0–19 Years	95	5.3	55	2	3	3	5	7	19	47
20–34	76	7.9	74	2	3	4	9	18	29	40
35–49	82	9.7	150	1	2	5	11	24	40	60
50–64	85	14.3	370	2	3	7	16	43	68	>99
65+	53	8.5	74	2	3	5	9	22	31	33
GRAND TOTAL	391	8.3	138	2	3	4	8	21	32	68

01.3: INC BRAIN/CEREB MENINGES

Type of Patients	Observed Patients	Avg. Stay	Vari-ance	Percentiles 10th	25th	50th	75th	90th	95th	99th
1. SINGLE DX										
0–19 Years	19	5.0	13	1	3	3	7	10	10	14
20–34	23	4.8	48	2	3	3	4	6	6	36
35–49	26	3.4	7	1	2	3	4	10	10	11
50–64	38	3.6	4	1	2	3	5	6	8	9
65+	26	4.0	3	2	3	4	5	7	7	8
2. MULTIPLE DX										
0–19 Years	231	16.0	298	3	4	9	21	47	54	76
20–34	267	16.7	313	3	5	10	21	40	55	96
35–49	497	15.8	241	3	6	10	21	40	56	>99
50–64	1,058	13.1	182	3	5	8	17	29	42	98
65+	2,803	10.0	68	3	5	7	12	20	26	43
TOTAL SINGLE DX	132	4.1	13	1	2	3	5	7	10	14
TOTAL MULTIPLE DX	4,856	12.1	147	3	5	8	15	26	37	74
TOTAL										
0–19 Years	250	15.4	288	3	4	8	20	45	52	76
20–34	290	15.8	302	3	4	9	21	39	53	96
35–49	523	15.2	236	3	5	9	20	38	56	>99
50–64	1,096	12.8	179	3	5	8	16	29	40	94
65+	2,829	10.0	68	3	5	7	12	20	26	43
GRAND TOTAL	4,988	11.9	146	3	5	8	15	26	37	74

01.31: INC CEREBRAL MENINGES

Type of Patients	Observed Patients	Avg. Stay	Vari-ance	Percentiles 10th	25th	50th	75th	90th	95th	99th
1. SINGLE DX										
0–19 Years	13	6.1	15	1	3	6	10	14	14	14
20–34	19	5.3	57	2	3	3	5	6	36	36
35–49	24	3.5	8	1	2	3	4	10	10	11
50–64	34	3.7	4	1	2	3	5	6	8	9
65+	23	3.7	2	2	3	4	5	6	6	7
2. MULTIPLE DX										
0–19 Years	163	16.2	292	3	5	9	20	45	52	76
20–34	189	16.6	319	3	5	9	21	40	60	>99
35–49	358	13.8	178	3	5	9	18	34	49	>99
50–64	808	11.5	160	3	4	7	14	26	37	86
65+	2,520	9.6	64	3	5	7	12	19	25	42
TOTAL SINGLE DX	113	4.2	15	1	2	3	5	8	10	14
TOTAL MULTIPLE DX	4,038	11.1	125	3	5	7	13	23	33	65
TOTAL										
0–19 Years	176	15.7	282	3	5	9	20	45	52	76
20–34	208	15.6	305	3	4	8	21	39	56	96
35–49	382	13.1	173	3	5	7	18	34	48	>99
50–64	842	11.2	156	3	4	7	14	25	37	86
65+	2,543	9.5	64	3	4	7	12	19	24	42
GRAND TOTAL	4,151	10.9	123	3	4	7	13	23	33	65

LOS by Diagnosis and Operation, Western Region, 45th Edition

13

Western Region, October 2007–September 2008 Data, by Operation

01.5: EXC/DESTR BRAIN/MENINGES

Type of Patients	Observed Patients	Avg. Stay	Vari-ance	10th	25th	50th	75th	90th	95th	99th
1. SINGLE DX										
0–19 Years	87	4.3	8	1	2	3	6	9	10	13
20–34	99	3.9	7	2	2	3	5	6	7	23
35–49	154	3.6	5	2	2	3	4	6	8	10
50–64	160	3.5	5	2	2	3	4	6	7	15
65+	39	4.6	12	1	2	3	6	10	14	16
2. MULTIPLE DX										
0–19 Years	732	10.0	135	2	3	6	12	23	36	76
20–34	718	6.9	46	2	3	5	8	14	19	35
35–49	1,465	7.1	58	2	3	5	8	14	21	36
50–64	2,637	7.1	61	2	3	5	8	14	20	46
65+	1,951	7.5	46	2	3	6	9	15	19	34
TOTAL SINGLE DX	539	3.9	7	2	2	3	5	7	9	13
TOTAL MULTIPLE DX	7,503	7.8	73	2	3	5	9	16	23	46
TOTAL										
0–19 Years	819	9.4	126	2	3	6	11	22	35	73
20–34	817	6.5	42	2	3	4	8	14	19	33
35–49	1,619	6.7	54	2	3	5	8	14	20	35
50–64	2,797	6.9	58	2	3	5	8	14	19	44
65+	1,990	7.5	45	2	3	6	9	15	19	34
GRAND TOTAL	8,042	7.5	69	2	3	5	9	15	22	44

01.51: EXC CEREB MENINGEAL LES

Type of Patients	Observed Patients	Avg. Stay	Vari-ance	10th	25th	50th	75th	90th	95th	99th
1. SINGLE DX										
0–19 Years	3	2.9	4	1	2	2	6	6	6	6
20–34	13	3.7	5	1	2	3	5	6	8	8
35–49	50	3.5	4	2	2	3	4	6	7	10
50–64	59	3.8	8	1	2	3	4	7	11	16
65+	13	3.2	4	1	2	3	4	6	8	8
2. MULTIPLE DX										
0–19 Years	22	11.9	150	2	3	8	12	32	42	42
20–34	75	6.6	36	2	3	4	8	17	19	33
35–49	364	6.4	51	2	3	4	7	13	17	35
50–64	637	6.5	46	2	3	5	8	13	18	37
65+	536	7.3	48	2	3	5	9	15	20	39
TOTAL SINGLE DX	138	3.6	6	2	2	3	4	6	8	15
TOTAL MULTIPLE DX	1,634	6.9	52	2	3	5	8	14	19	39
TOTAL										
0–19 Years	25	10.9	141	2	3	6	12	32	42	42
20–34	88	6.1	33	2	3	4	7	15	19	33
35–49	414	6.1	46	2	3	4	7	12	17	34
50–64	696	6.3	44	2	3	4	7	13	17	36
65+	549	7.2	48	2	3	5	9	14	19	39
GRAND TOTAL	1,772	6.7	49	2	3	4	8	13	19	37

01.39: BRAIN INCISION NEC

Type of Patients	Observed Patients	Avg. Stay	Vari-ance	10th	25th	50th	75th	90th	95th	99th
1. SINGLE DX										
0–19 Years	6	2.9	3	1	2	3	3	7	7	7
20–34	4	2.5	<1	2	2	2	3	3	3	3
35–49	2	2.5	<1	2	2	2	3	3	3	3
50–64	4	3.5	2	2	3	4	5	5	5	5
65+	3	6.0	7	3	3	7	8	8	8	8
2. MULTIPLE DX										
0–19 Years	61	13.8	232	3	3	7	25	31	47	>99
20–34	77	17.0	305	3	6	10	21	40	52	89
35–49	139	21.0	368	4	8	14	27	54	65	94
50–64	250	18.2	222	5	8	14	24	42	58	>99
65+	283	13.8	87	4	7	12	18	28	34	46
TOTAL SINGLE DX	19	3.3	3	2	2	3	3	7	7	8
TOTAL MULTIPLE DX	810	16.5	216	4	7	12	22	36	48	>99
TOTAL										
0–19 Years	67	13.0	224	3	3	6	23	31	47	>99
20–34	81	16.2	299	3	5	10	19	39	44	89
35–49	141	20.7	367	4	8	13	27	53	64	94
50–64	254	17.9	221	5	8	14	24	42	53	>99
65+	286	13.7	87	4	7	12	18	28	34	46
GRAND TOTAL	829	16.2	215	3	6	12	22	35	48	>99

01.4: THALAMUS/GLOBUS PALL OPS

Type of Patients	Observed Patients	Avg. Stay	Vari-ance	10th	25th	50th	75th	90th	95th	99th
1. SINGLE DX										
0–19 Years	0									
20–34	0									
35–49	0									
50–64	2	1.0	0	1	1	1	1	1	1	1
65+	0									
2. MULTIPLE DX										
0–19 Years	2	3.6	34	1	1	1	1	14	14	14
20–34	0									
35–49	1	1.0	0	1	1	1	1	1	1	1
50–64	1	1.0	0	1	1	1	1	1	1	1
65+	11	1.4	<1	1	1	1	2	2	3	3
TOTAL SINGLE DX	2	1.0	0	1	1	1	1	1	1	1
TOTAL MULTIPLE DX	15	1.9	9	1	1	1	1	3	14	14
TOTAL										
0–19 Years	2	3.6	34	1	1	1	1	14	14	14
20–34	0									
35–49	1	1.0	0	1	1	1	1	1	1	1
50–64	3	1.0	<1	1	1	1	1	1	1	1
65+	11	1.4	<1	1	1	1	2	2	3	3
GRAND TOTAL	17	1.8	8	1	1	1	1	2	3	14

LOS by Diagnosis and Operation, Western Region, 45th Edition

Western Region, October 2007–September 2008 Data, by Operation

01.53: BRAIN LOBECTOMY

Type of Patients	Observed Patients	Avg. Stay	Variance	Percentiles						
				10th	25th	50th	75th	90th	95th	99th
1. SINGLE DX										
0–19 Years	7	8.5	16	3	4	10	13	13	13	13
20–34	6	4.2	1	3	3	5	5	6	6	6
35–49	13	4.9	3	3	4	4	6	8	8	8
50–64	4	3.2	2	2	2	3	3	5	5	5
65+	0									
2. MULTIPLE DX										
0–19 Years	32	8.0	55	2	3	5	11	21	30	31
20–34	32	6.4	35	2	3	3	7	15	16	31
35–49	37	9.2	115	3	3	6	12	18	25	63
50–64	47	7.6	39	3	3	5	11	14	22	30
65+	32	10.0	29	5	5	9	13	16	18	27
TOTAL SINGLE DX	30	6.0	11	3	3	5	8	13	13	13
TOTAL MULTIPLE DX	180	8.1	55	3	3	5	11	16	22	31
TOTAL										
0–19 Years	39	8.1	49	2	3	5	11	15	21	30
20–34	38	6.0	31	3	3	4	6	14	16	31
35–49	50	8.1	89	3	3	5	9	17	18	63
50–64	51	7.3	38	3	3	5	10	14	22	30
65+	32	10.0	29	5	5	9	13	16	18	27
GRAND TOTAL	210	7.8	50	3	3	5	11	16	21	31

01.6: EXCISION OF SKULL LESION

Type of Patients	Observed Patients	Avg. Stay	Variance	Percentiles						
				10th	25th	50th	75th	90th	95th	99th
1. SINGLE DX										
0–19 Years	39	1.6	2	1	1	1	1	4	4	7
20–34	12	2.0	2	1	1	1	2	4	5	5
35–49	8	1.4	<1	1	1	1	2	3	3	3
50–64	11	2.4	4	1	1	2	3	3	8	8
65+	1	1.0	0	1	1	1	1	1	1	1
2. MULTIPLE DX										
0–19 Years	41	5.8	126	1	1	2	4	12	33	52
20–34	29	5.2	89	1	2	2	4	9	16	51
35–49	51	3.3	9	1	1	2	4	7	11	14
50–64	74	4.4	23	1	1	3	6	10	12	25
65+	63	5.1	39	1	2	4	5	9	19	38
TOTAL SINGLE DX	71	1.7	2	1	1	1	2	4	5	7
TOTAL MULTIPLE DX	258	4.9	61	1	1	2	5	9	16	52
TOTAL										
0–19 Years	80	3.8	71	1	1	1	3	7	12	52
20–34	41	4.3	65	1	1	2	4	7	9	51
35–49	59	3.0	8	1	1	2	4	7	11	14
50–64	85	4.1	21	1	1	3	6	9	10	25
65+	64	5.1	39	1	2	4	5	9	19	38
GRAND TOTAL	329	4.0	47	1	1	2	4	8	12	51

01.59: EXC/DESTR BRAIN LES NEC

Type of Patients	Observed Patients	Avg. Stay	Variance	Percentiles						
				10th	25th	50th	75th	90th	95th	99th
1. SINGLE DX										
0–19 Years	76	4.0	6	1	2	3	6	8	9	10
20–34	80	3.9	8	2	2	3	5	6	7	23
35–49	91	3.5	5	2	2	3	4	6	8	13
50–64	97	3.4	4	2	2	3	4	6	7	13
65+	26	5.2	15	2	3	4	6	12	14	16
2. MULTIPLE DX										
0–19 Years	655	9.7	135	2	3	6	11	23	36	76
20–34	611	7.0	47	2	3	5	8	14	19	38
35–49	1,061	7.2	59	2	3	5	8	15	22	40
50–64	1,952	7.3	66	2	3	5	9	15	20	49
65+	1,382	7.6	44	2	3	6	9	15	19	32
TOTAL SINGLE DX	370	3.8	6	2	2	3	5	7	8	13
TOTAL MULTIPLE DX	5,661	7.9	77	2	3	5	9	16	23	51
TOTAL										
0–19 Years	731	9.2	125	2	3	5	10	22	35	76
20–34	691	6.6	44	2	3	5	8	13	19	35
35–49	1,152	6.9	56	2	3	4	8	14	21	36
50–64	2,049	7.1	64	2	3	5	9	14	20	47
65+	1,408	7.5	44	2	3	6	9	15	19	31
GRAND TOTAL	6,031	7.6	73	2	3	5	9	16	23	48

02.0: CRANIOPLASTY

Type of Patients	Observed Patients	Avg. Stay	Variance	Percentiles						
				10th	25th	50th	75th	90th	95th	99th
1. SINGLE DX										
0–19 Years	270	2.7	2	1	2	3	3	4	5	7
20–34	35	2.5	3	1	1	3	3	6	6	7
35–49	31	2.0	2	1	1	2	2	3	5	9
50–64	30	2.4	2	1	2	2	2	5	6	7
65+	4	1.3	<1	1	1	1	2	2	2	2
2. MULTIPLE DX										
0–19 Years	623	5.3	54	2	2	3	5	9	18	42
20–34	404	6.7	90	2	2	3	7	17	25	40
35–49	368	6.7	83	1	2	3	7	15	27	43
50–64	411	6.5	88	1	2	3	8	16	24	53
65+	136	6.6	104	1	2	3	8	14	21	68
TOTAL SINGLE DX	370	2.6	2	1	2	3	3	4	5	7
TOTAL MULTIPLE DX	1,942	5.9	71	1	2	3	6	12	21	43
TOTAL										
0–19 Years	893	4.4	39	1	2	3	4	7	12	35
20–34	439	6.4	84	1	2	3	7	15	25	40
35–49	399	6.3	78	1	2	3	7	14	26	43
50–64	441	6.2	83	1	2	3	7	15	22	53
65+	140	6.4	102	1	2	3	7	13	21	68
GRAND TOTAL	2,312	5.2	58	1	2	3	5	10	18	41

LOS by Diagnosis and Operation, Western Region, 45th Edition

Western Region, October 2007–September 2008 Data, by Operation

02.01: OPENING CRANIAL SUTURE

Type of Patients	Observed Patients	Avg. Stay	Variance	10th	25th	50th	75th	90th	95th	99th
1. SINGLE DX										
0–19 Years	76	2.9	<1	2	2	3	3	4	4	6
20–34	0									
35–49	0									
50–64	0									
65+	0									
2. MULTIPLE DX										
0–19 Years	74	4.2	12	2	3	4	4	5	10	19
20–34	1	9.0	0	9	9	9	9	9	9	19
35–49	1	3.0	0	3	3	3	3	3	3	3
50–64	0									
65+	1	2.0	0	2	2	2	2	2	2	2
TOTAL SINGLE DX	76	2.9	<1	2	2	3	3	4	4	6
TOTAL MULTIPLE DX	77	4.2	12	2	3	4	4	5	10	19
TOTAL										
0–19 Years	150	3.5	7	2	2	3	4	5	5	19
20–34	1	9.0	0	9	9	9	9	9	9	9
35–49	1	3.0	0	3	3	3	3	3	3	3
50–64	0									
65+	1	2.0	0	2	2	2	2	2	2	2
GRAND TOTAL	153	3.5	7	2	2	3	4	5	5	19

02.02: ELEVATION SKULL FX FRAG

Type of Patients	Observed Patients	Avg. Stay	Variance	10th	25th	50th	75th	90th	95th	99th
1. SINGLE DX										
0–19 Years	33	2.7	4	1	1	2	4	5	8	8
20–34	4	4.3	7	2	2	6	7	7	7	7
35–49	4	5.0	8	3	3	3	9	9	9	9
50–64	1	2.0	0	2	2	2	2	2	2	2
65+	0									
2. MULTIPLE DX										
0–19 Years	139	8.0	91	2	2	4	10	21	23	36
20–34	190	9.3	127	2	3	5	12	22	35	44
35–49	97	10.4	133	2	3	6	11	27	34	71
50–64	80	12.3	177	2	4	8	17	30	37	82
65+	15	9.4	48	3	4	8	12	18	29	29
TOTAL SINGLE DX	42	2.9	4	1	1	2	4	5	8	9
TOTAL MULTIPLE DX	521	9.4	120	2	3	5	12	21	32	44
TOTAL										
0–19 Years	172	6.8	76	1	2	4	8	18	21	36
20–34	194	9.2	125	2	3	5	12	21	35	44
35–49	101	10.2	129	2	3	6	11	26	32	43
50–64	81	12.1	176	2	4	7	16	25	34	82
65+	15	9.4	48	3	4	8	12	18	29	29
GRAND TOTAL	563	8.7	112	2	3	5	11	21	30	44

02.03: CRAN BONE FLAP FORMATION

Type of Patients	Observed Patients	Avg. Stay	Variance	10th	25th	50th	75th	90th	95th	99th
1. SINGLE DX										
0–19 Years	23	3.2	2	1	3	3	4	5	6	7
20–34	3	2.3	1	1	1	3	3	3	3	3
35–49	3	2.0	<1	1	1	2	3	3	3	3
50–64	2	3.5	4	2	2	5	5	5	5	5
65+	0									
2. MULTIPLE DX										
0–19 Years	67	5.9	75	2	3	4	5	8	24	55
20–34	29	6.1	180	1	2	2	4	7	38	66
35–49	34	6.8	78	2	2	3	6	20	30	38
50–64	29	4.4	20	1	1	3	6	9	16	20
65+	12	3.9	12	1	1	3	4	7	13	13
TOTAL SINGLE DX	31	3.1	2	1	2	3	4	5	6	7
TOTAL MULTIPLE DX	171	5.8	77	1	2	4	5	8	24	55
TOTAL										
0–19 Years	90	5.2	57	1	3	4	5	7	9	55
20–34	32	5.7	163	1	2	3	4	5	38	66
35–49	37	6.4	73	1	1	3	6	20	30	38
50–64	31	6.4	19	1	1	3	6	8	16	20
65+	12	3.9	12	1	1	3	4	7	13	13
GRAND TOTAL	202	5.2	63	1	2	4	5	7	16	55

02.04: BONE GRAFT TO SKULL

Type of Patients	Observed Patients	Avg. Stay	Variance	10th	25th	50th	75th	90th	95th	99th
1. SINGLE DX										
0–19 Years	9	2.9	<1	1	3	3	3	4	4	4
20–34	0									
35–49	1	2.0	0	2	2	2	2	2	2	2
50–64	1	2.0	0	2	2	2	2	2	2	2
65+	0									
2. MULTIPLE DX										
0–19 Years	44	3.8	15	1	3	3	4	5	7	13
20–34	8	3.8	10	1	1	3	7	10	10	10
35–49	11	2.5	5	1	2	2	3	6	8	8
50–64	15	6.5	171	1	1	2	5	10	53	53
65+	7	6.4	67	1	1	1	9	23	23	23
TOTAL SINGLE DX	11	2.8	<1	1	3	3	3	4	4	4
TOTAL MULTIPLE DX	85	4.1	30	1	2	3	4	7	8	42
TOTAL										
0–19 Years	53	3.7	12	1	3	3	4	5	7	13
20–34	8	3.8	10	1	1	3	7	10	10	10
35–49	12	2.5	5	1	1	2	2	6	8	8
50–64	16	6.3	161	1	2	2	5	10	53	53
65+	7	6.4	67	1	1	1	9	23	23	23
GRAND TOTAL	96	3.9	26	1	2	3	4	5	8	42

LOS by Diagnosis and Operation, Western Region, 45th Edition

Western Region, October 2007–September 2008 Data, by Operation

02.05: SKULL PLATE INSERTION

Type of Patients	Observed Patients	Avg. Stay	Variance	Percentiles						
				10th	25th	50th	75th	90th	95th	99th
1. SINGLE DX										
0–19 Years	6	2.3	1	1	1	2	3	4	4	4
20–34	7	1.3	<1	1	1	1	2	2	2	2
35–49	5	1.4	<1	1	1	1	2	2	2	2
50–64	3	1.3	<1	1	1	1	2	2	2	2
65+	1	1.0	0	1	1	1	1	1	1	1
2. MULTIPLE DX										
0–19 Years	14	3.9	13	1	3	3	4	6	6	22
20–34	41	3.6	28	1	3	3	4	6	7	35
35–49	52	3.9	31	1	1	2	4	8	10	39
50–64	60	3.4	23	1	1	2	4	6	12	34
65+	21	4.7	33	1	2	3	5	8	15	26
TOTAL SINGLE DX	22	1.6	<1	1	1	1	2	3	3	4
TOTAL MULTIPLE DX	188	3.8	25	1	1	3	4	6	9	34
TOTAL										
0–19 Years	20	3.7	11	1	2	3	4	6	6	22
20–34	48	3.2	25	1	1	2	3	6	7	35
35–49	57	3.7	29	1	1	2	4	8	10	39
50–64	63	3.3	22	1	1	2	3	6	7	34
65+	22	4.5	32	1	2	3	5	8	15	26
GRAND TOTAL	210	3.6	23	1	1	2	4	6	9	34

02.06: CRANIAL OSTEOPLASTY NEC

Type of Patients	Observed Patients	Avg. Stay	Variance	Percentiles						
				10th	25th	50th	75th	90th	95th	99th
1. SINGLE DX										
0–19 Years	122	2.4	1	1	1	3	3	4	4	6
20–34	21	2.5	3	1	1	2	3	5	6	6
35–49	18	1.6	<1	1	1	2	2	2	2	2
50–64	23	2.4	2	1	1	2	3	4	6	7
65+	2	1.5	<1	1	1	2	2	2	2	2
2. MULTIPLE DX										
0–19 Years	278	4.7	51	1	2	3	4	7	13	42
20–34	124	4.0	23	1	1	2	4	8	10	27
35–49	164	5.6	69	1	2	3	6	11	17	58
50–64	206	5.3	65	1	2	3	6	10	21	52
65+	71	7.4	167	1	2	3	8	15	21	77
TOTAL SINGLE DX	186	2.4	2	1	1	2	3	4	4	6
TOTAL MULTIPLE DX	843	5.0	60	1	2	3	5	9	15	47
TOTAL										
0–19 Years	400	3.9	36	1	2	3	4	6	9	23
20–34	145	3.8	20	1	1	2	4	8	10	27
35–49	182	5.2	63	1	2	3	5	11	17	58
50–64	229	5.0	59	1	2	3	5	10	20	52
65+	73	7.3	163	1	2	3	7	15	21	77
GRAND TOTAL	1,029	4.4	47	1	2	3	4	7	13	42

02.1: CEREBRAL MENINGES REPAIR

Type of Patients	Observed Patients	Avg. Stay	Variance	Percentiles						
				10th	25th	50th	75th	90th	95th	99th
1. SINGLE DX										
0–19 Years	24	2.8	2	1	2	2	4	5	5	6
20–34	20	3.1	1	2	2	3	3	4	5	6
35–49	12	3.5	4	2	2	3	5	6	7	7
50–64	8	4.1	9	1	2	4	4	11	11	11
65+	1	3.0	0	3	3	3	3	3	3	3
2. MULTIPLE DX										
0–19 Years	136	7.2	103	2	3	4	7	21	22	43
20–34	142	5.6	29	2	3	4	7	12	15	28
35–49	153	5.8	69	2	3	4	6	10	16	43
50–64	132	7.5	64	2	3	4	9	19	24	34
65+	57	8.6	68	1	3	5	12	22	26	32
TOTAL SINGLE DX	65	3.2	3	1	2	3	4	5	6	11
TOTAL MULTIPLE DX	620	6.8	74	2	3	4	7	16	22	42
TOTAL										
0–19 Years	160	6.9	96	2	2	4	7	20	22	43
20–34	162	5.3	26	2	2	3	6	11	15	28
35–49	165	5.6	65	2	3	4	6	9	14	43
50–64	140	7.3	61	2	3	4	9	19	24	34
65+	58	8.5	67	1	3	5	12	22	26	32
GRAND TOTAL	685	6.5	69	2	3	4	7	15	22	35

02.12: REP CEREBRAL MENING NEC

Type of Patients	Observed Patients	Avg. Stay	Variance	Percentiles						
				10th	25th	50th	75th	90th	95th	99th
1. SINGLE DX										
0–19 Years	21	2.8	2	1	2	2	4	4	5	6
20–34	20	3.1	1	2	2	3	3	4	5	6
35–49	12	3.5	4	2	2	3	5	6	7	7
50–64	8	4.1	9	1	2	4	4	11	11	11
65+	0									
2. MULTIPLE DX										
0–19 Years	127	6.9	102	2	3	4	7	16	22	66
20–34	137	5.5	28	2	3	4	6	12	15	28
35–49	150	5.7	70	2	3	4	6	10	14	43
50–64	128	7.6	65	2	3	4	9	19	24	34
65+	53	8.3	68	1	3	5	10	22	26	32
TOTAL SINGLE DX	61	3.2	3	1	2	3	4	5	6	11
TOTAL MULTIPLE DX	595	6.6	73	2	3	4	7	13	22	42
TOTAL										
0–19 Years	148	6.5	95	2	2	4	6	15	21	43
20–34	157	5.2	26	2	3	3	6	11	15	28
35–49	162	5.5	65	2	3	4	5	9	13	43
50–64	136	7.4	62	2	3	4	8	19	24	34
65+	53	8.3	68	1	3	5	10	22	26	32
GRAND TOTAL	656	6.3	69	2	3	4	7	13	21	35

LOS by Diagnosis and Operation, Western Region, 45th Edition

Western Region, October 2007–September 2008 Data, by Operation

02.2: VENTRICULOSTOMY

Type of Patients	Observed Patients	Avg. Stay	Variance	10th	25th	50th	75th	90th	95th	99th
1. SINGLE DX										
0–19 Years	21	2.7	5	1	1	2	3	8	8	8
20–34	11	4.1	11	1	1	4	6	7	12	12
35–49	4	2.5	3	1	1	2	5	5	5	5
50–64	6	3.0	5	1	1	2	4	7	7	7
65+	1	1.0	0	1	1	1	1	1	1	1
2. MULTIPLE DX										
0–19 Years	340	16.9	341	2	4	11	23	48	65	>99
20–34	270	16.3	168	3	6	13	24	35	45	>99
35–49	333	18.4	293	1	6	14	26	43	61	>99
50–64	445	20.1	332	2	6	15	27	45	62	93
65+	318	15.6	166	2	6	12	22	31	38	56
TOTAL SINGLE DX	43	2.9	6	1	1	2	4	7	8	12
TOTAL MULTIPLE DX	1,706	17.5	285	2	6	13	24	41	58	98
TOTAL										
0–19 Years	361	16.1	333	2	3	10	21	48	64	>99
20–34	281	15.8	168	2	6	12	24	34	45	>99
35–49	337	18.2	292	1	6	14	25	42	61	>99
50–64	451	19.9	331	1	7	15	27	45	62	93
65+	319	15.5	166	2	6	12	22	31	38	56
GRAND TOTAL	1,749	17.1	283	2	5	12	24	39	58	97

02.3: EXTRACRANIAL VENT SHUNT

Type of Patients	Observed Patients	Avg. Stay	Variance	10th	25th	50th	75th	90th	95th	99th
1. SINGLE DX										
0–19 Years	54	2.0	4	1	1	1	2	4	4	4
20–34	17	4.7	45	1	1	1	4	17	24	24
35–49	15	2.1	4	1	1	2	3	4	8	8
50–64	15	1.9	2	1	1	2	2	4	6	6
65+	31	2.2	2	1	1	2	3	4	5	6
2. MULTIPLE DX										
0–19 Years	420	8.4	190	1	2	3	8	25	47	>99
20–34	183	8.5	188	1	2	4	8	17	39	81
35–49	229	9.9	176	1	5	5	13	30	40	>99
50–64	354	8.6	149	1	2	4	10	22	36	69
65+	828	5.3	46	1	2	3	6	13	18	35
TOTAL SINGLE DX	132	2.3	8	1	1	2	2	4	5	22
TOTAL MULTIPLE DX	2,014	7.6	139	1	2	3	8	19	36	88
TOTAL										
0–19 Years	474	7.7	173	1	1	3	7	24	44	>99
20–34	200	8.2	177	1	2	4	8	17	39	72
35–49	244	9.4	168	1	2	4	12	30	38	>99
50–64	369	8.3	145	1	2	4	9	22	34	69
65+	859	5.2	45	1	2	3	6	13	17	35
GRAND TOTAL	2,146	7.2	131	1	2	3	7	18	34	87

02.34: VENT SHUNT TO ABD CAVITY

Type of Patients	Observed Patients	Avg. Stay	Variance	10th	25th	50th	75th	90th	95th	99th
1. SINGLE DX										
0–19 Years	50	1.8	1	1	1	1	2	4	4	4
20–34	15	4.1	39	1	1	1	4	12	24	24
35–49	14	2.0	4	1	1	1	3	3	8	8
50–64	15	1.9	2	1	1	2	2	4	6	6
65+	29	2.0	1	1	1	2	2	4	5	5
2. MULTIPLE DX										
0–19 Years	368	7.6	177	1	1	3	7	21	43	>99
20–34	163	7.1	140	1	2	3	7	13	39	72
35–49	205	9.7	186	1	2	4	11	30	38	78
50–64	310	7.1	103	1	2	3	8	16	29	56
65+	790	4.9	35	1	2	3	6	12	16	29
TOTAL SINGLE DX	123	2.0	5	1	1	1	2	4	4	12
TOTAL MULTIPLE DX	1,836	6.8	119	1	2	3	7	16	29	75
TOTAL										
0–19 Years	418	6.9	160	1	1	3	6	18	42	>99
20–34	178	6.9	132	1	2	4	7	13	32	72
35–49	219	9.2	177	1	2	4	10	27	37	78
50–64	325	6.8	99	1	2	3	8	15	26	56
65+	819	4.8	34	1	2	3	6	12	16	29
GRAND TOTAL	1,959	6.4	112	1	1	3	6	15	27	73

02.39: OPS TO ESTAB VENT DRAIN

Type of Patients	Observed Patients	Avg. Stay	Variance	10th	25th	50th	75th	90th	95th	99th
1. SINGLE DX										
0–19 Years	4	7.0	100	2	2	2	22	22	22	22
20–34	2	8.9	126	1	1	1	17	17	17	17
35–49	0									
50–64	0									
65+										
2. MULTIPLE DX										
0–19 Years	28	15.3	191	1	5	12	26	61	>99	>99
20–34	8	29.4	746	4	12	23	56	81	81	81
35–49	14	14.7	110	4	15	15	30	33	>99	>99
50–64	25	27.4	426	9	15	22	42	69	89	>99
65+	18	21.0	219	1	9	19	28	45	54	54
TOTAL SINGLE DX	6	7.7	86	1	2	2	17	22	22	22
TOTAL MULTIPLE DX	93	19.6	292	3	7	16	30	56	>99	>99
TOTAL										
0–19 Years	32	14.8	187	1	5	11	25	41	>99	>99
20–34	10	25.4	670	1	6	17	38	81	81	81
35–49	14	14.7	110	4	6	15	30	33	>99	>99
50–64	25	27.4	426	9	15	22	42	69	89	>99
65+	18	21.0	219	1	9	19	28	45	54	54
GRAND TOTAL	99	19.0	288	2	7	16	29	54	>99	>99

LOS by Diagnosis and Operation, Western Region, 45th Edition

Western Region, October 2007–September 2008 Data, by Operation

02.4: VENT SHUNT REV/RMVL

Type of Patients	Observed Patients	Avg. Stay	Vari-ance	Percentiles						
				10th	25th	50th	75th	90th	95th	99th
1. SINGLE DX										
0–19 Years	24	1.3	<1	1	1	1	1	2	2	6
20–34	12	2.5	4	1	1	2	3	5	8	8
35–49	7	2.4	4	1	1	1	5	5	5	5
50–64	3	3.3	2	2	2	3	5	5	5	5
65+	3	3.0	12	1	1	1	7	7	7	7
2. MULTIPLE DX										
0–19 Years	1,030	4.8	56	1	1	2	4	12	16	42
20–34	347	4.8	39	1	1	3	5	12	16	35
35–49	236	7.6	129	1	2	4	8	17	24	76
50–64	211	6.8	76	1	2	4	8	16	22	38
65+	208	6.4	68	1	2	3	8	15	22	45
TOTAL SINGLE DX	49	1.8	2	1	1	1	2	4	5	8
TOTAL MULTIPLE DX	2,032	5.2	61	1	1	2	5	12	18	43
TOTAL										
0–19 Years	1,054	4.7	55	1	1	2	4	12	16	42
20–34	359	4.8	38	1	1	3	5	12	16	35
35–49	243	7.5	126	1	2	4	7	16	24	76
50–64	214	6.8	75	1	2	4	8	16	22	38
65+	211	6.3	67	1	2	3	7	14	22	45
GRAND TOTAL	2,081	5.1	60	1	1	2	5	12	18	42

02.42: REPL VENTRICULAR SHUNT

Type of Patients	Observed Patients	Avg. Stay	Vari-ance	Percentiles						
				10th	25th	50th	75th	90th	95th	99th
1. SINGLE DX										
0–19 Years	20	1.4	<1	1	1	1	2	2	3	6
20–34	11	2.0	2	1	1	2	3	4	5	5
35–49	7	2.4	4	1	1	1	5	5	5	5
50–64	3	3.3	2	2	2	3	5	5	5	5
65+	3	3.0	12	1	1	1	7	7	7	7
2. MULTIPLE DX										
0–19 Years	953	4.3	45	1	1	2	4	11	15	37
20–34	296	4.4	33	1	1	3	5	10	14	35
35–49	183	7.1	112	1	2	4	7	15	21	84
50–64	147	6.6	91	1	2	4	8	17	23	43
65+	147	5.1	51	1	1	3	6	12	16	37
TOTAL SINGLE DX	44	1.8	2	1	1	1	2	4	5	7
TOTAL MULTIPLE DX	1,726	4.6	50	1	1	2	4	11	15	38
TOTAL										
0–19 Years	973	4.3	45	1	1	2	4	10	15	37
20–34	307	4.3	32	1	1	3	5	10	14	35
35–49	190	6.9	109	1	2	4	7	14	21	84
50–64	150	6.6	90	1	2	3	7	16	23	43
65+	150	5.1	50	1	1	2	6	12	16	37
GRAND TOTAL	1,770	4.6	49	1	1	2	4	11	15	37

02.43: RMVL VENTRICULAR SHUNT

Type of Patients	Observed Patients	Avg. Stay	Vari-ance	Percentiles						
				10th	25th	50th	75th	90th	95th	99th
1. SINGLE DX										
0–19 Years	4	1.0	0	1	1		1	1	1	1
20–34	1	8.0	0	8	8	8	8	8	8	8
35–49	0									
50–64	0									
65+	0									
2. MULTIPLE DX										
0–19 Years	70	10.8	171	1	1	7	13	26	32	64
20–34	36	10.0	88	1	3	7	15	26	30	38
35–49	43	11.1	217	1	3	6	13	24	30	76
50–64	42	8.6	50	2	3	7	12	17	22	30
65+	39	11.4	126	2	3	8	18	24	45	45
TOTAL SINGLE DX	5	1.6	4	1	1	1	1	1	8	8
TOTAL MULTIPLE DX	230	10.6	148	1	2	7	13	25	32	64
TOTAL										
0–19 Years	74	10.4	167	1	1	7	13	25	32	64
20–34	37	10.0	86	1	3	7	14	26	30	38
35–49	43	11.1	217	1	3	6	13	24	30	76
50–64	42	8.6	50	2	3	7	12	17	22	30
65+	39	11.4	126	2	3	8	18	24	45	45
GRAND TOTAL	235	10.3	146	1	2	7	13	24	32	64

02.9: SKULL & BRAIN OPS NEC

Type of Patients	Observed Patients	Avg. Stay	Vari-ance	Percentiles						
				10th	25th	50th	75th	90th	95th	99th
1. SINGLE DX										
0–19 Years	17	4.0	19	1	1	2	2	13	13	13
20–34	27	4.8	9	1	2	4	4	9	10	11
35–49	21	2.4	3	1	1	1	4	4	6	6
50–64	49	2.2	5	1	1	1	2	4	9	12
65+	34	1.4	<1	1	1	1	1	2	3	5
2. MULTIPLE DX										
0–19 Years	108	10.5	94	2	4	8	14	22	30	32
20–34	198	11.4	149	2	3	7	14	27	35	65
35–49	184	7.5	62	1	2	5	10	21	25	44
50–64	374	5.8	72	1	1	3	7	15	19	48
65+	495	4.5	50	1	1	2	5	10	16	36
TOTAL SINGLE DX	148	2.8	8	1	1	2	3	6	9	13
TOTAL MULTIPLE DX	1,359	7.1	84	1	1	4	9	17	25	40
TOTAL										
0–19 Years	125	9.9	91	2	3	7	13	21	30	32
20–34	225	10.6	137	2	3	7	13	26	33	65
35–49	205	6.9	59	1	1	4	9	18	24	38
50–64	423	5.4	65	1	1	4	6	14	18	47
65+	529	4.3	47	1	1	2	5	10	16	31
GRAND TOTAL	1,507	6.7	78	1	1	3	8	17	23	39

LOS by Diagnosis and Operation, Western Region, 45th Edition

Western Region, October 2007–September 2008 Data, by Operation

02.93: IMPL/REPL IC NEURSTIM LD

Type of Patients	Observed Patients	Avg. Stay	Vari-ance	Percentiles						
				10th	25th	50th	75th	90th	95th	99th
1. SINGLE DX										
0–19 Years	2	10.8	24	2	13	13	13	13	13	13
20–34	11	6.4	13	2	2	8	9	10	11	11
35–49	16	2.1	3	1	1	1	3	4	6	6
50–64	44	2.0	5	1	1	1	2	3	9	12
65+	32	1.3	<1	1	1	1	1	2	2	3
2. MULTIPLE DX										
0–19 Years	39	15.6	71	6	10	14	21	30	32	37
20–34	57	11.4	90	1	4	9	14	22	35	35
35–49	85	5.3	48	1	1	2	7	13	21	38
50–64	219	2.9	18	1	1	1	2	7	13	19
65+	298	1.8	3	1	1	1	2	4	5	11
TOTAL SINGLE DX	105	2.7	10	1	1	1	2	9	11	13
TOTAL MULTIPLE DX	698	5.0	50	1	1	2	6	14	21	33
TOTAL										
0–19 Years	41	15.3	69	6	10	13	20	30	32	37
20–34	68	10.6	81	1	4	9	14	22	35	35
35–49	101	4.8	43	1	1	2	6	11	17	28
50–64	263	2.7	16	1	1	1	2	7	12	19
65+	330	1.8	3	1	1	1	2	3	5	11
GRAND TOTAL	803	4.7	46	1	1	1	5	14	20	32

02.94: INSERT/REPL SKULL TONGS

Type of Patients	Observed Patients	Avg. Stay	Vari-ance	Percentiles						
				10th	25th	50th	75th	90th	95th	99th
1. SINGLE DX										
0–19 Years	10	2.4	2	1	1	2	3	4	6	6
20–34	10	3.3	5	1	2	3	4	7	7	7
35–49	2	2.5	2	1	2	3	4	4	4	4
50–64	5	4.0	0	3	3	4	4	6	6	6
65+	1	1.0		1	1	1	1	1	1	1
2. MULTIPLE DX										
0–19 Years	42	10.3	171	3	5	7	11	16	27	90
20–34	120	12.6	192	2	3	8	17	28	36	68
35–49	72	10.6	83	3	4	6	17	24	28	>99
50–64	122	10.6	135	3	4	6	12	20	35	62
65+	171	9.2	102	2	4	6	10	18	26	64
TOTAL SINGLE DX	28	2.9	3	1	1	3	4	6	7	7
TOTAL MULTIPLE DX	527	10.6	135	2	4	7	13	23	32	65
TOTAL										
0–19 Years	52	8.6	145	2	4	5	9	16	17	90
20–34	130	11.9	184	2	3	7	16	27	36	68
35–49	74	10.4	82	3	4	6	17	24	28	>99
50–64	127	10.3	132	3	4	6	12	20	35	62
65+	172	9.1	102	2	4	6	10	18	26	64
GRAND TOTAL	555	10.2	130	2	4	6	12	22	31	65

03.0: SPINAL CANAL EXPLORATION

Type of Patients	Observed Patients	Avg. Stay	Vari-ance	Percentiles						
				10th	25th	50th	75th	90th	95th	99th
1. SINGLE DX										
0–19 Years	45	2.7	6	1	1	2	3	4	7	14
20–34	80	2.3	3	1	1	2	3	5	7	8
35–49	278	1.7	2	1	1	1	2	3	4	6
50–64	454	1.7	2	1	1	1	2	3	4	8
65+	316	1.8	2	1	1	1	2	3	4	5
2. MULTIPLE DX										
0–19 Years	373	7.6	120	2	3	4	7	18	37	61
20–34	463	5.2	52	1	1	3	6	12	18	41
35–49	1,905	3.9	42	1	1	2	4	8	14	39
50–64	5,712	3.3	25	1	1	2	3	6	10	26
65+	9,303	3.2	13	1	1	2	4	6	9	18
TOTAL SINGLE DX	1,173	1.8	2	1	1	1	2	3	4	7
TOTAL MULTIPLE DX	17,756	3.5	27	1	1	2	4	7	11	27
TOTAL										
0–19 Years	418	7.2	112	2	2	4	6	16	33	61
20–34	543	4.8	46	1	1	3	5	11	16	36
35–49	2,183	3.7	37	1	1	2	4	7	13	35
50–64	6,166	3.1	24	1	1	2	3	6	9	26
65+	9,619	3.2	13	1	1	2	4	6	9	18
GRAND TOTAL	18,929	3.4	25	1	1	2	4	7	10	26

03.02: REOPEN LAMINECTOMY SITE

Type of Patients	Observed Patients	Avg. Stay	Vari-ance	Percentiles						
				10th	25th	50th	75th	90th	95th	99th
1. SINGLE DX										
0–19 Years	0									
20–34	2	5.0	8	3	3	3	7	7	7	7
35–49	5	1.6	<1	1	1	1	3	3	3	3
50–64	5	1.2	<1	1	1	1	1	2	2	2
65+	3	1.0	0	1	1	1	1	1	1	1
2. MULTIPLE DX										
0–19 Years	5	9.4	31	4	4	8	16	16	16	16
20–34	18	5.8	18	1	3	4	10	12	15	15
35–49	71	4.8	42	1	2	6	6	9	16	41
50–64	110	6.3	81	1	2	3	7	14	21	49
65+	132	4.9	18	1	2	4	7	10	14	20
TOTAL SINGLE DX	15	1.8	3	1	1	1	2	3	7	7
TOTAL MULTIPLE DX	336	5.5	44	1	2	4	7	12	16	41
TOTAL										
0–19 Years	5	9.4	31	4	4	8	16	16	16	16
20–34	20	5.7	17	1	3	4	9	12	15	15
35–49	76	4.6	40	1	1	3	5	9	16	41
50–64	115	6.1	79	1	2	3	7	13	21	49
65+	135	4.8	18	1	2	4	6	10	14	20
GRAND TOTAL	351	5.4	43	1	2	4	6	11	16	41

Western Region, October 2007–September 2008 Data, by Operation

03.09: SPINAL CANAL EXPL NEC

Type of Patients	Observed Patients	Avg. Stay	Variance	10th	25th	50th	75th	90th	95th	99th
1. SINGLE DX										
0–19 Years	44	2.7	6	1	2	2	3	4	7	14
20–34	77	2.2	3	1	1	2	3	5	6	8
35–49	273	1.7	2	1	1	1	2	3	4	6
50–64	449	1.7	2	1	1	1	2	3	4	6
65+	313	1.8	2	1	1	1	2	3	4	5
2. MULTIPLE DX										
0–19 Years	362	7.6	122	2	2	4	6	18	37	61
20–34	442	5.2	54	1	1	3	6	12	18	41
35–49	1,830	3.9	42	1	1	2	4	8	14	39
50–64	5,598	3.2	24	1	1	2	3	6	9	26
65+	9,166	3.2	13	1	1	2	4	6	9	18
TOTAL SINGLE DX	1,156	1.8	2	1	1	1	2	3	4	7
TOTAL MULTIPLE DX	17,398	3.5	26	1	1	2	4	7	10	27
TOTAL										
0–19 Years	406	7.2	114	2	2	4	6	16	33	61
20–34	519	4.7	47	1	1	2	5	11	16	36
35–49	2,103	3.6	37	1	1	2	3	7	13	34
50–64	6,047	3.1	23	1	1	2	3	6	9	25
65+	9,479	3.1	13	1	1	2	4	6	8	17
GRAND TOTAL	18,554	3.4	25	1	1	2	4	6	10	26

03.1: INTRASPIN NERVE ROOT DIV

Type of Patients	Observed Patients	Avg. Stay	Variance	10th	25th	50th	75th	90th	95th	99th
1. SINGLE DX										
0–19 Years	3	3.3	<1	3	3	3	4	4	4	4
20–34	0									
35–49	0									
50–64	0									
65+	1	2.0	0	2	2	2	2	2	2	2
2. MULTIPLE DX										
0–19 Years	6	7.9	16	4	4	5	11	13	13	13
20–34	0									
35–49	9	2.8	3	1	1	3	3	6	6	6
50–64	2	1.0	<1	1	1	1	1	1	1	1
65+										
TOTAL SINGLE DX	4	3.0	<1	2	2	3	3	4	4	4
TOTAL MULTIPLE DX	17	5.8	18	1	3	5	11	13	13	13
TOTAL										
0–19 Years	9	7.2	16	3	4	5	11	13	13	13
20–34	0									
35–49	9	2.8	3	1	1	3	3	6	6	6
50–64	9	2.8	<1	1	1	3	3	6	6	6
65+	3	1.3	<1	1	1	1	2	2	2	2
GRAND TOTAL	21	5.5	17	1	3	4	11	13	13	13

03.2: CHORDOTOMY

Type of Patients	Observed Patients	Avg. Stay	Variance	10th	25th	50th	75th	90th	95th	99th
1. SINGLE DX										
0–19 Years	0									
20–34	1	1.0	0	1	1	1	1	1	1	1
35–49	1									
50–64	1	2.0	0	2	2	2	2	2	2	2
65+	0									
2. MULTIPLE DX										
0–19 Years	16	7.6	329	2	2	3	4	6	84	84
20–34	1	4.0	0	4	4	4	4	4	4	4
35–49	4	3.3	7	1	2	3	3	7	7	7
50–64	2	5.5	4	4	4	4	7	7	7	7
65+	5	8.8	11	3	9	10	11	11	11	11
TOTAL SINGLE DX	2	1.5	<1	1	1	1	2	2	2	2
TOTAL MULTIPLE DX	28	7.0	207	2	3	3	7	11	12	84
TOTAL										
0–19 Years	16	7.6	329	2	2	3	4	6	84	84
20–34	1	4.0	0	4	4	4	4	4	4	4
35–49	5	2.8	6	1	1	2	3	7	7	7
50–64	3	4.3	6	2	2	4	7	7	7	7
65+	5	8.8	11	3	9	10	11	11	11	11
GRAND TOTAL	30	6.7	196	2	2	3	6	11	12	84

03.3: DXTIC PX ON SPINAL CANAL

Type of Patients	Observed Patients	Avg. Stay	Variance	10th	25th	50th	75th	90th	95th	99th
1. SINGLE DX										
0–19 Years	2,919	2.6	3	1	2	2	3	4	5	10
20–34	443	2.6	3	1	2	2	3	5	6	10
35–49	238	2.9	5	1	1	2	4	5	6	14
50–64	82	2.9	11	1	1	2	3	4	6	26
65+	15	3.3	4	2	2	3	5	6	7	7
2. MULTIPLE DX										
0–19 Years	13,915	4.5	26	1	2	3	5	9	13	26
20–34	4,917	4.3	19	1	2	3	5	8	12	22
35–49	6,097	5.0	29	1	2	4	6	10	14	26
50–64	6,098	5.8	36	2	3	5	7	12	16	32
65+	5,767	6.6	34	2	3	5	8	13	17	30
TOTAL SINGLE DX	3,697	2.6	3	1	2	2	3	4	5	10
TOTAL MULTIPLE DX	36,794	4.9	28	1	2	3	6	10	14	27
TOTAL										
0–19 Years	16,834	4.1	23	1	2	3	4	8	12	24
20–34	5,360	4.1	17	1	2	3	5	8	11	21
35–49	6,335	4.9	29	1	2	4	6	10	13	26
50–64	6,180	5.8	36	1	2	4	7	12	16	32
65+	5,782	6.5	34	2	3	5	8	13	17	30
GRAND TOTAL	40,491	4.7	26	1	2	3	5	9	13	26

LOS by Diagnosis and Operation, Western Region, 45th Edition

Western Region, October 2007–September 2008 Data, by Operation

03.31: SPINAL TAP

Type of Patients	Observed Patients	Avg. Stay	Vari-ance	Percentiles						
				10th	25th	50th	75th	90th	95th	99th
1. SINGLE DX										
0–19 Years	2,919	2.6	3	1	2	2	3	4	5	10
20–34	443	2.6	3	1	2	2	3	4	6	10
35–49	237	2.9	5	1	2	2	4	5	6	14
50–64	82	2.9	11	1	3	2	3	4	6	26
65+	15	3.3	4	2	2	3	5	6	7	7
2. MULTIPLE DX										
0–19 Years	13,905	4.5	26	1	2	3	5	9	13	26
20–34	4,903	4.3	18	1	2	3	5	8	12	21
35–49	6,075	5.0	28	1	2	4	6	10	13	26
50–64	6,043	5.7	35	1	2	4	7	12	16	31
65+	5,709	6.5	34	2	3	5	8	13	17	30
TOTAL SINGLE DX	3,696	2.6	3	1	2	2	3	4	5	10
TOTAL MULTIPLE DX	36,635	4.9	28	1	2	3	6	10	14	27
TOTAL										
0–19 Years	16,824	4.1	23	1	2	3	4	8	12	24
20–34	5,346	4.1	17	1	2	3	5	8	11	21
35–49	6,312	4.9	27	1	2	3	6	10	13	26
50–64	6,125	5.7	35	1	2	4	7	11	16	31
65+	5,724	6.5	34	2	3	5	8	13	17	29
GRAND TOTAL	40,331	4.7	26	1	2	3	5	9	13	26

03.32: SPINAL CORD/MENINGES BX

Type of Patients	Observed Patients	Avg. Stay	Vari-ance	Percentiles						
				10th	25th	50th	75th	90th	95th	99th
1. SINGLE DX										
0–19 Years	0									
20–34	0									
35–49	0									
65+	0									
2. MULTIPLE DX										
0–19 Years	8	4.7	26	1	2	2	5	15	15	15
20–34	10	11.3	127	3	3	6	16	22	38	38
35–49	21	14.9	437	3	4	7	9	52	62	76
50–64	46	11.8	127	3	6	8	15	21	32	62
65+	43	10.1	54	3	4	8	14	22	24	30
TOTAL SINGLE DX	0									
TOTAL MULTIPLE DX	128	10.6	140	2	4	7	14	21	30	62
TOTAL										
0–19 Years	8	4.7	26	1	2	2	5	15	15	15
20–34	10	11.3	127	3	3	6	16	22	38	38
35–49	21	14.9	437	3	4	7	9	52	62	76
50–64	46	11.8	127	3	6	8	15	21	32	62
65+	43	10.1	54	3	4	8	14	22	24	30
GRAND TOTAL	128	10.6	140	2	4	7	14	21	30	62

03.4: EXC SPINAL CORD LESION

Type of Patients	Observed Patients	Avg. Stay	Vari-ance	Percentiles						
				10th	25th	50th	75th	90th	95th	99th
1. SINGLE DX										
0–19 Years	27	3.0	3	1	2	2	4	5	5	10
20–34	24	4.3	5	2	3	4	6	7	8	10
35–49	34	3.4	6	1	2	3	4	6	9	12
50–64	44	3.6	3	2	3	3	4	6	8	9
65+	8	2.1	2	1	1	2	4	4	4	4
2. MULTIPLE DX										
0–19 Years	175	7.0	86	1	2	4	7	15	20	68
20–34	97	8.0	81	2	3	6	9	16	28	44
35–49	251	7.2	88	2	3	4	7	15	20	51
50–64	520	6.4	58	1	3	5	8	13	17	45
65+	406	7.1	56	1	3	5	9	14	21	34
TOTAL SINGLE DX	137	3.4	4	1	2	3	4	6	8	10
TOTAL MULTIPLE DX	1,449	6.9	70	1	3	5	8	14	20	53
TOTAL										
0–19 Years	202	6.5	78	1	2	4	7	15	18	54
20–34	121	7.3	68	2	3	5	8	13	22	44
35–49	285	6.8	80	1	3	4	7	13	20	51
50–64	564	6.2	54	1	3	4	7	12	17	45
65+	414	7.0	55	1	3	5	9	14	21	34
GRAND TOTAL	1,586	6.6	65	1	3	4	7	13	19	49

03.5: SPINAL CORD PLASTIC OPS

Type of Patients	Observed Patients	Avg. Stay	Vari-ance	Percentiles						
				10th	25th	50th	75th	90th	95th	99th
1. SINGLE DX										
0–19 Years	40	2.5	3	1	1	2	3	5	6	9
20–34	11	5.7	18	2	2	5	9	11	15	15
35–49	19	3.5	4	1	2	3	4	8	8	8
50–64	21	3.9	6	2	2	3	5	8	9	10
65+	6	2.3	3	1	1	2	2	6	6	6
2. MULTIPLE DX										
0–19 Years	402	6.4	82	2	2	3	6	15	22	53
20–34	232	9.3	91	2	4	7	12	17	27	55
35–49	261	8.5	91	2	3	6	10	18	28	72
50–64	277	8.4	81	2	3	5	10	18	25	52
65+	272	8.6	75	2	4	5	11	19	23	52
TOTAL SINGLE DX	97	3.1	6	1	2	2	4	6	8	11
TOTAL MULTIPLE DX	1,444	7.6	84	2	3	5	9	17	25	53
TOTAL										
0–19 Years	442	6.1	77	1	3	3	6	14	21	53
20–34	243	9.1	88	2	4	6	11	17	26	55
35–49	280	8.2	86	2	3	5	9	17	28	72
50–64	298	8.1	77	2	3	5	10	18	24	45
65+	278	8.5	74	2	3	5	11	19	23	52
GRAND TOTAL	1,541	7.3	81	2	3	4	8	16	25	53

LOS by Diagnosis and Operation, Western Region, 45th Edition

Western Region, October 2007–September 2008 Data, by Operation

03.51: SPINAL MENINGOCELE REP

Type of Patients	Observed Patients	Avg. Stay	Vari-ance	Percentiles						
				10th	25th	50th	75th	90th	95th	99th
1. SINGLE DX										
0–19 Years	4	3.1	2	1	2	4	4	4	6	6
20–34	1	2.0	0	2	2	2	2	2	2	2
35–49	0									
50–64	2	3.0	2	2	2	4	4	4	4	4
65+	0									
2. MULTIPLE DX										
0–19 Years	16	9.1	66	4	4	6	10	23	32	32
20–34	12	4.5	8	1	1	5	6	8	9	9
35–49	24	4.5	11	1	2	4	6	7	9	16
50–64	27	4.9	26	1	2	3	5	10	20	22
65+	20	4.6	9	2	2	4	5	11	12	12
TOTAL SINGLE DX	**7**	**3.0**	**2**	**2**	**2**	**2**	**4**	**4**	**6**	**6**
TOTAL MULTIPLE DX	**99**	**5.7**	**30**	**1**	**3**	**4**	**6**	**10**	**18**	**32**
TOTAL										
0–19 Years	20	7.5	55	2	4	5	6	18	32	32
20–34	13	4.3	8	1	2	5	6	8	9	9
35–49	24	4.5	11	1	2	4	6	7	9	16
50–64	29	4.8	24	2	2	3	5	10	20	22
65+	20	4.6	9	2	2	4	5	11	12	12
GRAND TOTAL	**106**	**5.4**	**28**	**1**	**2**	**4**	**6**	**10**	**16**	**32**

03.53: VERTEBRAL FX REPAIR

Type of Patients	Observed Patients	Avg. Stay	Vari-ance	Percentiles						
				10th	25th	50th	75th	90th	95th	99th
1. SINGLE DX										
0–19 Years	6	4.3	14	1	1	4	8	9	9	9
20–34	4	6.7	16	2	2	5	9	11	11	11
35–49	4	4.8	6	3	3	5	8	8	8	8
50–64	4	5.5	12	2	3	5	8	8	8	8
65+	2	2.0	0	2	2	2	2	2	2	2
2. MULTIPLE DX										
0–19 Years	51	10.0	78	2	5	9	12	22	27	53
20–34	141	11.3	119	3	5	8	14	25	38	67
35–49	121	12.5	144	3	6	9	16	28	47	>99
50–64	110	12.2	129	4	6	9	14	25	41	74
65+	155	10.2	100	2	4	7	13	21	36	62
TOTAL SINGLE DX	**18**	**4.8**	**11**	**1**	**2**	**5**	**8**	**9**	**11**	**11**
TOTAL MULTIPLE DX	**578**	**11.3**	**117**	**3**	**5**	**8**	**14**	**24**	**38**	**74**
TOTAL										
0–19 Years	57	9.4	75	1	5	8	11	22	27	53
20–34	145	11.2	116	3	5	8	14	25	38	67
35–49	125	12.2	141	3	5	8	16	28	47	>99
50–64	112	12.1	128	4	5	9	13	25	41	74
65+	157	10.1	100	2	4	7	13	21	36	62
GRAND TOTAL	**596**	**11.1**	**115**	**2**	**5**	**8**	**14**	**24**	**37**	**72**

03.59: SPINAL STRUCT REPAIR NEC

Type of Patients	Observed Patients	Avg. Stay	Vari-ance	Percentiles						
				10th	25th	50th	75th	90th	95th	99th
1. SINGLE DX										
0–19 Years	29	2.1	2	1	1	2	2	4	5	6
20–34	6	5.7	23	2	2	5	6	15	15	15
35–49	15	3.1	3	2	2	3	4	9	8	8
50–64	17	3.8	7	1	2	3	5	9	10	10
65+	4	2.5	6	1	1	1	2	6	6	6
2. MULTIPLE DX										
0–19 Years	255	4.6	53	1	2	3	4	8	14	50
20–34	79	6.3	35	2	3	5	7	13	16	43
35–49	116	5.2	21	2	2	4	7	9	16	25
50–64	140	6.1	35	2	3	5	7	12	15	26
65+	97	6.8	38	2	3	5	8	15	19	37
TOTAL SINGLE DX	**71**	**2.8**	**5**	**1**	**2**	**2**	**4**	**5**	**6**	**15**
TOTAL MULTIPLE DX	**687**	**5.2**	**45**	**2**	**2**	**3**	**5**	**10**	**15**	**44**
TOTAL										
0–19 Years	284	4.5	50	1	2	3	4	7	14	50
20–34	85	6.2	34	2	3	5	7	13	15	43
35–49	131	4.9	19	2	3	4	6	8	16	25
50–64	157	5.8	32	2	3	5	7	12	14	26
65+	101	6.7	37	2	3	5	8	15	19	29
GRAND TOTAL	**758**	**5.0**	**43**	**1**	**2**	**3**	**5**	**10**	**15**	**43**

03.6: SPINAL CORD ADHESIOLYSIS

Type of Patients	Observed Patients	Avg. Stay	Vari-ance	Percentiles						
				10th	25th	50th	75th	90th	95th	99th
1. SINGLE DX										
0–19 Years	73	1.1	<1	1	1	1	1	1	1	3
20–34	2	1.0	0	1	1	1	1	1	1	1
35–49	2	2.5	<1	2	2	3	3	3	3	3
50–64	0									
65+	0									
2. MULTIPLE DX										
0–19 Years	102	1.7	7	1	1	1	2	2	3	14
20–34	13	2.2	1	1	1	2	2	4	5	5
35–49	24	3.2	6	1	1	2	5	7	8	9
50–64	24	3.5	6	1	2	2	5	8	8	8
65+	49	4.5	22	1	2	3	7	12	12	25
TOTAL SINGLE DX	**77**	**1.1**	**<1**	**1**	**1**	**1**	**1**	**1**	**2**	**3**
TOTAL MULTIPLE DX	**212**	**2.7**	**11**	**1**	**1**	**2**	**3**	**7**	**9**	**14**
TOTAL										
0–19 Years	175	1.4	4	1	1	1	1	2	3	14
20–34	15	2.0	1	1	1	2	2	4	5	5
35–49	26	3.2	6	1	2	2	4	7	8	9
50–64	24	3.5	6	1	2	2	5	8	8	8
65+	49	4.5	22	1	1	3	7	12	12	25
GRAND TOTAL	**289**	**2.3**	**8**	**1**	**1**	**1**	**2**	**5**	**8**	**14**

LOS by Diagnosis and Operation, Western Region, 45th Edition

Western Region, October 2007–September 2008 Data, by Operation

03.7: SPINAL THECAL SHUNT

Type of Patients	Observed Patients	Avg. Stay	Variance	Percentiles						
				10th	25th	50th	75th	90th	95th	99th
1. SINGLE DX										
0–19 Years	2	1.8	<1	1	2	2	2	2	2	2
20–34	10	2.0	1	1	1	2	3	4	4	4
35–49	2	6.5	4	5	5	8	8	8	8	8
50–64	6	1.8	1	1	1	1	2	4	4	4
65+	2	1.0	0	1	1	1	1	1	1	1
2. MULTIPLE DX										
0–19 Years	32	6.5	39	1	2	4	11	15	26	>99
20–34	40	6.4	35	1	2	5	8	12	14	28
35–49	56	5.0	28	1	2	3	6	11	14	32
50–64	47	5.6	68	1	2	3	6	14	20	46
65+	30	5.3	20	2	3	4	5	9	17	19
TOTAL SINGLE DX	22	2.2	3	1	1	2	2	4	5	8
TOTAL MULTIPLE DX	205	5.9	39	1	2	4	8	14	20	>99
TOTAL										
0–19 Years	34	6.3	38	1	2	4	10	15	26	>99
20–34	50	5.5	31	1	2	4	7	12	14	28
35–49	58	5.1	27	1	2	3	6	11	14	32
50–64	53	5.2	62	1	2	3	5	10	20	46
65+	32	5.0	20	2	3	4	5	9	17	19
GRAND TOTAL	227	5.5	37	1	2	4	7	14	19	>99

03.71: SUBARACH-PERITON SHUNT

Type of Patients	Observed Patients	Avg. Stay	Variance	Percentiles						
				10th	25th	50th	75th	90th	95th	99th
1. SINGLE DX										
0–19 Years	2	1.8	<1	1	2	2	2	2	2	2
20–34	8	1.8	1	1	1	2	2	4	4	4
35–49	0									
50–64	3	1.0	0	1	1	1	1	1	1	1
65+	2	1.0	0	1	1	1	1	1	1	1
2. MULTIPLE DX										
0–19 Years	21	7.4	49	1	2	4	13	15	26	26
20–34	32	6.1	27	1	2	4	9	12	14	25
35–49	38	5.2	35	1	1	3	6	13	15	32
50–64	30	4.8	40	1	1	3	6	10	14	33
65+	17	5.2	21	2	3	4	5	16	17	17
TOTAL SINGLE DX	15	1.6	<1	1	1	1	2	2	4	4
TOTAL MULTIPLE DX	138	6.1	38	1	2	4	9	14	16	32
TOTAL										
0–19 Years	23	7.0	48	1	2	3	13	15	26	26
20–34	40	5.3	25	1	2	4	8	11	13	25
35–49	38	5.2	35	1	2	3	6	13	15	32
50–64	33	4.5	37	1	1	2	4	10	14	33
65+	19	4.8	21	2	2	3	5	16	17	17
GRAND TOTAL	153	5.7	37	1	2	3	8	14	15	32

03.8: DESTR INJECT-SPINE CANAL

Type of Patients	Observed Patients	Avg. Stay	Variance	Percentiles						
				10th	25th	50th	75th	90th	95th	99th
1. SINGLE DX										
0–19 Years	0									
20–34	0									
35–49	0									
50–64	0									
65+										
2. MULTIPLE DX										
0–19 Years	4	14.7	414	3	3	4	4	49	49	49
20–34	2	9.0	125	1	1	17	17	17	17	17
35–49	2	11.5	85	5	5	12	18	18	18	18
50–64	0									
65+	3	17.0	142	5	5	17	29	29	29	29
TOTAL SINGLE DX	0									
TOTAL MULTIPLE DX	11	14.2	311	3	3	4	18	49	49	49
TOTAL										
0–19 Years	4	14.7	414	3	3	4	4	49	49	49
20–34	2	9.0	125	1	1	17	17	17	17	17
35–49	2	11.5	85	5	5	12	18	18	18	18
50–64	0									
65+	3	17.0	142	5	5	17	29	29	29	29
GRAND TOTAL	11	14.2	311	3	3	4	18	49	49	49

03.9: SPINAL CORD OPS NEC

Type of Patients	Observed Patients	Avg. Stay	Variance	Percentiles						
				10th	25th	50th	75th	90th	95th	99th
1. SINGLE DX										
0–19 Years	50	3.0	5	1	1	2	5	6	6	12
20–34	176	1.8	2	1	1	2	2	3	4	8
35–49	64	2.8	4	1	1	2	4	6	7	10
50–64	42	2.5	4	1	1	2	3	5	6	8
65+	15	3.1	5	1	1	3	5	5	9	9
2. MULTIPLE DX										
0–19 Years	718	7.5	82	2	3	4	7	17	27	52
20–34	909	4.2	25	1	2	3	5	8	14	34
35–49	1,164	4.5	26	1	2	3	5	9	12	24
50–64	1,355	4.8	28	1	2	4	6	9	13	28
65+	2,091	5.3	17	1	3	4	7	10	13	20
TOTAL SINGLE DX	347	2.3	3	1	1	2	3	5	6	9
TOTAL MULTIPLE DX	6,237	5.4	37	1	2	4	6	10	15	32
TOTAL										
0–19 Years	768	7.3	79	2	3	4	7	17	27	48
20–34	1,085	3.9	23	1	2	2	4	7	12	29
35–49	1,228	4.4	25	1	2	3	5	9	11	24
50–64	1,397	4.8	27	1	2	3	6	9	13	28
65+	2,106	5.3	17	1	3	4	7	10	12	20
GRAND TOTAL	6,584	5.3	36	1	2	4	6	10	15	32

LOS by Diagnosis and Operation, Western Region, 45th Edition

Western Region, October 2007–September 2008 Data, by Operation

03.90: INSERT SPINAL CANAL CATH

Type of Patients	Observed Patients	Avg. Stay	Variance	10th	25th	50th	75th	90th	95th	99th
1. SINGLE DX										
0–19 Years	8	3.6	5	1	2	2	6	6	6	6
20–34	46	1.7	1	1	1	1	2	3	3	7
35–49	4	4.0	12	1	1	1	7	7	7	7
50–64	8	3.3	7	1	1	2	6	8	8	8
65+	4	1.3	<1	1	1	1	2	2	2	2
2. MULTIPLE DX										
0–19 Years	65	6.0	104	1	2	3	7	10	18	53
20–34	157	4.1	28	1	2	2	4	7	15	29
35–49	151	4.5	68	1	2	3	5	8	10	65
50–64	225	5.2	33	1	2	3	7	12	14	32
65+	232	4.8	23	1	2	4	6	10	15	24
TOTAL SINGLE DX	70	2.2	3	1	1	2	2	6	7	8
TOTAL MULTIPLE DX	830	4.9	46	1	2	3	6	10	15	29
TOTAL										
0–19 Years	73	5.8	97	1	2	3	7	10	18	53
20–34	203	3.6	23	1	1	2	3	7	14	26
35–49	155	4.5	67	1	2	3	5	8	10	65
50–64	233	5.2	32	1	2	3	7	11	14	32
65+	236	4.8	23	1	2	3	6	10	15	24
GRAND TOTAL	900	4.7	43	1	2	3	6	10	14	29

03.91: INJECT ANES-SPINAL CANAL

Type of Patients	Observed Patients	Avg. Stay	Variance	10th	25th	50th	75th	90th	95th	99th
1. SINGLE DX										
0–19 Years	24	1.9	<1	1	1	2	2	3	3	4
20–34	102	1.6	<1	1	1	2	2	2	3	3
35–49	19	2.1	2	1	1	2	2	3	7	7
50–64	8	3.4	2	1	3	4	4	5	5	5
65+	3	2.7	<1	2	2	3	3	3	3	3
2. MULTIPLE DX										
0–19 Years	36	5.1	37	1	2	3	3	15	15	28
20–34	187	2.7	5	1	2	2	3	5	7	13
35–49	142	5.0	24	1	2	4	6	9	12	32
50–64	179	5.8	56	1	2	4	6	9	16	44
65+	430	5.6	13	2	3	5	7	10	12	19
TOTAL SINGLE DX	156	1.8	<1	1	1	2	2	3	3	5
TOTAL MULTIPLE DX	974	5.0	23	1	2	4	6	10	12	22
TOTAL										
0–19 Years	60	3.9	25	1	2	2	3	15	15	28
20–34	289	2.3	3	1	1	2	3	4	5	12
35–49	161	4.7	22	1	2	4	6	9	12	32
50–64	187	5.7	54	1	3	4	6	9	14	44
65+	433	5.6	13	2	3	5	7	10	12	19
GRAND TOTAL	1,130	4.5	21	1	2	3	6	9	11	20

03.92: INJECT SPINAL CANAL NEC

Type of Patients	Observed Patients	Avg. Stay	Variance	10th	25th	50th	75th	90th	95th	99th
1. SINGLE DX										
0–19 Years	10	4.3	12	1	1	5	6	9	12	12
20–34	8	3.6	5	1	2	4	5	8	8	8
35–49	24	3.5	5	1	2	3	4	6	9	10
50–64	13	2.6	2	1	2	2	3	4	6	6
65+	4	5.2	7	3	3	4	5	9	9	9
2. MULTIPLE DX										
0–19 Years	531	8.0	79	2	3	5	8	21	28	43
20–34	240	6.4	51	2	3	4	6	13	21	35
35–49	427	5.2	19	2	3	4	6	9	13	24
50–64	542	5.5	26	2	3	4	6	10	15	29
65+	1,173	5.8	15	2	3	5	7	10	13	20
TOTAL SINGLE DX	59	3.6	6	1	2	3	5	6	9	12
TOTAL MULTIPLE DX	2,913	6.4	42	2	3	5	7	12	19	34
TOTAL										
0–19 Years	541	7.9	78	2	3	5	8	20	28	43
20–34	248	6.3	50	2	3	4	6	13	21	35
35–49	451	5.1	19	2	3	4	6	9	12	24
50–64	555	5.4	26	2	3	4	6	10	15	29
65+	1,177	5.8	15	2	3	5	7	10	13	20
GRAND TOTAL	2,972	6.4	42	2	3	5	7	12	19	34

03.93: IMPL/REPL SP NEURSTIM LD

Type of Patients	Observed Patients	Avg. Stay	Variance	10th	25th	50th	75th	90th	95th	99th
1. SINGLE DX										
0–19 Years	0									
20–34	3	1.3	<1	1	1	1	2	2	2	2
35–49	8	2.3	3	1	1	1	4	6	6	6
50–64	7	1.3	<1	1	1	1	2	2	2	2
65+	1	1.0	0	1	1	1	1	1	1	1
2. MULTIPLE DX										
0–19 Years	1	1.0	0	1	1	1	1	1	1	1
20–34	48	2.7	19	1	1	1	2	4	11	24
35–49	170	2.2	4	1	1	2	3	4	6	9
50–64	224	2.6	11	1	1	2	3	5	7	15
65+	153	2.5	7	1	1	1	3	6	7	16
TOTAL SINGLE DX	19	1.7	2	1	1	1	2	4	6	6
TOTAL MULTIPLE DX	596	2.5	8	1	1	2	3	5	7	16
TOTAL										
0–19 Years	1	1.0	0	1	1	1	1	1	1	1
20–34	51	2.7	18	1	1	1	2	3	11	24
35–49	178	2.2	4	1	1	2	3	4	6	9
50–64	231	2.6	10	1	1	2	3	5	7	15
65+	154	2.5	7	1	1	1	3	6	7	16
GRAND TOTAL	615	2.5	8	1	1	2	3	5	7	15

LOS by Diagnosis and Operation, Western Region, 45th Edition

25

Western Region, October 2007–September 2008 Data, by Operation

03.94: RMVL SP NEUROSTIM LEAD

Type of Patients	Observed Patients	Avg. Stay	Vari-ance	10th	25th	50th	75th	90th	95th	99th
1. SINGLE DX										
0–19 Years	0									
20–34	1	5.0	0	5	5	5	5	5	5	5
35–49	3	3.3	10	1	1	2	7	7	7	7
50–64	2	2.0	2	1	1	2	3	3	3	3
65+	1	1.0	0	1	1	1	1	1	1	1
2. MULTIPLE DX										
0–19 Years	1	2.0	0	2	2	2	2	2	2	2
20–34	15	5.7	28	1	2	4	6	17	17	17
35–49	63	4.1	15	1	1	3	5	7	13	19
50–64	54	3.6	5	1	1	3	5	7	8	10
65+	51	3.9	13	1	1	3	5	7	12	19
TOTAL SINGLE DX	7	2.9	5	1	1	2	5	7	7	7
TOTAL MULTIPLE DX	184	4.0	13	1	1	3	5	7	13	19
TOTAL										
0–19 Years	1	2.0	0	2	2	2	2	2	2	2
20–34	16	5.6	27	1	2	5	6	17	17	17
35–49	66	4.1	14	1	1	3	5	7	13	19
50–64	56	3.5	5	1	1	3	5	7	8	10
65+	52	3.8	13	1	1	3	5	7	12	19
GRAND TOTAL	191	4.0	13	1	1	3	5	7	13	19

03.95: SPINAL BLOOD PATCH

Type of Patients	Observed Patients	Avg. Stay	Vari-ance	10th	25th	50th	75th	90th	95th	99th
1. SINGLE DX										
0–19 Years	7	3.1	3	1	1	4	5	5	5	5
20–34	13	1.5	<1	1	1	2	2	2	2	2
35–49	4	2.0	2	1	1	1	4	4	4	4
50–64	2	1.5	<1	1	1	2	2	2	2	2
65+	1	5.0	0	5	5	5	5	5	5	5
2. MULTIPLE DX										
0–19 Years	41	3.4	3	2	2	3	4	7	7	7
20–34	216	3.4	8	1	2	3	4	6	9	15
35–49	139	3.5	8	1	2	3	4	7	9	16
50–64	58	4.0	6	1	2	3	6	8	9	11
65+	11	4.3	6	2	2	4	6	7	9	9
TOTAL SINGLE DX	27	2.2	2	1	1	2	2	5	5	5
TOTAL MULTIPLE DX	465	3.5	7	1	2	3	4	7	9	14
TOTAL										
0–19 Years	48	3.4	3	2	2	3	4	7	7	7
20–34	229	3.3	8	1	2	3	4	6	9	15
35–49	143	3.5	8	1	2	3	4	7	9	16
50–64	60	3.9	6	1	2	3	6	8	9	11
65+	12	4.3	6	2	2	4	6	7	9	9
GRAND TOTAL	492	3.5	7	1	2	3	4	7	9	14

03.97: REV SPINAL THECAL SHUNT

Type of Patients	Observed Patients	Avg. Stay	Vari-ance	10th	25th	50th	75th	90th	95th	99th
1. SINGLE DX										
0–19 Years	0									
20–34	0									
35–49	1	1.0	0						1	1
50–64	2	1.0	0						1	1
65+	0									
2. MULTIPLE DX										
0–19 Years	21	8.9	207	1	2	3	9	26	60	60
20–34	34	3.0	3	1	1	3	4	6	6	7
35–49	46	5.0	48	1	1	3	5	13	19	40
50–64	50	4.1	19	1	1	3	5	9	12	25
65+	26	4.5	15	1	1	3	8	10	11	14
TOTAL SINGLE DX	3	1.0	0	1	1	1	1	1	1	1
TOTAL MULTIPLE DX	177	5.6	82	1	1	3	6	11	19	60
TOTAL										
0–19 Years	21	8.9	207	1	2	3	9	26	60	60
20–34	34	3.0	3	1	1	3	4	6	6	7
35–49	47	4.9	47	1	1	3	5	13	19	40
50–64	52	4.0	19	1	1	2	5	9	12	25
65+	26	4.5	15	1	1	3	8	10	11	14
GRAND TOTAL	180	5.5	81	1	1	3	6	11	19	60

04.0: PERIPH NERVE INC/DIV/EXC

Type of Patients	Observed Patients	Avg. Stay	Vari-ance	10th	25th	50th	75th	90th	95th	99th
1. SINGLE DX										
0–19 Years	3	1.2	<1	1	1	1	1	2	2	2
20–34	17	2.7	2	1	1	2	4	5	5	5
35–49	23	2.0	2	1	2	2	3	4	4	5
50–64	39	2.5	2	1	1	2	3	4	5	5
65+	9	3.1	7	1	1	2	3	8	8	8
2. MULTIPLE DX										
0–19 Years	28	3.2	2	1	2	3	4	5	6	9
20–34	80	3.9	9	1	2	3	5	8	10	14
35–49	143	4.7	44	1	3	3	5	8	13	23
50–64	239	4.4	15	1	2	3	5	8	11	27
65+	108	4.6	20	1	2	4	5	9	11	22
TOTAL SINGLE DX	91	2.4	2	1	1	2	3	4	5	8
TOTAL MULTIPLE DX	598	4.3	20	1	2	3	5	8	11	22
TOTAL										
0–19 Years	31	3.0	2	1	2	3	3	5	6	9
20–34	97	3.7	8	1	2	3	5	7	10	14
35–49	166	4.3	39	1	2	3	5	7	10	23
50–64	278	4.2	13	1	2	3	5	7	11	27
65+	117	4.4	19	1	2	4	5	8	11	22
GRAND TOTAL	689	4.1	19	1	2	3	5	7	10	21

Western Region, October 2007–September 2008 Data, by Operation

04.01: EXC ACOUSTIC NEUROMA

Type of Patients	Observed Patients	Avg. Stay	Variance	Percentiles						
				10th	25th	50th	75th	90th	95th	99th
1. SINGLE DX										
0–19 Years	0									
20–34	9	3.5	2	1	3	4	4	5	5	5
35–49	4	3.5	<1	2	4	4	4	4	4	4
50–64	21	3.2	1	2	2	3	4	5	5	5
65+	2	2.5	<1	2	2	2	3	3	3	3
2. MULTIPLE DX										
0–19 Years	6	4.2	3	3	3	4	4	9	9	9
20–34	38	5.4	9	3	3	4	6	10	13	14
35–49	65	6.0	74	3	3	4	6	9	15	69
50–64	144	4.7	10	3	3	4	5	7	11	14
65+	51	6.3	31	3	3	4	7	11	16	34
TOTAL SINGLE DX	36	3.3	1	2	2	3	4	5	5	5
TOTAL MULTIPLE DX	304	5.3	27	3	3	4	6	9	12	22
TOTAL										
0–19 Years	6	4.2	3	3	3	4	4	9	9	9
20–34	47	5.0	8	3	3	4	6	9	12	14
35–49	69	5.9	70	3	3	4	6	9	15	69
50–64	165	4.5	9	3	3	4	5	7	10	14
65+	53	6.1	30	3	3	4	7	11	16	34
GRAND TOTAL	340	5.1	25	3	3	4	5	8	11	22

04.07: PERIPH/CRAN NERV EXC NEC

Type of Patients	Observed Patients	Avg. Stay	Variance	Percentiles						
				10th	25th	50th	75th	90th	95th	99th
1. SINGLE DX										
0–19 Years	3	1.2	<1	1	1	1	1	2	2	2
20–34	8	1.9	2	1	1	1	2	5	5	5
35–49	18	1.7	1	1	1	1	3	3	5	5
50–64	16	1.6	1	1	1	2	2	3	3	3
65+	5	4.2	10	1	2	3	7	8	8	8
2. MULTIPLE DX										
0–19 Years	19	3.2	2	2	2	3	3	5	6	6
20–34	28	2.5	6	1	1	2	3	5	7	13
35–49	57	3.9	22	1	1	3	5	8	21	23
50–64	70	4.3	28	1	1	2	5	9	15	27
65+	43	3.1	6	1	1	2	4	7	8	10
TOTAL SINGLE DX	50	1.9	2	1	1	1	2	3	5	8
TOTAL MULTIPLE DX	217	3.6	15	1	1	3	4	7	9	23
TOTAL										
0–19 Years	22	2.9	2	1	2	3	3	5	6	6
20–34	36	2.4	5	1	1	2	3	5	7	13
35–49	75	3.4	18	1	1	2	4	6	9	23
50–64	86	3.8	24	1	1	2	4	9	14	27
65+	48	3.2	6	1	1	2	4	7	8	10
GRAND TOTAL	267	3.3	13	1	1	2	4	6	9	21

04.1: DXTIC PX PERIPH NERV

Type of Patients	Observed Patients	Avg. Stay	Variance	Percentiles						
				10th	25th	50th	75th	90th	95th	99th
1. SINGLE DX										
0–19 Years	1	5.0	0	5	5	5	5	5	5	5
20–34	0									
35–49	3	1.7	1	1	1	1	3	3	3	3
50–64	1	1.0	0	1	1	1	1	1	1	1
65+	0									
2. MULTIPLE DX										
0–19 Years	2	9.8	16	8	8	8	8	17	17	17
20–34	6	29.6	534	5	5	20	52	56	56	56
35–49	10	9.0	44	3	5	5	13	17	23	23
50–64	13	18.9	399	5	7	13	21	43	76	76
65+	10	13.3	189	3	5	7	23	45	45	45
TOTAL SINGLE DX	5	3.3	4	1	1	5	5	5	5	5
TOTAL MULTIPLE DX	41	15.8	270	3	5	8	20	43	52	76
TOTAL										
0–19 Years	3	7.7	14	5	5	8	8	17	17	17
20–34	6	29.6	534	4	5	20	52	56	56	56
35–49	13	7.3	43	1	3	5	9	17	23	23
50–64	14	17.6	391	3	6	12	21	43	76	76
65+	10	13.3	189	3	5	7	23	45	45	45
GRAND TOTAL	46	13.9	249	3	5	7	17	41	52	76

04.2: DESTR PERIPH/CRAN NERVES

Type of Patients	Observed Patients	Avg. Stay	Variance	Percentiles						
				10th	25th	50th	75th	90th	95th	99th
1. SINGLE DX										
0–19 Years	0									
20–34	0									
35–49	0									
50–64	0									
65+	2	1.0	0	1	1	1	1	1	1	1
2. MULTIPLE DX										
0–19 Years	0									
20–34	0									
35–49	6	7.7	32	3	5	6	7	19	19	19
50–64	8	2.0	3	1	1	1	2	6	6	6
65+	7	4.0	17	1	1	2	7	12	12	12
TOTAL SINGLE DX	2	1.0	0	1	1	1	1	1	1	1
TOTAL MULTIPLE DX	21	4.3	20	1	1	2	6	7	12	19
TOTAL										
0–19 Years	0									
20–34	0									
35–49	6	7.7	32	3	5	6	7	19	19	19
50–64	8	2.0	3	1	1	1	2	6	6	6
65+	9	3.3	15	1	1	1	4	12	12	12
GRAND TOTAL	23	4.0	19	1	1	2	6	7	12	19

LOS by Diagnosis and Operation, Western Region, 45th Edition

Western Region, October 2007–September 2008 Data, by Operation

04.3: CRAN/PERIPH NERVE SUTURE

Type of Patients	Observed Patients	Avg. Stay	Variance	Percentiles						
				10th	25th	50th	75th	90th	95th	99th
1. SINGLE DX										
0–19 Years	3	1.0	0	1	1	1	1	1	1	1
20–34	3	2.7	4	1	1	2	5	5	5	5
35–49	3	2.4	2	1	1	2	4	4	4	4
50–64	0									
65+	0									
2. MULTIPLE DX										
0–19 Years	24	2.2	5	1	1	1	2	4	8	10
20–34	100	2.6	4	1	1	2	4	5	7	11
35–49	39	2.6	4	1	1	2	4	6	7	9
50–64	36	3.4	20	1	1	1	3	10	17	20
65+	4	1.0	0	1	1	1	1	1	1	1
TOTAL SINGLE DX	9	2.0	2	1	1	1	2	5	5	5
TOTAL MULTIPLE DX	203	2.7	7	1	1	2	3	5	8	13
TOTAL										
0–19 Years	27	2.0	5	1	1	1	2	4	8	10
20–34	103	2.6	4	1	1	2	4	5	6	10
35–49	42	2.6	4	1	1	2	4	6	6	9
50–64	36	3.4	20	1	1	1	3	10	17	20
65+	4	1.0	0	1	1	1	1	1	1	1
GRAND TOTAL	212	2.7	7	1	1	2	3	5	8	13

04.41: DECOMP TRIGEMINAL ROOT

Type of Patients	Observed Patients	Avg. Stay	Variance	Percentiles						
				10th	25th	50th	75th	90th	95th	99th
1. SINGLE DX										
0–19 Years	2	3.8	<1	3	4	4	4	4	4	4
20–34	9	3.3	<1	1	2	3	4	6	6	6
35–49	11	2.2	<1	1	2	2	3	3	4	4
50–64	14	2.5	1	1	2	2	3	3	5	5
65+	6	1.8	<1	1	2	2	2	2	2	2
2. MULTIPLE DX										
0–19 Years	0									
20–34	19	3.0	5	2	2	2	4	5	5	11
35–49	34	3.2	2	2	2	3	3	5	6	7
50–64	120	2.9	2	2	2	3	3	4	5	7
65+	78	3.1	4	1	2	3	3	5	7	13
TOTAL SINGLE DX	42	2.6	1	1	2	2	3	4	5	6
TOTAL MULTIPLE DX	251	3.0	3	2	2	3	3	5	5	10
TOTAL										
0–19 Years	2	3.8	<1	3	4	4	4	4	4	4
20–34	28	3.1	4	1	2	3	4	5	6	11
35–49	45	3.0	2	2	2	3	4	5	6	7
50–64	134	3.0	2	2	2	3	3	4	5	7
65+	84	3.0	4	1	2	3	3	5	7	13
GRAND TOTAL	293	3.0	2	2	2	3	3	5	5	10

04.4: PERIPH NERV ADHESIOLYSIS

Type of Patients	Observed Patients	Avg. Stay	Variance	Percentiles						
				10th	25th	50th	75th	90th	95th	99th
1. SINGLE DX										
0–19 Years	9	2.1	2	1	1	1	4	4	4	4
20–34	18	2.8	2	1	1	3	4	5	6	6
35–49	20	2.1	<1	1	1	2	3	4	4	4
50–64	36	2.2	<1	1	2	2	3	3	4	5
65+	8	1.6	<1	1	1	2	2	2	2	2
2. MULTIPLE DX										
0–19 Years	34	3.3	16	1	1	1	4	7	16	16
20–34	116	3.3	15	1	1	1	4	7	11	14
35–49	144	4.2	32	1	1	3	4	8	15	25
50–64	330	2.8	6	1	1	2	3	5	7	12
65+	161	3.1	7	1	2	2	4	6	8	13
TOTAL SINGLE DX	91	2.2	1	1	1	2	3	4	4	6
TOTAL MULTIPLE DX	785	3.2	13	1	1	2	4	6	9	16
TOTAL										
0–19 Years	43	3.0	13	1	1	2	4	7	16	16
20–34	134	3.3	13	1	1	2	4	7	10	14
35–49	164	4.0	29	1	1	2	4	8	15	25
50–64	366	2.7	6	1	1	2	3	5	7	12
65+	169	3.1	7	1	2	2	3	6	7	13
GRAND TOTAL	876	3.1	12	1	1	2	3	6	8	16

04.42: CRANIAL NERVE DECOMP NEC

Type of Patients	Observed Patients	Avg. Stay	Variance	Percentiles						
				10th	25th	50th	75th	90th	95th	99th
1. SINGLE DX										
0–19 Years	3	3.0	3	1	1	4	4	4	4	4
20–34	3	4.0	0	4	4	4	4	4	4	4
35–49	13	3.7	<1	3	3	4	4	4	4	4
50–64	13	2.5	<1	1	1	2	3	4	4	5
65+	1	1.0	0	1	1	1	1	1	1	1
2. MULTIPLE DX										
0–19 Years	7	2.9	1	2	2	3	4	5	5	5
20–34	18	4.3	10	1	2	3	7	10	12	12
35–49	14	5.5	38	2	2	4	5	15	23	23
50–64	55	2.8	2	1	2	3	3	7	7	12
65+	22	3.6	4	1	2	3	5	7	7	8
TOTAL SINGLE DX	23	2.9	1	2	2	3	4	4	4	4
TOTAL MULTIPLE DX	116	3.5	8	1	2	3	4	7	8	15
TOTAL										
0–19 Years	10	2.9	1	2	2	3	4	4	5	5
20–34	21	4.3	9	1	2	3	5	8	10	12
35–49	17	5.2	32	2	2	4	4	15	23	23
50–64	68	2.8	2	2	2	2	3	5	5	9
65+	23	3.4	4	1	2	3	5	7	7	8
GRAND TOTAL	139	3.4	7	1	2	3	4	5	8	15

LOS by Diagnosis and Operation, Western Region, 45th Edition

Western Region, October 2007–September 2008 Data, by Operation

04.43: CARPAL TUNNEL RELEASE

Type of Patients	Observed Patients	Avg. Stay	Variance	Percentiles						
				10th	25th	50th	75th	90th	95th	99th
1. SINGLE DX										
0–19 Years	1	1.0	0	1	1	1	1	1	1	1
20–34	0									
35–49	0									
50–64	3	1.3	<1	1	1	1	2	2	2	2
65+	0									
2. MULTIPLE DX										
0–19 Years	9	2.5	3	1	1	2	3	5	6	6
20–34	39	3.7	10	1	2	2	5	8	12	14
35–49	46	5.6	62	1	1	3	6	15	16	48
50–64	76	3.3	17	1	1	2	3	8	12	28
65+	45	3.4	16	1	1	2	4	7	8	24
TOTAL SINGLE DX	4	1.3	<1	1	1	1	1	2	2	2
TOTAL MULTIPLE DX	215	3.8	25	1	1	2	5	8	12	24
TOTAL										
0–19 Years	10	2.4	3	1	1	2	3	5	6	6
20–34	39	3.7	10	1	2	2	5	8	12	14
35–49	46	5.6	62	1	1	3	6	15	16	48
50–64	79	3.2	17	1	1	2	3	8	12	28
65+	45	3.4	16	1	1	2	4	7	8	24
GRAND TOTAL	219	3.8	25	1	1	2	5	8	12	24

04.5: CRAN OR PERIPH NERV GRFT

Type of Patients	Observed Patients	Avg. Stay	Variance	Percentiles						
				10th	25th	50th	75th	90th	95th	99th
1. SINGLE DX										
0–19 Years	2	1.0	0	1	1	1	1	1	1	1
20–34	3	2.0	<1	1	1	2	3	3	3	3
35–49	0									
50–64	0									
65+	0									
2. MULTIPLE DX										
0–19 Years	11	1.6	2	1	1	1	2	4	4	6
20–34	17	1.8	4	1	1	1	2	5	8	8
35–49	5	1.8	<1	1	1	2	2	3	3	3
50–64	7	4.8	13	1	2	4	8	11	11	11
65+	3	1.7	<1	1	1	2	2	2	2	2
TOTAL SINGLE DX	5	1.6	<1	1	1	1	2	3	3	3
TOTAL MULTIPLE DX	43	2.1	4	1	1	1	2	5	8	11
TOTAL										
0–19 Years	13	1.6	1	1	1	1	2	4	4	6
20–34	20	1.9	3	1	1	1	2	5	8	8
35–49	5	1.8	<1	1	1	2	2	3	3	3
50–64	7	4.8	13	1	2	4	8	11	11	11
65+	3	1.7	<1	1	1	2	2	2	2	2
GRAND TOTAL	48	2.0	4	1	1	1	2	4	6	11

04.49: PERIPH NERV ADHESIO NEC

Type of Patients	Observed Patients	Avg. Stay	Variance	Percentiles						
				10th	25th	50th	75th	90th	95th	99th
1. SINGLE DX										
0–19 Years	3	1.0	0	1	1	1	1	1	1	1
20–34	6	1.3	<1	1	1	1	2	2	2	2
35–49	6	1.2	<1	1	1	1	1	2	2	2
50–64	6	1.3	<1	1	1	1	1	3	3	3
65+	1	1.0	0	1	1	1	1	1	1	1
2. MULTIPLE DX										
0–19 Years	15	3.9	28	1	1	1	7	16	16	16
20–34	39	2.8	27	1	1	1	2	4	9	33
35–49	44	3.4	23	1	1	2	3	6	10	25
50–64	75	2.1	4	1	1	2	2	5	7	12
65+	16	1.9	1	1	1	2	2	3	5	5
TOTAL SINGLE DX	22	1.2	<1	1	1	1	1	2	2	3
TOTAL MULTIPLE DX	189	2.8	16	1	1	1	3	6	8	21
TOTAL										
0–19 Years	18	3.2	23	1	1	1	2	16	16	16
20–34	45	2.6	24	1	1	1	3	3	8	33
35–49	50	3.1	20	1	1	2	3	6	10	25
50–64	81	2.1	4	1	1	2	2	5	6	12
65+	17	1.8	1	1	1	2	2	3	5	5
GRAND TOTAL	211	2.6	14	1	1	1	2	5	8	21

04.6: PERIPH NERVES TRANSPOS

Type of Patients	Observed Patients	Avg. Stay	Variance	Percentiles						
				10th	25th	50th	75th	90th	95th	99th
1. SINGLE DX										
0–19 Years	0									
20–34	2	1.0	0	1	1	1	1	1	1	1
35–49	1	3.0	0	3	3	3	3	3	3	3
50–64	0									
65+	1	1.0	0	1	1	1	1	1	1	1
2. MULTIPLE DX										
0–19 Years	8	1.4	2	1	1	1	1	2	6	6
20–34	5	1.4	<1	1	1	1	1	3	3	3
35–49	20	1.6	2	1	1	1	2	2	2	7
50–64	24	2.2	5	1	1	1	2	5	7	10
65+	9	4.0	20	1	1	3	4	15	15	15
TOTAL SINGLE DX	4	1.5	1	1	1	1	3	3	3	3
TOTAL MULTIPLE DX	66	2.0	5	1	1	1	2	4	7	15
TOTAL										
0–19 Years	8	1.4	2	1	1	1	1	2	6	6
20–34	7	1.3	<1	1	1	1	1	3	3	3
35–49	21	1.7	2	1	1	1	2	2	3	7
50–64	24	2.2	5	1	1	2	2	5	7	10
65+	10	3.7	18	1	1	2	4	6	15	15
GRAND TOTAL	70	2.0	5	1	1	1	2	4	7	15

LOS by Diagnosis and Operation, Western Region, 45th Edition

Western Region, October 2007–September 2008 Data, by Operation

04.81: ANES INJECT PERIPH NERVE

Type of Patients	Observed Patients	Avg. Stay	Variance	Percentiles						
				10th	25th	50th	75th	90th	95th	99th
1. SINGLE DX										
0–19 Years	0									
20–34	2	3.0	2	2	2	3	4	4	4	4
35–49	3	3.3	2	2	2	3	5	5	5	5
50–64	2	2.0	0	2	2	2	2	2	2	2
65+	0									
2. MULTIPLE DX										
0–19 Years	13	13.1	206	1	4	5	19	44	44	44
20–34	51	5.4	32	2	2	4	5	12	14	36
35–49	67	5.3	16	2	3	4	6	11	15	19
50–64	89	5.2	18	1	2	4	7	11	11	28
65+	120	6.1	18	2	3	5	8	12	15	21
TOTAL SINGLE DX	7	2.9	1	2	2	2	4	5	5	5
TOTAL MULTIPLE DX	340	6.2	39	2	3	4	7	12	18	44
TOTAL										
0–19 Years	13	13.1	206	1	4	5	19	44	44	44
20–34	53	5.3	31	2	3	4	5	12	14	36
35–49	70	5.2	16	2	3	4	6	11	15	19
50–64	91	5.1	18	1	2	4	7	10	11	28
65+	120	6.1	18	2	3	5	8	12	15	21
GRAND TOTAL	347	6.1	38	2	3	4	7	12	18	44

04.9: OTH PERIPH NERVE OPS

Type of Patients	Observed Patients	Avg. Stay	Variance	Percentiles						
				10th	25th	50th	75th	90th	95th	99th
1. SINGLE DX										
0–19 Years	13	1.0	0	1	1	1	1	1	1	1
20–34	7	2.0	5	1	1	1	2	7	7	7
35–49	10	1.6	<1	1	1	1	2	4	4	4
50–64	20	1.5	0	1	1	1	2	4	4	4
65+	3	1.0	0	1	1	1	1	1	1	1
2. MULTIPLE DX										
0–19 Years	52	1.4	2	1	1	1	1	2	4	8
20–34	53	3.4	16	1	1	2	4	7	8	27
35–49	82	4.0	125	1	1	1	3	5	9	94
50–64	134	2.2	5	1	1	1	2	5	7	12
65+	71	2.4	6	1	1	1	2	6	8	12
TOTAL SINGLE DX	53	1.4	1	1	1	1	1	2	4	7
TOTAL MULTIPLE DX	392	2.6	30	1	1	1	2	5	8	17
TOTAL										
0–19 Years	65	1.3	1	1	1	1	1	2	4	8
20–34	60	3.2	15	1	1	2	4	7	8	27
35–49	92	3.7	112	1	1	1	3	5	9	94
50–64	154	2.1	5	1	1	1	2	5	6	12
65+	74	2.3	6	1	1	1	2	6	8	12
GRAND TOTAL	445	2.4	27	1	1	1	2	5	7	17

04.7: OTHER PERIPH NEUROPLASTY

Type of Patients	Observed Patients	Avg. Stay	Variance	Percentiles						
				10th	25th	50th	75th	90th	95th	99th
1. SINGLE DX										
0–19 Years	1	1.0	0	1	1	1	1	1	1	1
20–34	1	1.0	0	1	1	1	1	1	1	1
35–49	3	1.7	1	1	1	1	3	3	3	3
50–64	0									
65+	0									
2. MULTIPLE DX										
0–19 Years	8	3.2	4	1	2	2	5	7	7	7
20–34	20	3.9	13	1	2	3	3	11	12	12
35–49	15	2.9	7	1	1	2	3	4	12	12
50–64	14	1.8	1	1	1	1	2	4	4	4
65+	2	1.5	<1	1	1	1	2	2	2	2
TOTAL SINGLE DX	5	1.4	<1	1	1	1	1	3	3	3
TOTAL MULTIPLE DX	59	3.0	7	1	1	2	3	7	11	12
TOTAL										
0–19 Years	9	3.1	5	1	1	2	5	7	7	7
20–34	21	3.8	12	1	2	3	3	11	11	12
35–49	18	2.7	6	1	1	2	3	4	12	12
50–64	14	1.8	1	1	1	1	2	4	4	4
65+	2	1.5	<1	1	1	1	2	2	2	2
GRAND TOTAL	64	2.9	7	1	1	2	3	5	11	12

04.8: PERIPHERAL NERVE INJECT

Type of Patients	Observed Patients	Avg. Stay	Variance	Percentiles						
				10th	25th	50th	75th	90th	95th	99th
1. SINGLE DX										
0–19 Years	0									
20–34	2	3.0	2	2	2	3	4	4	4	4
35–49	3	3.3	2	2	2	3	5	5	5	5
50–64	2	2.0	0	2	2	2	2	2	2	2
65+	0									
2. MULTIPLE DX										
0–19 Years	13	13.1	206	1	4	5	19	44	44	44
20–34	51	5.4	32	2	2	4	5	12	14	36
35–49	69	5.2	16	1	3	4	6	11	15	19
50–64	89	5.2	18	1	2	4	7	11	11	28
65+	120	6.1	18	1	3	5	8	12	15	21
TOTAL SINGLE DX	7	2.9	1	2	2	2	4	5	5	5
TOTAL MULTIPLE DX	342	6.2	39	2	3	4	7	12	18	44
TOTAL										
0–19 Years	13	13.1	206	1	4	5	19	44	44	44
20–34	53	5.3	31	2	3	4	5	12	14	36
35–49	72	5.1	16	1	3	4	6	11	15	19
50–64	91	5.1	18	1	2	4	7	10	11	28
65+	120	6.1	18	2	3	5	8	12	15	21
GRAND TOTAL	349	6.1	38	2	3	4	7	12	18	44

LOS by Diagnosis and Operation, Western Region, 45th Edition

Western Region, October 2007–September 2008 Data, by Operation

04.92: IMPL PERIPH NEUROSTIM LD

Type of Patients	Observed Patients	Avg. Stay	Vari-ance	Percentiles						
				10th	25th	50th	75th	90th	95th	99th
1. SINGLE DX										
0–19 Years	12	1.0	0	1	1	1	1	1	1	1
20–34	6	2.2	6	1	1	1	2	7	7	7
35–49	9	1.3	<1	1	1	1	1	3	3	3
50–64	20	1.5	<1	1	1	1	2	4	4	4
65+	3	1.0	0	1	1	1	1	1	1	1
2. MULTIPLE DX										
0–19 Years	49	1.4	2	1	1	1	1	2	4	8
20–34	42	2.5	4	1	1	2	4	6	7	8
35–49	69	4.1	148	1	1	1	3	5	9	94
50–64	111	1.9	4	1	1	1	2	4	6	8
65+	61	2.1	5	1	1	1	2	5	6	12
TOTAL SINGLE DX	**50**	**1.4**	**1**	**1**	**1**	**1**	**1**	**2**	**4**	**7**
TOTAL MULTIPLE DX	**332**	**2.3**	**32**	**1**	**1**	**1**	**2**	**4**	**6**	**12**
TOTAL										
0–19 Years	61	1.3	1	1	1	1	1	2	4	8
20–34	48	2.5	4	1	1	2	4	6	7	8
35–49	78	3.8	132	1	1	1	3	4	9	94
50–64	131	1.9	3	1	1	1	2	4	6	8
65+	64	2.0	5	1	1	1	2	5	6	12
GRAND TOTAL	**382**	**2.2**	**28**	**1**	**1**	**1**	**2**	**4**	**6**	**12**

05.0: SYMPATH NERVE DIVISION

Type of Patients	Observed Patients	Avg. Stay	Vari-ance	Percentiles						
				10th	25th	50th	75th	90th	95th	99th
1. SINGLE DX										
0–19 Years	0									
20–34	0									
35–49	0									
50–64	0									
65+	0									
2. MULTIPLE DX										
0–19 Years	0									
20–34	0									
35–49	0									
50–64	0									
65+	0									
TOTAL SINGLE DX	**0**									
TOTAL MULTIPLE DX	**0**									
TOTAL										
0–19 Years	0									
20–34	0									
35–49	0									
50–64	0									
65+	0									
GRAND TOTAL	**0**									

05.1: SYMPATH NERVE DXTIC PX

Type of Patients	Observed Patients	Avg. Stay	Vari-ance	Percentiles						
				10th	25th	50th	75th	90th	95th	99th
1. SINGLE DX										
0–19 Years	0									
20–34	0									
35–49	0									
50–64	0									
65+	0									
2. MULTIPLE DX										
0–19 Years	0									
20–34	0									
35–49	1	1.0	0	1	1	1	1	1	1	1
50–64	2	8.5	82	2	2	9	15	15	15	15
65+	1	5.0	0	5	5	5	5	5	5	5
TOTAL SINGLE DX	**0**									
TOTAL MULTIPLE DX	**4**	**5.8**	**41**	**1**	**2**	**4**	**10**	**15**	**15**	**15**
TOTAL										
0–19 Years	0									
20–34	0									
35–49	1	1.0	0	1	1	1	1	1	1	1
50–64	2	8.5	82	2	2	9	15	15	15	15
65+	1	5.0	0	5	5	5	5	5	5	5
GRAND TOTAL	**4**	**5.8**	**41**	**1**	**2**	**4**	**10**	**15**	**15**	**15**

05.2: SYMPATHECTOMY

Type of Patients	Observed Patients	Avg. Stay	Vari-ance	Percentiles						
				10th	25th	50th	75th	90th	95th	99th
1. SINGLE DX										
0–19 Years	4	1.0	<1	1	1	1	1	1	1	1
20–34	13	1.3	<1	1	1	1	1	3	3	3
35–49	7	1.0	0	1	1	1	1	1	1	1
50–64	1	3.0	0	3	3	3	3	3	3	3
65+	0									
2. MULTIPLE DX										
0–19 Years	7	1.4	<1	1	1	1	2	2	2	2
20–34	29	1.9	4	1	1	1	2	3	6	10
35–49	18	2.2	3	1	1	2	3	4	7	7
50–64	18	5.6	47	3	3	11	11	21	21	21
65+	5	3.4	<1	3	3	3	4	4	4	4
TOTAL SINGLE DX	**25**	**1.2**	**<1**	**1**	**1**	**1**	**1**	**3**	**3**	**3**
TOTAL MULTIPLE DX	**77**	**2.9**	**15**	**1**	**1**	**1**	**3**	**6**	**11**	**21**
TOTAL										
0–19 Years	11	1.3	<1	1	1	1	2	2	2	2
20–34	42	1.7	3	1	1	1	2	3	3	10
35–49	25	1.9	2	1	1	2	2	4	4	7
50–64	19	5.4	45	1	1	2	11	21	21	21
65+	5	3.4	<1	3	3	3	4	4	4	4
GRAND TOTAL	**102**	**2.5**	**12**	**1**	**1**	**1**	**3**	**4**	**10**	**21**

LOS by Diagnosis and Operation, Western Region, 45th Edition

Western Region, October 2007–September 2008 Data, by Operation

05.3: SYMPATH NERVE INJECTION

Type of Patients	Observed Patients	Avg. Stay	Vari-ance	Percentiles						
				10th	25th	50th	75th	90th	95th	99th
1. SINGLE DX										
0–19 Years	0									
20–34	0									
35–49	2	4.0	2	3	3	5	5	5	5	5
50–64	0									
65+	0									
2. MULTIPLE DX										
0–19 Years	7	8.4	38	3	4	9	9	11	25	25
20–34	18	9.9	35	2	5	10	13	16	27	27
35–49	32	6.4	25	1	2	5	11	12	18	20
50–64	41	6.2	29	2	2	4	8	11	18	22
65+	51	6.9	20	2	3	6	9	11	17	22
TOTAL SINGLE DX	2	4.0	2	3	3	5	5	5	5	5
TOTAL MULTIPLE DX	149	7.1	27	2	3	6	10	13	18	25
TOTAL										
0–19 Years	7	8.4	38	3	4	9	9	11	25	25
20–34	18	9.9	35	2	5	10	13	16	27	27
35–49	34	6.3	24	1	2	5	10	12	18	20
50–64	41	6.2	29	2	2	4	8	11	18	22
65+	51	6.9	20	2	3	6	9	11	17	22
GRAND TOTAL	151	7.0	27	2	3	6	10	13	18	25

05.31: ANES INJECT SYMPATH NERV

Type of Patients	Observed Patients	Avg. Stay	Vari-ance	Percentiles						
				10th	25th	50th	75th	90th	95th	99th
1. SINGLE DX										
0–19 Years	0									
20–34	0									
35–49	2	4.0	2	3	3	5	5	5	5	5
50–64	0									
65+	0									
2. MULTIPLE DX										
0–19 Years	7	8.4	38	3	4	9	9	11	25	25
20–34	16	9.9	37	2	6	10	13	16	27	27
35–49	27	6.7	30	1	2	5	11	14	18	22
50–64	39	6.0	26	2	2	4	8	11	21	22
65+	45	7.2	21	2	4	7	9	12	17	22
TOTAL SINGLE DX	2	4.0	2	3	3	5	5	5	5	5
TOTAL MULTIPLE DX	134	7.2	28	2	3	6	10	13	20	25
TOTAL										
0–19 Years	7	8.4	38	3	4	9	9	11	25	25
20–34	16	9.9	37	2	6	10	13	16	27	27
35–49	29	6.5	28	1	2	5	11	14	18	20
50–64	39	6.0	26	2	2	4	8	11	21	22
65+	45	7.2	21	2	4	7	9	12	17	22
GRAND TOTAL	136	7.2	28	2	3	6	10	13	18	25

05.8: OTH SYMPATH NERVE OPS

Type of Patients	Observed Patients	Avg. Stay	Vari-ance	Percentiles						
				10th	25th	50th	75th	90th	95th	99th
1. SINGLE DX										
0–19 Years	0									
20–34	0									
35–49	0									
50–64	0									
65+	0									
2. MULTIPLE DX										
0–19 Years	1	11.0	0	11	11	11	11	11	11	11
20–34	0									
35–49	0									
50–64	1	8.0	0	8	8	8	8	8	8	8
65+	0									
TOTAL SINGLE DX	0									
TOTAL MULTIPLE DX	2	10.0	3	8	8	11	11	11	11	11
TOTAL										
0–19 Years	1	11.0	0	11	11	11	11	11	11	11
20–34	0									
35–49	0									
50–64	1	8.0	0	8	8	8	8	8	8	8
65+	0									
GRAND TOTAL	2	10.0	3	8	8	11	11	11	11	11

05.9: OTHER NERVOUS SYSTEM OPS

Type of Patients	Observed Patients	Avg. Stay	Vari-ance	Percentiles						
				10th	25th	50th	75th	90th	95th	99th
1. SINGLE DX										
0–19 Years	0									
20–34	0									
35–49	0									
50–64	0									
65+	0									
2. MULTIPLE DX										
0–19 Years	0									
20–34	0									
35–49	0									
50–64	0									
65+	0									
TOTAL SINGLE DX	0									
TOTAL MULTIPLE DX	0									
TOTAL										
0–19 Years	0									
20–34	0									
35–49	0									
50–64	0									
65+	0									
GRAND TOTAL	0									

LOS by Diagnosis and Operation, Western Region, 45th Edition

Western Region, October 2007–September 2008 Data, by Operation

06.0: THYROID FIELD INCISION

Type of Patients	Observed Patients	Avg. Stay	Variance	10th	25th	50th	75th	90th	95th	99th
						Percentiles				
1. SINGLE DX										
0–19 Years	9	3.7	3	2	3	3	6	6	6	6
20–34	11	1.7	<1	1	1	1	3	3	3	3
35–49	2	1.0	0	1	1	1	1	1	1	1
50–64	0									
65+	1	3.0	0	3	3	3	3	3	3	3
2. MULTIPLE DX										
0–19 Years	23	3.7	6	2	2	3	4	8	8	12
20–34	41	5.1	87	1	2	2	4	9	13	54
35–49	34	4.6	20	1	1	3	5	12	14	16
50–64	41	4.9	34	1	2	2	7	11	12	33
65+	56	8.2	142	1	2	4	9	14	40	62
TOTAL SINGLE DX	**23**	**2.8**	**3**	**1**	**1**	**3**	**3**	**6**	**6**	**6**
TOTAL MULTIPLE DX	**195**	**5.6**	**68**	**1**	**2**	**3**	**7**	**12**	**14**	**43**
TOTAL										
0–19 Years	32	3.7	5	2	2	3	4	6	8	12
20–34	52	4.4	71	1	1	2	3	9	13	54
35–49	36	4.4	20	1	1	3	5	12	14	16
50–64	41	4.9	34	1	1	3	7	11	12	33
65+	57	8.1	140	1	2	4	8	14	40	62
GRAND TOTAL	**218**	**5.2**	**61**	**1**	**2**	**3**	**6**	**11**	**14**	**43**

06.1: THYROID/PARATHY DXTIC PX

Type of Patients	Observed Patients	Avg. Stay	Variance	10th	25th	50th	75th	90th	95th	99th
						Percentiles				
1. SINGLE DX										
0–19 Years	1	3.0	0	3	3	3	3	3	3	3
20–34	3	3.3	4	1	1	4	5	5	5	5
35–49	0									
50–64	1	2.0	0	2	2	2	2	2	2	2
65+	1	1.0	0	1	1	1	1	1	1	1
2. MULTIPLE DX										
0–19 Years	7	4.8	15	1	1	4	8	8	15	15
20–34	16	4.7	20	1	1	3	8	12	15	15
35–49	52	4.3	15	1	2	3	6	8	9	22
50–64	124	6.4	38	2	3	5	8	11	18	28
65+	242	6.8	25	2	4	6	8	12	16	28
TOTAL SINGLE DX	**6**	**2.8**	**2**	**1**	**2**	**3**	**3**	**5**	**5**	**5**
TOTAL MULTIPLE DX	**441**	**6.2**	**27**	**2**	**3**	**5**	**8**	**12**	**16**	**28**
TOTAL										
0–19 Years	8	4.4	12	1	1	4	5	8	8	15
20–34	19	4.5	18	1	1	3	5	12	15	15
35–49	52	4.3	15	1	2	3	6	8	9	22
50–64	125	6.4	38	2	3	5	8	11	18	28
65+	243	6.7	25	2	4	6	8	12	16	28
GRAND TOTAL	**447**	**6.2**	**27**	**2**	**3**	**5**	**8**	**12**	**16**	**28**

06.09: INC THYROID FIELD NEC

Type of Patients	Observed Patients	Avg. Stay	Variance	10th	25th	50th	75th	90th	95th	99th
						Percentiles				
1. SINGLE DX										
0–19 Years	5	2.9	3	1	2	3	3	6	6	6
20–34	10	1.7	<1	1	1	1	3	3	3	3
35–49	1	1.0	0	1	1	1	1	1	1	1
50–64	0									
65+	0									
2. MULTIPLE DX										
0–19 Years	17	3.5	4	2	2	3	4	8	8	8
20–34	33	5.5	106	1	2	2	4	10	31	54
35–49	24	4.9	22	1	1	2	5	13	14	16
50–64	31	4.7	41	1	1	2	7	11	14	33
65+	28	10.0	238	1	2	4	9	40	43	62
TOTAL SINGLE DX	**16**	**2.1**	**2**	**1**	**1**	**2**	**3**	**3**	**6**	**6**
TOTAL MULTIPLE DX	**133**	**5.7**	**86**	**1**	**2**	**3**	**5**	**12**	**16**	**54**
TOTAL										
0–19 Years	22	3.4	4	2	2	3	3	8	8	8
20–34	43	4.6	84	1	1	2	3	9	13	54
35–49	25	4.7	22	1	1	3	5	13	14	16
50–64	31	4.7	41	1	1	2	7	11	14	33
65+	28	10.0	238	1	2	4	9	40	43	62
GRAND TOTAL	**149**	**5.3**	**78**	**1**	**1**	**3**	**5**	**11**	**14**	**54**

06.11: CLOSED THYROID BIOPSY

Type of Patients	Observed Patients	Avg. Stay	Variance	10th	25th	50th	75th	90th	95th	99th
						Percentiles				
1. SINGLE DX										
0–19 Years	1	3.0	0	3	3	3	3	3	3	3
20–34	3	3.3	4	1	1	4	5	5	5	5
35–49	0									
50–64	1	2.0	0	2	2	2	2	2	2	2
65+	0									
2. MULTIPLE DX										
0–19 Years	7	4.8	15	1	1	4	8	8	15	15
20–34	13	4.6	14	1	2	3	5	12	12	12
35–49	44	4.4	13	1	2	3	6	8	9	22
50–64	107	6.2	20	2	3	5	8	11	14	21
65+	217	6.8	20	3	4	6	8	12	16	26
TOTAL SINGLE DX	**5**	**3.0**	**1**	**1**	**3**	**3**	**3**	**3**	**5**	**5**
TOTAL MULTIPLE DX	**388**	**6.2**	**20**	**2**	**3**	**5**	**8**	**11**	**14**	**26**
TOTAL										
0–19 Years	8	4.4	12	1	1	4	5	8	8	15
20–34	16	4.3	12	1	2	3	5	12	12	12
35–49	44	4.4	13	1	2	3	6	8	9	22
50–64	108	6.2	20	2	3	5	8	11	14	21
65+	217	6.8	20	3	4	6	8	12	16	26
GRAND TOTAL	**393**	**6.2**	**20**	**2**	**3**	**5**	**8**	**11**	**14**	**22**

LOS by Diagnosis and Operation, Western Region, 45th Edition

Western Region, October 2007–September 2008 Data, by Operation

06.2: UNILAT THYROID LOBECTOMY

Type of Patients	Observed Patients	Avg. Stay	Variance	10th	25th	50th	75th	90th	95th	99th
1. SINGLE DX										
0–19 Years	41	1.1	<1	1	1	1	1	2	2	3
20–34	206	1.2	<1	1	1	1	1	2	2	3
35–49	343	1.2	<1	1	1	1	2	2	2	3
50–64	236	1.3	<1	1	1	1	1	2	2	5
65+	67	1.2	<1	1	1	1	1	2	2	3
2. MULTIPLE DX										
0–19 Years	26	1.1	<1	1	1	1	1	2	2	2
20–34	280	1.4	<1	1	1	1	1	2	3	5
35–49	733	1.4	1	1	1	1	1	2	3	5
50–64	1,169	1.4	2	1	1	1	1	2	3	6
65+	877	1.8	11	1	1	1	2	2	3	15
TOTAL SINGLE DX	893	1.2	<1	1	1	1	1	2	2	3
TOTAL MULTIPLE DX	3,085	1.5	4	1	1	1	1	2	3	7
TOTAL										
0–19 Years	67	1.1	<1	1	1	1	1	2	2	2
20–34	486	1.3	<1	1	1	1	1	2	2	4
35–49	1,076	1.3	1	1	1	1	1	2	3	5
50–64	1,405	1.4	2	1	1	1	1	2	3	6
65+	944	1.7	10	1	1	1	2	2	3	15
GRAND TOTAL	3,978	1.4	3	1	1	1	1	2	3	6

06.3: OTHER PART THYROIDECTOMY

Type of Patients	Observed Patients	Avg. Stay	Variance	10th	25th	50th	75th	90th	95th	99th
1. SINGLE DX										
0–19 Years	8	1.0	0	1	1	1	1	1	1	1
20–34	62	1.2	<1	1	1	1	1	2	2	5
35–49	109	1.2	<1	1	1	1	1	2	2	3
50–64	104	1.2	<1	1	1	1	1	2	2	3
65+	26	1.3	<1	1	1	1	1	2	3	3
2. MULTIPLE DX										
0–19 Years	15	2.0	6	1	1	1	1	4	5	14
20–34	121	2.1	33	1	1	1	2	2	5	28
35–49	238	1.9	16	1	1	1	2	3	5	25
50–64	428	2.4	42	1	1	1	2	3	4	36
65+	280	3.1	38	1	1	1	2	6	16	38
TOTAL SINGLE DX	309	1.2	<1	1	1	1	1	2	2	3
TOTAL MULTIPLE DX	1,082	2.4	33	1	1	1	2	3	7	35
TOTAL										
0–19 Years	23	1.6	4	1	1	1	1	4	4	14
20–34	183	1.8	22	1	1	1	1	2	3	28
35–49	347	1.7	11	1	1	1	1	3	3	13
50–64	532	2.2	34	1	1	1	2	3	4	34
65+	306	3.0	35	1	1	1	2	6	16	35
GRAND TOTAL	1,391	2.2	26	1	1	1	2	3	5	29

06.31: EXCISION THYROID LESION

Type of Patients	Observed Patients	Avg. Stay	Variance	10th	25th	50th	75th	90th	95th	99th
1. SINGLE DX										
0–19 Years	3	1.0	0	1	1	1	1	1	1	1
20–34	8	1.0	0	1	1	1	1	1	1	1
35–49	6	1.3	<1	1	1	1	2	2	2	2
50–64	7	1.0	0	1	1	1	1	1	1	1
65+	1	1.0	0	1	1	1	1	1	1	1
2. MULTIPLE DX										
0–19 Years	2	3.0	8	1	1	3	5	5	5	5
20–34	7	12.9	479	1	1	1	28	57	57	57
35–49	21	1.7	5	1	1	1	1	2	3	11
50–64	46	3.7	127	1	1	1	2	2	4	70
65+	35	3.7	43	1	1	1	3	9	18	34
TOTAL SINGLE DX	25	1.1	<1	1	1	1	1	1	2	2
TOTAL MULTIPLE DX	111	3.9	98	1	1	1	2	4	18	57
TOTAL										
0–19 Years	5	1.5	2	1	1	1	1	5	5	5
20–34	15	6.5	243	1	1	1	1	28	57	57
35–49	27	1.6	4	1	1	1	2	2	3	11
50–64	53	3.3	110	1	1	1	2	2	4	70
65+	36	3.6	42	1	1	1	3	9	18	34
GRAND TOTAL	136	3.3	80	1	1	1	2	4	15	57

06.39: PART THYROIDECTOMY NEC

Type of Patients	Observed Patients	Avg. Stay	Variance	10th	25th	50th	75th	90th	95th	99th
1. SINGLE DX										
0–19 Years	5	1.0	0	1	1	1	1	1	1	1
20–34	54	1.2	<1	1	1	1	1	2	2	5
35–49	103	1.2	<1	1	1	1	1	2	2	3
50–64	97	1.3	<1	1	1	1	1	2	3	3
65+	25	1.3	<1	1	1	1	1	2	3	3
2. MULTIPLE DX										
0–19 Years	13	1.9	6	1	1	1	1	4	4	14
20–34	114	1.4	2	1	1	1	2	2	4	8
35–49	217	2.0	17	1	1	1	2	3	5	25
50–64	382	2.2	32	1	1	1	2	3	4	34
65+	245	3.1	38	1	1	1	2	6	16	38
TOTAL SINGLE DX	284	1.2	<1	1	1	1	1	2	2	3
TOTAL MULTIPLE DX	971	2.3	26	1	1	1	2	3	6	33
TOTAL										
0–19 Years	18	1.6	4	1	1	1	1	4	4	14
20–34	168	1.4	1	1	1	1	1	2	3	8
35–49	320	1.7	12	1	1	1	2	3	3	13
50–64	479	2.0	25	1	1	1	2	3	4	17
65+	270	2.9	34	1	1	1	2	4	16	38
GRAND TOTAL	1,255	2.0	20	1	1	1	2	3	4	25

LOS by Diagnosis and Operation, Western Region, 45th Edition

Western Region, October 2007–September 2008 Data, by Operation

06.4: COMPLETE THYROIDECTOMY

Type of Patients	Observed Patients	Avg. Stay	Vari-ance	10th	25th	50th	75th	90th	95th	99th
1. SINGLE DX										
0–19 Years	33	1.4	<1	1	1	1	2	2	3	3
20–34	214	1.4	<1	1	1	1	2	2	3	3
35–49	364	1.5	<1	1	1	1	2	2	3	7
50–64	288	1.4	<1	1	1	1	2	2	3	5
65+	60	1.3	<1	1	1	1	1	2	2	3
2. MULTIPLE DX										
0–19 Years	66	3.8	69	1	2	2	4	8	10	21
20–34	622	2.0	4	1	1	1	2	4	5	9
35–49	1,386	1.9	5	1	1	1	2	3	5	8
50–64	1,822	1.9	6	1	1	1	2	3	4	10
65+	1,079	2.2	9	1	1	1	2	4	6	15
TOTAL SINGLE DX	**959**	**1.4**	**<1**	**1**	**1**	**1**	**2**	**2**	**3**	**5**
TOTAL MULTIPLE DX	**4,975**	**2.0**	**7**	**1**	**1**	**1**	**2**	**3**	**5**	**11**
TOTAL										
0–19 Years	99	3.0	45	1	1	2	2	5	9	21
20–34	836	1.8	3	1	1	1	2	3	5	9
35–49	1,750	1.8	4	1	1	1	2	3	4	8
50–64	2,110	1.8	5	1	1	1	2	3	4	9
65+	1,139	2.1	8	1	1	1	2	4	6	15
GRAND TOTAL	**5,934**	**1.9**	**6**	**1**	**1**	**1**	**2**	**3**	**5**	**10**

06.5: SUBSTERNAL THYROIDECTOMY

Type of Patients	Observed Patients	Avg. Stay	Vari-ance	10th	25th	50th	75th	90th	95th	99th
1. SINGLE DX										
0–19 Years	2	1.0	0	1	1	1	1	1	1	1
20–34	14	1.1	<1	1	1	1	1	1	2	2
35–49	34	1.3	<1	1	1	1	1	2	3	3
50–64	29	1.7	2	1	1	1	2	2	3	3
65+	10	1.6	<1	1	1	1	2	2	3	3
2. MULTIPLE DX										
0–19 Years	8	2.9	1	2	2	3	4	5	5	5
20–34	40	2.4	5	1	1	2	3	4	7	13
35–49	76	1.7	5	1	1	1	2	3	4	6
50–64	158	2.3	16	1	1	1	2	4	6	18
65+	124	4.4	41	1	1	2	4	10	15	34
TOTAL SINGLE DX	**89**	**1.4**	**<1**	**1**	**1**	**1**	**2**	**2**	**3**	**9**
TOTAL MULTIPLE DX	**406**	**2.9**	**20**	**1**	**1**	**2**	**3**	**5**	**10**	**21**
TOTAL										
0–19 Years	10	2.6	2	2	2	2	4	5	5	5
20–34	54	2.0	4	1	1	1	3	4	7	13
35–49	110	1.6	4	1	1	1	2	3	4	6
50–64	187	2.2	14	1	1	1	2	4	6	18
65+	134	4.2	38	1	1	2	4	10	15	34
GRAND TOTAL	**495**	**2.6**	**17**	**1**	**1**	**2**	**2**	**4**	**8**	**18**

06.51: PART SUBSTERN THYROIDECT

Type of Patients	Observed Patients	Avg. Stay	Vari-ance	10th	25th	50th	75th	90th	95th	99th
1. SINGLE DX										
0–19 Years	0		0							
20–34	5	1.0	0	1	1	1	1	1	1	1
35–49	9	1.1	<1	1	1	1	1	2	2	2
50–64	4	1.3	<1	1	1	1	1	2	2	2
65+	1	2.0	0	2	2	2	2	2	2	2
2. MULTIPLE DX										
0–19 Years	0									
20–34	11	2.1	3	1	1	2	2	3	7	7
35–49	15	1.7	1	1	1	1	2	4	5	5
50–64	34	3.4	60	1	1	2	3	4	14	45
65+	28	5.9	103	1	1	2	3	18	34	42
TOTAL SINGLE DX	**19**	**1.2**	**<1**	**1**	**1**	**1**	**1**	**2**	**2**	**2**
TOTAL MULTIPLE DX	**88**	**3.7**	**58**	**1**	**1**	**1**	**2**	**7**	**18**	**45**
TOTAL										
0–19 Years	0									
20–34	16	1.8	2	1	1	1	2	3	7	7
35–49	24	1.5	1	1	1	1	2	2	4	5
50–64	38	3.2	54	1	1	2	2	4	14	45
65+	29	5.7	100	1	1	2	3	18	34	42
GRAND TOTAL	**107**	**3.3**	**49**	**1**	**1**	**1**	**2**	**5**	**14**	**42**

06.52: TOT SUBSTERN THYROIDECT

Type of Patients	Observed Patients	Avg. Stay	Vari-ance	10th	25th	50th	75th	90th	95th	99th
1. SINGLE DX										
0–19 Years	2	1.0	0	1	1	1	1	1	1	1
20–34	9	1.1	<1	1	1	1	1	2	2	2
35–49	25	1.3	<1	1	1	1	1	2	3	3
50–64	25	1.8	3	1	1	1	2	3	3	3
65+	8	1.5	<1	1	1	1	2	3	3	3
2. MULTIPLE DX										
0–19 Years	8	2.9	1	2	2	3	4	5	5	5
20–34	29	2.5	5	1	1	2	3	4	4	13
35–49	60	1.7	1	1	1	1	2	3	4	6
50–64	122	2.0	4	1	1	1	2	4	5	7
65+	91	3.9	23	1	1	2	4	10	13	30
TOTAL SINGLE DX	**69**	**1.4**	**1**	**1**	**1**	**1**	**2**	**2**	**3**	**9**
TOTAL MULTIPLE DX	**310**	**2.6**	**9**	**1**	**1**	**2**	**3**	**5**	**7**	**15**
TOTAL										
0–19 Years	10	2.6	2	1	2	2	4	5	5	5
20–34	38	2.1	4	1	1	1	3	4	4	13
35–49	85	1.6	1	1	1	1	2	3	4	6
50–64	147	2.0	4	1	1	2	2	3	5	9
65+	99	3.7	21	1	1	2	4	10	13	30
GRAND TOTAL	**379**	**2.4**	**8**	**1**	**1**	**2**	**2**	**4**	**7**	**15**

LOS by Diagnosis and Operation, Western Region, 45th Edition

Western Region, October 2007–September 2008 Data, by Operation

06.6: LINGUAL THYROID EXCISION

Type of Patients	Observed Patients	Avg. Stay	Vari-ance	Percentiles						
				10th	25th	50th	75th	90th	95th	99th
1. SINGLE DX										
0–19 Years	0									
20–34	0									
35–49	0									
50–64	1	2.0	0	2	2	2	2	2	2	2
65+	1	2.0	0	2	2	2	2	2	2	2
2. MULTIPLE DX										
0–19 Years	0									
20–34	0									
35–49	1	2.0	0	2	2	2	2	2	2	2
50–64	1	11.0	0	11	11	11	11	11	11	11
65+	0									
TOTAL SINGLE DX	2	2.0	0	2	2	2	2	2	2	2
TOTAL MULTIPLE DX	2	6.5	39	2	2	2	11	11	11	11
TOTAL										
0–19 Years	0									
20–34	0									
35–49	1	2.0	0	2	2	2	2	2	2	2
50–64	2	6.5	40	2	2	11	11	11	11	11
65+	1	2.0	0	2	2	2	2	2	2	2
GRAND TOTAL	4	4.3	20	2	2	2	2	11	11	11

06.7: THYROGLOSSAL DUCT EXC

Type of Patients	Observed Patients	Avg. Stay	Vari-ance	Percentiles						
				10th	25th	50th	75th	90th	95th	99th
1. SINGLE DX										
0–19 Years	99	1.2	<1	1	1	1	2	2	2	3
20–34	10	1.2	<1	1	1	1	1	1	3	3
35–49	7	1.3	<1	1	1	1	2	2	2	2
50–64	7	1.1	<1	1	1	1	1	2	2	2
65+	0									
2. MULTIPLE DX										
0–19 Years	32	2.2	5	1	1	1	2	3	9	9
20–34	12	1.3	<1	1	1	1	1	2	3	3
35–49	22	1.3	<1	1	1	1	2	2	3	3
50–64	23	1.4	<1	1	1	1	2	3	3	4
65+	12	2.2	4	1	1	1	2	5	7	7
TOTAL SINGLE DX	123	1.2	<1	1	1	1	1	2	2	3
TOTAL MULTIPLE DX	101	1.9	4	1	1	1	2	3	9	9
TOTAL										
0–19 Years	131	1.4	2	1	1	1	1	2	3	9
20–34	22	1.2	<1	1	1	1	1	2	3	3
35–49	29	1.3	<1	1	1	1	1	2	2	3
50–64	30	1.4	<1	1	1	1	2	3	3	4
65+	12	2.2	4	1	1	1	2	5	7	7
GRAND TOTAL	224	1.4	2	1	1	1	1	2	3	9

06.8: PARATHYROIDECTOMY

Type of Patients	Observed Patients	Avg. Stay	Vari-ance	Percentiles						
				10th	25th	50th	75th	90th	95th	99th
1. SINGLE DX										
0–19 Years	0									
20–34	8	1.8	1	1	1	1	2	4	4	4
35–49	14	1.1	<1	1	1	1	1	2	2	2
50–64	45	1.1	<1	1	1	1	1	1	2	3
65+	23	1.2	<1	1	1	1	1	2	2	3
2. MULTIPLE DX										
0–19 Years	11	4.6	17	1	1	5	7	9	15	15
20–34	149	4.0	21	1	1	2	5	10	13	24
35–49	374	2.9	11	1	1	2	3	7	10	15
50–64	922	2.1	8	1	1	1	2	4	7	16
65+	933	1.9	8	1	1	1	2	3	6	19
TOTAL SINGLE DX	90	1.2	<1	1	1	1	1	2	2	4
TOTAL MULTIPLE DX	2,389	2.3	10	1	1	1	2	5	8	17
TOTAL										
0–19 Years	11	4.6	17	1	1	5	7	9	15	15
20–34	157	3.9	21	1	1	2	4	9	13	24
35–49	388	2.9	10	1	1	1	3	7	10	15
50–64	967	2.0	8	1	1	1	2	4	7	16
65+	956	1.9	8	1	1	1	2	3	6	19
GRAND TOTAL	2,479	2.3	9	1	1	1	2	5	8	17

06.81: TOTAL PARATHYROIDECTOMY

Type of Patients	Observed Patients	Avg. Stay	Vari-ance	Percentiles						
				10th	25th	50th	75th	90th	95th	99th
1. SINGLE DX										
0–19 Years	0									
20–34	1	3.0	0	3	3	3	3	3	3	3
35–49	1	1.0	0	1	1	1	1	1	1	1
50–64	6	1.2	<1	1	1	1	1	2	2	2
65+	5	1.2	<1	1	1	1	1	2	2	2
2. MULTIPLE DX										
0–19 Years	3	6.7	4	5	5	6	9	9	9	9
20–34	34	6.2	37	1	2	4	8	14	17	29
35–49	62	4.9	23	1	2	3	6	13	13	27
50–64	124	2.7	12	1	1	2	3	7	9	18
65+	102	2.0	6	1	1	1	2	3	4	12
TOTAL SINGLE DX	13	1.3	<1	1	1	1	1	2	3	3
TOTAL MULTIPLE DX	325	3.3	17	1	1	2	3	8	12	19
TOTAL										
0–19 Years	3	6.7	4	5	5	6	9	9	9	9
20–34	35	6.1	37	1	2	3	8	14	17	29
35–49	63	4.9	23	1	2	3	6	13	13	27
50–64	130	2.7	12	1	1	1	3	7	9	18
65+	107	2.0	6	1	1	1	2	3	4	12
GRAND TOTAL	338	3.2	16	1	1	2	3	8	12	19

LOS by Diagnosis and Operation, Western Region, 45th Edition

Western Region, October 2007–September 2008 Data, by Operation

06.89: OTHER PARATHYROIDECTOMY

Type of Patients	Observed Patients	Avg. Stay	Vari-ance	Percentiles						
				10th	25th	50th	75th	90th	95th	99th
1. SINGLE DX										
0–19 Years	0									
20–34	7	1.6	1	1	1	1	2	4	4	4
35–49	13	1.2	<1	1	1	1	1	2	2	2
50–64	39	1.1	<1	1	1	1	1	1	2	3
65+	18	1.2	<1	1	1	1	1	2	3	3
2. MULTIPLE DX										
0–19 Years	8	4.1	20	1	1	1	7	8	15	15
20–34	115	3.4	15	1	1	2	4	9	11	18
35–49	312	2.5	7	1	1	1	3	6	8	14
50–64	798	2.0	7	1	1	1	2	3	7	16
65+	831	1.9	8	1	1	1	2	3	6	19
TOTAL SINGLE DX	77	1.2	<1	1	1	1	1	2	2	4
TOTAL MULTIPLE DX	2,064	2.1	8	1	1	1	2	4	7	17
TOTAL										
0–19 Years	8	4.1	20	1	1	1	7	8	15	15
20–34	122	3.2	14	1	1	2	4	8	11	18
35–49	325	2.5	7	1	1	1	3	6	8	14
50–64	837	1.9	7	1	1	1	2	3	7	15
65+	849	1.9	8	1	1	1	2	3	6	19
GRAND TOTAL	2,141	2.1	8	1	1	1	2	4	7	17

06.9: THYROID/PARATHY OPS NEC

Type of Patients	Observed Patients	Avg. Stay	Vari-ance	Percentiles						
				10th	25th	50th	75th	90th	95th	99th
1. SINGLE DX										
0–19 Years	0									
20–34	1	2.0	0	2	2	2	2	2	2	2
35–49	2	1.5	<1	1	1	1	2	2	2	2
50–64	2	1.5	<1	1	1	1	2	2	2	2
65+	2	1.0	0	1	1	1	1	1	1	1
2. MULTIPLE DX										
0–19 Years	1	7.0	0	7	7	7	7	7	7	7
20–34	6	7.7	31	3	4	4	9	18	18	18
35–49	20	5.3	137	1	1	2	4	9	54	54
50–64	26	3.9	49	1	1	2	3	9	11	36
65+	24	8.5	168	1	1	2	6	34	35	36
TOTAL SINGLE DX	7	1.4	<1	1	1	1	2	2	2	2
TOTAL MULTIPLE DX	77	6.0	107	1	1	2	4	18	35	54
TOTAL										
0–19 Years	1	7.0	0	7	7	7	7	7	7	7
20–34	7	6.9	31	2	3	4	3	18	18	18
35–49	22	4.9	125	1	1	2	3	7	9	54
50–64	28	3.8	46	1	1	2	3	9	11	36
65+	26	7.9	159	1	1	2	6	34	35	36
GRAND TOTAL	84	5.7	100	1	1	2	4	11	34	54

07.0: ADRENAL FIELD EXPL

Type of Patients	Observed Patients	Avg. Stay	Vari-ance	Percentiles						
				10th	25th	50th	75th	90th	95th	99th
1. SINGLE DX										
0–19 Years	0									
20–34	0									
35–49	0									
50–64	0									
65+	0									
2. MULTIPLE DX										
0–19 Years	0									
20–34	0									
35–49	0									
50–64	0									
65+	0									
TOTAL SINGLE DX	0									
TOTAL MULTIPLE DX	0									
TOTAL										
0–19 Years	0									
20–34	0									
35–49	0									
50–64	0									
65+	0									
GRAND TOTAL	0									

07.1: OTH ENDOCRINE DXTIC PX

Type of Patients	Observed Patients	Avg. Stay	Vari-ance	Percentiles						
				10th	25th	50th	75th	90th	95th	99th
1. SINGLE DX										
0–19 Years	0									
20–34	1	3.0	0	3	3	3	3	3	3	3
35–49	0									
50–64	2	2.0	0	2	2	2	2	2	2	2
65+	0									
2. MULTIPLE DX										
0–19 Years	12	11.0	85	1	3	6	17	29	29	29
20–34	8	5.3	14	1	4	5	6	11	11	11
35–49	21	4.8	24	1	2	4	5	10	11	23
50–64	51	6.7	44	2	3	5	9	13	15	39
65+	57	6.4	21	2	3	5	7	13	16	22
TOTAL SINGLE DX	3	2.3	<1	2	2	2	3	3	3	3
TOTAL MULTIPLE DX	149	7.2	44	2	3	5	9	17	19	29
TOTAL										
0–19 Years	12	11.0	85	1	3	6	17	29	29	29
20–34	9	5.0	12	1	3	4	6	11	11	11
35–49	21	4.8	24	1	2	4	5	10	11	23
50–64	53	6.5	43	2	3	5	8	13	15	39
65+	57	6.4	21	2	3	5	7	13	16	22
GRAND TOTAL	152	7.1	44	2	3	5	9	16	19	29

LOS by Diagnosis and Operation, Western Region, 45th Edition

Western Region, October 2007–September 2008 Data, by Operation

07.11: CLSD ADRENAL GLAND BX

Type of Patients	Observed Patients	Avg. Stay	Variance	Percentiles						
				10th	25th	50th	75th	90th	95th	99th
1. SINGLE DX										
0–19 Years	0									
20–34	0									
35–49	0									
50–64	2	2.0	0	2	2	2	2	2	2	2
65+	0									
2. MULTIPLE DX										
0–19 Years	0									
20–34	3	6.0	25	1	1	6	11	11	11	11
35–49	8	5.6	11	2	3	6	10	11	11	11
50–64	37	7.4	55	2	3	5	9	15	27	39
65+	52	6.2	20	2	3	5	7	12	15	22
TOTAL SINGLE DX	2	2.0	0	2	2	2	2	2	2	2
TOTAL MULTIPLE DX	100	6.6	32	2	3	5	8	13	15	39
TOTAL										
0–19 Years	0									
20–34	3	6.0	25	1	1	6	11	11	11	11
35–49	8	5.6	11	2	3	6	10	11	11	11
50–64	39	7.2	53	2	3	5	9	15	27	39
65+	52	6.2	20	2	3	5	7	12	15	22
GRAND TOTAL	102	6.5	32	2	3	5	8	12	15	27

07.2: PARTIAL ADRENALECTOMY

Type of Patients	Observed Patients	Avg. Stay	Variance	Percentiles						
				10th	25th	50th	75th	90th	95th	99th
1. SINGLE DX										
0–19 Years	9	4.2	7	1	2	4	8	8	8	8
20–34	9	2.0	2	1	1	2	2	5	5	5
35–49	12	2.1	<1	1	1	2	3	3	3	3
50–64	12	2.0	0	1	1	1	1	4	5	5
65+	1	1.0		1	1	1	1	1	1	1
2. MULTIPLE DX										
0–19 Years	49	10.2	211	2	4	5	10	29	71	>99
20–34	63	3.7	21	1	2	3	5	6	6	35
35–49	186	3.9	35	1	2	3	5	7	10	29
50–64	343	3.5	9	1	2	3	5	6	8	14
65+	195	4.7	34	1	2	3	5	8	14	37
TOTAL SINGLE DX	43	2.9	5	1	1	2	4	8	8	8
TOTAL MULTIPLE DX	836	4.8	54	1	2	3	5	8	13	64
TOTAL										
0–19 Years	58	9.4	186	2	4	5	9	21	71	>99
20–34	72	3.5	19	1	1	3	4	5	6	35
35–49	198	3.8	33	1	1	2	4	7	10	29
50–64	355	3.4	9	1	2	3	5	6	8	14
65+	196	4.7	34	1	2	3	5	8	14	37
GRAND TOTAL	879	4.7	51	1	2	3	5	8	12	50

07.22: UNILATERAL ADRENALECTOMY

Type of Patients	Observed Patients	Avg. Stay	Variance	Percentiles						
				10th	25th	50th	75th	90th	95th	99th
1. SINGLE DX										
0–19 Years	6	4.6	11	1	1	4	8	8	8	8
20–34	8	1.6	<1	1	1	1	2	3	3	3
35–49	7	2.0	<1	1	1	2	3	3	3	3
50–64	11	2.1	2	1	1	1	3	4	5	5
65+	1	1.0	0	1	1	1	1	1	1	1
2. MULTIPLE DX										
0–19 Years	33	8.2	109	2	4	5	9	29	50	>99
20–34	53	3.7	25	1	2	3	4	5	7	35
35–49	169	3.8	37	1	1	2	4	6	9	29
50–64	307	3.4	9	1	2	3	4	6	8	12
65+	176	4.6	34	1	2	3	5	8	14	37
TOTAL SINGLE DX	33	2.8	6	1	1	2	3	8	8	8
TOTAL MULTIPLE DX	738	4.3	34	1	2	3	5	7	11	50
TOTAL										
0–19 Years	39	7.7	98	2	4	5	8	16	50	>99
20–34	61	3.4	22	1	1	2	4	5	6	35
35–49	176	3.7	35	1	2	3	4	6	9	29
50–64	318	3.3	9	1	2	3	4	6	8	12
65+	177	4.6	34	1	2	3	5	8	14	37
GRAND TOTAL	771	4.2	33	1	2	3	5	7	11	50

07.3: BILATERAL ADRENALECTOMY

Type of Patients	Observed Patients	Avg. Stay	Variance	Percentiles						
				10th	25th	50th	75th	90th	95th	99th
1. SINGLE DX										
0–19 Years	0									
20–34	0									
35–49	1	2.0	0	2	2	2	2	2	2	2
50–64	0									
65+	0									
2. MULTIPLE DX										
0–19 Years	0									
20–34	5	5.0	3	3	4	4	7	7	7	7
35–49	10	5.3	39	1	2	3	6	22	22	22
50–64	15	3.5	3	2	2	3	5	6	8	8
65+	5	5.2	7	3	3	4	5	8	8	8
TOTAL SINGLE DX	1	2.0	0	2	2	2	2	2	2	2
TOTAL MULTIPLE DX	35	4.5	14	2	3	3	6	8	8	22
TOTAL										
0–19 Years	0									
20–34	5	5.0	3	3	4	4	7	7	7	7
35–49	11	5.0	36	1	2	3	6	7	22	22
50–64	15	3.5	3	2	2	3	5	6	8	8
65+	5	5.2	7	3	3	4	5	8	8	8
GRAND TOTAL	36	4.4	13	2	2	3	6	8	8	22

LOS by Diagnosis and Operation, Western Region, 45th Edition

Western Region, October 2007–September 2008 Data, by Operation

07.6: HYPOPHYSECTOMY

Type of Patients	Observed Patients	Avg. Stay	Vari-ance	Percentiles						
				10th	25th	50th	75th	90th	95th	99th
1. SINGLE DX										
0–19 Years	10	2.0	<1	1	1	2	3	3	3	3
20–34	35	2.5	2	1	1	2	3	5	6	6
35–49	34	3.0	6	1	2	3	4	4	11	12
50–64	38	2.8	2	2	2	2	3	5	6	9
65+	8	2.0	2	1	1	2	2	4	4	4
2. MULTIPLE DX										
0–19 Years	65	8.8	177	2	4	5	7	16	20	71
20–34	214	4.6	31	2	2	3	5	8	14	42
35–49	343	4.6	22	2	2	3	5	8	12	21
50–64	578	4.5	24	2	2	3	5	9	14	29
65+	361	5.1	47	2	2	3	5	10	15	29
TOTAL SINGLE DX	125	2.7	3	1	2	2	3	4	5	11
TOTAL MULTIPLE DX	1,561	5.0	44	2	2	3	5	9	15	30
TOTAL										
0–19 Years	75	8.3	168	2	3	5	7	16	19	71
20–34	249	4.3	28	1	2	3	4	7	12	42
35–49	377	4.5	21	2	2	3	5	8	12	21
50–64	616	4.4	23	2	2	3	5	8	13	28
65+	369	5.0	47	2	2	3	5	9	15	29
GRAND TOTAL	1,686	4.9	41	2	2	3	5	9	14	30

07.61: EXC PIT LES-TRANSFRONTAL

Type of Patients	Observed Patients	Avg. Stay	Vari-ance	Percentiles						
				10th	25th	50th	75th	90th	95th	99th
1. SINGLE DX										
0–19 Years	0									
20–34	2	2.5	4	1	1	4	4	4	4	4
35–49	1	4.0	0	4	4	4	4	4	4	4
50–64	0									
65+	0									
2. MULTIPLE DX										
0–19 Years	17	15.9	405	5	5	8	16	71	71	71
20–34	14	15.5	251	3	4	9	19	42	48	48
35–49	20	8.1	51	2	3	6	12	17	22	29
50–64	37	11.2	108	3	3	7	17	28	40	41
65+	23	11.9	355	2	3	5	15	24	35	89
TOTAL SINGLE DX	3	3.0	3	1	1	4	4	4	4	4
TOTAL MULTIPLE DX	111	12.6	244	3	4	7	15	28	42	71
TOTAL										
0–19 Years	17	15.9	405	5	5	8	16	71	71	71
20–34	16	13.9	238	3	4	6	19	42	48	48
35–49	21	7.9	49	2	3	6	12	17	22	29
50–64	37	11.2	108	3	3	7	17	28	40	41
65+	23	11.9	355	2	3	5	15	24	35	89
GRAND TOTAL	114	12.4	240	3	4	6	15	28	42	71

07.4: OTHER ADRENAL OPERATIONS

Type of Patients	Observed Patients	Avg. Stay	Vari-ance	Percentiles						
				10th	25th	50th	75th	90th	95th	99th
1. SINGLE DX										
0–19 Years	0									
20–34	0									
35–49	0									
50–64	0									
65+	0									
2. MULTIPLE DX										
0–19 Years	0									
20–34	0									
35–49	0									
50–64	1	3.0	0	3	3	3	3	3	3	3
65+	1	4.0	0	4	4	4	4	4	4	4
TOTAL SINGLE DX	0									
TOTAL MULTIPLE DX	2	3.5	<1	3	3	4	4	4	4	4
TOTAL										
0–19 Years	0									
20–34	0									
35–49	0									
50–64	1	3.0	0	3	3	3	3	3	3	3
65+	1	4.0	0	4	4	4	4	4	4	4
GRAND TOTAL	2	3.5	<1	3	3	4	4	4	4	4

07.5: PINEAL GLAND OPERATIONS

Type of Patients	Observed Patients	Avg. Stay	Vari-ance	Percentiles						
				10th	25th	50th	75th	90th	95th	99th
1. SINGLE DX										
0–19 Years	1	5.0	0							
20–34	0									
35–49	1	4.0	0							
50–64	0									
65+	0									
2. MULTIPLE DX										
0–19 Years	5	21.4	144	10	10	12	30	37	37	37
20–34	4	15.2	137	5	5	6	29	29	29	29
35–49	3	7.0	37	3	3	4	4	14	14	14
50–64	4	16.3	82	6	14	17	17	28	28	28
65+	0									
TOTAL SINGLE DX	2	4.8	<1	4	5	5	5	5	5	5
TOTAL MULTIPLE DX	16	18.3	135	5	10	14	30	37	37	37
TOTAL										
0–19 Years	6	18.3	159	5	10	12	30	37	37	37
20–34	4	15.2	137	5	5	6	29	29	29	29
35–49	4	6.3	27	3	3	4	4	14	14	14
50–64	4	16.3	82	6	14	17	17	28	28	28
65+	0									
GRAND TOTAL	18	16.3	138	5	6	12	29	37	37	37

LOS by Diagnosis and Operation, Western Region, 45th Edition

Western Region, October 2007–September 2008 Data, by Operation

07.62: EXC PIT LES-TRANSSPHEN

Type of Patients	Observed Patients	Avg. Stay	Variance	10th	25th	50th	75th	90th	95th	99th
1. SINGLE DX										
0–19 Years	7	2.2	<1	1	2	2	3	3	3	3
20–34	25	2.6	2	1	2	2	3	5	6	6
35–49	20	3.4	9	1	2	2	4	11	12	12
50–64	23	2.6	1	2	2	2	3	4	5	6
65+	7	2.1	2	1	1	2	4	4	4	4
2. MULTIPLE DX										
0–19 Years	34	4.8	5	2	4	4	6	7	9	13
20–34	155	3.8	8	1	2	3	4	6	10	16
35–49	249	4.3	10	2	2	3	4	8	11	17
50–64	379	3.9	11	2	2	3	4	7	10	20
65+	268	4.2	12	2	2	3	5	8	11	20
TOTAL SINGLE DX	82	2.7	3	1	2	2	3	4	6	12
TOTAL MULTIPLE DX	1,085	4.1	10	2	2	3	5	7	10	18
TOTAL										
0–19 Years	41	4.6	5	2	3	4	6	7	9	13
20–34	180	3.6	8	1	2	3	4	6	8	16
35–49	269	4.2	10	2	2	3	5	8	11	17
50–64	402	3.8	10	2	2	3	4	7	10	19
65+	275	4.1	12	2	2	3	5	8	11	20
GRAND TOTAL	1,167	4.0	10	2	2	3	5	7	10	18

07.65: TOT EXC PIT-TRANSSPHEN

Type of Patients	Observed Patients	Avg. Stay	Variance	10th	25th	50th	75th	90th	95th	99th
1. SINGLE DX										
0–19 Years	2	1.5	<1	1	1	2	2	2	2	2
20–34	7	2.2	3	1	1	2	3	5	5	5
35–49	12	2.3	1	1	1	2	4	4	4	4
50–64	15	3.0	4	2	2	3	3	5	9	9
65+	1	1.0	0	1	1	1	1	1	1	1
2. MULTIPLE DX										
0–19 Years	11	9.7	216	2	3	6	10	19	19	76
20–34	41	3.7	6	2	2	3	4	7	12	>99
35–49	71	4.8	55	2	2	3	5	7	10	64
50–64	139	4.1	18	2	2	3	4	7	11	29
65+	66	6.3	69	2	2	3	6	14	22	53
TOTAL SINGLE DX	37	2.5	2	1	1	2	3	4	5	9
TOTAL MULTIPLE DX	328	5.1	51	2	2	3	5	10	14	53
TOTAL										
0–19 Years	13	9.1	205	2	2	4	10	19	19	76
20–34	48	3.5	6	1	2	3	4	7	12	>99
35–49	83	4.5	48	2	2	3	5	6	9	64
50–64	154	4.0	17	2	2	3	4	7	11	29
65+	67	6.3	68	2	2	3	6	14	22	53
GRAND TOTAL	365	4.8	47	2	2	3	5	9	12	53

07.7: OTHER HYPOPHYSIS OPS

Type of Patients	Observed Patients	Avg. Stay	Variance	10th	25th	50th	75th	90th	95th	99th
1. SINGLE DX										
0–19 Years	1	2.0	0	2	2	2	2	2	2	2
20–34	2	3.0	0	3	3	3	3	3	3	3
35–49	0									
50–64	1	3.0	0	3	3	3	3	3	3	3
65+	0									
2. MULTIPLE DX										
0–19 Years	4	6.4	6	2	7	7	8	8	8	8
20–34	4	5.5	17	2	2	2	8	10	10	10
35–49	2	3.5	<1	3	3	4	4	4	4	4
50–64	5	7.6	90	1	2	3	8	24	24	24
65+	3	9.9	131	1	1	6	23	23	23	23
TOTAL SINGLE DX	4	2.8	<1	2	2	3	3	3	3	3
TOTAL MULTIPLE DX	18	6.7	34	2	2	7	8	10	23	24
TOTAL										
0–19 Years	5	6.0	7	2	2	7	8	8	8	8
20–34	6	4.7	12	2	2	3	4	10	10	10
35–49	2	3.5	<1	3	3	4	4	4	4	4
50–64	6	6.8	75	1	2	3	8	24	24	24
65+	3	9.9	131	1	1	6	23	23	23	23
GRAND TOTAL	22	6.1	31	2	2	6	8	10	23	24

07.8: THYMECTOMY

Type of Patients	Observed Patients	Avg. Stay	Variance	10th	25th	50th	75th	90th	95th	99th
1. SINGLE DX										
0–19 Years	7	2.6	<1	2	2	2	3	4	5	5
20–34	14	2.9	4	1	1	3	4	4	8	8
35–49	10	2.9	<1	2	2	3	3	4	4	4
50–64	9	3.1	<1	2	2	3	4	5	5	5
65+	3	3.0	<1	2	2	3	4	4	4	4
2. MULTIPLE DX										
0–19 Years	13	7.7	31	1	3	8	14	17	>99	>99
20–34	70	6.3	61	2	3	4	6	11	26	43
35–49	68	4.6	13	2	3	4	5	9	14	18
50–64	117	5.0	19	2	3	4	6	8	13	17
65+	106	5.1	20	3	3	4	5	9	12	21
TOTAL SINGLE DX	43	2.8	2	1	2	3	4	4	5	8
TOTAL MULTIPLE DX	374	5.4	27	2	3	4	6	10	15	38
TOTAL										
0–19 Years	20	5.9	27	1	2	3	9	17	17	>99
20–34	84	5.8	53	1	3	4	5	9	24	43
35–49	78	4.4	11	2	3	4	5	8	14	18
50–64	126	4.9	18	2	3	4	5	8	12	17
65+	109	5.0	20	2	3	4	5	9	12	21
GRAND TOTAL	417	5.1	25	2	3	4	5	10	14	38

LOS by Diagnosis and Operation, Western Region, 45th Edition

Western Region, October 2007–September 2008 Data, by Operation

07.82: TOT EXCISION THYMUS NEC

Type of Patients	Observed Patients	Avg. Stay	Variance	Percentiles						
				10th	25th	50th	75th	90th	95th	99th
1. SINGLE DX										
0–19 Years	3	2.8	2	2	2	2	4	5	5	5
20–34	5	3.2	<1	2	3	3	4	5	5	5
35–49	5	3.2	<1	2	3	3	4	4	4	4
50–64	2	4.5	<1	4	4	5	5	5	5	5
65+	1	4.0	0	4	4	4	4	4	4	4
2. MULTIPLE DX										
0–19 Years	9	9.0	32	3	3	8	17	17	>99	>99
20–34	42	6.4	60	2	3	4	7	11	24	43
35–49	36	5.0	14	2	3	4	5	11	16	16
50–64	66	5.2	25	2	3	4	6	8	12	38
65+	57	5.1	27	2	3	4	5	9	11	37
TOTAL SINGLE DX	16	3.3	1	2	2	3	4	5	5	5
TOTAL MULTIPLE DX	210	5.8	32	2	3	4	6	12	17	43
TOTAL										
0–19 Years	12	7.7	32	2	3	8	14	17	>99	>99
20–34	47	6.1	55	2	3	4	6	11	24	43
35–49	41	4.8	12	2	3	4	5	9	14	16
50–64	68	5.2	24	2	3	4	6	8	12	38
65+	58	5.1	27	2	3	4	5	9	11	37
GRAND TOTAL	226	5.6	30	2	3	4	6	11	17	43

08.0: EYELID INCISION

Type of Patients	Observed Patients	Avg. Stay	Variance	Percentiles						
				10th	25th	50th	75th	90th	95th	99th
1. SINGLE DX										
0–19 Years	7	2.5	1	1	1	2	4	4	4	4
20–34	1	1.0	0	1	1	1	1	1	1	1
35–49	2	2.0	2	1	1	2	3	3	3	3
50–64	0									
65+	0									
2. MULTIPLE DX										
0–19 Years	23	3.7	3	1	2	4	4	6	6	8
20–34	33	4.6	18	2	2	4	5	6	17	22
35–49	31	4.9	19	2	2	4	6	8	11	24
50–64	21	3.6	3	2	2	3	5	5	7	8
65+	9	4.8	5	2	3	6	7	7	7	7
TOTAL SINGLE DX	10	2.4	1	1	1	2	4	4	4	4
TOTAL MULTIPLE DX	117	4.3	11	2	2	4	5	7	8	22
TOTAL										
0–19 Years	30	3.3	3	1	2	4	4	6	6	8
20–34	34	4.5	17	2	2	4	5	6	17	22
35–49	33	4.7	18	2	2	4	5	8	11	24
50–64	21	3.6	3	2	2	3	5	5	7	8
65+	9	4.8	5	2	3	6	7	7	7	7
GRAND TOTAL	127	4.0	10	2	2	4	5	6	8	22

07.9: OTHER THYMUS OPERATIONS

Type of Patients	Observed Patients	Avg. Stay	Variance	Percentiles						
				10th	25th	50th	75th	90th	95th	99th
1. SINGLE DX										
0–19 Years	0									
20–34	0									
35–49	0									
50–64	0									
65+	1	1.0	0	1	1	1	1	1	1	1
2. MULTIPLE DX										
0–19 Years	1	4.0	0	4	4	4	4	4	4	4
20–34	5	3.0	2	2	2	3	3	5	5	5
35–49	9	1.7	<1	1	1	2	2	2	2	2
50–64	9	2.1	9	1	1	1	1	10	10	10
65+	5	3.0	3	1	2	3	4	5	5	5
TOTAL SINGLE DX	1	1.0	0	1	1	1	1	1	1	1
TOTAL MULTIPLE DX	23	2.5	4	1	1	2	3	5	5	10
TOTAL										
0–19 Years	1	4.0	0	4	4	4	4	4	4	4
20–34	5	3.0	2	2	2	3	3	5	5	5
35–49	9	1.7	<1	1	1	2	2	2	2	2
50–64	9	2.1	9	1	1	1	1	10	10	10
65+	6	2.7	3	1	2	2	4	5	5	5
GRAND TOTAL	24	2.5	4	1	1	2	3	5	5	10

08.09: OTHER EYELID INCISION

Type of Patients	Observed Patients	Avg. Stay	Variance	Percentiles						
				10th	25th	50th	75th	90th	95th	99th
1. SINGLE DX										
0–19 Years	7	2.5	1	1	1	2	4	4	4	4
20–34	1	1.0	0	1	1	1	1	1	1	1
35–49	2	2.0	2	1	1	2	3	3	3	3
50–64	0									
65+	0									
2. MULTIPLE DX										
0–19 Years	23	3.7	3	1	2	4	4	6	6	8
20–34	33	4.6	18	2	2	4	5	6	17	22
35–49	31	4.9	19	2	2	4	6	8	11	24
50–64	21	3.6	3	2	2	3	5	5	7	8
65+	9	4.8	5	2	3	6	7	7	7	7
TOTAL SINGLE DX	10	2.4	1	1	1	2	4	4	4	4
TOTAL MULTIPLE DX	117	4.3	11	2	2	4	5	7	8	22
TOTAL										
0–19 Years	30	3.3	3	1	2	4	4	6	6	8
20–34	34	4.5	17	2	2	4	5	6	17	22
35–49	33	4.7	18	2	2	4	5	8	11	24
50–64	21	3.6	3	2	2	3	5	5	7	8
65+	9	4.8	5	2	3	6	7	7	7	7
GRAND TOTAL	127	4.0	10	2	2	4	5	6	8	22

Western Region, October 2007–September 2008 Data, by Operation

08.1: DXTIC PX ON EYELID

Type of Patients	Observed Patients	Avg. Stay	Variance	10th	25th	50th	75th	90th	95th	99th
1. SINGLE DX										
0–19 Years	0									
20–34	0									
35–49	0									
50–64	0									
65+	0									
2. MULTIPLE DX										
0–19 Years	0									
20–34	0									
35–49	1	3.0	0	3	3	3	3	3	3	3
50–64	0									
65+	4	6.0	28	1	2	9	9	12	12	12
TOTAL SINGLE DX	0									
TOTAL MULTIPLE DX	5	5.4	23	1	2	3	9	12	12	12
TOTAL										
0–19 Years	0									
20–34	0									
35–49	1	3.0	0	3	3	3	3	3	3	3
50–64	0									
65+	4	6.0	28	1	2	9	9	12	12	12
GRAND TOTAL	5	5.4	23	1	2	3	9	12	12	12

08.2: EXC/DESTR EYELID LESION

Type of Patients	Observed Patients	Avg. Stay	Variance	10th	25th	50th	75th	90th	95th	99th
1. SINGLE DX										
0–19 Years	4	1.0	0	1	1	1	1	1	1	1
20–34	0									
35–49	1	1.0	0	1	1	1	1	1	1	1
50–64	1	1.0	0	1	1	1	1	1	1	1
65+	1									
2. MULTIPLE DX										
0–19 Years	16	2.4	4	1	1	2	2	5	7	7
20–34	15	2.9	6	1	1	2	5	7	8	8
35–49	6	9.3	255	1	2	4	4	42	42	42
50–64	15	3.4	6	1	1	3	5	6	9	9
65+	16	3.2	8	1	1	2	6	7	10	10
TOTAL SINGLE DX	6	1.0	0	1	1	1	1	1	1	1
TOTAL MULTIPLE DX	68	3.2	21	1	1	2	4	7	7	42
TOTAL										
0–19 Years	20	2.2	3	1	1	1	2	5	7	7
20–34	15	2.9	6	1	1	2	5	7	8	8
35–49	6	9.3	255	1	2	4	4	42	42	42
50–64	16	3.3	6	1	1	3	5	6	9	9
65+	17	3.1	8	1	1	2	4	7	10	10
GRAND TOTAL	74	3.0	20	1	1	2	4	7	7	10

08.3: PTOSIS/LID RETRACT REP

Type of Patients	Observed Patients	Avg. Stay	Variance	10th	25th	50th	75th	90th	95th	99th
1. SINGLE DX										
0–19 Years	3	1.0	0	1	1	1	1	1	1	1
20–34	0									
35–49	0									
50–64	0									
65+	0									
2. MULTIPLE DX										
0–19 Years	4	13.8	272	1	1	1	33	33	33	33
20–34	1	1.0	0	1	1	1	1	1	1	1
35–49	6	5.9	26	1	2	6	11	13	13	13
50–64	12	1.3	<1	1	1	1	2	2	2	2
65+	5	2.4	7	1	1	1	2	7	7	7
TOTAL SINGLE DX	3	1.0	0	1	1	1	1	1	1	1
TOTAL MULTIPLE DX	28	6.0	109	1	1	1	2	33	33	33
TOTAL										
0–19 Years	7	10.9	237	1	1	1	33	33	33	33
20–34	1	1.0	0	1	1	1	1	1	1	1
35–49	6	5.9	26	1	2	6	11	13	13	13
50–64	12	1.3	<1	1	1	1	2	2	2	2
65+	5	2.4	7	1	1	1	2	7	7	7
GRAND TOTAL	31	5.6	102	1	1	1	2	33	33	33

08.4: ENTROPION/ECTROPION REP

Type of Patients	Observed Patients	Avg. Stay	Variance	10th	25th	50th	75th	90th	95th	99th
1. SINGLE DX										
0–19 Years	0									
20–34	0									
35–49	0									
50–64	0									
65+	0									
2. MULTIPLE DX										
0–19 Years	3	1.2	<1	1	1	1	1	2	2	2
20–34	2	1.0	0	1	1	1	1	1	1	1
35–49	0	94.0	0	94	94	94	94	94	94	94
50–64	0									
65+	5	5.2	5	3	3	5	7	8	8	8
TOTAL SINGLE DX	0									
TOTAL MULTIPLE DX	11	9.2	597	1	1	1	5	8	94	94
TOTAL										
0–19 Years	3	1.2	<1	1	1	1	1	2	2	2
20–34	2	1.0	0	1	1	1	1	1	1	1
35–49	1	94.0	0	94	94	94	94	94	94	94
50–64	0									
65+	5	5.2	5	3	3	5	7	8	8	8
GRAND TOTAL	11	9.2	597	1	1	1	5	8	94	94

LOS by Diagnosis and Operation, Western Region, 45th Edition

Western Region, October 2007–September 2008 Data, by Operation

08.5: OTH ADJUST LID POSITION

Type of Patients	Observed Patients	Avg. Stay	Variance	Percentiles						
				10th	25th	50th	75th	90th	95th	99th
1. SINGLE DX										
0–19 Years	2	1.0	0	1	1	1	1	1	1	1
20–34	2	1.5	<1	1	1	2	2	2	2	2
35–49	0									
50–64	0									
65+	0									
2. MULTIPLE DX										
0–19 Years	21	6.3	89	1	1	2	6	31	31	31
20–34	22	2.5	7	1	1	1	3	6	8	11
35–49	20	7.1	70	1	2	3	9	14	35	35
50–64	32	8.9	101	1	2	5	15	22	31	44
65+	24	5.6	21	1	2	4	9	11	14	18
TOTAL SINGLE DX	4	1.3	<1	1	1	1	2	2	2	2
TOTAL MULTIPLE DX	119	6.3	66	1	1	2	8	16	31	35
TOTAL										
0–19 Years	23	6.0	86	1	1	2	6	31	31	31
20–34	24	2.5	6	1	1	2	2	6	8	11
35–49	20	7.1	70	1	2	3	9	14	35	35
50–64	32	8.9	101	1	2	5	15	22	31	44
65+	24	5.6	21	1	2	4	9	11	14	18
GRAND TOTAL	123	6.2	65	1	1	2	8	16	31	35

08.6: EYELID RECONST W GRAFT

Type of Patients	Observed Patients	Avg. Stay	Variance	Percentiles						
				10th	25th	50th	75th	90th	95th	99th
1. SINGLE DX										
0–19 Years	1	1.0	0	1	1	1	1	1	1	1
20–34	1	1.0	0	1	1	1	1	1	1	1
35–49	1	1.0	0	1	1	1	1	1	1	1
50–64	2	1.5	<1	1	1	2	2	2	2	2
65+	0									
2. MULTIPLE DX										
0–19 Years	9	6.0	90	1	1	1	4	24	24	24
20–34	10	2.5	2	1	1	2	3	5	5	5
35–49	3	6.4	70	1	1	2	16	16	16	16
50–64	7	2.3	4	1	1	1	4	6	6	6
65+	13	2.8	10	1	1	2	3	3	13	13
TOTAL SINGLE DX	5	1.2	<1	1	1	1	1	2	2	2
TOTAL MULTIPLE DX	42	4.0	41	1	1	1	3	13	24	24
TOTAL										
0–19 Years	10	5.8	87	1	1	1	2	24	24	24
20–34	11	2.4	2	1	1	1	3	5	5	5
35–49	4	5.0	54	1	1	2	16	16	16	16
50–64	9	2.1	3	1	1	1	4	6	6	6
65+	13	2.8	10	1	1	2	3	3	13	13
GRAND TOTAL	47	3.8	38	1	1	1	3	13	24	24

08.7: OTHER EYELID RECONST

Type of Patients	Observed Patients	Avg. Stay	Variance	Percentiles						
				10th	25th	50th	75th	90th	95th	99th
1. SINGLE DX										
0–19 Years	3	1.2	<1	1	1	1	1	2	2	2
20–34	2	1.0	0	1	1	1	1	1	1	1
35–49	0									
50–64	0									
65+	0									
2. MULTIPLE DX										
0–19 Years	9	2.4	9	1	1	2	1	9	9	9
20–34	14	1.9	1	1	1	2	2	4	5	5
35–49	14	4.3	44	1	1	3	4	5	27	27
50–64	12	1.9	2	1	1	1	3	4	5	5
65+	12	2.3	2	1	1	2	3	4	6	6
TOTAL SINGLE DX	5	1.1	<1	1	1	1	1	2	2	2
TOTAL MULTIPLE DX	61	2.6	12	1	1	1	3	5	9	27
TOTAL										
0–19 Years	12	2.2	8	1	1	1	1	9	9	9
20–34	16	1.8	1	1	1	1	2	4	5	5
35–49	14	4.3	44	1	1	3	4	5	27	27
50–64	12	1.9	2	1	1	1	3	4	5	5
65+	12	2.3	2	1	1	2	3	4	6	6
GRAND TOTAL	66	2.4	11	1	1	1	3	5	9	27

08.8: OTHER REPAIR OF EYELID

Type of Patients	Observed Patients	Avg. Stay	Variance	Percentiles						
				10th	25th	50th	75th	90th	95th	99th
1. SINGLE DX										
0–19 Years	7	1.0	0	1	1	1	1	1	1	1
20–34	2	1.0	0	1	1	1	1	1	1	1
35–49	2	2.0	2	1	1	1	3	3	3	3
50–64	0									
65+	0									
2. MULTIPLE DX										
0–19 Years	159	1.6	1	1	1	1	2	3	3	6
20–34	259	2.0	3	1	1	1	2	4	7	9
35–49	271	2.8	21	1	1	2	3	5	7	16
50–64	297	3.5	26	1	2	3	4	7	10	39
65+	547	3.6	13	1	2	3	4	7	9	18
TOTAL SINGLE DX	11	1.2	<1	1	1	1	1	1	3	3
TOTAL MULTIPLE DX	1,533	2.9	14	1	1	2	3	6	8	17
TOTAL										
0–19 Years	166	1.6	1	1	1	1	2	3	3	6
20–34	261	2.0	3	1	1	1	2	4	5	9
35–49	273	2.8	21	1	1	2	3	5	7	16
50–64	297	3.5	26	1	2	2	4	7	10	39
65+	547	3.6	13	1	2	3	4	7	9	18
GRAND TOTAL	1,544	2.9	14	1	1	2	3	5	8	17

LOS by Diagnosis and Operation, Western Region, 45th Edition

Western Region, October 2007–September 2008 Data, by Operation

08.81: LINEAR REP EYELID LAC

Type of Patients	Observed Patients	Avg. Stay	Variance	Percentiles						
				10th	25th	50th	75th	90th	95th	99th
1. SINGLE DX										
0–19 Years	4	1.0	0	1	1	1	1	1	1	1
20–34	0									
35–49	2	2.0	2	1	1	1	3	3	3	3
50–64	0									
65+	0									
2. MULTIPLE DX										
0–19 Years	142	1.6	1	1	1	1	2	3	3	6
20–34	246	2.0	3	1	1	1	2	4	5	9
35–49	265	2.8	22	1	1	2	3	5	7	16
50–64	289	3.5	26	1	2	2	4	6	10	39
65+	536	3.6	13	1	2	3	4	7	9	18
TOTAL SINGLE DX	6	1.3	<1	1	1	1	1	3	3	3
TOTAL MULTIPLE DX	1,478	2.9	14	1	1	2	3	6	8	17
TOTAL										
0–19 Years	146	1.6	1	1	1	1	2	3	3	6
20–34	246	2.0	3	1	1	1	2	4	5	9
35–49	267	2.8	22	1	1	2	3	5	7	16
50–64	289	3.5	26	1	2	2	4	6	10	39
65+	536	3.6	13	1	2	3	4	7	9	18
GRAND TOTAL	1,484	2.9	14	1	1	2	3	6	8	17

08.9: OTHER EYELID OPERATIONS

Type of Patients	Observed Patients	Avg. Stay	Variance	Percentiles						
				10th	25th	50th	75th	90th	95th	99th
1. SINGLE DX										
0–19 Years	0									
20–34	0									
35–49	0									
50–64	0									
65+	0									
2. MULTIPLE DX										
0–19 Years	1	1.0	0	1	1	1	1	1	1	1
20–34	4	2.5	6	1	1	2	6	6	6	6
35–49	2	36.0	>999	1	1	36	71	71	71	71
50–64	4	8.5	70	3	4	5	6	21	21	21
65+	2	1.5	<1	1	1	2	2	2	2	2
TOTAL SINGLE DX	0									
TOTAL MULTIPLE DX	13	9.3	376	1	1	2	6	21	71	71
TOTAL										
0–19 Years	1	1.0	0	1	1	1	1	1	1	1
20–34	4	2.5	6	1	1	2	6	6	6	6
35–49	2	36.0	>999	1	1	36	71	71	71	71
50–64	4	8.5	70	3	4	5	6	21	21	21
65+	2	1.5	<1	1	1	2	2	2	2	2
GRAND TOTAL	13	9.3	376	1	1	2	6	21	71	71

09.0: LACRIMAL GLAND INCISION

Type of Patients	Observed Patients	Avg. Stay	Variance	Percentiles						
				10th	25th	50th	75th	90th	95th	99th
1. SINGLE DX										
0–19 Years	0									
20–34	0									
35–49	0									
50–64	0									
65+	0									
2. MULTIPLE DX										
0–19 Years	2	6.0	2	5	5	6	7	7	7	7
20–34	0									
35–49	1	6.0	0	6	6	6	6	6	6	6
50–64	0									
65+	2	2.5	4	1	1	1	4	4	4	4
TOTAL SINGLE DX	0									
TOTAL MULTIPLE DX	5	4.6	5	1	4	5	6	7	7	7
TOTAL										
0–19 Years	2	6.0	2	5	5	6	7	7	7	7
20–34	0									
35–49	1	6.0	0	6	6	6	6	6	6	6
50–64	0									
65+	2	2.5	4	1	1	1	4	4	4	4
GRAND TOTAL	5	4.6	5	1	4	5	6	7	7	7

09.1: LACRIMAL SYSTEM DXTIC PX

Type of Patients	Observed Patients	Avg. Stay	Variance	Percentiles						
				10th	25th	50th	75th	90th	95th	99th
1. SINGLE DX										
0–19 Years	0									
20–34	0									
35–49	0									
50–64	0									
65+	1	4.0	0	4	4	4	4	4	4	4
2. MULTIPLE DX										
0–19 Years	1	8.0	0	8	8	8	8	8	8	8
20–34	0									
35–49	0									
50–64	0									
65+	3	3.0	<1	2	2	3	4	4	4	4
TOTAL SINGLE DX	1	4.0	0	4	4	4	4	4	4	4
TOTAL MULTIPLE DX	4	5.9	7	2	3	8	8	8	8	8
TOTAL										
0–19 Years	1	8.0	0	8	8	8	8	8	8	8
20–34	0									
35–49	0									
50–64	0									
65+	4	3.3	<1	2	3	4	4	4	4	4
GRAND TOTAL	5	5.7	7	2	4	8	8	8	8	8

LOS by Diagnosis and Operation, Western Region, 45th Edition

Western Region, October 2007–September 2008 Data, by Operation

09.2: LACRIMAL GLAND LES EXC

Type of Patients	Observed Patients	Avg. Stay	Variance	10th	25th	50th	75th	90th	95th	99th
1. SINGLE DX										
0–19 Years	0									
20–34	0									
35–49	0									
50–64	1	1.0	0	1	1	1	1	1	1	1
65+	0									
2. MULTIPLE DX										
0–19 Years	1	5.0	0	5	5	5	5	5	5	5
20–34	0									
35–49	0									
50–64	0									
65+	0									
TOTAL SINGLE DX	1	1.0	0	1	1	1	1	1	1	1
TOTAL MULTIPLE DX	1	5.0	0	5	5	5	5	5	5	5
TOTAL										
0–19 Years	1	5.0	0	5	5	5	5	5	5	5
20–34	0									
35–49	0									
50–64	1	1.0	0	1	1	1	1	1	1	1
65+	0									
GRAND TOTAL	2	3.6	6	1	1	5	5	5	5	5

09.3: OTHER LACRIMAL GLAND OPS

Type of Patients	Observed Patients	Avg. Stay	Variance	10th	25th	50th	75th	90th	95th	99th
1. SINGLE DX										
0–19 Years	0									
20–34	0									
35–49	0									
50–64	0									
65+	0									
2. MULTIPLE DX										
0–19 Years	0									
20–34	0									
35–49	0									
50–64	0									
65+	0									
TOTAL SINGLE DX	0									
TOTAL MULTIPLE DX	0									
TOTAL										
0–19 Years	0									
20–34	0									
35–49	0									
50–64	0									
65+	0									
GRAND TOTAL	0									

09.4: LACRIMAL PASSAGE MANIP

Type of Patients	Observed Patients	Avg. Stay	Variance	10th	25th	50th	75th	90th	95th	99th
1. SINGLE DX										
0–19 Years	10	1.9	2	1	1	1	2	4	4	4
20–34	0									
35–49	0									
50–64	0									
65+	1	1.0	0	1	1	1	1	1	1	1
2. MULTIPLE DX										
0–19 Years	42	4.8	33	1	1	3	5	9	14	29
20–34	4	5.5	27	2	2	5	13	13	13	13
35–49	0									
50–64	4	4.0	10	1	2	5	8	8	8	8
65+	1	1.0	0	1	1	1	1	1	1	1
TOTAL SINGLE DX	11	1.9	2	1	1	1	2	4	4	4
TOTAL MULTIPLE DX	51	4.8	31	1	1	3	5	9	13	29
TOTAL										
0–19 Years	52	4.2	27	1	1	3	5	7	10	29
20–34	4	5.5	27	2	2	5	13	13	13	13
35–49	0									
50–64	4	4.0	10	1	2	5	8	8	8	8
65+	2	1.0	0	1	1	1	1	1	1	1
GRAND TOTAL	62	4.2	26	1	1	3	5	8	10	29

09.5: INC LACRIMAL SAC/PASSG

Type of Patients	Observed Patients	Avg. Stay	Variance	10th	25th	50th	75th	90th	95th	99th
1. SINGLE DX										
0–19 Years	0									
20–34	0									
35–49	0									
50–64	0									
65+										
2. MULTIPLE DX										
0–19 Years	4	3.3	2	2	3	3	3	6	6	6
20–34	2	3.0	0	3	3	3	3	3	3	3
35–49	7	4.9	4	2	3	5	7	8	8	8
50–64	5	13.1	288	3	3	7	9	43	43	43
65+	4	2.0	1	1	1	1	3	3	3	3
TOTAL SINGLE DX	0									
TOTAL MULTIPLE DX	22	5.4	66	2	3	3	5	8	9	43
TOTAL										
0–19 Years	4	3.3	2	2	3	3	3	6	6	6
20–34	2	3.0	0	3	3	3	3	3	3	3
35–49	7	4.9	4	2	3	5	7	8	8	8
50–64	5	13.1	288	3	3	7	9	43	43	43
65+	4	2.0	1	1	1	1	3	3	3	3
GRAND TOTAL	22	5.4	66	2	3	3	5	8	9	43

LOS by Diagnosis and Operation, Western Region, 45th Edition

Western Region, October 2007–September 2008 Data, by Operation

09.6: LACRIMAL SAC/PASSAGE EXC

Type of Patients	Observed Patients	Avg. Stay	Vari-ance	10th	25th	50th	75th	90th	95th	99th
1. SINGLE DX										
0–19 Years	0									
20–34	0									
35–49	0									
50–64	0									
65+	0									
2. MULTIPLE DX										
0–19 Years	3	4.4	8	2	2	3	8	8	8	8
20–34	0									
35–49	0									
50–64	1	7.0	0	7	7	7	7	7	7	7
65+	1	6.0	0	6	6	6	6	6	6	6
TOTAL SINGLE DX	0									
TOTAL MULTIPLE DX	5	4.7	7	2	2	3	8	8	8	8
TOTAL										
0–19 Years	3	4.4	8	2	2	3	8	8	8	8
20–34	0									
35–49	0									
50–64	1	7.0	0	7	7	7	7	7	7	7
65+	1	6.0	0	6	6	6	6	6	6	6
GRAND TOTAL	5	4.7	7	2	2	3	8	8	8	8

09.7: CANALICULUS/PUNCTUM REP

Type of Patients	Observed Patients	Avg. Stay	Vari-ance	10th	25th	50th	75th	90th	95th	99th
1. SINGLE DX										
0–19 Years	6	1.0	0	1	1	1	1	1	1	1
20–34	1	3.0	0	3	3	3	3	3	3	3
35–49	1	1.0	0	1	1	1	1	1	1	1
50–64	0									
65+	0									
2. MULTIPLE DX										
0–19 Years	10	2.5	12	1	1	1	2	12	12	12
20–34	8	3.0	8	1	1	2	5	9	9	9
35–49	5	1.8	1	1	1	1	3	3	3	3
50–64	5	3.4	11	1	1	1	7	7	7	7
65+	2	2.0	2	1	1	2	3	3	3	3
TOTAL SINGLE DX	8	1.2	<1	1	1	1	1	3	3	3
TOTAL MULTIPLE DX	30	2.6	8	1	1	1	3	7	9	12
TOTAL										
0–19 Years	16	1.9	7	1	1	2	2	3	12	12
20–34	9	3.0	7	1	1	3	3	9	9	9
35–49	6	1.7	7	1	1	1	3	3	3	3
50–64	5	3.4	11	1	1	1	7	7	7	7
65+	2	2.0	2	1	1	2	3	3	3	3
GRAND TOTAL	38	2.3	6	1	1	1	3	7	9	12

09.8: NL FISTULIZATION

Type of Patients	Observed Patients	Avg. Stay	Vari-ance	10th	25th	50th	75th	90th	95th	99th
1. SINGLE DX										
0–19 Years	1	1.0	0	1	1	1	1	1	1	1
20–34	0									
35–49	0									
50–64	1	1.0	0	1	1	1	1	1	1	1
65+	0									
2. MULTIPLE DX										
0–19 Years	0									
20–34	3	3.2	4	1	1	2	5	5	5	5
35–49	5	4.6	41	1	2	2	2	16	16	16
50–64	6	2.4	3	1	1	3	3	5	5	5
65+	8	2.9	2	1	2	3	5	5	5	5
TOTAL SINGLE DX	2	1.0	0	1	1	1	1	1	1	1
TOTAL MULTIPLE DX	21	3.2	10	1	2	2	5	5	5	16
TOTAL										
0–19 Years	1	1.0	0	1	1	1	1	1	1	1
20–34	3	3.2	4	1	1	2	5	5	5	5
35–49	5	4.6	41	1	2	2	2	16	16	16
50–64	6	2.2	3	1	1	3	3	5	5	5
65+	8	2.9	2	1	2	3	5	5	5	5
GRAND TOTAL	23	3.0	10	1	1	2	3	5	5	16

09.9: OTH LACRIMAL SYST OPS

Type of Patients	Observed Patients	Avg. Stay	Vari-ance	10th	25th	50th	75th	90th	95th	99th
1. SINGLE DX										
0–19 Years	0									
20–34	0									
35–49	0									
50–64	0									
65+	0									
2. MULTIPLE DX										
0–19 Years	3	2.3	2	1	1	2	4	4	4	4
20–34	0									
35–49	3	1.7	1	1	1	1	3	3	3	3
50–64	2	1.0	0	1	1	1	1	1	1	1
65+	0									
TOTAL SINGLE DX	0									
TOTAL MULTIPLE DX	8	1.8	1	1	1	1	2	4	4	4
TOTAL										
0–19 Years	3	2.3	2	1	1	2	4	4	4	4
20–34	0									
35–49	3	1.7	1	1	1	1	3	3	3	3
50–64	2	1.0	0	1	1	1	1	1	1	1
65+	0									
GRAND TOTAL	8	1.8	1	1	1	1	2	4	4	4

LOS by Diagnosis and Operation, Western Region, 45th Edition

Western Region, October 2007–September 2008 Data, by Operation

10.0: INC/RMVL FB-CONJUNCTIVA

Type of Patients	Observed Patients	Avg. Stay	Vari-ance	Percentiles						
				10th	25th	50th	75th	90th	95th	99th
1. SINGLE DX										
0–19 Years	0									
20–34	0									
35–49	0									
50–64	0									
65+	0									
2. MULTIPLE DX										
0–19 Years	2	1.0	0	1	1	1	1	1	1	1
20–34	1	1.0	0	1	1	1	1	1	1	1
35–49	0									
50–64	0									
65+	0									
TOTAL SINGLE DX	0									
TOTAL MULTIPLE DX	3	1.0	0	1	1	1	1	1	1	1
TOTAL										
0–19 Years	2	1.0	0	1	1	1	1	1	1	1
20–34	1	1.0	0	1	1	1	1	1	1	1
35–49	0									
50–64	0									
65+	0									
GRAND TOTAL	3	1.0	0	1	1	1	1	1	1	1

10.1: CONJUNCTIVA INCISION NEC

Type of Patients	Observed Patients	Avg. Stay	Vari-ance	Percentiles						
				10th	25th	50th	75th	90th	95th	99th
1. SINGLE DX										
0–19 Years	0									
20–34	0									
35–49	0									
50–64	0									
65+	0									
2. MULTIPLE DX										
0–19 Years	1	1.0	0	1	1	1	1	1	1	1
20–34	3	1.0	0	1	1	1	1	1	1	1
35–49	1	3.0	0	3	3	3	3	3	3	3
50–64	3	1.3	<1	1	1	1	2	2	2	2
65+	4	2.3	4	1	1	1	5	5	5	5
TOTAL SINGLE DX	0									
TOTAL MULTIPLE DX	12	1.5	1	1	1	1	2	3	5	5
TOTAL										
0–19 Years	1	1.0	0	1	1	1	1	1	1	1
20–34	3	1.0	0	1	1	1	1	1	1	1
35–49	1	3.0	0	3	3	3	3	3	3	3
50–64	3	1.3	<1	1	1	1	2	2	2	2
65+	4	2.3	4	1	1	1	5	5	5	5
GRAND TOTAL	12	1.5	1	1	1	1	2	3	5	5

10.2: CONJUNCTIVA DXTIC PX

Type of Patients	Observed Patients	Avg. Stay	Vari-ance	Percentiles						
				10th	25th	50th	75th	90th	95th	99th
1. SINGLE DX										
0–19 Years	0									
20–34	0									
35–49	0									
50–64	0									
65+	0									
2. MULTIPLE DX										
0–19 Years	3	14.9	42	5	8	19	19	19	19	19
20–34	1	6.0	0	6	6	6	6	6	6	6
35–49	0									
50–64	0									
65+	0									
TOTAL SINGLE DX	0									
TOTAL MULTIPLE DX	4	13.6	46	5	6	19	19	19	19	19
TOTAL										
0–19 Years	3	14.9	42	5	8	19	19	19	19	19
20–34	1	6.0	0	6	6	6	6	6	6	6
35–49	0									
50–64	0									
65+	0									
GRAND TOTAL	4	13.6	46	5	6	19	19	19	19	19

10.3: EXC/DESTR CONJUNCT LES

Type of Patients	Observed Patients	Avg. Stay	Vari-ance	Percentiles						
				10th	25th	50th	75th	90th	95th	99th
1. SINGLE DX										
0–19 Years	0									
20–34	0									
35–49	0									
50–64	0									
65+	0									
2. MULTIPLE DX										
0–19 Years	1	1.0	0	1	1	1	1	1	1	1
20–34	0									
35–49	0									
50–64	0									
65+	0									
TOTAL SINGLE DX	0									
TOTAL MULTIPLE DX	1	1.0	0	1	1	1	1	1	1	1
TOTAL										
0–19 Years	1	1.0	0	1	1	1	1	1	1	1
20–34	0									
35–49	0									
50–64	0									
65+	0									
GRAND TOTAL	1	1.0	0	1	1	1	1	1	1	1

LOS by Diagnosis and Operation, Western Region, 45th Edition

Western Region, October 2007–September 2008 Data, by Operation

10.4: CONJUNCTIVOPLASTY

Type of Patients	Observed Patients	Avg. Stay	Vari-ance	Percentiles						
				10th	25th	50th	75th	90th	95th	99th
1. SINGLE DX										
0–19 Years	0									
20–34	0									
35–49	0									
50–64	0									
65+	0									
2. MULTIPLE DX										
0–19 Years	1	5.0	0	5	5	5	5	5	5	5
20–34	0									
35–49	1	2.0	0	2	2	2	2	2	2	2
50–64	0									
65+	1	1.0	0	1	1	1	1	1	1	1
TOTAL SINGLE DX	0									
TOTAL MULTIPLE DX	3	3.8	3	1	2	5	5	5	5	5
TOTAL										
0–19 Years	1	5.0	0	5	5	5	5	5	5	5
20–34	0									
35–49	1	2.0	0	2	2	2	2	2	2	2
50–64	0									
65+	1	1.0	0	1	1	1	1	1	1	1
GRAND TOTAL	3	3.8	3	1	2	5	5	5	5	5

10.5: CONJUNCT/LID ADHESIO

Type of Patients	Observed Patients	Avg. Stay	Vari-ance	Percentiles						
				10th	25th	50th	75th	90th	95th	99th
1. SINGLE DX										
0–19 Years	0									
20–34	0									
35–49	0									
50–64	0									
65+	0									
2. MULTIPLE DX										
0–19 Years	0									
20–34	0									
35–49	0									
50–64	1	2.0	0	2	2	2	2	2	2	2
65+	1	2.0	0	2	2	2	2	2	2	2
TOTAL SINGLE DX	0									
TOTAL MULTIPLE DX	2	2.0	0	2	2	2	2	2	2	2
TOTAL										
0–19 Years	0									
20–34	0									
35–49	0									
50–64	1	2.0	0	2	2	2	2	2	2	2
65+	1	2.0	0	2	2	2	2	2	2	2
GRAND TOTAL	2	2.0	0	2	2	2	2	2	2	2

10.6: REPAIR CONJUNCT LAC

Type of Patients	Observed Patients	Avg. Stay	Vari-ance	Percentiles						
				10th	25th	50th	75th	90th	95th	99th
1. SINGLE DX										
0–19 Years	1	2.0	0	2	2	2	2	2	2	2
20–34	0									
35–49	1	1.0	0	1	1	1	1	1	1	1
50–64	1	1.0	0	1	1	1	1	1	1	1
65+	0									
2. MULTIPLE DX										
0–19 Years	1	3.0	0	3	3	3	3	3	3	3
20–34	3	1.3	<1	1	1	1	2	2	2	2
35–49	3	1.7	1	1	1	1	3	3	3	3
50–64	3	3.7	6	1	1	4	6	6	6	6
65+	2	1.5	<1	1	1	2	2	2	2	2
TOTAL SINGLE DX	3	1.7	<1	1	1	2	2	2	2	2
TOTAL MULTIPLE DX	12	2.3	2	1	1	2	3	4	6	6
TOTAL										
0–19 Years	2	2.5	<1	2	2	3	3	3	3	3
20–34	3	1.3	<1	1	1	1	2	2	2	2
35–49	4	1.5	<1	1	1	1	1	3	3	3
50–64	4	3.0	6	1	1	3	4	6	6	6
65+	2	1.5	<1	1	1	2	2	2	2	2
GRAND TOTAL	15	2.1	2	1	1	2	3	3	4	6

10.9: OTHER CONJUNCTIVAL OPS

Type of Patients	Observed Patients	Avg. Stay	Vari-ance	Percentiles						
				10th	25th	50th	75th	90th	95th	99th
1. SINGLE DX										
0–19 Years	0									
20–34	1	1.0	0	1	1	1	1	1	1	1
35–49	0									
50–64	0									
65+	0									
2. MULTIPLE DX										
0–19 Years	3	3.7	6	1	1	4	6	6	6	6
20–34	2	1.0	0	1	1	1	1	1	1	1
35–49	3	8.3	32	2	2	10	13	13	13	13
50–64	2	1.0	0	1	1	1	1	1	1	1
65+	10	7.1	103	2	2	3	6	35	35	35
TOTAL SINGLE DX	1	1.0	0	1	1	1	1	1	1	1
TOTAL MULTIPLE DX	20	5.6	61	1	1	3	6	13	35	35
TOTAL										
0–19 Years	3	3.7	6	1	1	4	6	6	6	6
20–34	3	1.0	0	1	1	1	1	1	1	1
35–49	3	8.3	32	2	2	10	13	13	13	13
50–64	2	1.0	0	1	1	1	1	1	1	1
65+	10	7.1	103	2	2	3	6	35	35	35
GRAND TOTAL	21	5.4	59	1	1	3	6	10	13	35

LOS by Diagnosis and Operation, Western Region, 45th Edition

48

11.0: MAGNET REMOVAL CORNEA FB

Type of Patients	Observed Patients	Avg. Stay	Variance	Percentiles						
				10th	25th	50th	75th	90th	95th	99th
1. SINGLE DX										
0–19 Years	0									
20–34	0									
35–49	0									
50–64	0									
65+	0									
2. MULTIPLE DX										
0–19 Years	0									
20–34	0									
35–49	0									
50–64	0									
65+	0									
TOTAL SINGLE DX	**0**									
TOTAL MULTIPLE DX	**0**									
TOTAL										
0–19 Years	0									
20–34	0									
35–49	0									
50–64	0									
65+	0									
GRAND TOTAL	**0**									

11.1: CORNEAL INCISION

Type of Patients	Observed Patients	Avg. Stay	Variance	Percentiles						
				10th	25th	50th	75th	90th	95th	99th
1. SINGLE DX										
0–19 Years	0									
20–34	0									
35–49	0									
50–64	0									
65+	0									
2. MULTIPLE DX										
0–19 Years	1	5.0	0	5	5	5	5	5	5	5
20–34	1	1.0	0	1	1	1	1	1	1	1
35–49	0									
50–64	1	22.0	0	22	22	22	22	22	22	22
65+	1	10.0	0	10	10	10	10	10	10	10
TOTAL SINGLE DX	**0**									
TOTAL MULTIPLE DX	**4**	**9.5**	**83**	**1**	**1**	**5**	**22**	**22**	**22**	**22**
TOTAL										
0–19 Years	1	5.0	0	5	5	5	5	5	5	5
20–34	1	1.0	0	1	1	1	1	1	1	1
35–49	0									
50–64	1	22.0	0	22	22	22	22	22	22	22
65+	1	10.0	0	10	10	10	10	10	10	10
GRAND TOTAL	**4**	**9.5**	**83**	**1**	**1**	**5**	**22**	**22**	**22**	**22**

11.2: DXTIC PX ON CORNEA

Type of Patients	Observed Patients	Avg. Stay	Variance	Percentiles						
				10th	25th	50th	75th	90th	95th	99th
1. SINGLE DX										
0–19 Years	0									
20–34	0									
35–49	0									
50–64	0									
65+	0									
2. MULTIPLE DX										
0–19 Years	0									
20–34	2	7.9	71	2	2	2	14	14	14	14
35–49	1	1.0	0	1	1	1	1	1	1	1
50–64	2	5.5	13	3	3	6	8	8	8	8
65+	2	2.0	0	2	2	2	2	2	2	2
TOTAL SINGLE DX	**0**									
TOTAL MULTIPLE DX	**7**	**4.5**	**22**	**1**	**2**	**2**	**8**	**14**	**14**	**14**
TOTAL										
0–19 Years	0									
20–34	2	7.9	71	2	2	2	14	14	14	14
35–49	1	1.0	0	1	1	1	1	1	1	1
50–64	2	5.5	13	3	3	6	8	8	8	8
65+	2	2.0	0	2	2	2	2	2	2	2
GRAND TOTAL	**7**	**4.5**	**22**	**1**	**2**	**2**	**8**	**14**	**14**	**14**

11.3: EXCISION OF PTERYGIUM

Type of Patients	Observed Patients	Avg. Stay	Variance	Percentiles						
				10th	25th	50th	75th	90th	95th	99th
1. SINGLE DX										
0–19 Years	0									
20–34	0									
35–49	0									
50–64	0									
65+	0									
2. MULTIPLE DX										
0–19 Years	0									
20–34	0									
35–49	0									
50–64	1	1.0	0	1	1	1	1	1	1	1
65+	0									
TOTAL SINGLE DX	**0**									
TOTAL MULTIPLE DX	**1**	**1.0**	**0**	**1**	**1**	**1**	**1**	**1**	**1**	**1**
TOTAL										
0–19 Years	0									
20–34	0									
35–49	0									
50–64	1	1.0	0	1	1	1	1	1	1	1
65+	0									
GRAND TOTAL	**1**	**1.0**	**0**	**1**	**1**	**1**	**1**	**1**	**1**	**1**

LOS by Diagnosis and Operation, Western Region, 45th Edition

49

Western Region, October 2007–September 2008 Data, by Operation

11.4: EXC/DESTR CORNEAL LESION

Type of Patients	Observed Patients	Avg. Stay	Variance	Percentiles						
				10th	25th	50th	75th	90th	95th	99th
1. SINGLE DX										
0–19 Years	0									
20–34	0									
35–49	0									
50–64	0									
65+	0									
2. MULTIPLE DX										
0–19 Years	1	5.0	0	5	5	5	5	5	5	5
20–34	0									
35–49	1	5.0	0	5	5	5	5	5	5	5
50–64	1	7.0	0	7	7	7	7	7	7	7
65+	1	1.0	0	1	1	1	1	1	1	1
TOTAL SINGLE DX	0									
TOTAL MULTIPLE DX	4	4.5	6	1	1	5	7	7	7	7
TOTAL										
0–19 Years	1	5.0	0	5	5	5	5	5	5	5
20–34	0									
35–49	1	5.0	0	5	5	5	5	5	5	5
50–64	1	7.0	0	7	7	7	7	7	7	7
65+	1	1.0	0	1	1	1	1	1	1	1
GRAND TOTAL	4	4.5	6	1	1	5	7	7	7	7

11.5: CORNEAL REPAIR

Type of Patients	Observed Patients	Avg. Stay	Variance	Percentiles						
				10th	25th	50th	75th	90th	95th	99th
1. SINGLE DX										
0–19 Years	32	1.9	1	1	1	2	2	4	4	4
20–34	19	1.6	<1	1	1	1	2	3	3	3
35–49	12	1.2	<1	1	1	1	1	2	2	2
50–64	3	1.0	0	1	1	1	1	1	1	1
65+	1	2.0	0	2	2	2	2	2	2	2
2. MULTIPLE DX										
0–19 Years	31	2.7	2	1	2	2	3	4	7	7
20–34	35	1.6	1	1	1	1	2	3	3	7
35–49	29	2.7	31	1	1	1	3	3	4	31
50–64	15	2.4	8	1	1	2	2	5	12	12
65+	26	3.2	7	2	2	2	5	7	9	10
TOTAL SINGLE DX	67	1.7	<1	1	1	1	2	3	4	4
TOTAL MULTIPLE DX	136	2.5	8	1	1	2	3	4	7	12
TOTAL										
0–19 Years	63	2.3	2	1	1	2	3	4	4	7
20–34	54	1.6	1	1	1	1	2	3	3	7
35–49	41	2.3	22	1	1	1	3	3	3	31
50–64	18	2.2	7	1	1	1	2	5	12	12
65+	27	3.1	6	1	2	2	5	7	9	10
GRAND TOTAL	203	2.2	6	1	1	2	3	4	5	10

11.51: SUTURE OF CORNEAL LAC

Type of Patients	Observed Patients	Avg. Stay	Variance	Percentiles						
				10th	25th	50th	75th	90th	95th	99th
1. SINGLE DX										
0–19 Years	29	2.0	1	1	1	2	3	4	4	4
20–34	17	1.6	<1	1	1	1	2	3	3	3
35–49	10	1.1	<1	1	1	1	1	2	2	2
50–64	3	1.0	0	1	1	1	1	1	1	1
65+	0									
2. MULTIPLE DX										
0–19 Years	26	2.8	2	1	2	2	3	4	7	7
20–34	29	1.6	2	1	1	1	2	3	3	7
35–49	25	1.8	<1	1	1	1	3	3	3	4
50–64	11	1.6	1	1	1	1	2	2	5	5
65+	15	4.4	7	2	2	4	6	9	10	10
TOTAL SINGLE DX	59	1.8	<1	1	1	1	2	4	4	4
TOTAL MULTIPLE DX	106	2.4	3	1	1	2	3	4	7	9
TOTAL										
0–19 Years	55	2.4	2	1	1	2	3	4	4	7
20–34	46	1.6	1	1	1	1	2	3	3	7
35–49	35	1.6	<1	1	1	1	3	3	3	4
50–64	14	1.5	1	1	1	1	2	2	5	5
65+	15	4.4	7	2	2	4	6	9	10	10
GRAND TOTAL	165	2.2	2	1	1	2	3	4	5	7

11.6: CORNEAL TRANSPLANT

Type of Patients	Observed Patients	Avg. Stay	Variance	Percentiles						
				10th	25th	50th	75th	90th	95th	99th
1. SINGLE DX										
0–19 Years	2	1.0	0	1	1	1	1	1	1	1
20–34	1	3.0	0	3	3	3	3	3	3	3
35–49	0									
50–64	1	1.0	0	1	1	1	1	1	1	1
65+	3	1.0	0	1	1	1	1	1	1	1
2. MULTIPLE DX										
0–19 Years	4	2.2	2	1	1	1	4	4	4	4
20–34	4	2.8	6	1	1	3	6	6	6	6
35–49	7	6.8	229	1	1	1	2	41	41	41
50–64	8	3.1	10	1	1	2	3	10	10	10
65+	27	2.4	6	1	1	1	3	5	8	12
TOTAL SINGLE DX	7	1.3	<1	1	1	1	1	3	3	3
TOTAL MULTIPLE DX	50	3.1	32	1	1	1	3	6	10	41
TOTAL										
0–19 Years	6	2.0	2	1	1	1	4	4	4	4
20–34	5	2.8	4	1	1	3	6	6	6	6
35–49	7	6.8	229	1	1	1	1	41	41	41
50–64	9	2.9	10	1	1	2	3	5	8	10
65+	30	2.3	6	1	1	1	3	5	8	12
GRAND TOTAL	57	2.9	29	1	1	1	3	5	8	41

LOS by Diagnosis and Operation, Western Region, 45th Edition

Western Region, October 2007–September 2008 Data, by Operation

11.7: OTHER CORNEA RECONST

Type of Patients	Observed Patients	Avg. Stay	Vari-ance	Percentiles						
				10th	25th	50th	75th	90th	95th	99th
1. SINGLE DX										
0–19 Years	0									
20–34	0									
35–49	0									
50–64	0									
65+	0									
2. MULTIPLE DX										
0–19 Years	0									
20–34	2	6.5	12	4	4	4	9	9	9	9
35–49	1	1.0	0	1	1	1	1	1	1	1
50–64	2	3.5	4	2	2	4	5	5	5	5
65+	1	2.0	0	2	2	2	2	2	2	2
TOTAL SINGLE DX	0									
TOTAL MULTIPLE DX	6	3.8	9	1	2	4	5	9	9	9
TOTAL										
0–19 Years	0									
20–34	2	6.5	12	4	4	4	9	9	9	9
35–49	1	1.0	0	1	1	1	1	1	1	1
50–64	2	3.5	4	2	2	4	5	5	5	5
65+	1	2.0	0	2	2	2	2	2	2	2
GRAND TOTAL	6	3.8	9	1	2	4	5	9	9	9

11.9: OTHER CORNEAL OPERATIONS

Type of Patients	Observed Patients	Avg. Stay	Vari-ance	Percentiles						
				10th	25th	50th	75th	90th	95th	99th
1. SINGLE DX										
0–19 Years	0									
20–34	0									
35–49	0									
50–64	0									
65+	0									
2. MULTIPLE DX										
0–19 Years	0									
20–34	0									
35–49	2	2.0	2	1	1	2	3	3	3	3
50–64	1	3.0	0	3	3	3	3	3	3	3
65+	1	1.0	0	1	1	1	1	1	1	1
TOTAL SINGLE DX	0									
TOTAL MULTIPLE DX	4	2.0	1	1	1	2	3	3	3	3
TOTAL										
0–19 Years	0									
20–34	0									
35–49	2	2.0	2	1	1	2	3	3	3	3
50–64	1	3.0	0	3	3	3	3	3	3	3
65+	1	1.0	0	1	1	1	1	1	1	1
GRAND TOTAL	4	2.0	1	1	1	2	3	3	3	3

12.0: RMVL INOC FB ANT SEGMENT

Type of Patients	Observed Patients	Avg. Stay	Vari-ance	Percentiles						
				10th	25th	50th	75th	90th	95th	99th
1. SINGLE DX										
0–19 Years	0									
20–34	1	1.0	0	1	1	1	1	1	1	1
35–49	0									
50–64	0									
65+	0									
2. MULTIPLE DX										
0–19 Years	0									
20–34	3	1.0	0	1	1	1	1	1	1	1
35–49	2	1.0	0	1	1	1	1	1	1	1
50–64	2	2.5	4	1	1	3	4	4	4	4
65+	0									
TOTAL SINGLE DX	1	1.0	0	1	1	1	1	1	1	1
TOTAL MULTIPLE DX	7	1.4	1	1	1	1	1	4	4	4
TOTAL										
0–19 Years	0									
20–34	4	1.0	0	1	1	1	1	1	1	1
35–49	2	1.0	0	1	1	1	1	1	1	1
50–64	2	2.5	4	1	1	3	4	4	4	4
65+	0									
GRAND TOTAL	8	1.4	1	1	1	1	1	4	4	4

12.1: IRIDOTOMY/SMP IRIDECTOMY

Type of Patients	Observed Patients	Avg. Stay	Vari-ance	Percentiles						
				10th	25th	50th	75th	90th	95th	99th
1. SINGLE DX										
0–19 Years	0									
20–34	0									
35–49	1	1.0	0	1	1	1	1	1	1	1
50–64	1	1.0	0	1	1	1	1	1	1	1
65+	0									
2. MULTIPLE DX										
0–19 Years	1	2.0	0	2	2	2	2	2	2	2
20–34	1	2.0	0	2	2	2	2	2	2	2
35–49	3	4.0	3	4	4	4	4	4	4	4
50–64	6	3.2	5	1	2	2	3	7	7	7
65+	13	3.6	12	1	1	2	5	10	11	11
TOTAL SINGLE DX	2	1.0	0	1	1	1	1	1	1	1
TOTAL MULTIPLE DX	22	3.4	8	1	1	2	4	7	10	11
TOTAL										
0–19 Years	1	2.0	0	2	2	2	2	2	2	2
20–34	1	2.0	0	2	1	2	2	2	2	2
35–49	3	3.0	3	1	1	4	4	4	4	4
50–64	6	2.8	5	1	1	2	3	7	7	7
65+	13	3.6	12	1	1	2	5	10	11	11
GRAND TOTAL	24	3.2	8	1	1	2	4	7	10	11

LOS by Diagnosis and Operation, Western Region, 45th Edition

Western Region, October 2007–September 2008 Data, by Operation

12.2: ANTERIOR SEG DXTIC PX

Type of Patients	Observed Patients	Avg. Stay	Variance	Percentiles						
				10th	25th	50th	75th	90th	95th	99th
1. SINGLE DX										
0–19 Years	0									
20–34	0									
35–49	0									
50–64	0									
65+	0									
2. MULTIPLE DX										
0–19 Years	0									
20–34	2	1.0	0	1	1	1	1	1	1	1
35–49	1	1.0	0	1	1	1	1	1	1	1
50–64	5	6.9	35	1	2	5	12	14	14	14
65+	5	5.8	11	3	3	5	7	11	11	11
TOTAL SINGLE DX	0									
TOTAL MULTIPLE DX	13	5.1	21	1	1	3	7	12	14	14
TOTAL										
0–19 Years	0									
20–34	2	1.0	0	1	1	1	1	1	1	1
35–49	1	1.0	0	1	1	1	1	1	1	1
50–64	5	6.9	35	1	2	5	12	14	14	14
65+	5	5.8	11	3	3	5	7	11	11	11
GRAND TOTAL	13	5.1	21	1	1	3	7	12	14	14

12.3: IRIDOPLASTY/COREOPLASTY

Type of Patients	Observed Patients	Avg. Stay	Variance	Percentiles						
				10th	25th	50th	75th	90th	95th	99th
1. SINGLE DX										
0–19 Years	0									
20–34	0									
35–49	0									
50–64	0									
65+	0									
2. MULTIPLE DX										
0–19 Years	3	1.0	0	1	1	1	1	1	1	1
20–34	0									
35–49	0									
50–64	0									
65+	2	1.5	<1	1	1	2	2	2	2	2
TOTAL SINGLE DX	0									
TOTAL MULTIPLE DX	5	1.2	<1	1	1	1	1	2	2	2
TOTAL										
0–19 Years	3	1.0	0	1	1	1	1	1	1	1
20–34	0									
35–49	0									
50–64	0									
65+	2	1.5	<1	1	1	2	2	2	2	2
GRAND TOTAL	5	1.2	<1	1	1	1	1	2	2	2

12.4: DESTR IRIS/CIL BODY LES

Type of Patients	Observed Patients	Avg. Stay	Variance	Percentiles						
				10th	25th	50th	75th	90th	95th	99th
1. SINGLE DX										
0–19 Years	0									
20–34	0									
35–49	0									
50–64	0									
65+	0									
2. MULTIPLE DX										
0–19 Years	0									
20–34	0									
35–49	0									
50–64	0									
65+	0									
TOTAL SINGLE DX	0									
TOTAL MULTIPLE DX	0									
TOTAL										
0–19 Years	0									
20–34	0									
35–49	0									
50–64	0									
65+	0									
GRAND TOTAL	0									

12.5: INOC CIRCULAT FACILITAT

Type of Patients	Observed Patients	Avg. Stay	Variance	Percentiles						
				10th	25th	50th	75th	90th	95th	99th
1. SINGLE DX										
0–19 Years	0									
20–34	0									
35–49	0									
50–64	1	1.0	0	1	1	1	1	1	1	1
65+	0									
2. MULTIPLE DX										
0–19 Years	0									
20–34	0									
35–49	0									
50–64	0									
65+	1	1.0	0	1	1	1	1	1	1	1
TOTAL SINGLE DX	1	1.0	0	1	1	1	1	1	1	1
TOTAL MULTIPLE DX	1	1.0	0	1	1	1	1	1	1	1
TOTAL										
0–19 Years	0									
20–34	0									
35–49	0									
50–64	1	1.0	0	1	1	1	1	1	1	1
65+	1	1.0	0	1	1	1	1	1	1	1
GRAND TOTAL	2	1.0	0	1	1	1	1	1	1	1

LOS by Diagnosis and Operation, Western Region, 45th Edition

Western Region, October 2007–September 2008 Data, by Operation

12.6: SCLERAL FISTULIZATION

Type of Patients	Observed Patients	Avg. Stay	Variance	Percentiles						
				10th	25th	50th	75th	90th	95th	99th
1. SINGLE DX										
0–19 Years	0									
20–34	1	1.0	0	1	1	1	1	1	1	1
35–49	1	1.0	0	1	1	1	1	1	1	1
50–64	0									
65+	0									
2. MULTIPLE DX										
0–19 Years	3	1.0	0	1	1	1	1	1	1	1
20–34	4	4.8	30	2	2	2	13	13	13	13
35–49	11	3.7	50	1	1	1	2	4	25	25
50–64	20	4.0	59	1	1	1	1	6	35	35
65+	11	1.9	3	1	1	1	3	3	7	7
TOTAL SINGLE DX	**2**	**1.0**	**0**	**1**	**1**	**1**	**1**	**1**	**1**	**1**
TOTAL MULTIPLE DX	**49**	**3.2**	**36**	**1**	**1**	**1**	**2**	**6**	**13**	**35**
TOTAL										
0–19 Years	3	1.0	0	1	1	1	1	1	1	1
20–34	5	4.0	25	1	2	2	2	13	13	13
35–49	12	3.5	47	1	1	1	2	4	25	25
50–64	20	4.0	59	1	1	1	1	6	35	35
65+	11	1.9	3	1	1	1	3	3	7	7
GRAND TOTAL	**51**	**3.1**	**35**	**1**	**1**	**1**	**2**	**6**	**13**	**35**

12.7: ELEVAT INOC PRESS RELIEF

Type of Patients	Observed Patients	Avg. Stay	Variance	Percentiles						
				10th	25th	50th	75th	90th	95th	99th
1. SINGLE DX										
0–19 Years	0									
20–34	0									
35–49	0									
50–64	0									
65+	0									
2. MULTIPLE DX										
0–19 Years	0									
20–34	1	5.0	0	5	5	5	5	5	5	5
35–49	4	2.7	2	1	1	2	4	4	4	4
50–64	2	4.5	4	3	3	6	6	6	6	6
65+	4	2.2	2	1	1	1	3	4	4	4
TOTAL SINGLE DX	**0**									
TOTAL MULTIPLE DX	**11**	**3.1**	**3**	**1**	**1**	**3**	**4**	**5**	**6**	**6**
TOTAL										
0–19 Years	0									
20–34	1	5.0	0	5	5	5	5	5	5	5
35–49	4	2.7	2	1	1	2	4	4	4	4
50–64	2	4.5	4	3	3	6	6	6	6	6
65+	4	2.2	2	1	1	1	3	4	4	4
GRAND TOTAL	**11**	**3.1**	**3**	**1**	**1**	**3**	**4**	**5**	**6**	**6**

12.8: OPERATIONS ON SCLERA

Type of Patients	Observed Patients	Avg. Stay	Variance	Percentiles						
				10th	25th	50th	75th	90th	95th	99th
1. SINGLE DX										
0–19 Years	4	2.5	2	1	1	2	3	4	4	4
20–34	2	2.0	2	1	1	1	3	3	3	3
35–49	3	2.3	2	1	1	2	4	4	4	4
50–64	1	1.0	0	1	1	1	1	1	1	1
65+	1	2.0	0	2	2	2	2	2	2	2
2. MULTIPLE DX										
0–19 Years	5	3.3	3	1	2	5	5	>99	>99	>99
20–34	16	3.1	11	1	1	2	3	8	13	13
35–49	16	1.9	3	1	1	1	2	5	7	7
50–64	9	2.3	2	1	1	2	3	5	5	5
65+	12	2.8	6	1	2	2	5	6	8	8
TOTAL SINGLE DX	**11**	**2.2**	**1**	**1**	**1**	**2**	**3**	**4**	**4**	**4**
TOTAL MULTIPLE DX	**58**	**2.6**	**5**	**1**	**1**	**2**	**3**	**6**	**8**	**>99**
TOTAL										
0–19 Years	9	3.0	3	1	2	3	5	5	>99	>99
20–34	18	3.0	10	1	1	2	3	8	13	13
35–49	19	2.0	3	1	1	1	2	5	7	7
50–64	10	2.2	2	1	1	2	3	5	5	5
65+	13	2.7	5	1	1	2	3	6	8	8
GRAND TOTAL	**69**	**2.6**	**5**	**1**	**1**	**2**	**3**	**5**	**8**	**>99**

12.9: OTH ANTERIOR SEGMENT OPS

Type of Patients	Observed Patients	Avg. Stay	Variance	Percentiles						
				10th	25th	50th	75th	90th	95th	99th
1. SINGLE DX										
0–19 Years	2	6.0	0	6	6	6	6	6	6	6
20–34	0									
35–49	0									
50–64	0									
65+										
2. MULTIPLE DX										
0–19 Years	7	5.5	5	2	4	7	7	7	7	7
20–34	1	4.0	0	4	4	4	4	4	4	4
35–49	8	4.4	23	2	2	3	4	16	16	16
50–64	2	5.0	32	1	1	5	9	9	9	9
65+	10	5.9	32	1	2	5	8	16	16	16
TOTAL SINGLE DX	**2**	**6.0**	**0**	**6**	**6**	**6**	**6**	**6**	**6**	**6**
TOTAL MULTIPLE DX	**28**	**5.3**	**17**	**1**	**2**	**4**	**7**	**9**	**16**	**16**
TOTAL										
0–19 Years	9	5.6	4	2	4	7	7	7	7	7
20–34	1	4.0	0	4	4	4	4	4	4	4
35–49	8	4.4	23	2	2	3	4	16	16	16
50–64	2	5.0	32	1	1	5	9	9	9	9
65+	10	5.9	32	1	2	5	8	16	16	16
GRAND TOTAL	**30**	**5.3**	**16**	**1**	**2**	**4**	**7**	**9**	**16**	**16**

LOS by Diagnosis and Operation, Western Region, 45th Edition

Western Region, October 2007–September 2008 Data, by Operation

13.0: REMOVAL FB FROM LENS

Type of Patients	Observed Patients	Avg. Stay	Variance	10th	25th	50th	75th	90th	95th	99th
1. SINGLE DX										
0–19 Years	0									
20–34	0									
35–49	0									
50–64	0									
65+										
2. MULTIPLE DX										
0–19 Years	0									
20–34	0									
35–49	0									
50–64	1	1.0	0	1	1	1	1	1	1	1
65+	0									
TOTAL SINGLE DX	0									
TOTAL MULTIPLE DX	1	1.0	0	1	1	1	1	1	1	1
TOTAL										
0–19 Years	0									
20–34	0									
35–49	0									
50–64	1	1.0	0	1	1	1	1	1	1	1
65+	0									
GRAND TOTAL	1	1.0	0	1	1	1	1	1	1	1

13.1: INTRACAP LENS EXTRACTION

Type of Patients	Observed Patients	Avg. Stay	Variance	10th	25th	50th	75th	90th	95th	99th
1. SINGLE DX										
0–19 Years	1	2.0	0	2	2	2	2	2	2	2
20–34	0									
35–49	0									
50–64	0									
65+	0									
2. MULTIPLE DX										
0–19 Years	6	3.2	72	1	1	2	2	2	34	34
20–34	1	2.0	0	2	2	2	2	2	2	2
35–49	9	3.8	15	1	1	3	3	11	11	11
50–64	3	9.3	81	1	1	8	19	19	19	19
65+										
TOTAL SINGLE DX	1	2.0	0	2	2	2	2	2	2	2
TOTAL MULTIPLE DX	19	4.0	52	1	1	1	3	11	19	34
TOTAL										
0–19 Years	7	3.1	67	1	1	1	2	2	34	34
20–34	1	2.0	0	2	2	2	2	2	2	2
35–49	9	3.8	15	1	1	3	3	11	11	11
50–64	3	9.3	81	1	1	8	19	19	19	19
65+										
GRAND TOTAL	20	3.9	50	1	1	1	3	11	19	34

13.2: LIN EXTRACAPS LENS EXTR

Type of Patients	Observed Patients	Avg. Stay	Variance	10th	25th	50th	75th	90th	95th	99th
1. SINGLE DX										
0–19 Years	0									
20–34	0									
35–49	0									
50–64	0									
65+										
2. MULTIPLE DX										
0–19 Years	0									
20–34	0									
35–49	0									
50–64	1	1.0	0	1	1	1	1	1	1	1
65+	0									
TOTAL SINGLE DX	0									
TOTAL MULTIPLE DX	1	1.0	0	1	1	1	1	1	1	1
TOTAL										
0–19 Years	0									
20–34	0									
35–49	0									
50–64	1	1.0	0	1	1	1	1	1	1	1
65+	0									
GRAND TOTAL	1	1.0	0	1	1	1	1	1	1	1

13.3: SIMP ASP LENS EXTRACTION

Type of Patients	Observed Patients	Avg. Stay	Variance	10th	25th	50th	75th	90th	95th	99th
1. SINGLE DX										
0–19 Years	0									
20–34	0									
35–49	0									
50–64	0									
65+										
2. MULTIPLE DX										
0–19 Years	2	4.5	24	1	1	1	8	8	8	8
20–34	0									
35–49	1	1.0	0	1	1	1	1	1	1	1
50–64	0									
65+	1	1.0	0	1	1	1	1	1	1	1
TOTAL SINGLE DX	0									
TOTAL MULTIPLE DX	4	2.7	12	1	1	1	1	8	8	8
TOTAL										
0–19 Years	2	4.5	24	1	1	1	8	8	8	8
20–34	0									
35–49	1	1.0	0	1	1	1	1	1	1	1
50–64	0									
65+	1	1.0	0	1	1	1	1	1	1	1
GRAND TOTAL	4	2.7	12	1	1	1	1	8	8	8

LOS by Diagnosis and Operation, Western Region, 45th Edition

Western Region, October 2007–September 2008 Data, by Operation

13.4: FRAG-ASP EXTRACAPS LENS

Type of Patients	Observed Patients	Avg. Stay	Vari-ance	10th	25th	50th	75th	90th	95th	99th
1. SINGLE DX										
0–19 Years	0									
20–34	0									
35–49	0									
50–64	1	1.0	0	1	1		1	1	1	1
65+	1	1.0	0	1	1		1	1	1	1
2. MULTIPLE DX										
0–19 Years	0									
20–34	2	2.5	<1	2	2	2	3	3	3	3
35–49	3	11.3	185	2	2	5	27	27	27	27
50–64	21	3.2	51	1	1	1	2	3	3	34
65+	44	3.3	110	1	1	1	2	3	4	70
TOTAL SINGLE DX	2	1.0	0	1	1	1	1	1	1	1
TOTAL MULTIPLE DX	70	3.6	92	1	1	1	2	3	12	70
TOTAL										
0–19 Years	0									
20–34	2	2.5	<1	2	2	2	3	3	3	3
35–49	3	11.3	185	2	2	5	27	27	27	27
50–64	22	3.1	49	1	1	1	2	3	3	34
65+	45	3.2	108	1	1	1	2	3	4	70
GRAND TOTAL	72	3.5	89	1	1	1	2	3	12	70

13.5: OTH EXTRACAPS LENS EXTR

Type of Patients	Observed Patients	Avg. Stay	Vari-ance	10th	25th	50th	75th	90th	95th	99th
1. SINGLE DX										
0–19 Years	1	1.0	0	1	1	1	1	1	1	1
20–34	0									
35–49	0									
50–64	0									
65+	1	1.0	0	1	1	1	1	1	1	1
2. MULTIPLE DX										
0–19 Years	2	1.0	0	1	1	1	1	1	1	1
20–34	1	1.0	0	1	1	1	1	1	1	1
35–49	1	3.0	0	3	3	3	3	3	3	3
50–64	3	1.0	0	1	1	1	>99	>99	>99	>99
65+	3	7.4	87	1	1	3	18	18	18	18
TOTAL SINGLE DX	2	1.0	0	1	1	1	1	1	1	1
TOTAL MULTIPLE DX	10	2.6	22	1	1	1	3	18	>99	>99
TOTAL										
0–19 Years	3	1.0	0	1	1	1	1	1	1	1
20–34	1	1.0	0	1	1	1	1	1	1	1
35–49	1	3.0	0	3	3	3	3	3	3	3
50–64	3	1.0	0	1	1	1	>99	>99	>99	>99
65+	4	5.8	68	1	1	3	18	18	18	18
GRAND TOTAL	12	2.4	19	1	1	1	1	18	>99	>99

13.6: OTH CATARACT EXTRACTION

Type of Patients	Observed Patients	Avg. Stay	Vari-ance	10th	25th	50th	75th	90th	95th	99th
1. SINGLE DX										
0–19 Years	4	1.9	<1	1	1	2	3	3	3	3
20–34	0									
35–49	0									
50–64	0									
65+	0									
2. MULTIPLE DX										
0–19 Years	2	7.0	187	1	1	1	1	32	32	32
20–34	0									
35–49	1	1.0	0	1	1	1	1	1	1	1
50–64	3	2.0	<1	1	1	2	3	3	3	3
65+	3	13.6	374	1	1	4	36	36	36	36
TOTAL SINGLE DX	4	1.9	<1	1	1	2	3	3	3	3
TOTAL MULTIPLE DX	9	6.9	158	1	1	1	3	32	36	36
TOTAL										
0–19 Years	6	3.6	61	1	1	3	3	3	32	32
20–34	0									
35–49	1	1.0	0	1	1	1	1	1	1	1
50–64	3	2.0	<1	1	1	2	3	3	3	3
65+	3	13.6	374	1	1	4	36	36	36	36
GRAND TOTAL	13	4.6	90	1	1	1	3	4	32	36

13.7: INSERT PROSTHETIC LENS

Type of Patients	Observed Patients	Avg. Stay	Vari-ance	10th	25th	50th	75th	90th	95th	99th
1. SINGLE DX										
0–19 Years	0									
20–34	0									
35–49	0									
50–64	0									
65+	0									
2. MULTIPLE DX										
0–19 Years	0									
20–34	0									
35–49	0									
50–64	0									
65+	0									
TOTAL SINGLE DX	0									
TOTAL MULTIPLE DX	0									
TOTAL										
0–19 Years	0									
20–34	0									
35–49	0									
50–64	0									
65+	0									
GRAND TOTAL	0									

LOS by Diagnosis and Operation, Western Region, 45th Edition

Western Region, October 2007–September 2008 Data, by Operation

13:8: IMPLANTED LENS REMOVAL

Type of Patients	Observed Patients	Avg. Stay	Variance	10th	25th	50th	75th	90th	95th	99th
1. SINGLE DX										
0–19 Years	0									
20–34	0									
35–49	0									
50–64	0									
65+	1	1.0	0	1	1	1	1	1	1	1
2. MULTIPLE DX										
0–19 Years	0									
20–34	0									
35–49	0									
50–64	0									
65+	0									
TOTAL SINGLE DX	1	1.0	0	1	1	1	1	1	1	1
TOTAL MULTIPLE DX	0									
TOTAL										
0–19 Years	0									
20–34	0									
35–49	0									
50–64	0									
65+	1	1.0	0	1	1	1	1	1	1	1
GRAND TOTAL	1	1.0	0	1	1	1	1	1	1	1

13.9: OTHER OPERATIONS ON LENS

Type of Patients	Observed Patients	Avg. Stay	Variance	10th	25th	50th	75th	90th	95th	99th
1. SINGLE DX										
0–19 Years	0									
20–34	0									
35–49	0									
50–64	0									
65+	0									
2. MULTIPLE DX										
0–19 Years	0									
20–34	0									
35–49	0									
50–64	1	1.0	0	1	1	1	1	1	1	1
65+	1	1.0	0	1	1	1	1	1	1	1
TOTAL SINGLE DX	0									
TOTAL MULTIPLE DX	2	1.0	0	1	1	1	1	1	1	1
TOTAL										
0–19 Years	0									
20–34	0									
35–49	0									
50–64	1	1.0	0	1	1	1	1	1	1	1
65+	1	1.0	0	1	1	1	1	1	1	1
GRAND TOTAL	2	1.0	0	1	1	1	1	1	1	1

14.0: RMVL OF POST SEGMENT FB

Type of Patients	Observed Patients	Avg. Stay	Variance	10th	25th	50th	75th	90th	95th	99th
1. SINGLE DX										
0–19 Years	0									
20–34	0									
35–49	1	1.0	0	1	1	1	1	1	1	1
50–64	0									
65+	0									
2. MULTIPLE DX										
0–19 Years	1	1.0	0	1	1	1	1	1	1	1
20–34	1	1.0	0	1	1	1	1	1	1	1
35–49	4	1.5	<1	1	1	1	2	2	2	2
50–64	0									
65+	0									
TOTAL SINGLE DX	1	1.0	0	1	1	1	1	1	1	1
TOTAL MULTIPLE DX	6	1.3	<1	1	1	1	2	2	2	2
TOTAL										
0–19 Years	1	1.0	0	1	1	1	1	1	1	1
20–34	1	1.0	0	1	1	1	1	1	1	1
35–49	5	1.4	<1	1	1	1	2	2	2	2
50–64	0									
65+	0									
GRAND TOTAL	7	1.3	<1	1	1	1	2	2	2	2

14.1: DXTIC PX POSTERIOR SEG

Type of Patients	Observed Patients	Avg. Stay	Variance	10th	25th	50th	75th	90th	95th	99th
1. SINGLE DX										
0–19 Years	0									
20–34	0									
35–49	0									
50–64	0									
65+	0									
2. MULTIPLE DX										
0–19 Years	0									
20–34	0									
35–49	0									
50–64	2	9.5	<1	9	9	10	10	10	10	10
65+	3	7.7	33	1	1	11	11	11	11	11
TOTAL SINGLE DX	0									
TOTAL MULTIPLE DX	5	8.4	18	1	9	10	11	11	11	11
TOTAL										
0–19 Years	0									
20–34	0									
35–49	0									
50–64	2	9.5	<1	9	9	10	10	10	10	10
65+	3	7.7	33	1	1	11	11	11	11	11
GRAND TOTAL	5	8.4	18	1	9	10	11	11	11	11

LOS by Diagnosis and Operation, Western Region, 45th Edition

Western Region, October 2007–September 2008 Data, by Operation

14.2: RETINA-CHOROID LES DESTR

Type of Patients	Observed Patients	Avg. Stay	Variance	Percentiles						
				10th	25th	50th	75th	90th	95th	99th
1. SINGLE DX										
0–19 Years	3	1.7	1	1	1	1	3	3	3	3
20–34	0									
35–49	0									
50–64	0									
65+	1	2.0	0	2	2	2	2	2	2	2
2. MULTIPLE DX										
0–19 Years	36	11.2	692	1	1	1	7	>99	>99	>99
20–34	0									
35–49	3	6.0	12	4	4	4	10	10	10	10
50–64	1	40.0	0	40	40	40	40	40	40	40
65+	0									
TOTAL SINGLE DX	4	1.7	<1	1	1	1	2	3	3	3
TOTAL MULTIPLE DX	40	11.4	662	1	1	1	10	>99	>99	>99
TOTAL										
0–19 Years	39	10.8	662	1	1	1	7	>99	>99	>99
20–34	0									
35–49	3	6.0	12	4	4	4	10	10	10	10
50–64	1	40.0	0	40	40	40	40	40	40	40
65+	1	2.0	0	2	2	2	2	2	2	2
GRAND TOTAL	44	10.9	627	1	1	1	7	>99	>99	>99

14.3: REPAIR OF RETINAL TEAR

Type of Patients	Observed Patients	Avg. Stay	Variance	Percentiles						
				10th	25th	50th	75th	90th	95th	99th
1. SINGLE DX										
0–19 Years	1	3.0	0	3	3	3	3	3	3	3
20–34	0									
35–49	0									
50–64	0									
65+	0									
2. MULTIPLE DX										
0–19 Years	1	1.0	0	1	1	1	1	1	1	1
20–34	2	1.5	<1	1	1	2	2	2	2	2
35–49	2	3.0	2	2	2	3	4	4	4	4
50–64	1	1.0	0	1	1	1	1	1	1	1
65+	0									
TOTAL SINGLE DX	1	3.0	0	3	3	3	3	3	3	3
TOTAL MULTIPLE DX	6	1.6	1	1	1	1	2	3	4	4
TOTAL										
0–19 Years	2	1.4	<1	1	1	1	1	3	3	3
20–34	2	1.5	<1	1	1	2	2	2	2	2
35–49	2	3.0	2	2	2	3	4	4	4	4
50–64	1	1.0	0	1	1	1	1	1	1	1
65+	0									
GRAND TOTAL	7	1.7	1	1	1	1	2	4	4	4

14.4: REP RETINA DETACH/BUCKLE

Type of Patients	Observed Patients	Avg. Stay	Variance	Percentiles						
				10th	25th	50th	75th	90th	95th	99th
1. SINGLE DX										
0–19 Years	1	1.0	0	1	1	1	1	1	1	1
20–34	6	1.2	<1	1	1	1	1	2	2	2
35–49	6	1.3	<1	1	1	1	2	2	2	2
50–64	25	1.4	3	1	1	1	1	2	2	9
65+	3	1.7	1	1	1	1	3	3	3	3
2. MULTIPLE DX										
0–19 Years	7	1.4	<1	1	1	1	2	3	>99	>99
20–34	14	2.2	4	1	1	1	2	5	8	8
35–49	26	1.9	1	1	1	1	3	3	4	4
50–64	51	1.8	2	1	1	1	2	4	5	6
65+	23	1.5	<1	1	1	1	2	3	3	5
TOTAL SINGLE DX	41	1.4	2	1	1	1	1	2	2	9
TOTAL MULTIPLE DX	121	1.8	2	1	1	1	2	4	5	8
TOTAL										
0–19 Years	8	1.4	<1	1	1	1	2	3	>99	>99
20–34	20	1.9	3	1	1	1	2	4	5	8
35–49	32	1.8	<1	1	1	1	2	3	4	4
50–64	76	1.7	2	1	1	1	2	4	5	9
65+	26	1.5	<1	1	1	1	2	3	3	5
GRAND TOTAL	162	1.7	2	1	1	1	2	3	4	9

14.49: SCLERAL BUCKLING NEC

Type of Patients	Observed Patients	Avg. Stay	Variance	Percentiles						
				10th	25th	50th	75th	90th	95th	99th
1. SINGLE DX										
0–19 Years	1	1.0	0	1	1	1	1	1	1	1
20–34	6	1.2	<1	1	1	1	1	2	2	2
35–49	6	1.3	<1	1	1	1	2	2	2	2
50–64	22	1.5	3	1	1	1	1	2	2	9
65+	3	1.7	1	1	1	1	3	3	3	3
2. MULTIPLE DX										
0–19 Years	6	1.4	<1	1	1	1	2	3	>99	>99
20–34	13	2.3	5	1	1	1	2	5	8	8
35–49	24	1.9	1	1	1	1	3	3	4	4
50–64	46	1.8	1	1	1	1	2	4	4	5
65+	20	1.5	1	1	1	1	2	3	5	5
TOTAL SINGLE DX	38	1.4	2	1	1	1	1	2	3	9
TOTAL MULTIPLE DX	109	1.8	2	1	1	1	2	4	5	8
TOTAL										
0–19 Years	7	1.4	<1	1	1	1	2	3	>99	>99
20–34	19	1.9	3	1	1	1	2	3	5	8
35–49	30	1.8	1	1	1	1	2	3	4	4
50–64	68	1.7	2	1	1	1	2	4	4	9
65+	23	1.5	<1	1	1	1	2	3	3	5
GRAND TOTAL	147	1.7	2	1	1	1	2	3	4	9

LOS by Diagnosis and Operation, Western Region, 45th Edition

Western Region, October 2007–September 2008 Data, by Operation

14.5: OTH REPAIR RETINA DETACH

Type of Patients	Observed Patients	Avg. Stay	Vari-ance	Percentiles						
				10th	25th	50th	75th	90th	95th	99th
1. SINGLE DX										
0–19 Years	0									
20–34	0									
35–49	0									
50–64	3	1.0	0	1	1		1	1	1	1
65+	2	1.0	0	1	1		1	1	1	1
2. MULTIPLE DX										
0–19 Years	10	2.9	6	1	1	2	7	7	>99	>99
20–34	5	2.6	2	1	2	2	3	5	5	5
35–49	14	1.8	4	1	1	1	2	3	8	8
50–64	27	1.9	2	1	1	1	3	4	5	6
65+	24	3.1	18	1	1	1	4	7	11	18
TOTAL SINGLE DX	5	1.0	0	1	1		1	1	1	1
TOTAL MULTIPLE DX	75	2.5	7	1	1	1	3	7	7	>99
TOTAL										
0–19 Years	10	2.9	6	1	1	2	7	7	>99	>99
20–34	5	2.6	2	1	2	2	3	5	5	5
35–49	14	1.8	4	1	1	1	2	3	8	8
50–64	27	1.8	2	1	1	1	2	4	5	6
65+	24	2.9	17	1	1	1	4	7	11	18
GRAND TOTAL	80	2.4	7	1	1	1	3	7	7	>99

14.6: RMVL PROSTH MAT POST SEG

Type of Patients	Observed Patients	Avg. Stay	Vari-ance	Percentiles						
				10th	25th	50th	75th	90th	95th	99th
1. SINGLE DX										
0–19 Years	0									
20–34	1	3.0	0	3	3	3	3	3	3	3
35–49	0									
50–64	0									
65+										
2. MULTIPLE DX										
0–19 Years	0									
20–34	2	2.0	0	2	2	2	2	2	2	2
35–49	3	7.4	50	1	1	6	15	15	15	15
50–64	1	1.0	0	1	1	1	1	1	1	1
65+										
TOTAL SINGLE DX	1	3.0	0	3	3	3	3	3	3	3
TOTAL MULTIPLE DX	6	4.5	30	1	1	2	6	15	15	15
TOTAL										
0–19 Years	1	3.0	0	3	3	3	3	3	3	3
20–34	2	2.0	0	2	2	2	2	2	2	2
35–49	3	7.4	50	1	1	6	15	15	15	15
50–64	1	1.0	0	1	1	1	1	1	1	1
65+										
GRAND TOTAL	7	4.3	25	1	1	2	6	15	15	15

14.7: OPERATIONS ON VITREOUS

Type of Patients	Observed Patients	Avg. Stay	Vari-ance	Percentiles						
				10th	25th	50th	75th	90th	95th	99th
1. SINGLE DX										
0–19 Years	2	1.0	0	1	1	1	1	1	1	1
20–34	4	2.7	6	1	1	1	3	6	6	6
35–49	1	1.0	0	1	1	1	1	1	1	1
50–64	7	1.1	<1	1	1	1	1	2	2	2
65+	3	2.3	1	1	1	3	3	3	3	3
2. MULTIPLE DX										
0–19 Years	24	10.4	339	1	1	1	20	48	48	>99
20–34	19	7.8	107	1	1	4	9	26	36	36
35–49	48	4.3	38	1	1	2	6	9	9	41
50–64	88	4.6	43	1	1	2	6	12	15	42
65+	74	3.3	16	1	1	2	4	7	13	22
TOTAL SINGLE DX	17	1.6	2	1	1	1	1	3	3	6
TOTAL MULTIPLE DX	253	5.4	93	1	1	2	6	13	24	48
TOTAL										
0–19 Years	26	9.5	312	1	1	1	10	48	48	>99
20–34	23	6.9	92	1	1	3	8	24	26	36
35–49	49	4.3	38	1	1	2	6	9	9	41
50–64	95	4.3	41	1	1	2	6	12	15	42
65+	77	3.3	15	1	1	2	4	7	13	22
GRAND TOTAL	270	5.1	87	1	1	2	5	12	23	48

14.74: MECH VITRECTOMY NEC

Type of Patients	Observed Patients	Avg. Stay	Vari-ance	Percentiles						
				10th	25th	50th	75th	90th	95th	99th
1. SINGLE DX										
0–19 Years	1	1.0	0	1	1	1	1	1	1	1
20–34	3	1.7	1	1	1	1	3	3	3	3
35–49	1	1.0	0	1	1	1	1	1	1	1
50–64	6	1.2	<1	1	1	1	1	2	2	2
65+	2	2.0	2	1	1	1	3	3	3	3
2. MULTIPLE DX										
0–19 Years	16	7.8	272	1	1	1	10	20	84	>99
20–34	14	5.9	96	1	1	2	8	16	36	36
35–49	35	3.4	9	1	1	1	6	9	9	10
50–64	69	4.5	50	1	1	2	5	12	23	42
65+	55	2.8	16	1	1	1	3	6	9	22
TOTAL SINGLE DX	13	1.4	<1	1	1	1	1	3	3	3
TOTAL MULTIPLE DX	189	4.4	72	1	1	1	4	10	20	42
TOTAL										
0–19 Years	17	7.6	265	1	1	1	4	20	84	>99
20–34	17	5.1	81	1	1	1	6	16	36	36
35–49	36	3.3	9	1	1	2	6	9	9	10
50–64	75	4.2	47	1	1	1	5	12	23	42
65+	57	2.8	15	1	1	1	3	6	9	22
GRAND TOTAL	202	4.3	68	1	1	1	4	10	20	42

LOS by Diagnosis and Operation, Western Region, 45th Edition

Western Region, October 2007–September 2008 Data, by Operation

14.9: OTHER POST SEGMENT OPS

Type of Patients	Observed Patients	Avg. Stay	Variance	Percentiles						
				10th	25th	50th	75th	90th	95th	99th
1. SINGLE DX										
0–19 Years	0									
20–34	0									
35–49	0									
50–64	0									
65+	0									
2. MULTIPLE DX										
0–19 Years	2	2.2	<1	2	2	2	2	3	3	3
20–34	3	1.7	<1	1	1	2	2	2	2	2
35–49	6	2.8	6	1	1	2	6	6	6	6
50–64	4	1.3	<1	1	1	1	1	2	2	2
65+	6	4.2	25	1	1	2	5	14	14	14
TOTAL SINGLE DX	0									
TOTAL MULTIPLE DX	21	2.6	8	1	1	2	2	6	6	14
TOTAL										
0–19 Years	2	2.2	<1	2	2	2	2	3	3	3
20–34	3	1.7	<1	1	1	2	2	2	2	2
35–49	6	2.8	6	1	1	2	6	6	6	6
50–64	4	1.3	<1	1	1	1	1	2	2	2
65+	6	4.2	25	1	1	2	5	14	14	14
GRAND TOTAL	21	2.6	8	1	1	2	2	6	6	14

15.0: EXOC MUSC-TEND DXTIC PX

Type of Patients	Observed Patients	Avg. Stay	Variance	Percentiles						
				10th	25th	50th	75th	90th	95th	99th
1. SINGLE DX										
0–19 Years	1	1.0	0	1	1	1	1	1	1	1
20–34	0									
35–49	0									
50–64	0									
65+	0									
2. MULTIPLE DX										
0–19 Years	0									
20–34	0									
35–49	0									
50–64	0									
65+	0									
TOTAL SINGLE DX	1	1.0	0	1	1	1	1	1	1	1
TOTAL MULTIPLE DX	0									
TOTAL										
0–19 Years	1	1.0	0	1	1	1	1	1	1	1
20–34	0									
35–49	0									
50–64	0									
65+	0									
GRAND TOTAL	1	1.0	0	1	1	1	1	1	1	1

15.1: 1 EXOC MUSC OPS W DETACH

Type of Patients	Observed Patients	Avg. Stay	Variance	Percentiles						
				10th	25th	50th	75th	90th	95th	99th
1. SINGLE DX										
0–19 Years	0									
20–34	0									
35–49	0									
50–64	0									
65+	0									
2. MULTIPLE DX										
0–19 Years	11	1.2	<1	1	1	1	1	2	2	>99
20–34	2	2.5	<1	2	2	3	3	3	3	3
35–49	2	3.0	8	1	1	1	5	5	5	5
50–64	1	1.0	0	1	1	1	1	1	1	1
65+	0									
TOTAL SINGLE DX	0									
TOTAL MULTIPLE DX	16	1.4	<1	1	1	1	1	2	5	>99
TOTAL										
0–19 Years	11	1.2	<1	1	1	1	1	2	2	>99
20–34	2	2.5	<1	2	2	3	3	3	3	3
35–49	2	3.0	8	1	1	1	5	5	5	5
50–64	1	1.0	0	1	1	1	1	1	1	1
65+	0									
GRAND TOTAL	16	1.4	<1	1	1	1	1	2	5	>99

15.2: OTH OPS ON 1 EXOC MUSCLE

Type of Patients	Observed Patients	Avg. Stay	Variance	Percentiles						
				10th	25th	50th	75th	90th	95th	99th
1. SINGLE DX										
0–19 Years	0									
20–34	0									
35–49	0									
50–64	0									
65+	0									
2. MULTIPLE DX										
0–19 Years	0									
20–34	0									
35–49	0									
50–64	0									
65+	0									
TOTAL SINGLE DX	0									
TOTAL MULTIPLE DX	0									
TOTAL										
0–19 Years	0									
20–34	0									
35–49	0									
50–64	0									
65+	0									
GRAND TOTAL	0									

LOS by Diagnosis and Operation, Western Region, 45th Edition

Western Region, October 2007–September 2008 Data, by Operation

15.3: TEMP DETACH >1 EXOC MUSC

Type of Patients	Observed Patients	Avg. Stay	Vari-ance	Percentiles						
				10th	25th	50th	75th	90th	95th	99th
1. SINGLE DX										
0–19 Years	0									
20–34	0									
35–49	0									
50–64	0									
65+	0									
2. MULTIPLE DX										
0–19 Years	4	1.0	0	1	1	1	1	1	1	1
20–34	0									
35–49	1	1.0	0	1	1	1	1	1	1	1
50–64	1	1.0	0	1	1	1	1	1	1	1
65+	1	1.0	0	1	1	1	1	1	1	1
TOTAL SINGLE DX	0									
TOTAL MULTIPLE DX	7	1.0	0	1	1	1	1	1	1	1
TOTAL										
0–19 Years	4	1.0	0	1	1	1	1	1	1	1
20–34	0									
35–49	1	1.0	0	1	1	1	1	1	1	1
50–64	1	1.0	0	1	1	1	1	1	1	1
65+	1	1.0	0	1	1	1	1	1	1	1
GRAND TOTAL	7	1.0	0	1	1	1	1	1	1	1

15.4: OTH OPS ON >1 EXOC MUSC

Type of Patients	Observed Patients	Avg. Stay	Vari-ance	Percentiles						
				10th	25th	50th	75th	90th	95th	99th
1. SINGLE DX										
0–19 Years	0									
20–34	0									
35–49	0									
50–64	0									
65+	0									
2. MULTIPLE DX										
0–19 Years	0									
20–34	0									
35–49	0									
50–64	0									
65+	0									
TOTAL SINGLE DX	0									
TOTAL MULTIPLE DX	0									
TOTAL										
0–19 Years	0									
20–34	0									
35–49	0									
50–64	0									
65+	0									
GRAND TOTAL	0									

15.5: EXOC MUSC TRANSPOSITION

Type of Patients	Observed Patients	Avg. Stay	Vari-ance	Percentiles						
				10th	25th	50th	75th	90th	95th	99th
1. SINGLE DX										
0–19 Years	0									
20–34	0									
35–49	0									
50–64	0									
65+	0									
2. MULTIPLE DX										
0–19 Years	0									
20–34	0									
35–49	0									
50–64	0									
65+	0									
TOTAL SINGLE DX	0									
TOTAL MULTIPLE DX	0									
TOTAL										
0–19 Years	0									
20–34	0									
35–49	0									
50–64	0									
65+	0									
GRAND TOTAL	0									

15.6: REV EXOC MUSCLE SURGERY

Type of Patients	Observed Patients	Avg. Stay	Vari-ance	Percentiles						
				10th	25th	50th	75th	90th	95th	99th
1. SINGLE DX										
0–19 Years	0									
20–34	0									
35–49	0									
50–64	0									
65+	0									
2. MULTIPLE DX										
0–19 Years	0									
20–34	0									
35–49	0									
50–64	0									
65+	0									
TOTAL SINGLE DX	0									
TOTAL MULTIPLE DX	0									
TOTAL										
0–19 Years	0									
20–34	0									
35–49	0									
50–64	0									
65+	0									
GRAND TOTAL	0									

LOS by Diagnosis and Operation, Western Region, 45th Edition

Western Region, October 2007–September 2008 Data, by Operation

15.7: EXOC MUSCLE INJURY REP

Type of Patients	Observed Patients	Avg. Stay	Vari-ance	10th	25th	50th	75th	90th	95th	99th
1. SINGLE DX										
0–19 Years	0									
20–34	0									
35–49	0									
50–64	0									
65+	0									
2. MULTIPLE DX										
0–19 Years	0									
20–34	3	2.0	3	1	1	1	4	4	4	4
35–49	3	2.7	4	1	1	2	5	5	5	5
50–64	0									
65+	3	6.7	9	4	4	6	10	10	10	10
TOTAL SINGLE DX	0									
TOTAL MULTIPLE DX	9	3.8	9	1	1	4	5	10	10	10
TOTAL										
0–19 Years	0									
20–34	3	2.0	3	1	1	1	4	4	4	4
35–49	3	2.7	4	1	1	2	5	5	5	5
50–64	0									
65+	3	6.7	9	4	4	6	10	10	10	10
GRAND TOTAL	9	3.8	9	1	1	4	5	10	10	10

15.9: OTH EXOC MUSC-TEND OPS

Type of Patients	Observed Patients	Avg. Stay	Vari-ance	10th	25th	50th	75th	90th	95th	99th
1. SINGLE DX										
0–19 Years	0									
20–34	0									
35–49	0									
50–64	0									
65+	0									
2. MULTIPLE DX										
0–19 Years	0									
20–34	0									
35–49	0									
50–64	0									
65+	0									
TOTAL SINGLE DX	0									
TOTAL MULTIPLE DX	0									
TOTAL										
0–19 Years	0									
20–34	0									
35–49	0									
50–64	0									
65+	0									
GRAND TOTAL	0									

16.0: ORBITOTOMY

Type of Patients	Observed Patients	Avg. Stay	Vari-ance	10th	25th	50th	75th	90th	95th	99th
1. SINGLE DX										
0–19 Years	1	1.0	0	1	1	1	1	1	1	1
20–34	0									
35–49	5	3.4	4	1	2	4	4	6	6	6
50–64	2	1.5	<1	1	1	2	2	2	2	2
65+	0									
2. MULTIPLE DX										
0–19 Years	67	8.1	69	2	4	5	9	21	21	41
20–34	35	3.9	7	1	2	3	6	8	10	11
35–49	28	4.3	12	1	1	4	7	9	12	13
50–64	47	4.5	20	1	1	3	6	9	14	23
65+	29	6.1	34	1	2	5	6	18	19	24
TOTAL SINGLE DX	8	2.6	3	1	1	2	4	6	6	6
TOTAL MULTIPLE DX	206	6.3	44	1	2	4	8	14	21	41
TOTAL										
0–19 Years	68	8.1	69	2	4	5	9	21	21	41
20–34	35	3.9	7	1	2	3	6	8	10	11
35–49	33	4.1	11	1	1	4	6	9	12	13
50–64	49	4.4	19	1	1	3	6	9	14	23
65+	29	6.1	34	1	2	5	6	18	19	24
GRAND TOTAL	214	6.1	44	1	2	4	7	13	21	41

16.09: ORBITOTOMY NEC

Type of Patients	Observed Patients	Avg. Stay	Vari-ance	10th	25th	50th	75th	90th	95th	99th
1. SINGLE DX										
0–19 Years	1	1.0	0	1	1	1	1	1	1	1
20–34	0									
35–49	4	4.0	3	2	2	4	6	6	6	6
50–64	1	2.0	0	2	2	2	2	2	2	2
65+	0									
2. MULTIPLE DX										
0–19 Years	63	8.5	70	3	4	5	9	21	21	41
20–34	28	4.3	8	1	2	4	6	8	10	11
35–49	24	4.3	13	1	1	4	7	9	12	13
50–64	42	4.4	19	1	1	3	6	9	11	23
65+	23	6.2	34	1	2	5	6	16	19	24
TOTAL SINGLE DX	6	3.2	3	1	2	4	4	6	6	6
TOTAL MULTIPLE DX	180	6.6	47	1	3	4	8	15	21	41
TOTAL										
0–19 Years	64	8.5	70	2	4	5	9	21	21	41
20–34	28	4.3	8	1	2	4	6	8	10	11
35–49	28	4.2	12	1	1	3	6	9	12	13
50–64	43	4.3	18	1	1	3	6	9	11	23
65+	23	6.2	34	1	2	5	6	16	19	24
GRAND TOTAL	186	6.5	46	1	3	4	8	14	21	41

LOS by Diagnosis and Operation, Western Region, 45th Edition

61

Western Region, October 2007–September 2008 Data, by Operation

16.1: RMVL PENETR FB EYE NOS

Type of Patients	Observed Patients	Avg. Stay	Vari-ance	10th	25th	50th	75th	90th	95th	99th
1. SINGLE DX										
0–19 Years	0									
20–34	0									
35–49	0									
50–64	0									
65+	0									
2. MULTIPLE DX										
0–19 Years	1	3.0	0	3	3	3	3	3	3	3
20–34	2	5.5	24	2	2	9	9	9	9	9
35–49	1	5.0	0	5	5	5	5	5	5	5
50–64	3	3.7	1	3	3	3	5	5	5	5
65+	0									
TOTAL SINGLE DX	0									
TOTAL MULTIPLE DX	7	4.3	6	2	3	3	5	9	9	9
TOTAL										
0–19 Years	1	3.0	0	3	3	3	3	3	3	3
20–34	2	5.5	24	2	2	9	9	9	9	9
35–49	1	5.0	0	5	5	5	5	5	5	5
50–64	3	3.7	1	3	3	3	5	5	5	5
65+	0									
GRAND TOTAL	7	4.3	6	2	3	3	5	9	9	9

16.2: ORBIT & EYEBALL DXTIC PX

Type of Patients	Observed Patients	Avg. Stay	Vari-ance	10th	25th	50th	75th	90th	95th	99th
1. SINGLE DX										
0–19 Years	3	2.4	2	1	1	2	4	4	4	4
20–34	0									
35–49	0									
50–64	0									
65+	0									
2. MULTIPLE DX										
0–19 Years	10	8.1	87	2	3	6	6	21	37	37
20–34	3	3.3	6	1	1	3	6	6	6	6
35–49	7	11.6	193	1	1	11	14	40	40	40
50–64	6	2.7	6	1	1	2	4	7	7	7
65+	10	5.9	40	1	1	3	8	15	19	19
TOTAL SINGLE DX	3	2.4	2	1	1	2	4	4	4	4
TOTAL MULTIPLE DX	36	7.1	78	1	1	4	7	17	21	40
TOTAL										
0–19 Years	13	6.1	63	1	2	4	6	17	21	37
20–34	3	3.3	6	1	1	3	6	6	6	6
35–49	7	11.6	193	1	1	11	14	40	40	40
50–64	6	2.7	6	1	1	2	4	7	7	7
65+	10	5.9	40	1	1	3	8	15	19	19
GRAND TOTAL	39	6.2	67	1	1	3	6	15	21	40

16.3: EVISCERATION OF EYEBALL

Type of Patients	Observed Patients	Avg. Stay	Vari-ance	10th	25th	50th	75th	90th	95th	99th
1. SINGLE DX										
0–19 Years	1	1.0	0	1	1	1	1	1	1	1
20–34	0									
35–49	1	1.0	0	1	1	1	1	1	1	1
50–64	0									
65+	1	1.0	0	1	1	1	1	1	1	1
2. MULTIPLE DX										
0–19 Years	3	2.1	1	1	1	3	3	3	3	3
20–34	5	2.2	3	1	1	2	2	5	5	5
35–49	10	2.8	3	1	2	2	4	4	7	7
50–64	7	8.4	166	1	1	1	20	33	33	33
65+	19	4.8	47	1	1	2	6	14	29	29
TOTAL SINGLE DX	3	1.0	0	1	1	1	1	1	1	1
TOTAL MULTIPLE DX	44	4.1	43	1	1	2	3	8	20	33
TOTAL										
0–19 Years	4	2.0	1	1	1	1	3	3	3	3
20–34	5	2.2	3	1	1	2	2	5	5	5
35–49	11	2.6	3	1	2	2	4	4	7	7
50–64	7	8.4	166	1	1	1	20	33	33	33
65+	20	4.6	45	1	1	2	6	14	29	29
GRAND TOTAL	47	4.0	41	1	1	2	3	8	20	33

16.4: ENUCLEATION OF EYEBALL

Type of Patients	Observed Patients	Avg. Stay	Vari-ance	10th	25th	50th	75th	90th	95th	99th
1. SINGLE DX										
0–19 Years	5	1.7	<1	1	1	2	2	2	3	3
20–34	1	1.0	0	1	1	1	1	1	1	1
35–49	1	2.0	0	2	2	2	2	2	2	2
50–64	0									
65+	0									
2. MULTIPLE DX										
0–19 Years	15	2.9	4	1	2	2	3	4	8	8
20–34	14	4.8	38	1	1	2	6	17	19	19
35–49	8	3.0	9	1	1	2	3	10	10	10
50–64	19	7.0	61	1	1	5	10	24	28	28
65+	25	5.1	27	1	1	3	7	14	14	19
TOTAL SINGLE DX	7	1.7	<1	1	1	2	2	2	3	3
TOTAL MULTIPLE DX	81	4.4	25	1	2	2	5	12	14	24
TOTAL										
0–19 Years	20	2.6	3	1	2	2	3	4	8	8
20–34	15	4.5	36	1	1	2	6	17	19	19
35–49	9	2.9	8	1	1	2	3	10	10	10
50–64	19	7.0	61	1	1	5	10	24	28	28
65+	25	5.1	27	1	1	3	7	14	14	19
GRAND TOTAL	88	4.0	23	1	1	2	4	10	14	24

LOS by Diagnosis and Operation, Western Region, 45th Edition

Western Region, October 2007–September 2008 Data, by Operation

16.5: EXENTERATION OF ORBIT

Type of Patients	Observed Patients	Avg. Stay	Variance	10th	25th	50th	75th	90th	95th	99th
1. SINGLE DX										
0–19 Years	0									
20–34	0									
35–49	0									
50–64	2	4.0	2	3	3	3	5	5	5	5
65+	0									
2. MULTIPLE DX										
0–19 Years	1	3.0	0	3	3	3	3	3	3	3
20–34	2	15.0	195	5	5	5	25	25	25	25
35–49	1	6.0	0	6	6	6	6	6	6	6
50–64	13	6.9	57	1	3	5	6	17	28	28
65+	22	4.8	48	1	1	3	6	7	9	34
TOTAL SINGLE DX	2	4.0	2	3	3	3	5	5	5	5
TOTAL MULTIPLE DX	39	6.0	56	1	2	3	6	17	28	34
TOTAL										
0–19 Years	1	3.0	0	3	3	3	3	3	3	3
20–34	2	15.0	195	5	5	5	25	25	25	25
35–49	1	6.0	0	6	6	6	6	6	6	6
50–64	15	6.5	50	1	3	5	6	17	28	28
65+	22	4.8	48	1	1	3	6	7	9	34
GRAND TOTAL	41	5.9	53	1	2	3	6	9	25	34

16.6: 2ND PX POST RMVL EYEBALL

Type of Patients	Observed Patients	Avg. Stay	Variance	10th	25th	50th	75th	90th	95th	99th
1. SINGLE DX										
0–19 Years	0									
20–34	0									
35–49	0									
50–64	0									
65+	0									
2. MULTIPLE DX										
0–19 Years	3	1.5	<1	1	1	1	2	2	2	2
20–34	3	1.0	0	1	1	1	1	1	1	1
35–49	4	1.0	0	1	1	1	1	1	1	1
50–64	4	2.5	9	1	1	1	4	7	7	7
65+	3	2.3	2	1	1	2	4	4	4	4
TOTAL SINGLE DX	0									
TOTAL MULTIPLE DX	17	1.6	2	1	1	1	2	2	4	7
TOTAL										
0–19 Years	3	1.5	<1	1	1	1	2	2	2	2
20–34	3	1.0	0	1	1	1	1	1	1	1
35–49	4	1.0	0	1	1	1	1	1	1	1
50–64	4	2.5	9	1	1	1	4	7	7	7
65+	3	2.3	2	1	1	2	4	4	4	4
GRAND TOTAL	17	1.6	2	1	1	1	2	2	4	7

16.7: OCULAR/ORBITAL IMPL RMVL

Type of Patients	Observed Patients	Avg. Stay	Variance	10th	25th	50th	75th	90th	95th	99th
1. SINGLE DX										
0–19 Years	2	3.2	<1	3	3	3	3	4	4	4
20–34	0									
35–49	0									
50–64	1	2.0	0	2	2	2	2	2	2	2
65+	0									
2. MULTIPLE DX										
0–19 Years	1	2.0	0	2	2	2	2	2	2	2
20–34	1	1.0	0	1	1	1	1	1	1	1
35–49	3	6.0	28	2	2	4	12	12	12	12
50–64	3	2.3	2	1	1	3	2	4	4	4
65+	4	4.5	33	1	1	3	13	13	13	13
TOTAL SINGLE DX	3	3.0	<1	2	3	3	3	4	4	4
TOTAL MULTIPLE DX	12	3.8	18	1	1	2	4	12	13	13
TOTAL										
0–19 Years	3	3.0	0	2	3	3	3	4	4	4
20–34	1	1.0	0	1	1	1	1	1	1	1
35–49	3	6.0	28	2	2	4	12	12	12	12
50–64	3	2.3	2	1	1	3	2	4	4	4
65+	4	4.5	33	1	1	3	13	13	13	13
GRAND TOTAL	15	3.6	12	1	2	3	4	12	13	13

16.8: EYEBALL/ORBIT INJ REPAIR

Type of Patients	Observed Patients	Avg. Stay	Variance	10th	25th	50th	75th	90th	95th	99th
1. SINGLE DX										
0–19 Years	10	1.5	<1	1	1	1	2	3	3	3
20–34	9	1.2	<1	1	1	1	1	2	2	2
35–49	3	2.0	1	1	1	2	3	3	3	3
50–64	4	1.3	<1	1	1	1	1	2	2	2
65+	2	1.0	0	1	1	1	1	1	1	1
2. MULTIPLE DX										
0–19 Years	33	1.9	2	1	1	2	2	4	4	7
20–34	37	2.4	5	1	1	1	3	5	7	11
35–49	28	2.3	4	1	1	1	4	5	10	>99
50–64	30	5.3	55	1	1	3	6	19	19	36
65+	61	2.9	8	1	1	2	4	5	10	13
TOTAL SINGLE DX	28	1.4	<1	1	1	1	2	3	3	3
TOTAL MULTIPLE DX	189	2.9	13	1	1	2	4	6	9	19
TOTAL										
0–19 Years	43	1.8	2	1	1	1	2	3	4	7
20–34	46	2.2	4	1	1	1	3	5	6	11
35–49	31	2.3	4	1	1	1	5	5	10	>99
50–64	34	4.8	50	1	1	2	5	9	19	36
65+	63	2.8	7	1	1	2	4	5	10	13
GRAND TOTAL	217	2.7	12	1	1	2	3	5	9	19

LOS by Diagnosis and Operation, Western Region, 45th Edition

Western Region, October 2007–September 2008 Data, by Operation

16.82: REPAIR EYEBALL RUPTURE

Type of Patients	Observed Patients	Avg. Stay	Variance	Percentiles						
				10th	25th	50th	75th	90th	95th	99th
1. SINGLE DX										
0–19 Years	10	1.5	<1	1	1	1	2	3	3	3
20–34	8	1.1	<1	1	1	1	1	2	2	2
35–49	3	2.0	1	1	1	2	3	3	3	3
50–64	4	1.3	<1	1	1	1	1	2	2	2
65+	2	1.0	0	1	1	1	1	1	1	1
2. MULTIPLE DX										
0–19 Years	24	1.9	2	1	1	2	2	3	4	7
20–34	32	2.2	3	1	1	1	3	5	6	7
35–49	21	2.4	5	1	1	2	4	5	10	>99
50–64	26	4.5	24	1	1	3	6	9	19	19
65+	53	3.0	9	1	1	2	4	8	10	13
TOTAL SINGLE DX	27	1.4	<1	1	1	1	2	3	3	3
TOTAL MULTIPLE DX	156	2.8	9	1	1	2	3	6	9	19
TOTAL										
0–19 Years	34	1.8	1	1	1	1	2	3	4	7
20–34	40	2.0	2	1	1	1	2	5	5	7
35–49	24	2.3	4	1	1	2	3	5	10	>99
50–64	30	4.0	22	1	1	2	5	9	19	19
65+	55	2.9	8	1	1	2	4	8	10	13
GRAND TOTAL	183	2.6	8	1	1	1	3	5	9	19

16.9: OTHER EYE & ORBIT OPS

Type of Patients	Observed Patients	Avg. Stay	Variance	Percentiles						
				10th	25th	50th	75th	90th	95th	99th
1. SINGLE DX										
0–19 Years	1	1.0	0	1	1	1	1	1	1	1
20–34	2	1.0	0	1	1	1	1	1	1	1
35–49	2	1.5	<1	1	1	2	2	2	2	2
50–64	1	1.0	0	1	1	1	1	1	1	1
65+	0									
2. MULTIPLE DX										
0–19 Years	20	5.0	194	1	1	2	5	6	6	91
20–34	11	3.5	5	1	1	3	6	7	7	7
35–49	14	2.9	9	1	1	3	3	4	13	13
50–64	17	4.5	21	1	1	3	6	13	17	17
65+	14	4.5	11	1	1	5	6	9	12	12
TOTAL SINGLE DX	6	1.2	<1	1	1	1	1	2	2	2
TOTAL MULTIPLE DX	76	4.4	89	1	1	3	5	7	12	91
TOTAL										
0–19 Years	21	4.9	189	1	1	2	5	6	6	91
20–34	13	3.1	5	1	1	2	4	7	7	7
35–49	16	2.8	8	1	1	2	3	4	13	13
50–64	18	4.3	21	1	1	3	6	13	17	17
65+	14	4.5	11	1	1	5	6	9	12	12
GRAND TOTAL	82	4.2	84	1	1	2	5	7	9	17

18.0: EXTERNAL EAR INCISION

Type of Patients	Observed Patients	Avg. Stay	Variance	Percentiles						
				10th	25th	50th	75th	90th	95th	99th
1. SINGLE DX										
0–19 Years	13	3.5	4	1	2	3	4	7	7	7
20–34	1	1.5	<1	1	1	2	2	2	2	2
35–49	1	1.0	0	1	1	1	1	1	1	1
50–64	0									
65+	0									
2. MULTIPLE DX										
0–19 Years	34	2.7	2	1	2	2	4	4	5	9
20–34	28	6.8	120	2	3	4	7	9	17	60
35–49	18	3.7	3	1	2	4	5	6	6	6
50–64	22	4.0	9	2	2	3	5	8	11	13
65+	7	4.9	6	2	2	5	6	9	9	9
TOTAL SINGLE DX	16	3.2	4	1	2	2	4	7	7	7
TOTAL MULTIPLE DX	109	3.8	27	1	2	3	4	6	8	17
TOTAL										
0–19 Years	47	2.8	3	1	2	2	4	4	7	9
20–34	30	6.4	113	2	3	4	7	8	17	60
35–49	19	3.6	3	1	2	4	5	6	6	6
50–64	22	4.0	9	2	2	3	5	8	11	13
65+	7	4.9	6	2	2	5	6	9	9	9
GRAND TOTAL	125	3.8	24	1	2	3	4	6	8	17

18.09: EXTERNAL EAR INC NEC

Type of Patients	Observed Patients	Avg. Stay	Variance	Percentiles						
				10th	25th	50th	75th	90th	95th	99th
1. SINGLE DX										
0–19 Years	11	3.6	4	1	2	4	4	7	7	7
20–34	2	1.5	<1	1	1	2	2	2	2	2
35–49	1	1.0	0	1	1	1	1	1	1	1
50–64	0									
65+	0									
2. MULTIPLE DX										
0–19 Years	32	2.7	2	1	2	2	4	4	5	9
20–34	27	6.7	124	2	3	4	7	8	17	60
35–49	16	3.6	3	1	2	3	5	6	6	13
50–64	16	3.8	7	1	2	3	5	8	11	11
65+	5	4.6	3	2	4	5	6	6	6	6
TOTAL SINGLE DX	14	3.3	5	1	2	2	4	7	7	7
TOTAL MULTIPLE DX	96	3.8	29	1	2	3	4	6	7	17
TOTAL										
0–19 Years	43	2.9	3	1	2	2	4	4	7	9
20–34	29	6.3	117	2	3	4	6	7	7	60
35–49	17	3.4	4	1	2	3	5	6	6	13
50–64	16	3.8	7	1	2	3	5	8	11	11
65+	5	4.6	3	2	4	5	6	6	6	6
GRAND TOTAL	110	3.7	25	1	2	3	4	6	7	17

LOS by Diagnosis and Operation, Western Region, 45th Edition

Western Region, October 2007–September 2008 Data, by Operation

18.1: EXTERNAL EAR DXTIC PX

Type of Patients	Observed Patients	Avg. Stay	Variance	10th	25th	50th	75th	90th	95th	99th
1. SINGLE DX										
0–19 Years	1	2.0	0	2	2	2	2	2	2	2
20–34	0									
35–49	0									
50–64	0									
65+	0									
2. MULTIPLE DX										
0–19 Years	9	4.0	11	1	1	3	7	7	7	13
20–34	5	7.8	38	3	3	4	14	15	15	15
35–49	5	6.8	51	1	3	4	7	19	19	19
50–64	15	7.3	28	2	3	8	12	14	18	18
65+	12	8.0	23	3	4	8	13	16	16	16
TOTAL SINGLE DX	1	2.0	0	2	2	2	2	2	2	2
TOTAL MULTIPLE DX	46	6.2	25	1	3	4	8	14	16	19
TOTAL										
0–19 Years	10	3.9	11	1	1	2	7	7	7	13
20–34	5	7.8	38	3	3	4	14	15	15	15
35–49	5	6.8	51	1	3	4	7	19	19	19
50–64	15	7.3	28	2	3	8	12	14	18	18
65+	12	8.0	23	3	4	8	13	16	16	16
GRAND TOTAL	47	6.2	25	1	2	4	8	14	16	19

18.29: DESTR EXT EAR LES NEC

Type of Patients	Observed Patients	Avg. Stay	Variance	10th	25th	50th	75th	90th	95th	99th
1. SINGLE DX										
0–19 Years	4	1.6	<1	1	1	2	2	2	2	2
20–34	1	2.0	0	2	2	2	2	2	2	2
35–49	0									
50–64	0									
65+	0									
2. MULTIPLE DX										
0–19 Years	121	2.7	6	1	2	2	3	4	9	15
20–34	2	1.0	<1	1	1	1	1	1	1	1
35–49	8	5.4	41	1	1	3	14	17	17	17
50–64	6	7.2	22	2	5	6	8	16	16	16
65+	15	4.1	9	1	2	5	5	10	>99	>99
TOTAL SINGLE DX	5	1.6	<1	1	1	2	2	2	2	2
TOTAL MULTIPLE DX	152	3.1	9	1	2	2	3	6	11	17
TOTAL										
0–19 Years	125	2.6	6	1	2	2	3	4	9	15
20–34	3	1.3	<1	1	1	1	2	2	2	2
35–49	8	5.4	41	1	1	3	14	17	17	17
50–64	6	7.2	22	2	5	6	8	16	16	16
65+	15	4.1	9	1	2	5	5	10	>99	>99
GRAND TOTAL	157	3.0	9	1	2	2	3	6	11	17

18.2: EXC/DESTR EXT EAR LESION

Type of Patients	Observed Patients	Avg. Stay	Variance	10th	25th	50th	75th	90th	95th	99th
1. SINGLE DX										
0–19 Years	5	1.4	<1	1	1	1	2	2	2	2
20–34	1	2.0	0	2	2	2	2	2	2	2
35–49	1	1.0	0	1	1	1	1	1	1	1
50–64	0									
65+	0									
2. MULTIPLE DX										
0–19 Years	124	2.6	6	1	1	2	3	4	9	15
20–34	2	1.0	<1	1	1	1	1	1	1	1
35–49	6	5.4	41	1	1	3	14	17	17	17
50–64	6	7.2	22	2	5	6	8	16	18	18
65+	15	4.1	9	1	2	5	5	10	>99	>99
TOTAL SINGLE DX	7	1.4	<1	1	1	1	2	2	2	2
TOTAL MULTIPLE DX	155	3.0	9	1	1	2	3	6	11	17
TOTAL										
0–19 Years	129	2.5	6	1	1	2	3	4	8	15
20–34	3	1.3	<1	1	1	2	2	2	2	2
35–49	9	4.9	38	1	1	2	4	17	17	17
50–64	6	7.2	22	2	5	6	8	16	18	18
65+	15	4.1	9	1	2	5	5	10	>99	>99
GRAND TOTAL	162	2.9	8	1	1	2	3	5	11	16

18.3: OTHER EXTERNAL EAR EXC

Type of Patients	Observed Patients	Avg. Stay	Variance	10th	25th	50th	75th	90th	95th	99th
1. SINGLE DX										
0–19 Years	2	2.0	0	2	2	2	2	2	2	2
20–34	2	1.0	0	1	1	1	1	1	1	1
35–49	0									
50–64	1	1.0	0	1	1	1	1	1	1	1
65+	1	3.0	0	3	3	3	3	3	3	3
2. MULTIPLE DX										
0–19 Years	1	8.0	0	8	8	8	8	8	8	8
20–34	5	3.0	0	3	3	3	3	3	3	3
35–49	5	1.8	<1	1	1	2	2	3	3	3
50–64	14	2.1	5	1	1	1	3	4	9	9
65+	29	4.6	22	1	1	4	6	13	15	19
TOTAL SINGLE DX	6	1.8	<1	1	2	2	2	2	3	3
TOTAL MULTIPLE DX	50	3.9	16	1	1	2	6	8	13	19
TOTAL										
0–19 Years	3	4.0	9	2	2	2	8	8	8	8
20–34	5	1.7	<1	1	1	1	2	3	3	3
35–49	5	1.8	<1	1	1	2	2	3	3	3
50–64	15	2.0	5	1	1	1	3	4	9	9
65+	30	4.6	21	1	1	4	6	13	15	19
GRAND TOTAL	56	3.5	14	1	1	2	5	8	9	19

LOS by Diagnosis and Operation, Western Region, 45th Edition

Western Region, October 2007–September 2008 Data, by Operation

18.4: SUTURE EXT EAR LAC

Type of Patients	Observed Patients	Avg. Stay	Vari-ance	Percentiles						
				10th	25th	50th	75th	90th	95th	99th
1. SINGLE DX										
0–19 Years	1	1.0	0	1	1	1	1	1	1	1
20–34	2	1.0	0	1	1	1	1	1	1	1
35–49	1	1.0	0	1	1	1	1	1	1	1
50–64	0									
65+	0									
2. MULTIPLE DX										
0–19 Years	51	4.5	44	1	1	3	5	8	18	47
20–34	91	2.6	10	1	1	2	3	5	9	24
35–49	47	3.2	11	1	1	2	4	7	8	17
50–64	53	4.4	97	1	1	2	4	7	10	72
65+	100	4.0	12	1	2	3	5	8	10	25
TOTAL SINGLE DX	4	1.0	0	1	1	1	1	1	1	1
TOTAL MULTIPLE DX	342	3.7	30	1	1	2	4	7	10	24
TOTAL										
0–19 Years	52	4.4	43	1	1	3	5	8	8	47
20–34	93	2.6	10	1	1	2	3	5	9	24
35–49	48	3.2	11	1	1	2	4	7	8	17
50–64	53	4.4	97	1	1	2	4	7	10	72
65+	100	4.0	12	1	2	3	5	8	10	25
GRAND TOTAL	346	3.6	30	1	1	2	4	7	10	24

18.5: CORRECTION PROMINENT EAR

Type of Patients	Observed Patients	Avg. Stay	Vari-ance	Percentiles						
				10th	25th	50th	75th	90th	95th	99th
1. SINGLE DX										
0–19 Years	6	1.2	<1	1	1	1	1	1	2	2
20–34	0									
35–49	0									
50–64	0									
65+	0									
2. MULTIPLE DX										
0–19 Years	3	1.0	0	1	1	1	1	1	1	1
20–34	0									
35–49	0									
50–64	0									
65+	0									
TOTAL SINGLE DX	6	1.2	<1	1	1	1	1	2	2	2
TOTAL MULTIPLE DX	3	1.0	0	1	1	1	1	1	1	1
TOTAL										
0–19 Years	9	1.1	<1	1	1	1	1	2	2	2
20–34	0									
35–49	0									
50–64	0									
65+	0									
GRAND TOTAL	9	1.1	<1	1	1	1	1	2	2	2

18.6: EXT AUDIT CANAL RECONST

Type of Patients	Observed Patients	Avg. Stay	Vari-ance	Percentiles						
				10th	25th	50th	75th	90th	95th	99th
1. SINGLE DX										
0–19 Years	7	1.4	<1	1	1	1	2	2	2	2
20–34	1	1.0	0	1	1	1	1	1	1	1
35–49	1	39.0	0	39	39	39	39	39	39	39
50–64	0									
65+	1	1.0	0	1	1	1	1	1	1	1
2. MULTIPLE DX										
0–19 Years	11	2.1	6	1	1	1	2	3	11	11
20–34	5	2.8	12	1	1	1	2	11	11	11
35–49	2	6.5	<1	6	6	7	7	7	7	7
50–64	7	3.1	16	1	1	1	4	12	12	12
65+	6	4.0	30	1	1	1	4	15	15	15
TOTAL SINGLE DX	10	3.5	83	1	1	1	2	2	39	39
TOTAL MULTIPLE DX	31	2.9	12	1	1	1	3	7	12	15
TOTAL										
0–19 Years	18	1.7	3	1	1	1	2	2	3	11
20–34	6	2.6	11	1	1	1	2	11	11	11
35–49	3	17.4	349	6	6	7	39	39	39	39
50–64	7	3.1	16	1	1	1	4	12	12	12
65+	7	3.6	27	1	1	1	4	15	15	15
GRAND TOTAL	41	3.1	32	1	1	1	2	7	12	39

18.7: OTH PLASTIC REP EXT EAR

Type of Patients	Observed Patients	Avg. Stay	Vari-ance	Percentiles						
				10th	25th	50th	75th	90th	95th	99th
1. SINGLE DX										
0–19 Years	84	2.0	1	1	1	2	3	4	4	5
20–34	3	2.7	2	1	2	3	4	4	4	4
35–49	1	2.0	0	2	2	2	2	2	2	2
50–64	1	1.0	0	1	1	1	1	1	1	1
65+	1	3.0	0	3	3	3	3	3	3	3
2. MULTIPLE DX										
0–19 Years	83	2.2	2	1	1	2	3	4	4	6
20–34	25	2.2	3	1	1	1	3	5	5	7
35–49	9	7.2	101	2	2	2	5	27	27	27
50–64	15	3.7	13	1	1	2	5	12	12	12
65+	19	6.1	48	1	1	3	8	21	23	23
TOTAL SINGLE DX	90	2.0	1	1	1	2	3	4	4	5
TOTAL MULTIPLE DX	151	2.8	11	1	1	2	3	5	6	22
TOTAL										
0–19 Years	167	2.1	2	1	1	2	3	4	4	5
20–34	28	2.3	3	1	1	2	3	5	5	7
35–49	10	6.7	93	1	1	2	5	27	27	27
50–64	16	3.6	13	1	1	2	5	12	12	12
65+	20	6.0	46	1	1	3	7	18	21	23
GRAND TOTAL	241	2.4	6	1	1	2	3	4	5	18

19.0: STAPES MOBILIZATION

Type of Patients	Observed Patients	Avg. Stay	Variance	Percentiles						
				10th	25th	50th	75th	90th	95th	99th
1. SINGLE DX										
0–19 Years	0									
20–34	0									
35–49	0									
50–64	0									
65+	0									
2. MULTIPLE DX										
0–19 Years	0									
20–34	0									
35–49	1	1.0	0	1	1	1	1	1	1	1
50–64	1	1.0	0	1	1	1	1	1	1	1
65+	1	1.0	0	1	1	1	1	1	1	1
TOTAL SINGLE DX	**0**									
TOTAL MULTIPLE DX	**3**	**1.0**	**0**	**1**	**1**	**1**	**1**	**1**	**1**	**1**
TOTAL										
0–19 Years	0									
20–34	0									
35–49	1	1.0	0	1	1	1	1	1	1	1
50–64	1	1.0	0	1	1	1	1	1	1	1
65+	1	1.0	0	1	1	1	1	1	1	1
GRAND TOTAL	**3**	**1.0**	**0**	**1**	**1**	**1**	**1**	**1**	**1**	**1**

19.1: STAPEDECTOMY

Type of Patients	Observed Patients	Avg. Stay	Variance	Percentiles						
				10th	25th	50th	75th	90th	95th	99th
1. SINGLE DX										
0–19 Years	0									
20–34	1	1.0	0	1	1	1	1	1	1	1
35–49	2	1.5	<1	1	1	2	2	2	2	2
50–64	2	1.0	0	1	1	1	1	1	1	1
65+	0									
2. MULTIPLE DX										
0–19 Years	1	1.0	0	1	1	1	1	1	1	1
20–34	0									
35–49	12	1.2	<1	1	1	1	2	2	2	2
50–64	15	1.5	<1	1	1	1	2	3	3	3
65+	2	1.5	<1	1	1	1	2	2	2	2
TOTAL SINGLE DX	**5**	**1.2**	**<1**	**1**	**1**	**1**	**1**	**2**	**2**	**2**
TOTAL MULTIPLE DX	**30**	**1.4**	**<1**	**1**	**1**	**1**	**2**	**2**	**3**	**3**
TOTAL										
0–19 Years	1	1.0	0	1	1	1	1	1	1	1
20–34	1	1.0	0	1	1	1	1	1	1	1
35–49	14	1.2	<1	1	1	1	1	2	2	2
50–64	17	1.5	<1	1	1	1	2	3	3	3
65+	2	1.5	<1	1	1	1	2	2	2	2
GRAND TOTAL	**35**	**1.3**	**<1**	**1**	**1**	**1**	**2**	**2**	**3**	**3**

18.79: PLASTIC REP EXT EAR NEC

Type of Patients	Observed Patients	Avg. Stay	Variance	Percentiles						
				10th	25th	50th	75th	90th	95th	99th
1. SINGLE DX										
0–19 Years	39	1.5	<1	1	1	1	2	3	4	4
20–34	1	3.0	0	3	3	3	3	3	3	3
35–49	0									
50–64	1	1.0	0	1	1	1	1	1	1	1
65+	1	3.0	0	3	3	3	3	3	3	3
2. MULTIPLE DX										
0–19 Years	45	1.9	1	1	1	1	2	4	4	7
20–34	22	2.4	3	1	1	2	3	5	5	7
35–49	9	7.2	101	1	1	2	5	27	27	27
50–64	12	3.3	10	1	1	2	5	5	12	12
65+	18	5.3	37	1	1	3	7	18	23	23
TOTAL SINGLE DX	**42**	**1.5**	**<1**	**1**	**1**	**1**	**2**	**3**	**4**	**4**
TOTAL MULTIPLE DX	**106**	**2.8**	**14**	**1**	**1**	**2**	**3**	**5**	**7**	**23**
TOTAL										
0–19 Years	84	1.7	1	1	1	1	2	3	4	5
20–34	23	2.4	3	1	1	2	3	5	5	7
35–49	9	7.2	101	1	1	2	5	27	27	27
50–64	13	3.1	9	1	1	2	4	5	12	12
65+	19	5.2	35	1	1	3	7	18	23	23
GRAND TOTAL	**148**	**2.3**	**9**	**1**	**1**	**1**	**2**	**4**	**5**	**22**

18.9: OTHER EXT EAR OPERATIONS

Type of Patients	Observed Patients	Avg. Stay	Variance	Percentiles						
				10th	25th	50th	75th	90th	95th	99th
1. SINGLE DX										
0–19 Years	0									
20–34	0									
35–49	0									
50–64	0									
65+	0									
2. MULTIPLE DX										
0–19 Years	1	2.0	0	2	2	2	2	2	2	2
20–34	1	2.0	0	2	2	2	2	2	2	2
35–49	0									
50–64	0									
65+	1	10.0	0	10	10	10	10	10	10	10
TOTAL SINGLE DX	**0**									
TOTAL MULTIPLE DX	**3**	**4.7**	**21**	**2**	**2**	**2**	**10**	**10**	**10**	**10**
TOTAL										
0–19 Years	1	2.0	0	2	2	2	2	2	2	2
20–34	1	2.0	0	2	2	2	2	2	2	2
35–49	0									
50–64	0									
65+	1	10.0	0	10	10	10	10	10	10	10
GRAND TOTAL	**3**	**4.7**	**21**	**2**	**2**	**2**	**10**	**10**	**10**	**10**

LOS by Diagnosis and Operation, Western Region, 45th Edition

Western Region, October 2007–September 2008 Data, by Operation

19.2: STAPEDECTOMY REVISION

Type of Patients	Observed Patients	Avg. Stay	Vari-ance	Percentiles						
				10th	25th	50th	75th	90th	95th	99th
1. SINGLE DX										
0–19 Years	0									
20–34	0									
35–49	0									
50–64	0									
65+	0									
2. MULTIPLE DX										
0–19 Years	0									
20–34	0									
35–49	1	1.0	0	1	1	1	1	1	1	1
50–64	3	2.3	2	1	1	2	4	4	4	4
65+	1	1.0	0	1	1	1	1	1	1	1
TOTAL SINGLE DX	0									
TOTAL MULTIPLE DX	5	1.8	2	1	1	1	2	4	4	4
TOTAL										
0–19 Years	0									
20–34	0									
35–49	1	1.0	0	1	1	1	1	1	1	1
50–64	3	2.3	2	1	1	2	4	4	4	4
65+	1	1.0	0	1	1	1	1	1	1	1
GRAND TOTAL	5	1.8	2	1	1	1	2	4	4	4

19.3: OSSICULAR CHAIN OPS NEC

Type of Patients	Observed Patients	Avg. Stay	Vari-ance	Percentiles						
				10th	25th	50th	75th	90th	95th	99th
1. SINGLE DX										
0–19 Years	0									
20–34	0									
35–49	0									
50–64	0									
65+	1	1.0	0	1	1	1	1	1	1	1
2. MULTIPLE DX										
0–19 Years	1	1.0	0	1	1	1	1	1	1	1
20–34	2	1.5	<1	1	1	1	2	2	2	2
35–49	2	1.0	0	1	1	1	1	1	1	1
50–64	2	1.5	<1	1	1	1	2	2	2	2
65+	3	2.3	1	1	1	3	3	3	3	3
TOTAL SINGLE DX	1	1.0	0	1	1	1	1	1	1	1
TOTAL MULTIPLE DX	10	1.6	<1	1	1	1	2	3	3	3
TOTAL										
0–19 Years	1	1.0	0	1	1	1	1	1	1	1
20–34	2	1.5	<1	1	1	1	2	2	2	2
35–49	2	1.0	0	1	1	1	2	2	2	2
50–64	2	1.5	<1	1	1	1	2	2	2	2
65+	4	2.0	1	1	1	3	3	3	3	3
GRAND TOTAL	11	1.5	<1	1	1	1	2	3	3	3

19.4: MYRINGOPLASTY

Type of Patients	Observed Patients	Avg. Stay	Vari-ance	Percentiles						
				10th	25th	50th	75th	90th	95th	99th
1. SINGLE DX										
0–19 Years	1	3.0	0	3	3	3	3	3	3	3
20–34	1	1.0	0	1	1	1	1	1	1	1
35–49	1	1.0	0	1	1	1	1	1	1	1
50–64	2	1.0	0	1	1	1	1	1	1	1
65+	0									
2. MULTIPLE DX										
0–19 Years	20	1.8	3	1	1	1	1	5	5	6
20–34	5	2.6	4	1	1	2	3	6	6	6
35–49	10	2.9	15	1	1	1	2	6	13	13
50–64	15	3.9	8	1	1	4	5	9	10	10
65+	13	3.3	11	1	1	1	4	8	12	12
TOTAL SINGLE DX	5	1.4	<1	1	1	1	1	3	3	3
TOTAL MULTIPLE DX	63	2.5	7	1	1	1	4	6	8	13
TOTAL										
0–19 Years	21	1.8	3	1	1	1	1	5	5	6
20–34	6	2.3	4	1	1	2	3	6	6	6
35–49	11	2.7	14	1	1	1	2	6	13	13
50–64	17	3.5	8	1	1	2	5	9	10	10
65+	13	3.3	11	1	1	1	4	8	12	12
GRAND TOTAL	68	2.5	6	1	1	1	4	6	8	13

19.5: OTHER TYMPANOPLASTY

Type of Patients	Observed Patients	Avg. Stay	Vari-ance	Percentiles						
				10th	25th	50th	75th	90th	95th	99th
1. SINGLE DX										
0–19 Years	3	1.0	0	1	1	1	1	1	1	1
20–34	1	1.0	0	1	1	1	1	1	1	1
35–49	1	1.0	0	1	1	1	1	1	1	1
50–64	0									
65+	0									
2. MULTIPLE DX										
0–19 Years	15	1.4	2	1	1	1	1	2	2	9
20–34	3	2.4	5	1	1	1	5	5	5	5
35–49	8	1.4	<1	1	1	1	2	2	2	2
50–64	13	1.1	<1	1	1	1	1	1	2	2
65+	7	1.1	<1	1	1	1	1	2	2	2
TOTAL SINGLE DX	5	1.0	0	1	1	1	1	1	1	1
TOTAL MULTIPLE DX	46	1.3	1	1	1	1	1	2	2	9
TOTAL										
0–19 Years	18	1.3	2	1	1	1	1	2	2	9
20–34	4	2.0	4	1	1	1	5	5	5	5
35–49	9	1.3	<1	1	1	1	2	2	2	2
50–64	13	1.1	<1	1	1	1	1	1	2	2
65+	7	1.1	<1	1	1	1	1	2	2	2
GRAND TOTAL	51	1.3	1	1	1	1	1	2	2	9

LOS by Diagnosis and Operation, Western Region, 45th Edition

19.6: TYMPANOPLASTY REVISION

Type of Patients	Observed Patients	Avg. Stay	Vari-ance	Percentiles						
				10th	25th	50th	75th	90th	95th	99th
1. SINGLE DX										
0–19 Years	0									
20–34	0									
35–49	0									
50–64	0									
65+	0									
2. MULTIPLE DX										
0–19 Years	3	1.5	<1	1	1	1	2	2	2	2
20–34	5	1.4	<1	1	1	1	1	3	3	3
35–49	3	2.7	8	1	1	1	6	6	6	6
50–64	3	2.0	<1	1	1	2	3	3	3	3
65+	2	7.0	2	6	6	8	8	8	8	8
TOTAL SINGLE DX	0									
TOTAL MULTIPLE DX	16	2.2	4	1	1	1	2	6	6	8
TOTAL										
0–19 Years	3	1.5	<1	1	1	1	2	2	2	2
20–34	5	1.4	<1	1	1	1	1	3	3	3
35–49	3	2.7	8	1	1	1	6	6	6	6
50–64	3	2.0	<1	1	1	2	3	3	3	3
65+	2	7.0	2	6	6	8	8	8	8	8
GRAND TOTAL	16	2.2	4	1	1	1	2	6	6	8

20.0: MYRINGOTOMY

Type of Patients	Observed Patients	Avg. Stay	Vari-ance	Percentiles						
				10th	25th	50th	75th	90th	95th	99th
1. SINGLE DX										
0–19 Years	17	2.2	1	1	1	2	3	4	4	4
20–34	2	4.0	18	1	1	1	7	7	7	7
35–49	0									
50–64	3	1.7	1	1	1	1	3	3	3	3
65+	0									
2. MULTIPLE DX										
0–19 Years	510	3.9	37	1	1	2	4	10	14	30
20–34	26	5.4	21	1	1	4	7	11	13	20
35–49	53	6.9	50	1	3	4	9	15	23	31
50–64	55	7.7	96	1	4	6	9	14	18	>99
65+	41	7.4	31	1	3	6	11	14	16	25
TOTAL SINGLE DX	22	2.3	2	1	1	2	3	4	4	7
TOTAL MULTIPLE DX	685	4.3	40	1	1	2	5	11	15	31
TOTAL										
0–19 Years	527	3.9	36	1	1	2	4	10	14	30
20–34	28	5.3	20	1	1	4	7	11	13	20
35–49	53	6.9	50	1	3	4	9	15	23	31
50–64	58	7.4	93	1	3	6	9	14	18	>99
65+	41	7.4	31	1	3	6	11	14	16	25
GRAND TOTAL	707	4.3	39	1	1	2	5	11	14	31

19.9: MIDDLE EAR REPAIR NEC

Type of Patients	Observed Patients	Avg. Stay	Vari-ance	Percentiles						
				10th	25th	50th	75th	90th	95th	99th
1. SINGLE DX										
0–19 Years	0									
20–34	0									
35–49	1	2.0	0	2	2	2	2	2	2	2
50–64	1	3.0	0	3	3	3	3	3	3	3
65+	0									
2. MULTIPLE DX										
0–19 Years	0									
20–34	1	1.0	0	1	1	1	1	1	1	1
35–49	3	2.3	2	1	1	2	4	4	4	4
50–64	3	3.0	4	1	1	3	5	5	5	5
65+	0									
TOTAL SINGLE DX	2	2.5	<1	2	2	2	3	3	3	3
TOTAL MULTIPLE DX	7	2.4	3	1	1	2	4	5	5	5
TOTAL										
0–19 Years	0									
20–34	1	1.0	0	1	1	1	2	2	2	2
35–49	4	2.3	2	1	2	2	2	4	4	4
50–64	4	3.0	3	1	1	3	3	5	5	5
65+	0									
GRAND TOTAL	9	2.4	2	1	1	2	3	5	5	5

20.01: MYRINGOTOMY W INTUBATION

Type of Patients	Observed Patients	Avg. Stay	Vari-ance	Percentiles						
				10th	25th	50th	75th	90th	95th	99th
1. SINGLE DX										
0–19 Years	16	2.4	<1	1	2	2	3	4	4	4
20–34	2	4.0	18	1	1	1	7	7	7	7
35–49	0									
50–64	3	1.7	1	1	1	1	3	3	3	3
65+	0									
2. MULTIPLE DX										
0–19 Years	495	3.9	37	1	1	2	4	10	14	30
20–34	24	5.7	21	1	3	5	8	11	13	20
35–49	49	7.3	52	1	3	4	10	16	23	31
50–64	49	7.8	106	1	2	6	11	15	18	>99
65+	38	7.3	32	1	3	6	11	15	19	25
TOTAL SINGLE DX	21	2.4	2	1	1	2	3	4	4	7
TOTAL MULTIPLE DX	655	4.3	41	1	1	2	5	11	14	31
TOTAL										
0–19 Years	511	3.9	36	1	1	2	4	10	13	30
20–34	26	5.6	20	1	2	5	7	11	13	20
35–49	49	7.3	52	1	3	4	10	16	23	31
50–64	52	7.5	102	1	3	6	10	13	18	>99
65+	38	7.3	32	1	2	6	11	15	19	25
GRAND TOTAL	676	4.3	40	1	1	2	5	10	14	31

LOS by Diagnosis and Operation, Western Region, 45th Edition

Western Region, October 2007–September 2008 Data, by Operation

20.1: TYMPANOSTOMY TUBE RMVL

Type of Patients	Observed Patients	Avg. Stay	Vari-ance	Percentiles						
				10th	25th	50th	75th	90th	95th	99th
1. SINGLE DX										
0–19 Years	0									
20–34	0									
35–49	0									
50–64	0									
65+	0									
2. MULTIPLE DX										
0–19 Years	1	6.0	0	6	6	6	6	6	6	6
20–34	1	10.0	0	10	10	10	10	10	10	10
35–49	0									
50–64	2	9.5	141	1	1	1	18	18	18	18
65+	1	5.0	0	5	5	5	5	5	5	5
TOTAL SINGLE DX	0									
TOTAL MULTIPLE DX	5	8.0	41	1	5	6	10	18	18	18
TOTAL										
0–19 Years	1	6.0	0	6	6	6	6	6	6	6
20–34	1	10.0	0	10	10	10	10	10	10	10
35–49	0									
50–64	2	9.5	141	1	1	1	18	18	18	18
65+	1	5.0	0	5	5	5	5	5	5	5
GRAND TOTAL	5	8.0	41	1	5	6	10	18	18	18

20.2: MASTOID & MID EAR INC

Type of Patients	Observed Patients	Avg. Stay	Vari-ance	Percentiles						
				10th	25th	50th	75th	90th	95th	99th
1. SINGLE DX										
0–19 Years	0									
20–34	0									
35–49	2	1.0	0	1	1	1	1	1	1	1
50–64	0									
65+	0									
2. MULTIPLE DX										
0–19 Years	10	4.2	4	2	4	4	5	8	8	9
20–34	2	2.5	<1	2	2	2	3	3	3	3
35–49	9	1.6	2	1	1	1	1	5	5	5
50–64	6	3.3	32	1	1	1	1	15	15	15
65+	5	7.1	115	1	1	3	4	26	26	26
TOTAL SINGLE DX	2	1.0	0	1	1	1	1	1	1	1
TOTAL MULTIPLE DX	32	3.8	20	1	1	3	4	8	9	26
TOTAL										
0–19 Years	10	4.2	4	2	4	4	5	8	8	9
20–34	2	2.5	<1	2	2	2	3	3	3	3
35–49	11	1.5	1	1	1	1	1	2	5	5
50–64	6	3.3	32	1	1	1	1	15	15	15
65+	5	7.1	115	1	1	3	4	26	26	26
GRAND TOTAL	34	3.7	19	1	1	2	4	8	9	26

20.3: MID & INNER EAR DXTIC PX

Type of Patients	Observed Patients	Avg. Stay	Vari-ance	Percentiles						
				10th	25th	50th	75th	90th	95th	99th
1. SINGLE DX										
0–19 Years	0									
20–34	0									
35–49	0									
50–64	0									
65+	0									
2. MULTIPLE DX										
0–19 Years	3	15.6	226	6	6	6	32	38	38	38
20–34	0									
35–49	0									
50–64	0									
65+	2	1.5	<1	1	1	2	2	2	2	2
TOTAL SINGLE DX	0									
TOTAL MULTIPLE DX	5	12.1	204	1	6	6	6	38	38	38
TOTAL										
0–19 Years	3	15.6	226	6	6	6	32	38	38	38
20–34	0									
35–49	0									
50–64	0									
65+	2	1.5	<1	1	1	2	2	2	2	2
GRAND TOTAL	5	12.1	204	1	6	6	6	38	38	38

20.4: MASTOIDECTOMY

Type of Patients	Observed Patients	Avg. Stay	Vari-ance	Percentiles						
				10th	25th	50th	75th	90th	95th	99th
1. SINGLE DX										
0–19 Years	3	4.0	9	1	1	4	7	7	7	7
20–34	1	1.0	0	1	1	1	1	1	1	1
35–49	0									
50–64	0									
65+	0									
2. MULTIPLE DX										
0–19 Years	38	7.9	156	1	1	4	9	17	31	56
20–34	16	4.6	4	1	3	5	6	8	8	8
35–49	20	4.0	18	1	1	2	6	10	17	17
50–64	40	7.4	126	1	1	2	9	24	38	46
65+	42	5.0	49	1	1	3	7	11	13	42
TOTAL SINGLE DX	4	3.3	8	1	1	4	7	7	7	7
TOTAL MULTIPLE DX	156	6.6	103	1	1	3	7	14	31	56
TOTAL										
0–19 Years	41	7.8	151	1	1	4	8	17	31	56
20–34	17	4.5	5	1	3	5	6	6	8	8
35–49	20	4.0	18	1	1	2	6	10	17	17
50–64	40	7.4	126	1	1	2	9	24	38	46
65+	42	5.0	49	1	1	3	7	11	13	42
GRAND TOTAL	160	6.5	102	1	1	3	7	14	31	56

Western Region, October 2007–September 2008 Data, by Operation

20.5: OTH MIDDLE EAR EXCISION

Type of Patients	Observed Patients	Avg. Stay	Variance	10th	25th	50th	75th	90th	95th	99th
1. SINGLE DX										
0–19 Years	1	1.0	0	1	1	1	1	1	1	1
20–34	1	1.0	0	1	1	1	1	1	1	1
35–49	0									
50–64	2	1.5	<1	1	1	1	2	2	2	2
65+	0									
2. MULTIPLE DX										
0–19 Years	8	8.1	301	1	2	2	3	54	54	54
20–34	3	2.3	1	1	1	3	3	3	3	3
35–49	6	4.0	14	1	1	1	6	10	10	10
50–64	5	3.7	<1	3	3	4	4	4	4	4
65+	6	9.0	206	1	2	4	7	38	38	38
TOTAL SINGLE DX	4	1.1	<1	1	1	1	1	2	2	2
TOTAL MULTIPLE DX	26	6.2	141	1	1	3	4	10	38	54
TOTAL										
0–19 Years	9	5.9	212	1	1	2	3	4	54	54
20–34	4	2.0	1	1	1	1	3	3	3	3
35–49	6	4.0	14	1	1	1	6	10	10	10
50–64	5	2.8	2	1	2	3	4	4	4	4
65+	6	9.0	206	1	2	4	7	38	38	38
GRAND TOTAL	30	5.2	116	1	1	2	4	7	38	54

20.6: FENESTRATION INNER EAR

Type of Patients	Observed Patients	Avg. Stay	Variance	10th	25th	50th	75th	90th	95th	99th
1. SINGLE DX										
0–19 Years	0									
20–34	0									
35–49	0									
50–64	0									
65+	0									
2. MULTIPLE DX										
0–19 Years	0									
20–34	0									
35–49	0									
50–64	1	3.0	0	3	3	3	3	3	3	3
65+	0									
TOTAL SINGLE DX	0									
TOTAL MULTIPLE DX	1	3.0	0	3	3	3	3	3	3	3
TOTAL										
0–19 Years	0									
20–34	0									
35–49	0									
50–64	1	3.0	0	3	3	3	3	3	3	3
65+	0									
GRAND TOTAL	1	3.0	0	3	3	3	3	3	3	3

20.7: INC/EXC/DESTR INNER EAR

Type of Patients	Observed Patients	Avg. Stay	Variance	10th	25th	50th	75th	90th	95th	99th
1. SINGLE DX										
0–19 Years	0									
20–34	1	1.0	0	1	1	1	1	1	1	1
35–49	4	1.8	2	1	1	1	4	4	4	4
50–64	4	3.8	<1	3	4	4	4	4	4	4
65+	1	1.0	0	1	1	1	1	1	1	1
2. MULTIPLE DX										
0–19 Years	2	7.0	5	3	8	8	8	8	8	8
20–34	3	2.3	<1	2	2	2	3	3	3	3
35–49	12	3.4	6	1	1	3	5	8	8	8
50–64	14	2.7	1	1	2	3	3	4	5	5
65+	18	4.0	14	1	2	3	4	9	17	17
TOTAL SINGLE DX	10	2.4	2	1	1	1	4	4	4	4
TOTAL MULTIPLE DX	49	3.7	8	1	2	3	4	8	8	17
TOTAL										
0–19 Years	2	7.0	5	3	8	8	8	8	8	8
20–34	4	2.0	<1	1	1	2	3	3	3	3
35–49	16	3.0	6	1	1	3	4	8	8	8
50–64	18	2.9	1	1	2	3	4	4	5	5
65+	19	3.8	14	1	2	3	4	9	17	17
GRAND TOTAL	59	3.5	8	1	2	3	4	8	8	17

20.8: EUSTACHIAN TUBE OPS

Type of Patients	Observed Patients	Avg. Stay	Variance	10th	25th	50th	75th	90th	95th	99th
1. SINGLE DX										
0–19 Years	0									
20–34	0									
35–49	0									
50–64	0									
65+	0									
2. MULTIPLE DX										
0–19 Years	1	3.0	0	3	3	3	3	3	3	3
20–34	0									
35–49	0									
50–64	1	3.0	0	3	3	3	3	3	3	3
65+	0									
TOTAL SINGLE DX	0									
TOTAL MULTIPLE DX	2	3.0	0	3	3	3	3	3	3	3
TOTAL										
0–19 Years	1	3.0	0	3	3	3	3	3	3	3
20–34	0									
35–49	0									
50–64	1	3.0	0	3	3	3	3	3	3	3
65+	0									
GRAND TOTAL	2	3.0	0	3	3	3	3	3	3	3

LOS by Diagnosis and Operation, Western Region, 45th Edition

Western Region, October 2007–September 2008 Data, by Operation

20.9: OTHER ME & IE OPS

Type of Patients	Observed Patients	Avg. Stay	Variance	10th	25th	50th	75th	90th	95th	99th
1. SINGLE DX										
0–19 Years	11	1.1	<1	1	1	1	1	2	2	2
20–34	2	2.0	2	1	1	3	3	3	3	3
35–49	2	1.5	<1	1	1	2	2	2	2	2
50–64	1	2.0	0	2	2	2	2	2	2	2
65+	2	1.5	<1	1	1	2	2	2	2	2
2. MULTIPLE DX										
0–19 Years	32	1.3	1	1	1	1	1	1	2	7
20–34	2	1.0	0	1	1	1	1	1	1	1
35–49	12	1.9	2	1	1	1	3	4	5	5
50–64	18	1.8	1	1	1	1	2	4	4	4
65+	25	2.5	5	1	1	2	3	7	7	10
TOTAL SINGLE DX	18	1.2	<1	1	1	1	1	2	2	3
TOTAL MULTIPLE DX	89	1.6	2	1	1	1	1	3	5	7
TOTAL										
0–19 Years	43	1.3	1	1	1	1	1	2	2	7
20–34	4	1.5	<1	1	1	1	1	3	3	3
35–49	14	1.9	2	1	1	1	3	4	5	5
50–64	19	1.8	1	1	1	1	2	4	4	4
65+	27	2.4	5	1	1	2	3	7	7	10
GRAND TOTAL	107	1.5	2	1	1	1	1	3	4	7

21.0: CONTROL OF EPISTAXIS

Type of Patients	Observed Patients	Avg. Stay	Variance	10th	25th	50th	75th	90th	95th	99th
1. SINGLE DX										
0–19 Years	4	1.1	<1	1	1	1	1	2	2	2
20–34	9	2.2	2	1	1	2	3	4	4	4
35–49	15	1.3	<1	1	1	2	2	2	3	3
50–64	8	1.9	2	1	1	1	3	5	5	5
65+	4	4.8	6	2	2	4	8	8	8	8
2. MULTIPLE DX										
0–19 Years	55	5.2	32	1	1	3	7	14	14	16
20–34	107	4.4	46	1	1	2	4	8	17	36
35–49	246	3.7	13	1	1	3	5	7	9	22
50–64	503	4.1	24	1	2	3	5	8	13	26
65+	1,442	3.9	15	1	2	3	5	8	11	20
TOTAL SINGLE DX	40	1.9	2	1	1	1	2	4	5	8
TOTAL MULTIPLE DX	2,353	4.0	19	1	2	3	5	8	12	22
TOTAL										
0–19 Years	59	4.9	30	1	1	3	7	14	14	16
20–34	116	4.2	43	1	1	3	4	8	17	36
35–49	261	3.6	13	1	1	3	5	7	9	22
50–64	511	4.1	24	1	2	3	5	8	13	26
65+	1,446	4.0	15	2	2	3	5	8	11	20
GRAND TOTAL	2,393	4.0	18	1	1	3	5	8	12	22

21.01: ANT NAS PACK FOR EPISTX

Type of Patients	Observed Patients	Avg. Stay	Variance	10th	25th	50th	75th	90th	95th	99th
1. SINGLE DX										
0–19 Years	2	1.2	<1	1	1	1	1	2	2	2
20–34	1	1.0	0	1	1	1	1	1	1	1
35–49	2	1.0	0	1	1	1	1	1	1	1
50–64	1	3.0	0	3	3	3	3	3	3	3
65+	0									
2. MULTIPLE DX										
0–19 Years	22	6.5	52	1	2	5	7	10	16	40
20–34	44	5.0	46	1	2	2	5	11	18	36
35–49	105	3.8	16	1	1	2	5	8	9	22
50–64	217	4.4	24	1	2	3	5	11	14	28
65+	653	3.9	15	1	2	3	5	8	12	19
TOTAL SINGLE DX	6	1.3	<1	1	1	1	1	3	3	3
TOTAL MULTIPLE DX	1,041	4.1	20	1	2	3	5	8	12	23
TOTAL										
0–19 Years	24	5.7	48	1	1	5	6	10	16	40
20–34	45	4.9	45	1	2	2	5	11	18	36
35–49	107	3.7	16	1	1	2	5	8	9	22
50–64	218	4.4	24	1	2	3	5	11	14	28
65+	653	3.9	15	1	2	3	5	8	12	19
GRAND TOTAL	1,047	4.1	19	1	2	3	5	8	12	23

21.02: POST NAS PACK FOR EPISTX

Type of Patients	Observed Patients	Avg. Stay	Variance	10th	25th	50th	75th	90th	95th	99th
1. SINGLE DX										
0–19 Years	1	1.0	0	1	1	1	1	1	1	1
20–34	1	4.0	0	4	4	4	4	4	4	4
35–49	3	1.7	1	1	1	1	3	3	3	3
50–64	2	3.0	8	1	1	3	5	5	5	5
65+	1	2.0	0	2	2	2	2	2	2	2
2. MULTIPLE DX										
0–19 Years	4	3.5	9	1	1	3	7	7	7	7
20–34	17	2.9	6	1	1	3	3	5	11	11
35–49	51	3.5	14	1	2	2	5	6	6	8
50–64	107	3.6	14	1	2	3	4	6	8	17
65+	289	3.4	7	1	2	3	4	7	9	13
TOTAL SINGLE DX	8	2.3	2	1	1	1	3	5	5	5
TOTAL MULTIPLE DX	468	3.4	8	1	2	3	4	6	8	15
TOTAL										
0–19 Years	5	3.0	8	1	1	1	5	7	7	7
20–34	18	3.0	5	1	2	3	4	5	11	11
35–49	54	3.3	3	1	1	2	5	6	6	8
50–64	109	3.6	14	1	2	3	4	6	8	17
65+	290	3.4	7	1	2	3	4	7	9	13
GRAND TOTAL	476	3.4	8	1	2	3	4	6	8	15

LOS by Diagnosis and Operation, Western Region, 45th Edition

Western Region, October 2007–September 2008 Data, by Operation

21.03: CAUT TO CNTRL EPISTAXIS

Type of Patients	Observed Patients	Avg. Stay	Vari-ance	Percentiles 10th	25th	50th	75th	90th	95th	99th
1. SINGLE DX										
0–19 Years	1	1.0	0	1	1	1	1	1	1	1
20–34	5	1.6	<1	1	1	1	2	3	3	3
35–49	9	1.2	<1	1	1	1	1	2	2	2
50–64	5	1.2	<1	1	1	1	1	2	2	2
65+	2	6.0	8	4	4	8	8	8	8	8
2. MULTIPLE DX										
0–19 Years	24	4.5	24	1	1	2	5	14	14	15
20–34	37	4.2	70	1	1	2	4	8	24	48
35–49	72	3.6	17	1	1	2	4	7	9	30
50–64	121	3.6	12	1	1	2	5	7	10	18
65+	400	4.3	20	1	2	3	5	8	11	24
TOTAL SINGLE DX	22	1.7	3	1	1	1	2	3	4	8
TOTAL MULTIPLE DX	654	4.1	21	1	1	3	5	8	12	24
TOTAL										
0–19 Years	25	4.4	23	1	1	2	5	14	14	15
20–34	42	3.9	62	1	1	2	3	5	8	48
35–49	81	3.3	16	1	1	2	4	7	9	30
50–64	126	3.5	12	1	1	2	5	7	10	18
65+	402	4.3	20	1	2	3	5	8	11	23
GRAND TOTAL	676	4.0	21	1	1	3	5	8	12	23

21.09: EPISTAXIS CONTROL NEC

Type of Patients	Observed Patients	Avg. Stay	Vari-ance	Percentiles 10th	25th	50th	75th	90th	95th	99th
1. SINGLE DX										
0–19 Years	0									
20–34	1	4.0	0	4	4	4	4	4	4	4
35–49	1	1.0	0	1	1	1	1	1	1	1
50–64	0									
65+	0									
2. MULTIPLE DX										
0–19 Years	4	7.3	14	1	8	8	10	14	14	15
20–34	3	8.0	62	2	2	5	17	8	24	48
35–49	16	4.5	16	1	1	3	7	7	9	14
50–64	34	6.0	101	1	1	3	6	7	10	54
65+	69	4.7	18	1	2	3	6	8	11	22
TOTAL SINGLE DX	2	2.5	5	1	1	3	4	4	4	4
TOTAL MULTIPLE DX	126	5.2	41	1	2	3	6	8	12	26
TOTAL										
0–19 Years	4	7.3	14	1	8	8	10	14	14	10
20–34	4	7.0	46	2	2	5	17	17	17	17
35–49	17	4.3	15	1	1	3	7	12	14	14
50–64	34	6.0	101	1	1	3	6	15	26	54
65+	69	4.7	18	1	2	3	6	8	11	22
GRAND TOTAL	128	5.1	40	1	2	3	6	11	15	26

21.1: NOSE INCISION

Type of Patients	Observed Patients	Avg. Stay	Vari-ance	Percentiles 10th	25th	50th	75th	90th	95th	99th
1. SINGLE DX										
0–19 Years	6	2.8	18	1	1	1	2	14	14	14
20–34	5	2.8	4	1	1	3	3	6	6	6
35–49	6	2.8	2	1	2	3	4	5	5	5
50–64	1	1.0	0	1	1	1	1	1	1	1
65+	0									
2. MULTIPLE DX										
0–19 Years	23	2.8	3	2	2	2	4	4	8	9
20–34	26	3.2	3	1	2	3	4	5	6	7
35–49	49	3.8	4	2	3	3	4	7	8	10
50–64	49	4.3	7	2	3	4	5	7	8	17
65+	21	4.0	7	1	2	4	5	6	10	11
TOTAL SINGLE DX	18	2.7	9	1	1	2	3	5	6	14
TOTAL MULTIPLE DX	168	3.7	5	1	2	3	4	7	8	11
TOTAL										
0–19 Years	29	2.8	6	1	1	2	3	4	8	14
20–34	31	3.1	3	1	2	3	4	5	6	7
35–49	55	3.7	4	2	2	3	4	7	8	10
50–64	50	4.2	7	2	3	4	5	7	8	17
65+	21	4.0	7	1	2	4	5	6	10	11
GRAND TOTAL	186	3.6	5	1	2	3	4	6	8	14

21.2: NASAL DIAGNOSTIC PX

Type of Patients	Observed Patients	Avg. Stay	Vari-ance	Percentiles 10th	25th	50th	75th	90th	95th	99th
1. SINGLE DX										
0–19 Years	6	1.3	<1	1	1	1	1	1	4	4
20–34	3	4.0	7	2	2	3	7	7	7	7
35–49	0									
50–64	0									
65+	1	1.0	0	1	1	1	1	1	1	1
2. MULTIPLE DX										
0–19 Years	25	5.0	17	1	2	3	7	10	16	16
20–34	13	7.4	27	2	4	6	8	17	17	17
35–49	11	7.2	96	2	2	3	6	13	35	35
50–64	14	6.0	59	1	1	4	7	16	29	29
65+	30	4.7	5	2	3	4	6	7	9	11
TOTAL SINGLE DX	10	1.8	3	1	1	1	1	4	7	7
TOTAL MULTIPLE DX	93	5.5	27	1	2	4	7	11	16	29
TOTAL										
0–19 Years	31	4.3	16	1	1	3	6	10	16	16
20–34	16	6.8	25	2	3	6	8	17	17	17
35–49	11	7.2	96	2	2	3	6	13	35	35
50–64	14	6.0	59	1	1	4	7	16	29	29
65+	31	4.6	6	2	3	4	6	7	9	11
GRAND TOTAL	103	5.1	26	1	2	4	6	10	16	29

LOS by Diagnosis and Operation, Western Region, 45th Edition

73

Western Region, October 2007–September 2008 Data, by Operation

21.21: RHINOSCOPY

Type of Patients	Observed Patients	Avg. Stay	Variance	10th	25th	50th	75th	90th	95th	99th
1. SINGLE DX										
0–19 Years	3	1.0	0	1	1	1	1	1	1	1
20–34	0									
35–49	0									
50–64	0									
65+	0									
2. MULTIPLE DX										
0–19 Years	22	4.1	19	1	2	3	4	16	16	16
20–34	8	6.3	25	1	3	6	8	17	17	17
35–49	8	8.7	126	2	2	3	6	35	35	35
50–64	11	6.9	72	1	1	4	7	16	29	29
65+	25	4.1	3	2	3	4	5	6	7	9
TOTAL SINGLE DX	3	1.0	0	1	1	1	1	1	1	1
TOTAL MULTIPLE DX	74	5.1	31	1	2	3	6	13	16	35
TOTAL										
0–19 Years	25	3.5	17	1	1	2	4	7	16	16
20–34	8	6.3	25	1	3	6	8	17	17	17
35–49	8	8.7	126	2	2	3	6	35	35	35
50–64	11	6.9	72	1	1	4	7	16	29	29
65+	25	4.1	3	2	3	4	5	6	7	9
GRAND TOTAL	77	4.7	30	1	2	3	5	9	16	35

21.3: NASAL LESION DESTR/EXC

Type of Patients	Observed Patients	Avg. Stay	Variance	10th	25th	50th	75th	90th	95th	99th
1. SINGLE DX										
0–19 Years	6	1.3	<1	1	1	1	2	2	2	2
20–34	0									
35–49	1	1.0	0	1	1	1	1	1	1	1
50–64	2	1.0	0	1	1	1	1	1	1	1
65+	1	2.0	0	2	2	2	2	2	2	2
2. MULTIPLE DX										
0–19 Years	15	1.8	1	1	1	1	2	3	4	4
20–34	3	4.3	2	3	3	4	6	6	6	6
35–49	6	2.2	4	1	1	1	3	6	6	6
50–64	6	3.0	8	1	1	2	4	8	8	8
65+	24	3.5	8	2	1	3	5	8	9	10
TOTAL SINGLE DX	10	1.3	<1	1	1	1	2	2	2	2
TOTAL MULTIPLE DX	54	2.5	4	1	1	2	3	6	7	10
TOTAL										
0–19 Years	21	1.6	<1	1	1	1	2	3	4	4
20–34	3	4.3	2	3	3	4	6	6	6	6
35–49	7	2.0	4	1	1	1	3	6	6	6
50–64	8	2.5	6	1	1	2	3	8	8	8
65+	25	3.5	8	1	1	3	5	8	9	10
GRAND TOTAL	64	2.2	4	1	1	1	3	4	6	9

21.4: RESECTION OF NOSE

Type of Patients	Observed Patients	Avg. Stay	Variance	10th	25th	50th	75th	90th	95th	99th
1. SINGLE DX										
0–19 Years	0									
20–34	0									
35–49	0									
50–64	0									
65+	1	1.0	0	1	1	1	1	1	1	1
2. MULTIPLE DX										
0–19 Years	1	1.0	0	1	1	1	1	1	1	1
20–34	1	4.0	0	4	4	4	4	4	4	4
35–49	1	4.0	0	4	4	4	4	4	4	4
50–64	12	4.9	59	1	1	1	4	9	28	28
65+	16	3.0	6	1	1	2	5	6	9	9
TOTAL SINGLE DX	1	1.0	0	1	1	1	1	1	1	1
TOTAL MULTIPLE DX	31	3.7	26	1	1	2	4	7	9	28
TOTAL										
0–19 Years	1	1.0	0	1	1	1	1	1	1	1
20–34	1	4.0	0	4	4	4	4	4	4	4
35–49	1	4.0	0	4	4	4	4	4	4	4
50–64	12	4.9	59	1	1	1	4	9	28	28
65+	17	2.9	6	1	1	2	4	6	9	9
GRAND TOTAL	32	3.6	25	1	1	2	4	7	9	28

21.5: SUBMUC NAS SEPTUM RESECT

Type of Patients	Observed Patients	Avg. Stay	Variance	10th	25th	50th	75th	90th	95th	99th
1. SINGLE DX										
0–19 Years	2	2.6	<1	1	3	3	3	3	3	3
20–34	0									
35–49	0									
50–64	0									
65+	0									
2. MULTIPLE DX										
0–19 Years	8	1.3	1	1	1	1	1	2	6	6
20–34	20	2.4	9	1	1	1	2	4	11	11
35–49	62	1.6	2	1	1	1	2	3	4	9
50–64	51	2.5	39	1	1	1	3	4	6	44
65+	27	3.9	52	1	1	2	3	7	15	37
TOTAL SINGLE DX	2	2.6	<1	1	3	3	3	3	3	3
TOTAL MULTIPLE DX	168	2.3	21	1	1	1	2	4	6	37
TOTAL										
0–19 Years	10	1.6	2	1	1	1	2	3	3	6
20–34	20	2.4	9	1	1	1	2	4	11	11
35–49	62	1.6	2	1	1	1	2	3	4	9
50–64	51	2.5	39	1	1	1	3	4	6	44
65+	27	3.9	52	1	1	2	3	7	15	37
GRAND TOTAL	170	2.3	20	1	1	1	2	4	6	37

LOS by Diagnosis and Operation, Western Region, 45th Edition

74

Western Region, October 2007–September 2008 Data, by Operation

21.6: TURBINECTOMY

Type of Patients	Observed Patients	Avg. Stay	Vari-ance	Percentiles						
				10th	25th	50th	75th	90th	95th	99th
1. SINGLE DX										
0–19 Years	0									
20–34	0									
35–49	1	1.0	0	1	1	1	1	1	1	1
50–64	0									
65+	0									
2. MULTIPLE DX										
0–19 Years	8	25.1	456	1	1	35	49	49	49	49
20–34	18	2.2	5	1	1	1	3	5	9	9
35–49	26	1.6	<1	1	1	1	2	3	4	4
50–64	41	2.2	12	1	1	1	2	3	8	21
65+	19	4.0	22	1	1	2	5	9	21	21
TOTAL SINGLE DX	**1**	**1.0**	**0**	**1**	**1**	**1**	**1**	**1**	**1**	**1**
TOTAL MULTIPLE DX	**112**	**5.1**	**116**	**1**	**1**	**1**	**3**	**9**	**35**	**49**
TOTAL										
0–19 Years	8	25.1	456	1	1	35	49	49	49	49
20–34	18	2.2	5	1	1	1	3	5	9	9
35–49	27	1.6	<1	1	1	1	2	3	4	4
50–64	41	2.2	12	1	1	1	2	3	8	21
65+	19	4.0	22	1	1	2	5	9	21	21
GRAND TOTAL	**113**	**5.1**	**115**	**1**	**1**	**1**	**3**	**9**	**35**	**49**

21.7: NASAL FRACTURE REDUCTION

Type of Patients	Observed Patients	Avg. Stay	Vari-ance	Percentiles						
				10th	25th	50th	75th	90th	95th	99th
1. SINGLE DX										
0–19 Years	4	1.2	<1	1	1	1	1	2	2	2
20–34	8	1.1	<1	1	1	1	1	2	2	2
35–49	4	1.3	<1	1	1	1	2	2	2	2
50–64	2	1.0	0	1	1	1	1	1	1	1
65+	0									
2. MULTIPLE DX										
0–19 Years	38	2.6	4	1	1	2	4	5	7	10
20–34	93	2.7	5	1	1	2	4	6	7	13
35–49	60	3.1	22	1	1	2	3	5	16	29
50–64	57	3.9	22	1	1	2	4	7	16	24
65+	31	4.2	8	1	2	4	6	9	10	10
TOTAL SINGLE DX	**18**	**1.2**	**<1**	**1**	**1**	**1**	**1**	**2**	**2**	**2**
TOTAL MULTIPLE DX	**279**	**3.2**	**12**	**1**	**1**	**2**	**4**	**6**	**9**	**23**
TOTAL										
0–19 Years	42	2.5	4	1	1	2	4	5	7	10
20–34	101	2.6	5	1	1	2	4	5	6	12
35–49	64	3.0	20	1	1	2	3	4	6	29
50–64	59	3.8	22	1	1	2	4	7	16	24
65+	31	4.2	8	1	2	4	6	9	10	10
GRAND TOTAL	**297**	**3.0**	**12**	**1**	**1**	**2**	**4**	**6**	**9**	**20**

21.71: CLSD REDUCTION NASAL FX

Type of Patients	Observed Patients	Avg. Stay	Vari-ance	Percentiles						
				10th	25th	50th	75th	90th	95th	99th
1. SINGLE DX										
0–19 Years	4	1.2	<1	1	1	1	2	2	2	2
20–34	5	1.0	0	1	1	1	1	1	1	1
35–49	2	1.5	<1	1	1	2	2	2	2	2
50–64	2	1.0	0	1	1	1	1	1	1	1
65+	0									
2. MULTIPLE DX										
0–19 Years	23	3.1	5	1	1	3	4	5	8	10
20–34	58	2.8	5	1	1	2	4	6	7	12
35–49	28	3.7	37	1	2	2	3	4	20	29
50–64	32	4.2	23	1	2	3	4	7	16	24
65+	25	4.0	8	1	2	3	6	9	9	10
TOTAL SINGLE DX	**13**	**1.2**	**<1**	**1**	**1**	**1**	**1**	**2**	**2**	**2**
TOTAL MULTIPLE DX	**166**	**3.4**	**14**	**1**	**1**	**2**	**4**	**6**	**9**	**24**
TOTAL										
0–19 Years	27	2.9	4	1	1	2	4	5	8	10
20–34	63	2.7	5	1	1	2	4	5	6	12
35–49	30	3.5	35	1	1	3	3	4	20	29
50–64	34	4.0	22	1	2	3	4	7	16	24
65+	25	4.0	8	1	2	3	6	9	9	10
GRAND TOTAL	**179**	**3.3**	**13**	**1**	**1**	**2**	**4**	**6**	**9**	**24**

21.72: OPEN REDUCTION NASAL FX

Type of Patients	Observed Patients	Avg. Stay	Vari-ance	Percentiles						
				10th	25th	50th	75th	90th	95th	99th
1. SINGLE DX										
0–19 Years	0									
20–34	3	1.3	<1	1	1	1	2	2	2	2
35–49	2	1.0	0	1	1	1	1	1	1	1
50–64	0									
65+	0									
2. MULTIPLE DX										
0–19 Years	15	1.8	3	1	1	1	2	5	7	7
20–34	35	2.6	6	1	1	1	3	6	7	13
35–49	32	2.6	8	1	1	2	3	5	6	16
50–64	25	3.4	22	1	1	2	4	7	10	23
65+	6	4.8	8	1	4	4	5	10	10	10
TOTAL SINGLE DX	**5**	**1.2**	**<1**	**1**	**1**	**1**	**1**	**2**	**2**	**2**
TOTAL MULTIPLE DX	**113**	**2.8**	**10**	**1**	**1**	**1**	**3**	**6**	**7**	**16**
TOTAL										
0–19 Years	15	1.8	3	1	1	1	2	5	7	7
20–34	38	2.5	6	1	1	1	3	6	7	13
35–49	34	2.5	8	1	1	1	3	5	6	16
50–64	25	3.4	22	1	1	2	4	7	10	23
65+	6	4.8	8	1	4	4	5	10	10	10
GRAND TOTAL	**118**	**2.7**	**10**	**1**	**1**	**1**	**3**	**6**	**7**	**16**

LOS by Diagnosis and Operation, Western Region, 45th Edition

Western Region, October 2007–September 2008 Data, by Operation

21.8: NASAL REP & PLASTIC OPS

Type of Patients	Observed Patients	Avg. Stay	Variance	10th	25th	50th	75th	90th	95th	99th
1. SINGLE DX										
0–19 Years	27	1.1	<1	1	1	1	1	1	1	4
20–34	5	1.8	3	1	1	1	1	5	5	5
35–49	3	2.7	8	1	1	1	6	6	6	6
50–64	8	2.3	10	1	1	2	2	10	10	10
65+	3	1.7	<1	1	1	2	2	2	2	2
2. MULTIPLE DX										
0–19 Years	172	1.8	6	1	1	1	2	3	6	15
20–34	170	1.8	4	1	1	1	2	4	6	14
35–49	265	1.9	3	1	1	1	2	4	5	7
50–64	320	2.0	4	1	1	1	2	4	5	12
65+	273	2.8	9	1	1	2	4	6	9	16
TOTAL SINGLE DX	46	1.3	2	1	1	1	1	1	2	10
TOTAL MULTIPLE DX	1,200	2.1	6	1	1	1	2	4	6	14
TOTAL										
0–19 Years	199	1.7	6	1	1	1	1	3	4	15
20–34	175	1.8	4	1	1	1	2	4	6	14
35–49	268	1.9	3	1	1	1	2	4	5	7
50–64	328	2.0	4	1	1	1	2	4	5	12
65+	276	2.8	9	1	1	2	4	6	9	16
GRAND TOTAL	1,246	2.0	5	1	1	1	2	4	6	14

21.88: SEPTOPLASTY NEC

Type of Patients	Observed Patients	Avg. Stay	Variance	10th	25th	50th	75th	90th	95th	99th
1. SINGLE DX										
0–19 Years	3	1.0	0	1	1	1	1	1	1	1
20–34	2	1.0	0	1	1	1	1	1	1	1
35–49	1	1.0	0	1	1	1	1	1	1	1
50–64	5	1.2	<1	1	1	1	1	2	2	2
65+	1	2.0	0	2	2	2	2	2	2	2
2. MULTIPLE DX										
0–19 Years	21	1.8	6	1	1	1	1	4	5	13
20–34	70	2.2	7	1	1	1	2	6	7	14
35–49	166	1.7	3	1	1	1	2	3	4	7
50–64	186	1.7	2	1	1	1	2	3	4	11
65+	82	2.0	6	1	1	2	2	4	6	15
TOTAL SINGLE DX	12	1.1	<1	1	1	1	1	2	2	2
TOTAL MULTIPLE DX	525	1.8	4	1	1	1	2	3	5	13
TOTAL										
0–19 Years	24	1.6	5	1	1	1	1	2	5	13
20–34	72	2.2	7	1	1	1	2	5	7	14
35–49	167	1.7	3	1	1	1	2	3	4	7
50–64	191	1.7	2	1	1	1	2	3	4	11
65+	83	2.0	6	1	1	1	2	4	6	15
GRAND TOTAL	537	1.8	4	1	1	1	2	3	5	13

21.81: NASAL LACERATION SUTURE

Type of Patients	Observed Patients	Avg. Stay	Variance	10th	25th	50th	75th	90th	95th	99th
1. SINGLE DX										
0–19 Years	3	1.0	0	1	1	1	1	1	1	1
20–34	0									
35–49	1	1.0	0	1	1	1	1	1	1	1
50–64	0									
65+	0									
2. MULTIPLE DX										
0–19 Years	33	1.6	1	1	1	1	2	3	4	6
20–34	63	1.7	2	1	1	1	2	3	4	8
35–49	53	2.6	4	1	1	2	3	5	7	10
50–64	84	2.4	6	1	1	2	3	4	5	18
65+	128	3.5	10	1	1	3	4	6	9	16
TOTAL SINGLE DX	4	1.0	0	1	1	1	1	1	1	1
TOTAL MULTIPLE DX	361	2.6	7	1	1	2	3	5	7	15
TOTAL										
0–19 Years	36	1.6	1	1	1	1	2	3	3	6
20–34	63	1.7	2	1	1	1	2	3	4	8
35–49	54	2.5	4	1	1	2	3	5	7	10
50–64	84	2.4	6	1	1	2	3	4	5	18
65+	128	3.5	10	1	1	3	4	6	9	16
GRAND TOTAL	365	2.6	7	1	1	2	3	5	7	15

21.89: NASAL REPAIR NEC

Type of Patients	Observed Patients	Avg. Stay	Variance	10th	25th	50th	75th	90th	95th	99th
1. SINGLE DX										
0–19 Years	6	1.3	<1	1	1	1	1	1	4	4
20–34	2	3.0	8	1	1	1	5	5	5	5
35–49	0									
50–64	1	1.0	0	1	1	1	1	1	1	1
65+	2	1.5	<1	1	1	1	2	2	2	2
2. MULTIPLE DX										
0–19 Years	27	4.5	28	1	1	3	3	14	15	26
20–34	13	1.2	<1	1	1	1	1	2	2	2
35–49	13	1.9	3	1	1	1	3	4	4	4
50–64	21	2.3	3	1	1	1	3	6	6	6
65+	36	3.0	15	1	1	1	2	10	11	18
TOTAL SINGLE DX	11	1.5	1	1	1	1	1	4	5	5
TOTAL MULTIPLE DX	110	3.3	17	1	1	2	3	10	14	18
TOTAL										
0–19 Years	33	4.0	25	1	1	2	3	12	15	26
20–34	15	1.4	1	1	1	1	1	2	5	5
35–49	13	1.9	1	1	1	1	3	4	4	4
50–64	22	2.3	3	1	1	1	3	6	6	6
65+	38	2.9	14	1	1	1	2	10	11	18
GRAND TOTAL	121	3.1	16	1	1	1	3	10	14	18

LOS by Diagnosis and Operation, Western Region, 45th Edition

Western Region, October 2007–September 2008 Data, by Operation

21.9: OTHER NASAL OPERATIONS

Type of Patients	Observed Patients	Avg. Stay	Variance	10th	25th	50th	75th	90th	95th	99th
1. SINGLE DX										
0–19 Years	0									
20–34	1	1.0	0						1	1
35–49	0									
50–64	0									
65+	0									
2. MULTIPLE DX										
0–19 Years	5	6.8	66	1	1	3	4	21	21	21
20–34	2	1.0	0	1	1	1	1	1	1	1
35–49	0									
50–64	2	1.5	<1	1	1	1	2	2	2	2
65+	1	3.0	0	3	3	3	3	3	3	3
TOTAL SINGLE DX	1	1.0	0	1	1	1	1	1	1	1
TOTAL MULTIPLE DX	10	5.7	56	1	1	3	4	21	21	21
TOTAL										
0–19 Years	5	6.8	66	1	1	3	4	21	21	21
20–34	3	1.0	0	1	1	1	1	1	1	1
35–49	0									
50–64	2	1.5	<1	1	1	1	2	2	2	2
65+	1	3.0	0	3	3	3	3	3	3	3
GRAND TOTAL	11	5.5	54	1	1	3	4	21	21	21

22.1: NASAL SINUS DXTIC PX

Type of Patients	Observed Patients	Avg. Stay	Variance	10th	25th	50th	75th	90th	95th	99th
1. SINGLE DX										
0–19 Years	1	1.0	0	1	1	1	1	1	1	1
20–34	0									
35–49	2	1.0	0	1	1	1	1	1	1	1
50–64	1	1.0	0	1	1	1	1	1	1	1
65+	0									
2. MULTIPLE DX										
0–19 Years	12	13.5	166	3	4	8	30	30	39	43
20–34	4	12.7	10	8	8	14	15	15	15	15
35–49	12	4.3	4	2	3	5	6	6	8	8
50–64	15	6.3	29	2	2	5	8	11	22	22
65+	19	6.8	28	2	3	5	9	16	22	22
TOTAL SINGLE DX	4	1.0	0	1	1	1	1	1	1	1
TOTAL MULTIPLE DX	62	8.7	77	2	3	6	9	22	30	43
TOTAL										
0–19 Years	13	13.0	165	3	4	8	30	30	39	43
20–34	4	12.7	10	8	8	14	15	15	15	15
35–49	14	3.8	5	1	2	4	6	6	8	8
50–64	16	6.0	29	2	3	5	8	11	22	22
65+	19	6.8	28	2	3	5	9	16	22	22
GRAND TOTAL	66	8.3	76	2	3	5	9	22	30	43

22.0: NASAL SINUS ASP & LAVAGE

Type of Patients	Observed Patients	Avg. Stay	Variance	10th	25th	50th	75th	90th	95th	99th
1. SINGLE DX										
0–19 Years	1	4.0	0	4	4	4	4	4	4	4
20–34	1	1.0	0	1	1	1	1	1	1	1
35–49	0									
50–64	1	6.0	0	6	6	6	6	6	6	6
65+	0									
2. MULTIPLE DX										
0–19 Years	12	8.4	39	3	4	5	13	18	18	18
20–34	1	5.0	0	5	5	5	5	5	5	5
35–49	5	3.8	4	1	5	5	5	5	5	5
50–64	5	4.6	4	2	4	4	6	7	7	7
65+	4	4.5	4	3	3	5	7	7	7	7
TOTAL SINGLE DX	3	3.8	3	1	4	4	4	6	6	6
TOTAL MULTIPLE DX	28	6.5	26	3	3	4	7	18	18	18
TOTAL										
0–19 Years	13	7.6	34	3	4	4	13	18	18	18
20–34	2	3.0	8	1	1	3	5	5	5	5
35–49	6	3.8	4	1	3	3	5	7	7	7
50–64	6	4.8	3	2	4	4	6	7	7	7
65+	4	4.5	4	3	3	5	7	7	7	7
GRAND TOTAL	31	6.1	23	3	3	4	7	18	18	18

22.19: NASAL SINUS DXTIC PX NEC

Type of Patients	Observed Patients	Avg. Stay	Variance	10th	25th	50th	75th	90th	95th	99th
1. SINGLE DX										
0–19 Years	1	1.0	0	1	1	1	1	1	1	1
20–34	0									
35–49	0									
50–64	0									
65+										
2. MULTIPLE DX										
0–19 Years	7	8.8	176	2	3	4	4	43	43	43
20–34	3	12.3	14	8	8	14	15	15	15	15
35–49	6	5.0	2	3	4	6	6	6	6	6
50–64	9	7.1	40	2	3	4	8	22	22	22
65+	14	4.6	5	2	3	4	7	7	9	9
TOTAL SINGLE DX	1	1.0	0	1	1	1	1	1	1	1
TOTAL MULTIPLE DX	39	6.7	50	2	3	4	7	11	15	43
TOTAL										
0–19 Years	8	8.0	162	1	3	4	4	43	43	43
20–34	3	12.3	14	8	8	14	15	15	15	15
35–49	6	5.0	2	4	4	6	6	6	6	6
50–64	9	7.1	40	2	3	6	7	7	9	9
65+	14	4.6	5	2	3	4	7	7	9	9
GRAND TOTAL	40	6.5	49	2	3	4	7	11	15	43

LOS by Diagnosis and Operation, Western Region, 45th Edition

77

Western Region, October 2007–September 2008 Data, by Operation

22.2: INTRANASAL ANTROTOMY

Type of Patients	Observed Patients	Avg. Stay	Variance	Percentiles						
				10th	25th	50th	75th	90th	95th	99th
1. SINGLE DX										
0–19 Years	0									
20–34	1	1.0	0	1	1	1	1	1	1	1
35–49	0									
50–64	0									
65+	0									
2. MULTIPLE DX										
0–19 Years	7	7.3	30	2	2	12	14	>99	>99	>99
20–34	2	6.0	9	5	5	7	7	7	7	7
35–49	4	4.3	5	1	1	5	6	6	6	6
50–64	7	3.6	6	1	2	2	6	7	7	7
65+	8	5.5	12	1	3	7	8	11	11	11
TOTAL SINGLE DX	**1**	**1.0**	**0**	**1**	**1**	**1**	**1**	**1**	**1**	**1**
TOTAL MULTIPLE DX	**28**	**5.7**	**18**	**2**	**2**	**5**	**12**	**>99**	**>99**	**>99**
TOTAL										
0–19 Years	7	7.3	30	2	2	12	14	>99	>99	>99
20–34	3	4.4	9	2	1	5	7	7	7	7
35–49	4	4.3	5	1	1	5	6	6	6	6
50–64	7	3.6	6	1	2	2	6	7	7	7
65+	8	5.5	12	1	3	7	8	11	11	11
GRAND TOTAL	**29**	**5.6**	**18**	**2**	**2**	**5**	**11**	**>99**	**>99**	**>99**

22.3: EXT MAXILLARY ANTROTOMY

Type of Patients	Observed Patients	Avg. Stay	Variance	Percentiles						
				10th	25th	50th	75th	90th	95th	99th
1. SINGLE DX										
0–19 Years	0									
20–34	1	1.0	0	1	1	1	1	1	1	1
35–49	1	1.0	0	1	1	1	1	1	1	1
50–64	0									
65+	0									
2. MULTIPLE DX										
0–19 Years	3	30.1	162	5	27	37	37	37	37	37
20–34	9	3.2	15	1	1	1	3	5	13	13
35–49	5	2.8	2	1	2	3	3	5	5	5
50–64	15	4.9	23	1	1	2	7	12	17	17
65+	4	2.8	12	1	1	1	8	8	8	8
TOTAL SINGLE DX	**2**	**1.0**	**0**	**1**	**1**	**1**	**1**	**1**	**1**	**1**
TOTAL MULTIPLE DX	**36**	**7.9**	**128**	**1**	**1**	**3**	**8**	**37**	**37**	**37**
TOTAL										
0–19 Years	3	30.1	162	5	27	37	37	37	37	37
20–34	10	3.0	14	1	1	1	3	5	13	13
35–49	6	2.5	2	1	1	3	3	5	5	5
50–64	15	4.9	23	1	1	2	7	12	17	17
65+	4	2.8	12	1	1	1	8	8	8	8
GRAND TOTAL	**38**	**7.6**	**124**	**1**	**1**	**3**	**7**	**27**	**37**	**37**

22.4: FRONT SINUSOT & SINUSECT

Type of Patients	Observed Patients	Avg. Stay	Variance	Percentiles						
				10th	25th	50th	75th	90th	95th	99th
1. SINGLE DX										
0–19 Years	0									
20–34	2	3.0	0	3	3	3	3	3	3	3
35–49	3	2.7	2	1	1	3	4	4	4	4
50–64	1	1.0	0	1	1	1	1	1	1	1
65+	0									
2. MULTIPLE DX										
0–19 Years	19	8.4	115	1	3	4	11	37	37	37
20–34	26	9.8	86	2	3	7	14	19	35	35
35–49	30	3.9	15	1	1	2	4	13	14	14
50–64	34	4.2	40	1	2	3	6	7	9	37
65+	22	3.5	6	1	2	3	4	7	8	10
TOTAL SINGLE DX	**6**	**2.5**	**1**	**1**	**1**	**3**	**3**	**4**	**4**	**4**
TOTAL MULTIPLE DX	**131**	**6.1**	**63**	**1**	**2**	**4**	**7**	**13**	**25**	**37**
TOTAL										
0–19 Years	19	8.4	115	1	3	4	11	37	37	37
20–34	28	9.3	83	2	3	5	14	19	35	35
35–49	33	3.8	14	1	1	3	4	13	14	14
50–64	35	4.1	39	1	2	3	6	7	9	37
65+	22	3.5	6	1	2	3	4	7	8	10
GRAND TOTAL	**137**	**6.0**	**61**	**1**	**2**	**3**	**7**	**13**	**25**	**37**

22.5: OTHER NASAL SINUSOTOMY

Type of Patients	Observed Patients	Avg. Stay	Variance	Percentiles						
				10th	25th	50th	75th	90th	95th	99th
1. SINGLE DX										
0–19 Years	1	1.0	0	1	1	1	1	1	1	1
20–34	0									
35–49	0									
50–64	0									
65+	0									
2. MULTIPLE DX										
0–19 Years	10	14.2	360	2	3	8	14	58	58	58
20–34	13	9.7	91	3	4	8	8	23	37	37
35–49	13	6.2	36	1	1	4	9	16	18	18
50–64	19	9.3	148	1	1	4	13	25	49	49
65+	16	9.5	237	1	2	4	9	22	63	63
TOTAL SINGLE DX	**1**	**1.0**	**0**	**1**	**1**	**1**	**1**	**1**	**1**	**1**
TOTAL MULTIPLE DX	**71**	**10.5**	**203**	**1**	**3**	**6**	**11**	**22**	**58**	**63**
TOTAL										
0–19 Years	11	13.8	353	2	3	8	14	58	58	58
20–34	13	9.7	91	3	4	8	8	23	37	37
35–49	13	6.2	36	1	1	4	9	16	18	18
50–64	19	9.3	148	1	1	4	13	25	49	49
65+	16	9.5	237	1	2	4	9	22	63	63
GRAND TOTAL	**72**	**10.4**	**202**	**1**	**2**	**5**	**10**	**22**	**58**	**63**

LOS by Diagnosis and Operation, Western Region, 45th Edition

Western Region, October 2007–September 2008 Data, by Operation

22.6: OTHER NASAL SINUSECTOMY

Type of Patients	Observed Patients	Avg. Stay	Variance	Percentiles						
				10th	25th	50th	75th	90th	95th	99th
1. SINGLE DX										
0–19 Years	9	2.4	1	1	2	2	3	4	4	4
20–34	3	1.0	0	1	1	1	1	1	1	1
35–49	12	2.1	3	1	1	2	2	3	7	7
50–64	6	1.5	<1	1	1	1	2	3	3	3
65+	1	1.0	0	1	1	1	1	1	1	1
2. MULTIPLE DX										
0–19 Years	143	9.6	133	1	4	6	13	18	27	>99
20–34	81	9.0	124	1	2	6	14	17	20	71
35–49	97	5.1	56	1	1	3	6	10	14	55
50–64	180	5.2	79	1	1	2	5	14	18	56
65+	141	4.9	48	1	1	2	6	12	15	42
TOTAL SINGLE DX	31	2.0	2	1	1	2	2	4	4	7
TOTAL MULTIPLE DX	642	7.3	103	1	1	4	10	15	22	71
TOTAL										
0–19 Years	152	9.3	130	1	4	6	13	17	27	>99
20–34	84	8.8	122	1	2	6	13	16	20	71
35–49	109	4.7	51	1	1	3	6	10	13	43
50–64	186	5.1	77	1	1	2	5	14	18	56
65+	142	4.9	48	1	1	2	6	12	15	42
GRAND TOTAL	673	7.1	100	1	1	4	9	15	21	71

22.62: EXC MAX SINUS LESION NEC

Type of Patients	Observed Patients	Avg. Stay	Variance	Percentiles						
				10th	25th	50th	75th	90th	95th	99th
1. SINGLE DX										
0–19 Years	5	2.7	1	2	2	2	4	4	4	4
20–34	1	1.0	0	1	1	1	1	1	1	1
35–49	7	1.9	<1	1	1	2	2	3	3	3
50–64	0									
65+	0									
2. MULTIPLE DX										
0–19 Years	44	10.2	44	1	5	11	15	22	27	>99
20–34	24	8.9	38	1	3	7	14	16	19	20
35–49	36	5.7	83	1	1	4	7	10	13	55
50–64	55	6.4	104	1	1	3	6	17	21	58
65+	49	6.1	56	1	1	4	8	13	21	42
TOTAL SINGLE DX	13	2.3	1	1	2	2	3	4	4	4
TOTAL MULTIPLE DX	208	8.1	65	1	2	6	13	17	22	>99
TOTAL										
0–19 Years	49	9.6	45	1	4	9	14	22	27	>99
20–34	25	8.6	38	1	2	7	14	16	19	20
35–49	43	5.1	71	1	1	3	6	10	13	55
50–64	55	6.4	104	1	1	3	6	17	21	58
65+	49	6.1	56	1	1	4	8	13	21	42
GRAND TOTAL	221	7.7	63	1	2	5	13	17	22	>99

22.63: ETHMOIDECTOMY

Type of Patients	Observed Patients	Avg. Stay	Variance	Percentiles						
				10th	25th	50th	75th	90th	95th	99th
1. SINGLE DX										
0–19 Years	2	2.5	<1	2	2	3	3	3	3	3
20–34	2	1.0	0	1	1	1	1	1	1	1
35–49	4	1.3	<1	1	1	1	2	2	2	2
50–64	2	1.0	0	1	1	1	1	1	1	1
65+	1	1.0	0	1	1	1	1	1	1	1
2. MULTIPLE DX										
0–19 Years	79	9.9	214	3	3	5	11	18	43	81
20–34	46	8.7	200	1	2	4	10	17	31	71
35–49	47	4.1	41	1	1	3	4	8	11	43
50–64	94	4.7	79	1	1	1	5	10	18	56
65+	65	3.8	25	1	1	2	4	9	14	24
TOTAL SINGLE DX	11	1.4	<1	1	1	1	2	2	3	3
TOTAL MULTIPLE DX	331	7.1	144	1	1	4	8	14	22	71
TOTAL										
0–19 Years	81	9.8	213	1	3	5	10	18	43	81
20–34	48	8.4	194	1	2	4	9	17	31	71
35–49	51	3.9	38	1	1	2	4	7	11	43
50–64	96	4.7	77	1	1	2	5	10	18	56
65+	66	3.8	24	1	1	2	4	9	14	24
GRAND TOTAL	342	7.0	141	1	1	4	8	14	22	71

22.7: NASAL SINUS REPAIR

Type of Patients	Observed Patients	Avg. Stay	Variance	Percentiles						
				10th	25th	50th	75th	90th	95th	99th
1. SINGLE DX										
0–19 Years	1	2.0	0	2	2	2	2	2	2	2
20–34	0									
35–49	0									
50–64	0									
65+	0									
2. MULTIPLE DX										
0–19 Years	1	1.0	0	1	1	1	1	1	1	1
20–34	0									
35–49	5	5.5	4	4	4	7	7	7	7	7
50–64	4	9.0	64	3	3	7	10	20	20	20
65+	3	5.4	34	1	1	3	12	12	12	12
TOTAL SINGLE DX	1	2.0	0	2	2	2	2	2	2	2
TOTAL MULTIPLE DX	10	5.2	33	1	1	3	7	12	20	20
TOTAL										
0–19 Years	2	1.2	<1	1	1	1	1	2	2	2
20–34	0									
35–49	2	5.5	4	4	4	7	7	7	7	7
50–64	4	9.0	64	3	3	7	10	20	20	20
65+	3	5.4	34	1	1	3	12	12	12	12
GRAND TOTAL	11	4.9	31	1	1	3	7	12	20	20

LOS by Diagnosis and Operation, Western Region, 45th Edition

Western Region, October 2007–September 2008 Data, by Operation

22.9: OTHER NASAL SINUS OPS

Type of Patients	Observed Patients	Avg. Stay	Vari-ance	10th	25th	50th	75th	90th	95th	99th
1. SINGLE DX										
0–19 Years	0									
20–34	0									
35–49	0									
50–64	0									
65+	0									
2. MULTIPLE DX										
0–19 Years	2	7.5	<1	7	7	8	8	8	8	8
20–34	1	14.0	0	14	14	14	14	14	14	14
35–49	0									
50–64	1	10.0	0	10	10	10	10	10	10	10
65+	2	6.0	0	6	6	6	6	6	6	6
TOTAL SINGLE DX	0									
TOTAL MULTIPLE DX	6	8.4	7	6	7	8	8	14	14	14
TOTAL										
0–19 Years	2	7.5	<1	7	7	8	8	8	8	8
20–34	1	14.0	0	14	14	14	14	14	14	14
35–49	0									
50–64	1	10.0	0	10	10	10	10	10	10	10
65+	2	6.0	0	6	6	6	6	6	6	6
GRAND TOTAL	6	8.4	7	6	7	8	8	14	14	14

23.09: TOOTH EXTRACTION NEC

Type of Patients	Observed Patients	Avg. Stay	Vari-ance	10th	25th	50th	75th	90th	95th	99th
1. SINGLE DX										
0–19 Years	3	2.0	0	2	2	2	2	2	2	2
20–34	1	2.0	0	2	2	2	2	2	2	2
35–49	1	3.0	0	3	3	3	3	3	3	3
50–64	1	1.0	0	1	1	1	1	1	1	1
65+	0									
2. MULTIPLE DX										
0–19 Years	124	2.9	8	1	2	2	3	6	6	13
20–34	48	5.1	69	1	2	3	4	8	18	43
35–49	44	6.7	149	1	2	4	7	11	14	81
50–64	42	12.6	320	1	3	7	15	55	59	>99
65+	46	12.6	372	1	3	6	12	30	76	80
TOTAL SINGLE DX	6	2.0	<1	1	2	2	2	3	3	3
TOTAL MULTIPLE DX	304	5.6	112	1	2	3	5	11	16	76
TOTAL										
0–19 Years	127	2.9	8	1	1	2	3	6	6	13
20–34	49	5.1	68	1	2	3	4	8	18	43
35–49	45	6.6	146	1	2	3	7	11	14	81
50–64	43	12.3	315	1	2	6	12	55	59	>99
65+	46	12.6	372	1	3	6	12	30	76	80
GRAND TOTAL	310	5.5	110	1	2	3	5	11	16	76

23.0: FORCEPS TOOTH EXTRACTION

Type of Patients	Observed Patients	Avg. Stay	Vari-ance	10th	25th	50th	75th	90th	95th	99th
1. SINGLE DX										
0–19 Years	3	2.0	0	2	2	2	2	2	2	2
20–34	1	2.0	0	2	2	2	2	2	2	2
35–49	1	3.0	0	3	3	3	3	3	3	3
50–64	1	1.0	0	1	1	1	1	1	1	1
65+	0									
2. MULTIPLE DX										
0–19 Years	156	2.8	8	1	1	2	3	5	6	16
20–34	51	4.9	66	1	2	3	4	8	18	43
35–49	45	6.7	146	1	2	4	7	11	14	81
50–64	43	12.5	313	1	2	7	12	55	59	>99
65+	47	12.4	367	1	3	6	12	30	76	80
TOTAL SINGLE DX	6	2.0	<1	1	2	2	2	3	3	3
TOTAL MULTIPLE DX	342	5.0	94	1	1	2	5	9	15	71
TOTAL										
0–19 Years	159	2.8	8	1	1	2	3	5	6	16
20–34	52	4.9	65	1	2	3	4	8	18	43
35–49	46	6.6	143	1	2	4	7	11	14	81
50–64	44	12.2	309	1	2	7	12	55	59	>99
65+	47	12.4	367	1	3	6	12	30	76	80
GRAND TOTAL	348	4.9	93	1	1	2	4	9	15	71

23.1: SURG REMOVAL OF TOOTH

Type of Patients	Observed Patients	Avg. Stay	Vari-ance	10th	25th	50th	75th	90th	95th	99th
1. SINGLE DX										
0–19 Years	3	3.4	1	1	3	4	4	4	4	4
20–34	4	1.5	<1	1	1	2	2	2	2	2
35–49	0									
50–64	0									
65+	1	1.0	0	1	1	1	1	1	1	1
2. MULTIPLE DX										
0–19 Years	52	2.9	14	1	1	2	3	7	8	25
20–34	50	8.0	147	1	1	3	7	35	39	42
35–49	49	4.8	22	1	2	3	6	11	16	20
50–64	59	6.4	67	1	2	4	8	13	21	51
65+	34	7.3	69	1	3	5	9	15	25	43
TOTAL SINGLE DX	8	2.5	2	1	1	2	4	4	4	4
TOTAL MULTIPLE DX	244	5.5	62	1	1	3	6	11	20	42
TOTAL										
0–19 Years	55	2.9	13	1	1	2	3	7	8	25
20–34	54	7.6	139	1	1	3	7	35	39	42
35–49	49	4.8	22	1	2	3	6	11	16	20
50–64	59	6.4	67	1	2	4	8	13	21	51
65+	35	7.1	68	1	2	5	9	15	25	43
GRAND TOTAL	252	5.4	60	1	1	3	6	11	20	42

LOS by Diagnosis and Operation, Western Region, 45th Edition

Western Region, October 2007–September 2008 Data, by Operation

23.19: SURG TOOTH EXTRACT NEC

Type of Patients	Observed Patients	Avg. Stay	Variance	Percentiles						
				10th	25th	50th	75th	90th	95th	99th
1. SINGLE DX										
0–19 Years	3	3.4	1	1	3	4	4	4	4	4
20–34	4	1.5	<1	1	1	2	2	2	2	2
35–49	0									
50–64	0									
65+	1	1.0	0	1	1	1	1	1	1	1
2. MULTIPLE DX										
0–19 Years	51	2.9	14	1	1	2	3	7	8	25
20–34	50	8.0	147	1	1	2	7	35	39	42
35–49	48	4.9	22	1	2	3	6	11	16	20
50–64	57	6.5	69	1	2	4	8	13	21	51
65+	34	7.3	69	1	3	5	9	15	25	43
TOTAL SINGLE DX	**8**	**2.5**	**2**	**1**	**1**	**2**	**4**	**4**	**4**	**4**
TOTAL MULTIPLE DX	**240**	**5.6**	**62**	**1**	**1**	**3**	**6**	**12**	**21**	**42**
TOTAL										
0–19 Years	54	2.9	13	1	1	2	3	7	8	25
20–34	54	7.6	139	1	1	2	7	35	39	42
35–49	48	4.9	22	1	2	3	6	11	16	20
50–64	57	6.5	69	1	2	4	8	13	21	51
65+	35	7.1	68	1	3	5	9	15	25	43
GRAND TOTAL	**248**	**5.4**	**60**	**1**	**1**	**3**	**6**	**11**	**20**	**42**

23.2: TOOTH RESTOR BY FILLING

Type of Patients	Observed Patients	Avg. Stay	Variance	Percentiles						
				10th	25th	50th	75th	90th	95th	99th
1. SINGLE DX										
0–19 Years	0									
20–34	0									
35–49	0									
50–64	0									
65+										
2. MULTIPLE DX										
0–19 Years	16	2.4	12	1	1	1	2	4	13	13
20–34	1	9.0	0	9	9	9	9	9	9	9
35–49	0									
50–64	0									
65+	0									
TOTAL SINGLE DX	**0**									
TOTAL MULTIPLE DX	**17**	**2.6**	**12**	**1**	**1**	**1**	**2**	**9**	**13**	**13**
TOTAL										
0–19 Years	16	2.4	12	1	1	1	2	4	13	13
20–34	1	9.0	0	9	9	9	9	9	9	9
35–49	0									
50–64	0									
65+	0									
GRAND TOTAL	**17**	**2.6**	**12**	**1**	**1**	**1**	**2**	**9**	**13**	**13**

23.3: TOOTH RESTOR BY INLAY

Type of Patients	Observed Patients	Avg. Stay	Variance	Percentiles						
				10th	25th	50th	75th	90th	95th	99th
1. SINGLE DX										
0–19 Years	0									
20–34	0									
35–49	0									
50–64	0									
65+	0									
2. MULTIPLE DX										
0–19 Years	0									
20–34	0									
35–49	0									
50–64	0									
65+	0									
TOTAL SINGLE DX	**0**									
TOTAL MULTIPLE DX	**0**									
TOTAL										
0–19 Years	0									
20–34	0									
35–49	0									
50–64	0									
65+	0									
GRAND TOTAL	**0**									

23.4: OTHER DENTAL RESTORATION

Type of Patients	Observed Patients	Avg. Stay	Variance	Percentiles						
				10th	25th	50th	75th	90th	95th	99th
1. SINGLE DX										
0–19 Years	2	1.0	0	1	1	1	1	1	1	1
20–34	0									
35–49	0									
50–64	0									
65+										
2. MULTIPLE DX										
0–19 Years	28	4.3	24	1	1	2	6	14	18	18
20–34	2	7.1	71	1	1	13	13	13	13	13
35–49	1	1.0	0	1	1	1	1	1	1	1
50–64	0									
65+	0									
TOTAL SINGLE DX	**2**	**1.0**	**0**	**1**	**1**	**1**	**1**	**1**	**1**	**1**
TOTAL MULTIPLE DX	**31**	**4.4**	**25**	**1**	**1**	**2**	**6**	**14**	**18**	**18**
TOTAL										
0–19 Years	30	4.2	24	1	1	2	6	14	18	18
20–34	2	7.1	71	1	1	13	13	13	13	13
35–49	1	1.0	0	1	1	1	1	1	1	1
50–64	0									
65+	0									
GRAND TOTAL	**33**	**4.2**	**24**	**1**	**1**	**2**	**6**	**14**	**18**	**18**

LOS by Diagnosis and Operation, Western Region, 45th Edition

Western Region, October 2007–September 2008 Data, by Operation

23.5: TOOTH IMPLANTATION

Type of Patients	Observed Patients	Avg. Stay	Variance	10th	25th	50th	75th	90th	95th	99th
1. SINGLE DX										
0–19 Years	0									
20–34	0									
35–49	0									
50–64	0									
65+	0									
2. MULTIPLE DX										
0–19 Years	0									
20–34	1	2.0	0	2	2	2	2	2	2	2
35–49	1	2.0	0	2	2	2	2	2	2	2
50–64	0									
65+	0									
TOTAL SINGLE DX	0									
TOTAL MULTIPLE DX	2	2.0	0	2	2	2	2	2	2	2
TOTAL										
0–19 Years	0									
20–34	1	2.0	0	2	2	2	2	2	2	2
35–49	1	2.0	0	2	2	2	2	2	2	2
50–64	0									
65+	0									
GRAND TOTAL	2	2.0	0	2	2	2	2	2	2	2

23.6: PROSTHETIC DENTAL IMPL

Type of Patients	Observed Patients	Avg. Stay	Variance	10th	25th	50th	75th	90th	95th	99th
1. SINGLE DX										
0–19 Years	0									
20–34	0									
35–49	0									
50–64	0									
65+										
2. MULTIPLE DX										
0–19 Years	0									
20–34	0									
35–49	0									
50–64	0									
65+	1	1.0	0	1	1	1	1	1	1	1
TOTAL SINGLE DX	0									
TOTAL MULTIPLE DX	1	1.0	0	1	1	1	1	1	1	1
TOTAL										
0–19 Years	0									
20–34	0									
35–49	0									
50–64	0									
65+	1	1.0	0	1	1	1	1	1	1	1
GRAND TOTAL	1	1.0	0	1	1	1	1	1	1	1

23.7: ROOT CANAL TX & APICOECT

Type of Patients	Observed Patients	Avg. Stay	Variance	10th	25th	50th	75th	90th	95th	99th
1. SINGLE DX										
0–19 Years	0									
20–34	0									
35–49	0									
50–64	0									
65+	0									
2. MULTIPLE DX										
0–19 Years	1	1.0	0	1	1	1	1	1	1	1
20–34	1	1.0	0	1	1	1	1	1	1	1
35–49	0									
50–64	1	1.0	0	1	1	1	1	1	1	1
65+	1	2.0	0	2	2	2	2	2	2	2
TOTAL SINGLE DX	0									
TOTAL MULTIPLE DX	4	1.1	<1	1	1	1	1	2	2	2
TOTAL										
0–19 Years	1	1.0	0	1	1	1	1	1	1	1
20–34	1	1.0	0	1	1	1	1	1	1	1
35–49	0									
50–64	1	1.0	0	1	1	1	1	1	1	1
65+	1	2.0	0	2	2	2	2	2	2	2
GRAND TOTAL	4	1.1	<1	1	1	1	1	2	2	2

24.0: GUM OR ALVEOLAR INCISION

Type of Patients	Observed Patients	Avg. Stay	Variance	10th	25th	50th	75th	90th	95th	99th
1. SINGLE DX										
0–19 Years	10	3.0	4	1	1	3	4	6	6	6
20–34	8	2.3	<1	1	2	2	2	4	4	4
35–49	10	2.0	2	1	1	1	3	3	5	5
50–64	1	2.0	0	2	2	2	2	2	2	2
65+	0									
2. MULTIPLE DX										
0–19 Years	42	2.8	1	1	2	3	3	4	5	5
20–34	76	2.9	4	1	2	2	4	5	6	13
35–49	49	3.1	5	1	2	3	4	6	8	11
50–64	46	3.5	5	1	2	3	5	6	8	10
65+	21	3.5	8	1	2	3	4	6	8	13
TOTAL SINGLE DX	29	2.5	2	1	1	2	3	5	6	6
TOTAL MULTIPLE DX	234	3.1	4	1	2	3	4	6	7	11
TOTAL										
0–19 Years	52	2.8	2	1	2	3	3	4	5	6
20–34	84	2.9	4	1	2	2	4	5	6	13
35–49	59	2.9	4	1	2	2	4	6	8	11
50–64	47	3.5	5	1	2	3	5	6	8	10
65+	21	3.5	8	1	2	3	4	6	8	13
GRAND TOTAL	263	3.0	4	1	2	2	4	6	6	11

Western Region, October 2007–September 2008 Data, by Operation

24.1: TOOTH & GUM DXTIC PX

Type of Patients	Observed Patients	Avg. Stay	Variance	10th	25th	50th	75th	90th	95th	99th
1. SINGLE DX										
0–19 Years	0									
20–34	0									
35–49	0									
50–64	0									
65+	0									
2. MULTIPLE DX										
0–19 Years	1	16.0	0	16	16	16	16	16	16	16
20–34	0									
35–49	2	12.5	216	2	2	2	23	23	23	23
50–64	2	6.5	40	2	2	11	11	11	11	11
65+	2	2.0	2	1	1	3	3	3	3	3
TOTAL SINGLE DX	**0**									
TOTAL MULTIPLE DX	**7**	**10.6**	**63**	**2**	**2**	**16**	**16**	**16**	**23**	**23**
TOTAL										
0–19 Years	1	16.0	0	16	16	16	16	16	16	16
20–34	0									
35–49	2	12.5	216	2	2	2	23	23	23	23
50–64	2	6.5	40	2	2	11	11	11	11	11
65+	2	2.0	2	1	1	3	3	3	3	3
GRAND TOTAL	**7**	**10.6**	**63**	**2**	**2**	**16**	**16**	**16**	**23**	**23**

24.2: GINGIVOPLASTY

Type of Patients	Observed Patients	Avg. Stay	Variance	10th	25th	50th	75th	90th	95th	99th
1. SINGLE DX										
0–19 Years	0									
20–34	0									
35–49	0									
50–64	0									
65+	0									
2. MULTIPLE DX										
0–19 Years	0									
20–34	1	2.0	0	2	2	2	2	2	2	2
35–49	2	2.0	0	2	2	2	2	2	2	2
50–64	0									
65+	1	14.0	0	14	14	14	14	14	14	14
TOTAL SINGLE DX	**0**									
TOTAL MULTIPLE DX	**4**	**5.0**	**36**	**2**	**2**	**2**	**14**	**14**	**14**	**14**
TOTAL										
0–19 Years	0									
20–34	1	2.0	0	2	2	2	2	2	2	2
35–49	2	2.0	0	2	2	2	2	2	2	2
50–64	0									
65+	1	14.0	0	14	14	14	14	14	14	14
GRAND TOTAL	**4**	**5.0**	**36**	**2**	**2**	**2**	**14**	**14**	**14**	**14**

24.3: OTHER OPERATIONS ON GUMS

Type of Patients	Observed Patients	Avg. Stay	Variance	10th	25th	50th	75th	90th	95th	99th
1. SINGLE DX										
0–19 Years	2	1.0	0	1	1	1	1	1	1	1
20–34	0									
35–49	0									
50–64	0									
65+	1	2.0	0	2	2	2	2	2	2	2
2. MULTIPLE DX										
0–19 Years	12	2.9	5	1	1	2	4	8	8	8
20–34	2	1.5	<1	1	1	2	2	2	2	2
35–49	1	1.0	0	1	1	1	1	1	1	1
50–64	6	2.3	5	1	1	2	2	7	7	7
65+	4	6.5	81	1	2	3	3	20	20	20
TOTAL SINGLE DX	**3**	**1.1**	**<1**	**1**	**1**	**1**	**1**	**2**	**2**	**2**
TOTAL MULTIPLE DX	**25**	**3.1**	**14**	**1**	**1**	**2**	**4**	**7**	**8**	**20**
TOTAL										
0–19 Years	14	2.3	4	1	1	1	4	5	8	8
20–34	2	1.5	<1	1	1	2	2	2	2	2
35–49	1	1.0	0	1	1	1	1	1	1	1
50–64	6	2.3	5	1	2	2	2	7	7	7
65+	5	5.6	65	1	2	2	3	20	20	20
GRAND TOTAL	**28**	**2.7**	**11**	**1**	**1**	**1**	**3**	**5**	**8**	**20**

24.4: EXC OF DENTAL LES OF JAW

Type of Patients	Observed Patients	Avg. Stay	Variance	10th	25th	50th	75th	90th	95th	99th
1. SINGLE DX										
0–19 Years	1	1.0	0	1	1	1	1	1	1	1
20–34	4	1.0	0	1	1	1	1	1	1	1
35–49	0									
50–64	0									
65+	0									
2. MULTIPLE DX										
0–19 Years	18	1.7	3	1	1	1	1	4	6	7
20–34	9	2.2	<1	1	2	2	3	4	4	4
35–49	8	3.5	4	1	3	4	6	6	6	6
50–64	8	2.4	3	1	1	2	5	5	5	5
65+	9	2.4	3	1	1	2	3	5	5	5
TOTAL SINGLE DX	**5**	**1.0**	**0**	**1**	**1**	**1**	**1**	**1**	**1**	**1**
TOTAL MULTIPLE DX	**48**	**2.1**	**3**	**1**	**1**	**1**	**3**	**5**	**5**	**7**
TOTAL										
0–19 Years	19	1.6	2	1	1	1	1	4	6	7
20–34	13	1.9	<1	1	1	2	2	3	4	4
35–49	8	3.5	4	1	3	4	6	6	6	6
50–64	8	2.4	3	1	1	2	5	5	5	5
65+	9	2.4	3	1	1	2	3	5	5	5
GRAND TOTAL	**53**	**2.0**	**2**	**1**	**1**	**1**	**3**	**5**	**5**	**7**

LOS by Diagnosis and Operation, Western Region, 45th Edition

Western Region, October 2007–September 2008 Data, by Operation

24.5: ALVEOLOPLASTY

Type of Patients	Observed Patients	Avg. Stay	Variance	Percentiles						
				10th	25th	50th	75th	90th	95th	99th
1. SINGLE DX										
0–19 Years	4	1.0	0	1	1	1	1	1	1	1
20–34	0									
35–49	0									
50–64	1	2.0	0	2	2	2	2	2	2	2
65+	0									
2. MULTIPLE DX										
0–19 Years	6	1.0	0	1	1	1	1	1	1	1
20–34	3	1.0	0	1	1	1	1	1	1	1
35–49	13	6.8	71	1	3	4	4	13	32	32
50–64	22	9.1	143	1	1	4	18	34	45	>99
65+	34	5.9	45	1	2	2	8	17	20	24
TOTAL SINGLE DX	5	1.2	<1	1	1	1	1	2	2	2
TOTAL MULTIPLE DX	78	6.1	72	1	1	2	8	20	24	>99
TOTAL										
0–19 Years	10	1.0	0	1	1	1	1	1	1	1
20–34	3	1.0	0	1	1	1	1	1	1	1
35–49	13	6.8	71	1	3	4	4	13	32	32
50–64	23	8.8	139	1	1	4	18	34	45	>99
65+	34	5.9	45	1	2	2	8	17	20	24
GRAND TOTAL	83	5.8	70	1	1	2	7	20	24	>99

24.6: EXPOSURE OF TOOTH

Type of Patients	Observed Patients	Avg. Stay	Variance	Percentiles						
				10th	25th	50th	75th	90th	95th	99th
1. SINGLE DX										
0–19 Years	0									
20–34	0									
35–49	0									
50–64	0									
65+	0									
2. MULTIPLE DX										
0–19 Years	2	2.5	<1	2	2	3	3	3	3	3
20–34	0									
35–49	0									
50–64	0									
65+	0									
TOTAL SINGLE DX	0									
TOTAL MULTIPLE DX	2	2.5	<1	2	2	3	3	3	3	3
TOTAL										
0–19 Years	2	2.5	<1	2	2	3	3	3	3	3
20–34	0									
35–49	0									
50–64	0									
65+	0									
GRAND TOTAL	2	2.5	<1	2	2	3	3	3	3	3

24.7: APPL ORTHODONT APPLIANCE

Type of Patients	Observed Patients	Avg. Stay	Variance	Percentiles						
				10th	25th	50th	75th	90th	95th	99th
1. SINGLE DX										
0–19 Years	0									
20–34	0									
35–49	0									
50–64	0									
65+	0									
2. MULTIPLE DX										
0–19 Years	2	1.7	1	1	1	1	3	3	3	3
20–34	1	3.0	0	3	3	3	3	3	3	3
35–49	0									
50–64	1	1.0	0	1	1	1	1	1	1	1
65+	0									
TOTAL SINGLE DX	0									
TOTAL MULTIPLE DX	4	1.8	1	1	1	1	3	3	3	3
TOTAL										
0–19 Years	2	1.7	1	1	1	1	3	3	3	3
20–34	1	3.0	0	3	3	3	3	3	3	3
35–49	0									
50–64	1	1.0	0	1	1	1	1	1	1	1
65+	0									
GRAND TOTAL	4	1.8	1	1	1	1	3	3	3	3

24.8: OTHER ORTHODONTIC OP

Type of Patients	Observed Patients	Avg. Stay	Variance	Percentiles						
				10th	25th	50th	75th	90th	95th	99th
1. SINGLE DX										
0–19 Years	2	1.0	0	1	1	1	1	1	1	1
20–34	0									
35–49	1	4.0	0	4	4	4	4	4	4	4
50–64	0									
65+	0									
2. MULTIPLE DX										
0–19 Years	0									
20–34	0									
35–49	2	9.5	59	4	4	4	15	15	15	15
50–64	0									
65+	0									
TOTAL SINGLE DX	3	2.0	3	1	1	1	4	4	4	4
TOTAL MULTIPLE DX	2	9.5	59	4	4	4	15	15	15	15
TOTAL										
0–19 Years	2	1.0	0	1	1	1	1	1	1	1
20–34	0									
35–49	3	7.7	40	4	4	4	15	15	15	15
50–64	0									
65+	0									
GRAND TOTAL	5	5.0	33	1	1	1	4	15	15	15

LOS by Diagnosis and Operation, Western Region, 45th Edition

Western Region, October 2007–September 2008 Data, by Operation

24.9: OTHER DENTAL OPERATION

Type of Patients	Observed Patients	Avg. Stay	Variance	10th	25th	50th	75th	90th	95th	99th
1. SINGLE DX										
0–19 Years	0									
20–34	0									
35–49	0									
50–64	1	3.0	0	3	3	3	3	3	3	3
65+	0									
2. MULTIPLE DX										
0–19 Years	1	1.0	0	1	1	1	1	1	1	1
20–34	3	3.3	10	1	1	2	7	7	7	7
35–49	0									
50–64	1	20.0	0	20	20	20	20	20	20	20
65+	0									
TOTAL SINGLE DX	1	3.0	0	3	3	3	3	3	3	3
TOTAL MULTIPLE DX	5	4.1	43	1	1	1	2	20	20	20
TOTAL										
0–19 Years	1	1.0	0	1	1	1	1	1	1	1
20–34	3	3.3	10	1	1	2	7	7	7	7
35–49	0									
50–64	2	11.4	143	3	3	3	20	20	20	20
65+	0									
GRAND TOTAL	6	4.0	38	1	1	1	3	20	20	20

25.0: DXTIC PX ON TONGUE

Type of Patients	Observed Patients	Avg. Stay	Variance	10th	25th	50th	75th	90th	95th	99th
1. SINGLE DX										
0–19 Years	0									
20–34	0									
35–49	1	2.0	0	2	2	2	2	2	2	2
50–64	2	1.0	0	1	1	1	1	1	1	1
65+	1	2.0	0	2	2	2	2	2	2	2
2. MULTIPLE DX										
0–19 Years	4	7.2	126	2	3	3	4	33	33	33
20–34	5	2.2	2	1	1	2	3	4	4	4
35–49	14	7.0	84	1	1	5	7	13	37	37
50–64	34	4.7	30	1	1	3	7	10	15	28
65+	32	5.5	22	1	2	5	8	13	14	20
TOTAL SINGLE DX	4	1.5	<1	1	1	2	2	2	2	2
TOTAL MULTIPLE DX	89	5.4	40	1	2	3	7	12	15	37
TOTAL										
0–19 Years	4	7.2	126	2	3	3	4	33	33	33
20–34	5	2.2	2	1	1	2	3	4	4	4
35–49	15	6.7	80	1	2	4	7	13	37	37
50–64	36	4.5	29	1	1	2	7	10	15	28
65+	33	5.4	21	1	2	4	8	13	14	20
GRAND TOTAL	93	5.3	39	1	1	3	7	12	15	37

25.1: EXC/DESTR TONGUE LES

Type of Patients	Observed Patients	Avg. Stay	Variance	10th	25th	50th	75th	90th	95th	99th
1. SINGLE DX										
0–19 Years	4	1.0	0	1	1	1	1	1	1	1
20–34	1	1.0	0	1	1	1	1	1	1	1
35–49	1	2.0	0	2	2	2	2	2	2	2
50–64	2	1.0	0	1	1	1	1	1	1	1
65+	1	1.0	0	1	1	1	1	1	1	1
2. MULTIPLE DX										
0–19 Years	13	12.8	615	1	1	3	8	82	82	82
20–34	7	1.7	<1	1	1	1	3	3	3	3
35–49	5	1.8	<1	1	1	2	2	3	3	3
50–64	26	3.2	25	1	1	1	2	8	11	24
65+	26	3.8	16	1	2	2	6	11	14	14
TOTAL SINGLE DX	9	1.1	<1	1	1	1	1	1	2	2
TOTAL MULTIPLE DX	77	6.7	257	1	1	2	4	8	24	82
TOTAL										
0–19 Years	17	10.3	507	1	1	3	8	28	82	82
20–34	8	1.6	<1	1	1	1	3	3	3	3
35–49	6	1.8	<1	1	1	2	2	3	3	3
50–64	28	3.0	23	1	1	1	2	8	11	24
65+	27	3.7	16	1	2	2	6	11	14	14
GRAND TOTAL	86	6.0	227	1	1	2	3	8	24	82

25.2: PARTIAL GLOSSECTOMY

Type of Patients	Observed Patients	Avg. Stay	Variance	10th	25th	50th	75th	90th	95th	99th
1. SINGLE DX										
0–19 Years	0									
20–34	2	3.0	0	3	3	3	3	3	3	3
35–49	7	1.7	1	1	1	1	2	4	4	4
50–64	13	1.2	<1	1	1	1	1	2	2	2
65+	4	2.3	4	1	1	2	2	5	5	5
2. MULTIPLE DX										
0–19 Years	11	6.6	23	1	2	6	12	15	15	15
20–34	7	4.5	14	1	1	4	8	10	10	10
35–49	31	3.8	13	1	1	3	5	9	10	16
50–64	84	4.4	19	1	1	2	6	9	15	20
65+	118	3.9	17	1	1	2	5	9	13	22
TOTAL SINGLE DX	26	1.6	1	1	1	1	2	3	4	5
TOTAL MULTIPLE DX	251	4.4	18	1	1	3	6	10	15	20
TOTAL										
0–19 Years	11	6.6	23	1	2	6	12	15	15	15
20–34	9	4.1	11	1	1	3	6	10	10	10
35–49	38	3.5	12	1	1	2	5	9	10	16
50–64	97	3.9	18	1	1	2	6	8	15	20
65+	122	3.8	16	1	2	2	5	8	13	22
GRAND TOTAL	277	4.1	17	1	1	2	6	10	14	19

LOS by Diagnosis and Operation, Western Region, 45th Edition

Western Region, October 2007–September 2008 Data, by Operation

25.3: COMPLETE GLOSSECTOMY

Type of Patients	Observed Patients	Avg. Stay	Variance	Percentiles						
				10th	25th	50th	75th	90th	95th	99th
1. SINGLE DX										
0–19 Years	0									
20–34	0									
35–49	0									
50–64	0									
65+	0									
2. MULTIPLE DX										
0–19 Years	0									
20–34	0									
35–49	1	16.0	0	16	16	16	16	16	16	16
50–64	6	11.3	57	2	8	10	13	25	25	25
65+	1	12.0	0	12	12	12	12	12	12	12
TOTAL SINGLE DX	**0**									
TOTAL MULTIPLE DX	**8**	**12.0**	**44**	**2**	**10**	**10**	**13**	**25**	**25**	**25**
TOTAL										
0–19 Years	0									
20–34	0									
35–49	1	16.0	0	16	16	16	16	16	16	16
50–64	6	11.3	57	2	8	10	13	25	25	25
65+	1	12.0	0	12	12	12	12	12	12	12
GRAND TOTAL	**8**	**12.0**	**44**	**2**	**10**	**10**	**13**	**25**	**25**	**25**

25.4: RADICAL GLOSSECTOMY

Type of Patients	Observed Patients	Avg. Stay	Variance	Percentiles						
				10th	25th	50th	75th	90th	95th	99th
1. SINGLE DX										
0–19 Years	0									
20–34	0									
35–49	0									
50–64	0									
65+	0									
2. MULTIPLE DX										
0–19 Years	0									
20–34	0									
35–49	2	5.5	12	3	3	8	8	8	8	8
50–64	5	10.0	76	1	2	12	13	22	22	22
65+	3	13.7	37	7	7	15	19	19	19	19
TOTAL SINGLE DX	**0**									
TOTAL MULTIPLE DX	**10**	**10.2**	**52**	**1**	**3**	**12**	**15**	**22**	**22**	**22**
TOTAL										
0–19 Years	0									
20–34	0									
35–49	2	5.5	12	3	3	8	8	8	8	8
50–64	5	10.0	76	1	2	12	13	22	22	22
65+	3	13.7	37	7	7	15	19	19	19	19
GRAND TOTAL	**10**	**10.2**	**52**	**1**	**3**	**12**	**15**	**22**	**22**	**22**

25.5: REPAIR OF TONGUE

Type of Patients	Observed Patients	Avg. Stay	Variance	Percentiles						
				10th	25th	50th	75th	90th	95th	99th
1. SINGLE DX										
0–19 Years	8	1.1	<1	1	1	1	1	1	1	2
20–34	2	1.0	0	1	1	1	1	1	1	1
35–49	2	1.5	<1	1	1	2	2	2	2	2
50–64	1	1.0	0	1	1	1	1	1	1	1
65+	0									
2. MULTIPLE DX										
0–19 Years	21	3.8	51	1	1	1	4	7	16	33
20–34	17	3.6	15	1	1	2	4	11	12	12
35–49	29	2.9	8	1	1	2	3	6	8	15
50–64	37	3.4	51	1	1	2	3	6	9	44
65+	12	3.7	8	1	2	3	4	7	11	11
TOTAL SINGLE DX	**13**	**1.1**	**<1**	**1**	**1**	**1**	**1**	**1**	**2**	**2**
TOTAL MULTIPLE DX	**116**	**3.5**	**33**	**1**	**1**	**2**	**3**	**7**	**12**	**33**
TOTAL										
0–19 Years	29	2.9	35	1	1	1	2	4	14	33
20–34	19	3.3	14	1	1	1	4	11	12	12
35–49	31	2.8	8	1	1	2	3	5	8	15
50–64	38	3.3	49	1	1	2	3	6	9	44
65+	12	3.7	8	1	2	3	4	7	11	11
GRAND TOTAL	**129**	**3.1**	**28**	**1**	**1**	**1**	**3**	**6**	**11**	**33**

25.9: OTHER TONGUE OPERATIONS

Type of Patients	Observed Patients	Avg. Stay	Variance	Percentiles						
				10th	25th	50th	75th	90th	95th	99th
1. SINGLE DX										
0–19 Years	5	1.4	<1	1	1	1	2	2	2	2
20–34	1	1.0	0	1	1	1	1	1	1	1
35–49	0									
50–64	1	1.0	0	1	1	1	1	1	1	1
65+	0									
2. MULTIPLE DX										
0–19 Years	831	2.6	6	1	2	2	3	4	5	13
20–34	2	3.0	0	3	3	3	3	3	3	3
35–49	4	1.5	<1	1	1	1	2	2	2	2
50–64	5	2.8	2	1	2	3	3	5	5	5
65+	0									
TOTAL SINGLE DX	**7**	**1.3**	**<1**	**1**	**1**	**1**	**2**	**2**	**2**	**2**
TOTAL MULTIPLE DX	**842**	**2.6**	**6**	**1**	**2**	**2**	**3**	**4**	**5**	**13**
TOTAL										
0–19 Years	836	2.6	6	1	2	2	3	4	5	13
20–34	3	2.3	<1	1	1	3	3	3	3	3
35–49	4	1.5	<1	1	1	1	2	2	2	2
50–64	6	2.5	2	1	1	3	3	5	5	5
65+	0									
GRAND TOTAL	**849**	**2.6**	**6**	**1**	**2**	**2**	**3**	**4**	**5**	**13**

LOS by Diagnosis and Operation, Western Region, 45th Edition

Western Region, October 2007–September 2008 Data, by Operation

25.91: LINGUAL FRENOTOMY

Type of Patients	Observed Patients	Avg. Stay	Vari-ance	10th	25th	50th	75th	90th	95th	99th
1. SINGLE DX										
0–19 Years	4	1.5	<1	1	1	2	2	2	2	2
20–34	0									
35–49	0									
50–64	0									
65+	0									
2. MULTIPLE DX										
0–19 Years	666	2.5	6	1	2	2	3	4	4	11
20–34	0									
35–49	0									
50–64	0									
65+	0									
TOTAL SINGLE DX	4	1.5	<1	1	1	2	2	2	2	2
TOTAL MULTIPLE DX	666	2.5	6	1	2	2	3	4	4	11
TOTAL										
0–19 Years	670	2.5	6	1	2	2	3	4	4	11
20–34	0									
35–49	0									
50–64	0									
65+	0									
GRAND TOTAL	670	2.5	6	1	2	2	3	4	4	11

26.0: INC SALIVARY GLAND/DUCT

Type of Patients	Observed Patients	Avg. Stay	Vari-ance	10th	25th	50th	75th	90th	95th	99th
1. SINGLE DX										
0–19 Years	7	5.0	4	3	4	5	5	9	9	9
20–34	1	3.0	0	3	3	3	3	3	3	3
35–49	1	2.0	0	2	2	2	2	2	2	2
50–64	5	2.0	<1	1	1	2	3	3	3	3
65+	1	1.0	0	1	1	1	1	1	1	1
2. MULTIPLE DX										
0–19 Years	10	8.3	82	2	3	4	9	25	25	25
20–34	8	2.1	<1	1	2	3	3	3	3	3
35–49	19	4.2	11	1	2	3	5	12	12	12
50–64	13	4.7	36	1	1	3	4	9	23	23
65+	23	7.2	27	2	3	6	8	16	16	18
TOTAL SINGLE DX	15	4.0	5	1	2	4	5	7	9	9
TOTAL MULTIPLE DX	73	5.9	38	1	2	4	6	15	23	25
TOTAL										
0–19 Years	17	6.9	49	2	3	5	6	25	25	25
20–34	9	2.2	<1	1	2	2	3	3	3	3
35–49	20	4.1	10	1	2	3	4	9	12	12
50–64	18	3.9	27	1	1	3	4	9	23	23
65+	24	7.0	27	2	3	6	8	16	18	18
GRAND TOTAL	88	5.5	31	1	2	4	6	12	18	25

25.92: LINGUAL FRENECTOMY

Type of Patients	Observed Patients	Avg. Stay	Vari-ance	10th	25th	50th	75th	90th	95th	99th
1. SINGLE DX										
0–19 Years	0									
20–34	0									
35–49	0									
50–64	0									
65+	0									
2. MULTIPLE DX										
0–19 Years	160	2.8	5	1	2	2	3	4	5	16
20–34	0									
35–49	0									
50–64	0									
65+	0									
TOTAL SINGLE DX	0									
TOTAL MULTIPLE DX	160	2.8	5	1	2	2	3	4	5	16
TOTAL										
0–19 Years	160	2.8	5	1	2	2	3	4	5	16
20–34	0									
35–49	0									
50–64	0									
65+	0									
GRAND TOTAL	160	2.8	5	1	2	2	3	4	5	16

26.1: SALIVARY GLAND DXTIC PX

Type of Patients	Observed Patients	Avg. Stay	Vari-ance	10th	25th	50th	75th	90th	95th	99th
1. SINGLE DX										
0–19 Years	1	3.0	0	3	3	3	3	3	3	3
20–34	0									
35–49	0									
50–64	0									
2. MULTIPLE DX										
0–19 Years	6	7.9	31	2	2	8	8	17	17	17
20–34	5	13.1	144	2	4	11	16	32	32	32
35–49	15	3.5	9	1	1	2	4	7	12	12
50–64	21	7.1	256	1	2	4	5	7	10	76
65+	30	6.6	19	2	4	5	9	14	15	19
TOTAL SINGLE DX	1	3.0	0	3	3	3	3	3	3	3
TOTAL MULTIPLE DX	77	6.8	82	1	2	4	8	15	17	76
TOTAL										
0–19 Years	7	7.7	30	2	3	8	8	17	17	17
20–34	5	13.1	144	2	4	11	16	32	32	32
35–49	15	3.5	9	1	1	2	4	7	12	12
50–64	21	7.1	256	1	2	4	5	7	10	76
65+	30	6.6	19	2	4	5	9	14	15	19
GRAND TOTAL	78	6.8	82	1	2	4	8	15	17	76

LOS by Diagnosis and Operation, Western Region, 45th Edition

87

Western Region, October 2007–September 2008 Data, by Operation

26.2: EXC OF SG LESION

Type of Patients	Observed Patients	Avg. Stay	Variance	10th	25th	50th	75th	90th	95th	99th
1. SINGLE DX										
0–19 Years	11	1.1	<1	1	1	1	1	2	2	2
20–34	11	1.8	1	1	1	1	3	3	4	4
35–49	2	1.0	0	1	1	1	1	1	1	1
50–64	10	1.1	<1	1	1	1	1	1	2	2
65+	4	1.0	0	1	1	1	1	1	1	1
2. MULTIPLE DX										
0–19 Years	11	2.2	1	1	1	2	3	4	4	4
20–34	10	1.4	<1	1	1	1	2	2	2	2
35–49	13	2.2	8	1	1	1	1	5	11	11
50–64	25	1.5	<1	1	1	1	2	2	3	6
65+	26	2.5	11	1	1	1	2	7	11	14
TOTAL SINGLE DX	38	1.2	<1	1	1	1	1	2	3	4
TOTAL MULTIPLE DX	85	2.0	5	1	1	1	2	4	6	14
TOTAL										
0–19	22	1.6	<1	1	1	1	2	3	4	4
20–34	21	1.6	<1	1	1	1	2	3	3	4
35–49	15	2.1	7	1	1	1	1	5	11	11
50–64	35	1.4	<1	1	1	1	2	2	3	6
65+	30	2.3	10	1	1	1	2	7	11	14
GRAND TOTAL	123	1.7	3	1	1	1	2	3	4	11

26.3: SIALOADENECTOMY

Type of Patients	Observed Patients	Avg. Stay	Variance	10th	25th	50th	75th	90th	95th	99th
1. SINGLE DX										
0–19 Years	20	1.6	<1	1	1	1	2	3	3	4
20–34	44	1.4	<1	1	1	1	1	3	3	5
35–49	59	1.3	<1	1	1	1	1	2	3	4
50–64	86	1.4	<1	1	1	1	2	2	3	4
65+	28	1.1	<1	1	1	1	1	1	2	2
2. MULTIPLE DX										
0–19 Years	22	2.5	11	1	1	1	2	11	11	11
20–34	53	1.8	1	1	1	1	2	3	4	6
35–49	132	1.7	1	1	1	1	2	3	4	5
50–64	327	1.7	3	1	1	1	2	3	4	10
65+	345	1.8	4	1	1	1	2	3	4	14
TOTAL SINGLE DX	237	1.4	<1	1	1	1	1	2	3	4
TOTAL MULTIPLE DX	879	1.8	4	1	1	1	2	3	4	11
TOTAL										
0–19	42	2.1	6	1	1	1	2	3	11	11
20–34	97	1.6	1	1	1	1	2	3	4	6
35–49	191	1.5	1	1	1	1	2	3	4	5
50–64	413	1.6	2	1	1	1	2	3	4	9
65+	373	1.8	4	1	1	1	2	3	4	14
GRAND TOTAL	1,116	1.7	3	1	1	1	2	3	4	10

26.29: SALIVARY LES EXC NEC

Type of Patients	Observed Patients	Avg. Stay	Variance	10th	25th	50th	75th	90th	95th	99th
1. SINGLE DX										
0–19 Years	11	1.1	<1	1	1	1	1	2	2	2
20–34	10	1.8	1	1	1	1	3	4	4	4
35–49	2	1.0	0	1	1	1	1	1	1	1
50–64	10	1.1	<1	1	1	1	1	1	2	2
65+	4	1.0	0	1	1	1	1	1	1	1
2. MULTIPLE DX										
0–19 Years	10	2.2	1	1	1	2	2	4	4	4
20–34	10	1.4	<1	1	1	1	2	2	2	2
35–49	13	2.2	8	1	1	1	1	5	11	11
50–64	25	1.5	<1	1	1	1	2	2	3	6
65+	26	2.5	11	1	1	1	2	7	11	14
TOTAL SINGLE DX	37	1.2	<1	1	1	1	1	2	3	4
TOTAL MULTIPLE DX	84	2.0	5	1	1	1	2	4	6	14
TOTAL										
0–19	21	1.6	<1	1	1	1	2	3	4	4
20–34	20	1.6	<1	1	1	1	2	3	4	4
35–49	15	2.1	7	1	1	1	1	5	11	11
50–64	35	1.4	<1	1	1	1	1	2	3	6
65+	30	2.3	10	1	1	1	2	7	11	14
GRAND TOTAL	121	1.7	3	1	1	1	2	3	4	11

26.30: SIALOADENECTOMY NOS

Type of Patients	Observed Patients	Avg. Stay	Variance	10th	25th	50th	75th	90th	95th	99th
1. SINGLE DX										
0–19 Years	5	1.1	<1	1	1	1	1	2	2	2
20–34	10	1.3	<1	1	1	1	1	2	3	3
35–49	11	1.4	<1	1	1	2	2	2	2	3
50–64	18	1.2	<1	1	1	1	1	1	1	2
65+	5	1.0	0	1	1	1	1	1	1	1
2. MULTIPLE DX										
0–19 Years	6	1.3	<1	1	1	1	1	2	3	3
20–34	9	2.4	1	1	2	2	3	4	4	4
35–49	23	1.6	1	1	1	1	2	2	4	4
50–64	50	1.7	6	1	1	1	2	2	4	17
65+	64	1.7	4	1	1	1	2	2	3	15
TOTAL SINGLE DX	49	1.2	<1	1	1	1	1	2	2	3
TOTAL MULTIPLE DX	152	1.7	3	1	1	1	2	3	4	15
TOTAL										
0–19	11	1.2	<1	1	1	1	1	2	2	3
20–34	19	1.8	1	1	1	1	3	4	4	4
35–49	34	1.5	<1	1	1	1	2	2	4	4
50–64	68	1.6	4	1	1	1	2	2	3	17
65+	69	1.6	3	1	1	1	2	2	3	15
GRAND TOTAL	201	1.6	3	1	1	1	2	2	3	6

LOS by Diagnosis and Operation, Western Region, 45th Edition

Western Region, October 2007–September 2008 Data, by Operation

26.31: PARTIAL SIALOADENECTOMY

Type of Patients	Observed Patients	Avg. Stay	Vari-ance	Percentiles						
				10th	25th	50th	75th	90th	95th	99th
1. SINGLE DX										
0–19 Years	4	1.5	<1	1	1	1	2	2	2	2
20–34	18	1.5	1	1	1	1	2	3	5	5
35–49	27	1.2	<1	1	1	1	1	2	3	3
50–64	43	1.4	<1	1	1	1	2	3	3	4
65+	18	1.1	<1	1	1	1	1	1	2	2
2. MULTIPLE DX										
0–19 Years	7	1.0	0	1	1	1	1	1	1	1
20–34	33	1.6	<1	1	1	1	2	3	3	4
35–49	62	1.6	<1	1	1	1	2	3	4	5
50–64	175	1.6	3	1	1	1	2	3	4	10
65+	149	1.7	3	1	1	1	2	3	4	8
TOTAL SINGLE DX	**110**	**1.3**	**<1**	**1**	**1**	**1**	**1**	**2**	**3**	**4**
TOTAL MULTIPLE DX	**426**	**1.6**	**2**	**1**	**1**	**1**	**2**	**3**	**4**	**8**
TOTAL										
0–19 Years	11	1.2	<1	1	1	1	1	2	2	2
20–34	51	1.6	<1	1	1	1	2	3	3	5
35–49	89	1.5	<1	1	1	1	2	3	4	5
50–64	218	1.6	2	1	1	1	2	3	4	9
65+	167	1.6	3	1	1	1	2	3	4	8
GRAND TOTAL	**536**	**1.6**	**2**	**1**	**1**	**1**	**2**	**3**	**4**	**8**

26.32: COMPLETE SIALOADENECTOMY

Type of Patients	Observed Patients	Avg. Stay	Vari-ance	Percentiles						
				10th	25th	50th	75th	90th	95th	99th
1. SINGLE DX										
0–19 Years	11	1.8	1	1	1	1	3	3	4	4
20–34	16	1.4	<1	1	1	1	1	3	4	4
35–49	21	1.3	<1	1	1	1	1	2	2	4
50–64	25	1.4	<1	1	1	1	2	2	2	3
65+	5	1.2	<1	1	1	1	1	2	2	2
2. MULTIPLE DX										
0–19 Years	9	4.1	19	1	1	2	11	11	11	11
20–34	11	1.9	2	1	1	1	3	3	6	6
35–49	47	1.8	2	1	1	1	2	3	5	9
50–64	102	1.8	2	1	1	1	2	3	5	7
65+	132	2.1	7	1	1	1	2	4	6	14
TOTAL SINGLE DX	**78**	**1.4**	**<1**	**1**	**1**	**1**	**2**	**3**	**3**	**4**
TOTAL MULTIPLE DX	**301**	**2.0**	**5**	**1**	**1**	**1**	**2**	**4**	**6**	**11**
TOTAL										
0–19 Years	20	2.9	11	1	1	1	3	11	11	11
20–34	27	1.6	2	1	1	1	2	3	4	6
35–49	68	1.6	2	1	1	1	2	3	4	9
50–64	127	1.7	2	1	1	1	2	3	4	7
65+	137	2.0	6	1	1	1	2	4	6	14
GRAND TOTAL	**379**	**1.9**	**4**	**1**	**1**	**1**	**2**	**3**	**5**	**11**

26.4: SG & DUCT REPAIR

Type of Patients	Observed Patients	Avg. Stay	Vari-ance	Percentiles						
				10th	25th	50th	75th	90th	95th	99th
1. SINGLE DX										
0–19 Years	0									
20–34	0									
35–49	0									
50–64	0									
65+	0									
2. MULTIPLE DX										
0–19 Years	2	1.4	<1	1	1	1	2	2	2	2
20–34	2	2.5	4	1	1	1	4	4	4	4
35–49	2	2.0	2	1	1	2	3	3	3	3
50–64	2	1.5	<1	1	1	2	2	2	2	2
65+	3	8.7	134	1	1	3	22	22	22	22
TOTAL SINGLE DX	**0**									
TOTAL MULTIPLE DX	**11**	**3.5**	**36**	**1**	**1**	**2**	**3**	**4**	**22**	**22**
TOTAL										
0–19 Years	2	1.4	<1	1	1	1	2	2	2	2
20–34	2	2.5	4	1	1	1	4	4	4	4
35–49	2	2.0	2	1	1	2	3	3	3	3
50–64	2	1.5	<1	1	1	2	2	2	2	2
65+	3	8.7	134	1	1	3	22	22	22	22
GRAND TOTAL	**11**	**3.5**	**36**	**1**	**1**	**2**	**3**	**4**	**22**	**22**

26.9: OTH SALIVARY OPERATIONS

Type of Patients	Observed Patients	Avg. Stay	Vari-ance	Percentiles						
				10th	25th	50th	75th	90th	95th	99th
1. SINGLE DX										
0–19 Years	0									
20–34	1	7.0	0	7	7	7	7	7	7	7
35–49	0									
50–64	0									
65+	0									
2. MULTIPLE DX										
0–19 Years	5	11.5	370	1	2	6	6	53	53	53
20–34	2	1.5	<1	1	1	1	2	2	2	2
50–64	4	2.3	2	1	2	2	2	4	4	4
65+	7	2.9	1	2	2	2	4	5	5	5
TOTAL SINGLE DX	**1**	**7.0**	**0**	**7**	**7**	**7**	**7**	**7**	**7**	**7**
TOTAL MULTIPLE DX	**18**	**6.7**	**187**	**1**	**2**	**2**	**5**	**6**	**53**	**53**
TOTAL										
0–19 Years	5	11.5	370	1	2	6	6	53	53	53
20–34	3	3.3	10	1	1	2	7	7	7	7
50–64	4	2.3	2	1	2	2	2	4	4	4
65+	7	2.9	1	2	2	2	4	5	5	5
GRAND TOTAL	**19**	**6.7**	**179**	**1**	**2**	**2**	**6**	**7**	**53**	**53**

LOS by Diagnosis and Operation, Western Region, 45th Edition

Western Region, October 2007–September 2008 Data, by Operation

27.0: DRAIN FACE & MOUTH FLOOR

Type of Patients	Observed Patients	Avg. Stay	Vari-ance	Percentiles						
				10th	25th	50th	75th	90th	95th	99th
1. SINGLE DX										
0–19 Years	16	3.8	7	2	2	3	4	10	10	10
20–34	24	2.5	7	1	2	2	2	3	4	15
35–49	13	2.5	3	1	1	2	3	5	6	6
50–64	4	3.8	3	2	2	3	6	6	6	6
65+	3	2.0	<1	1	1	2	3	3	3	3
2. MULTIPLE DX										
0–19 Years	156	3.4	4	1	2	3	4	6	7	8
20–34	370	4.3	22	1	2	3	5	8	10	23
35–49	314	4.6	29	1	2	4	5	8	13	26
50–64	243	5.2	40	2	2	4	6	10	12	16
65+	123	6.0	27	2	3	4	7	12	18	24
TOTAL SINGLE DX	60	3.1	6	1	2	2	4	5	10	15
TOTAL MULTIPLE DX	1,206	4.5	24	1	2	3	5	8	11	23
TOTAL										
0–19 Years	172	3.5	4	1	2	3	4	6	8	10
20–34	394	4.2	22	1	2	3	5	8	10	23
35–49	327	4.5	28	1	2	3	5	7	13	26
50–64	247	5.2	39	2	2	4	6	10	12	16
65+	126	5.9	27	2	3	4	7	12	18	24
GRAND TOTAL	1,266	4.4	24	1	2	3	5	8	11	23

27.1: INCISION OF PALATE

Type of Patients	Observed Patients	Avg. Stay	Vari-ance	Percentiles						
				10th	25th	50th	75th	90th	95th	99th
1. SINGLE DX										
0–19 Years	0									
20–34	1	1.0	0	1	1	1	1	1	1	1
35–49	0									
50–64	0									
65+	0									
2. MULTIPLE DX										
0–19 Years	7	2.8	3	2	2	2	3	6	6	6
20–34	6	3.9	9	2	2	3	3	10	10	10
35–49	4	3.5	9	2	2	3	8	8	8	8
50–64	2	2.0	2	1	1	1	2	3	3	3
65+	2	1.5	<1	1	1	1	2	2	2	2
TOTAL SINGLE DX	1	1.0	0	1	1	1	1	1	1	1
TOTAL MULTIPLE DX	21	3.0	5	1	2	2	3	6	8	10
TOTAL										
0–19 Years	7	2.8	3	2	2	2	3	6	6	6
20–34	7	3.4	9	2	2	3	3	10	10	10
35–49	4	3.5	9	2	2	2	8	8	8	8
50–64	2	2.0	2	1	1	1	2	3	3	3
65+	2	1.5	<1	1	1	1	2	2	2	2
GRAND TOTAL	22	2.9	5	1	2	2	3	6	8	10

27.2: ORAL CAVITY DXTIC PX

Type of Patients	Observed Patients	Avg. Stay	Vari-ance	Percentiles						
				10th	25th	50th	75th	90th	95th	99th
1. SINGLE DX										
0–19 Years	1	6.0	0	6	6	6	6	6	6	6
20–34	0									
35–49	0									
50–64	1	2.0	0	2	2	2	2	2	2	2
65+	0									
2. MULTIPLE DX										
0–19 Years	3	28.5	153	4	27	35	35	35	35	35
20–34	4	4.8	17	1	4	4	8	10	10	10
35–49	15	8.2	110	2	4	6	8	10	45	45
50–64	15	12.1	164	3	4	7	15	31	49	49
65+	19	9.2	105	1	3	5	9	31	37	37
TOTAL SINGLE DX	2	4.0	8	2	2	6	6	6	6	6
TOTAL MULTIPLE DX	56	11.4	151	2	4	6	13	35	37	49
TOTAL										
0–19 Years	4	25.3	200	4	6	35	35	35	35	35
20–34	4	4.8	17	1	2	4	8	10	10	10
35–49	15	8.2	110	2	4	6	8	10	45	45
50–64	16	11.5	159	2	3	7	14	31	49	49
65+	19	9.2	105	1	3	5	9	31	37	37
GRAND TOTAL	58	11.1	148	2	4	6	10	35	35	49

27.3: EXC BONY PALATE LES/TISS

Type of Patients	Observed Patients	Avg. Stay	Vari-ance	Percentiles						
				10th	25th	50th	75th	90th	95th	99th
1. SINGLE DX										
0–19 Years	3	1.2	<1	1	1	1	1	3	3	3
20–34	1	1.0	0	1	1	1	1	1	1	1
35–49	1	1.0	0	1	1	1	1	1	1	1
50–64	2	2.0	2	1	1	1	3	3	3	3
65+	1	1.0	0	1	1	1	1	1	1	1
2. MULTIPLE DX										
0–19 Years	1	1.0	0	1	1	1	1	1	1	1
20–34	1	3.0	0	3	3	3	3	3	3	3
35–49	1	31.0	0	31	31	31	31	31	31	31
50–64	9	4.9	57	1	1	1	6	24	24	31
65+	31	4.9	21	1	1	3	8	9	12	20
TOTAL SINGLE DX	8	1.3	<1	1	1	1	1	3	3	3
TOTAL MULTIPLE DX	43	5.4	42	1	1	2	8	12	20	31
TOTAL										
0–19 Years	4	1.2	<1	1	1	1	1	1	3	3
20–34	2	2.0	2	1	1	3	3	3	3	3
35–49	2	16.1	439	1	1	31	31	31	31	31
50–64	11	4.4	47	1	1	1	6	7	24	24
65+	32	4.8	20	1	1	3	8	9	12	20
GRAND TOTAL	51	4.4	35	1	1	1	7	9	20	31

LOS by Diagnosis and Operation, Western Region, 45th Edition

Western Region, October 2007–September 2008 Data, by Operation

27.4: OTHER EXCISION OF MOUTH

Type of Patients	Observed Patients	Avg. Stay	Vari-ance	10th	25th	50th	75th	90th	95th	99th
1. SINGLE DX										
0–19 Years	8	1.3	<1	1	1	1	2	2	2	2
20–34	3	1.7	1	1	1	1	3	3	3	3
35–49	4	2.7	5	1	1	2	2	6	6	6
50–64	5	1.4	<1	1	1	1	2	2	2	2
65+	0									
2. MULTIPLE DX										
0–19 Years	26	3.3	18	1	1	2	3	5	17	17
20–34	16	2.4	3	1	1	2	4	5	6	6
35–49	32	3.9	18	1	1	2	5	9	15	19
50–64	47	5.4	66	1	1	3	4	14	30	36
65+	98	4.8	39	1	1	3	6	10	22	35
TOTAL SINGLE DX	20	1.5	<1	1	1	1	2	2	3	6
TOTAL MULTIPLE DX	219	4.3	35	1	1	2	4	9	17	31
TOTAL										
0–19 Years	34	2.6	13	1	1	2	3	4	17	17
20–34	19	2.3	3	1	1	2	3	5	6	6
35–49	36	3.8	17	1	1	2	5	9	15	19
50–64	52	5.0	61	1	1	3	4	14	30	36
65+	98	4.8	39	1	1	3	6	10	22	35
GRAND TOTAL	239	3.9	31	1	1	2	4	8	15	31

27.49: EXCISION OF MOUTH NEC

Type of Patients	Observed Patients	Avg. Stay	Vari-ance	10th	25th	50th	75th	90th	95th	99th
1. SINGLE DX										
0–19 Years	5	1.6	<1	1	1	2	2	2	2	2
20–34	2	1.0	0	1	1	1	1	1	1	1
35–49	3	1.7	<1	1	1	2	2	2	2	2
50–64	4	1.5	<1	1	1	1	2	2	2	2
65+	0									
2. MULTIPLE DX										
0–19 Years	7	2.4	<1	1	2	3	3	3	3	3
20–34	4	1.5	<1	1	1	1	1	3	3	3
35–49	14	5.2	32	1	1	2	8	15	19	19
50–64	35	6.4	84	1	1	3	7	18	31	36
65+	65	5.3	53	1	1	3	7	11	23	35
TOTAL SINGLE DX	14	1.5	<1	1	1	2	2	2	2	2
TOTAL MULTIPLE DX	125	5.1	52	1	1	3	5	12	23	35
TOTAL										
0–19 Years	12	2.0	<1	1	1	2	3	3	3	3
20–34	6	1.3	<1	1	1	1	1	3	3	3
35–49	17	4.6	28	1	1	2	5	15	19	19
50–64	39	5.9	78	1	1	2	6	18	31	36
65+	65	5.3	53	1	1	3	7	11	23	35
GRAND TOTAL	139	4.6	46	1	1	2	4	11	22	35

27.5: MOUTH PLASTIC REPAIR

Type of Patients	Observed Patients	Avg. Stay	Vari-ance	10th	25th	50th	75th	90th	95th	99th
1. SINGLE DX										
0–19 Years	210	1.1	<1	1	1	1	1	2	2	4
20–34	4	1.0	0	1	1	1	1	1	1	1
35–49	4	3.3	10	1	1	2	8	8	8	8
50–64	2	1.5	<1	1	1	2	2	2	2	2
65+	0									
2. MULTIPLE DX										
0–19 Years	494	1.5	3	1	1	1	1	2	3	7
20–34	195	2.5	10	1	1	1	3	5	8	15
35–49	189	3.2	25	1	1	2	3	6	10	27
50–64	189	3.0	18	1	1	2	3	5	7	17
65+	276	3.3	10	1	1	3	4	6	9	18
TOTAL SINGLE DX	220	1.2	<1	1	1	1	1	2	2	4
TOTAL MULTIPLE DX	1,343	2.1	9	1	1	1	2	4	6	15
TOTAL										
0–19 Years	704	1.3	2	1	1	1	1	2	3	6
20–34	199	2.4	10	1	1	1	3	5	8	15
35–49	193	3.2	25	1	1	2	3	6	10	27
50–64	191	3.0	17	1	1	2	3	5	7	17
65+	276	3.3	10	1	1	3	4	6	9	18
GRAND TOTAL	1,563	1.9	8	1	1	1	2	3	5	13

27.51: SUTURE OF LIP LACERATION

Type of Patients	Observed Patients	Avg. Stay	Vari-ance	10th	25th	50th	75th	90th	95th	99th
1. SINGLE DX										
0–19 Years	11	1.1	<1	1	1	1	1	2	2	2
20–34	1	1.0	0	1	1	1	1	1	1	1
35–49	0									
50–64	0									
65+	0									
2. MULTIPLE DX										
0–19 Years	100	1.6	1	1	1	1	2	3	4	5
20–34	155	2.3	10	1	1	1	3	4	7	18
35–49	147	3.1	25	1	1	2	3	6	9	20
50–64	145	2.9	20	1	1	2	3	5	7	17
65+	241	3.1	6	1	1	3	4	6	7	13
TOTAL SINGLE DX	12	1.1	<1	1	1	1	1	1	2	2
TOTAL MULTIPLE DX	788	2.7	12	1	1	2	3	5	7	15
TOTAL										
0–19 Years	111	1.5	<1	1	1	1	2	3	4	5
20–34	156	2.3	10	1	1	1	3	4	7	18
35–49	147	3.1	25	1	1	2	3	6	9	20
50–64	145	2.9	20	1	1	2	3	5	7	17
65+	241	3.1	6	1	1	3	4	6	7	13
GRAND TOTAL	800	2.7	12	1	1	2	3	5	7	15

LOS by Diagnosis and Operation, Western Region, 45th Edition

Western Region, October 2007–September 2008 Data, by Operation

27.54: REPAIR OF CLEFT LIP

Type of Patients	Observed Patients	Avg. Stay	Variance	10th	25th	50th	75th	90th	95th	99th
1. SINGLE DX										
0–19 Years	186	1.1	<1	1	1	1	1	2	2	3
20–34	0									
35–49	0									
50–64	0									
65+	0									
2. MULTIPLE DX										
0–19 Years	341	1.3	3	1	1	1	1	2	2	6
20–34	4	1.1	<1	1	1	1	1	2	2	2
35–49	1	1.0	0	1	1	1	1	1	1	1
50–64	0									
65+	0									
TOTAL SINGLE DX	186	1.1	<1	1	1	1	1	2	2	3
TOTAL MULTIPLE DX	346	1.3	3	1	1	1	1	2	2	6
TOTAL										
0–19 Years	527	1.2	2	1	1	1	1	2	2	4
20–34	4	1.1	<1	1	1	1	1	2	2	2
35–49	1	1.0	0	1	1	1	1	1	1	1
50–64	0									
65+	0									
GRAND TOTAL	532	1.2	2	1	1	1	1	2	2	4

27.6: PALATOPLASTY

Type of Patients	Observed Patients	Avg. Stay	Variance	10th	25th	50th	75th	90th	95th	99th
1. SINGLE DX										
0–19 Years	283	1.4	<1	1	1	1	2	2	2	4
20–34	11	1.3	<1	1	1	1	2	2	2	2
35–49	23	1.3	<1	1	1	1	2	2	2	3
50–64	24	1.7	<1	1	1	1	2	3	3	4
65+	2	2.0	2	1	1	3	3	3	3	3
2. MULTIPLE DX										
0–19 Years	892	1.6	2	1	1	1	2	2	3	9
20–34	141	1.7	5	1	1	1	2	3	3	8
35–49	327	1.6	2	1	1	1	2	3	3	8
50–64	300	1.7	2	1	1	1	2	3	4	7
65+	51	1.6	1	1	1	1	2	3	4	7
TOTAL SINGLE DX	343	1.4	<1	1	1	1	2	2	3	4
TOTAL MULTIPLE DX	1,711	1.6	2	1	1	1	2	3	3	8
TOTAL										
0–19 Years	1,175	1.6	2	1	1	1	2	3	3	7
20–34	152	1.7	4	1	1	1	2	3	3	8
35–49	350	1.6	2	1	1	1	2	3	3	8
50–64	324	1.7	2	1	1	1	2	3	4	7
65+	53	1.6	1	1	1	1	2	3	4	7
GRAND TOTAL	2,054	1.6	2	1	1	1	2	3	3	7

27.59: MOUTH REPAIR NEC

Type of Patients	Observed Patients	Avg. Stay	Variance	10th	25th	50th	75th	90th	95th	99th
1. SINGLE DX										
0–19 Years	6	1.6	1	1	1	1	1	4	4	4
20–34	0									
35–49	1	1.0	0	1	1	1	1	1	1	1
50–64	0									
65+	0									
2. MULTIPLE DX										
0–19 Years	28	1.5	1	1	1	1	2	2	4	6
20–34	24	2.9	14	1	1	2	3	6	13	15
35–49	26	3.6	43	1	1	1	3	5	24	27
50–64	19	3.0	10	1	1	2	4	9	13	13
65+	18	3.8	7	1	2	3	5	9	10	10
TOTAL SINGLE DX	7	1.6	1	1	1	1	1	4	4	4
TOTAL MULTIPLE DX	115	2.7	14	1	1	1	3	5	9	24
TOTAL										
0–19 Years	34	1.5	1	1	1	1	2	3	4	6
20–34	24	2.9	14	1	1	2	3	6	13	15
35–49	27	3.5	41	1	1	1	3	5	24	27
50–64	19	3.0	10	1	1	2	4	9	13	13
65+	18	3.8	7	1	2	3	5	9	10	10
GRAND TOTAL	122	2.5	12	1	1	1	3	5	9	24

27.62: CLEFT PALATE CORRECTION

Type of Patients	Observed Patients	Avg. Stay	Variance	10th	25th	50th	75th	90th	95th	99th
1. SINGLE DX										
0–19 Years	213	1.4	<1	1	1	1	2	2	2	4
20–34	1	2.0	0	2	2	2	2	2	2	2
35–49	3	1.7	1	1	1	1	3	3	3	3
50–64	0									
65+	0									
2. MULTIPLE DX										
0–19 Years	617	1.7	3	1	1	1	2	3	3	10
20–34	0									
35–49	0									
50–64	0									
65+	1	1.0	0	1	1	1	1	1	1	1
TOTAL SINGLE DX	217	1.4	<1	1	1	1	2	2	2	4
TOTAL MULTIPLE DX	618	1.7	3	1	1	1	2	3	3	10
TOTAL										
0–19 Years	830	1.6	2	1	1	1	2	3	3	9
20–34	1	2.0	0	2	2	2	2	2	2	2
35–49	3	1.7	1	1	1	1	3	3	3	3
50–64	0									
65+	1	1.0	0	1	1	1	1	1	1	1
GRAND TOTAL	835	1.6	2	1	1	1	2	3	3	9

LOS by Diagnosis and Operation, Western Region, 45th Edition

Western Region, October 2007–September 2008 Data, by Operation

27.63: REV CLEFT PALATE REPAIR

Type of Patients	Observed Patients	Avg. Stay	Vari-ance	Percentiles						
				10th	25th	50th	75th	90th	95th	99th
1. SINGLE DX										
0–19 Years	37	1.3	<1	1	1	1	2	2	2	3
20–34	2	1.0	0	1	1	1	1	1	1	1
35–49	1	1.0	0	1	1	1	1	1	1	1
50–64	1	2.0	0	2	2	2	2	2	2	2
65+	0									
2. MULTIPLE DX										
0–19 Years	210	1.4	<1	1	1	1	2	2	3	4
20–34	10	2.0	4	1	1	1	2	4	8	8
35–49	0									
50–64	2	1.5	<1	1	1	1	2	2	2	2
65+	0									
TOTAL SINGLE DX	**41**	**1.3**	**<1**	**1**	**1**	**1**	**2**	**2**	**2**	**3**
TOTAL MULTIPLE DX	**222**	**1.4**	**1**	**1**	**1**	**1**	**2**	**2**	**3**	**4**
TOTAL										
0–19 Years	247	1.4	<1	1	1	1	2	2	3	4
20–34	12	1.9	4	1	1	1	2	4	8	8
35–49	1	1.0	0	1	1	1	1	1	1	1
50–64	3	1.7	<1	1	1	2	2	2	2	2
65+	0									
GRAND TOTAL	**263**	**1.4**	**<1**	**1**	**1**	**1**	**2**	**2**	**3**	**4**

27.69: OTHER PLASTIC REP PALATE

Type of Patients	Observed Patients	Avg. Stay	Vari-ance	Percentiles						
				10th	25th	50th	75th	90th	95th	99th
1. SINGLE DX										
0–19 Years	18	2.0	2	1	1	2	2	6	6	6
20–34	8	1.3	<1	1	1	1	1	2	2	2
35–49	19	1.3	<1	1	1	1	2	2	2	2
50–64	23	1.7	<1	1	1	1	2	3	3	3
65+	2	2.0	2	1	1	3	3	3	3	3
2. MULTIPLE DX										
0–19 Years	62	1.9	6	1	1	1	3	3	4	5
20–34	127	1.5	<1	1	1	1	2	2	3	4
35–49	327	1.6	2	1	1	1	2	3	3	8
50–64	298	1.7	2	1	1	1	2	3	4	9
65+	49	1.6	1	1	1	1	2	3	4	7
TOTAL SINGLE DX	**70**	**1.7**	**1**	**1**	**1**	**1**	**2**	**3**	**4**	**6**
TOTAL MULTIPLE DX	**863**	**1.6**	**2**	**1**	**1**	**1**	**2**	**3**	**4**	**7**
TOTAL										
0–19 Years	80	1.9	5	1	1	1	2	3	4	6
20–34	135	1.5	<1	1	1	1	2	2	3	4
35–49	346	1.6	2	1	1	1	2	3	3	8
50–64	321	1.7	2	1	1	1	2	3	4	7
65+	51	1.6	1	1	1	1	2	3	4	7
GRAND TOTAL	**933**	**1.6**	**2**	**1**	**1**	**1**	**2**	**3**	**4**	**7**

27.7: OPERATIONS ON UVULA

Type of Patients	Observed Patients	Avg. Stay	Vari-ance	Percentiles						
				10th	25th	50th	75th	90th	95th	99th
1. SINGLE DX										
0–19 Years	0									
20–34	0									
35–49	0									
50–64	0									
65+	0									
2. MULTIPLE DX										
0–19 Years	0									
20–34	2	4.0	2	3	3	3	5	5	5	5
35–49	3	1.7	1	1	1	1	3	3	3	3
50–64	5	1.2	<1	1	1	1	1	2	2	2
65+	0									
TOTAL SINGLE DX	**0**									
TOTAL MULTIPLE DX	**10**	**1.9**	**2**	**1**	**1**	**1**	**3**	**3**	**5**	**5**
TOTAL										
0–19 Years	0									
20–34	2	4.0	2	3	3	3	5	5	5	5
35–49	3	1.7	1	1	1	1	3	3	3	3
50–64	5	1.2	<1	1	1	1	1	2	2	2
65+	0									
GRAND TOTAL	**10**	**1.9**	**2**	**1**	**1**	**1**	**3**	**3**	**5**	**5**

27.9: OTH OPS ON MOUTH & FACE

Type of Patients	Observed Patients	Avg. Stay	Vari-ance	Percentiles						
				10th	25th	50th	75th	90th	95th	99th
1. SINGLE DX										
0–19 Years	3	1.5	1	1	1	1	1	4	4	4
20–34	4	1.8	<1	1	1	1	2	3	3	3
35–49	0									
50–64	0									
65+	0									
2. MULTIPLE DX										
0–19 Years	27	2.4	2	1	2	2	3	4	6	6
20–34	37	3.6	6	2	2	3	4	7	11	11
35–49	21	3.8	3	2	2	3	5	6	6	8
50–64	10	4.1	9	1	2	4	7	11	11	11
65+	13	4.4	7	2	3	4	7	7	10	10
TOTAL SINGLE DX	**7**	**1.6**	**1**	**1**	**1**	**1**	**2**	**4**	**4**	**4**
TOTAL MULTIPLE DX	**108**	**3.3**	**5**	**1**	**2**	**3**	**4**	**6**	**7**	**11**
TOTAL										
0–19 Years	30	2.3	2	1	1	2	3	4	6	6
20–34	41	3.4	6	1	2	3	4	6	9	11
35–49	21	3.8	3	2	2	4	5	6	6	8
50–64	10	4.1	9	1	2	4	5	11	11	11
65+	13	4.4	7	2	3	3	7	7	10	10
GRAND TOTAL	**115**	**3.2**	**4**	**1**	**2**	**3**	**4**	**6**	**7**	**11**

LOS by Diagnosis and Operation, Western Region, 45th Edition

Western Region, October 2007–September 2008 Data, by Operation

27.92: MOUTH STRUCT INC NOS

Type of Patients	Observed Patients	Avg. Stay	Vari-ance	Percentiles						
				10th	25th	50th	75th	90th	95th	99th
1. SINGLE DX										
0–19 Years	3	1.5	1	1	1	1	1	4	4	4
20–34	4	1.8	<1	1	1	1	2	3	3	3
35–49	0									
50–64	0									
65+	0									
2. MULTIPLE DX										
0–19 Years	23	2.5	2	1	2	2	3	5	6	6
20–34	37	3.6	6	2	2	3	4	7	11	11
35–49	21	3.8	3	2	2	3	5	6	6	8
50–64	9	4.0	10	2	2	4	4	11	11	11
65+	12	4.6	7	2	3	3	7	7	10	10
TOTAL SINGLE DX	7	1.6	1	1	1	1	2	4	4	4
TOTAL MULTIPLE DX	102	3.3	5	1	2	3	4	6	7	11
TOTAL										
0–19 Years	26	2.4	2	1	1	2	3	4	6	6
20–34	41	3.4	6	1	2	3	5	6	9	11
35–49	21	3.8	3	2	2	3	5	6	6	8
50–64	9	4.0	10	1	2	4	4	11	11	11
65+	12	4.6	7	2	3	3	7	7	10	10
GRAND TOTAL	109	3.2	5	1	2	3	4	6	7	11

28.0: TONSIL/PERITONSILLAR I&D

Type of Patients	Observed Patients	Avg. Stay	Vari-ance	Percentiles						
				10th	25th	50th	75th	90th	95th	99th
1. SINGLE DX										
0–19 Years	208	1.9	1	1	1	2	2	4	5	5
20–34	98	1.6	<1	1	1	1	2	3	4	5
35–49	33	1.9	2	1	1	1	2	3	4	7
50–64	9	2.3	2	1	1	2	3	4	4	4
65+	3	2.7	2	1	1	3	4	4	4	4
2. MULTIPLE DX										
0–19 Years	429	3.4	10	1	2	3	4	6	8	15
20–34	301	2.6	9	1	1	2	3	5	6	13
35–49	170	3.3	20	1	1	2	3	7	12	19
50–64	131	5.3	45	1	1	3	6	11	17	35
65+	57	8.0	63	1	2	5	13	23	28	>99
TOTAL SINGLE DX	351	1.9	1	1	1	2	2	4	4	5
TOTAL MULTIPLE DX	1,088	3.6	17	1	2	2	4	7	10	21
TOTAL										
0–19 Years	637	3.0	7	1	1	2	4	5	7	15
20–34	399	2.4	7	1	1	2	3	4	5	10
35–49	203	3.1	17	1	1	2	3	6	10	18
50–64	140	5.1	42	1	1	3	6	11	17	35
65+	60	7.8	61	1	2	4	12	20	28	>99
GRAND TOTAL	1,439	3.1	13	1	2	2	4	6	8	19

28.1: TONSIL&ADENOID DXTIC PX

Type of Patients	Observed Patients	Avg. Stay	Vari-ance	Percentiles						
				10th	25th	50th	75th	90th	95th	99th
1. SINGLE DX										
0–19 Years	1	1.0	0	1	1	1	1	1	1	1
20–34	1	2.0	0	2	2	2	2	2	2	2
35–49	0									
50–64	0									
2. MULTIPLE DX										
0–19 Years	3	2.0	<1	1	1	2	3	3	3	3
20–34	5	4.4	3	2	3	5	6	6	6	6
35–49	12	5.1	12	1	3	5	7	10	12	12
50–64	19	6.8	92	1	1	4	8	18	41	41
65+	10	6.0	58	1	1	3	9	22	22	22
TOTAL SINGLE DX	2	1.5	<1	1	1	1	2	2	2	2
TOTAL MULTIPLE DX	49	5.7	50	1	1	3	6	15	18	41
TOTAL										
0–19 Years	4	1.8	<1	1	1	1	2	3	3	3
20–34	5	4.0	4	2	2	5	6	6	6	6
35–49	12	5.1	12	1	3	5	7	10	12	12
50–64	19	6.8	92	1	1	4	8	18	41	41
65+	10	6.0	58	1	1	3	9	22	22	22
GRAND TOTAL	51	5.5	49	1	1	3	6	12	18	41

28.2: TONSILLECTOMY

Type of Patients	Observed Patients	Avg. Stay	Vari-ance	Percentiles						
				10th	25th	50th	75th	90th	95th	99th
1. SINGLE DX										
0–19 Years	56	2.9	26	1	1	1	3	4	5	25
20–34	38	1.3	<1	1	1	1	1	2	3	4
35–49	8	1.5	<1	1	1	1	1	4	4	4
50–64	10	1.1	<1	1	1	1	2	2	2	2
65+	1	2.0	0	2	2	2	2	2	2	2
2. MULTIPLE DX										
0–19 Years	292	1.9	2	1	1	1	2	4	5	9
20–34	199	2.0	3	1	1	1	2	4	5	11
35–49	190	2.3	10	1	1	1	2	4	8	21
50–64	100	2.1	12	1	1	1	2	4	5	35
65+	24	5.4	71	1	2	3	5	14	24	37
TOTAL SINGLE DX	113	2.3	16	1	1	1	2	3	4	25
TOTAL MULTIPLE DX	805	2.1	7	1	1	1	2	4	5	11
TOTAL										
0–19 Years	348	2.0	6	1	1	1	2	4	5	10
20–34	237	1.9	2	1	1	1	2	4	5	8
35–49	198	2.3	10	1	1	1	2	4	8	21
50–64	110	2.1	11	1	1	1	2	4	5	6
65+	25	5.3	68	1	1	2	5	14	24	37
GRAND TOTAL	918	2.1	8	1	1	1	2	4	5	12

LOS by Diagnosis and Operation, Western Region, 45th Edition

Western Region, October 2007–September 2008 Data, by Operation

28.3: T&A

Type of Patients	Observed Patients	Avg. Stay	Variance	10th	25th	50th	75th	90th	95th	99th
1. SINGLE DX										
0–19 Years	215	1.2	<1	1	1	1	1	2	3	5
20–34	3	1.0	0	1	1	1	1	1	1	1
35–49	1	1.0	0	1	1	1	1	1	1	1
50–64	0									
65+	0									
2. MULTIPLE DX										
0–19 Years	1,834	1.9	10	1	1	1	2	3	5	14
20–34	47	1.9	7	1	1	1	1	3	5	15
35–49	16	1.9	4	1	1	1	2	5	8	8
50–64	2	1.5	<1	1	1	2	2	2	2	2
65+	1	1.0	0	1	1	1	1	1	1	1
TOTAL SINGLE DX	219	1.2	<1	1	1	1	1	2	3	5
TOTAL MULTIPLE DX	1,900	1.9	10	1	1	1	2	3	5	14
TOTAL										
0–19 Years	2,049	1.8	9	1	1	1	2	3	5	13
20–34	50	1.8	7	1	1	1	1	2	5	15
35–49	17	1.9	4	1	1	1	2	5	8	8
50–64	2	1.5	<1	1	1	2	2	2	2	2
65+	1	1.0	0	1	1	1	1	1	1	1
GRAND TOTAL	2,119	1.8	9	1	1	1	2	3	5	13

28.4: EXCISION OF TONSIL TAG

Type of Patients	Observed Patients	Avg. Stay	Variance	10th	25th	50th	75th	90th	95th	99th
1. SINGLE DX										
0–19 Years	0									
20–34	0									
35–49	0									
50–64	0									
65+	0									
2. MULTIPLE DX										
0–19 Years	0									
20–34	1	3.0	0	3	3	3	3	3	3	3
35–49	0									
50–64	0									
65+	0									
TOTAL SINGLE DX	0									
TOTAL MULTIPLE DX	1	3.0	0	3	3	3	3	3	3	3
TOTAL										
0–19 Years	0									
20–34	1	3.0	0	3	3	3	3	3	3	3
35–49	0									
50–64	0									
65+	0									
GRAND TOTAL	1	3.0	0	3	3	3	3	3	3	3

28.5: EXCISION LINGUAL TONSIL

Type of Patients	Observed Patients	Avg. Stay	Variance	10th	25th	50th	75th	90th	95th	99th
1. SINGLE DX										
0–19 Years	0									
20–34	0									
35–49	1	1.0	0	1	1	1	1	1	1	1
50–64	0									
65+	0									
2. MULTIPLE DX										
0–19 Years	13	1.0	0	1	1	1	1	1	1	1
20–34	2	2.0	2	1	1	3	3	3	3	3
35–49	2	1.0	0	1	1	1	1	1	1	1
50–64	2	2.0	2	1	1	3	3	3	3	3
65+	1	1.0	0	1	1	1	1	1	1	1
TOTAL SINGLE DX	1	1.0	0	1	1	1	1	1	1	1
TOTAL MULTIPLE DX	20	1.1	<1	1	1	1	1	1	3	3
TOTAL										
0–19 Years	13	1.0	0	1	1	1	1	1	1	1
20–34	2	2.0	2	1	1	3	3	3	3	3
35–49	3	1.0	0	1	1	1	1	1	1	1
50–64	2	2.0	2	1	1	3	3	3	3	3
65+	1	1.0	0	1	1	1	1	1	1	1
GRAND TOTAL	21	1.1	<1	1	1	1	1	1	3	3

28.6: ADENOIDECTOMY

Type of Patients	Observed Patients	Avg. Stay	Variance	10th	25th	50th	75th	90th	95th	99th
1. SINGLE DX										
0–19 Years	5	1.6	2	1	1	1	1	4	4	4
20–34	0									
35–49	0									
50–64	1	1.0	0	1	1	1	1	1	1	1
65+	0									
2. MULTIPLE DX										
0–19 Years	80	3.0	37	1	1	1	2	8	10	43
20–34	2	1.0	0	1	1	1	1	1	1	1
35–49	2	1.0	0	1	1	1	1	1	1	1
50–64	0									
65+	0									
TOTAL SINGLE DX	6	1.5	1	1	1	1	1	4	4	4
TOTAL MULTIPLE DX	84	3.0	36	1	1	1	2	8	10	43
TOTAL										
0–19 Years	85	3.0	35	1	1	1	2	7	10	43
20–34	2	1.0	0	1	1	1	1	1	1	1
35–49	2	1.0	0	1	1	1	1	1	1	1
50–64	1	1.0	0	1	1	1	1	1	1	1
65+	0									
GRAND TOTAL	90	2.9	35	1	1	1	2	7	10	43

LOS by Diagnosis and Operation, Western Region, 45th Edition

Western Region, October 2007–September 2008 Data, by Operation

28.7: HEMOR CONTROL POST T&A

Type of Patients	Observed Patients	Avg. Stay	Vari-ance	Percentiles						
				10th	25th	50th	75th	90th	95th	99th
1. SINGLE DX										
0–19 Years	176	1.1	<1	1	1	1	1	2	2	3
20–34	79	1.1	<1	1	1	1	1	2	2	3
35–49	19	1.0	0	1	1	1	1	1	1	1
50–64	5	1.0	0	1	1	1	1	1	1	1
65+	0									
2. MULTIPLE DX										
0–19 Years	150	1.8	5	1	1	1	2	3	4	7
20–34	67	1.8	3	1	1	1	2	3	4	12
35–49	36	1.5	<1	1	1	1	2	3	3	5
50–64	14	2.0	3	1	1	1	2	5	6	6
65+	6	2.7	3	1	1	2	5	5	5	5
TOTAL SINGLE DX	279	1.1	<1	1	1	1	1	2	2	3
TOTAL MULTIPLE DX	273	1.8	4	1	1	1	2	3	4	7
TOTAL										
0–19 Years	326	1.4	2	1	1	1	1	2	3	4
20–34	146	1.4	1	1	1	1	1	2	3	7
35–49	55	1.3	<1	1	1	1	1	2	3	5
50–64	19	1.7	2	1	1	1	2	5	6	6
65+	6	2.7	3	1	1	2	5	5	5	5
GRAND TOTAL	552	1.4	2	1	1	1	1	2	3	5

28.9: OTHER TONSIL/ADENOID OPS

Type of Patients	Observed Patients	Avg. Stay	Vari-ance	Percentiles						
				10th	25th	50th	75th	90th	95th	99th
1. SINGLE DX										
0–19 Years	2	1.0	0	1	1	1	1	1	1	1
20–34	0									
35–49	1	1.0	0	1	1	1	1	1	1	1
50–64	0									
65+	0									
2. MULTIPLE DX										
0–19 Years	4	3.4	4	3	3	3	3	3	9	9
20–34	0									
35–49	4	1.5	<1	1	1	2	2	2	2	2
50–64	5	4.8	35	1	1	2	5	15	15	15
65+	6	6.0	20	1	4	5	8	14	14	14
TOTAL SINGLE DX	3	1.0	0	1	1	1	1	1	1	1
TOTAL MULTIPLE DX	19	4.0	14	1	2	3	4	9	14	15
TOTAL										
0–19 Years	6	2.6	4	1	1	3	3	3	9	9
20–34	0									
35–49	5	1.4	<1	1	1	1	2	2	2	2
50–64	5	4.8	35	1	1	2	5	15	15	15
65+	6	6.0	20	1	4	5	8	14	14	14
GRAND TOTAL	22	3.4	13	1	1	3	4	8	14	15

29.0: PHARYNGOTOMY

Type of Patients	Observed Patients	Avg. Stay	Vari-ance	Percentiles						
				10th	25th	50th	75th	90th	95th	99th
1. SINGLE DX										
0–19 Years	7	2.0	<1	1	2	2	2	3	3	3
20–34	3	4.0	9	1	1	4	7	7	7	7
35–49	4	3.5	4	1	1	3	4	6	6	6
50–64	0									
65+	0									
2. MULTIPLE DX										
0–19 Years	8	3.6	1	2	3	4	4	5	5	5
20–34	8	5.5	29	2	2	5	7	18	18	18
35–49	13	5.0	13	2	3	4	6	10	14	14
50–64	11	6.8	156	1	2	5	5	6	44	44
65+	4	6.5	15	3	5	5	12	12	12	12
TOTAL SINGLE DX	14	2.7	3	1	2	2	3	6	7	7
TOTAL MULTIPLE DX	44	5.3	44	2	2	4	5	10	14	44
TOTAL										
0–19 Years	15	2.9	2	1	2	3	4	4	5	5
20–34	11	5.1	23	2	3	4	7	7	18	18
35–49	17	4.7	11	1	2	4	6	10	14	14
50–64	11	6.8	156	1	2	3	5	6	44	44
65+	4	6.5	15	3	5	5	12	12	12	12
GRAND TOTAL	58	4.6	35	1	2	3	5	7	12	44

29.1: PHARYNGEAL DXTIC PX

Type of Patients	Observed Patients	Avg. Stay	Vari-ance	Percentiles						
				10th	25th	50th	75th	90th	95th	99th
1. SINGLE DX										
0–19 Years	4	1.3	<1	1	1	1	2	2	2	2
20–34	3	2.0	<1	1	1	2	3	3	3	3
35–49	3	2.0	0	2	2	1	1	1	1	1
50–64	1	1.0	0	1	1	1	1	1	1	1
65+	1	1.0	0	1	1	1	1	1	1	1
2. MULTIPLE DX										
0–19 Years	44	5.2	39	1	2	3	6	17	19	36
20–34	38	3.5	19	1	1	2	4	7	12	26
35–49	46	4.1	32	2	2	3	3	11	15	31
50–64	95	4.9	19	1	2	3	6	11	14	22
65+	130	5.6	25	2	2	4	7	12	15	27
TOTAL SINGLE DX	12	1.5	<1	1	1	1	2	2	3	3
TOTAL MULTIPLE DX	353	5.0	27	1	2	3	6	12	16	27
TOTAL										
0–19 Years	48	4.9	37	1	2	3	4	13	17	36
20–34	41	3.4	18	1	1	2	3	5	8	26
35–49	49	4.0	30	1	1	2	3	11	15	31
50–64	96	4.9	19	1	2	3	6	11	14	22
65+	131	5.6	25	2	2	4	7	12	15	27
GRAND TOTAL	365	4.8	26	1	2	3	6	11	15	26

LOS by Diagnosis and Operation, Western Region, 45th Edition

Western Region, October 2007–September 2008 Data, by Operation

29.11: PHARYNGOSCOPY

Type of Patients	Observed Patients	Avg. Stay	Variance	Percentiles						
				10th	25th	50th	75th	90th	95th	99th
1. SINGLE DX										
0–19 Years	4	1.3	<1	1	1	1	2	2	2	2
20–34	3	2.0	<1	1	1	2	3	3	3	3
35–49	3	2.0	0	2	2	2	2	2	2	2
50–64	1	1.0	0	1	1	1	1	1	1	1
65+	0									
2. MULTIPLE DX										
0–19 Years	40	5.1	38	1	2	3	6	13	17	36
20–34	34	3.6	21	1	1	2	4	7	12	26
35–49	38	3.0	12	1	1	2	3	7	14	18
50–64	60	3.7	8	1	2	3	5	8	10	14
65+	95	5.3	22	2	2	4	7	12	16	27
TOTAL SINGLE DX	11	1.6	<1	1	1	2	2	2	3	3
TOTAL MULTIPLE DX	267	4.5	22	1	2	3	5	9	15	26
TOTAL										
0–19 Years	44	4.7	36	1	2	3	4	13	17	36
20–34	37	3.5	20	1	1	2	3	7	12	26
35–49	41	3.0	12	1	1	2	3	7	7	18
50–64	61	3.7	8	1	2	3	5	8	8	14
65+	95	5.3	22	2	2	4	7	12	16	27
GRAND TOTAL	278	4.3	22	1	2	3	5	9	15	24

29.3: EXC/DESTR PHARYNGEAL LES

Type of Patients	Observed Patients	Avg. Stay	Variance	Percentiles						
				10th	25th	50th	75th	90th	95th	99th
1. SINGLE DX										
0–19 Years	7	3.4	4	1	1	3	5	6	6	6
20–34	2	1.5	<1	1	1	2	2	2	2	2
35–49	2	2.0	2	1	1	2	3	3	3	3
50–64	9	1.9	1	1	1	1	3	3	3	3
65+	8	2.4	<1	1	2	2	3	4	4	4
2. MULTIPLE DX										
0–19 Years	10	3.7	6	1	1	5	5	7	8	8
20–34	9	3.8	8	1	2	3	4	9	9	9
35–49	19	4.2	18	1	1	2	6	11	17	17
50–64	59	4.6	38	1	1	3	5	11	11	43
65+	188	4.8	59	1	1	2	5	11	18	53
TOTAL SINGLE DX	28	2.5	2	1	1	2	3	5	5	6
TOTAL MULTIPLE DX	285	4.6	47	1	1	2	5	10	16	43
TOTAL										
0–19 Years	17	3.6	5	1	1	5	5	7	7	8
20–34	11	3.4	8	1	1	2	4	8	9	9
35–49	21	4.0	16	1	1	2	5	8	11	17
50–64	68	4.2	34	1	1	3	4	10	11	43
65+	196	4.7	57	1	1	2	5	11	18	53
GRAND TOTAL	313	4.4	43	1	1	2	5	10	16	39

29.2: EXC BRANCHIAL CLEFT CYST

Type of Patients	Observed Patients	Avg. Stay	Variance	Percentiles						
				10th	25th	50th	75th	90th	95th	99th
1. SINGLE DX										
0–19 Years	15	1.6	<1	1	1	1	2	2	2	2
20–34	15	1.5	<1	1	1	1	2	3	3	3
35–49	6	1.7	<1	1	1	2	2	2	2	2
50–64	3	1.0	0	1	1	1	1	1	1	1
65+	0									
2. MULTIPLE DX										
0–19 Years	14	5.4	58	1	1	2	4	23	23	23
20–34	8	4.0	9	1	1	2	6	9	9	9
35–49	11	1.9	4	1	1	1	2	2	8	8
50–64	15	1.7	2	1	1	1	2	4	5	5
65+	6	1.2	<1	1	1	1	1	2	2	2
TOTAL SINGLE DX	39	1.5	<1	1	1	1	2	3	4	4
TOTAL MULTIPLE DX	54	3.5	28	1	1	1	4	7	23	23
TOTAL										
0–19 Years	29	3.2	28	1	1	1	2	4	23	23
20–34	23	2.3	5	1	1	1	3	6	7	9
35–49	17	1.8	3	1	1	1	2	3	8	8
50–64	18	1.6	1	1	1	1	1	4	5	5
65+	6	1.2	<1	1	1	1	1	2	2	2
GRAND TOTAL	93	2.5	16	1	1	1	2	4	7	23

29.32: PHAR DIVERTICULECTOMY

Type of Patients	Observed Patients	Avg. Stay	Variance	Percentiles						
				10th	25th	50th	75th	90th	95th	99th
1. SINGLE DX										
0–19 Years	0									
20–34	0									
35–49	1	1.0	0	1	1	1	1	1	1	1
50–64	7	2.1	1	1	1	3	3	3	3	3
65+	4	2.3	<1	1	1	2	3	3	3	3
2. MULTIPLE DX										
0–19 Years	0									
20–34	0									
35–49	2	3.0	8	1	1	5	5	5	5	5
50–64	20	3.5	9	1	1	3	4	9	11	11
65+	87	4.6	36	1	1	2	5	13	18	31
TOTAL SINGLE DX	12	2.1	<1	1	1	2	3	3	3	3
TOTAL MULTIPLE DX	109	4.4	31	1	1	2	5	12	18	24
TOTAL										
0–19 Years	0									
20–34	0									
35–49	3	2.3	5	1	1	1	5	5	5	5
50–64	27	3.2	7	1	1	3	4	9	9	11
65+	91	4.5	35	1	1	2	5	12	18	31
GRAND TOTAL	121	4.1	28	1	1	2	4	11	17	24

LOS by Diagnosis and Operation, Western Region, 45th Edition

Western Region, October 2007–September 2008 Data, by Operation

29.4: PLASTIC OP ON PHARYNX

Type of Patients	Observed Patients	Avg. Stay	Vari-ance	10th	25th	50th	75th	90th	95th	99th
1. SINGLE DX										
0–19 Years	16	1.6	<1	1	1	1	2	2	2	4
20–34	1	1.0	0	1	1	1	1	1	1	1
35–49	0									
50–64	2	1.5	<1	1	1	1	2	2	2	2
65+	0									
2. MULTIPLE DX										
0–19 Years	95	1.6	1	1	1	1	2	3	4	6
20–34	15	2.0	3	1	1	1	3	4	7	7
35–49	24	1.5	<1	1	1	1	2	3	3	4
50–64	24	2.2	4	1	1	2	3	3	4	10
65+	9	1.9	2	1	1	1	2	5	5	5
TOTAL SINGLE DX	19	1.5	<1	1	1	1	2	2	2	4
TOTAL MULTIPLE DX	167	1.7	2	1	1	1	2	3	4	6
TOTAL										
0–19 Years	111	1.6	1	1	1	1	2	3	4	6
20–34	16	1.9	3	1	1	1	2	4	7	7
35–49	24	1.5	<1	1	1	1	2	3	3	4
50–64	26	2.1	3	1	1	2	2	3	4	10
65+	9	1.9	2	1	1	1	2	5	5	5
GRAND TOTAL	186	1.7	1	1	1	1	2	3	4	6

29.5: OTHER PHARYNGEAL REPAIR

Type of Patients	Observed Patients	Avg. Stay	Vari-ance	10th	25th	50th	75th	90th	95th	99th
1. SINGLE DX										
0–19 Years	4	1.3	<1	1	1	1	1	3	3	3
20–34	0									
35–49	1	1.0	0	1	1	1	1	1	1	1
50–64	0									
65+	0									
2. MULTIPLE DX										
0–19 Years	8	2.7	9	1	1	1	2	8	10	10
20–34	7	9.6	49	1	3	9	14	22	22	22
35–49	7	4.2	15	1	1	3	8	11	11	11
50–64	7	8.6	38	1	5	7	13	20	20	20
65+	12	9.5	119	1	3	7	12	19	40	40
TOTAL SINGLE DX	5	1.2	<1	1	1	1	1	3	3	3
TOTAL MULTIPLE DX	41	6.7	55	1	1	5	9	14	20	40
TOTAL										
0–19 Years	12	2.1	6	1	1	1	2	8	10	10
20–34	7	9.6	49	1	3	9	14	22	22	22
35–49	8	3.8	15	1	1	3	8	11	11	11
50–64	7	8.6	38	1	5	7	13	20	20	20
65+	12	9.5	119	1	3	7	12	19	40	40
GRAND TOTAL	46	5.9	51	1	1	3	8	13	20	40

29.9: OTHER PHARYNGEAL OPS

Type of Patients	Observed Patients	Avg. Stay	Vari-ance	10th	25th	50th	75th	90th	95th	99th
1. SINGLE DX										
0–19 Years	0									
20–34	0									
35–49	1	3.0	0	3	3	3	3	3	3	3
50–64	0									
65+	0									
2. MULTIPLE DX										
0–19 Years	1	2.0	0	2	2	2	2	2	2	2
20–34	0									
35–49	1	3.0	0	3	3	3	3	3	3	3
50–64	0									
65+	1	2.0	0	2	2	2	2	2	2	2
TOTAL SINGLE DX	1	3.0	0	3	3	3	3	3	3	3
TOTAL MULTIPLE DX	3	2.3	<1	2	2	2	3	3	3	3
TOTAL										
0–19 Years	1	2.0	0	2	2	2	2	2	2	2
20–34	0									
35–49	2	3.0	0	3	3	3	3	3	3	3
50–64	0									
65+	1	2.0	0	2	2	2	2	2	2	2
GRAND TOTAL	4	2.5	<1	2	2	2	3	3	3	3

30.0: EXC/DESTR LES LARYNX

Type of Patients	Observed Patients	Avg. Stay	Vari-ance	10th	25th	50th	75th	90th	95th	99th
1. SINGLE DX										
0–19 Years	16	2.0	4	1	1	1	2	4	7	7
20–34	2	2.0	0	2	2	2	2	2	2	2
35–49	2	1.0	0	1	1	1	1	1	1	1
50–64	1	2.0	0	2	2	2	2	2	2	2
65+	0									
2. MULTIPLE DX										
0–19 Years	130	5.9	95	1	1	2	6	18	26	46
20–34	9	2.6	6	1	1	2	2	8	8	8
35–49	32	3.0	15	1	1	2	3	6	6	22
50–64	59	4.6	101	1	1	2	4	9	14	74
65+	63	3.4	17	1	1	2	4	8	11	21
TOTAL SINGLE DX	21	2.0	3	1	1	1	2	4	7	7
TOTAL MULTIPLE DX	293	5.2	80	1	1	2	5	13	24	46
TOTAL										
0–19 Years	146	5.5	87	1	1	2	6	16	26	46
20–34	11	2.5	5	1	1	2	2	5	8	8
35–49	34	2.9	14	1	1	1	3	6	6	22
50–64	60	4.5	100	1	1	2	4	9	14	74
65+	63	3.4	17	1	1	2	4	8	11	21
GRAND TOTAL	314	4.9	75	1	1	2	5	13	22	46

LOS by Diagnosis and Operation, Western Region, 45th Edition

Western Region, October 2007–September 2008 Data, by Operation

30.09: EXC/DESTR LARYNX LES NEC

Type of Patients	Observed Patients	Avg. Stay	Vari-ance	10th	25th	50th	75th	90th	95th	99th
1. SINGLE DX										
0–19 Years	16	2.0	4	1	1	1	2	4	7	7
20–34	2	2.0	0	2	2	2	2	2	2	2
35–49	2	1.0	0	1	1	1	1	1	1	1
50–64	1	2.0	0	2	2	2	2	2	2	2
65+	0									
2. MULTIPLE DX										
0–19 Years	124	5.6	87	1	1	2	6	16	26	46
20–34	9	2.6	6	1	1	2	2	8	8	8
35–49	32	3.0	15	1	1	2	3	6	6	22
50–64	56	4.6	106	1	1	2	4	9	14	74
65+	63	3.4	17	1	1	2	4	8	11	21
TOTAL SINGLE DX	21	2.0	3	1	1	1	2	4	7	7
TOTAL MULTIPLE DX	284	5.0	74	1	1	2	5	13	24	46
TOTAL										
0–19 Years	140	5.2	79	1	1	1	5	13	26	46
20–34	11	2.5	5	1	1	2	2	5	8	8
35–49	34	2.9	14	1	1	1	3	6	6	22
50–64	57	4.6	105	1	1	2	4	9	14	74
65+	63	3.4	17	1	1	2	4	8	11	21
GRAND TOTAL	305	4.7	69	1	1	2	4	12	22	46

30.2: PARTIAL LARYNGECTOMY NEC

Type of Patients	Observed Patients	Avg. Stay	Vari-ance	10th	25th	50th	75th	90th	95th	99th
1. SINGLE DX										
0–19 Years	2	1.5	<1	1	1	2	2	2	2	2
20–34	1	2.0	0	2	1	1	2	2	2	2
35–49	1	2.0	0	1	1	1	1	1	1	1
50–64	4	1.0	0	1	1	1	1	1	1	1
65+	1	2.0	0	2	2	2	2	2	2	2
2. MULTIPLE DX										
0–19 Years	18	7.7	54	1	1	4	15	19	19	19
20–34	9	6.0	31	1	2	5	9	17	17	17
35–49	10	6.0	30	1	2	3	7	18	18	18
50–64	21	5.1	17	1	2	4	7	9	10	18
65+	29	4.6	12	1	2	4	7	11	11	13
TOTAL SINGLE DX	9	1.4	<1	1	1	1	2	2	2	2
TOTAL MULTIPLE DX	87	6.2	34	1	1	4	10	15	19	19
TOTAL										
0–19 Years	20	6.9	51	1	1	2	15	19	19	19
20–34	10	5.6	29	1	2	5	9	17	17	17
35–49	11	5.6	29	1	1	3	7	12	18	18
50–64	25	4.4	17	1	2	3	7	9	10	18
65+	30	4.5	12	1	2	4	7	10	11	13
GRAND TOTAL	96	5.7	33	1	1	3	8	15	19	19

30.1: HEMILARYNGECTOMY

Type of Patients	Observed Patients	Avg. Stay	Vari-ance	10th	25th	50th	75th	90th	95th	99th
1. SINGLE DX										
0–19 Years	0									
20–34	0									
35–49	0									
50–64	0									
65+	0									
2. MULTIPLE DX										
0–19 Years	0									
20–34	0									
35–49	2	6.0	49	1	1	1	11	11	11	11
50–64	0									
65+	5	9.0	53	1	2	10	15	17	17	17
TOTAL SINGLE DX	0									
TOTAL MULTIPLE DX	7	8.1	46	1	1	10	15	17	17	17
TOTAL										
0–19 Years	0									
20–34	0									
35–49	2	6.0	49	1	1	1	11	11	11	11
50–64	0									
65+	5	9.0	53	1	2	10	15	17	17	17
GRAND TOTAL	7	8.1	46	1	1	10	15	17	17	17

30.3: COMPLETE LARYNGECTOMY

Type of Patients	Observed Patients	Avg. Stay	Vari-ance	10th	25th	50th	75th	90th	95th	99th
1. SINGLE DX										
0–19 Years	0									
20–34	0									
35–49	2	21.0	0	21	21	21	21	21	21	21
50–64	1	4.0	0	4	4	4	4	4	4	4
65+	0									
2. MULTIPLE DX										
0–19 Years	0									
20–34	1	8.0	0	8	8	8	8	8	8	8
35–49	8	22.7	353	7	8	13	31	60	60	60
50–64	53	14.6	115	7	8	10	16	30	36	52
65+	79	13.3	94	6	7	10	16	27	35	55
TOTAL SINGLE DX	3	15.4	95	4	4	21	21	21	21	21
TOTAL MULTIPLE DX	141	14.3	118	6	8	10	17	28	36	55
TOTAL										
0–19 Years	0									
20–34	1	8.0	0	8	8	8	8	8	8	8
35–49	10	22.3	275	7	8	17	31	38	60	60
50–64	54	14.4	115	6	8	10	16	30	36	52
65+	79	13.3	94	6	7	10	16	27	35	55
GRAND TOTAL	144	14.3	117	6	8	10	17	28	36	55

LOS by Diagnosis and Operation, Western Region, 45th Edition

Western Region, October 2007–September 2008 Data, by Operation

30.4: RADICAL LARYNGECTOMY

Type of Patients	Observed Patients	Avg. Stay	Variance	10th	25th	50th	75th	90th	95th	99th
1. SINGLE DX										
0–19 Years	0									
20–34	0									
35–49	1	15.0	0	15	15	15	15	15	15	15
50–64	1	3.0	0	3	3	3	3	3	3	3
65+	3	7.4	9	4	4	8	10	10	10	10
2. MULTIPLE DX										
0–19 Years	0									
20–34	3	7.7	2	6	6	8	9	9	9	9
35–49	20	14.7	169	6	7	9	15	43	45	45
50–64	81	13.5	179	7	7	10	14	22	33	96
65+	64	11.8	31	7	8	10	15	20	24	28
TOTAL SINGLE DX	5	8.0	23	3	4	8	10	15	15	15
TOTAL MULTIPLE DX	168	12.9	118	7	7	9	15	22	31	69
TOTAL										
0–19 Years	0									
20–34	3	7.7	2	6	6	8	9	9	9	9
35–49	21	14.7	160	6	7	9	15	43	43	45
50–64	82	13.4	178	7	7	10	14	22	33	96
65+	67	11.6	30	7	8	10	15	20	24	28
GRAND TOTAL	173	12.8	116	6	7	9	15	21	31	69

31.0: LARYNX INJECTION

Type of Patients	Observed Patients	Avg. Stay	Variance	10th	25th	50th	75th	90th	95th	99th
1. SINGLE DX										
0–19 Years	1	1.0	0	1	1	1	1	1	1	1
20–34	1	2.0	0	2	2	2	2	2	2	2
35–49	2	1.0	0	1	1	1	1	1	1	1
50–64	1	1.0	0	1	1	1	1	1	1	1
65+	0									
2. MULTIPLE DX										
0–19 Years	2	4.5	24	1	1	1	8	8	8	8
20–34	1	1.0	0	1	1	1	1	1	1	1
35–49	1	1.0		1	1	1	1	1	1	1
50–64	8	5.7	28	2	2	6	10	16	16	16
65+	16	5.4	40	1	1	2	7	14	22	22
TOTAL SINGLE DX	5	1.2	<1	1	1	1	1	2	2	2
TOTAL MULTIPLE DX	28	5.1	32	1	1	2	7	14	16	22
TOTAL										
0–19 Years	3	3.3	16	1	1	2	8	8	8	8
20–34	2	1.5	<1	1	1	2	2	2	2	2
35–49	3	1.0	0	1	1	1	1	1	1	1
50–64	9	5.1	27	1	1	2	7	16	16	16
65+	16	5.4	40	1	1	2	7	14	22	22
GRAND TOTAL	33	4.5	29	1	1	2	7	13	16	22

31.1: TEMPORARY TRACHEOSTOMY

Type of Patients	Observed Patients	Avg. Stay	Variance	10th	25th	50th	75th	90th	95th	99th
1. SINGLE DX										
0–19 Years	1	9.0	0	9	9	9	9	9	9	9
20–34	3	6.3	5	5	5	5	5	9	9	9
35–49	10	5.6	4	3	4	6	7	8	8	8
50–64	13	6.7	16	2	4	7	8	11	16	16
65+	4	7.3	18	3	5	7	13	13	13	13
2. MULTIPLE DX										
0–19 Years	216	31.5	555	7	14	27	59	98	>99	>99
20–34	375	27.1	356	7	11	24	39	60	79	>99
35–49	841	26.2	318	7	13	23	36	52	68	>99
50–64	1,788	24.1	314	6	11	20	33	52	69	>99
65+	2,139	23.6	242	7	13	21	31	46	59	>99
TOTAL SINGLE DX	31	6.5	10	3	4	6	8	10	13	16
TOTAL MULTIPLE DX	5,359	25.0	313	7	12	22	34	53	72	>99
TOTAL										
0–19 Years	217	31.5	555	7	14	27	59	98	>99	>99
20–34	378	27.0	357	7	11	24	38	59	79	>99
35–49	851	26.0	320	7	13	23	36	52	68	>99
50–64	1,801	24.0	314	6	11	20	32	52	69	>99
65+	2,143	23.5	242	7	13	21	31	46	59	>99
GRAND TOTAL	5,390	24.9	313	7	12	21	34	53	72	>99

31.2: PERMANENT TRACHEOSTOMY

Type of Patients	Observed Patients	Avg. Stay	Variance	10th	25th	50th	75th	90th	95th	99th
1. SINGLE DX										
0–19 Years	0									
20–34	1	4.0	0	4	4	4	4	4	4	4
35–49	0									
50–64	0									
65+	1	3.0	0	3	3	3	3	3	3	3
2. MULTIPLE DX										
0–19 Years	31	29.7	453	7	17	25	42	82	>99	>99
20–34	49	30.9	437	10	15	27	39	79	88	>99
35–49	133	27.0	371	6	13	22	36	56	79	>99
50–64	334	24.2	349	6	10	20	33	54	70	>99
65+	440	24.5	261	8	13	22	32	52	66	>99
TOTAL SINGLE DX	2	3.5	<1	3	3	3	4	4	4	4
TOTAL MULTIPLE DX	987	25.3	326	7	13	22	34	55	75	>99
TOTAL										
0–19 Years	31	29.7	453	7	17	25	42	82	>99	>99
20–34	50	30.4	443	7	15	27	39	79	88	>99
35–49	133	27.0	371	6	13	22	36	56	79	>99
50–64	334	24.2	349	6	10	20	33	54	70	>99
65+	441	24.5	262	8	13	22	32	52	66	>99
GRAND TOTAL	989	25.3	326	7	13	22	34	55	75	>99

LOS by Diagnosis and Operation, Western Region, 45th Edition

Western Region, October 2007–September 2008 Data, by Operation

31.4: LARYNX/TRACHEA DXTIC PX

Type of Patients	Observed Patients	Avg. Stay	Variance	10th	25th	50th	75th	90th	95th	99th
1. SINGLE DX										
0–19 Years	60	1.5	<1	1	1	1	2	2	3	5
20–34	19	1.9	2	1	1	1	2	4	7	7
35–49	10	2.4	2	1	1	2	3	4	6	6
50–64	15	1.7	3	1	1	1	2	3	8	8
65+	2	4.0	2	3	3	5	5	5	5	5
2. MULTIPLE DX										
0–19 Years	415	5.8	68	1	1	3	7	12	23	40
20–34	150	2.9	8	1	1	2	3	6	8	16
35–49	251	4.1	18	1	1	3	5	8	12	23
50–64	424	4.9	29	1	2	3	6	10	14	29
65+	604	6.1	35	1	2	4	8	12	17	28
TOTAL SINGLE DX	106	1.6	1	1	1	1	2	3	4	7
TOTAL MULTIPLE DX	1,844	5.3	43	1	2	3	6	11	17	31
TOTAL										
0–19 Years	475	5.2	61	1	1	2	5	12	22	40
20–34	169	2.8	8	1	1	2	3	6	7	16
35–49	261	4.0	17	1	1	3	5	8	12	23
50–64	439	4.8	29	1	1	3	6	10	14	29
65+	606	6.1	34	1	2	4	8	12	17	27
GRAND TOTAL	1,950	5.0	41	1	1	3	6	10	16	31

31.42: LARYNGOSCOPY/TRACHEOSCPY

Type of Patients	Observed Patients	Avg. Stay	Variance	10th	25th	50th	75th	90th	95th	99th
1. SINGLE DX										
0–19 Years	60	1.5	<1	1	1	1	2	2	3	5
20–34	17	1.4	<1	1	1	1	2	3	3	3
35–49	8	1.8	<1	1	1	2	2	3	3	3
50–64	13	1.9	4	1	1	1	2	3	8	8
65+	2	4.0	2	3	3	5	5	5	5	5
2. MULTIPLE DX										
0–19 Years	402	5.8	69	1	1	3	7	13	23	40
20–34	147	2.8	8	1	1	2	3	5	7	16
35–49	218	3.7	11	1	1	3	5	8	10	15
50–64	351	4.7	26	1	2	3	6	9	14	29
65+	534	6.1	31	1	2	4	8	12	18	27
TOTAL SINGLE DX	100	1.5	1	1	1	1	2	2	3	5
TOTAL MULTIPLE DX	1,652	5.3	42	1	2	3	6	11	17	31
TOTAL										
0–19 Years	462	5.2	62	1	1	2	5	12	22	40
20–34	164	2.7	7	1	1	2	3	5	6	16
35–49	226	3.7	11	1	1	3	5	7	10	15
50–64	364	4.6	25	1	2	3	6	9	14	29
65+	536	6.1	31	1	2	4	8	12	18	27
GRAND TOTAL	1,752	5.0	40	1	1	3	6	10	16	31

31.29: OTHER PERM TRACHEOSTOMY

Type of Patients	Observed Patients	Avg. Stay	Variance	10th	25th	50th	75th	90th	95th	99th
1. SINGLE DX										
0–19 Years	0									
20–34	1	4.0	0	4	4	4	4	4	4	4
35–49	0									
50–64	0									
65+	1	3.0	0	3	3	3	3	3	3	3
2. MULTIPLE DX										
0–19 Years	31	29.7	453	7	17	25	42	82	>99	>99
20–34	49	30.9	437	10	15	27	39	79	88	>99
35–49	130	26.9	377	6	13	22	36	56	79	>99
50–64	325	23.9	344	6	10	20	32	54	70	>99
65+	435	24.6	264	8	13	22	32	52	66	>99
TOTAL SINGLE DX	2	3.5	<1	3	3	3	4	4	4	4
TOTAL MULTIPLE DX	970	25.2	326	7	12	22	34	55	76	>99
TOTAL										
0–19 Years	31	29.7	453	7	17	25	42	82	>99	>99
20–34	50	30.4	443	9	15	27	39	79	88	>99
35–49	130	26.9	377	6	13	22	36	56	79	>99
50–64	325	23.9	344	6	10	20	32	54	70	>99
65+	436	24.5	265	8	13	22	32	52	66	>99
GRAND TOTAL	972	25.2	326	7	12	22	34	55	76	>99

31.3: INC LARYNX/TRACHEA NEC

Type of Patients	Observed Patients	Avg. Stay	Variance	10th	25th	50th	75th	90th	95th	99th
1. SINGLE DX										
0–19 Years	1	1.0	0	1	1	1	1	1	1	1
20–34	0									
35–49	0									
50–64	1	3.0	0	3	3	3	3	3	3	3
65+	0									
2. MULTIPLE DX										
0–19 Years	4	3.0	13	1	1	2	2	11	11	11
20–34	2	5.0	0	5	5	5	5	5	5	5
35–49	9	11.1	79	2	7	8	14	30	30	30
50–64	14	7.6	75	1	1	5	12	19	31	31
65+	11	8.4	144	1	1	3	17	39	>99	>99
TOTAL SINGLE DX	2	1.4	<1	1	1	1	1	3	3	3
TOTAL MULTIPLE DX	40	7.7	82	1	2	4	11	22	31	>99
TOTAL										
0–19 Years	5	2.3	9	1	1	1	2	2	11	11
20–34	2	5.0	0	5	5	5	5	5	5	5
35–49	9	11.1	79	2	7	8	14	30	30	30
50–64	15	7.3	71	1	1	4	12	19	31	31
65+	11	8.4	144	1	1	3	17	39	>99	>99
GRAND TOTAL	42	7.0	78	1	1	3	9	20	31	>99

LOS by Diagnosis and Operation, Western Region, 45th Edition

Western Region, October 2007–September 2008 Data, by Operation

31.43: CLOSED LARYNX BIOPSY

Type of Patients	Observed Patients	Avg. Stay	Vari-ance	Percentiles						
				10th	25th	50th	75th	90th	95th	99th
1. SINGLE DX										
0–19 Years	0									
20–34	2	5.5	4	4	4	4	7	7	7	7
35–49	2	5.0	2	4	4	4	6	6	6	6
50–64	2	5.0	0	1	1	1	1	1	1	1
65+	0									
2. MULTIPLE DX										
0–19 Years	5	5.5	14	1	1	6	10	10	10	10
20–34	1	6.0	0	6	6	6	6	6	6	6
35–49	25	6.9	72	1	1	3	8	22	28	28
50–64	61	6.3	53	1	1	5	8	12	14	42
65+	44	5.0	21	1	1	4	6	13	15	19
TOTAL SINGLE DX	6	3.8	6	1	1	4	6	7	7	7
TOTAL MULTIPLE DX	136	5.9	42	1	1	4	8	13	16	37
TOTAL										
0–19 Years	5	5.5	14	1	1	6	10	10	10	10
20–34	3	5.7	2	4	4	6	7	7	7	7
35–49	27	6.8	67	1	1	3	8	22	28	28
50–64	63	6.1	52	1	1	5	8	12	14	42
65+	44	5.0	21	1	1	4	6	13	15	19
GRAND TOTAL	142	5.8	41	1	1	4	7	12	16	37

31.5: LOC EXC/DESTR LARYNX LES

Type of Patients	Observed Patients	Avg. Stay	Vari-ance	Percentiles						
				10th	25th	50th	75th	90th	95th	99th
1. SINGLE DX										
0–19 Years	2	3.0	5	1	1	3	5	5	5	5
20–34	1	5.0	0	5	5	5	5	5	5	5
35–49	0									
50–64	1	5.0	0	5	5	5	5	5	5	5
65+	0									
2. MULTIPLE DX										
0–19 Years	45	3.6	19	1	1	2	4	8	15	31
20–34	15	3.8	8	1	1	4	7	8	9	9
35–49	21	6.5	87	2	3	4	6	8	13	46
50–64	35	7.5	102	1	1	4	8	19	39	45
65+	48	11.1	308	1	3	6	10	35	71	>99
TOTAL SINGLE DX	4	3.4	4	1	1	5	5	5	5	5
TOTAL MULTIPLE DX	164	6.1	107	1	1	3	6	12	19	71
TOTAL										
0–19 Years	47	3.6	18	1	1	2	4	6	11	15
20–34	16	3.8	8	1	1	3	7	8	9	9
35–49	21	6.5	87	2	3	4	6	8	13	46
50–64	36	7.4	100	1	1	4	8	19	39	45
65+	48	11.1	308	1	3	6	10	35	71	>99
GRAND TOTAL	168	6.0	103	1	1	3	6	11	19	71

31.6: REPAIR OF LARYNX

Type of Patients	Observed Patients	Avg. Stay	Vari-ance	Percentiles						
				10th	25th	50th	75th	90th	95th	99th
1. SINGLE DX										
0–19 Years	8	3.0	6	1	1	2	5	8	8	8
20–34	1	1.0	0	1	1	2	1	1	1	1
35–49	6	3.8	5	1	2	4	5	7	7	7
50–64	6	1.5	<1	1	1	1	2	3	3	3
65+	1	1.0	0	1	1	1	1	1	1	1
2. MULTIPLE DX										
0–19 Years	61	10.4	155	1	2	5	18	30	38	>99
20–34	7	10.1	103	1	1	7	15	30	30	30
35–49	23	3.6	22	1	1	1	4	11	12	20
50–64	30	3.3	30	1	1	1	2	10	12	27
65+	42	2.3	26	1	1	1	1	2	7	30
TOTAL SINGLE DX	22	2.7	5	1	1	2	5	5	8	8
TOTAL MULTIPLE DX	163	7.4	115	1	1	2	8	27	32	>99
TOTAL										
0–19 Years	69	9.6	144	1	2	5	14	29	38	>99
20–34	8	8.9	98	1	1	7	15	30	30	30
35–49	29	3.6	18	1	1	1	4	11	12	20
50–64	36	3.0	25	1	1	1	2	10	12	27
65+	43	2.3	25	1	1	1	1	2	7	30
GRAND TOTAL	185	6.9	105	1	1	2	7	24	30	>99

31.69: OTHER LARYNGEAL REPAIR

Type of Patients	Observed Patients	Avg. Stay	Vari-ance	Percentiles						
				10th	25th	50th	75th	90th	95th	99th
1. SINGLE DX										
0–19 Years	8	3.0	6	1	1	2	5	8	8	8
20–34	0									
35–49	3	2.7	4	1	1	2	5	5	5	5
50–64	5	1.2	<1	1	1	1	1	2	2	2
65+	1	1.0	0	1	1	1	1	1	1	1
2. MULTIPLE DX										
0–19 Years	60	10.4	156	1	2	5	15	30	38	>99
20–34	6	6.7	29	1	1	7	10	15	15	15
35–49	18	1.8	1	1	1	1	3	4	4	4
50–64	26	2.6	30	1	1	1	1	4	12	27
65+	41	2.4	27	1	1	1	1	2	7	30
TOTAL SINGLE DX	17	2.5	5	1	1	2	5	5	8	8
TOTAL MULTIPLE DX	151	7.3	117	1	1	2	7	27	32	>99
TOTAL										
0–19 Years	68	9.5	144	1	2	4	14	29	38	>99
20–34	6	6.7	29	1	1	7	10	15	15	15
35–49	21	2.0	2	1	1	1	4	4	4	5
50–64	31	2.4	25	1	1	1	1	2	12	27
65+	42	2.3	26	1	1	1	1	2	7	30
GRAND TOTAL	168	6.8	108	1	1	2	7	24	30	>99

LOS by Diagnosis and Operation, Western Region, 45th Edition

Western Region, October 2007–September 2008 Data, by Operation

31.7: REPAIR OF TRACHEA

Type of Patients	Observed Patients	Avg. Stay	Variance	Percentiles						
				10th	25th	50th	75th	90th	95th	99th
1. SINGLE DX										
0–19 Years	9	2.0	4	1	1	1	1	5	5	9
20–34	1	3.0	0	3	3	3	3	3	3	3
35–49	1	2.0	0	2	2	2	2	2	2	2
50–64	0									
65+	0									
2. MULTIPLE DX										
0–19 Years	147	9.5	158	1	1	4	14	27	37	>99
20–34	38	11.6	340	1	3	7	9	33	67	94
35–49	71	13.0	215	2	3	9	16	28	47	84
50–64	134	12.6	208	1	3	8	17	31	37	88
65+	108	15.2	261	1	3	11	22	40	61	72
TOTAL SINGLE DX	11	2.1	4	1	1	1	2	5	5	9
TOTAL MULTIPLE DX	498	11.6	206	1	1	7	16	31	45	>99
TOTAL										
0–19 Years	156	8.9	150	1	1	3	13	26	37	>99
20–34	39	11.4	333	1	3	6	9	33	67	94
35–49	72	12.9	214	2	3	9	16	28	47	84
50–64	134	12.6	208	1	3	8	17	31	37	88
65+	108	15.2	261	1	3	11	22	40	61	72
GRAND TOTAL	509	11.2	201	1	1	6	15	30	43	>99

31.74: REVISION OF TRACHEOSTOMY

Type of Patients	Observed Patients	Avg. Stay	Variance	Percentiles						
				10th	25th	50th	75th	90th	95th	99th
1. SINGLE DX										
0–19 Years	1	1.0	0	1	1	1	1	1	1	1
20–34	0									
35–49	1	2.0	0	2	2	2	2	2	2	2
50–64	0									
65+	0									
2. MULTIPLE DX										
0–19 Years	16	6.0	241	1	1	3	3	9	14	79
20–34	14	18.6	807	1	2	3	26	67	94	94
35–49	41	14.7	176	2	5	10	20	31	47	50
50–64	82	15.1	218	2	5	11	21	33	41	>99
65+	81	17.5	301	1	5	13	24	45	63	>99
TOTAL SINGLE DX	2	1.5	<1	1	1	2	2	2	2	2
TOTAL MULTIPLE DX	234	15.1	280	1	3	9	20	37	53	94
TOTAL										
0–19 Years	17	5.8	232	1	1	2	3	9	14	79
20–34	14	18.6	807	1	2	3	26	67	94	94
35–49	42	14.4	175	2	4	10	20	31	47	50
50–64	82	15.1	218	2	5	11	21	33	41	>99
65+	81	17.5	301	1	5	13	24	45	63	>99
GRAND TOTAL	236	15.0	279	1	3	9	20	37	53	94

31.73: TRACH FISTULA CLOSE NEC

Type of Patients	Observed Patients	Avg. Stay	Variance	Percentiles						
				10th	25th	50th	75th	90th	95th	99th
1. SINGLE DX										
0–19 Years	5	1.1	<1	1	1	1	1	1	1	2
20–34	0									
35–49	0									
50–64	0									
65+	0									
2. MULTIPLE DX										
0–19 Years	79	11.1	224	1	1	4	19	37	69	>99
20–34	3	5.3	16	1	1	6	9	9	9	9
35–49	6	13.3	281	1	2	11	12	46	46	46
50–64	11	8.8	73	1	2	6	15	21	26	26
65+	12	6.7	56	1	1	5	11	13	26	26
TOTAL SINGLE DX	5	1.1	<1	1	1	1	1	1	2	2
TOTAL MULTIPLE DX	111	10.7	201	1	1	4	15	35	49	>99
TOTAL										
0–19 Years	84	10.2	212	1	1	3	15	35	61	>99
20–34	3	5.3	16	1	1	6	9	9	9	9
35–49	6	13.3	281	1	1	11	12	46	46	46
50–64	11	8.8	73	2	2	6	15	21	26	26
65+	12	6.7	56	1	1	5	11	13	26	26
GRAND TOTAL	116	9.9	192	1	1	3	15	35	46	>99

31.9: OTHER LARYNX/TRACHEA OPS

Type of Patients	Observed Patients	Avg. Stay	Variance	Percentiles						
				10th	25th	50th	75th	90th	95th	99th
1. SINGLE DX										
0–19 Years	3	5.7	4	4	4	5	8	8	8	8
20–34	4	1.5	<1	1	1	2	2	2	2	2
35–49	7	1.0	0	1	1	1	1	1	1	1
50–64	8	1.8	2	1	2	1	2	5	5	5
65+	1	1.0	0	1	1	1	1	1	1	1
2. MULTIPLE DX										
0–19 Years	56	14.1	445	1	2	5	26	63	98	>99
20–34	16	2.6	3	1	1	2	4	5	5	5
35–49	38	4.7	31	1	1	2	7	18	21	>99
50–64	65	4.4	32	1	1	2	7	11	13	>99
65+	57	6.3	135	1	1	2	8	13	20	83
TOTAL SINGLE DX	23	2.0	3	1	1	1	2	5	5	8
TOTAL MULTIPLE DX	232	8.6	236	1	1	3	8	31	66	>99
TOTAL										
0–19 Years	59	13.9	436	1	2	5	26	63	98	>99
20–34	20	2.4	2	1	1	2	3	5	5	5
35–49	45	4.1	28	1	1	2	4	18	21	>99
50–64	73	4.1	29	1	1	2	6	10	13	>99
65+	58	6.2	133	1	1	2	8	13	20	83
GRAND TOTAL	255	8.1	222	1	1	3	8	31	63	>99

LOS by Diagnosis and Operation, Western Region, 45th Edition

Western Region, October 2007–September 2008 Data, by Operation

31.99: TRACHEAL OPERATION NEC

Type of Patients	Observed Patients	Avg. Stay	Variance	10th	25th	50th	75th	90th	95th	99th
1. SINGLE DX										
0–19 Years	2	6.0	8	4	4	8	8	8	8	8
20–34	3	1.7	<1	1	1	2	2	2	2	2
35–49	5	1.0	0	1	1	1	1	1	1	1
50–64	2	1.0	0	1	1	1	1	1	1	1
65+	1	1.0	0	1	1	1	1	1	1	1
2. MULTIPLE DX										
0–19 Years	17	4.5	44	1	1	2	6	11	24	32
20–34	13	2.5	2	1	1	2	4	5	5	5
35–49	31	5.2	36	1	1	2	9	19	>99	>99
50–64	43	5.4	42	1	1	2	9	13	17	>99
65+	40	7.4	178	1	2	3	9	17	20	83
TOTAL SINGLE DX	13	1.9	4	1	1	1	2	4	8	8
TOTAL MULTIPLE DX	144	5.4	72	1	1	2	7	13	20	>99
TOTAL										
0–19 Years	19	4.6	42	1	1	2	6	11	24	32
20–34	16	2.3	2	1	1	2	4	5	5	5
35–49	36	4.6	33	1	1	2	8	19	>99	>99
50–64	45	5.2	41	1	1	2	9	13	17	>99
65+	41	7.3	174	1	2	3	8	13	18	83
GRAND TOTAL	157	5.2	68	1	1	2	6	13	20	>99

32.0: LOC EXC/DESTR BRONCH LES

Type of Patients	Observed Patients	Avg. Stay	Variance	10th	25th	50th	75th	90th	95th	99th
1. SINGLE DX										
0–19 Years	1	1.0	0	1	1	1	1	1	1	1
20–34	1	5.0	0	5	5	5	5	5	5	5
35–49	0									
50–64	1	8.0	0	8	8	8	8	8	8	8
65+	1	1.0	0	1	1	1	1	1	1	1
2. MULTIPLE DX										
0–19 Years	10	4.2	35	1	1	1	3	15	15	16
20–34	8	5.6	27	2	4	4	5	18	18	18
35–49	10	8.4	145	1	4	4	6	42	42	42
50–64	25	4.1	12	1	1	3	5	8	9	16
65+	32	4.4	14	1	2	3	5	11	13	13
TOTAL SINGLE DX	4	3.8	12	1	1	1	8	8	8	8
TOTAL MULTIPLE DX	85	4.8	33	1	1	3	6	13	15	42
TOTAL										
0–19 Years	11	4.1	33	1	1	1	3	15	15	16
20–34	9	5.6	24	2	4	4	5	18	18	18
35–49	10	8.4	145	1	4	4	6	42	42	42
50–64	26	4.2	12	1	1	3	6	8	9	16
65+	33	4.3	14	1	2	3	5	11	13	13
GRAND TOTAL	89	4.7	32	1	1	3	6	13	15	18

32.1: BRONCHIAL EXCISION NEC

Type of Patients	Observed Patients	Avg. Stay	Variance	10th	25th	50th	75th	90th	95th	99th
1. SINGLE DX										
0–19 Years	0									
20–34	0									
35–49	0									
50–64	0									
65+	0									
2. MULTIPLE DX										
0–19 Years	1	7.0	0	7	7	7	7	7	7	7
20–34	0									
35–49	4	5.0	0	5	4	5	5	5	5	5
50–64	3	6.0	7	5	4	5	9	9	9	9
65+	3	8.0	9	5	5	8	11	11	11	11
TOTAL SINGLE DX	0									
TOTAL MULTIPLE DX	8	6.8	4	5	5	7	8	9	11	11
TOTAL										
0–19 Years	1	7.0	0	7	7	7	7	7	7	7
20–34	0									
35–49	4	5.0	0	5	5	5	5	5	5	5
50–64	3	6.0	7	5	4	5	9	9	9	9
65+	3	8.0	9	5	5	8	11	11	11	11
GRAND TOTAL	8	6.8	4	5	5	7	8	9	11	11

32.2: LOC EXC/DESTR LUNG LES

Type of Patients	Observed Patients	Avg. Stay	Variance	10th	25th	50th	75th	90th	95th	99th
1. SINGLE DX										
0–19 Years	58	3.6	6	1	2	3	4	6	8	10
20–34	33	3.6	3	2	2	3	5	6	8	8
35–49	16	2.4	2	1	2	2	3	4	5	5
50–64	45	2.6	2	1	2	2	3	4	6	10
65+	23	2.8	3	1	1	3	4	5	5	7
2. MULTIPLE DX										
0–19 Years	316	8.5	115	2	3	6	9	16	29	83
20–34	338	7.9	79	2	3	5	9	16	23	>99
35–49	566	6.8	60	1	2	4	8	15	20	40
50–64	1,384	6.5	53	1	2	4	8	15	20	36
65+	1,902	6.7	46	1	3	4	8	14	19	36
TOTAL SINGLE DX	175	3.3	4	1	2	3	4	6	7	10
TOTAL MULTIPLE DX	4,506	6.9	62	1	3	4	8	15	21	46
TOTAL										
0–19 Years	374	7.7	101	2	3	5	8	15	28	83
20–34	371	7.5	74	2	3	5	9	16	23	>99
35–49	582	6.6	59	1	2	4	8	15	20	40
50–64	1,429	6.3	52	1	2	4	7	14	20	34
65+	1,925	6.6	46	1	3	4	8	14	19	34
GRAND TOTAL	4,681	6.8	60	1	3	4	8	14	20	45

LOS by Diagnosis and Operation, Western Region, 45th Edition

Western Region, October 2007–September 2008 Data, by Operation

32.20: THORSCPY EXC LUNG LES

Type of Patients	Observed Patients	Avg. Stay	Vari-ance	Percentiles						
				10th	25th	50th	75th	90th	95th	99th
1. SINGLE DX										
0–19 Years	41	3.9	8	1	2	3	5	8	10	17
20–34	27	3.5	4	2	2	3	4	6	8	8
35–49	12	2.4	2	1	1	3	3	4	5	5
50–64	39	2.5	3	1	1	2	3	4	7	10
65+	19	3.0	3	1	1	3	4	5	7	7
2. MULTIPLE DX										
0–19 Years	224	7.5	73	2	3	5	9	13	26	52
20–34	230	7.9	98	2	3	5	9	15	23	46
35–49	375	6.0	58	1	2	3	7	13	20	37
50–64	853	5.8	57	1	2	3	6	14	20	37
65+	1,135	6.0	42	1	2	4	7	14	18	33
TOTAL SINGLE DX	138	3.3	5	1	2	3	4	6	8	10
TOTAL MULTIPLE DX	2,817	6.3	57	1	2	4	7	14	20	41
TOTAL										
0–19 Years	265	7.0	65	2	3	4	8	13	23	46
20–34	257	7.5	90	2	3	5	9	13	23	46
35–49	387	5.9	56	1	2	3	7	13	19	37
50–64	892	5.7	55	1	2	3	6	14	20	37
65+	1,154	6.0	41	1	2	4	7	14	18	33
GRAND TOTAL	2,955	6.2	55	1	2	4	7	13	19	39

32.3: SEG RESECTION LUNG

Type of Patients	Observed Patients	Avg. Stay	Vari-ance	Percentiles						
				10th	25th	50th	75th	90th	95th	99th
1. SINGLE DX										
0–19 Years	10	4.1	2	2	3	4	6	6	6	6
20–34	3	7.0	7	4	4	8	9	9	9	9
35–49	2	5.0	2	4	4	4	6	6	6	6
50–64	6	2.3	1	1	1	3	3	4	4	4
65+	2	2.5	4	1	1	4	4	4	4	4
2. MULTIPLE DX										
0–19 Years	38	6.3	53	2	2	4	7	17	17	39
20–34	52	7.7	31	2	4	6	9	16	19	26
35–49	76	8.3	93	2	4	5	9	14	26	61
50–64	267	6.3	38	2	3	5	7	13	16	28
65+	500	6.8	26	2	4	5	8	13	18	25
TOTAL SINGLE DX	23	4.0	4	1	3	4	5	6	8	9
TOTAL MULTIPLE DX	933	6.8	37	2	3	5	8	13	18	29
TOTAL										
0–19 Years	48	5.8	42	2	3	4	6	11	17	39
20–34	55	7.7	30	2	4	6	9	16	19	26
35–49	78	8.2	91	2	4	5	9	14	26	61
50–64	273	6.2	37	2	3	5	7	12	16	28
65+	502	6.8	26	2	4	5	8	13	18	25
GRAND TOTAL	956	6.7	36	2	3	5	8	13	18	29

32.29: LOC EXC LUNG LES NEC

Type of Patients	Observed Patients	Avg. Stay	Vari-ance	Percentiles						
				10th	25th	50th	75th	90th	95th	99th
1. SINGLE DX										
0–19 Years	15	3.2	2	2	2	3	4	5	5	7
20–34	5	3.8	3	2	2	4	5	6	6	6
35–49	4	2.2	2	1	1	1	3	4	4	4
50–64	5	3.0	4	1	1	2	4	6	6	6
65+	4	2.3	<1	1	1	3	3	3	3	3
2. MULTIPLE DX										
0–19 Years	82	10.9	214	4	5	6	10	28	52	>99
20–34	88	8.0	48	3	4	6	10	21	30	>99
35–49	160	8.4	71	2	4	6	9	17	25	42
50–64	459	7.4	46	3	4	5	9	15	20	34
65+	642	7.8	43	3	4	5	9	15	21	33
TOTAL SINGLE DX	33	3.1	2	1	2	3	4	5	5	7
TOTAL MULTIPLE DX	1,431	8.1	69	3	4	5	9	16	23	57
TOTAL										
0–19 Years	97	9.5	184	3	4	6	8	26	52	>99
20–34	93	7.8	47	3	4	6	9	21	30	>99
35–49	164	8.2	70	2	4	6	10	17	25	42
50–64	464	7.4	46	3	4	5	9	15	20	34
65+	646	7.7	43	3	4	5	9	15	21	33
GRAND TOTAL	1,464	7.9	68	3	4	5	9	16	23	52

32.30: THORSCPY SEG LUNG RESECT

Type of Patients	Observed Patients	Avg. Stay	Vari-ance	Percentiles						
				10th	25th	50th	75th	90th	95th	99th
1. SINGLE DX										
0–19 Years	7	3.9	3	2	3	3	6	6	6	6
20–34	2	6.5	12	4	4	4	9	9	9	9
35–49	0									
50–64	3	2.7	2	1	1	3	4	4	4	4
65+	2	2.5	4	1	1	4	4	4	4	4
2. MULTIPLE DX										
0–19 Years	16	5.8	32	1	2	3	6	17	17	17
20–34	19	4.7	6	1	3	4	6	9	9	9
35–49	37	5.5	16	2	3	4	7	14	14	15
50–64	128	5.1	20	1	2	3	6	12	16	20
65+	249	6.0	30	2	3	4	7	13	20	26
TOTAL SINGLE DX	14	3.9	4	1	3	4	4	6	6	9
TOTAL MULTIPLE DX	449	5.7	25	2	3	4	7	12	17	25
TOTAL										
0–19 Years	23	5.1	22	1	2	4	6	17	17	17
20–34	21	4.9	7	2	3	4	7	9	9	9
35–49	37	5.5	16	2	3	4	7	14	14	15
50–64	131	5.0	20	1	2	3	6	12	16	20
65+	251	6.0	30	2	3	4	7	12	20	26
GRAND TOTAL	463	5.6	25	2	3	4	7	12	17	25

LOS by Diagnosis and Operation, Western Region, 45th Edition

Western Region, October 2007–September 2008 Data, by Operation

32.39: SEG RESECT LUNG NEC&NOS

Type of Patients	Observed Patients	Avg. Stay	Vari-ance	Percentiles						
				10th	25th	50th	75th	90th	95th	99th
1. SINGLE DX										
0–19 Years	3	4.5	<1	4	4	4	5	6	6	6
20–34	1	8.0	0	8	8	8	8	8	8	8
35–49	2	5.0	2	4	4	4	6	6	6	6
50–64	3	2.0	1	1	1	2	3	3	3	3
65+	0									
2. MULTIPLE DX										
0–19 Years	22	6.7	66	2	3	4	7	9	24	39
20–34	33	9.5	38	3	5	8	14	18	20	26
35–49	39	10.9	154	3	5	6	12	26	45	61
50–64	139	7.4	52	3	4	6	7	14	19	53
65+	251	7.5	21	4	5	6	9	13	18	25
TOTAL SINGLE DX	9	4.3	3	2	4	4	5	6	8	8
TOTAL MULTIPLE DX	484	7.8	45	3	4	6	8	14	20	39
TOTAL										
0–19 Years	25	6.4	58	2	3	4	7	9	24	39
20–34	34	9.5	37	3	5	8	14	18	20	26
35–49	41	10.6	148	3	5	6	12	25	39	61
50–64	142	7.3	51	3	4	6	7	13	16	53
65+	251	7.5	21	4	5	6	9	13	18	25
GRAND TOTAL	493	7.7	45	3	4	6	8	14	20	39

32.4: LUNG LOBECTOMY

Type of Patients	Observed Patients	Avg. Stay	Vari-ance	Percentiles						
				10th	25th	50th	75th	90th	95th	99th
1. SINGLE DX										
0–19 Years	32	3.9	6	2	2	3	4	6	6	15
20–34	2	5.5	<1	5	5	6	6	6	6	6
35–49	14	4.9	6	2	4	4	5	8	12	12
50–64	25	4.1	3	2	4	4	5	7	7	7
65+	12	4.6	4	1	4	5	6	7	7	7
2. MULTIPLE DX										
0–19 Years	82	11.7	188	3	4	6	14	29	33	93
20–34	79	9.1	52	4	5	6	11	21	22	42
35–49	291	8.3	75	3	4	6	9	16	22	53
50–64	1,323	8.0	43	3	4	6	9	14	19	38
65+	2,795	7.9	38	3	5	6	9	14	18	32
TOTAL SINGLE DX	85	4.2	5	2	3	4	5	7	9	12
TOTAL MULTIPLE DX	4,570	8.1	48	3	5	6	9	14	19	36
TOTAL										
0–19 Years	114	9.9	157	3	3	5	10	23	30	66
20–34	81	9.0	51	4	5	6	11	19	22	42
35–49	305	8.1	72	3	4	6	9	15	21	36
50–64	1,348	7.9	42	3	4	6	9	14	19	38
65+	2,807	7.9	38	3	5	6	9	14	17	32
GRAND TOTAL	4,655	8.0	47	3	4	6	9	14	19	35

32.41: THORSCPY LUNG LOBECTOMY

Type of Patients	Observed Patients	Avg. Stay	Vari-ance	Percentiles						
				10th	25th	50th	75th	90th	95th	99th
1. SINGLE DX										
0–19 Years	18	3.7	5	2	2	3	4	9	9	9
20–34	0									
35–49	2	5.5	12	3	3	8	8	8	8	8
50–64	7	3.0	2	1	1	3	4	5	5	5
65+	5	3.4	5	1	1	4	5	6	6	6
2. MULTIPLE DX										
0–19 Years	24	5.7	34	2	3	4	6	10	10	31
20–34	18	5.4	10	2	3	5	7	11	13	13
35–49	60	4.6	12	2	3	4	6	8	15	18
50–64	277	5.9	22	2	3	5	7	10	13	29
65+	644	6.1	24	2	3	5	7	11	15	24
TOTAL SINGLE DX	32	3.6	5	2	2	3	5	8	9	9
TOTAL MULTIPLE DX	1,023	5.9	23	2	3	5	7	10	14	27
TOTAL										
0–19 Years	42	4.9	23	2	3	3	5	9	10	31
20–34	18	5.4	10	2	3	5	7	11	13	13
35–49	62	4.7	12	2	3	4	6	8	11	18
50–64	284	5.8	21	2	3	5	7	10	13	29
65+	649	6.1	24	2	3	5	7	11	15	24
GRAND TOTAL	1,055	5.8	22	2	3	5	7	10	14	27

32.49: LUNG LOBECTOMY NEC

Type of Patients	Observed Patients	Avg. Stay	Vari-ance	Percentiles						
				10th	25th	50th	75th	90th	95th	99th
1. SINGLE DX										
0–19 Years	14	4.2	7	2	3	4	4	5	6	15
20–34	2	5.5	<1	5	5	6	6	6	6	6
35–49	12	4.8	6	3	4	4	4	6	12	12
50–64	18	4.6	2	3	4	4	5	7	7	7
65+	7	5.4	2	4	4	5	7	7	7	7
2. MULTIPLE DX										
0–19 Years	58	13.9	226	4	5	8	18	30	33	93
20–34	61	10.1	60	4	5	7	13	21	22	42
35–49	231	9.2	86	4	5	6	10	17	25	53
50–64	1,046	8.5	47	4	5	6	9	15	22	41
65+	2,151	8.5	41	4	5	7	9	14	19	35
TOTAL SINGLE DX	53	4.6	5	3	4	4	5	7	7	15
TOTAL MULTIPLE DX	3,547	8.7	54	4	5	7	10	15	21	39
TOTAL										
0–19 Years	72	12.6	208	3	5	7	15	29	33	93
20–34	63	10.0	59	4	5	6	13	21	22	42
35–49	243	9.0	83	4	5	6	10	17	24	53
50–64	1,064	8.5	47	4	5	6	9	15	21	41
65+	2,158	8.4	41	4	5	7	9	14	19	35
GRAND TOTAL	3,600	8.7	53	4	5	7	9	15	20	38

Western Region, October 2007–September 2008 Data, by Operation

32.5: PNEUMONECTOMY

Type of Patients	Observed Patients	Avg. Stay	Vari-ance	Percentiles						
				10th	25th	50th	75th	90th	95th	99th
1. SINGLE DX										
0–19 Years	0									
20–34	0									
35–49	1	5.0	0	5	5	5	5	5	5	5
50–64	0									
65+	0									
2. MULTIPLE DX										
0–19 Years	4	29.7	166	19	23	23	44	44	44	44
20–34	6	14.7	286	6	6	7	10	49	49	49
35–49	31	9.6	55	4	4	6	14	21	25	34
50–64	138	8.8	82	4	5	6	9	17	24	67
65+	145	8.8	84	4	5	6	9	13	21	52
TOTAL SINGLE DX	1	5.0	0	5	5	5	5	5	5	5
TOTAL MULTIPLE DX	324	9.6	99	4	5	6	10	20	27	67
TOTAL										
0–19 Years	4	29.7	166	19	23	23	44	44	44	44
20–34	6	14.7	286	6	6	7	10	49	49	49
35–49	32	9.5	54	4	4	6	10	21	25	34
50–64	138	8.8	82	4	5	6	9	17	24	67
65+	145	8.8	84	4	5	6	9	13	21	52
GRAND TOTAL	325	9.6	98	4	5	6	10	20	27	67

32.59: PNEUMONECTOMY NEC & NOS

Type of Patients	Observed Patients	Avg. Stay	Vari-ance	Percentiles						
				10th	25th	50th	75th	90th	95th	99th
1. SINGLE DX										
0–19 Years	0									
20–34	0									
35–49	1	5.0	0	5	5	5	5	5	5	5
50–64	0									
65+	0									
2. MULTIPLE DX										
0–19 Years	3	34.2	238	10	19	44	44	44	44	44
20–34	6	14.7	286	6	6	7	10	49	49	49
35–49	28	10.2	57	4	5	7	15	21	25	34
50–64	125	9.1	88	4	5	6	9	19	24	67
65+	138	8.8	87	4	5	6	9	13	21	52
TOTAL SINGLE DX	1	5.0	0	5	5	5	5	5	5	5
TOTAL MULTIPLE DX	300	9.7	103	4	5	7	10	19	30	67
TOTAL										
0–19 Years	3	34.2	238	10	19	44	44	44	44	44
20–34	6	14.7	286	6	6	7	10	49	49	49
35–49	29	10.1	56	4	6	7	14	21	25	34
50–64	125	9.1	88	4	5	6	9	19	24	67
65+	138	8.8	87	4	5	6	9	13	21	52
GRAND TOTAL	301	9.7	102	4	5	7	10	19	30	67

32.6: RAD DISSECT THOR STRUCT

Type of Patients	Observed Patients	Avg. Stay	Vari-ance	Percentiles						
				10th	25th	50th	75th	90th	95th	99th
1. SINGLE DX										
0–19 Years	0									
20–34	0									
35–49	1	1.0	0	1	1	1	1	1	1	1
50–64	0									
65+	0									
2. MULTIPLE DX										
0–19 Years	0									
20–34	0									
35–49	2	13.6	111	6	6	21	21	21	21	21
50–64	7	6.6	4	4	4	7	8	9	9	9
65+	14	14.0	349	4	7	8	12	20	76	76
TOTAL SINGLE DX	1	1.0	0	1	1	1	1	1	1	1
TOTAL MULTIPLE DX	23	11.7	225	4	6	7	11	20	21	76
TOTAL										
0–19 Years	0									
20–34	0									
35–49	3	9.4	108	1	1	6	21	21	21	21
50–64	7	6.6	4	4	4	7	8	9	9	9
65+	14	14.0	349	4	7	8	12	20	76	76
GRAND TOTAL	24	11.3	220	4	6	7	11	20	21	76

32.9: LUNG EXCISION NEC

Type of Patients	Observed Patients	Avg. Stay	Vari-ance	Percentiles						
				10th	25th	50th	75th	90th	95th	99th
1. SINGLE DX										
0–19 Years	0									
20–34	0									
35–49	0									
50–64	0									
65+	0									
2. MULTIPLE DX										
0–19 Years	0									
20–34	0									
35–49	0									
50–64	0									
65+	0									
TOTAL SINGLE DX	0									
TOTAL MULTIPLE DX	0									
TOTAL										
0–19 Years	0									
20–34	0									
35–49	0									
50–64	0									
65+	0									
GRAND TOTAL	0									

LOS by Diagnosis and Operation, Western Region, 45th Edition

Western Region, October 2007–September 2008 Data, by Operation

33.0: BRONCHUS INCISION

Type of Patients	Observed Patients	Avg. Stay	Variance	10th	25th	50th	75th	90th	95th	99th
1. SINGLE DX										
0–19 Years	0									
20–34	0									
35–49	0									
50–64	0									
65+	0									
2. MULTIPLE DX										
0–19 Years	1	2.0	0	2	2		2	2	2	2
20–34	0									
35–49	1	8.0	0	8	8		8	8	8	8
50–64	0									
65+	0									
TOTAL SINGLE DX	0									
TOTAL MULTIPLE DX	2	3.2	7	2	2	2	2	8	8	8
TOTAL										
0–19 Years	1	2.0	0	2	2	2	2	2	2	2
20–34	0									
35–49	1	8.0	0	8	8	8	8	8	8	8
50–64	0									
65+	0									
GRAND TOTAL	2	3.2	7	2	2	2	2	8	8	8

33.1: LUNG INCISION

Type of Patients	Observed Patients	Avg. Stay	Variance	10th	25th	50th	75th	90th	95th	99th
1. SINGLE DX										
0–19 Years	0									
20–34	0									
35–49	0									
50–64	0									
65+	0									
2. MULTIPLE DX										
0–19 Years	8	13.9	192	1	4	9	21	40	40	40
20–34	1	10.0	0	10	10	10	10	10	10	10
35–49	10	10.9	40	4	6	11	15	18	22	22
50–64	11	9.5	17	5	6	11	13	13	15	15
65+	16	14.5	71	6	9	11	24	26	28	28
TOTAL SINGLE DX	0									
TOTAL MULTIPLE DX	46	12.7	102	3	6	10	18	25	40	40
TOTAL										
0–19 Years	8	13.9	192	1	4	9	21	40	40	40
20–34	1	10.0	0	10	10	10	10	10	10	10
35–49	10	10.9	40	4	6	11	15	18	22	22
50–64	11	9.5	17	5	6	11	13	13	15	15
65+	16	14.5	71	6	9	11	24	26	28	28
GRAND TOTAL	46	12.7	102	3	6	10	18	25	40	40

33.2: BRONCHIAL/LUNG DXTIC PX

Type of Patients	Observed Patients	Avg. Stay	Variance	10th	25th	50th	75th	90th	95th	99th
1. SINGLE DX										
0–19 Years	76	2.1	4	1	1	1	2	4	6	11
20–34	32	4.5	33	1	1	2	5	11	22	22
35–49	24	2.2	3	1	1	2	3	4	5	8
50–64	26	2.7	4	1	1	2	3	5	8	8
65+	16	2.2	4	1	1	1	2	6	8	8
2. MULTIPLE DX										
0–19 Years	1,011	9.0	120	1	3	6	11	18	26	63
20–34	1,122	8.9	84	2	4	7	10	17	25	50
35–49	2,748	8.1	58	2	4	6	9	16	21	39
50–64	6,053	8.1	57	2	4	6	10	16	21	38
65+	11,011	8.2	40	2	4	7	10	15	20	32
TOTAL SINGLE DX	174	2.5	8	1	1	1	3	5	8	14
TOTAL MULTIPLE DX	21,945	8.3	57	2	4	6	10	16	21	39
TOTAL										
0–19 Years	1,087	8.6	116	1	2	6	11	18	26	63
20–34	1,154	8.8	83	2	4	6	10	17	24	50
35–49	2,772	8.0	58	2	4	6	9	15	21	39
50–64	6,079	8.1	57	2	4	6	10	16	21	38
65+	11,027	8.1	40	2	4	7	10	15	20	32
GRAND TOTAL	22,119	8.2	57	2	4	6	10	16	21	39

33.20: THORACOSCOPIC LUNG BX

Type of Patients	Observed Patients	Avg. Stay	Variance	10th	25th	50th	75th	90th	95th	99th
1. SINGLE DX										
0–19 Years	0									
20–34	3	2.7	<1	2	2	3	3	3	3	3
35–49	9	1.9	<1	1	1	2	2	3	3	3
50–64	9	1.6	<1	1	1	1	2	3	3	3
65+	7	2.9	3	1	2	2	4	6	6	6
2. MULTIPLE DX										
0–19 Years	45	12.5	156	2	3	8	19	39	53	>99
20–34	35	11.2	222	1	3	9	14	17	25	92
35–49	138	8.5	152	1	2	4	8	20	34	67
50–64	312	6.7	78	1	2	3	8	18	23	48
65+	312	7.1	75	2	2	4	8	18	27	40
TOTAL SINGLE DX	28	2.1	1	1	1	2	3	3	4	6
TOTAL MULTIPLE DX	842	8.1	108	1	2	4	10	20	28	60
TOTAL										
0–19 Years	45	12.5	156	2	3	8	19	39	53	>99
20–34	38	10.6	211	1	2	8	14	17	22	92
35–49	147	8.1	145	1	2	3	8	19	30	67
50–64	321	6.6	77	1	2	3	8	18	21	48
65+	319	7.0	74	1	2	4	8	18	27	40
GRAND TOTAL	870	7.9	106	1	2	4	10	20	28	60

LOS by Diagnosis and Operation, Western Region, 45th Edition

Western Region, October 2007–September 2008 Data, by Operation

33.21: BRONCHOSCOPY THRU STOMA

Type of Patients	Observed Patients	Avg. Stay	Vari-ance	Percentiles						
				10th	25th	50th	75th	90th	95th	99th
1. SINGLE DX										
0–19 Years	0									
20–34	0									
35–49	0									
50–64	0									
65+	0									
2. MULTIPLE DX										
0–19 Years	25	5.6	39	1	2	3	8	11	11	42
20–34	15	3.6	7	1	1	3	6	8	8	8
35–49	22	5.3	22	1	2	4	7	9	16	19
50–64	31	5.7	29	1	2	3	9	15	18	19
65+	39	6.7	50	2	3	4	7	15	28	32
TOTAL SINGLE DX	0									
TOTAL MULTIPLE DX	132	5.7	35	1	2	4	8	11	16	32
TOTAL										
0–19 Years	25	5.6	39	1	2	3	8	11	11	42
20–34	15	3.6	7	1	1	3	6	8	8	8
35–49	22	5.3	22	1	2	4	7	9	16	19
50–64	31	5.7	29	1	2	3	9	15	18	19
65+	39	6.7	50	2	3	4	7	15	28	32
GRAND TOTAL	132	5.7	35	1	2	4	8	11	16	32

33.22: FIBER-OPTIC BRONCHOSCOPY

Type of Patients	Observed Patients	Avg. Stay	Vari-ance	Percentiles						
				10th	25th	50th	75th	90th	95th	99th
1. SINGLE DX										
0–19 Years	12	2.7	3	1	1	3	4	4	4	7
20–34	5	1.4	<1	1	1	1	1	3	3	3
35–49	1	1.0	0	1	1	1	1	1	1	1
50–64	1	1.0	0	1	1	1	1	1	1	1
65+	0									
2. MULTIPLE DX										
0–19 Years	95	8.4	169	1	2	4	9	18	42	63
20–34	45	8.2	67	2	3	6	9	16	19	45
35–49	113	5.8	24	1	3	4	9	13	16	19
50–64	211	7.7	36	1	3	6	11	16	20	27
65+	410	9.0	64	2	4	7	12	17	25	41
TOTAL SINGLE DX	19	2.4	2	1	1	2	3	4	4	7
TOTAL MULTIPLE DX	874	8.2	73	1	3	6	10	16	23	42
TOTAL										
0–19 Years	107	7.8	154	1	2	4	8	17	32	63
20–34	50	7.5	64	1	3	6	9	15	19	45
35–49	114	5.7	23	1	2	4	9	13	16	19
50–64	212	7.6	36	1	3	6	11	16	20	27
65+	410	9.0	64	2	4	7	12	17	25	41
GRAND TOTAL	893	8.0	72	1	3	6	10	16	23	42

33.23: BRONCHOSCOPY NEC

Type of Patients	Observed Patients	Avg. Stay	Vari-ance	Percentiles						
				10th	25th	50th	75th	90th	95th	99th
1. SINGLE DX										
0–19 Years	46	1.5	1	1	1	1	1	2	3	6
20–34	5	1.0	0	1	1	1	1	1	1	1
35–49	0									
50–64	2	2.0	2	1	1	3	3	3	3	3
65+	4	1.0	0	1	1	1	1	1	1	1
2. MULTIPLE DX										
0–19 Years	178	5.0	33	1	1	3	7	12	14	31
20–34	54	7.3	76	1	2	5	9	15	25	53
35–49	94	8.2	46	1	4	6	10	18	24	34
50–64	158	6.8	35	1	3	5	8	15	19	26
65+	255	8.7	48	2	4	7	12	19	22	33
TOTAL SINGLE DX	57	1.4	1	1	1	1	1	2	3	6
TOTAL MULTIPLE DX	739	6.7	43	1	2	5	9	14	19	31
TOTAL										
0–19 Years	224	4.2	28	1	1	2	5	11	14	31
20–34	59	6.8	73	1	2	5	9	15	25	53
35–49	94	8.2	46	1	3	6	10	18	24	34
50–64	160	6.7	35	1	3	5	8	14	18	26
65+	259	8.6	48	2	4	7	11	19	22	33
GRAND TOTAL	796	6.2	42	1	2	4	8	14	18	31

33.24: CLOSED BRONCHUS BIOPSY

Type of Patients	Observed Patients	Avg. Stay	Vari-ance	Percentiles						
				10th	25th	50th	75th	90th	95th	99th
1. SINGLE DX										
0–19 Years	16	3.9	12	1	2	2	6	11	11	11
20–34	14	3.7	10	1	1	3	5	9	9	9
35–49	6	1.2	<1	1	1	1	1	2	2	2
50–64	7	4.0	9	1	1	3	8	8	8	8
65+	0									
2. MULTIPLE DX										
0–19 Years	597	9.0	63	2	4	7	12	17	24	41
20–34	637	8.5	56	3	4	7	10	16	21	42
35–49	1,404	7.8	40	3	4	6	10	14	20	34
50–64	2,765	8.3	50	3	4	7	10	16	21	38
65+	5,023	8.7	40	3	5	7	11	16	20	32
TOTAL SINGLE DX	43	3.6	10	1	1	2	5	9	11	11
TOTAL MULTIPLE DX	10,426	8.5	47	3	4	7	11	16	21	36
TOTAL										
0–19 Years	613	8.9	63	2	4	7	12	17	24	41
20–34	651	8.4	56	3	4	7	10	16	21	42
35–49	1,410	7.8	40	3	4	6	10	14	20	34
50–64	2,772	8.3	50	3	4	7	10	16	21	38
65+	5,023	8.7	40	3	5	7	11	16	20	32
GRAND TOTAL	10,469	8.5	46	3	4	7	11	16	21	36

LOS by Diagnosis and Operation, Western Region, 45th Edition

Western Region, October 2007–September 2008 Data, by Operation

33.26: CLOSED LUNG BIOPSY

Type of Patients	Observed Patients	Avg. Stay	Variance	Percentiles						
				10th	25th	50th	75th	90th	95th	99th
1. SINGLE DX										
0–19 Years	1	3.0	0	3	3	3	3	3	3	3
20–34	1	22.0	0	22	22	22	22	22	22	22
35–49	2	1.5	<1	1	1	1	2	2	2	2
50–64	2	2.5	<1	2	2	3	3	3	3	3
65+	3	3.3	16	1	1	1	8	8	8	8
2. MULTIPLE DX										
0–19 Years	24	8.0	88	1	2	6	10	17	39	>99
20–34	75	6.9	51	2	3	6	8	12	19	50
35–49	251	6.7	52	2	3	5	8	13	17	39
50–64	928	6.6	42	2	3	5	8	13	18	35
65+	2,316	6.3	22	2	3	5	8	12	15	24
TOTAL SINGLE DX	9	4.7	46	1	1	2	3	22	22	22
TOTAL MULTIPLE DX	3,594	6.5	31	2	3	5	8	12	16	29
TOTAL										
0–19 Years	25	7.9	87	1	2	6	10	17	39	>99
20–34	76	7.1	53	2	3	6	8	14	22	50
35–49	253	6.7	52	2	3	5	8	13	17	39
50–64	930	6.6	42	2	3	5	8	13	18	35
65+	2,319	6.3	22	2	3	5	8	12	15	24
GRAND TOTAL	3,603	6.5	31	2	3	5	8	12	16	29

33.27: ENDOSCOPIC LUNG BIOPSY

Type of Patients	Observed Patients	Avg. Stay	Variance	Percentiles						
				10th	25th	50th	75th	90th	95th	99th
1. SINGLE DX										
0–19 Years	0									
20–34	4	12.6	61	3	11	14	22	22	22	22
35–49	4	3.0	3	1	1	4	5	5	5	5
50–64	2	4.0	2	3	3	3	5	5	5	5
65+	1	1.0	0	1	1	1	1	1	1	1
2. MULTIPLE DX										
0–19 Years	27	13.9	373	3	5	7	15	26	26	96
20–34	238	10.7	139	3	4	7	12	22	29	62
35–49	645	8.8	62	3	4	7	10	16	22	41
50–64	1,425	9.0	68	3	4	7	11	18	24	46
65+	2,374	8.7	39	3	5	7	11	16	20	31
TOTAL SINGLE DX	11	6.5	43	1	2	4	11	14	22	22
TOTAL MULTIPLE DX	4,709	8.9	60	3	4	7	11	17	22	39
TOTAL										
0–19 Years	27	13.9	373	3	5	7	15	26	26	96
20–34	242	10.7	138	3	4	7	12	22	29	62
35–49	649	8.7	62	3	4	7	10	16	22	41
50–64	1,427	9.0	68	3	4	7	11	18	24	46
65+	2,375	8.7	39	3	5	7	11	16	20	31
GRAND TOTAL	4,720	8.9	60	3	4	7	11	17	22	39

33.28: OPEN BIOPSY OF LUNG

Type of Patients	Observed Patients	Avg. Stay	Variance	Percentiles						
				10th	25th	50th	75th	90th	95th	99th
1. SINGLE DX										
0–19 Years	1	3.0	0	3	3	3	3	3	3	3
20–34	0									
35–49	2	6.0	8	4	4	8	8	8	8	8
50–64	3	3.0	<1	2	2	3	4	4	4	4
65+	1	1.0	0	1	1	1	1	1	1	1
2. MULTIPLE DX										
0–19 Years	20	34.4	>999	3	7	16	55	84	99	>99
20–34	23	13.4	162	2	4	10	15	35	42	48
35–49	81	13.9	205	3	4	8	20	31	36	88
50–64	216	10.2	113	2	4	6	14	22	31	55
65+	280	9.5	74	2	4	7	12	21	27	46
TOTAL SINGLE DX	7	3.6	5	1	2	3	4	8	8	8
TOTAL MULTIPLE DX	620	12.5	242	2	4	7	15	27	42	84
TOTAL										
0–19 Years	21	33.8	>999	3	7	14	55	84	99	>99
20–34	23	13.4	162	2	4	10	15	35	42	48
35–49	83	13.7	202	3	4	8	20	31	36	88
50–64	219	10.1	112	2	3	6	14	22	31	55
65+	281	9.4	74	2	4	7	12	20	27	46
GRAND TOTAL	627	12.4	240	2	4	7	15	27	42	84

33.3: SURG COLLAPSE OF LUNG

Type of Patients	Observed Patients	Avg. Stay	Variance	Percentiles						
				10th	25th	50th	75th	90th	95th	99th
1. SINGLE DX										
0–19 Years	3	2.7	1	2	2	2	4	4	4	4
20–34	2	1.5	<1	1	1	1	2	2	2	2
35–49	1	3.0	0	3	3	3	3	3	3	3
50–64	0									
65+	1	3.0	0	3	3	3	3	3	3	3
2. MULTIPLE DX										
0–19 Years	6	6.7	6	2	5	8	8	9	9	9
20–34	13	11.8	84	2	3	13	18	20	32	32
35–49	21	6.8	38	2	4	5	6	16	16	27
50–64	42	13.1	213	4	4	7	14	30	47	61
65+	96	9.1	50	3	5	7	10	20	27	35
TOTAL SINGLE DX	7	2.4	<1	1	2	2	3	4	4	4
TOTAL MULTIPLE DX	178	9.9	90	3	4	7	12	20	28	59
TOTAL										
0–19 Years	9	5.7	8	2	4	8	8	8	9	9
20–34	15	10.4	85	2	2	7	18	20	32	32
35–49	22	6.6	37	2	4	5	6	16	16	27
50–64	42	13.1	213	4	4	7	14	30	47	61
65+	97	9.1	50	3	5	7	10	20	27	35
GRAND TOTAL	185	9.6	89	2	4	7	11	20	28	59

LOS by Diagnosis and Operation, Western Region, 45th Edition

Western Region, October 2007–September 2008 Data, by Operation

33.39: SURG COLLAPS OF LUNG NEC

Type of Patients	Observed Patients	Avg. Stay	Vari-ance	Percentiles						
				10th	25th	50th	75th	90th	95th	99th
1. SINGLE DX										
0–19 Years	1	4.0	0	4	4	4	4	4	4	4
20–34	1	2.0	0	2	2	2	2	2	2	2
35–49	0									
50–64	0									
65+	1	3.0	0	3	3	3	3	3	3	3
2. MULTIPLE DX										
0–19 Years	1	5.0	0	5	5	5	5	5	5	5
20–34	8	14.6	97	2	5	13	20	32	32	32
35–49	11	7.4	58	1	4	5	7	16	27	27
50–64	26	11.9	86	4	5	8	14	27	30	37
65+	67	9.7	47	4	5	7	12	20	27	30
TOTAL SINGLE DX	3	3.0	<1	2	2	3	4	4	4	4
TOTAL MULTIPLE DX	113	10.3	62	4	5	7	13	24	28	32
TOTAL										
0–19 Years	2	4.5	<1	4	4	5	5	5	5	5
20–34	9	13.2	103	2	5	13	20	32	32	32
35–49	11	7.4	58	1	4	5	7	16	27	27
50–64	26	11.9	86	4	5	8	14	27	30	37
65+	68	9.6	47	4	5	7	12	20	27	30
GRAND TOTAL	116	10.1	61	4	5	7	13	24	28	32

33.5: LUNG TRANSPLANTATION

Type of Patients	Observed Patients	Avg. Stay	Vari-ance	Percentiles						
				10th	25th	50th	75th	90th	95th	99th
1. SINGLE DX										
0–19 Years	0									
20–34	0									
35–49	0									
50–64	0									
65+	0									
2. MULTIPLE DX										
0–19 Years	6	28.4	268	14	18	23	51	51	56	56
20–34	24	19.4	149	8	12	16	26	39	58	>99
35–49	22	14.5	34	10	11	13	17	26	29	>99
50–64	131	17.6	190	8	10	13	21	36	50	>99
65+	35	21.2	379	8	10	14	20	54	69	82
TOTAL SINGLE DX	0									
TOTAL MULTIPLE DX	218	19.0	214	8	10	14	23	44	56	>99
TOTAL										
0–19 Years	6	28.4	268	14	18	23	51	51	56	56
20–34	24	19.4	149	8	12	16	26	39	58	>99
35–49	22	14.5	34	10	11	13	17	26	29	>99
50–64	131	17.6	190	8	10	13	21	36	50	>99
65+	35	21.2	379	8	10	14	20	54	69	82
GRAND TOTAL	218	19.0	214	8	10	14	23	44	56	>99

33.4: LUNG & BRONCHUS REPAIR

Type of Patients	Observed Patients	Avg. Stay	Vari-ance	Percentiles						
				10th	25th	50th	75th	90th	95th	99th
1. SINGLE DX										
0–19 Years	0									
20–34	0									
35–49	0									
50–64	0									
65+	0									
2. MULTIPLE DX										
0–19 Years	3	7.8	13	6	6	6	8	15	15	15
20–34	25	13.0	130	5	6	9	14	22	37	54
35–49	6	25.9	>999	5	5	11	27	98	98	98
50–64	17	11.6	53	1	6	12	17	22	22	22
65+	13	14.4	38	7	11	13	20	22	27	27
TOTAL SINGLE DX	0									
TOTAL MULTIPLE DX	64	13.6	187	5	6	11	16	22	27	98
TOTAL										
0–19 Years	3	7.8	13	6	6	6	8	15	15	15
20–34	25	13.0	130	5	6	9	14	22	37	54
35–49	6	25.9	>999	5	5	11	27	98	98	98
50–64	17	11.6	53	1	6	12	17	22	22	22
65+	13	14.4	38	7	11	13	20	22	27	27
GRAND TOTAL	64	13.6	187	5	6	11	16	22	27	98

33.52: BILAT LUNG TRANSPLANT

Type of Patients	Observed Patients	Avg. Stay	Vari-ance	Percentiles						
				10th	25th	50th	75th	90th	95th	99th
1. SINGLE DX										
0–19 Years	0									
20–34	0									
35–49	0									
50–64	0									
65+	0									
2. MULTIPLE DX										
0–19 Years	6	28.4	268	14	18	23	51	51	56	56
20–34	22	20.0	152	8	12	16	26	39	58	>99
35–49	20	14.6	36	10	11	13	17	26	29	>99
50–64	94	19.4	218	9	11	15	24	37	92	>99
65+	13	27.6	553	11	14	18	25	66	82	82
TOTAL SINGLE DX	0									
TOTAL MULTIPLE DX	155	20.6	230	9	12	16	25	51	66	>99
TOTAL										
0–19 Years	6	28.4	268	14	18	23	51	51	56	56
20–34	22	20.0	152	8	12	16	26	39	58	>99
35–49	20	14.6	36	10	11	13	17	26	29	>99
50–64	94	19.4	218	9	11	15	24	37	92	>99
65+	13	27.6	553	11	14	18	25	66	82	82
GRAND TOTAL	155	20.6	230	9	12	16	25	51	66	>99

LOS by Diagnosis and Operation, Western Region, 45th Edition

Western Region, October 2007–September 2008 Data, by Operation

33.6: HEART-LUNG TRANSPLANT

Type of Patients	Observed Patients	Avg. Stay	Variance	10th	25th	50th	75th	90th	95th	99th
1. SINGLE DX										
0–19 Years	0									
20–34	0									
35–49	0									
50–64	0									
65+	0									
2. MULTIPLE DX										
0–19 Years	3	45.6	472	19	19	52	66	66	66	66
20–34	1	87.0	0	87	87	87	87	87	87	87
35–49	1	16.0	0	16	16	16	16	16	16	16
50–64	1	17.0	0	17	17	17	17	17	17	17
65+	0									
TOTAL SINGLE DX	0									
TOTAL MULTIPLE DX	6	43.8	730	16	19	52	66	87	87	87
TOTAL										
0–19 Years	3	45.6	472	19	19	52	66	66	66	66
20–34	1	87.0	0	87	87	87	87	87	87	87
35–49	1	16.0	0	16	16	16	16	16	16	16
50–64	1	17.0	0	17	17	17	17	17	17	17
65+	0									
GRAND TOTAL	6	43.8	730	16	19	52	66	87	87	87

33.7: ENDO INS/REPL/RMV RESP

Type of Patients	Observed Patients	Avg. Stay	Variance	10th	25th	50th	75th	90th	95th	99th
1. SINGLE DX										
0–19 Years	2	1.5	<1	1	1	2	2	2	2	2
20–34	0									
35–49	0									
50–64	0									
65+	0									
2. MULTIPLE DX										
0–19 Years	4	1.6	1	1	1	1	2	2	5	5
20–34	0									
35–49	0									
50–64	19	2.1	4	1	1	1	2	6	7	7
65+	10	2.1	4	1	1	1	2	7	7	7
TOTAL SINGLE DX	2	1.5	<1	1	1	2	2	2	2	2
TOTAL MULTIPLE DX	33	2.0	3	1	1	1	2	5	6	7
TOTAL										
0–19 Years	6	1.6	<1	1	1	1	2	2	2	5
20–34	0									
35–49	0									
50–64	19	2.1	4	1	1	1	2	6	7	7
65+	10	2.1	4	1	1	1	2	7	7	7
GRAND TOTAL	35	1.9	3	1	1	1	2	4	6	7

33.9: OTHER BRONCHIAL LUNG OPS

Type of Patients	Observed Patients	Avg. Stay	Variance	10th	25th	50th	75th	90th	95th	99th
1. SINGLE DX										
0–19 Years	0									
20–34	1	1.0	0	1	1	1	1	1	1	1
35–49	0									
50–64	1	1.0	0	1	1	1	1	1	1	1
65+	0									
2. MULTIPLE DX										
0–19 Years	23	16.5	150	4	7	13	27	30	41	42
20–34	20	7.9	42	2	3	6	10	18	26	26
35–49	23	6.6	17	3	4	6	8	12	15	18
50–64	45	9.6	145	2	3	6	10	22	36	66
65+	60	8.7	62	1	3	7	13	18	27	38
TOTAL SINGLE DX	2	1.0	0	1	1	1	1	1	1	1
TOTAL MULTIPLE DX	171	9.9	97	2	3	7	13	26	30	42
TOTAL										
0–19 Years	23	16.5	150	4	7	13	27	30	41	42
20–34	21	7.5	42	2	3	6	10	18	26	26
35–49	23	6.6	17	3	4	6	8	12	15	18
50–64	46	9.5	143	2	3	6	10	22	36	66
65+	60	8.7	62	1	3	7	13	18	27	38
GRAND TOTAL	173	9.8	97	2	3	7	13	26	30	42

33.93: PUNCTURE OF LUNG

Type of Patients	Observed Patients	Avg. Stay	Variance	10th	25th	50th	75th	90th	95th	99th
1. SINGLE DX										
0–19 Years	0									
20–34	0									
35–49	0									
50–64	1	1.0	0	1	1	1	1	1	1	1
65+	0									
2. MULTIPLE DX										
0–19 Years	21	15.3	153	4	7	11	28	37	41	42
20–34	9	7.6	28	2	3	7	10	18	18	18
35–49	9	7.2	7	3	6	7	8	12	12	12
50–64	21	10.4	115	3	4	6	12	25	36	40
65+	32	9.4	69	1	2	8	13	18	27	38
TOTAL SINGLE DX	1	1.0	0	1	1	1	1	1	1	1
TOTAL MULTIPLE DX	92	10.8	97	2	4	7	13	28	37	42
TOTAL										
0–19 Years	21	15.3	153	4	7	11	28	37	41	42
20–34	9	7.6	28	2	3	7	10	18	18	18
35–49	9	7.2	7	3	6	7	8	12	12	12
50–64	22	10.0	113	3	4	6	12	25	36	40
65+	32	9.4	69	1	2	8	13	18	27	38
GRAND TOTAL	93	10.7	97	2	4	7	13	28	37	42

LOS by Diagnosis and Operation, Western Region, 45th Edition

Western Region, October 2007–September 2008 Data, by Operation

34.0: INC CHEST WALL & PLEURA

Type of Patients	Observed Patients	Avg. Stay	Variance	Percentiles						
				10th	25th	50th	75th	90th	95th	99th
1. SINGLE DX										
0–19 Years	161	3.7	10	1	2	3	4	7	11	14
20–34	210	3.4	9	1	2	3	4	7	8	15
35–49	69	3.0	4	1	2	2	4	5	9	9
50–64	26	3.0	6	1	1	2	4	6	8	10
65+	12	3.6	9	1	1	2	4	7	11	11
2. MULTIPLE DX										
0–19 Years	757	8.9	79	2	4	6	11	18	24	49
20–34	1,210	5.4	26	2	3	4	6	10	14	26
35–49	1,588	6.7	45	2	3	5	8	13	18	35
50–64	2,417	7.3	50	2	3	5	9	15	20	36
65+	3,507	7.8	40	2	4	6	10	15	19	31
TOTAL SINGLE DX	478	3.5	9	1	2	3	4	7	10	14
TOTAL MULTIPLE DX	9,479	7.3	47	2	3	5	9	15	19	35
TOTAL										
0–19 Years	918	8.1	72	2	3	5	10	17	21	43
20–34	1,420	5.1	24	2	3	4	6	10	14	26
35–49	1,657	6.5	44	2	3	5	8	13	18	33
50–64	2,443	7.3	50	2	3	5	9	15	20	36
65+	3,519	7.8	40	2	4	6	10	15	19	31
GRAND TOTAL	9,957	7.1	46	2	3	5	9	14	19	34

34.01: CHEST WALL INCISION

Type of Patients	Observed Patients	Avg. Stay	Variance	Percentiles						
				10th	25th	50th	75th	90th	95th	99th
1. SINGLE DX										
0–19 Years	6	1.2	<1	1	1	1	1	2	3	3
20–34	5	1.5	1	1	1	1	1	4	4	4
35–49	1	5.0	0	5	5	5	5	5	5	5
50–64	1	1.0	0	1	1	1	1	1	1	1
65+	1	4.0	0	4	4	4	4	4	4	4
2. MULTIPLE DX										
0–19 Years	28	3.6	9	1	1	2	5	7	8	14
20–34	25	3.8	12	1	1	3	5	11	12	12
35–49	41	5.7	33	1	2	4	7	10	15	29
50–64	85	6.0	41	1	2	4	7	14	17	33
65+	98	5.3	23	1	2	4	7	12	17	21
TOTAL SINGLE DX	14	1.5	1	1	1	1	1	4	4	5
TOTAL MULTIPLE DX	277	5.2	27	1	2	4	7	12	15	29
TOTAL										
0–19 Years	34	3.0	7	1	1	2	4	7	8	14
20–34	30	3.2	10	1	1	2	4	7	12	12
35–49	42	5.6	32	1	2	5	7	10	15	29
50–64	86	6.0	41	1	2	4	7	14	17	33
65+	99	5.3	22	1	2	4	7	12	15	21
GRAND TOTAL	291	4.9	26	1	1	3	6	11	14	29

34.02: EXPLORATORY THORACOTOMY

Type of Patients	Observed Patients	Avg. Stay	Variance	Percentiles						
				10th	25th	50th	75th	90th	95th	99th
1. SINGLE DX										
0–19 Years	0									
20–34	2	2.5	4	1	1	1	4	4	4	4
35–49	0									
50–64	0									
65+	1	6.0	0	6	6	6	6	6	6	6
2. MULTIPLE DX										
0–19 Years	7	10.3	63	4	4	6	15	32	>99	>99
20–34	6	7.8	22	4	5	5	10	16	16	16
35–49	13	17.9	248	5	8	13	18	39	59	59
50–64	35	13.1	294	3	4	5	17	24	55	89
65+	43	10.0	68	3	5	7	12	21	32	35
TOTAL SINGLE DX	3	3.7	6	1	1	4	6	6	6	6
TOTAL MULTIPLE DX	104	11.8	158	3	5	7	15	24	35	89
TOTAL										
0–19 Years	7	10.3	63	4	4	6	15	32	>99	>99
20–34	8	6.5	23	1	3	5	10	16	16	16
35–49	13	17.9	248	5	8	13	18	39	59	59
50–64	35	13.1	294	3	4	5	17	24	55	89
65+	44	9.9	67	3	5	7	12	21	32	35
GRAND TOTAL	107	11.6	156	3	5	7	15	24	35	89

34.03: REOPEN THORACOTOMY SITE

Type of Patients	Observed Patients	Avg. Stay	Variance	Percentiles						
				10th	25th	50th	75th	90th	95th	99th
1. SINGLE DX										
0–19 Years	0									
20–34	0									
35–49	0									
50–64	0									
65+	0									
2. MULTIPLE DX										
0–19 Years	4	10.0	11	6	9	10	10	15	15	15
20–34	2	19.6	261	8	8	31	31	31	31	31
35–49	10	17.9	247	2	5	12	37	42	42	42
50–64	34	17.7	199	5	6	14	25	35	43	64
65+	39	13.6	115	3	6	12	20	31	42	>99
TOTAL SINGLE DX	0									
TOTAL MULTIPLE DX	89	14.9	144	4	6	11	19	35	42	64
TOTAL										
0–19 Years	4	10.0	11	6	9	10	10	15	15	15
20–34	2	19.6	261	8	8	31	31	31	31	31
35–49	10	17.9	247	2	5	12	37	42	42	42
50–64	34	17.7	199	5	6	14	25	35	43	64
65+	39	13.6	115	3	6	12	20	31	42	>99
GRAND TOTAL	89	14.9	144	4	6	11	19	35	42	64

LOS by Diagnosis and Operation, Western Region, 45th Edition

Western Region, October 2007–September 2008 Data, by Operation

34.04: INSERT INTERCOSTAL CATH

Type of Patients	Observed Patients	Avg. Stay	Variance	10th	25th	50th	75th	90th	95th	99th
1. SINGLE DX										
0–19 Years	121	3.7	9	1	2	3	4	7	10	14
20–34	155	3.6	11	1	2	3	4	7	9	16
35–49	50	2.8	4	1	2	3	3	5	9	9
50–64	14	3.0	6	1	2	2	4	6	10	10
65+	7	4.0	14	1	1	2	7	11	11	11
2. MULTIPLE DX										
0–19 Years	522	9.0	87	2	3	6	11	19	25	49
20–34	854	5.3	26	2	3	4	6	10	13	24
35–49	1,112	6.4	41	2	3	5	7	13	17	31
50–64	1,657	6.8	35	2	3	5	9	14	17	31
65+	2,486	7.5	36	2	4	6	10	15	18	28
TOTAL SINGLE DX	347	3.5	9	1	2	3	4	7	10	15
TOTAL MULTIPLE DX	6,631	7.0	42	2	3	5	9	14	18	31
TOTAL										
0–19 Years	643	8.1	78	2	3	5	10	17	23	43
20–34	1,009	5.0	24	2	3	4	6	9	12	24
35–49	1,162	6.3	40	2	3	4	7	13	17	31
50–64	1,671	6.8	35	2	3	5	9	14	17	31
65+	2,493	7.5	36	2	4	6	10	15	18	28
GRAND TOTAL	6,978	6.9	40	2	3	5	9	14	17	31

34.06: THORSCPY PLEURAL DRAIN

Type of Patients	Observed Patients	Avg. Stay	Variance	10th	25th	50th	75th	90th	95th	99th
1. SINGLE DX										
0–19 Years	3	4.0	3	2	2	4	6	6	6	6
20–34	5	5.4	15	2	2	4	9	10	10	10
35–49	0									
50–64	2	3.5	4	2	2	4	5	5	5	5
65+	1	2.0	0	2	2	2	2	2	2	2
2. MULTIPLE DX										
0–19 Years	31	9.6	25	4	5	9	13	18	19	19
20–34	30	10.2	69	3	4	8	15	26	30	32
35–49	58	9.1	39	3	4	8	12	18	23	26
50–64	116	11.6	135	2	4	8	13	28	37	57
65+	228	10.9	79	3	5	8	14	22	30	43
TOTAL SINGLE DX	11	4.3	8	2	2	4	6	9	10	10
TOTAL MULTIPLE DX	463	10.7	81	3	5	8	14	21	30	44
TOTAL										
0–19 Years	34	9.3	25	4	5	9	13	18	19	19
20–34	35	9.6	64	3	4	6	15	22	30	32
35–49	58	9.1	39	3	4	8	12	18	23	26
50–64	118	11.5	133	2	4	8	13	28	37	57
65+	229	10.9	79	3	5	8	14	22	30	43
GRAND TOTAL	474	10.5	80	3	4	8	14	21	30	44

34.09: PLEURAL INCISION NEC

Type of Patients	Observed Patients	Avg. Stay	Variance	10th	25th	50th	75th	90th	95th	99th
1. SINGLE DX										
0–19 Years	31	4.5	16	1	3	3	4	11	11	23
20–34	42	3.2	4	1	2	3	5	6	7	8
35–49	18	3.5	4	1	2	3	5	6	9	9
50–64	9	3.1	6	1	1	2	4	8	8	8
65+	2	1.5	<1	1	1	1	2	2	2	2
2. MULTIPLE DX										
0–19 Years	164	9.4	84	2	4	7	12	19	25	40
20–34	293	5.4	20	2	3	4	6	11	14	25
35–49	351	6.3	40	2	3	5	8	12	15	31
50–64	482	7.1	40	2	3	5	8	14	18	32
65+	609	7.8	34	2	4	7	10	15	19	28
TOTAL SINGLE DX	102	3.7	9	1	2	3	4	7	10	11
TOTAL MULTIPLE DX	1,899	7.2	42	2	3	5	9	14	19	31
TOTAL										
0–19 Years	195	8.6	76	2	3	6	11	17	21	40
20–34	335	5.2	18	2	3	4	6	10	14	22
35–49	369	6.2	38	2	3	5	8	12	15	31
50–64	491	7.1	40	2	3	5	8	13	18	32
65+	611	7.8	34	2	4	7	10	15	19	28
GRAND TOTAL	2,001	7.0	40	2	3	5	9	14	18	31

34.1: MEDIASTINUM INCISION

Type of Patients	Observed Patients	Avg. Stay	Variance	10th	25th	50th	75th	90th	95th	99th
1. SINGLE DX										
0–19 Years	0									
20–34	0									
35–49	0									
50–64	0									
65+	0									
2. MULTIPLE DX										
0–19 Years	5	7.2	9	4	5	8	10	10	14	14
20–34	11	12.8	128	4	4	7	24	27	35	35
35–49	8	13.1	84	1	4	14	18	30	30	30
50–64	23	11.1	122	1	4	7	12	29	32	39
65+	28	9.2	63	1	3	7	14	23	28	30
TOTAL SINGLE DX	0									
TOTAL MULTIPLE DX	75	10.1	78	2	4	7	12	27	30	39
TOTAL										
0–19 Years	5	7.2	9	4	5	8	10	10	14	14
20–34	11	12.8	128	4	4	7	24	27	35	35
35–49	8	13.1	84	1	4	14	18	30	30	30
50–64	23	11.1	122	1	4	7	12	29	32	39
65+	28	9.2	63	1	3	7	14	23	28	30
GRAND TOTAL	75	10.1	78	2	4	7	12	27	30	39

LOS by Diagnosis and Operation, Western Region, 45th Edition

Western Region, October 2007–September 2008 Data, by Operation

34.2: THORAX DXTIC PROCEDURES

Type of Patients	Observed Patients	Avg. Stay	Variance	Percentiles						
				10th	25th	50th	75th	90th	95th	99th
1. SINGLE DX										
0–19 Years	16	3.1	19	1	1	1	3	10	15	17
20–34	23	3.0	12	1	1	1	4	7	11	14
35–49	15	2.1	3	1	1	1	3	6	6	6
50–64	20	1.9	4	1	1	1	2	4	4	9
65+	10	2.2	3	1	1	1	3	5	6	6
2. MULTIPLE DX										
0–19 Years	77	10.6	101	2	4	8	13	18	27	53
20–34	154	8.6	71	2	3	6	11	20	29	38
35–49	302	6.8	45	1	2	5	9	14	19	34
50–64	680	6.9	51	1	2	5	10	15	21	35
65+	1,206	7.6	56	1	2	5	10	16	21	36
TOTAL SINGLE DX	84	2.6	10	1	1	1	3	6	10	17
TOTAL MULTIPLE DX	2,419	7.6	58	1	2	5	10	16	22	38
TOTAL										
0–19 Years	93	9.5	96	1	3	8	13	18	27	50
20–34	177	7.8	67	1	2	5	10	19	29	38
35–49	317	6.6	44	1	2	5	9	14	19	31
50–64	700	6.8	50	1	2	5	10	15	21	34
65+	1,216	7.6	55	1	2	5	10	16	21	36
GRAND TOTAL	2,503	7.4	57	1	2	5	10	16	21	38

34.20: THORACOSCOPIC PLEURAL BX

Type of Patients	Observed Patients	Avg. Stay	Variance	Percentiles						
				10th	25th	50th	75th	90th	95th	99th
1. SINGLE DX										
0–19 Years	0									
20–34	2	9.5	40	5	5	14	14	14	14	14
35–49	0									
50–64	5	2.6	2	1	2	2	4	4	4	4
65+	2	4.0	2	3	3	5	5	5	5	5
2. MULTIPLE DX										
0–19 Years	8	23.4	276	3	13	18	25	50	50	50
20–34	11	10.0	49	2	5	9	13	22	22	22
35–49	52	7.3	34	1	3	6	10	14	19	29
50–64	178	8.2	48	1	3	7	11	17	21	37
65+	409	8.3	50	2	3	6	11	17	24	34
TOTAL SINGLE DX	9	4.5	15	1	2	4	5	14	14	14
TOTAL MULTIPLE DX	658	8.6	60	2	3	6	11	18	24	36
TOTAL										
0–19 Years	8	23.4	276	3	13	18	25	50	50	50
20–34	13	9.9	44	2	5	9	13	22	22	22
35–49	52	7.3	34	1	3	7	10	14	19	29
50–64	183	8.1	48	1	3	7	11	17	21	37
65+	411	8.3	50	2	3	6	11	17	24	34
GRAND TOTAL	667	8.6	60	2	3	6	11	18	24	36

34.21: TRANSPLEURA THORACOSCOPY

Type of Patients	Observed Patients	Avg. Stay	Variance	Percentiles						
				10th	25th	50th	75th	90th	95th	99th
1. SINGLE DX										
0–19 Years	4	2.6	11	1	1	1	3	10	10	10
20–34	5	4.2	17	1	1	3	5	11	11	11
35–49	0									
50–64	2	1.5	<1	1	1	2	2	2	2	2
65+	1	1.0	0	1	1	1	1	1	1	1
2. MULTIPLE DX										
0–19 Years	20	10.6	48	4	5	7	14	27	27	27
20–34	22	13.7	137	3	5	10	18	30	32	47
35–49	39	10.3	83	3	5	8	13	26	28	44
50–64	94	10.4	90	3	4	8	12	21	28	58
65+	175	9.5	52	3	5	7	13	18	23	39
TOTAL SINGLE DX	12	2.9	11	1	1	1	3	10	11	11
TOTAL MULTIPLE DX	350	10.2	70	3	5	8	13	20	27	43
TOTAL										
0–19 Years	24	9.3	50	1	5	7	13	15	27	27
20–34	27	12.0	127	1	3	10	16	30	32	47
35–49	39	10.3	83	3	4	8	13	26	28	44
50–64	96	10.2	90	2	4	8	12	21	28	58
65+	176	9.5	52	3	5	7	13	18	23	39
GRAND TOTAL	362	9.9	69	3	4	7	13	19	27	43

34.22: MEDIASTINOSCOPY

Type of Patients	Observed Patients	Avg. Stay	Variance	Percentiles						
				10th	25th	50th	75th	90th	95th	99th
1. SINGLE DX										
0–19 Years	1	2.0	0	2	2	2	2	2	2	2
20–34	4	1.8	2	2	1	1	1	4	4	4
35–49	6	2.0	4	1	1	1	2	6	6	6
50–64	9	1.0	0	1	1	1	1	1	1	1
65+	3	3.0	7	1	1	2	6	6	6	6
2. MULTIPLE DX										
0–19 Years	5	3.7	5	1	2	2	6	6	6	6
20–34	32	9.3	83	1	3	7	10	23	32	38
35–49	112	6.2	38	1	1	4	9	14	18	29
50–64	216	4.9	36	1	1	3	7	12	18	29
65+	331	6.1	61	1	1	3	9	15	19	36
TOTAL SINGLE DX	23	1.7	2	1	1	1	2	4	6	6
TOTAL MULTIPLE DX	696	5.9	50	1	1	3	8	15	19	34
TOTAL										
0–19 Years	6	3.5	5	1	2	2	6	6	6	6
20–34	36	8.5	79	1	2	6	10	23	32	38
35–49	118	6.0	37	1	1	4	7	14	18	29
50–64	225	4.8	35	1	1	4	7	11	17	29
65+	334	6.1	60	1	1	3	9	15	19	36
GRAND TOTAL	719	5.7	49	1	1	3	8	15	19	32

LOS by Diagnosis and Operation, Western Region, 45th Edition

Western Region, October 2007–September 2008 Data, by Operation

34.23: CHEST WALL BIOPSY

Type of Patients	Observed Patients	Avg. Stay	Vari-ance	10th	25th	50th	75th	90th	95th	99th
1. SINGLE DX										
0–19 Years	0									
20–34	1	2.0	0	2	2	2	2	2	2	2
35–49	0									
50–64	0									
65+	0									
2. MULTIPLE DX										
0–19 Years	5	15.1	303	6	6	9	9	53	53	53
20–34	2	1.5	<1	1	1	2	2	2	2	2
35–49	14	5.5	25	2	3	3	5	16	16	16
50–64	26	7.7	54	2	3	5	9	19	28	29
65+	71	6.7	45	2	3	5	8	12	20	45
TOTAL SINGLE DX	1	2.0	0	2	2	2	2	2	2	2
TOTAL MULTIPLE DX	118	7.5	73	2	3	5	8	16	21	53
TOTAL										
0–19 Years	5	15.1	303	6	6	9	9	53	53	53
20–34	3	1.7	<1	1	1	2	2	2	2	2
35–49	14	5.5	25	2	3	3	5	16	16	16
50–64	26	7.7	54	2	3	5	9	19	28	29
65+	71	6.7	45	2	3	5	8	12	20	45
GRAND TOTAL	119	7.5	72	2	3	5	8	16	21	53

34.24: PLEURAL BIOPSY NEC

Type of Patients	Observed Patients	Avg. Stay	Vari-ance	10th	25th	50th	75th	90th	95th	99th
1. SINGLE DX										
0–19 Years	0									
20–34	1	1.0	0	1	1	1	1	1	1	1
35–49	1	6.0	0	6	6	6	6	6	6	6
50–64	0									
65+	2	1.0	0	1	1	1	1	1	1	1
2. MULTIPLE DX										
0–19 Years	2	11.2	3	8	12	12	12	12	12	12
20–34	10	5.8	6	3	4	6	8	9	10	10
35–49	15	6.7	18	1	4	5	11	14	14	14
50–64	36	6.1	17	1	3	5	9	13	14	16
65+	80	8.5	67	2	4	7	10	17	23	54
TOTAL SINGLE DX	4	2.3	6	1	1	1	6	6	6	6
TOTAL MULTIPLE DX	143	7.6	44	2	4	6	10	14	19	31
TOTAL										
0–19 Years	2	11.2	3	8	12	12	12	12	12	12
20–34	11	5.4	8	3	4	6	8	9	10	10
35–49	16	6.7	17	1	4	6	8	14	14	14
50–64	36	6.1	17	1	3	5	9	13	14	16
65+	82	8.3	66	2	3	7	10	17	23	54
GRAND TOTAL	147	7.5	44	1	3	6	10	13	19	31

34.25: CLOSED MEDIASTINAL BX

Type of Patients	Observed Patients	Avg. Stay	Vari-ance	10th	25th	50th	75th	90th	95th	99th
1. SINGLE DX										
0–19 Years	5	2.5	18	1	1	1	1	3	15	15
20–34	5	2.4	7	1	1	1	2	7	7	7
35–49	2	2.0	2	1	1	2	3	3	3	3
50–64	2	2.0	2	1	1	3	3	3	3	3
65+	1	1.0	0	1	1	1	1	1	1	1
2. MULTIPLE DX										
0–19 Years	18	6.3	17	1	3	7	9	10	13	18
20–34	45	5.7	21	1	3	5	7	13	17	20
35–49	39	4.5	17	1	1	3	7	10	15	18
50–64	68	6.2	40	1	2	5	8	11	14	44
65+	88	6.6	41	1	2	5	9	15	20	38
TOTAL SINGLE DX	15	2.3	11	1	1	1	2	3	7	15
TOTAL MULTIPLE DX	258	6.0	31	1	2	5	8	12	16	27
TOTAL										
0–19 Years	23	5.5	20	1	1	4	9	10	13	18
20–34	50	5.3	20	1	2	5	7	12	17	20
35–49	41	4.4	16	1	1	3	5	9	12	18
50–64	70	6.1	40	1	2	4	8	11	14	44
65+	89	6.6	41	1	2	5	9	15	20	38
GRAND TOTAL	273	5.8	30	1	2	4	8	12	15	25

34.26: OPEN MEDIASTINAL BIOPSY

Type of Patients	Observed Patients	Avg. Stay	Vari-ance	10th	25th	50th	75th	90th	95th	99th
1. SINGLE DX										
0–19 Years	6	4.3	30	1	1	2	4	17	17	17
20–34	5	1.6	<1	1	1	1	2	3	3	3
35–49	6	1.7	<1	1	1	1	2	3	3	3
50–64	1	1.0	0	1	1	1	1	1	1	1
65+	1	1.0	0	1	1	1	1	1	1	1
2. MULTIPLE DX										
0–19 Years	17	9.5	50	1	3	12	13	14	16	42
20–34	31	9.1	94	1	2	4	14	22	31	36
35–49	30	6.5	61	1	2	3	11	14	16	39
50–64	48	6.0	44	1	2	4	7	13	24	30
65+	39	5.7	60	1	1	3	6	13	24	42
TOTAL SINGLE DX	19	2.7	14	1	1	1	3	4	10	17
TOTAL MULTIPLE DX	165	7.4	60	1	2	4	12	14	24	42
TOTAL										
0–19 Years	23	8.7	50	1	2	10	13	14	17	42
20–34	36	8.0	87	1	1	3	12	22	31	36
35–49	36	5.7	54	1	1	3	7	14	16	39
50–64	49	5.9	43	1	2	4	7	13	24	30
65+	40	5.6	59	1	1	3	6	13	15	42
GRAND TOTAL	184	6.9	58	1	2	4	12	14	22	39

LOS by Diagnosis and Operation, Western Region, 45th Edition

Western Region, October 2007–September 2008 Data, by Operation

34.3: DESTR MEDIASTINUM LES

Type of Patients	Observed Patients	Avg. Stay	Variance	10th	25th	50th	75th	90th	95th	99th
1. SINGLE DX										
0–19 Years	13	3.7	8	1	2	3	4	7	12	12
20–34	9	2.4	2	1	1	3	4	5	5	5
35–49	9	3.2	2	1	2	3	4	5	5	5
50–64	5	3.4	2	2	2	3	5	5	5	5
65+	0									
2. MULTIPLE DX										
0–19 Years	30	5.9	38	2	3	4	7	23	23	>99
20–34	50	5.7	13	2	3	5	7	12	14	16
35–49	62	4.9	20	2	3	4	5	8	12	31
50–64	90	4.1	11	1	2	3	5	7	9	22
65+	69	5.4	20	1	3	4	7	11	16	22
TOTAL SINGLE DX	36	3.3	5	1	2	3	4	5	7	12
TOTAL MULTIPLE DX	301	5.1	21	1	3	4	6	10	18	>99
TOTAL										
0–19 Years	43	5.4	32	2	2	4	6	23	23	>99
20–34	59	5.2	13	1	3	5	7	12	14	16
35–49	71	4.6	18	2	3	4	5	7	12	31
50–64	95	4.1	11	1	3	3	5	7	9	22
65+	69	5.4	20	1	3	4	7	11	16	22
GRAND TOTAL	337	4.9	19	1	2	4	6	9	16	>99

34.4: EXC/DESTR CHEST WALL LES

Type of Patients	Observed Patients	Avg. Stay	Variance	10th	25th	50th	75th	90th	95th	99th
1. SINGLE DX										
0–19 Years	4	2.9	4	1	1	3	5	5	5	5
20–34	7	2.6	2	1	1	2	4	4	4	4
35–49	7	3.3	6	1	1	3	6	7	7	7
50–64	6	2.8	3	1	2	2	2	5	5	5
65+	1	2.0	0	2	2	2	2	2	2	2
2. MULTIPLE DX										
0–19 Years	33	7.1	14	2	5	6	9	12	14	15
20–34	24	5.0	10	2	3	5	6	9	11	14
35–49	42	5.2	32	1	2	3	7	10	13	29
50–64	105	5.2	23	1	2	4	7	12	16	24
65+	102	5.9	59	1	2	4	7	12	14	18
TOTAL SINGLE DX	25	2.9	3	1	1	2	5	5	6	7
TOTAL MULTIPLE DX	306	5.8	31	1	2	5	8	12	14	24
TOTAL										
0–19 Years	37	6.7	14	2	4	6	9	12	14	15
20–34	31	4.5	9	1	2	4	6	8	11	14
35–49	49	4.9	28	1	2	4	6	10	13	29
50–64	111	5.1	22	1	2	4	6	11	16	24
65+	103	5.8	59	1	2	4	7	12	14	18
GRAND TOTAL	331	5.6	30	1	2	5	7	12	14	24

34.5: PLEURECTOMY

Type of Patients	Observed Patients	Avg. Stay	Variance	10th	25th	50th	75th	90th	95th	99th
1. SINGLE DX										
0–19 Years	7	7.5	22	1	6	7	8	8	19	19
20–34	3	4.7	2	3	3	5	6	6	6	6
35–49	9	3.1	3	1	3	3	4	6	6	6
50–64	6	3.0	<1	2	2	3	4	4	4	4
65+	1	10.0	0	10	10	10	10	10	10	10
2. MULTIPLE DX										
0–19 Years	345	12.6	75	6	8	10	15	22	27	84
20–34	340	14.9	115	6	9	12	18	28	37	78
35–49	614	15.0	125	5	8	12	18	27	34	65
50–64	1,062	14.3	109	5	8	12	17	25	33	63
65+	1,063	13.7	82	5	8	12	17	24	31	47
TOTAL SINGLE DX	26	5.0	13	1	3	4	7	8	10	19
TOTAL MULTIPLE DX	3,424	14.0	99	5	8	12	17	25	32	61
TOTAL										
0–19 Years	352	12.6	74	6	8	10	15	21	27	84
20–34	343	14.9	115	6	9	12	18	28	37	78
35–49	623	14.8	125	5	8	12	18	27	33	65
50–64	1,068	14.2	109	5	8	12	17	25	33	63
65+	1,064	13.7	82	5	8	12	17	24	31	47
GRAND TOTAL	3,450	13.9	99	5	8	12	17	25	32	61

34.51: DECORTICATION OF LUNG

Type of Patients	Observed Patients	Avg. Stay	Variance	10th	25th	50th	75th	90th	95th	99th
1. SINGLE DX										
0–19 Years	0									
20–34	0									
35–49	1	6.0	0	6	6	6	6	6	6	6
50–64	0									
65+	0									
2. MULTIPLE DX										
0–19 Years	51	13.8	74	6	9	11	18	25	37	40
20–34	206	16.1	147	7	9	12	19	30	37	68
35–49	356	16.7	151	6	9	13	19	30	38	73
50–64	601	15.2	113	6	9	13	18	26	37	63
65+	566	15.3	87	6	9	14	19	26	33	54
TOTAL SINGLE DX	1	6.0	0	6	6	6	6	6	6	6
TOTAL MULTIPLE DX	1,780	15.6	115	6	9	13	19	27	35	62
TOTAL										
0–19 Years	51	13.8	74	6	9	11	18	25	37	40
20–34	206	16.1	147	7	9	12	19	30	37	68
35–49	357	16.7	151	6	9	13	19	30	38	73
50–64	601	15.2	113	6	9	13	18	26	37	63
65+	566	15.3	87	6	9	14	19	26	33	54
GRAND TOTAL	1,781	15.6	115	6	9	13	19	27	35	62

LOS by Diagnosis and Operation, Western Region, 45th Edition

117

Western Region, October 2007–September 2008 Data, by Operation

34.6: PLEURAL SCARIFICATION

Type of Patients	Observed Patients	Avg. Stay	Variance	Percentiles						
				10th	25th	50th	75th	90th	95th	99th
1. SINGLE DX										
0–19 Years	8	4.1	2	2	3	4	5	7	7	7
20–34	15	5.1	7	3	4	4	6	8	12	12
35–49	6	5.7	12	1	3	8	8	10	10	10
50–64	2	4.0	18	1	1	7	7	7	7	7
65+	0									
2. MULTIPLE DX										
0–19 Years	46	8.4	58	3	4	6	9	19	24	45
20–34	49	10.6	172	3	5	8	12	18	20	93
35–49	51	11.6	80	4	5	9	15	25	29	44
50–64	127	12.0	114	4	6	9	15	22	26	64
65+	247	10.7	67	3	5	9	14	21	25	47
TOTAL SINGLE DX	31	4.9	7	2	3	4	7	8	10	12
TOTAL MULTIPLE DX	520	10.7	88	3	5	8	14	21	25	48
TOTAL										
0–19 Years	54	8.0	54	3	4	5	7	16	24	45
20–34	64	9.3	138	3	4	7	11	17	19	93
35–49	57	11.0	75	4	5	8	14	25	29	44
50–64	129	11.9	113	4	6	9	15	22	26	64
65+	247	10.7	67	3	5	9	14	21	25	47
GRAND TOTAL	551	10.4	85	3	5	8	13	20	25	48

34.7: REPAIR OF CHEST WALL

Type of Patients	Observed Patients	Avg. Stay	Variance	Percentiles						
				10th	25th	50th	75th	90th	95th	99th
1. SINGLE DX										
0–19 Years	108	4.3	2	2	3	5	5	6	7	7
20–34	14	4.4	5	1	3	5	5	7	8	8
35–49	2	5.0	2	4	4	6	6	6	6	6
50–64	1	7.0	0	7	7	7	7	7	7	7
65+	0									
2. MULTIPLE DX										
0–19 Years	163	5.9	31	3	4	5	6	7	9	42
20–34	56	4.3	7	1	3	4	6	7	9	15
35–49	39	7.9	100	1	3	4	10	20	34	49
50–64	123	8.4	146	1	3	4	9	17	28	67
65+	105	9.7	82	2	4	7	11	24	27	49
TOTAL SINGLE DX	125	4.3	2	2	3	5	5	6	7	7
TOTAL MULTIPLE DX	486	6.8	60	2	4	5	7	11	19	42
TOTAL										
0–19 Years	271	5.3	20	3	4	5	6	7	8	31
20–34	70	4.3	7	1	3	4	6	7	8	15
35–49	41	7.7	95	1	2	4	10	15	25	49
50–64	124	8.4	144	1	3	4	9	17	28	67
65+	105	9.7	82	2	4	7	11	24	27	49
GRAND TOTAL	611	6.1	46	2	4	5	6	9	16	42

34.52: THORSCPY DECORT LUNG

Type of Patients	Observed Patients	Avg. Stay	Variance	Percentiles						
				10th	25th	50th	75th	90th	95th	99th
1. SINGLE DX										
0–19 Years	4	9.1	19	6	7	8	8	19	19	19
20–34	1	3.0	0	3	3	3	3	3	3	3
35–49	4	2.8	2	1	1	2	3	4	4	4
50–64	4	3.3	<1	2	2	3	4	4	4	4
65+	1	10.0	0	10	10	10	10	10	10	10
2. MULTIPLE DX										
0–19 Years	282	12.0	43	6	8	10	14	21	25	44
20–34	124	13.5	64	7	9	12	17	22	35	>99
35–49	238	13.1	81	5	8	11	16	24	28	65
50–64	407	13.9	103	5	8	12	17	24	31	57
65+	425	12.6	75	4	7	11	16	21	28	42
TOTAL SINGLE DX	14	5.9	18	2	3	4	8	10	19	19
TOTAL MULTIPLE DX	1,476	12.8	70	5	8	11	16	22	28	53
TOTAL										
0–19 Years	286	12.0	43	6	8	10	14	21	25	44
20–34	125	13.4	65	6	9	12	17	22	35	>99
35–49	242	12.9	82	5	8	11	16	24	28	65
50–64	411	13.8	103	5	8	11	17	24	31	57
65+	426	12.6	75	4	7	11	16	21	28	42
GRAND TOTAL	1,490	12.7	70	5	8	11	16	22	28	53

34.59: PLEURAL EXCISION NEC

Type of Patients	Observed Patients	Avg. Stay	Variance	Percentiles						
				10th	25th	50th	75th	90th	95th	99th
1. SINGLE DX										
0–19 Years	3	3.7	9	1	1	3	7	7	7	7
20–34	2	5.5	<1	5	5	6	6	6	6	6
35–49	4	2.8	3	1	2	2	3	5	5	5
50–64	2	2.5	<1	2	2	3	3	3	3	3
65+	0									
2. MULTIPLE DX										
0–19 Years	12	29.1	916	3	9	21	24	84	84	84
20–34	10	9.3	56	4	5	7	12	21	24	24
35–49	20	6.7	22	2	3	6	11	15	16	16
50–64	54	7.9	67	2	4	6	9	13	23	53
65+	72	8.3	26	3	4	7	11	15	19	22
TOTAL SINGLE DX	11	3.4	4	1	2	3	5	6	7	7
TOTAL MULTIPLE DX	168	10.3	172	3	4	7	12	21	23	84
TOTAL										
0–19 Years	15	25.6	865	3	7	17	22	84	84	84
20–34	12	8.7	48	4	5	6	12	21	24	24
35–49	24	6.1	21	1	2	4	8	13	15	16
50–64	56	7.7	66	2	3	5	9	13	23	53
65+	72	8.3	26	3	4	7	11	15	19	22
GRAND TOTAL	179	9.9	165	2	4	7	11	19	22	84

LOS by Diagnosis and Operation, Western Region, 45th Edition

Western Region, October 2007–September 2008 Data, by Operation

34.74: PECTUS DEFORMITY REPAIR

Type of Patients	Observed Patients	Avg. Stay	Variance	10th	25th	50th	75th	90th	95th	99th
1. SINGLE DX										
0–19 Years	101	4.5	2	3	3	5	5	6	7	7
20–34	9	4.9	3	3	4	5	7	7	7	7
35–49	2	5.0	2	4	4	6	6	6	6	6
50–64	0									
65+	0									
2. MULTIPLE DX										
0–19 Years	142	5.1	2	4	4	5	6	7	8	9
20–34	23	4.9	2	3	4	5	6	7	8	10
35–49	2	8.5	<1	8	8	8	9	9	9	9
50–64	3	3.7	1	3	3	3	5	5	5	5
65+	0									
TOTAL SINGLE DX	112	4.5	2	3	3	5	5	6	7	7
TOTAL MULTIPLE DX	170	5.1	2	3	4	5	6	7	8	9
TOTAL										
0–19 Years	243	4.8	2	3	4	5	6	7	7	9
20–34	32	4.9	3	3	4	5	6	7	8	10
35–49	4	6.8	5	4	6	7	8	9	9	9
50–64	3	3.7	1	3	3	3	5	5	5	5
65+	0									
GRAND TOTAL	282	4.8	2	3	4	5	6	7	7	9

34.8: OPERATIONS ON DIAPHRAGM

Type of Patients	Observed Patients	Avg. Stay	Variance	10th	25th	50th	75th	90th	95th	99th
1. SINGLE DX										
0–19 Years	0									
20–34	0									
35–49	2	1.5	<1	1	1	1	2	2	2	2
50–64	1	3.0	0	3	3	3	3	3	3	3
65+	0									
2. MULTIPLE DX										
0–19 Years	47	8.5	142	3	4	5	9	16	16	87
20–34	130	7.7	55	3	4	6	8	12	26	40
35–49	69	8.7	45	3	4	7	12	15	20	45
50–64	42	12.7	144	3	5	9	15	35	46	>99
65+	15	12.0	245	2	2	5	12	31	58	58
TOTAL SINGLE DX	3	2.0	1	1	1	2	3	3	3	3
TOTAL MULTIPLE DX	303	8.9	91	3	4	6	10	17	29	47
TOTAL										
0–19 Years	47	8.5	142	3	4	5	9	16	16	87
20–34	130	7.7	55	3	4	6	8	12	26	40
35–49	71	8.5	45	3	4	7	12	14	20	45
50–64	43	12.4	143	2	4	8	14	35	46	>99
65+	15	12.0	245	2	2	5	12	31	58	58
GRAND TOTAL	306	8.8	90	3	4	6	10	17	29	47

34.79: CHEST WALL REPAIR NEC

Type of Patients	Observed Patients	Avg. Stay	Variance	10th	25th	50th	75th	90th	95th	99th
1. SINGLE DX										
0–19 Years	1	5.0	0	5	5	5	5	5	5	5
20–34	1	8.0	0	8	8	8	8	8	8	8
35–49	0									
50–64	1	7.0	0	7	7	7	7	7	7	7
65+	0									
2. MULTIPLE DX										
0–19 Years	11	26.3	349	2	9	31	42	42	58	58
20–34	5	7.0	22	3	4	6	7	15	15	15
35–49	18	9.1	90	1	2	4	14	25	34	34
50–64	91	7.9	162	2	3	4	7	14	26	85
65+	77	8.6	67	2	3	6	10	20	25	50
TOTAL SINGLE DX	3	6.7	2	5	5	7	8	8	8	8
TOTAL MULTIPLE DX	202	9.5	148	2	3	5	10	24	37	58
TOTAL										
0–19 Years	12	24.8	355	2	5	27	42	42	58	58
20–34	6	7.2	18	3	4	6	7	15	15	15
35–49	18	9.1	90	1	2	4	14	25	34	34
50–64	92	7.9	160	2	3	4	7	14	26	85
65+	77	8.6	67	2	3	6	10	20	25	50
GRAND TOTAL	205	9.5	146	2	3	5	10	24	37	58

34.82: SUTURE DIAPHRAGM LAC

Type of Patients	Observed Patients	Avg. Stay	Variance	10th	25th	50th	75th	90th	95th	99th
1. SINGLE DX										
0–19 Years	0									
20–34	0									
35–49	1	1.0	0	1	1	1	1	1	1	1
50–64	0									
65+	0									
2. MULTIPLE DX										
0–19 Years	35	6.6	20	3	3	5	8	14	16	22
20–34	118	7.6	57	3	4	6	8	15	26	40
35–49	45	9.3	52	3	5	7	13	15	18	45
50–64	22	14.3	130	5	7	11	22	35	47	>99
65+	4	25.1	582	5	28	28	58	58	58	58
TOTAL SINGLE DX	1	1.0	0	1	1	1	1	1	1	1
TOTAL MULTIPLE DX	224	8.7	73	3	4	6	9	18	28	47
TOTAL										
0–19 Years	35	6.6	20	3	3	5	8	14	16	22
20–34	118	7.6	57	3	4	6	8	15	26	40
35–49	46	9.1	52	3	5	7	13	15	18	45
50–64	22	14.3	130	5	7	11	22	35	47	>99
65+	4	25.1	582	5	28	28	58	58	58	58
GRAND TOTAL	225	8.7	73	3	4	6	9	18	28	47

LOS by Diagnosis and Operation, Western Region, 45th Edition

Western Region, October 2007–September 2008 Data, by Operation

34.9: OTHER OPS ON THORAX

Type of Patients	Observed Patients	Avg. Stay	Vari-ance	Percentiles						
				10th	25th	50th	75th	90th	95th	99th
1. SINGLE DX										
0–19 Years	9	3.5	3	1	2	3	5	5	7	7
20–34	15	4.1	10	1	2	3	5	8	13	13
35–49	7	4.7	10	2	2	4	7	10	10	10
50–64	4	2.0	1	1	1	3	3	3	3	3
65+	7	1.7	4	1	1	1	1	6	6	6
2. MULTIPLE DX										
0–19 Years	203	8.7	67	3	4	6	11	16	28	37
20–34	491	7.2	31	2	3	6	9	13	18	31
35–49	1,637	7.1	40	2	3	6	9	14	18	29
50–64	4,492	6.5	37	2	3	5	8	13	17	31
65+	13,538	6.7	27	2	3	5	9	13	16	26
TOTAL SINGLE DX	42	3.5	7	1	1	3	5	7	8	13
TOTAL MULTIPLE DX	20,361	6.7	31	2	3	5	9	13	17	28
TOTAL										
0–19 Years	212	8.4	64	2	4	6	11	16	28	37
20–34	506	7.1	31	2	3	6	9	13	18	29
35–49	1,644	7.1	40	2	3	6	9	14	18	29
50–64	4,496	6.5	37	2	3	5	8	13	17	31
65+	13,545	6.7	27	2	3	5	9	13	16	26
GRAND TOTAL	20,403	6.7	31	2	3	5	9	13	17	28

34.91: THORACENTESIS

Type of Patients	Observed Patients	Avg. Stay	Vari-ance	Percentiles						
				10th	25th	50th	75th	90th	95th	99th
1. SINGLE DX										
0–19 Years	5	2.0	1	1	1	2	2	4	4	4
20–34	10	2.6	2	1	1	3	4	5	5	5
35–49	4	3.3	6	1	2	3	7	7	7	7
50–64	4	2.0	1	1	1	3	3	3	3	3
65+	7	1.7	4	1	1	1	1	6	6	6
2. MULTIPLE DX										
0–19 Years	193	8.9	71	2	4	6	11	17	28	37
20–34	476	7.2	32	2	3	6	9	14	18	31
35–49	1,583	7.0	39	2	3	6	9	14	18	29
50–64	4,337	6.5	36	2	3	5	8	13	17	30
65+	13,272	6.7	27	2	3	5	8	13	16	26
TOTAL SINGLE DX	30	2.3	3	1	1	2	3	5	6	7
TOTAL MULTIPLE DX	19,861	6.7	31	2	3	5	8	13	16	27
TOTAL										
0–19 Years	198	8.7	71	2	3	6	11	17	28	37
20–34	486	7.1	32	2	3	6	9	14	18	31
35–49	1,587	7.0	39	2	3	6	9	14	18	29
50–64	4,341	6.4	36	2	3	5	8	13	17	30
65+	13,279	6.6	27	2	3	5	8	13	16	26
GRAND TOTAL	19,891	6.7	31	2	3	5	8	13	16	27

34.92: INJECT INTO THOR CAVIT

Type of Patients	Observed Patients	Avg. Stay	Vari-ance	Percentiles						
				10th	25th	50th	75th	90th	95th	99th
1. SINGLE DX										
0–19 Years	4	4.3	2	3	3	4	5	7	7	7
20–34	5	7.2	14	3	5	7	8	13	13	13
35–49	3	6.7	9	4	4	6	10	10	10	10
50–64	0									
65+	0									
2. MULTIPLE DX										
0–19 Years	7	7.1	3	5	6	7	8	8	11	11
20–34	13	6.6	12	3	4	5	9	12	13	13
35–49	51	9.0	57	2	4	8	12	15	29	38
50–64	151	8.8	50	3	4	7	10	18	23	35
65+	262	8.5	29	3	4	7	11	16	19	28
TOTAL SINGLE DX	12	5.5	7	3	3	5	7	10	13	13
TOTAL MULTIPLE DX	484	8.6	37	3	4	7	11	16	21	34
TOTAL										
0–19 Years	11	5.9	4	3	4	6	7	8	8	11
20–34	18	6.8	12	3	4	5	9	13	13	13
35–49	54	8.9	55	3	4	8	12	15	29	38
50–64	151	8.8	50	3	4	7	10	18	23	35
65+	262	8.5	29	3	4	7	11	16	19	28
GRAND TOTAL	496	8.4	37	3	4	7	11	16	20	34

35.0: CLOSED HEART VALVOTOMY

Type of Patients	Observed Patients	Avg. Stay	Vari-ance	Percentiles						
				10th	25th	50th	75th	90th	95th	99th
1. SINGLE DX										
0–19 Years	0									
20–34	0									
35–49	0									
50–64	1	1.0	0	1	1	1	1	1	1	1
65+	0									
2. MULTIPLE DX										
0–19 Years	2	1.0	0	1	1	1	1	1	1	1
20–34	0									
35–49	0									
50–64	1	1.0	0	1	1	1	1	1	1	1
65+	3	6.6	52	2	2	3	15	15	15	15
TOTAL SINGLE DX	1	1.0	0	1	1	1	1	1	1	1
TOTAL MULTIPLE DX	6	3.8	30	1	1	1	3	15	15	15
TOTAL										
0–19 Years	2	1.0	0	1	1	1	1	1	1	1
20–34	0									
35–49	0									
50–64	2	1.0	0	1	1	1	1	1	1	1
65+	3	6.6	52	2	2	3	15	15	15	15
GRAND TOTAL	7	3.4	26	1	1	1	3	15	15	15

LOS by Diagnosis and Operation, Western Region, 45th Edition

Western Region, October 2007–September 2008 Data, by Operation

35.1: OPEN HEART VALVULOPLASTY

Type of Patients	Observed Patients	Avg. Stay	Vari-ance	Percentiles						
				10th	25th	50th	75th	90th	95th	99th
1. SINGLE DX										
0–19 Years	9	3.5	<1	3	3	4	4	4	4	4
20–34	1	6.0	0	6	6	6	6	6	6	6
35–49	5	4.0	<1	3	3	4	5	5	5	5
50–64	7	3.6	<1	2	3	4	4	5	5	5
65+	0									
2. MULTIPLE DX										
0–19 Years	295	8.5	93	3	4	5	8	18	31	79
20–34	56	12.0	283	3	4	5	13	23	47	95
35–49	205	8.7	67	4	4	6	10	17	24	49
50–64	729	8.7	52	4	5	6	10	17	22	38
65+	897	10.4	54	5	6	8	12	19	25	40
TOTAL SINGLE DX	22	3.7	<1	3	3	4	4	5	5	6
TOTAL MULTIPLE DX	2,182	9.3	71	4	5	7	11	18	25	47
TOTAL										
0–19 Years	304	8.3	90	3	4	5	8	18	28	79
20–34	57	11.9	276	3	4	5	13	23	47	95
35–49	210	8.6	66	4	4	6	9	16	24	49
50–64	736	8.7	52	4	5	6	10	17	22	38
65+	897	10.4	54	5	6	8	12	19	25	40
GRAND TOTAL	2,204	9.2	71	4	5	6	10	18	25	47

35.11: OPN AORTIC VALVULOPLASTY

Type of Patients	Observed Patients	Avg. Stay	Vari-ance	Percentiles						
				10th	25th	50th	75th	90th	95th	99th
1. SINGLE DX										
0–19 Years	7	3.5	<1	3	3	4	4	4	4	4
20–34	1	6.0	0	6	6	6	6	6	6	6
35–49	0									
50–64	0									
65+	0									
2. MULTIPLE DX										
0–19 Years	78	6.6	58	3	3	5	6	11	24	48
20–34	12	6.3	16	4	4	5	6	13	16	16
35–49	29	9.8	83	4	5	7	11	18	24	49
50–64	42	8.8	35	4	5	7	10	17	22	29
65+	58	9.8	43	5	6	8	11	17	23	46
TOTAL SINGLE DX	8	3.8	<1	3	3	4	4	4	6	6
TOTAL MULTIPLE DX	219	7.7	54	3	4	5	8	15	23	48
TOTAL										
0–19 Years	85	6.3	53	3	3	4	6	10	19	48
20–34	13	6.3	13	4	4	5	6	13	16	16
35–49	29	9.8	83	4	5	7	11	18	24	49
50–64	42	8.8	35	4	5	7	10	17	22	29
65+	58	9.8	43	5	6	8	11	17	23	46
GRAND TOTAL	227	7.5	52	3	4	5	8	13	19	48

35.12: OPN MITRAL VALVULOPLASTY

Type of Patients	Observed Patients	Avg. Stay	Vari-ance	Percentiles						
				10th	25th	50th	75th	90th	95th	99th
1. SINGLE DX										
0–19 Years	2	3.5	<1	3	3	4	4	4	4	4
20–34	0									
35–49	5	4.0	<1	3	3	4	5	5	5	5
50–64	7	3.6	<1	2	3	4	4	5	5	5
65+	0									
2. MULTIPLE DX										
0–19 Years	82	8.3	82	3	4	5	7	25	31	44
20–34	38	11.2	183	3	4	6	10	31	47	64
35–49	162	8.2	60	4	4	6	9	15	20	60
50–64	670	8.6	51	4	5	6	10	17	21	38
65+	814	10.4	56	5	6	8	12	19	25	40
TOTAL SINGLE DX	14	3.7	<1	3	3	4	4	5	5	5
TOTAL MULTIPLE DX	1,766	9.4	61	4	5	7	11	18	25	44
TOTAL										
0–19 Years	84	8.1	80	3	4	5	7	21	31	44
20–34	38	11.2	183	3	4	6	10	31	47	64
35–49	167	8.1	59	4	4	5	9	15	20	60
50–64	677	8.6	51	4	5	6	10	17	21	38
65+	814	10.4	56	5	6	8	12	19	25	40
GRAND TOTAL	1,780	9.3	60	4	5	7	11	18	25	44

35.14: OPN TRICUSP VALVULOPLAST

Type of Patients	Observed Patients	Avg. Stay	Vari-ance	Percentiles						
				10th	25th	50th	75th	90th	95th	99th
1. SINGLE DX										
0–19 Years	0									
20–34	0									
35–49	0									
50–64	0									
65+	0									
2. MULTIPLE DX										
0–19 Years	69	11.3	177	3	5	7	13	28	42	>99
20–34	6	23.0	>999	3	3	13	18	95	95	95
35–49	14	12.1	111	4	4	7	18	32	33	33
50–64	16	13.1	117	5	6	9	17	43	>99	>99
65+	22	11.1	27	6	8	10	12	17	23	24
TOTAL SINGLE DX	0									
TOTAL MULTIPLE DX	127	11.8	186	3	5	7	13	28	42	>99
TOTAL										
0–19 Years	69	11.3	177	3	5	7	13	28	42	>99
20–34	6	23.0	>999	3	3	13	18	95	95	95
35–49	14	12.1	111	4	4	7	18	32	33	33
50–64	16	13.1	117	5	6	9	17	43	>99	>99
65+	22	11.1	27	6	8	10	12	17	23	24
GRAND TOTAL	127	11.8	186	3	5	7	13	28	42	>99

LOS by Diagnosis and Operation, Western Region, 45th Edition

Western Region, October 2007–September 2008 Data, by Operation

35.2: HEART VALVE REPLACEMENT

Type of Patients	Observed Patients	Avg. Stay	Variance	10th	25th	50th	75th	90th	95th	99th
1. SINGLE DX										
0–19 Years	10	3.6	<1	3	3	3	4	5	5	5
20–34	8	5.0	2	3	5	5	5	8	8	8
35–49	8	4.1	<1	3	4	4	4	5	5	5
50–64	6	4.3	1	3	5	5	5	6	6	6
65+	2	22.3	607	5	5	5	40	40	40	40
2. MULTIPLE DX										
0–19 Years	259	8.4	101	3	4	5	8	18	30	53
20–34	242	10.4	111	4	5	6	11	24	34	56
35–49	755	9.9	59	4	5	7	12	19	25	37
50–64	2,687	10.2	76	4	5	7	12	19	26	48
65+	6,852	10.8	61	5	6	8	13	20	26	42
TOTAL SINGLE DX	34	4.9	29	3	3	4	5	5	6	40
TOTAL MULTIPLE DX	10,795	10.4	68	4	6	8	12	19	26	44
TOTAL										
0–19 Years	269	8.3	98	3	4	5	8	18	30	53
20–34	250	10.2	109	4	5	6	11	24	33	56
35–49	763	9.9	59	4	5	7	12	19	25	37
50–64	2,693	10.2	76	4	5	7	12	19	26	48
65+	6,854	10.8	61	5	6	8	13	20	26	42
GRAND TOTAL	10,829	10.4	68	4	6	8	12	19	26	44

35.21: REPL AORTIC VALVE-TISSUE

Type of Patients	Observed Patients	Avg. Stay	Variance	10th	25th	50th	75th	90th	95th	99th
1. SINGLE DX										
0–19 Years	3	3.0	1	2	2	3	4	4	4	4
20–34	4	4.5	1	3	3	5	5	5	5	5
35–49	4	4.3	<1	3	4	5	5	5	5	5
50–64	3	5.3	<1	5	5	5	6	6	6	6
65+	1	40.0	0	40	40	40	40	40	40	40
2. MULTIPLE DX										
0–19 Years	41	7.1	67	3	4	5	6	10	33	41
20–34	42	8.8	90	3	4	6	9	16	28	56
35–49	142	9.2	53	4	5	6	10	19	27	37
50–64	948	9.2	76	4	5	7	10	16	22	46
65+	4,172	10.3	56	5	6	8	12	18	24	41
TOTAL SINGLE DX	15	6.6	85	3	4	5	5	6	40	40
TOTAL MULTIPLE DX	5,345	10.0	60	5	6	7	12	18	24	41
TOTAL										
0–19 Years	44	6.9	66	3	4	5	6	10	33	41
20–34	46	8.5	84	3	4	5	9	14	28	56
35–49	146	8.9	52	4	5	6	10	19	27	37
50–64	951	9.2	75	4	5	7	10	16	22	46
65+	4,173	10.3	56	5	6	8	12	18	24	41
GRAND TOTAL	5,360	10.0	60	4	6	7	12	18	24	41

35.22: REPL AORTIC VALVE NEC

Type of Patients	Observed Patients	Avg. Stay	Variance	10th	25th	50th	75th	90th	95th	99th
1. SINGLE DX										
0–19 Years	1	4.0	0	4	4	4	4	4	4	4
20–34	3	6.0	3	5	5	5	8	8	8	8
35–49	3	3.7	<1	3	3	4	4	4	4	4
50–64	3	3.3	<1	3	3	3	4	4	4	4
65+	1	5.0	0	5	5	5	5	5	5	5
2. MULTIPLE DX										
0–19 Years	37	10.9	75	4	6	8	12	21	39	39
20–34	111	11.0	103	4	5	7	12	25	36	42
35–49	357	9.1	38	4	5	7	11	17	23	31
50–64	1,075	9.3	51	4	5	7	11	17	22	41
65+	1,674	10.5	54	5	6	8	13	20	24	41
TOTAL SINGLE DX	11	4.4	2	3	3	4	5	5	8	8
TOTAL MULTIPLE DX	3,254	10.0	54	4	6	8	12	19	24	40
TOTAL										
0–19 Years	38	10.8	74	4	6	8	12	21	39	39
20–34	114	10.9	101	4	5	7	12	25	34	42
35–49	360	9.0	38	4	5	7	11	17	23	31
50–64	1,078	9.3	51	4	5	7	11	17	22	41
65+	1,675	10.5	54	5	6	8	13	20	24	41
GRAND TOTAL	3,265	10.0	54	4	6	8	12	19	24	40

35.23: REPL MITRAL VALVE W TISS

Type of Patients	Observed Patients	Avg. Stay	Variance	10th	25th	50th	75th	90th	95th	99th
1. SINGLE DX										
0–19 Years	1	3.0	0	3	3	3	3	3	3	3
20–34	0									
35–49	0									
50–64	0									
65+	0									
2. MULTIPLE DX										
0–19 Years	1	5.0	0	5	5	5	5	5	5	5
20–34	7	28.5	698	10	12	19	35	85	85	85
35–49	50	11.0	30	6	7	9	14	18	23	25
50–64	217	14.5	151	6	7	10	17	29	41	70
65+	599	13.3	78	6	7	10	17	25	33	48
TOTAL SINGLE DX	1	3.0	0	3	3	3	3	3	3	3
TOTAL MULTIPLE DX	874	13.6	100	6	7	10	17	25	35	56
TOTAL										
0–19 Years	2	3.4	<1	3	3	3	5	5	5	5
20–34	7	28.5	698	10	12	19	35	85	85	85
35–49	50	11.0	30	6	7	9	14	18	23	25
50–64	217	14.5	151	6	7	10	17	29	41	70
65+	599	13.3	78	6	7	10	17	25	33	48
GRAND TOTAL	875	13.5	100	6	7	10	17	25	34	56

LOS by Diagnosis and Operation, Western Region, 45th Edition

122

Western Region, October 2007–September 2008 Data, by Operation

35.24: REPL MITRAL VALVE NEC

Type of Patients	Observed Patients	Avg. Stay	Variance	Percentiles						
				10th	25th	50th	75th	90th	95th	99th
1. SINGLE DX										
0–19 Years	1	5.0	0	5	5	5	5	5	5	5
20–34	0									
35–49	1	5.0	0	5	5	5	5	5	5	5
50–64	0									
65+	0									
2. MULTIPLE DX										
0–19 Years	27	15.2	178	4	7	11	18	26	53	54
20–34	33	13.6	117	6	7	9	15	26	39	55
35–49	163	11.7	66	5	6	9	15	22	27	64
50–64	419	12.2	85	5	7	10	14	23	30	50
65+	375	13.6	95	6	7	11	16	26	35	52
TOTAL SINGLE DX	2	5.0	0	5	5	5	5	5	5	5
TOTAL MULTIPLE DX	1,017	12.8	92	5	7	10	15	24	32	54
TOTAL										
0–19 Years	28	15.1	176	4	7	10	18	26	53	54
20–34	33	13.6	117	6	7	9	15	26	39	55
35–49	164	11.7	65	5	6	9	15	22	27	64
50–64	419	12.2	85	5	7	10	14	23	30	50
65+	375	13.6	95	6	7	11	16	26	35	52
GRAND TOTAL	1,019	12.8	92	5	7	10	15	24	32	54

35.3: TISS ADJ TO HRT VALV OPS

Type of Patients	Observed Patients	Avg. Stay	Variance	Percentiles						
				10th	25th	50th	75th	90th	95th	99th
1. SINGLE DX										
0–19 Years	1	3.0	0	3	3	3	3	3	3	3
20–34	0									
35–49	0									
50–64	0									
65+	0									
2. MULTIPLE DX										
0–19 Years	36	5.0	18	3	3	4	6	8	11	37
20–34	12	8.6	37	5	5	6	8	15	25	25
35–49	48	9.4	113	3	4	6	10	15	35	65
50–64	159	11.0	88	4	5	8	13	22	26	55
65+	256	11.6	59	5	6	9	15	21	27	40
TOTAL SINGLE DX	1	3.0	0	3	3	3	3	3	3	3
TOTAL MULTIPLE DX	511	10.1	70	4	5	7	12	20	25	47
TOTAL										
0–19 Years	37	4.9	18	3	3	6	6	6	11	37
20–34	12	8.6	37	5	5	6	8	15	25	25
35–49	48	9.4	113	3	4	6	10	15	35	65
50–64	159	11.0	88	4	5	8	13	22	26	55
65+	256	11.6	59	5	6	9	15	21	27	40
GRAND TOTAL	512	10.1	69	4	5	7	12	20	25	47

35.25: REPL PULMON VALVE W TISS

Type of Patients	Observed Patients	Avg. Stay	Variance	Percentiles						
				10th	25th	50th	75th	90th	95th	99th
1. SINGLE DX										
0–19 Years	3	4.0	<1	3	3	4	5	5	5	5
20–34	0									
35–49	0									
50–64	0									
65+	0									
2. MULTIPLE DX										
0–19 Years	90	7.4	119	3	3	4	6	11	18	74
20–34	28	5.7	13	3	4	5	5	11	11	23
35–49	12	11.4	203	4	5	6	9	16	55	55
50–64	8	5.9	2	4	5	6	7	8	8	8
65+	3	13.7	69	4	4	18	19	19	19	19
TOTAL SINGLE DX	3	4.0	<1	3	3	4	5	5	5	5
TOTAL MULTIPLE DX	141	7.3	104	3	4	4	6	11	18	74
TOTAL										
0–19 Years	93	7.2	114	3	3	4	6	11	18	74
20–34	28	5.7	13	3	4	5	5	11	11	23
35–49	12	11.4	203	4	5	6	9	16	55	55
50–64	8	5.9	2	4	5	6	7	8	8	8
65+	3	13.7	69	4	4	18	19	19	19	19
GRAND TOTAL	144	7.2	100	3	4	4	6	11	18	74

35.33: ANNULOPLASTY

Type of Patients	Observed Patients	Avg. Stay	Variance	Percentiles						
				10th	25th	50th	75th	90th	95th	99th
1. SINGLE DX										
0–19 Years	0									
20–34	0									
35–49	0									
50–64	0									
65+	0									
2. MULTIPLE DX										
0–19 Years	15	6.8	39	3	4	5	6	13	19	37
20–34	8	7.9	43	4	5	5	7	25	25	25
35–49	41	9.9	130	4	4	6	11	15	35	65
50–64	153	11.1	91	4	5	8	13	22	26	55
65+	254	11.6	59	5	6	9	15	21	27	40
TOTAL SINGLE DX	0									
TOTAL MULTIPLE DX	471	10.9	74	4	5	8	13	21	27	49
TOTAL										
0–19 Years	15	6.8	39	3	4	5	6	13	19	37
20–34	8	7.9	43	4	5	5	7	25	25	25
35–49	41	9.9	130	4	4	6	11	15	35	65
50–64	153	11.1	91	4	5	8	13	22	26	55
65+	254	11.6	59	5	6	9	15	21	27	40
GRAND TOTAL	471	10.9	74	4	5	8	13	21	27	49

LOS by Diagnosis and Operation, Western Region, 45th Edition

Western Region, October 2007–September 2008 Data, by Operation

35.4: SEPTAL DEFECT PRODUCTION

Type of Patients	Observed Patients	Avg. Stay	Vari-ance	10th	25th	50th	75th	90th	95th	99th
1. SINGLE DX										
0–19 Years	0									
20–34	0									
35–49	0									
50–64	0									
65+	0									
2. MULTIPLE DX										
0–19 Years	47	14.5	288	3	5	8	14	44	57	68
20–34	1	5.0	0	5	5	5	5	5	5	5
35–49	0									
50–64	2	13.5	<1	13	13	13	14	14	14	14
65+	0									
TOTAL SINGLE DX	0									
TOTAL MULTIPLE DX	50	14.4	281	3	5	8	14	44	57	68
TOTAL										
0–19 Years	47	14.5	288	3	5	8	14	44	57	68
20–34	1	5.0	0	5	5	5	5	5	5	5
35–49	0									
50–64	2	13.5	<1	13	13	13	14	14	14	14
65+	0									
GRAND TOTAL	50	14.4	281	3	5	8	14	44	57	68

35.5: PROSTH REP HEART SEPTA

Type of Patients	Observed Patients	Avg. Stay	Vari-ance	10th	25th	50th	75th	90th	95th	99th
1. SINGLE DX										
0–19 Years	77	1.1	<1	1	1	1	1	1	2	4
20–34	24	1.5	2	1	1	1	1	3	3	8
35–49	11	1.4	1	1	1	1	1	1	5	5
50–64	15	1.0	0	1	1	1	1	1	1	1
65+	3	1.0	0	1	1	1	1	1	1	1
2. MULTIPLE DX										
0–19 Years	291	6.4	64	1	1	4	7	16	21	45
20–34	59	2.1	6	1	1	1	1	5	8	14
35–49	129	1.7	4	1	1	1	2	4	5	9
50–64	209	2.6	19	1	1	1	2	7	10	22
65+	126	3.1	25	1	1	1	1	10	15	24
TOTAL SINGLE DX	130	1.2	<1	1	1	1	1	1	3	4
TOTAL MULTIPLE DX	814	4.7	47	1	1	2	5	12	18	36
TOTAL										
0–19 Years	368	5.4	56	1	1	3	6	14	20	42
20–34	83	1.9	5	1	1	1	1	4	8	14
35–49	140	1.7	4	1	1	1	2	4	5	9
50–64	224	2.5	18	1	1	1	1	7	8	22
65+	129	3.1	24	1	1	1	1	10	15	24
GRAND TOTAL	944	4.1	41	1	1	1	5	10	17	36

35.52: PROSTH REP ASD CLSD TECH

Type of Patients	Observed Patients	Avg. Stay	Vari-ance	10th	25th	50th	75th	90th	95th	99th
1. SINGLE DX										
0–19 Years	70	1.0	<1	1	1	1	1	1	1	2
20–34	23	1.4	2	1	1	1	1	2	3	8
35–49	10	1.0	0	1	1	1	1	1	1	1
50–64	15	1.0	0	1	1	1	1	1	1	1
65+	3	1.0	0	1	1	1	1	1	1	1
2. MULTIPLE DX										
0–19 Years	88	2.0	13	1	1	1	1	3	9	20
20–34	45	1.5	4	1	1	1	1	1	4	14
35–49	122	1.6	4	1	1	1	1	2	5	9
50–64	193	2.1	14	1	1	1	1	5	8	16
65+	115	2.5	15	1	1	1	1	6	11	19
TOTAL SINGLE DX	121	1.1	<1	1	1	1	1	1	1	2
TOTAL MULTIPLE DX	563	2.0	11	1	1	1	1	3	8	20
TOTAL										
0–19 Years	158	1.6	7	1	1	1	1	1	3	20
20–34	68	1.4	3	1	1	1	1	2	4	14
35–49	132	1.5	3	1	1	1	1	2	5	9
50–64	208	2.0	13	1	1	1	1	4	8	13
65+	118	2.4	15	1	1	1	1	6	11	19
GRAND TOTAL	684	1.8	9	1	1	1	1	2	6	17

35.53: OPEN PROSTH REP VSD

Type of Patients	Observed Patients	Avg. Stay	Vari-ance	10th	25th	50th	75th	90th	95th	99th
1. SINGLE DX										
0–19 Years	3	3.5	<1	2	3	4	4	4	4	4
20–34	0									
35–49	0									
50–64	0									
65+										
2. MULTIPLE DX										
0–19 Years	124	7.7	51	3	4	5	8	18	22	45
20–34	2	7.0	18	4	4	10	10	10	10	10
35–49	0									
50–64	5	15.4	60	7	10	13	22	25	25	25
65+	3	17.7	132	6	6	18	29	29	29	29
TOTAL SINGLE DX	3	3.5	<1	2	3	4	4	4	4	4
TOTAL MULTIPLE DX	134	7.9	53	3	4	5	9	18	22	45
TOTAL										
0–19 Years	127	7.6	50	3	4	5	8	18	22	45
20–34	2	7.0	18	4	4	10	10	10	10	10
35–49	0									
50–64	5	15.4	60	7	10	13	22	25	25	25
65+	3	17.7	132	6	6	18	29	29	29	29
GRAND TOTAL	137	7.8	52	3	4	5	8	18	22	45

LOS by Diagnosis and Operation, Western Region, 45th Edition

Western Region, October 2007–September 2008 Data, by Operation

35.6: TISS GRFT REP HRT SEPTA

Type of Patients	Observed Patients	Avg. Stay	Variance	Percentiles						
				10th	25th	50th	75th	90th	95th	99th
1. SINGLE DX										
0–19 Years	48	2.9	1	2	2	3	3	4	5	6
20–34	5	3.8	1	2	4	4	4	5	5	5
35–49	5	3.8	<1	3	3	4	4	5	5	5
50–64	1	5.0	0	5	5	5	5	5	5	5
65+	0									
2. MULTIPLE DX										
0–19 Years	455	6.7	79	2	3	4	6	13	23	66
20–34	31	4.4	2	3	3	4	5	6	7	9
35–49	28	5.6	8	3	3	5	7	10	11	13
50–64	32	6.7	14	4	4	6	8	11	12	21
65+	18	12.5	88	5	6	9	16	32	35	35
TOTAL SINGLE DX	59	3.0	1	2	2	3	3	4	5	6
TOTAL MULTIPLE DX	564	6.7	74	2	3	4	6	12	23	66
TOTAL										
0–19 Years	503	6.3	72	2	3	4	6	12	22	66
20–34	36	4.3	2	3	3	4	5	6	7	9
35–49	33	5.4	7	3	3	5	7	10	11	13
50–64	33	6.6	14	4	4	6	8	11	12	21
65+	18	12.5	88	5	6	9	16	32	35	35
GRAND TOTAL	623	6.3	69	2	3	4	6	12	21	66

35.61: REPAIR ASD W TISS GRAFT

Type of Patients	Observed Patients	Avg. Stay	Variance	Percentiles						
				10th	25th	50th	75th	90th	95th	99th
1. SINGLE DX										
0–19 Years	34	2.7	1	2	2	2	3	4	5	8
20–34	4	4.3	<1	4	4	4	5	5	5	5
35–49	5	3.8	<1	3	3	4	4	5	5	5
50–64	1	5.0	0	5	5	5	5	5	5	5
65+	0									
2. MULTIPLE DX										
0–19 Years	167	4.2	24	2	3	3	4	5	8	45
20–34	24	4.5	2	3	4	4	5	6	7	9
35–49	25	5.7	8	3	4	5	7	11	11	13
50–64	27	6.3	15	4	4	5	8	12	12	21
65+	13	8.2	12	5	6	7	9	14	16	16
TOTAL SINGLE DX	44	2.9	1	2	2	3	3	4	5	5
TOTAL MULTIPLE DX	256	4.5	22	2	3	3	5	7	11	45
TOTAL										
0–19 Years	201	3.9	21	2	2	3	4	5	8	45
20–34	28	4.5	2	4	4	4	5	6	7	9
35–49	30	5.5	7	3	3	5	7	10	11	13
50–64	28	6.3	15	3	4	5	8	12	12	21
65+	13	8.2	12	5	6	7	9	14	16	16
GRAND TOTAL	300	4.2	19	2	3	3	4	6	9	45

35.62: REPAIR VSD W TISS GRAFT

Type of Patients	Observed Patients	Avg. Stay	Variance	Percentiles						
				10th	25th	50th	75th	90th	95th	99th
1. SINGLE DX										
0–19 Years	13	3.5	1	2	3	3	4	5	5	6
20–34	1	2.0	0	2	2	2	2	2	2	2
35–49	0									
50–64	0									
65+	0									
2. MULTIPLE DX										
0–19 Years	191	7.4	106	3	3	4	7	14	26	66
20–34	3	3.7	0	3	3	3	5	5	5	5
35–49	1	2.0	0	2	2	2	2	2	2	2
50–64	2	7.0	0	7	7	7	7	7	7	7
65+	3	25.3	34	21	21	23	32	32	32	32
TOTAL SINGLE DX	14	3.5	1	2	3	3	4	5	5	6
TOTAL MULTIPLE DX	200	7.5	107	3	3	4	7	15	27	66
TOTAL										
0–19 Years	204	7.2	101	3	3	4	6	13	20	66
20–34	4	3.3	2	2	2	3	5	5	5	5
35–49	1	2.0	0	2	2	2	2	2	2	2
50–64	2	7.0	0	7	7	7	7	7	7	7
65+	3	25.3	34	21	21	23	32	32	32	32
GRAND TOTAL	214	7.3	102	3	3	4	6	14	23	66

35.63: REPAIR ECD W TISS GRAFT

Type of Patients	Observed Patients	Avg. Stay	Variance	Percentiles						
				10th	25th	50th	75th	90th	95th	99th
1. SINGLE DX										
0–19 Years	1	3.0	0	3	3	3	3	3	3	3
20–34	0									
35–49	0									
50–64	0									
65+										
2. MULTIPLE DX										
0–19 Years	96	9.3	99	3	4	6	10	22	39	>99
20–34	1	4.0	0	4	4	4	4	4	4	4
35–49	2	8.0	0	8	8	8	8	8	8	8
50–64	2	8.5	4	7	6	10	10	10	10	10
65+	2	20.7	414	6	6	35	35	35	35	35
TOTAL SINGLE DX	1	3.0	0	3	3	3	3	3	3	3
TOTAL MULTIPLE DX	102	9.4	99	3	4	6	10	22	35	>99
TOTAL										
0–19 Years	97	9.2	98	3	4	6	10	21	34	>99
20–34	1	4.0	0	4	4	4	4	4	4	4
35–49	2	8.0	0	8	8	8	8	8	8	8
50–64	2	8.5	4	7	6	10	10	10	10	10
65+	2	20.7	414	6	6	35	35	35	35	35
GRAND TOTAL	103	9.3	99	3	4	6	10	22	35	>99

LOS by Diagnosis and Operation, Western Region, 45th Edition

Western Region, October 2007–September 2008 Data, by Operation

35.7: HEART SEPTA REPAIR NEC

Type of Patients	Observed Patients	Avg. Stay	Vari-ance	10th	25th	50th	75th	90th	95th	99th
1. SINGLE DX										
0–19 Years	22	2.6	2	1	1	2	4	4	5	5
20–34	2	3.0	8	1	1	3	5	5	5	5
35–49	0									
50–64	0									
65+	1	2.0	0	2	2	2	2	2	2	2
2. MULTIPLE DX										
0–19 Years	199	7.9	101	2	3	4	8	19	28	66
20–34	15	5.6	23	1	2	4	7	13	18	18
35–49	42	5.6	37	1	2	4	6	13	15	31
50–64	74	5.7	22	1	3	5	7	11	13	31
65+	61	8.4	28	3	5	7	11	15	17	31
TOTAL SINGLE DX	25	2.6	2	1	1	2	4	4	5	5
TOTAL MULTIPLE DX	391	7.5	79	2	3	5	8	16	26	45
TOTAL										
0–19 Years	221	7.5	95	2	3	4	7	17	28	66
20–34	17	5.3	22	1	2	4	6	13	18	18
35–49	42	5.6	37	1	2	4	6	13	15	31
50–64	74	5.7	22	1	3	5	7	11	13	31
65+	62	8.3	28	3	5	7	11	15	17	31
GRAND TOTAL	416	7.2	75	2	3	4	8	14	26	45

35.71: REPAIR ASD NEC & NOS

Type of Patients	Observed Patients	Avg. Stay	Vari-ance	10th	25th	50th	75th	90th	95th	99th
1. SINGLE DX										
0–19 Years	17	2.1	1	1	1	2	3	4	4	4
20–34	2	3.0	8	1	1	3	5	5	5	5
35–49	0									
50–64	0									
65+	1	2.0	0	2	2	2	2	2	2	2
2. MULTIPLE DX										
0–19 Years	90	8.7	84	2	3	5	10	26	28	40
20–34	11	5.8	32	1	2	4	11	13	18	18
35–49	36	5.0	30	1	2	4	5	11	15	31
50–64	69	5.7	24	1	3	5	7	11	13	31
65+	55	8.3	29	3	5	7	11	15	17	31
TOTAL SINGLE DX	20	2.2	2	1	1	2	3	4	4	5
TOTAL MULTIPLE DX	261	7.6	59	2	3	5	9	17	28	40
TOTAL										
0–19 Years	107	7.9	78	2	3	4	9	26	28	40
20–34	13	5.4	28	1	2	4	5	13	18	18
35–49	36	4.8	30	1	2	4	5	11	15	31
50–64	69	5.7	24	1	3	5	7	11	13	31
65+	56	8.2	29	2	5	7	11	15	17	31
GRAND TOTAL	281	7.2	57	1	3	5	8	15	28	40

35.8: TOT REP CONG CARD ANOM

Type of Patients	Observed Patients	Avg. Stay	Vari-ance	10th	25th	50th	75th	90th	95th	99th
1. SINGLE DX										
0–19 Years	9	3.9	4	2	2	4	4	7	8	8
20–34	0									
35–49	0									
50–64	0									
65+										
2. MULTIPLE DX										
0–19 Years	363	13.4	204	4	5	8	14	30	49	78
20–34	7	10.6	112	1	4	10	11	33	33	33
35–49	5	5.6	6	3	4	5	7	9	9	9
50–64	2	6.5	4	5	5	5	8	8	8	8
65+	1	14.0	0	14	14	14	14	14	14	14
TOTAL SINGLE DX	9	3.9	4	2	2	4	4	7	8	8
TOTAL MULTIPLE DX	378	13.3	202	4	5	8	14	30	48	78
TOTAL										
0–19 Years	372	13.2	202	4	5	8	14	30	48	78
20–34	7	10.6	112	1	4	10	11	33	33	33
35–49	5	5.6	6	3	4	5	7	9	9	9
50–64	2	6.5	4	5	5	5	8	8	8	8
65+	1	14.0	0	14	14	14	14	14	14	14
GRAND TOTAL	387	13.2	200	4	5	8	14	30	46	78

35.81: TOT REP TETRALOGY FALLOT

Type of Patients	Observed Patients	Avg. Stay	Vari-ance	10th	25th	50th	75th	90th	95th	99th
1. SINGLE DX										
0–19 Years	9	3.9	4	2	2	4	4	7	8	8
20–34	0									
35–49	0									
50–64	0									
65+										
2. MULTIPLE DX										
0–19 Years	246	12.1	190	4	5	7	12	28	54	78
20–34	3	8.7	10	5	5	10	11	11	11	11
35–49	3	7.0	4	5	5	7	9	9	9	9
50–64	1	5.0	0	5	5	5	5	5	5	5
65+	1	14.0	0	14	14	14	14	14	14	14
TOTAL SINGLE DX	9	3.9	4	2	2	4	4	7	8	8
TOTAL MULTIPLE DX	254	12.0	188	4	5	7	12	28	54	78
TOTAL										
0–19 Years	255	11.9	187	4	5	7	12	27	53	78
20–34	3	8.7	10	5	5	10	11	11	11	11
35–49	3	7.0	4	5	5	7	9	9	9	9
50–64	1	5.0	0	5	5	5	5	5	5	5
65+	1	14.0	0	14	14	14	14	14	14	14
GRAND TOTAL	263	11.8	185	4	5	7	12	27	53	78

LOS by Diagnosis and Operation, Western Region, 45th Edition

Western Region, October 2007–September 2008 Data, by Operation

35.9: VALVES & SEPTA OPS NEC

Type of Patients	Observed Patients	Avg. Stay	Variance	10th	25th	50th	75th	90th	95th	99th
1. SINGLE DX										
0–19 Years	26	1.9	2	1	1	1	2	5	5	7
20–34	3	1.0	0	1	1	1	1	1	1	1
35–49	7	1.0	0	1	1	1	1	1	1	1
50–64	0									
65+	0									
2. MULTIPLE DX										
0–19 Years	412	10.6	198	1	3	6	11	27	39	93
20–34	22	5.3	19	1	1	5	9	10	12	15
35–49	15	4.6	31	1	1	1	6	17	17	17
50–64	49	5.2	101	1	1	2	5	12	17	67
65+	163	4.7	25	1	1	3	7	11	15	23
TOTAL SINGLE DX	36	1.7	2	1	1	1	2	4	5	7
TOTAL MULTIPLE DX	661	9.5	173	1	2	6	10	23	38	79
TOTAL										
0–19 Years	438	10.2	192	1	2	6	11	26	39	93
20–34	25	4.7	19	1	1	2	9	10	12	15
35–49	22	3.5	24	1	1	1	5	9	17	17
50–64	49	5.2	101	1	1	2	5	12	17	67
65+	163	4.7	25	1	1	3	7	11	15	23
GRAND TOTAL	697	9.1	167	1	2	5	10	21	35	79

35.92: CREAT CONDUIT RT VENT-PA

Type of Patients	Observed Patients	Avg. Stay	Variance	10th	25th	50th	75th	90th	95th	99th
1. SINGLE DX										
0–19 Years	1	3.0	0	3	3	3	3	3	3	3
20–34	0									
35–49	0									
50–64	0									
65+	0									
2. MULTIPLE DX										
0–19 Years	89	10.0	113	3	4	6	10	22	28	58
20–34	2	11.0	2	10	10	12	12	12	12	12
35–49	0									
50–64	0									
65+	0									
TOTAL SINGLE DX	1	3.0	0	3	3	3	3	3	3	3
TOTAL MULTIPLE DX	91	10.0	112	3	4	6	10	22	28	58
TOTAL										
0–19 Years	90	10.0	112	3	4	6	10	22	28	58
20–34	2	11.0	2	10	10	12	12	12	12	12
35–49	0									
50–64	0									
65+	0									
GRAND TOTAL	92	10.0	111	3	4	6	10	22	28	58

35.94: CREAT CONDUIT ATRIUM-PA

Type of Patients	Observed Patients	Avg. Stay	Variance	10th	25th	50th	75th	90th	95th	99th
1. SINGLE DX										
0–19 Years	5	4.8	3	3	4	4	6	7	7	7
20–34	0									
35–49	0									
50–64	0									
65+	0									
2. MULTIPLE DX										
0–19 Years	169	15.6	278	5	7	9	17	35	51	98
20–34	3	8.7	2	7	7	9	10	10	10	10
35–49	1	17.0	0	17	17	17	17	17	17	17
50–64	0									
65+	0									
TOTAL SINGLE DX	5	4.8	3	3	4	4	6	7	7	7
TOTAL MULTIPLE DX	173	15.5	275	5	7	9	17	35	46	98
TOTAL										
0–19 Years	174	15.4	276	5	7	9	17	35	46	98
20–34	3	8.7	2	7	7	9	10	10	10	10
35–49	1	17.0	0	17	17	17	17	17	17	17
50–64	0									
65+	0									
GRAND TOTAL	178	15.4	274	5	7	9	17	35	46	98

35.96: PERC VALVULOPLASTY

Type of Patients	Observed Patients	Avg. Stay	Variance	10th	25th	50th	75th	90th	95th	99th
1. SINGLE DX										
0–19 Years	19	1.2	<1	1	1	1	1	2	2	3
20–34	3	1.0	0	1	1	1	1	1	1	1
35–49	7	1.0	0	1	1	1	1	1	1	1
50–64	0									
65+	0									
2. MULTIPLE DX										
0–19 Years	110	4.6	122	1	1	1	2	7	29	51
20–34	12	2.9	17	1	1	1	2	8	15	15
35–49	10	2.3	7	1	1	1	2	5	9	9
50–64	37	5.1	132	1	1	1	3	12	21	67
65+	139	4.5	24	1	1	3	7	10	14	23
TOTAL SINGLE DX	29	1.2	<1	1	1	1	1	2	2	3
TOTAL MULTIPLE DX	308	4.5	89	1	1	1	4	10	17	51
TOTAL										
0–19 Years	129	4.1	107	1	1	1	2	6	19	51
20–34	15	2.4	14	1	1	1	2	8	15	15
35–49	17	1.8	4	1	1	1	1	5	9	9
50–64	37	5.1	132	1	1	1	3	12	21	67
65+	139	4.5	24	1	1	3	7	10	14	23
GRAND TOTAL	337	4.2	81	1	1	1	3	9	15	51

LOS by Diagnosis and Operation, Western Region, 45th Edition

Western Region, October 2007–September 2008 Data, by Operation

36.0: RMVL COR ART OBSTR/STENT

Type of Patients	Observed Patients	Avg. Stay	Vari-ance	Percentiles						
				10th	25th	50th	75th	90th	95th	99th
1. SINGLE DX										
0–19 Years	0									
20–34	0									
35–49	1	1.0	0	1	1	1	1	1	1	1
50–64	0									
65+	3	1.0	0	1	1	1	1	1	1	1
2. MULTIPLE DX										
0–19 Years	0									
20–34	4	14.6	274	4	4	10	39	39	39	39
35–49	66	2.7	4	1	1	3	3	4	5	14
50–64	267	2.8	11	1	1	2	3	5	10	22
65+	365	2.9	11	1	1	2	3	6	8	23
TOTAL SINGLE DX	4	1.0	0	1	1	1	1	1	1	1
TOTAL MULTIPLE DX	702	2.9	12	1	1	2	3	5	8	22
TOTAL										
0–19 Years	0									
20–34	4	14.6	274	4	4	10	39	39	39	39
35–49	67	2.7	4	1	1	3	3	4	5	14
50–64	267	2.8	11	1	1	2	3	5	10	22
65+	368	2.8	11	1	1	2	3	6	8	23
GRAND TOTAL	706	2.9	12	1	1	2	3	5	8	22

36.06: NON-DRUG-ELUT COR STENT

Type of Patients	Observed Patients	Avg. Stay	Vari-ance	Percentiles						
				10th	25th	50th	75th	90th	95th	99th
1. SINGLE DX										
0–19 Years	0									
20–34	0									
35–49	1	1.0	0	1	1	1	1	1	1	1
50–64	0									
65+	2	1.0	0	1	1	1	1	1	1	1
2. MULTIPLE DX										
0–19 Years	0									
20–34	0									
35–49	28	3.3	8	1	2	3	3	5	10	14
50–64	92	2.5	4	1	1	2	3	4	7	14
65+	133	3.0	11	1	1	2	3	6	10	18
TOTAL SINGLE DX	3	1.0	0	1	1	1	1	1	1	1
TOTAL MULTIPLE DX	253	2.8	8	1	1	2	3	5	7	15
TOTAL										
0–19 Years	0									
20–34	0									
35–49	29	3.2	7	1	2	3	3	5	10	14
50–64	92	2.5	4	1	1	2	3	4	7	14
65+	135	2.9	11	1	1	2	3	6	10	18
GRAND TOTAL	256	2.8	8	1	1	2	3	5	7	15

36.07: DRUG-ELUTING COR STENT

Type of Patients	Observed Patients	Avg. Stay	Vari-ance	Percentiles						
				10th	25th	50th	75th	90th	95th	99th
1. SINGLE DX										
0–19 Years	0									
20–34	0									
35–49	0									
50–64	0									
65+	1	1.0	0	1	1	1	1	1	1	1
2. MULTIPLE DX										
0–19 Years	0									
20–34	1	5.0	0	5	5	5	5	5	5	5
35–49	32	2.2	1	1	1	2	3	3	4	4
50–64	148	2.1	4	1	1	1	2	3	4	13
65+	205	2.2	3	1	1	2	3	4	6	8
TOTAL SINGLE DX	1	1.0	0	1	1	1	1	1	1	1
TOTAL MULTIPLE DX	386	2.1	3	1	1	2	3	4	5	10
TOTAL										
0–19 Years	0									
20–34	1	5.0	0	5	5	5	5	5	5	5
35–49	32	2.2	1	1	1	1	3	4	4	4
50–64	148	2.1	4	1	1	2	2	3	4	13
65+	206	2.2	3	1	1	2	3	4	6	8
GRAND TOTAL	387	2.1	3	1	1	2	3	4	5	10

36.1: HRT REVASC BYPASS ANAST

Type of Patients	Observed Patients	Avg. Stay	Vari-ance	Percentiles						
				10th	25th	50th	75th	90th	95th	99th
1. SINGLE DX										
0–19 Years	1	4.0	0	4	4	4	4	4	4	4
20–34	0									
35–49	4	5.0	5	2	5	6	7	7	7	7
50–64	10	5.2	5	3	4	5	5	9	9	9
65+	3	5.7	16	2	2	5	10	10	10	10
2. MULTIPLE DX										
0–19 Years	2	5.5	13	3	3	6	8	8	8	8
20–34	39	9.7	203	4	5	7	9	13	34	91
35–49	1,224	7.9	22	4	5	7	9	12	15	26
50–64	7,815	8.2	29	4	5	7	9	13	17	30
65+	11,258	9.3	37	5	6	8	11	15	20	34
TOTAL SINGLE DX	18	5.2	6	2	4	5	6	9	10	10
TOTAL MULTIPLE DX	20,338	8.8	34	4	5	7	10	14	19	32
TOTAL										
0–19 Years	3	5.0	7	3	3	4	8	8	8	8
20–34	39	9.7	203	4	5	7	8	13	34	91
35–49	1,228	7.9	22	4	5	7	9	12	15	26
50–64	7,825	8.2	29	4	5	7	9	13	17	30
65+	11,261	9.3	37	5	6	8	11	15	20	34
GRAND TOTAL	20,356	8.8	34	4	5	7	10	14	19	32

LOS by Diagnosis and Operation, Western Region, 45th Edition

Western Region, October 2007–September 2008 Data, by Operation

36.11: COR BYPASS-1 COR ART

Type of Patients	Observed Patients	Avg. Stay	Vari-ance	Percentiles						
				10th	25th	50th	75th	90th	95th	99th
1. SINGLE DX										
0–19 Years	1	4.0	0	4	4	4	4	4	4	4
20–34	0									
35–49	0									
50–64	2	3.0	0	2	2	2	2	2	2	2
65+	1	2.0	0	2	2	2	2	2	2	2
2. MULTIPLE DX										
0–19 Years	1	3.0	0	3	3	3	3	3	3	3
20–34	13	5.9	3	4	5	6	7	8	10	10
35–49	174	7.7	23	4	5	6	9	12	15	30
50–64	918	7.5	19	4	5	6	9	12	15	26
65+	1,432	9.0	42	4	6	7	10	15	20	34
TOTAL SINGLE DX	**4**	**3.0**	**1**	**2**	**2**	**4**	**4**	**4**	**4**	**4**
TOTAL MULTIPLE DX	**2,538**	**8.4**	**32**	**4**	**5**	**7**	**10**	**14**	**18**	**31**
TOTAL										
0–19 Years	2	3.5	<1	3	3	4	4	4	4	4
20–34	13	5.9	3	4	5	6	7	8	10	10
35–49	174	7.7	23	4	5	6	9	12	15	30
50–64	920	7.5	19	4	5	6	9	12	15	26
65+	1,433	9.0	42	4	6	7	10	15	20	34
GRAND TOTAL	**2,542**	**8.4**	**32**	**4**	**5**	**7**	**10**	**14**	**18**	**31**

36.12: COR BYPASS-2 COR ART

Type of Patients	Observed Patients	Avg. Stay	Vari-ance	Percentiles						
				10th	25th	50th	75th	90th	95th	99th
1. SINGLE DX										
0–19 Years	0									
20–34	0									
35–49	1	7.0	0	7	7	7	7	7	7	7
50–64	2	5.0	0	5	5	5	5	5	5	5
65+	0									
2. MULTIPLE DX										
0–19 Years	0									
20–34	8	7.3	10	5	5	6	9	14	14	14
35–49	327	7.9	27	4	5	7	9	12	15	31
50–64	2,290	8.1	26	4	5	7	9	14	18	29
65+	3,530	9.1	35	5	6	8	10	15	19	34
TOTAL SINGLE DX	**3**	**5.7**	**1**	**5**	**5**	**5**	**7**	**7**	**7**	**7**
TOTAL MULTIPLE DX	**6,155**	**8.7**	**32**	**4**	**5**	**7**	**10**	**14**	**18**	**32**
TOTAL										
0–19 Years	0									
20–34	8	7.3	10	5	5	6	9	14	14	14
35–49	328	7.9	27	4	5	7	9	12	15	31
50–64	2,292	8.1	26	4	5	7	9	14	18	29
65+	3,530	9.1	35	5	6	8	10	15	19	34
GRAND TOTAL	**6,158**	**8.7**	**32**	**4**	**5**	**7**	**10**	**14**	**18**	**32**

36.13: COR BYPASS-3 COR ART

Type of Patients	Observed Patients	Avg. Stay	Vari-ance	Percentiles						
				10th	25th	50th	75th	90th	95th	99th
1. SINGLE DX										
0–19 Years	0									
20–34	0									
35–49	2	5.5	<1	5	5	6	6	6	6	6
50–64	4	6.0	4	5	5	5	5	9	9	9
65+	2	7.5	12	5	5	5	10	10	10	10
2. MULTIPLE DX										
0–19 Years	0									
20–34	6	8.2	6	6	7	7	9	13	13	13
35–49	325	8.2	18	4	6	7	10	13	16	25
50–64	2,154	8.4	28	4	5	7	10	14	17	30
65+	3,147	9.5	38	5	6	8	11	16	20	36
TOTAL SINGLE DX	**8**	**6.2**	**4**	**5**	**5**	**5**	**6**	**10**	**10**	**10**
TOTAL MULTIPLE DX	**5,632**	**9.0**	**34**	**4**	**6**	**7**	**10**	**15**	**19**	**32**
TOTAL										
0–19 Years	0									
20–34	6	8.2	6	6	7	7	9	13	13	13
35–49	327	8.2	18	4	6	7	10	13	16	25
50–64	2,158	8.4	28	4	5	7	10	14	17	30
65+	3,149	9.5	38	5	6	8	11	16	20	36
GRAND TOTAL	**5,640**	**9.0**	**34**	**4**	**6**	**7**	**10**	**15**	**19**	**32**

36.14: COR BYPASS-4+ COR ART

Type of Patients	Observed Patients	Avg. Stay	Vari-ance	Percentiles						
				10th	25th	50th	75th	90th	95th	99th
1. SINGLE DX										
0–19 Years	0									
20–34	0									
35–49	0									
50–64	2	6.0	18	3	3	6	9	9	9	9
65+	0									
2. MULTIPLE DX										
0–19 Years	0									
20–34	4	13.3	192	5	6	8	34	34	34	34
35–49	199	8.2	28	4	5	7	9	13	16	26
50–64	1,177	8.5	28	5	6	8	10	14	17	30
65+	1,517	9.9	42	5	6	8	12	17	20	36
TOTAL SINGLE DX	**2**	**6.0**	**18**	**3**	**3**	**6**	**9**	**9**	**9**	**9**
TOTAL MULTIPLE DX	**2,897**	**9.2**	**36**	**5**	**6**	**8**	**11**	**15**	**19**	**33**
TOTAL										
0–19 Years	0									
20–34	4	13.3	192	5	6	8	34	34	34	34
35–49	199	8.2	28	4	5	7	9	13	16	26
50–64	1,179	8.5	28	5	6	8	10	14	17	30
65+	1,517	9.9	42	5	6	8	12	17	20	36
GRAND TOTAL	**2,899**	**9.2**	**36**	**5**	**6**	**8**	**11**	**15**	**19**	**33**

LOS by Diagnosis and Operation, Western Region, 45th Edition

Western Region, October 2007–September 2008 Data, by Operation

36.15: 1 INT MAM-COR ART BYPASS

Type of Patients	Observed Patients	Avg. Stay	Vari-ance	Percentiles						
				10th	25th	50th	75th	90th	95th	99th
1. SINGLE DX										
0–19 Years	0									
20–34	0									
35–49	1	2.0	0	2	2	2	2	2	2	2
50–64	0									
65+	0									
2. MULTIPLE DX										
0–19 Years	1	8.0	0	8	8	8	8	8	8	8
20–34	4	8.2	6	7	7	7	7	12	12	12
35–49	169	7.0	10	4	5	6	9	11	13	24
50–64	1,194	8.0	46	4	5	6	9	13	17	31
65+	1,549	8.9	32	4	6	7	11	15	19	34
TOTAL SINGLE DX	1	2.0	0	2	2	2	2	2	2	2
TOTAL MULTIPLE DX	2,917	8.4	37	4	5	7	10	14	18	33
TOTAL										
0–19 Years	1	8.0	0	8	8	8	8	8	8	8
20–34	4	8.2	6	7	7	7	7	12	12	12
35–49	170	7.0	10	4	5	6	9	11	13	24
50–64	1,194	8.0	46	4	5	6	9	13	17	31
65+	1,549	8.9	32	4	6	7	11	15	19	34
GRAND TOTAL	2,918	8.4	37	4	5	7	10	14	18	33

36.16: 2 INT MAM-COR ART BYPASS

Type of Patients	Observed Patients	Avg. Stay	Vari-ance	Percentiles						
				10th	25th	50th	75th	90th	95th	99th
1. SINGLE DX										
0–19 Years	0									
20–34	0									
35–49	0									
50–64	0									
65+	0									
2. MULTIPLE DX										
0–19 Years	0									
20–34	4	27.3	>999	3	4	8	51	91	91	91
35–49	29	7.8	24	5	5	6	9	11	20	27
50–64	76	7.1	14	4	5	6	8	12	15	21
65+	78	9.4	37	4	6	8	10	16	23	34
TOTAL SINGLE DX	0									
TOTAL MULTIPLE DX	187	8.6	63	4	5	7	10	14	19	34
TOTAL										
0–19 Years	0									
20–34	4	27.3	>999	3	4	8	51	91	91	91
35–49	29	7.8	24	5	5	6	9	11	20	27
50–64	76	7.1	14	4	5	6	8	12	15	21
65+	78	9.4	37	4	6	8	10	16	23	34
GRAND TOTAL	187	8.6	63	4	5	7	10	14	19	34

36.2: ARTERIAL IMPLANT REVASC

Type of Patients	Observed Patients	Avg. Stay	Vari-ance	Percentiles						
				10th	25th	50th	75th	90th	95th	99th
1. SINGLE DX										
0–19 Years	0									
20–34	0									
35–49	0									
50–64	0									
65+	0									
2. MULTIPLE DX										
0–19 Years	1	4.0	0	4	4	4	4	4	4	4
20–34	0									
35–49	0									
50–64	0									
65+	0									
TOTAL SINGLE DX	0									
TOTAL MULTIPLE DX	1	4.0	0	4	4	4	4	4	4	4
TOTAL										
0–19 Years	1	4.0	0	4	4	4	4	4	4	4
20–34	0									
35–49	0									
50–64	0									
65+	0									
GRAND TOTAL	1	4.0	0	4	4	4	4	4	4	4

36.3: OTHER HEART REVASC

Type of Patients	Observed Patients	Avg. Stay	Vari-ance	Percentiles						
				10th	25th	50th	75th	90th	95th	99th
1. SINGLE DX										
0–19 Years	0									
20–34	0									
35–49	0									
50–64	0									
65+	0									
2. MULTIPLE DX										
0–19 Years	0									
20–34	1	14.0	0	14	14	14	14	14	14	14
35–49	23	7.0	6	4	5	7	9	10	11	11
50–64	125	7.8	16	4	5	7	9	12	16	22
65+	143	9.5	29	5	6	7	12	16	20	29
TOTAL SINGLE DX	0									
TOTAL MULTIPLE DX	292	8.6	22	4	6	7	10	15	17	27
TOTAL										
0–19 Years	0									
20–34	1	14.0	0	14	14	14	14	14	14	14
35–49	23	7.0	6	4	5	7	9	10	11	11
50–64	125	7.8	16	4	5	7	9	12	16	22
65+	143	9.5	29	5	6	7	12	16	20	29
GRAND TOTAL	292	8.6	22	4	6	7	10	15	17	27

Western Region, October 2007–September 2008 Data, by Operation

36.31: OPEN TRANSMYO REVASC

Type of Patients	Observed Patients	Avg. Stay	Variance	Percentiles						
				10th	25th	50th	75th	90th	95th	99th
1. SINGLE DX										
0–19 Years	0									
20–34	0									
35–49	0									
50–64	0									
65+	0									
2. MULTIPLE DX										
0–19 Years	0									
20–34	1	14.0	0	14	14	14	14	14	14	14
35–49	20	7.4	6	4	6	8	8	10	11	11
50–64	112	7.8	17	4	5	7	9	12	16	22
65+	131	9.7	30	5	6	7	12	17	20	29
TOTAL SINGLE DX	0									
TOTAL MULTIPLE DX	264	8.7	24	4	6	7	10	15	19	27
TOTAL										
0–19 Years	0									
20–34	1	14.0	0	14	14	14	14	14	14	14
35–49	20	7.4	6	4	6	8	8	10	11	11
50–64	112	7.8	17	4	5	7	9	12	16	22
65+	131	9.7	30	5	6	7	12	17	20	29
GRAND TOTAL	264	8.7	24	4	6	7	10	15	19	27

36.99: HEART VESSEL OPS NEC

Type of Patients	Observed Patients	Avg. Stay	Variance	Percentiles						
				10th	25th	50th	75th	90th	95th	99th
1. SINGLE DX										
0–19 Years	3	3.7	<1	3	3	3	4	4	4	4
20–34	2	3.0	0	3	3	3	3	3	3	3
35–49	0									
50–64	0									
65+	0									
2. MULTIPLE DX										
0–19 Years	20	10.4	142	2	3	4	14	37	40	40
20–34	6	7.0	3	4	6	8	8	9	9	9
35–49	14	9.6	55	3	4	8	15	18	28	28
50–64	40	8.6	26	4	5	7	10	13	22	24
65+	55	10.5	46	5	6	9	13	18	19	44
TOTAL SINGLE DX	5	3.5	<1	3	3	3	4	4	4	4
TOTAL MULTIPLE DX	135	9.8	67	3	5	7	12	18	28	40
TOTAL										
0–19 Years	23	9.0	119	3	3	4	9	33	40	40
20–34	8	5.2	6	3	3	4	8	8	9	9
35–49	14	9.6	55	3	4	8	15	18	28	28
50–64	40	8.6	26	4	5	7	10	13	22	24
65+	55	10.5	46	5	6	9	13	18	19	44
GRAND TOTAL	140	9.2	64	3	4	7	12	18	27	40

36.9: OTHER HEART VESSEL OPS

Type of Patients	Observed Patients	Avg. Stay	Variance	Percentiles						
				10th	25th	50th	75th	90th	95th	99th
1. SINGLE DX										
0–19 Years	3	3.7	<1	3	3	4	4	4	4	4
20–34	2	3.0	0	3	3	3	3	3	3	3
35–49	0									
50–64	0									
65+	0									
2. MULTIPLE DX										
0–19 Years	21	10.4	130	3	3	6	13	37	40	40
20–34	6	7.0	3	4	6	8	8	9	9	9
35–49	16	8.7	55	4	5	5	15	18	28	28
50–64	44	8.8	35	4	5	7	10	15	22	30
65+	60	10.2	43	5	6	9	12	17	19	44
TOTAL SINGLE DX	5	3.5	<1	3	3	3	4	4	4	4
TOTAL MULTIPLE DX	147	9.7	65	3	4	7	12	18	28	40
TOTAL										
0–19 Years	24	9.0	112	3	3	4	10	18	40	40
20–34	8	5.2	6	3	3	4	8	8	9	9
35–49	16	8.7	55	3	4	5	15	18	28	28
50–64	44	8.8	35	4	5	7	10	15	22	30
65+	60	10.2	43	5	6	9	12	17	19	44
GRAND TOTAL	152	9.1	62	3	4	7	10	18	27	40

37.0: PERICARDIOCENTESIS

Type of Patients	Observed Patients	Avg. Stay	Variance	Percentiles						
				10th	25th	50th	75th	90th	95th	99th
1. SINGLE DX										
0–19 Years	2	3.0	8	1	1	5	5	5	5	5
20–34	2	3.0	2	2	2	3	4	4	4	4
35–49	3	3.3	1	2	2	4	4	4	4	4
50–64	0									
65+	0									
2. MULTIPLE DX										
0–19 Years	52	6.3	55	2	2	4	7	14	15	45
20–34	57	7.0	70	2	3	5	7	13	23	58
35–49	134	6.1	41	2	3	4	7	13	14	36
50–64	244	6.3	40	2	3	5	8	12	16	41
65+	320	6.8	27	2	3	5	9	13	18	27
TOTAL SINGLE DX	7	3.2	2	1	2	4	4	5	5	5
TOTAL MULTIPLE DX	807	6.5	39	2	3	5	8	13	16	28
TOTAL										
0–19 Years	54	6.2	54	2	2	4	7	14	15	45
20–34	59	6.8	68	2	3	4	7	13	23	58
35–49	137	6.1	40	2	4	4	7	13	14	36
50–64	244	6.3	40	2	3	5	8	12	16	41
65+	320	6.8	27	2	3	5	9	13	18	27
GRAND TOTAL	814	6.5	39	2	3	5	8	13	16	28

LOS by Diagnosis and Operation, Western Region, 45th Edition

Western Region, October 2007–September 2008 Data, by Operation

37.1: CARDIOTOMY & PERICARDIOT

Type of Patients	Observed Patients	Avg. Stay	Variance	Percentiles						
				10th	25th	50th	75th	90th	95th	99th
1. SINGLE DX										
0–19 Years	0									
20–34	1	4.0	0	4	4	4	4	4	4	4
35–49	2	2.0	2	1	1	1	3	3	3	3
50–64	4	2.5	<1	2	2	2	3	3	3	3
65+	0									
2. MULTIPLE DX										
0–19 Years	50	11.9	195	2	4	7	15	36	41	78
20–34	103	9.2	53	4	5	7	12	17	19	26
35–49	221	10.2	92	3	5	7	12	19	29	46
50–64	435	9.4	78	3	5	8	11	16	26	44
65+	566	9.7	58	3	5	8	12	18	25	39
TOTAL SINGLE DX	7	2.6	<1	1	2	3	3	4	4	4
TOTAL MULTIPLE DX	1,375	9.8	78	3	5	8	12	18	26	45
TOTAL										
0–19 Years	50	11.9	195	2	4	7	15	36	41	78
20–34	104	9.1	53	4	5	7	12	17	19	26
35–49	223	10.1	92	3	5	7	12	19	29	46
50–64	439	9.4	78	3	5	8	11	16	25	44
65+	566	9.7	58	3	5	8	12	18	25	39
GRAND TOTAL	1,382	9.8	78	3	5	7	12	18	26	45

37.2: DXTIC PX HRT/PERICARDIUM

Type of Patients	Observed Patients	Avg. Stay	Variance	Percentiles						
				10th	25th	50th	75th	90th	95th	99th
1. SINGLE DX										
0–19 Years	57	1.4	<1	1	1	1	1	3	3	5
20–34	62	1.4	<1	1	1	1	2	2	3	4
35–49	108	1.4	<1	1	1	1	2	3	3	3
50–64	115	1.5	<1	1	1	1	2	2	4	5
65+	51	1.6	2	1	1	1	2	2	6	7
2. MULTIPLE DX										
0–19 Years	512	4.2	61	1	1	1	4	11	17	41
20–34	1,145	4.1	28	1	1	3	5	8	12	26
35–49	8,343	3.1	10	1	1	2	4	6	8	15
50–64	19,923	3.4	14	1	2	3	4	7	9	17
65+	25,075	4.0	13	1	2	3	5	8	10	18
TOTAL SINGLE DX	393	1.4	<1	1	1	1	2	2	3	5
TOTAL MULTIPLE DX	54,998	3.6	14	1	1	3	4	7	10	18
TOTAL										
0–19 Years	569	3.9	56	1	1	1	4	10	17	41
20–34	1,207	4.0	27	1	1	2	4	8	12	26
35–49	8,451	3.1	10	1	1	2	4	6	8	15
50–64	20,038	3.4	14	1	2	3	4	7	9	17
65+	25,126	4.0	13	1	2	3	5	8	10	18
GRAND TOTAL	55,391	3.6	14	1	1	3	4	7	10	18

37.12: PERICARDIOTOMY

Type of Patients	Observed Patients	Avg. Stay	Variance	Percentiles						
				10th	25th	50th	75th	90th	95th	99th
1. SINGLE DX										
0–19 Years	0									
20–34	1	4.0	0	4	4	4	4	4	4	4
35–49	2	2.0	2	1	1	1	3	3	3	3
50–64	3	2.7	<1	2	2	3	3	3	3	3
65+	0									
2. MULTIPLE DX										
0–19 Years	45	12.7	228	2	4	8	16	36	43	78
20–34	98	9.3	55	3	5	7	12	17	21	60
35–49	215	10.3	95	3	5	7	12	19	31	46
50–64	421	9.3	80	3	5	7	11	16	26	44
65+	549	9.7	57	3	5	8	12	18	25	38
TOTAL SINGLE DX	6	2.7	1	1	2	3	3	4	4	4
TOTAL MULTIPLE DX	1,328	9.8	80	3	5	8	12	18	26	45
TOTAL										
0–19 Years	45	12.7	228	2	4	8	16	36	43	78
20–34	99	9.3	55	3	5	7	12	17	21	60
35–49	217	10.3	95	3	5	7	12	19	31	46
50–64	424	9.3	80	3	5	7	11	16	26	44
65+	549	9.7	57	3	5	8	12	18	25	38
GRAND TOTAL	1,334	9.8	80	3	5	7	12	18	26	45

37.20: NIPS

Type of Patients	Observed Patients	Avg. Stay	Variance	Percentiles						
				10th	25th	50th	75th	90th	95th	99th
1. SINGLE DX										
0–19 Years	0									
20–34	1	1.0	0	1	1	1	1	1	1	1
35–49	0									
50–64	0									
65+										
2. MULTIPLE DX										
0–19 Years	1	7.0	0	7	7	7	7	7	7	7
20–34	2	2.5	<1	2	2	3	3	3	3	3
35–49	6	4.5	4	2	3	4	5	8	8	8
50–64	20	4.2	7	2	2	4	6	9	10	10
65+	34	2.8	3	1	1	3	4	5	6	6
TOTAL SINGLE DX	1	1.0	0	1	1	1	1	1	1	1
TOTAL MULTIPLE DX	63	3.6	5	1	2	3	5	7	8	10
TOTAL										
0–19 Years	1	7.0	0	7	7	7	7	7	7	7
20–34	3	2.0	<1	2	2	3	3	3	3	3
35–49	6	4.5	4	2	3	4	5	8	8	8
50–64	20	4.2	7	2	2	4	6	9	10	10
65+	34	2.8	3	1	1	3	4	5	6	6
GRAND TOTAL	64	3.6	5	1	2	3	5	7	8	10

LOS by Diagnosis and Operation, Western Region, 45th Edition

Western Region, October 2007–September 2008 Data, by Operation

37.21: RT HEART CARDIAC CATH

Type of Patients	Observed Patients	Avg. Stay	Variance	Percentiles						
				10th	25th	50th	75th	90th	95th	99th
1. SINGLE DX										
0–19 Years	2	1.0	0	1	1	1	1	1	1	1
20–34	4	1.5	1	1	1	1	3	3	3	3
35–49	1	2.0	0	2	2	2	2	2	2	2
50–64	4	1.8	2	1	1	1	4	4	4	4
65+	0									
2. MULTIPLE DX										
0–19 Years	38	9.8	397	1	1	4	8	21	26	98
20–34	106	9.0	105	2	4	7	12	15	18	37
35–49	199	7.8	65	2	3	6	10	14	18	31
50–64	458	8.2	53	2	3	6	11	16	21	42
65+	472	7.6	47	2	3	6	10	17	21	30
TOTAL SINGLE DX	11	1.4	<1	1	1	1	1	3	4	4
TOTAL MULTIPLE DX	1,273	8.1	81	2	3	6	10	16	21	42
TOTAL										
0–19 Years	40	9.3	380	1	1	3	8	21	26	98
20–34	110	8.8	103	2	3	6	12	15	18	37
35–49	200	7.8	64	2	3	6	10	14	18	31
50–64	462	8.2	53	2	3	6	11	16	21	42
65+	472	7.6	47	2	3	6	10	17	21	30
GRAND TOTAL	1,284	8.1	81	1	3	6	10	16	21	42

37.22: LEFT HEART CARDIAC CATH

Type of Patients	Observed Patients	Avg. Stay	Variance	Percentiles						
				10th	25th	50th	75th	90th	95th	99th
1. SINGLE DX										
0–19 Years	10	2.1	1	1	1	2	3	3	4	4
20–34	31	1.6	<1	1	1	1	2	2	3	3
35–49	90	1.5	<1	1	1	1	2	2	3	3
50–64	83	1.5	1	1	1	1	2	2	4	6
65+	38	1.5	<1	1	1	1	2	2	3	6
2. MULTIPLE DX										
0–19 Years	47	3.7	16	1	1	2	3	9	14	17
20–34	764	2.9	7	1	1	2	3	6	8	12
35–49	7,040	2.7	7	1	1	2	4	5	7	13
50–64	16,616	3.0	9	1	1	2	4	6	8	14
65+	20,086	3.6	10	1	2	3	4	7	9	16
TOTAL SINGLE DX	252	1.5	<1	1	1	1	2	3	3	5
TOTAL MULTIPLE DX	44,553	3.2	9	1	1	2	4	6	8	14
TOTAL										
0–19 Years	57	3.5	14	1	1	2	3	8	14	17
20–34	795	2.8	7	1	1	2	3	5	7	12
35–49	7,130	2.7	7	1	1	2	3	5	7	13
50–64	16,699	3.0	9	1	1	2	4	6	8	14
65+	20,124	3.6	10	1	2	3	4	7	9	16
GRAND TOTAL	44,805	3.2	9	1	1	2	4	6	8	14

37.23: RT/LEFT HEART CARD CATH

Type of Patients	Observed Patients	Avg. Stay	Variance	Percentiles						
				10th	25th	50th	75th	90th	95th	99th
1. SINGLE DX										
0–19 Years	30	1.0	<1	1	1	1	1	1	1	2
20–34	4	1.5	<1	1	1	2	2	2	2	2
35–49	7	1.3	<1	1	1	1	2	2	2	2
50–64	4	1.8	<1	1	1	1	3	3	3	3
65+	6	3.0	8	1	1	1	6	7	7	7
2. MULTIPLE DX										
0–19 Years	354	3.4	32	1	1	3	3	8	15	30
20–34	159	5.8	47	1	3	4	7	10	24	37
35–49	863	4.9	17	1	2	4	6	9	12	19
50–64	2,342	5.3	26	1	2	4	7	10	14	25
65+	3,802	5.2	18	1	2	4	7	10	13	21
TOTAL SINGLE DX	51	1.2	<1	1	1	1	1	2	2	7
TOTAL MULTIPLE DX	7,520	5.0	23	1	2	4	6	10	13	24
TOTAL										
0–19 Years	384	3.2	30	1	1	4	3	7	14	30
20–34	163	5.7	46	1	2	4	7	10	20	37
35–49	870	4.8	17	1	2	4	6	9	12	19
50–64	2,346	5.3	26	1	2	4	7	10	14	25
65+	3,808	5.2	18	1	2	4	7	10	13	21
GRAND TOTAL	7,571	4.9	23	1	2	4	6	10	13	24

37.25: CARDIAC BIOPSY

Type of Patients	Observed Patients	Avg. Stay	Variance	Percentiles						
				10th	25th	50th	75th	90th	95th	99th
1. SINGLE DX										
0–19 Years	0									
20–34	0									
35–49	0									
50–64	0									
65+	0									
2. MULTIPLE DX										
0–19 Years	30	6.0	41	1	1	3	10	18	19	23
20–34	24	6.4	31	2	2	4	10	11	16	27
35–49	36	6.5	27	1	3	5	9	14	18	22
50–64	98	7.4	48	1	3	6	9	17	20	48
65+	34	6.1	25	1	3	5	7	14	19	20
TOTAL SINGLE DX	0									
TOTAL MULTIPLE DX	222	6.6	38	1	3	5	9	16	19	27
TOTAL										
0–19 Years	30	6.0	41	1	1	3	10	18	19	23
20–34	24	6.4	31	2	2	4	10	11	16	27
35–49	36	6.5	27	1	3	5	9	14	18	22
50–64	98	7.4	48	1	3	6	9	17	20	48
65+	34	6.1	25	1	3	5	7	14	19	20
GRAND TOTAL	222	6.6	38	1	3	5	9	16	19	27

LOS by Diagnosis and Operation, Western Region, 45th Edition

Western Region, October 2007–September 2008 Data, by Operation

37.26: CATH BASED INVAS EPS

Type of Patients	Observed Patients	Avg. Stay	Variance	10th	25th	50th	75th	90th	95th	99th
1. SINGLE DX										
0–19 Years	15	1.9	2	1	1	1	2	5	5	5
20–34	20	1.3	<1	1	1	1	1	3	4	4
35–49	10	1.2	<1	1	1	1	2	3	3	3
50–64	20	1.3	<1	1	1	1	2	2	3	3
65+	5	1.0	0	1	1	1	1	1	1	1
2. MULTIPLE DX										
0–19 Years	33	5.2	29	1	1	4	6	12	22	22
20–34	73	3.7	13	1	1	2	6	8	11	19
35–49	136	3.2	5	1	1	3	4	6	8	10
50–64	278	3.1	9	1	1	2	4	6	8	18
65+	460	4.2	15	1	1	3	5	9	13	17
TOTAL SINGLE DX	70	1.5	1	1	1	1	1	3	5	5
TOTAL MULTIPLE DX	980	3.8	13	1	1	3	5	8	11	19
TOTAL										
0–19 Years	48	4.1	23	1	1	2	5	12	12	22
20–34	93	3.2	11	1	1	1	4	8	10	19
35–49	146	3.1	5	1	1	2	4	6	7	10
50–64	298	3.0	8	1	1	2	4	6	8	18
65+	465	4.2	15	1	1	3	5	9	13	17
GRAND TOTAL	1,050	3.6	13	1	1	3	5	8	11	18

37.31: PERICARDIECTOMY

Type of Patients	Observed Patients	Avg. Stay	Variance	10th	25th	50th	75th	90th	95th	99th
1. SINGLE DX										
0–19 Years	1	2.0	0	2	2	2	2	2	2	2
20–34	1	1.0	0	1	1	1	1	2	1	1
35–49	2	1.5	<1	1	1	1	2	2	2	2
50–64	1	2.0	0	2	2	2	2	2	2	2
65+	0									
2. MULTIPLE DX										
0–19 Years	8	7.7	149	2	3	3	7	14	55	55
20–34	17	10.5	75	1	6	7	12	27	27	27
35–49	43	7.5	34	2	3	4	10	17	18	23
50–64	81	11.1	130	2	4	8	13	22	35	64
65+	70	11.4	64	4	6	9	16	27	30	>99
TOTAL SINGLE DX	5	1.6	<1	1	1	2	2	2	2	2
TOTAL MULTIPLE DX	219	10.2	90	2	4	7	13	22	29	55
TOTAL										
0–19 Years	9	7.4	142	2	2	3	7	14	55	55
20–34	18	9.9	75	1	5	7	12	27	27	27
35–49	45	7.2	34	2	3	4	10	17	18	23
50–64	82	11.0	130	2	4	7	13	22	35	64
65+	70	11.4	64	4	6	9	16	27	30	>99
GRAND TOTAL	224	10.0	90	2	4	7	12	22	29	55

37.3: PERICARDIECT/EXC HRT LES

Type of Patients	Observed Patients	Avg. Stay	Variance	10th	25th	50th	75th	90th	95th	99th
1. SINGLE DX										
0–19 Years	87	1.3	2	1	1	1	2	2	2	8
20–34	137	1.1	<1	1	1	1	1	1	2	4
35–49	176	1.2	<1	1	1	1	1	2	2	6
50–64	290	1.1	<1	1	1	1	1	1	2	3
65+	162	1.2	<1	1	1	1	1	1	2	5
2. MULTIPLE DX										
0–19 Years	174	3.8	22	1	1	3	5	7	9	22
20–34	377	2.8	21	1	1	1	2	6	11	26
35–49	971	2.8	13	1	1	1	3	6	9	19
50–64	3,194	2.8	15	1	1	1	3	7	9	19
65+	3,784	3.8	24	1	1	2	5	9	13	24
TOTAL SINGLE DX	852	1.2	<1	1	1	1	1	1	2	4
TOTAL MULTIPLE DX	8,500	3.3	20	1	1	1	4	8	11	22
TOTAL										
0–19 Years	261	3.1	18	1	1	1	4	6	9	19
20–34	514	2.4	16	1	1	1	2	6	8	17
35–49	1,147	2.6	11	1	1	1	3	6	8	18
50–64	3,484	2.7	14	1	1	1	3	6	9	18
65+	3,946	3.7	23	1	1	2	5	9	13	24
GRAND TOTAL	9,352	3.1	18	1	1	1	3	7	10	21

37.33: HEART LES EXC NEC-OPEN

Type of Patients	Observed Patients	Avg. Stay	Variance	10th	25th	50th	75th	90th	95th	99th
1. SINGLE DX										
0–19 Years	2	3.0	2	2	2	4	4	4	4	4
20–34	1	3.0	0	3	3	3	3	3	3	3
35–49	2	5.0	<1	4	4	4	6	6	6	6
50–64	7	2.5	<1	2	2	3	3	4	4	4
65+	1	2.0	0	2	2	2	2	2	2	2
2. MULTIPLE DX										
0–19 Years	46	5.4	14	3	3	5	6	9	13	22
20–34	23	11.2	102	4	6	7	16	16	21	55
35–49	81	6.7	25	3	3	6	7	11	15	32
50–64	305	7.0	28	3	4	6	9	13	15	30
65+	456	9.1	37	4	5	7	11	17	21	33
TOTAL SINGLE DX	13	2.9	2	2	2	3	4	4	6	6
TOTAL MULTIPLE DX	911	7.9	35	3	4	6	9	14	19	32
TOTAL										
0–19 Years	48	5.3	14	3	3	5	6	9	13	22
20–34	24	10.9	101	3	6	7	16	16	21	55
35–49	83	6.7	24	3	4	6	7	11	15	32
50–64	312	6.9	28	2	4	6	9	12	15	30
65+	457	9.1	37	4	5	7	11	17	21	33
GRAND TOTAL	924	7.9	34	3	4	6	9	14	19	32

Western Region, October 2007–September 2008 Data, by Operation

37.34: HEART LES EXC APPR NEC

Type of Patients	Observed Patients	Avg. Stay	Variance	Percentiles						
				10th	25th	50th	75th	90th	95th	99th
1. SINGLE DX										
0–19 Years	84	1.3	2	1	1	1	1	1	2	8
20–34	135	1.1	<1	1	1	1	1	1	2	4
35–49	172	1.2	<1	1	1	1	1	1	2	3
50–64	282	1.1	<1	1	1	1	1	1	2	3
65+	161	1.2	<1	1	1	1	1	1	2	5
2. MULTIPLE DX										
0–19 Years	118	2.4	11	1	1	1	3	5	7	19
20–34	335	1.8	3	1	1	1	2	4	6	9
35–49	838	2.1	7	1	1	1	2	4	7	13
50–64	2,781	2.0	6	1	1	1	2	4	6	12
65+	3,216	2.8	14	1	1	1	3	7	9	18
TOTAL SINGLE DX	834	1.1	<1	1	1	1	1	1	2	3
TOTAL MULTIPLE DX	7,288	2.4	10	1	1	1	3	5	8	15
TOTAL										
0–19 Years	202	1.9	8	1	1	1	2	4	5	16
20–34	470	1.6	2	1	1	1	1	3	5	9
35–49	1,010	1.9	6	1	1	1	2	4	6	12
50–64	3,063	1.9	5	1	1	1	2	4	6	11
65+	3,377	2.7	14	1	1	1	3	6	9	18
GRAND TOTAL	8,122	2.2	9	1	1	1	2	5	7	14

37.4: REP HEART & PERICARDIUM

Type of Patients	Observed Patients	Avg. Stay	Variance	Percentiles						
				10th	25th	50th	75th	90th	95th	99th
1. SINGLE DX										
0–19 Years	1	3.0	0	3	3	3	3	3	3	3
20–34	0									
35–49	0									
50–64	0									
65+	0									
2. MULTIPLE DX										
0–19 Years	17	6.7	20	3	4	5	8	10	18	21
20–34	28	9.0	27	4	5	8	11	15	22	22
35–49	20	8.4	21	5	5	7	10	16	21	21
50–64	16	9.3	44	4	5	9	16	19	26	26
65+	19	13.4	313	2	5	9	13	46	75	75
TOTAL SINGLE DX	1	3.0	0	3	3	3	3	3	3	3
TOTAL MULTIPLE DX	100	9.2	79	3	5	7	10	16	21	46
TOTAL										
0–19 Years	18	6.6	19	3	4	5	8	10	18	21
20–34	28	9.0	27	4	5	8	11	15	22	22
35–49	20	8.4	21	5	5	7	10	16	21	21
50–64	16	9.3	44	4	5	7	16	19	26	26
65+	19	13.4	313	2	5	9	13	46	75	75
GRAND TOTAL	101	9.1	78	3	5	7	10	16	21	46

37.5: HEART REPLACEMENT PX

Type of Patients	Observed Patients	Avg. Stay	Variance	Percentiles						
				10th	25th	50th	75th	90th	95th	99th
1. SINGLE DX										
0–19 Years	1	9.0	0	9	9	9	9	9	9	9
20–34	0									
35–49	0									
50–64	0									
65+	0									
2. MULTIPLE DX										
0–19 Years	37	28.1	700	7	11	22	61	>99	>99	>99
20–34	15	20.9	401	8	8	16	38	91	>99	>99
35–49	36	27.5	377	10	14	20	37	85	>99	>99
50–64	127	25.1	406	9	12	18	30	53	84	>99
65+	26	28.8	490	10	14	20	45	83	91	>99
TOTAL SINGLE DX	1	9.0	0	9	9	9	9	9	9	9
TOTAL MULTIPLE DX	241	26.4	502	9	11	19	43	89	>99	>99
TOTAL										
0–19 Years	38	27.9	697	7	10	20	61	>99	>99	>99
20–34	15	20.9	401	8	8	16	38	91	>99	>99
35–49	36	27.5	377	10	14	20	37	85	>99	>99
50–64	127	25.1	406	9	12	18	30	53	84	>99
65+	26	28.8	490	10	14	20	45	83	91	>99
GRAND TOTAL	242	26.3	501	9	11	19	43	89	>99	>99

37.51: HEART TRANSPLANTATION

Type of Patients	Observed Patients	Avg. Stay	Variance	Percentiles						
				10th	25th	50th	75th	90th	95th	99th
1. SINGLE DX										
0–19 Years	1	9.0	0	9	9	9	9	9	9	9
20–34	0									
35–49	0									
50–64	0									
65+	0									
2. MULTIPLE DX										
0–19 Years	37	28.1	700	7	11	22	61	>99	>99	>99
20–34	15	20.9	401	8	8	16	38	91	>99	>99
35–49	36	27.5	377	10	14	20	37	85	>99	>99
50–64	127	25.1	406	9	12	18	30	53	84	>99
65+	26	28.8	490	10	14	20	45	83	91	>99
TOTAL SINGLE DX	1	9.0	0	9	9	9	9	9	9	9
TOTAL MULTIPLE DX	241	26.4	502	9	11	19	43	89	>99	>99
TOTAL										
0–19 Years	38	27.9	697	7	10	20	61	>99	>99	>99
20–34	15	20.9	401	8	8	16	38	91	>99	>99
35–49	36	27.5	377	10	14	20	37	85	>99	>99
50–64	127	25.1	406	9	12	18	30	53	84	>99
65+	26	28.8	490	10	14	20	45	83	91	>99
GRAND TOTAL	242	26.3	501	9	11	19	43	89	>99	>99

LOS by Diagnosis and Operation, Western Region, 45th Edition

Western Region, October 2007–September 2008 Data, by Operation

37.66: INSERT IMPLANTABLE HAS

Type of Patients	Observed Patients	Avg. Stay	Variance	10th	25th	50th	75th	90th	95th	99th
1. SINGLE DX										
0–19 Years	0									
20–34	0									
35–49	0									
50–64	0									
65+										
2. MULTIPLE DX										
0–19 Years	2	39.0	70	33	33	33	45	45	45	45
20–34	4	49.0	662	30	31	49	85	85	85	85
35–49	17	38.5	334	17	28	34	50	67	73	73
50–64	29	43.9	417	19	30	47	60	76	88	>99
65+	19	34.7	231	20	23	33	48	64	67	>99
TOTAL SINGLE DX	0									
TOTAL MULTIPLE DX	71	40.3	351	19	29	36	52	73	85	>99
TOTAL										
0–19 Years	2	39.0	70	33	33	33	45	45	45	45
20–34	4	49.0	662	30	31	49	85	85	85	85
35–49	17	38.5	334	17	28	34	50	67	73	73
50–64	29	43.9	417	19	30	47	60	76	88	>99
65+	19	34.7	231	20	23	33	48	64	67	>99
GRAND TOTAL	71	40.3	351	19	29	36	52	73	85	>99

37.7: CARD LEAD PX/POCKET REV

Type of Patients	Observed Patients	Avg. Stay	Variance	10th	25th	50th	75th	90th	95th	99th
1. SINGLE DX										
0–19 Years	10	1.5	<1	1	1	1	2	2	2	3
20–34	14	1.1	<1	1	1	1	1	2	2	2
35–49	27	1.7	2	1	1	1	2	4	4	6
50–64	45	1.3	<1	1	1	1	1	2	2	3
65+	155	1.3	<1	1	1	1	1	2	3	6
2. MULTIPLE DX										
0–19 Years	122	4.1	35	1	1	3	4	7	12	35
20–34	140	3.6	19	1	1	2	4	8	12	25
35–49	501	4.3	23	1	1	3	5	9	14	22
50–64	2,300	4.4	28	1	1	3	5	9	13	28
65+	16,639	4.3	19	1	1	3	6	9	12	21
TOTAL SINGLE DX	251	1.3	<1	1	1	1	1	2	3	6
TOTAL MULTIPLE DX	19,702	4.3	20	1	1	3	6	9	12	22
TOTAL										
0–19 Years	132	3.9	33	1	1	3	4	6	12	35
20–34	154	3.4	18	1	1	3	4	8	12	25
35–49	528	4.1	22	1	1	3	5	9	13	22
50–64	2,345	4.4	28	1	1	3	6	9	13	27
65+	16,794	4.3	19	1	1	3	6	9	12	21
GRAND TOTAL	19,953	4.3	20	1	1	3	6	9	12	22

37.6: IMPL CIRCULATORY & HAS

Type of Patients	Observed Patients	Avg. Stay	Variance	10th	25th	50th	75th	90th	95th	99th
1. SINGLE DX										
0–19 Years	0									
20–34	0									
35–49	0									
50–64	1	5.0	0	5	5	5	5	5	5	5
65+	1	3.0	0	3	3	3	3	3	3	3
2. MULTIPLE DX										
0–19 Years	7	26.8	466	13	13	19	45	66	66	66
20–34	23	21.4	556	4	5	8	31	58	67	85
35–49	206	11.5	171	3	4	6	12	29	35	67
50–64	738	10.7	159	3	4	7	11	22	37	75
65+	877	10.6	83	3	5	8	13	20	30	48
TOTAL SINGLE DX	2	4.0	2	3	3	3	5	5	5	5
TOTAL MULTIPLE DX	1,851	11.0	134	3	4	7	13	22	34	66
TOTAL										
0–19 Years	7	26.8	466	13	13	19	45	66	66	66
20–34	23	21.4	556	4	5	8	31	58	67	85
35–49	206	11.5	171	3	4	6	12	29	35	67
50–64	739	10.6	159	3	4	7	11	22	37	75
65+	878	10.6	83	3	5	8	13	20	30	48
GRAND TOTAL	1,853	11.0	134	3	4	7	13	22	34	66

37.61: PULSATION BALLOON IMPL

Type of Patients	Observed Patients	Avg. Stay	Variance	10th	25th	50th	75th	90th	95th	99th
1. SINGLE DX										
0–19 Years	0									
20–34	0									
35–49	0									
50–64	1	5.0	0	5	5	5	5	5	5	5
65+	1	3.0	0	3	3	3	3	3	3	3
2. MULTIPLE DX										
0–19 Years	4	13.4	36	2	13	13	19	21	21	21
20–34	18	16.2	381	3	5	8	20	58	67	67
35–49	187	9.2	87	3	4	6	11	20	27	53
50–64	698	9.0	88	3	4	6	10	17	25	50
65+	842	10.0	66	3	5	8	13	19	25	40
TOTAL SINGLE DX	2	4.0	2	3	3	3	5	5	5	5
TOTAL MULTIPLE DX	1,749	9.6	81	3	4	7	12	19	25	46
TOTAL										
0–19 Years	4	13.4	36	2	13	13	19	21	21	21
20–34	18	16.2	381	3	5	8	20	58	67	67
35–49	187	9.2	87	3	4	6	11	20	27	53
50–64	699	9.0	88	3	4	6	10	17	25	50
65+	843	10.0	66	3	5	8	13	19	25	40
GRAND TOTAL	1,751	9.6	80	3	4	7	12	19	25	46

LOS by Diagnosis and Operation, Western Region, 45th Edition

Western Region, October 2007–September 2008 Data, by Operation

37.71: INSERT TV LEAD-VENTRICLE

Type of Patients	Observed Patients	Avg. Stay	Variance	10th	25th	50th	75th	90th	95th	99th
1. SINGLE DX										
0–19 Years	0									
20–34	0									
35–49	0									
50–64	0									
65+	6	1.0	0	1	1	1	1	1	1	1
2. MULTIPLE DX										
0–19 Years	2	4.0	18	1	1		7	7	7	7
20–34	2	2.5	<1	2	2	2	3	3	3	3
35–49	22	9.3	80	1	2	7	13	22	22	34
50–64	176	6.0	59	1	1	3	8	14	21	36
65+	2,634	5.2	23	1	2	4	7	10	14	22
TOTAL SINGLE DX	6	1.0	0	1	1	1	1	1	1	1
TOTAL MULTIPLE DX	2,836	5.2	26	1	2	4	7	11	14	23
TOTAL										
0–19 Years	2	4.0	18	1	1		7	7	7	7
20–34	2	2.5	<1	2	2	2	3	3	3	3
35–49	22	9.3	80	1	2	7	13	22	22	34
50–64	176	6.0	59	1	1	3	8	14	21	36
65+	2,640	5.1	23	1	2	4	7	10	14	22
GRAND TOTAL	2,842	5.2	26	1	1	4	7	11	14	23

37.72: INSERT TV LEAD-ATR&VENT

Type of Patients	Observed Patients	Avg. Stay	Variance	10th	25th	50th	75th	90th	95th	99th
1. SINGLE DX										
0–19 Years	4	1.9	<1	1	1	2	2	3	3	3
20–34	9	1.2	<1	1	1	1	1	2	2	2
35–49	20	1.8	2	1	1	1	2	4	6	6
50–64	34	1.3	<1	1	1	1	1	2	3	3
65+	118	1.3	<1	1	1	1	1	2	3	4
2. MULTIPLE DX										
0–19 Years	29	4.4	21	1	2	4	5	8	8	33
20–34	75	3.5	17	1	1	2	4	8	12	25
35–49	310	3.9	16	1	2	3	5	8	11	18
50–64	1,560	4.2	19	1	2	3	5	8	12	23
65+	11,923	4.2	17	1	2	3	5	9	11	20
TOTAL SINGLE DX	185	1.3	<1	1	1	1	1	2	3	6
TOTAL MULTIPLE DX	13,897	4.2	17	1	2	3	5	9	11	21
TOTAL										
0–19 Years	33	4.1	19	1	2	3	5	7	8	33
20–34	84	3.2	15	1	1	2	4	8	10	25
35–49	330	3.8	15	1	1	3	5	8	11	18
50–64	1,594	4.2	19	1	1	3	5	8	11	23
65+	12,041	4.2	17	1	2	3	5	9	11	20
GRAND TOTAL	14,082	4.1	17	1	1	3	5	8	11	21

37.73: INSERT TV LEAD-ATRIUM

Type of Patients	Observed Patients	Avg. Stay	Variance	10th	25th	50th	75th	90th	95th	99th
1. SINGLE DX										
0–19 Years	1	1.0	0	1	1	1	1	1	1	1
20–34	1	1.0	0	1	1	1	1	1	1	1
35–49	0									
50–64	0									
65+	0									
2. MULTIPLE DX										
0–19 Years	3	5.8	66				15	15	15	15
20–34	3	3.0	<1	2	2	3	4	4	4	4
35–49	9	5.5	50	1	1	1	8	21	21	21
50–64	18	8.4	148	1	2	5	6	36	43	43
65+	83	4.1	15	1	1	3	6	10	13	21
TOTAL SINGLE DX	2	1.0	0	1	1	1	1	1	1	1
TOTAL MULTIPLE DX	116	4.9	40	1	1	3	6	11	15	36
TOTAL										
0–19 Years	4	4.6	28	1	1		15	15	15	15
20–34	4	2.5	2	1	2	3	4	4	4	4
35–49	9	5.5	50	1	1	1	8	21	21	21
50–64	18	8.4	148	1	2	5	6	36	43	43
65+	83	4.1	15	1	1	3	6	10	13	21
GRAND TOTAL	118	4.8	38	1	1	3	6	11	14	36

37.74: INSERT EPICARDIAL LEAD

Type of Patients	Observed Patients	Avg. Stay	Variance	10th	25th	50th	75th	90th	95th	99th
1. SINGLE DX										
0–19 Years	4	1.5	<1	1	1	2	2	2	2	2
20–34	0									
35–49	1	1.0	0	1	1	1	1	1	1	1
50–64	0									
65+	0									
2. MULTIPLE DX										
0–19 Years	52	4.1	33	1	2	3	4	6	7	35
20–34	10	2.9	<1	1	3	3	3	4	5	5
35–49	16	7.5	27	2	3	5	11	16	19	19
50–64	50	4.9	25	2	3	3	5	10	18	24
65+	201	5.1	41	1	2	4	7	9	15	19
TOTAL SINGLE DX	5	1.5	<1	1	1	1	2	2	2	2
TOTAL MULTIPLE DX	329	4.8	35	1	2	3	5	8	14	35
TOTAL										
0–19 Years	56	3.9	31	1	2	3	4	6	6	35
20–34	10	2.9	<1	1	3	3	3	4	5	5
35–49	17	7.1	28	2	3	5	11	16	19	19
50–64	50	4.9	25	2	2	3	5	10	18	24
65+	201	5.1	41	1	2	4	7	9	15	19
GRAND TOTAL	334	4.7	34	1	2	3	5	8	14	35

LOS by Diagnosis and Operation, Western Region, 45th Edition

Western Region, October 2007–September 2008 Data, by Operation

37.75: REVISION CARDIAC LEAD

Type of Patients	Observed Patients	Avg. Stay	Variance	Percentiles						
				10th	25th	50th	75th	90th	95th	99th
1. SINGLE DX										
0–19 Years	0									
20–34	1	1.0	0	1	1	1	1	1	1	1
35–49	2	2.5	4	1	1	3	4	4	4	4
50–64	3	1.0	0	1	1	1	1	1	1	1
65+	8	1.3	<1	1	1	1	2	2	2	2
2. MULTIPLE DX										
0–19 Years	4	3.4	3	1	1	4	4	6	6	6
20–34	13	2.2	3	1	1	1	4	4	7	7
35–49	40	3.1	7	1	1	2	4	7	7	12
50–64	134	2.7	16	1	1	2	3	4	9	26
65+	457	3.2	17	1	1	2	4	7	11	24
TOTAL SINGLE DX	14	1.4	<1	1	1	1	1	2	4	4
TOTAL MULTIPLE DX	648	3.1	15	1	1	2	4	7	10	24
TOTAL										
0–19 Years	4	3.4	3	1	1	4	4	6	6	6
20–34	14	2.1	3	1	1	1	3	4	4	7
35–49	42	3.0	6	1	1	2	4	7	7	12
50–64	137	2.7	16	1	1	2	3	4	9	26
65+	465	3.2	16	1	1	2	4	7	10	24
GRAND TOTAL	662	3.1	15	1	1	2	4	7	10	24

37.76: REPL TRANSVENOUS LEAD

Type of Patients	Observed Patients	Avg. Stay	Variance	Percentiles						
				10th	25th	50th	75th	90th	95th	99th
1. SINGLE DX										
0–19 Years	1	1.0	0	1	1	1	1	1	1	1
20–34	2	1.0	0	1	1	1	1	1	1	1
35–49	4	1.3	<1	1	1	1	1	2	2	2
50–64	7	1.0	0	1	1	1	1	1	1	1
65+	18	1.5	1	1	1	1	2	3	5	5
2. MULTIPLE DX										
0–19 Years	16	1.5	<1	1	1	1	2	4	4	4
20–34	13	1.6	<1	1	1	1	2	3	3	3
35–49	30	2.2	7	1	1	1	2	4	11	12
50–64	114	2.5	16	1	1	1	3	4	7	21
65+	648	2.9	14	1	1	1	3	7	9	18
TOTAL SINGLE DX	32	1.3	<1	1	1	1	1	2	3	5
TOTAL MULTIPLE DX	821	2.7	13	1	1	1	3	6	9	18
TOTAL										
0–19 Years	17	1.5	<1	1	1	1	2	2	4	4
20–34	15	1.5	<1	1	1	1	2	3	3	3
35–49	34	2.1	7	1	1	1	2	4	11	12
50–64	121	2.5	15	1	1	1	3	4	5	21
65+	666	2.9	13	1	1	1	3	7	9	18
GRAND TOTAL	853	2.7	13	1	1	1	3	6	9	18

37.77: REMOVAL CARDIAC LEAD

Type of Patients	Observed Patients	Avg. Stay	Variance	Percentiles						
				10th	25th	50th	75th	90th	95th	99th
1. SINGLE DX										
0–19 Years	0									
20–34	1	1.0	0	1	1	1	1	1	1	1
35–49	0									
50–64	0									
65+	0									
2. MULTIPLE DX										
0–19 Years	2	12.2	<1	12	12	12	12	13	13	13
20–34	3	5.1	32	1	1	5	13	13	13	13
35–49	6	4.3	11	1	2	4	6	10	10	10
50–64	19	8.7	63	1	3	7	13	24	28	28
65+	46	9.4	73	1	4	6	11	23	32	34
TOTAL SINGLE DX	1	1.0	0	1	1	1	1	1	1	1
TOTAL MULTIPLE DX	76	8.8	61	1	3	6	12	20	24	34
TOTAL										
0–19 Years	2	12.2	<1	12	12	12	12	13	13	13
20–34	4	4.3	27	1	1	4	5	13	13	13
35–49	6	4.3	11	1	2	4	6	10	10	10
50–64	19	8.7	63	1	3	7	13	24	28	28
65+	46	9.4	73	1	4	6	11	23	32	34
GRAND TOTAL	77	8.7	61	1	3	6	12	20	24	34

37.78: INSERT TEMP TV PACER

Type of Patients	Observed Patients	Avg. Stay	Variance	Percentiles						
				10th	25th	50th	75th	90th	95th	99th
1. SINGLE DX										
0–19 Years	0									
20–34	0									
35–49	0									
50–64	0									
65+	0									
2. MULTIPLE DX										
0–19 Years	0									
20–34	2	15.5	<1	15	15	15	16	16	16	16
35–49	11	4.4	13	2	2	3	5	7	14	14
50–64	74	5.3	45	1	2	4	6	8	18	49
65+	226	6.0	16	2	3	5	8	11	14	23
TOTAL SINGLE DX	0									
TOTAL MULTIPLE DX	313	5.9	23	2	3	5	7	10	15	24
TOTAL										
0–19 Years	0									
20–34	2	15.5	<1	15	15	15	16	16	16	16
35–49	11	4.4	13	2	2	3	5	7	14	14
50–64	74	5.3	45	1	2	4	6	8	18	49
65+	226	6.0	16	2	3	5	8	11	14	23
GRAND TOTAL	313	5.9	23	2	3	5	7	10	15	24

LOS by Diagnosis and Operation, Western Region, 45th Edition

Western Region, October 2007–September 2008 Data, by Operation

37.79: REV CARDIAC DEV POCKET

Type of Patients	Observed Patients	Avg. Stay	Variance	10th	25th	50th	75th	90th	95th	99th
1. SINGLE DX										
0–19 Years	0									
20–34	0									
35–49	0									
50–64	1	2.0	0	2	2	2	2	2	2	2
65+	5	2.0	5	1	1	1	1	6	6	6
2. MULTIPLE DX										
0–19 Years	14	7.4	163	1	1	2	6	36	47	47
20–34	19	6.1	58	1	2	3	9	12	34	34
35–49	57	5.0	43	1	1	3	5	13	18	39
50–64	153	6.2	67	1	2	4	7	13	22	43
65+	406	4.8	23	1	2	3	6	10	14	25
TOTAL SINGLE DX	6	2.0	4	1	1	1	2	2	6	6
TOTAL MULTIPLE DX	649	5.3	40	1	2	3	6	11	16	34
TOTAL										
0–19 Years	14	7.4	163	1	1	2	6	36	47	47
20–34	19	6.1	58	1	2	3	9	12	34	34
35–49	57	5.0	43	1	2	3	5	13	18	39
50–64	154	6.2	66	1	2	4	7	13	22	43
65+	411	4.8	23	1	2	3	6	10	14	25
GRAND TOTAL	655	5.2	40	1	2	3	6	11	16	34

37.8: CARDIAC PACEMAKER DEV OP

Type of Patients	Observed Patients	Avg. Stay	Variance	10th	25th	50th	75th	90th	95th	99th
1. SINGLE DX										
0–19 Years	9	1.3	<1	1	1	1	2	2	2	2
20–34	5	1.6	<1	1	1	1	2	3	3	3
35–49	4	1.8	<1	1	1	2	3	3	3	3
50–64	19	1.3	<1	1	1	1	1	2	3	3
65+	87	1.1	<1	1	1	1	1	1	3	4
2. MULTIPLE DX										
0–19 Years	80	4.2	40	1	1	2	4	10	17	30
20–34	83	4.2	41	1	1	2	4	11	14	40
35–49	193	3.7	24	1	1	2	4	7	11	23
50–64	827	4.4	40	1	1	3	5	9	14	27
65+	6,734	3.9	16	1	1	3	5	8	11	19
TOTAL SINGLE DX	124	1.2	<1	1	1	1	1	2	2	3
TOTAL MULTIPLE DX	7,917	4.0	20	1	1	3	5	8	12	21
TOTAL										
0–19 Years	89	4.0	37	1	1	2	4	10	16	30
20–34	88	4.0	39	1	1	2	4	11	14	40
35–49	197	3.6	24	1	1	2	4	7	11	23
50–64	846	4.3	39	1	1	3	5	9	13	27
65+	6,821	3.9	16	1	1	3	5	8	11	19
GRAND TOTAL	8,041	3.9	19	1	1	3	5	8	12	21

37.80: INSERT PACEMAKER DEV NOS

Type of Patients	Observed Patients	Avg. Stay	Variance	10th	25th	50th	75th	90th	95th	99th
1. SINGLE DX										
0–19 Years	0									
20–34	0									
35–49	0									
50–64	0									
65+	0									
2. MULTIPLE DX										
0–19 Years	5	2.6	3	1	1	2	4	5	5	5
20–34	1	2.0	0	2	2	2	2	2	2	2
35–49	3	2.7	<1	2	2	3	3	3	3	3
50–64	3	1.3	<1	1	1	1	2	2	2	2
65+	57	4.1	58	1	1	2	4	7	11	56
TOTAL SINGLE DX	0									
TOTAL MULTIPLE DX	69	3.6	40	1	1	2	4	6	7	56
TOTAL										
0–19 Years	5	2.6	3	1	1	2	4	5	5	5
20–34	1	2.0	0	2	2	2	2	2	2	2
35–49	3	2.7	<1	2	2	3	3	3	3	3
50–64	3	1.3	<1	1	1	1	2	2	2	2
65+	57	4.1	58	1	1	2	4	7	11	56
GRAND TOTAL	69	3.6	40	1	1	2	4	6	7	56

37.81: INSERT SINGLE CHAMB DEV

Type of Patients	Observed Patients	Avg. Stay	Variance	10th	25th	50th	75th	90th	95th	99th
1. SINGLE DX										
0–19 Years	0									
20–34	0									
35–49	1	1.0	0	1	1	1	1	1	1	1
50–64	0									
65+	4	1.8	2	1	1	1	4	4	4	4
2. MULTIPLE DX										
0–19 Years	2	1.8	<1	1	2	2	2	2	2	2
20–34	1	1.0	0	1	1	1	1	1	1	1
35–49	8	5.1	6	3	3	3	7	9	9	9
50–64	15	5.7	33	1	1	4	9	18	18	18
65+	296	4.9	23	1	1	4	6	10	14	29
TOTAL SINGLE DX	5	1.6	2	1	1	1	1	2	2	4
TOTAL MULTIPLE DX	322	4.9	23	1	1	4	6	10	14	24
TOTAL										
0–19 Years	2	1.8	<1	1	2	2	2	2	2	2
20–34	1	1.0	0	1	1	1	1	1	1	1
35–49	9	4.7	7	1	3	3	7	7	9	9
50–64	15	5.7	33	1	1	4	9	18	18	18
65+	300	4.9	23	1	1	4	6	10	14	24
GRAND TOTAL	327	4.9	22	1	1	4	6	10	14	24

LOS by Diagnosis and Operation, Western Region, 45th Edition

Western Region, October 2007–September 2008 Data, by Operation

37.82: INSERT RATE-RESPON DEV

Type of Patients	Observed Patients	Avg. Stay	Variance	Percentiles						
				10th	25th	50th	75th	90th	95th	99th
1. SINGLE DX										
0–19 Years	0									
20–34	0									
35–49	0									
50–64	0									
65+	3	1.3	<1	1	1	1	1	2	2	2
TOTAL SINGLE DX	3	1.3	<1	1	1	1	2	2	2	2
2. MULTIPLE DX										
0–19 Years	3	4.4	37	1	1	1	7	16	16	16
20–34	2	4.5	<1	4	4	5	5	5	5	5
35–49	6	6.7	53	1	1	4	12	19	19	19
50–64	16	5.9	55	1	1	2	9	12	30	30
65+	289	4.3	16	1	1	3	6	9	11	19
TOTAL MULTIPLE DX	316	4.4	19	1	1	3	6	9	12	19
TOTAL										
0–19 Years	3	4.4	37	1	1	1	7	16	16	16
20–34	2	4.5	<1	4	4	5	5	5	5	5
35–49	6	6.7	53	1	1	4	12	19	19	19
50–64	16	5.9	55	1	1	2	9	12	30	30
65+	292	4.3	16	1	1	3	6	9	11	19
GRAND TOTAL	319	4.4	19	1	1	3	6	9	12	19

37.85: REPL W 1-CHAMBER DEVICE

Type of Patients	Observed Patients	Avg. Stay	Variance	Percentiles						
				10th	25th	50th	75th	90th	95th	99th
1. SINGLE DX										
0–19 Years	0									
20–34	0									
35–49	0									
50–64	0									
65+	1	1.0	0	1	1	1	1	1	1	1
TOTAL SINGLE DX	1	1.0	0	1	1	1	1	1	1	1
2. MULTIPLE DX										
0–19 Years	7	5.4	34	1	1	1	11	11	17	17
20–34	6	1.7	1	1	1	1	2	4	4	4
35–49	3	4.3	33	1	1	1	11	11	11	11
50–64	14	12.5	715	1	1	4	4	48	96	96
65+	115	3.7	15	1	1	2	5	8	12	20
TOTAL MULTIPLE DX	145	4.6	83	1	1	2	5	11	13	48
TOTAL										
0–19 Years	7	5.4	34	1	1	1	11	11	17	17
20–34	6	1.7	1	1	1	1	2	4	4	4
35–49	3	4.3	33	1	1	1	11	11	11	11
50–64	14	12.5	715	1	1	4	4	48	96	96
65+	116	3.7	15	1	1	2	5	8	12	20
GRAND TOTAL	146	4.6	83	1	1	2	5	11	13	48

37.83: INSERT DUAL-CHAMBER DEV

Type of Patients	Observed Patients	Avg. Stay	Variance	Percentiles						
				10th	25th	50th	75th	90th	95th	99th
1. SINGLE DX										
0–19 Years	5	1.6	<1	1	1	2	2	2	2	2
20–34	2	2.0	2	1	1	3	3	3	3	3
35–49	2	2.5	<1	2	2	3	3	3	3	3
50–64	14	1.3	<1	1	1	1	1	2	3	3
65+	54	1.1	<1	1	1	1	1	1	1	3
TOTAL SINGLE DX	77	1.2	<1	1	1	1	1	2	3	3
2. MULTIPLE DX										
0–19 Years	11	9.9	87	2	2	9	10	28	28	28
20–34	31	4.2	49	1	1	2	3	10	17	36
35–49	119	3.8	30	1	1	2	4	7	9	23
50–64	606	4.1	24	1	1	3	5	9	13	21
65+	4,443	3.9	13	1	1	3	5	8	11	17
TOTAL MULTIPLE DX	5,210	4.0	15	1	1	3	5	8	11	18
TOTAL										
0–19 Years	16	7.8	77	2	2	4	10	28	28	28
20–34	33	4.1	46	1	1	2	3	10	17	36
35–49	121	3.7	30	1	1	2	4	7	8	23
50–64	620	4.1	24	1	1	3	5	8	12	21
65+	4,497	3.9	13	1	1	3	5	8	11	17
GRAND TOTAL	5,287	3.9	15	1	1	3	5	8	11	18

37.86: REPL W RATE-RESPON DEV

Type of Patients	Observed Patients	Avg. Stay	Variance	Percentiles						
				10th	25th	50th	75th	90th	95th	99th
1. SINGLE DX										
0–19 Years	0									
20–34	0									
35–49	1	1.0	0	1	1	1	1	1	1	1
50–64	1	2.0	0	2	2	2	2	2	2	2
65+	0									
TOTAL SINGLE DX	2	1.5	<1	1	1	2	2	2	2	2
2. MULTIPLE DX										
0–19 Years	3	1.0	0	1	1	1	1	1	1	1
20–34	0									
35–49	2	1.0	0	1	1	1	1	1	1	1
50–64	13	3.7	8	1	2	3	3	9	9	9
65+	124	3.3	17	1	1	1	4	7	12	20
TOTAL MULTIPLE DX	142	3.2	15	1	1	2	4	7	10	20
TOTAL										
0–19 Years	3	1.0	0	1	1	1	1	1	1	1
20–34	0									
35–49	3	1.0	0	1	1	1	3	9	9	9
50–64	14	3.6	7	1	2	3	3	7	12	20
65+	124	3.3	17	1	1	1	4	7	12	20
GRAND TOTAL	144	3.2	15	1	1	2	4	7	10	20

LOS by Diagnosis and Operation, Western Region, 45th Edition

Western Region, October 2007–September 2008 Data, by Operation

37.87: REPL W DUAL-CHAMB DEVICE

Type of Patients	Observed Patients	Avg. Stay	Variance	Percentiles						
				10th	25th	50th	75th	90th	95th	99th
1. SINGLE DX										
0–19 Years	4	1.0	0	1	1	1	1	1	1	1
20–34	2	1.5	<1	1	1	1	2	2	2	2
35–49	0									
50–64	4	1.0	0	1	1	1	1	1	1	1
65+	24	1.1	<1	1	1	1	1	2	2	2
2. MULTIPLE DX										
0–19 Years	41	2.0	2	1	1	1	2	4	4	7
20–34	34	3.7	18	1	1	2	5	14	14	14
35–49	44	2.5	5	1	1	2	3	5	5	11
50–64	126	3.6	30	1	1	2	4	7	9	23
65+	1,241	3.2	16	1	1	2	4	7	10	18
TOTAL SINGLE DX	34	1.1	<1	1	1	1	1	2	2	2
TOTAL MULTIPLE DX	1,486	3.1	16	1	1	2	4	7	10	18
TOTAL										
0–19 Years	45	1.9	2	1	1	1	2	4	4	7
20–34	36	3.6	17	1	1	2	5	14	14	14
35–49	44	2.5	5	1	1	2	3	5	5	11
50–64	130	3.5	29	1	1	2	4	7	9	23
65+	1,265	3.1	16	1	1	2	4	7	10	18
GRAND TOTAL	1,520	3.1	16	1	1	2	4	7	9	18

37.89: REV/RMVL PACEMAKER DEV

Type of Patients	Observed Patients	Avg. Stay	Variance	Percentiles						
				10th	25th	50th	75th	90th	95th	99th
1. SINGLE DX										
0–19 Years	0									
20–34	1	1.0	0	1	1	1	1	1	1	1
35–49	0									
50–64	0									
65+	1	1.0	0	1	1	1	1	1	1	1
2. MULTIPLE DX										
0–19 Years	8	9.8	146	1	1	3	16	30	30	30
20–34	8	7.2	130	1	1	3	10	11	40	40
35–49	8	5.4	40	1	1	2	4	18	18	18
50–64	34	8.6	72	2	3	6	11	21	27	39
65+	169	8.0	52	1	3	6	11	18	23	36
TOTAL SINGLE DX	2	1.0	0	1	1	1	1	1	1	1
TOTAL MULTIPLE DX	227	8.1	64	1	3	5	11	19	27	39
TOTAL										
0–19 Years	8	9.8	146	1	1	3	16	30	30	30
20–34	9	6.7	122	1	1	2	6	11	40	40
35–49	8	5.4	40	1	1	2	4	18	18	18
50–64	34	8.6	72	2	3	6	11	21	27	39
65+	170	7.9	52	1	3	6	11	18	23	36
GRAND TOTAL	229	8.0	64	1	3	5	11	18	27	39

37.9: HRT/PERICARDIUM OPS NEC

Type of Patients	Observed Patients	Avg. Stay	Variance	Percentiles						
				10th	25th	50th	75th	90th	95th	99th
1. SINGLE DX										
0–19 Years	4	1.0	0	1	1	1	1	1	1	1
20–34	9	1.1	<1	1	1	1	1	2	2	2
35–49	9	1.1	<1	1	1	1	1	2	2	2
50–64	28	1.7	2	1	1	1	1	4	5	7
65+	23	1.2	<1	1	1	1	1	2	2	3
2. MULTIPLE DX										
0–19 Years	77	4.1	24	1	1	3	5	9	16	39
20–34	237	5.6	60	1	1	3	7	13	15	48
35–49	851	4.9	32	1	1	3	7	11	14	25
50–64	2,725	4.9	38	1	1	3	6	11	16	29
65+	4,615	4.5	26	1	1	2	6	11	15	24
TOTAL SINGLE DX	73	1.3	1	1	1	1	1	2	4	7
TOTAL MULTIPLE DX	8,505	4.7	32	1	1	3	6	11	15	27
TOTAL										
0–19 Years	81	4.0	23	1	1	2	5	9	13	39
20–34	246	5.4	59	1	1	3	7	12	15	48
35–49	860	4.8	32	1	1	3	7	11	14	25
50–64	2,753	4.8	38	1	1	3	6	11	16	29
65+	4,638	4.5	26	1	1	2	6	11	15	24
GRAND TOTAL	8,578	4.7	32	1	1	2	6	11	15	27

37.94: IMPL/REPL AICD TOT SYST

Type of Patients	Observed Patients	Avg. Stay	Variance	Percentiles						
				10th	25th	50th	75th	90th	95th	99th
1. SINGLE DX										
0–19 Years	4	1.0	0	1	1	1	1	1	1	1
20–34	5	1.2	<1	1	1	1	1	2	2	2
35–49	6	1.0	0	1	1	1	1	1	1	1
50–64	24	1.5	2	1	1	1	1	4	4	7
65+	20	1.2	<1	1	1	1	1	2	3	3
2. MULTIPLE DX										
0–19 Years	60	4.4	28	1	1	3	5	10	16	39
20–34	201	5.9	64	1	1	4	8	13	15	48
35–49	746	5.1	32	1	1	4	7	11	14	25
50–64	2,426	5.1	40	1	1	3	7	12	16	31
65+	3,979	4.8	28	1	1	3	7	11	15	25
TOTAL SINGLE DX	59	1.3	<1	1	1	1	1	2	3	7
TOTAL MULTIPLE DX	7,412	4.9	33	1	1	3	7	11	15	27
TOTAL										
0–19 Years	64	4.2	27	1	1	3	5	10	16	39
20–34	206	5.8	63	1	1	4	8	13	15	48
35–49	752	5.1	32	1	1	3	7	11	14	25
50–64	2,450	5.1	40	1	1	3	7	12	16	31
65+	3,999	4.8	28	1	1	3	7	11	15	25
GRAND TOTAL	7,471	4.9	33	1	1	3	7	11	15	27

LOS by Diagnosis and Operation, Western Region, 45th Edition

Western Region, October 2007–September 2008 Data, by Operation

37.97: REPLACE AICD LEAD ONLY

Type of Patients	Observed Patients	Avg. Stay	Variance	Percentiles						
				10th	25th	50th	75th	90th	95th	99th
1. SINGLE DX										
0–19 Years	0									
20–34	1	1.0	0	1	1	1	1	1	1	1
35–49	1	2.0	0	2	2	2	2	2	2	2
50–64	2	4.5	<1	4	4	4	5	5	5	5
65+	0									
2. MULTIPLE DX										
0–19 Years	2	1.0	0	1	1	1	1	1	1	1
20–34	8	1.9	2	1	1	1	3	4	4	4
35–49	41	2.5	6	1	1	1	3	5	9	11
50–64	89	2.8	19	1	1	1	3	5	8	38
65+	160	2.6	6	1	1	1	4	6	7	10
TOTAL SINGLE DX	4	3.0	3	1	1	2	4	5	5	5
TOTAL MULTIPLE DX	300	2.6	10	1	1	1	3	5	7	12
TOTAL										
0–19 Years	2	1.0	0	1	1	1	1	1	1	1
20–34	9	1.8	1	1	1	1	3	4	4	4
35–49	42	2.5	6	1	1	1	3	5	9	11
50–64	91	2.8	19	1	1	1	3	5	8	38
65+	160	2.6	6	1	1	1	4	6	7	10
GRAND TOTAL	304	2.6	10	1	1	1	3	5	7	11

37.98: REPL AICD GENERATOR ONLY

Type of Patients	Observed Patients	Avg. Stay	Variance	Percentiles						
				10th	25th	50th	75th	90th	95th	99th
1. SINGLE DX										
0–19 Years	0									
20–34	3	1.0	0	1	1	1	1	1	1	1
35–49	2	1.0	0	1	1	1	1	1	1	1
50–64	2	1.0	0	1	1	1	1	1	1	1
65+	3	1.0	0	1	1	1	1	1	1	1
2. MULTIPLE DX										
0–19 Years	8	3.3	11	1	1	2	3	9	9	9
20–34	22	2.8	21	1	1	1	3	4	8	22
35–49	50	3.2	20	1	1	1	4	7	10	27
50–64	163	2.7	10	1	1	1	3	6	9	16
65+	389	3.1	17	1	1	1	3	7	11	22
TOTAL SINGLE DX	10	1.0	0	1	1	1	1	1	1	1
TOTAL MULTIPLE DX	632	3.0	15	1	1	1	3	7	11	21
TOTAL										
0–19 Years	8	3.3	11	1	1	2	3	9	9	9
20–34	25	2.6	18	1	1	1	2	4	8	22
35–49	52	3.1	19	1	1	1	4	6	10	27
50–64	165	2.6	10	1	1	1	3	6	9	16
65+	392	3.0	17	1	1	1	3	7	11	22
GRAND TOTAL	642	2.9	15	1	1	1	3	7	11	21

38.0: INCISION OF VESSEL

Type of Patients	Observed Patients	Avg. Stay	Variance	Percentiles						
				10th	25th	50th	75th	90th	95th	99th
1. SINGLE DX										
0–19 Years	0									
20–34	2	1.0	0	1	1	1	1	1	1	1
35–49	2	6.0	8	4	4	8	8	8	8	8
50–64	2	2.0	0	1	1	1	3	3	3	3
65+	1	2.0	0	2	2	2	2	2	2	2
2. MULTIPLE DX										
0–19 Years	13	15.4	234	3	6	10	19	46	46	>99
20–34	41	12.4	136	2	3	10	19	25	31	>99
35–49	131	9.4	89	2	3	6	12	22	34	43
50–64	331	7.4	53	2	3	5	9	15	21	45
65+	838	6.9	36	2	3	5	9	14	19	30
TOTAL SINGLE DX	7	2.9	7	1	1	2	4	8	8	8
TOTAL MULTIPLE DX	1,354	7.5	54	2	3	6	9	15	22	46
TOTAL										
0–19 Years	13	15.4	234	3	6	10	19	46	46	>99
20–34	43	11.9	136	1	3	10	19	25	31	>99
35–49	133	9.3	88	2	3	6	12	22	34	43
50–64	333	7.3	53	2	3	5	9	15	21	45
65+	839	6.9	36	2	3	5	9	14	19	30
GRAND TOTAL	1,361	7.5	53	2	3	6	9	15	22	46

38.03: UPPER LIMB VESSEL INC

Type of Patients	Observed Patients	Avg. Stay	Variance	Percentiles						
				10th	25th	50th	75th	90th	95th	99th
1. SINGLE DX										
0–19 Years	0									
20–34	0									
35–49	0									
50–64	1	3.0	0	3	3	3	3	3	3	3
65+	0									
2. MULTIPLE DX										
0–19 Years	5	7.9	48	3	3	4	10	19	19	19
20–34	18	8.9	59	1	3	6	15	23	23	23
35–49	44	8.3	76	1	2	6	10	22	29	38
50–64	98	6.9	63	1	2	4	9	15	21	47
65+	237	5.6	31	1	2	4	7	11	16	25
TOTAL SINGLE DX	1	3.0	0	3	3	3	3	3	3	3
TOTAL MULTIPLE DX	402	6.4	46	1	2	4	8	14	19	33
TOTAL										
0–19 Years	5	7.9	48	3	3	4	10	19	19	19
20–34	18	8.9	59	1	3	6	15	23	23	23
35–49	44	8.3	76	1	3	6	10	22	29	38
50–64	99	6.8	63	1	2	4	9	15	21	47
65+	237	5.6	31	1	2	4	7	11	16	25
GRAND TOTAL	403	6.4	46	1	2	4	8	14	19	33

LOS by Diagnosis and Operation, Western Region, 45th Edition

Western Region, October 2007–September 2008 Data, by Operation

38.06: ABDOMINAL ART INCISION

Type of Patients	Observed Patients	Avg. Stay	Vari-ance	10th	25th	50th	75th	90th	95th	99th
1. SINGLE DX										
0–19 Years	0									
20–34	0									
35–49	0									
50–64	1	1.0	0	1	1	1	1	1	1	1
65+	0									
2. MULTIPLE DX										
0–19 Years	1	46.0	0	46	46	46	46	>99	>99	>99
20–34	1	25.0	0	25	25	25	25	25	25	25
35–49	12	11.6	215	1	2	4	13	34	48	48
50–64	30	6.9	24	2	3	7	9	14	23	>99
65+	57	9.7	44	2	5	8	12	20	25	26
TOTAL SINGLE DX	1	1.0	0	1	1	1	1	1	1	1
TOTAL MULTIPLE DX	101	10.6	109	2	4	8	13	25	46	>99
TOTAL										
0–19 Years	1	46.0	0	46	46	46	46	>99	>99	>99
20–34	1	25.0	0	25	25	25	25	25	25	25
35–49	12	11.6	215	1	2	4	13	34	48	48
50–64	31	6.7	25	2	2	7	9	14	23	>99
65+	57	9.7	44	2	5	8	12	20	25	26
GRAND TOTAL	102	10.6	109	2	4	8	13	25	46	>99

38.1: ENDARTERECTOMY

Type of Patients	Observed Patients	Avg. Stay	Vari-ance	10th	25th	50th	75th	90th	95th	99th
1. SINGLE DX										
0–19 Years	0									
20–34	0									
35–49	3									
50–64	54	2.7	<1	2	2	3	3	3	3	3
65+	193	1.5	2	1	1	1	1	2	3	11
2. MULTIPLE DX										
0–19 Years	1	3.0	0	3	3	3	3	3	3	3
20–34	5	2.8	3	1	1	3	4	5	5	5
35–49	235	4.0	29	1	1	2	4	9	14	20
50–64	3,192	2.9	16	1	1	1	3	7	9	19
65+	12,462	2.8	12	1	1	2	3	6	9	17
TOTAL SINGLE DX	250	1.3	<1	1	1	1	1	2	2	4
TOTAL MULTIPLE DX	15,895	2.8	13	1	1	2	3	6	9	18
TOTAL										
0–19 Years	1	3.0	0	3	3	3	3	3	3	3
20–34	5	2.8	3	1	1	3	4	5	5	5
35–49	238	4.0	28	1	1	2	4	9	14	20
50–64	3,246	2.9	15	1	1	1	3	7	9	19
65+	12,655	2.7	12	1	1	1	3	6	9	17
GRAND TOTAL	16,145	2.8	13	1	1	1	3	6	9	18

38.08: LOWER LIMB ARTERY INC

Type of Patients	Observed Patients	Avg. Stay	Vari-ance	10th	25th	50th	75th	90th	95th	99th
1. SINGLE DX										
0–19 Years	0									
20–34	1	1.0	0	1	1	1	1	1	1	1
35–49	1	8.0	0	8	8	8	8	8	8	8
50–64	1		0							
65+	0									
2. MULTIPLE DX										
0–19 Years	1	9.0	0	9	9	9	9	9	9	9
20–34	12	16.4	260	3	4	11	19	62	>99	>99
35–49	48	9.4	76	2	4	6	13	17	30	43
50–64	145	7.2	43	2	3	5	9	14	17	35
65+	467	7.2	37	2	3	6	9	14	19	30
TOTAL SINGLE DX	2	4.5	24	1	1	5	8	8	8	8
TOTAL MULTIPLE DX	673	7.5	46	2	3	6	9	15	20	36
TOTAL										
0–19 Years	1	9.0	0	9	9	9	9	9	9	9
20–34	13	15.2	256	3	4	6	10	62	>99	>99
35–49	49	9.4	75	2	4	5	13	17	30	43
50–64	145	7.2	43	2	3	5	9	14	17	35
65+	467	7.2	37	2	3	6	9	14	19	30
GRAND TOTAL	675	7.5	46	2	3	6	9	15	20	36

38.12: HEAD/NK ENDARTERECT NEC

Type of Patients	Observed Patients	Avg. Stay	Vari-ance	10th	25th	50th	75th	90th	95th	99th
1. SINGLE DX										
0–19 Years	0									
20–34	0									
35–49	0									
50–64	49	1.3	<1	1	1	1	1	2	3	4
65+	185	1.2	<1	1	1	1	1	2	2	3
2. MULTIPLE DX										
0–19 Years	0									
20–34	1	1.0	0	1	1	1	1	1	1	1
35–49	147	3.0	14	1	1	1	3	8	13	18
50–64	2,611	2.4	9	1	1	1	2	5	8	15
65+	10,823	2.4	9	1	1	1	2	5	8	14
TOTAL SINGLE DX	234	1.2	<1	1	1	1	1	2	2	3
TOTAL MULTIPLE DX	13,582	2.4	9	1	1	1	2	5	8	15
TOTAL										
0–19 Years	0									
20–34	1	1.0	0	1	1	1	1	1	1	1
35–49	147	3.0	14	1	1	1	3	8	13	18
50–64	2,660	2.4	9	1	1	1	2	5	8	15
65+	11,008	2.4	9	1	1	1	2	5	8	14
GRAND TOTAL	13,816	2.4	9	1	1	1	2	5	8	14

LOS by Diagnosis and Operation, Western Region, 45th Edition

Western Region, October 2007–September 2008 Data, by Operation

38.16: ABDOMINAL ENDARTERECTOMY

Type of Patients	Observed Patients	Avg. Stay	Vari-ance	Percentiles						
				10th	25th	50th	75th	90th	95th	99th
1. SINGLE DX										
0–19 Years	0									
20–34	0									
35–49	2	3.0	0	3	3	3	3	3	3	3
50–64	0									
65+	1	4.0	0	4	4	4	4	4	4	4
2. MULTIPLE DX										
0–19 Years	0									
20–34	1	4.0	0	4	4	4	4	4	4	4
35–49	17	4.1	9	1	3	4	5	9	11	11
50–64	125	5.8	40	2	2	4	6	13	17	28
65+	402	5.8	34	1	2	4	7	13	18	29
TOTAL SINGLE DX	3	3.3	<1	3	3	3	4	4	4	4
TOTAL MULTIPLE DX	545	5.7	35	1	2	4	7	13	17	29
TOTAL										
0–19 Years	0									
20–34	1	4.0	0	4	4	4	4	4	4	4
35–49	19	4.0	8	1	2	3	5	9	11	11
50–64	125	5.8	40	2	3	4	6	13	17	28
65+	403	5.8	34	1	2	4	7	13	18	29
GRAND TOTAL	548	5.7	35	1	2	4	7	13	17	29

38.2: DXTIC BLOOD VESSELS PX

Type of Patients	Observed Patients	Avg. Stay	Vari-ance	Percentiles						
				10th	25th	50th	75th	90th	95th	99th
1. SINGLE DX										
0–19 Years	0									
20–34	0									
35–49	0									
50–64	2	5.0	31	1	1	1	9	9	9	9
65+	2	3.5	12	1	1	1	6	6	6	6
2. MULTIPLE DX										
0–19 Years	1	5.0	0	5	5	5	5	5	5	5
20–34	5	3.8	5	1	2	5	5	6	6	6
35–49	34	6.7	25	3	4	5	8	12	20	24
50–64	146	6.5	35	2	3	5	8	11	17	37
65+	416	6.9	44	2	4	5	8	13	16	32
TOTAL SINGLE DX	4	4.2	15	1	1	1	6	9	9	9
TOTAL MULTIPLE DX	602	6.8	40	2	3	5	8	12	16	32
TOTAL										
0–19 Years	1	5.0	0	5	5	5	5	5	5	5
20–34	5	3.8	5	1	2	5	5	6	6	6
35–49	34	6.7	25	3	4	5	8	12	20	24
50–64	148	6.5	34	2	3	5	8	11	17	37
65+	418	6.9	44	2	4	5	8	13	16	32
GRAND TOTAL	606	6.8	40	2	3	5	8	12	16	32

38.18: LOWER LIMB ENDARTERECT

Type of Patients	Observed Patients	Avg. Stay	Vari-ance	Percentiles						
				10th	25th	50th	75th	90th	95th	99th
1. SINGLE DX										
0–19 Years	0									
20–34	0									
35–49	0									
50–64	5	3.6	17	2	2	2	2	11	11	11
65+	7	1.9	1	1	1	2	2	4	4	4
2. MULTIPLE DX										
0–19 Years	0									
20–34	2	4.0	2	3	3	4	5	5	5	5
35–49	55	5.6	51	2	2	3	5	14	20	44
50–64	399	4.8	42	1	2	3	5	10	15	29
65+	1,182	4.7	25	1	2	3	6	10	15	24
TOTAL SINGLE DX	12	2.6	8	1	1	2	2	4	11	11
TOTAL MULTIPLE DX	1,638	4.8	30	1	2	3	6	10	15	26
TOTAL										
0–19 Years	0									
20–34	2	4.0	2	3	3	4	5	5	5	5
35–49	55	5.6	51	2	2	3	5	14	20	44
50–64	404	4.8	42	1	2	3	5	10	15	28
65+	1,189	4.7	25	1	2	3	6	10	15	24
GRAND TOTAL	1,650	4.7	30	1	2	3	6	10	15	26

38.21: BLOOD VESSEL BIOPSY

Type of Patients	Observed Patients	Avg. Stay	Vari-ance	Percentiles						
				10th	25th	50th	75th	90th	95th	99th
1. SINGLE DX										
0–19 Years	0									
20–34	0									
35–49	0									
50–64	2	5.0	31	1	1	1	9	9	9	9
65+	2	3.5	12	1	1	1	6	6	6	6
2. MULTIPLE DX										
0–19 Years	1	5.0	0	5	5	5	5	5	5	5
20–34	3	4.0	3	2	2	5	5	5	5	5
35–49	33	6.4	24	3	4	5	7	11	20	24
50–64	144	6.6	35	2	3	5	8	11	17	37
65+	412	6.8	42	2	4	5	8	12	15	32
TOTAL SINGLE DX	4	4.2	15	1	1	1	6	9	9	9
TOTAL MULTIPLE DX	593	6.7	39	2	3	5	8	12	15	33
TOTAL										
0–19 Years	1	5.0	0	5	5	5	5	5	5	5
20–34	3	4.0	3	2	2	5	5	5	5	5
35–49	33	6.4	24	3	4	5	7	11	20	24
50–64	146	6.5	35	2	3	5	8	11	17	37
65+	414	6.8	42	2	4	5	8	12	15	32
GRAND TOTAL	597	6.7	39	2	3	5	8	12	15	33

LOS by Diagnosis and Operation, Western Region, 45th Edition

Western Region, October 2007–September 2008 Data, by Operation

38.3: VESSEL RESECT W ANAST

Type of Patients	Observed Patients	Avg. Stay	Vari-ance	10th	25th	50th	75th	90th	95th	99th
1. SINGLE DX										
0–19 Years	3	2.4	<1	2	2	2	3	3	3	3
20–34	0									
35–49	0									
50–64	1	5.0	0			5	5	5	5	5
65+	0									
2. MULTIPLE DX										
0–19 Years	111	7.6	72	3	3	5	7	16	24	41
20–34	14	7.5	38	2	4	5	17	19	>99	>99
35–49	28	6.9	100	1	2	4	7	13	17	53
50–64	59	7.5	83	1	2	5	10	18	28	55
65+	126	9.3	81	1	3	7	11	19	27	50
TOTAL SINGLE DX	4	2.7	<1	2	2	2	3	3	5	5
TOTAL MULTIPLE DX	338	8.0	76	2	3	5	9	17	24	53
TOTAL										
0–19 Years	114	7.4	71	3	3	5	7	16	24	41
20–34	14	7.5	38	2	4	5	17	19	>99	>99
35–49	28	6.9	100	1	2	4	7	13	17	53
50–64	60	7.5	81	1	2	5	10	18	28	55
65+	126	9.3	81	1	3	7	11	19	27	50
GRAND TOTAL	342	7.9	75	2	3	5	9	17	24	53

38.4: VESSEL RESECT W REPL

Type of Patients	Observed Patients	Avg. Stay	Vari-ance	10th	25th	50th	75th	90th	95th	99th
1. SINGLE DX										
0–19 Years	2	3.0	8	1	1	1	5	5	5	5
20–34	4	4.1	8	1	2	4	7	7	7	7
35–49	2	5.0	2	4	4	5	6	6	6	6
50–64	4	3.0	3	1	1	2	4	5	5	5
65+	5	2.6	4	1	1	2	3	6	6	6
2. MULTIPLE DX										
0–19 Years	49	12.2	243	3	5	7	12	36	38	97
20–34	49	8.4	34	3	5	6	11	17	20	26
35–49	160	9.2	104	2	4	6	12	17	26	68
50–64	522	10.0	98	3	5	7	12	21	27	57
65+	1,368	9.7	69	3	5	7	11	19	25	43
TOTAL SINGLE DX	17	3.4	5	1	1	3	5	7	7	7
TOTAL MULTIPLE DX	2,148	9.8	86	3	5	7	12	20	26	51
TOTAL										
0–19 Years	51	12.0	240	3	5	7	12	35	38	97
20–34	53	8.0	33	3	4	6	11	17	20	26
35–49	162	9.1	103	2	4	6	12	17	21	68
50–64	526	9.9	98	3	5	7	12	21	27	57
65+	1,373	9.7	69	3	5	7	11	19	25	43
GRAND TOTAL	2,165	9.8	86	3	5	7	11	20	26	51

38.34: AORTA RESECTION W ANAST

Type of Patients	Observed Patients	Avg. Stay	Vari-ance	10th	25th	50th	75th	90th	95th	99th
1. SINGLE DX										
0–19 Years	2	2.8	<1	2	3	3	3	3	3	3
20–34	0									
35–49	0									
50–64	0									
65+	0									
2. MULTIPLE DX										
0–19 Years	90	7.6	82	3	4	5	7	16	32	41
20–34	1	5.0	0	5	5	5	5	5	5	5
35–49	12	4.0	0	4	4	4	4	4	4	4
50–64	12	11.3	69	6	6	8	14	18	34	34
65+	67	12.1	65	6	7	10	16	21	29	50
TOTAL SINGLE DX	2	2.8	<1	2	3	3	3	3	3	3
TOTAL MULTIPLE DX	172	8.7	80	3	4	6	9	18	29	41
TOTAL										
0–19 Years	92	7.5	80	3	3	5	7	16	32	41
20–34	1	5.0	0	5	5	5	5	5	5	5
35–49	12	4.0	0	4	4	4	4	4	4	4
50–64	12	11.3	69	6	6	8	14	18	34	34
65+	67	12.1	65	6	7	10	16	21	29	50
GRAND TOTAL	174	8.6	80	3	4	6	9	18	29	41

38.44: ABD AORTA RESECT W REPL

Type of Patients	Observed Patients	Avg. Stay	Vari-ance	10th	25th	50th	75th	90th	95th	99th
1. SINGLE DX										
0–19 Years	0									
20–34	0									
35–49	0									
50–64	1	1.0	0	1	1	1	1	1	1	1
65+	2	3.5	12	1	1	1	6	6	6	6
2. MULTIPLE DX										
0–19 Years	0									
20–34	4	7.2	11	3	3	7	8	11	11	11
35–49	33	12.7	180	4	5	9	14	18	39	77
50–64	258	10.0	79	4	5	7	11	22	26	51
65+	971	10.3	61	5	6	8	12	20	25	43
TOTAL SINGLE DX	3	2.6	8	1	1	1	6	6	6	6
TOTAL MULTIPLE DX	1,266	10.3	68	5	6	8	12	20	26	47
TOTAL										
0–19 Years	0									
20–34	4	7.2	11	3	3	7	8	11	11	11
35–49	33	12.7	180	4	5	9	14	18	39	77
50–64	259	10.0	79	4	5	7	11	22	26	51
65+	973	10.3	61	5	6	8	12	20	25	43
GRAND TOTAL	1,269	10.3	68	5	6	8	12	20	26	47

LOS by Diagnosis and Operation, Western Region, 45th Edition

Western Region, October 2007–September 2008 Data, by Operation

38.45: THOR VESS RESECT W REPL

Type of Patients	Observed Patients	Avg. Stay	Variance	10th	25th	50th	75th	90th	95th	99th
1. SINGLE DX										
0–19 Years	1	5.0	0	5	5	5	5	5	5	5
20–34	1	7.0	0	7	7	7	7	7	7	7
35–49	1	4.0	0	4	4	4	4	4	4	4
50–64	0									
65+	0									
2. MULTIPLE DX										
0–19 Years	42	12.8	263	3	5	7	12	37	38	>99
20–34	24	8.2	35	4	4	6	11	15	24	26
35–49	66	10.3	104	4	5	7	13	20	21	68
50–64	152	12.7	157	4	6	9	15	26	34	63
65+	139	13.4	130	5	7	9	16	24	33	60
TOTAL SINGLE DX	3	5.7	2	4	4	5	7	7	7	7
TOTAL MULTIPLE DX	423	12.4	157	4	5	8	14	25	37	68
TOTAL										
0–19 Years	43	12.8	261	3	5	7	12	37	38	>99
20–34	25	8.1	33	4	4	6	9	15	24	26
35–49	67	10.2	103	4	5	7	13	20	21	68
50–64	152	12.7	157	4	6	9	15	26	34	63
65+	139	13.4	130	5	7	9	16	24	33	60
GRAND TOTAL	426	12.3	156	4	5	8	14	25	37	68

38.48: LEG ARTERY RESECT W REPL

Type of Patients	Observed Patients	Avg. Stay	Variance	10th	25th	50th	75th	90th	95th	99th
1. SINGLE DX										
0–19 Years	1	1.0	0	1	1	1	1	1	1	1
20–34	1	1.0	0	1	1	1	1	1	1	1
35–49	1	6.0	0	6	6	6	6	6	6	6
50–64	1	6.0	0	2	2	2	2	2	2	2
65+	3	2.0	<1	1	1	2	3	3	3	3
2. MULTIPLE DX										
0–19 Years	2	6.0	2	5	5	6	7	7	7	7
20–34	13	6.9	38	2	3	5	6	17	18	18
35–49	22	7.5	54	2	3	5	9	13	27	29
50–64	60	7.0	37	2	2	3	8	12	19	36
65+	157	5.0	25	1	2	4	6	11	14	26
TOTAL SINGLE DX	7	2.3	3	1	1	2	3	6	6	6
TOTAL MULTIPLE DX	254	5.6	31	1	2	4	7	12	17	29
TOTAL										
0–19 Years	3	4.3	9	1	1	5	7	7	7	7
20–34	14	6.5	37	1	3	5	6	17	18	18
35–49	23	7.4	52	2	3	6	9	13	27	29
50–64	61	5.9	37	2	2	3	8	12	18	36
65+	160	5.0	25	1	2	4	6	11	14	26
GRAND TOTAL	261	5.5	30	1	2	4	7	12	17	29

38.5: LIG&STRIP VARICOSE VEINS

Type of Patients	Observed Patients	Avg. Stay	Variance	10th	25th	50th	75th	90th	95th	99th
1. SINGLE DX										
0–19 Years	0									
20–34	2	1.5	<1	1	1	2	2	2	2	2
35–49	9	1.2	<1	1	1	1	1	2	2	2
50–64	6	1.7	<1	1	1	1	2	3	3	3
65+	2	1.5	<1	1	1	1	2	2	2	2
2. MULTIPLE DX										
0–19 Years	2	1.0	0	1	1	1	1	1	1	1
20–34	7	3.3	21	1	1	1	5	13	13	13
35–49	30	2.7	6	1	1	2	3	7	8	11
50–64	58	3.0	12	1	1	1	4	8	12	18
65+	51	3.0	9	1	1	2	4	6	10	13
TOTAL SINGLE DX	19	1.4	<1	1	1	1	2	2	3	3
TOTAL MULTIPLE DX	148	2.9	9	1	1	1	4	7	10	13
TOTAL										
0–19 Years	2	1.0	0	1	1	1	1	1	1	1
20–34	9	2.9	16	1	1	1	2	13	13	13
35–49	39	2.4	5	1	1	1	3	7	8	11
50–64	64	2.9	11	1	1	1	3	7	9	18
65+	53	3.0	8	1	1	2	4	6	10	13
GRAND TOTAL	167	2.7	9	1	1	1	3	6	9	13

38.59: LOWER LIMB VV LIG&STRIP

Type of Patients	Observed Patients	Avg. Stay	Variance	10th	25th	50th	75th	90th	95th	99th
1. SINGLE DX										
0–19 Years	0									
20–34	2	1.5	<1	1	1	2	2	2	2	2
35–49	8	1.3	<1	1	1	1	1	2	2	2
50–64	6	1.7	<1	1	1	1	2	3	3	3
65+	2	1.5	<1	1	1	1	2	2	2	2
2. MULTIPLE DX										
0–19 Years	1	1.0	0	1	1	1	1	1	1	1
20–34	6	3.7	23	1	1	1	5	13	13	13
35–49	30	2.7	6	1	1	2	3	7	8	11
50–64	56	2.7	8	1	1	1	4	6	9	13
65+	50	3.0	9	1	1	2	4	6	10	13
TOTAL SINGLE DX	18	1.4	<1	1	1	1	2	2	3	3
TOTAL MULTIPLE DX	143	2.9	8	1	1	1	4	7	9	13
TOTAL										
0–19 Years	1	1.0	0	1	1	1	1	1	1	1
20–34	8	3.1	18	1	1	1	5	13	13	13
35–49	38	2.4	5	1	1	1	3	6	8	11
50–64	62	2.6	7	1	1	1	3	5	8	13
65+	52	2.9	8	1	1	2	4	6	10	13
GRAND TOTAL	161	2.7	8	1	1	1	3	6	9	13

Western Region, October 2007–September 2008 Data, by Operation

38.6: OTHER VESSEL EXCISION

Type of Patients	Observed Patients	Avg. Stay	Variance	10th	25th	50th	75th	90th	95th	99th
1. SINGLE DX										
0–19 Years	4	1.9	<1	1	1	1	3	3	3	3
20–34	2	3.0	2	2	2	2	4	4	4	4
35–49	8	1.8	<1	1	1	2	2	3	3	3
50–64	2	2.0	2	1	1	2	3	3	3	3
65+	3	1.7	<1	1	1	2	2	2	2	2
2. MULTIPLE DX										
0–19 Years	37	10.3	191	3	4	6	9	37	46	85
20–34	36	7.8	124	1	3	4	8	15	41	48
35–49	55	8.9	62	2	3	7	12	23	27	30
50–64	96	7.7	72	1	2	5	10	18	25	61
65+	111	7.2	47	1	2	5	9	17	22	30
TOTAL SINGLE DX	19	1.9	<1	1	1	2	3	3	3	4
TOTAL MULTIPLE DX	335	8.3	95	1	3	6	9	18	27	46
TOTAL										
0–19 Years	41	9.4	178	3	3	6	8	13	46	85
20–34	38	7.6	118	1	3	4	8	15	41	48
35–49	63	8.0	60	2	3	5	11	20	27	30
50–64	98	7.6	71	1	2	5	10	18	25	61
65+	114	7.1	47	1	2	5	9	17	22	30
GRAND TOTAL	354	7.9	91	1	3	5	9	17	27	46

38.63: UP LIMB VESSEL EXC NEC

Type of Patients	Observed Patients	Avg. Stay	Variance	10th	25th	50th	75th	90th	95th	99th
1. SINGLE DX										
0–19 Years	1	1.0	0	1	1	1	1	1	1	1
20–34	1	2.0	0	2	2	2	2	2	2	2
35–49	0									
50–64	2	2.0	2	1	1	1	3	3	3	3
65+	0									
2. MULTIPLE DX										
0–19 Years	1	3.0	0	3	3	3	3	3	3	3
20–34	24	8.0	139	1	3	4	8	15	41	48
35–49	30	10.4	73	1	3	8	14	27	27	30
50–64	42	6.8	96	1	1	4	9	14	17	61
65+	46	8.1	53	1	2	7	10	19	22	30
TOTAL SINGLE DX	4	1.8	<1	1	1	1	2	3	3	3
TOTAL MULTIPLE DX	143	8.1	84	1	2	5	10	19	27	48
TOTAL										
0–19 Years	2	2.0	2	1	1	1	3	3	3	3
20–34	25	7.8	135	2	2	4	8	15	41	48
35–49	30	10.4	73	2	3	8	14	27	27	30
50–64	44	6.5	92	1	1	4	9	14	17	61
65+	46	8.1	53	2	2	7	10	19	22	30
GRAND TOTAL	147	8.0	82	1	2	5	9	19	27	48

38.7: INTERRUPTION VENA CAVA

Type of Patients	Observed Patients	Avg. Stay	Variance	10th	25th	50th	75th	90th	95th	99th
1. SINGLE DX										
0–19 Years	4	3.0	2	2	2	3	5	5	5	5
20–34	3	5.7	2	4	4	6	7	7	7	7
35–49	4	3.3	7	1	2	3	5	7	7	7
50–64	4	3.5	6	1	1	2	5	6	6	6
65+	2	1.0	0	1	1	1	1	1	1	1
2. MULTIPLE DX										
0–19 Years	42	10.4	54	2	6	8	15	24	31	>99
20–34	298	13.9	211	3	5	9	16	33	50	78
35–49	890	10.4	122	2	4	7	12	23	32	70
50–64	2,052	10.7	130	2	4	7	13	24	35	65
65+	5,305	9.0	66	3	4	7	11	18	25	41
TOTAL SINGLE DX	17	3.4	5	1	2	3	5	7	7	7
TOTAL MULTIPLE DX	8,587	9.7	93	2	4	7	12	21	29	54
TOTAL										
0–19 Years	46	9.8	54	2	5	8	15	24	31	>99
20–34	301	13.8	209	3	5	8	16	33	47	78
35–49	894	10.4	121	2	4	7	12	23	32	70
50–64	2,056	10.7	130	2	4	7	13	24	35	65
65+	5,307	9.0	66	3	4	7	11	18	25	41
GRAND TOTAL	8,604	9.7	93	2	4	7	12	21	29	54

38.8: OTHER SURG VESSEL OCCL

Type of Patients	Observed Patients	Avg. Stay	Variance	10th	25th	50th	75th	90th	95th	99th
1. SINGLE DX										
0–19 Years	20	1.8	2	1	1	1	2	5	5	5
20–34	10	1.5	<1	1	1	1	2	2	4	4
35–49	9	1.5	1	1	1	1	1	4	4	4
50–64	6	1.8	3	1	1	1	2	5	5	5
65+	3	3.0	7	1	1	2	6	6	6	6
2. MULTIPLE DX										
0–19 Years	461	31.8	>999	2	5	41	98	>99	>99	>99
20–34	154	6.4	97	1	1	3	7	14	20	50
35–49	162	6.8	62	1	2	4	8	18	25	35
50–64	215	5.7	54	1	2	3	7	14	17	44
65+	216	7.4	43	1	2	5	11	16	22	27
TOTAL SINGLE DX	48	1.8	2	1	1	1	2	4	5	6
TOTAL MULTIPLE DX	1,208	19.3	772	1	3	8	63	>99	>99	>99
TOTAL										
0–19 Years	481	30.5	>999	2	4	36	96	>99	>99	>99
20–34	164	6.1	93	1	1	3	7	13	18	50
35–49	171	6.6	60	1	1	4	8	17	25	35
50–64	221	5.6	53	1	1	3	7	13	17	44
65+	219	7.3	43	1	2	5	10	16	21	27
GRAND TOTAL	1,256	18.6	753	1	2	7	58	>99	>99	>99

LOS by Diagnosis and Operation, Western Region, 45th Edition

Western Region, October 2007–September 2008 Data, by Operation

38.82: OCCL HEAD/NECK VESS NEC

Type of Patients	Observed Patients	Avg. Stay	Variance	Percentiles						
				10th	25th	50th	75th	90th	95th	99th
1. SINGLE DX										
0–19 Years	2	4.8	<1	4	5	5	5	5	5	5
20–34	1	2.0	0	2	2	2	2	2	2	2
35–49	2	1.0	0	1	1	1	1	1	1	1
50–64	1	5.0	0	5	5	5	5	5	5	5
65+	1	6.0	0	6	6	6	6	6	6	6
2. MULTIPLE DX										
0–19 Years	14	9.4	281	2	3	5	9	13	13	86
20–34	36	6.8	104	1	1	2	7	13	34	50
35–49	31	3.7	17	1	1	3	4	7	10	22
50–64	45	4.0	21	1	1	3	6	10	16	>99
65+	34	6.5	36	1	2	4	11	13	23	24
TOTAL SINGLE DX	7	3.9	3	1	2	5	5	5	6	6
TOTAL MULTIPLE DX	160	5.8	79	1	1	3	7	13	22	86
TOTAL										
0–19 Years	16	8.6	234	2	3	5	8	13	13	86
20–34	37	6.6	102	1	1	2	7	13	34	50
35–49	33	3.5	16	1	1	2	4	7	10	22
50–64	46	4.0	21	1	1	3	6	10	16	>99
65+	35	6.5	35	1	2	4	11	13	23	24
GRAND TOTAL	167	5.7	75	1	1	3	6	13	16	86

38.85: OCCL THORACIC VESS NEC

Type of Patients	Observed Patients	Avg. Stay	Variance	Percentiles						
				10th	25th	50th	75th	90th	95th	99th
1. SINGLE DX										
0–19 Years	15	1.3	<1	1	1	1	1	2	3	3
20–34	2	1.0	0	1	1	1	1	1	1	1
35–49	0									
50–64	0									
65+	0									
2. MULTIPLE DX										
0–19 Years	402	35.3	>999	2	6	58	>99	>99	>99	>99
20–34	20	13.2	383	1	4	9	14	34	90	90
35–49	14	5.7	27	1	2	5	6	11	21	21
50–64	13	4.5	17	1	2	3	7	10	13	13
65+	15	9.5	66	1	2	8	15	22	27	27
TOTAL SINGLE DX	17	1.3	<1	1	1	1	1	2	3	3
TOTAL MULTIPLE DX	464	33.1	>999	2	5	46	99	>99	>99	>99
TOTAL										
0–19 Years	417	34.1	>999	2	5	52	>99	>99	>99	>99
20–34	22	12.1	360	1	4	9	11	18	34	90
35–49	14	5.7	27	1	1	5	6	11	21	21
50–64	13	4.5	17	1	1	3	7	10	13	13
65+	15	9.5	66	1	2	8	15	22	27	27
GRAND TOTAL	481	31.9	>999	2	5	42	98	>99	>99	>99

38.83: OCCL UPPER LIMB VESS NEC

Type of Patients	Observed Patients	Avg. Stay	Variance	Percentiles						
				10th	25th	50th	75th	90th	95th	99th
1. SINGLE DX										
0–19 Years	1	1.0	0	1	1	1	1	1	1	1
20–34	2	1.0	0	1	1	1	1	1	1	1
35–49	0	1.0	0	1	1	1	1	1	1	1
50–64	0									
65+										
2. MULTIPLE DX										
0–19 Years	13	3.5	19	1	1	2	5	5	20	20
20–34	30	2.5	5	1	1	1	4	6	8	8
35–49	29	6.0	38	1	1	4	7	17	18	27
50–64	42	3.9	14	1	1	2	6	9	11	17
65+	48	7.1	49	1	2	4	11	16	20	36
TOTAL SINGLE DX	5	1.0	0	1	1	1	1	1	1	1
TOTAL MULTIPLE DX	162	4.9	30	1	1	3	6	11	17	27
TOTAL										
0–19 Years	14	3.4	18	1	1	2	4	5	20	20
20–34	32	2.4	5	1	1	1	4	6	8	8
35–49	31	5.7	37	1	1	3	7	15	18	27
50–64	42	3.9	14	1	1	2	6	9	11	17
65+	48	7.1	49	1	2	4	11	16	20	36
GRAND TOTAL	167	4.8	30	1	1	2	6	11	17	27

38.86: SURG OCCL ABD ARTERY NEC

Type of Patients	Observed Patients	Avg. Stay	Variance	Percentiles						
				10th	25th	50th	75th	90th	95th	99th
1. SINGLE DX										
0–19 Years	0									
20–34	2	3.0	2	2	2	4	4	4	4	4
35–49	1	1.0	0	1	1	1	1	1	1	1
50–64	1	2.0	0	2	2	2	2	2	2	2
65+										
2. MULTIPLE DX										
0–19 Years	7	4.7	7	3	4	4	4	5	12	12
20–34	29	6.9	58	2	2	5	8	14	22	39
35–49	50	8.3	88	1	2	5	9	24	32	35
50–64	56	9.1	129	1	2	5	11	17	43	52
65+	70	7.7	43	1	4	6	10	17	23	34
TOTAL SINGLE DX	4	2.3	2	1	1	2	4	4	4	4
TOTAL MULTIPLE DX	212	7.9	76	1	3	5	9	18	24	43
TOTAL										
0–19 Years	7	4.7	7	3	4	4	4	5	12	12
20–34	29	6.9	58	2	2	5	8	14	22	39
35–49	52	8.1	85	2	2	5	9	23	32	35
50–64	57	9.0	128	1	2	5	10	17	43	52
65+	71	7.6	43	1	3	6	10	16	23	34
GRAND TOTAL	216	7.8	75	1	2	5	9	17	24	43

LOS by Diagnosis and Operation, Western Region, 45th Edition

Western Region, October 2007–September 2008 Data, by Operation

38.9: PUNCTURE OF VESSEL

Type of Patients	Observed Patients	Avg. Stay	Vari-ance	Percentiles						
				10th	25th	50th	75th	90th	95th	99th
1. SINGLE DX										
0–19 Years	250	5.4	13	1	3	5	7	10	13	17
20–34	116	4.8	21	2	2	4	6	8	12	26
35–49	68	3.7	11	1	2	3	4	9	10	18
50–64	73	3.4	6	1	1	3	5	7	8	14
65+	19	3.4	3	1	2	3	5	6	6	6
2. MULTIPLE DX										
0–19 Years	7,995	13.7	207	3	5	9	17	32	45	79
20–34	6,963	7.3	47	2	3	5	9	14	19	37
35–49	13,849	7.2	43	2	3	5	9	14	19	34
50–64	22,927	7.5	46	2	4	6	9	14	19	34
65+	35,593	7.9	34	3	4	6	10	15	18	29
TOTAL SINGLE DX	**526**	**5.0**	**14**	**1**	**2**	**4**	**7**	**9**	**12**	**19**
TOTAL MULTIPLE DX	**87,327**	**8.4**	**67**	**2**	**4**	**6**	**10**	**16**	**22**	**44**
TOTAL										
0–19 Years	8,245	13.3	201	3	5	8	16	31	44	77
20–34	7,079	7.2	47	2	3	5	9	14	19	37
35–49	13,917	7.2	43	2	3	5	9	14	19	34
50–64	23,000	7.5	45	2	4	6	9	14	19	34
65+	35,612	7.9	34	3	4	6	10	15	18	29
GRAND TOTAL	**87,853**	**8.4**	**66**	**2**	**4**	**6**	**10**	**16**	**22**	**44**

38.91: ARTERIAL CATHETERIZATION

Type of Patients	Observed Patients	Avg. Stay	Vari-ance	Percentiles						
				10th	25th	50th	75th	90th	95th	99th
1. SINGLE DX										
0–19 Years	6	1.7	<1	1	1	2	2	2	4	4
20–34	5	3.2	3	1	2	4	4	5	5	5
35–49	4	3.5	19	1	1	1	10	10	10	10
50–64	4	5.7	10	1	1	7	8	8	8	8
65+	2	2.0	0	2	2	2	2	2	2	2
2. MULTIPLE DX										
0–19 Years	1,781	20.8	434	3	6	12	31	53	70	97
20–34	135	5.4	25	2	3	4	7	10	15	27
35–49	308	5.5	19	2	3	5	7	12	14	18
50–64	530	6.2	34	2	3	5	8	13	17	26
65+	778	6.0	22	1	3	5	8	11	14	24
TOTAL SINGLE DX	**21**	**2.8**	**6**	**1**	**1**	**2**	**4**	**7**	**8**	**10**
TOTAL MULTIPLE DX	**3,532**	**13.6**	**292**	**2**	**4**	**7**	**15**	**38**	**53**	**88**
TOTAL										
0–19 Years	1,787	20.7	433	3	6	12	30	53	70	97
20–34	140	5.3	24	2	3	4	6	10	15	27
35–49	312	5.5	19	2	3	4	7	11	14	18
50–64	534	6.2	34	1	3	5	8	13	17	26
65+	780	6.0	22	1	3	5	8	11	14	24
GRAND TOTAL	**3,553**	**13.5**	**291**	**2**	**4**	**7**	**15**	**38**	**53**	**88**

38.92: UMBILICAL VEIN CATH

Type of Patients	Observed Patients	Avg. Stay	Vari-ance	Percentiles						
				10th	25th	50th	75th	90th	95th	99th
1. SINGLE DX										
0–19 Years	2	5.8	<1	5	6	6	6	6	6	6
20–34	0									
35–49	0									
50–64	0									
65+	0									
2. MULTIPLE DX										
0–19 Years	1,119	16.6	292	3	5	10	23	42	56	94
20–34	0									
35–49	1	8.0	0	8	8	8	8	8	8	8
50–64	0									
65+	2	7.5	4	6	6	6	9	9	9	9
TOTAL SINGLE DX	**2**	**5.8**	**<1**	**5**	**6**	**6**	**6**	**6**	**6**	**6**
TOTAL MULTIPLE DX	**1,122**	**16.6**	**291**	**3**	**5**	**10**	**23**	**42**	**56**	**94**
TOTAL										
0–19 Years	1,121	16.5	291	3	5	10	23	42	56	94
20–34	0									
35–49	1	8.0	0	8	8	8	8	8	8	8
50–64	0									
65+	2	7.5	4	6	6	6	9	9	9	9
GRAND TOTAL	**1,124**	**16.5**	**290**	**3**	**5**	**10**	**23**	**42**	**56**	**94**

38.93: VENOUS CATHETER NEC

Type of Patients	Observed Patients	Avg. Stay	Vari-ance	Percentiles						
				10th	25th	50th	75th	90th	95th	99th
1. SINGLE DX										
0–19 Years	238	5.6	13	1	3	5	7	10	13	17
20–34	101	5.1	22	1	2	4	6	8	12	26
35–49	59	3.9	11	1	2	3	5	9	11	18
50–64	65	3.4	6	1	2	3	5	6	7	14
65+	15	3.3	3	2	2	3	5	6	6	6
2. MULTIPLE DX										
0–19 Years	4,825	12.1	137	3	5	9	15	26	35	62
20–34	6,132	7.3	47	2	3	5	9	14	20	37
35–49	11,990	7.2	42	2	4	6	9	14	19	34
50–64	19,015	7.6	46	2	4	6	9	14	19	35
65+	29,723	7.8	32	3	4	6	10	14	18	28
TOTAL SINGLE DX	**478**	**5.1**	**14**	**1**	**2**	**4**	**7**	**10**	**13**	**19**
TOTAL MULTIPLE DX	**71,685**	**8.1**	**52**	**3**	**4**	**6**	**10**	**15**	**21**	**38**
TOTAL										
0–19 Years	5,063	11.7	132	3	5	8	14	25	35	59
20–34	6,233	7.3	46	2	3	5	9	14	20	37
35–49	12,049	7.2	42	2	3	5	9	14	19	34
50–64	19,080	7.5	46	2	4	6	9	14	19	35
65+	29,738	7.8	32	3	4	6	10	14	18	28
GRAND TOTAL	**72,163**	**8.1**	**52**	**3**	**4**	**6**	**10**	**15**	**21**	**38**

Western Region, October 2007–September 2008 Data, by Operation

38.94: VENOUS CUTDOWN

Type of Patients	Observed Patients	Avg. Stay	Variance	10th	25th	50th	75th	90th	95th	99th
1. SINGLE DX										
0–19 Years	0									
20–34	1	1.0	0	1	1	1	1	1	1	1
35–49	0									
50–64	0									
65+	0									
2. MULTIPLE DX										
0–19 Years	32	14.8	183	1	4	12	19	37	37	59
20–34	13	10.7	57	2	5	11	14	18	29	29
35–49	12	6.8	18	3	3	6	11	13	15	15
50–64	26	7.7	40	3	4	6	10	14	18	32
65+	31	10.9	119	4	5	6	11	28	37	46
TOTAL SINGLE DX	1	1.0	0	1	1	1	1	1	1	1
TOTAL MULTIPLE DX	114	11.7	126	2	4	7	14	32	37	46
TOTAL										
0–19 Years	32	14.8	183	1	4	12	19	37	37	59
20–34	14	10.0	60	1	4	8	14	18	29	29
35–49	12	6.8	18	1	3	6	11	13	15	15
50–64	26	7.7	40	3	4	6	10	14	18	32
65+	31	10.9	119	4	5	6	11	28	37	46
GRAND TOTAL	115	11.6	126	2	4	7	14	32	37	46

38.98: ARTERIAL PUNCTURE NEC

Type of Patients	Observed Patients	Avg. Stay	Variance	10th	25th	50th	75th	90th	95th	99th
1. SINGLE DX										
0–19 Years	1	5.0	0	5	5	5	5	5	5	5
20–34	1	2.0	0	2	2	2	2	2	2	2
35–49	0									
50–64	0									
65+	1	5.0	0	5	5	5	5	5	5	5
2. MULTIPLE DX										
0–19 Years	62	7.3	75	2	3	4	10	14	19	56
20–34	62	3.0	13	1	2	2	3	4	6	29
35–49	105	4.1	9	1	2	3	5	7	9	17
50–64	191	3.9	6	2	2	3	5	7	10	13
65+	482	5.0	11	2	3	4	6	9	11	18
TOTAL SINGLE DX	3	4.0	3	2	2	5	5	5	5	5
TOTAL MULTIPLE DX	902	4.7	16	2	2	4	6	9	12	18
TOTAL										
0–19 Years	63	7.3	74	2	3	4	9	14	19	56
20–34	63	3.0	13	1	2	2	3	4	6	29
35–49	105	4.1	9	1	2	3	5	7	9	17
50–64	191	3.9	6	2	2	3	5	7	10	13
65+	483	5.0	11	2	3	4	6	9	11	18
GRAND TOTAL	905	4.7	16	2	2	4	6	9	12	18

38.95: VENOUS CATH FOR RD

Type of Patients	Observed Patients	Avg. Stay	Variance	10th	25th	50th	75th	90th	95th	99th
1. SINGLE DX										
0–19 Years	1	1.0	0	1	1	1	1	1	1	1
20–34	2	7.5	<1	7	7	8	8	8	8	8
35–49	0									
50–64	0									
65+	1	6.0	0	6	6	6	6	6	6	6
2. MULTIPLE DX										
0–19 Years	143	6.4	38	1	2	4	10	15	19	29
20–34	604	7.6	42	2	3	6	10	15	19	33
35–49	1,395	7.8	60	2	3	6	10	16	21	40
50–64	3,081	7.9	46	2	4	6	10	16	21	33
65+	4,499	8.8	50	2	4	7	11	17	22	37
TOTAL SINGLE DX	4	3.5	11	1	1	1	7	8	8	8
TOTAL MULTIPLE DX	9,722	8.3	49	2	4	6	10	16	21	35
TOTAL										
0–19 Years	144	6.3	38	1	2	4	9	15	19	29
20–34	606	7.6	42	2	3	6	10	15	19	33
35–49	1,395	7.8	60	2	3	6	10	16	21	40
50–64	3,081	7.9	46	2	4	6	10	16	21	33
65+	4,500	8.8	50	2	4	7	11	17	22	37
GRAND TOTAL	9,726	8.2	49	2	4	6	10	16	21	35

38.99: VENOUS PUNCTURE NEC

Type of Patients	Observed Patients	Avg. Stay	Variance	10th	25th	50th	75th	90th	95th	99th
1. SINGLE DX										
0–19 Years	2	4.3	9	3	3	3	3	10	10	10
20–34	6	1.5	<1	1	1	2	2	2	2	2
35–49	5	1.8	<1	1	1	1	2	2	2	2
50–64	4	1.0	0	1	1	1	1	1	1	1
65+	0									
2. MULTIPLE DX										
0–19 Years	33	9.6	105	2	3	6	10	26	28	60
20–34	17	13.0	548	2	2	3	10	37	96	96
35–49	38	4.9	27	2	2	3	6	11	23	23
50–64	84	5.9	50	2	2	4	7	11	17	57
65+	78	5.0	12	2	3	4	6	10	11	21
TOTAL SINGLE DX	17	2.2	4	1	1	2	3	3	3	10
TOTAL MULTIPLE DX	250	6.8	82	2	2	4	8	12	23	57
TOTAL										
0–19 Years	35	9.2	100	2	3	6	10	26	28	60
20–34	23	10.0	426	1	2	2	8	25	37	96
35–49	43	4.5	25	1	2	2	6	9	11	23
50–64	88	5.7	49	1	2	4	7	11	17	57
65+	78	5.0	12	2	3	4	6	10	11	21
GRAND TOTAL	267	6.5	78	2	2	4	8	12	23	37

LOS by Diagnosis and Operation, Western Region, 45th Edition

Western Region, October 2007–September 2008 Data, by Operation

39.0: SYSTEMIC TO PA SHUNT

Type of Patients	Observed Patients	Avg. Stay	Variance	Percentiles						
				10th	25th	50th	75th	90th	95th	99th
1. SINGLE DX										
0–19 Years	0									
20–34	0									
35–49	0									
50–64	0									
65+	0									
2. MULTIPLE DX										
0–19 Years	133	25.3	480	5	8	17	36	60	73	91
20–34	0									
35–49	0									
50–64	0									
65+	0									
TOTAL SINGLE DX	0									
TOTAL MULTIPLE DX	133	25.3	480	5	8	17	36	60	73	91
TOTAL										
0–19 Years	133	25.3	480	5	8	17	36	60	73	91
20–34	0									
35–49	0									
50–64	0									
65+	0									
GRAND TOTAL	133	25.3	480	5	8	17	36	60	73	91

39.1: INTRA-ABD VENOUS SHUNT

Type of Patients	Observed Patients	Avg. Stay	Variance	Percentiles						
				10th	25th	50th	75th	90th	95th	99th
1. SINGLE DX										
0–19 Years	0									
20–34	1	1.0	0	1	1	1	1	1	1	1
35–49	0									
50–64	0									
65+	0									
2. MULTIPLE DX										
0–19 Years	13	14.8	119	6	7	8	29	34	34	35
20–34	21	8.9	55	1	5	8	12	13	18	35
35–49	188	9.1	57	1	4	8	11	19	23	38
50–64	352	8.6	71	1	3	7	11	17	24	37
65+	134	7.2	28	1	2	7	10	14	17	25
TOTAL SINGLE DX	1	1.0	0	1	1	1	1	1	1	1
TOTAL MULTIPLE DX	708	8.7	62	1	4	7	11	17	24	35
TOTAL										
0–19 Years	13	14.8	119	6	7	8	29	34	34	35
20–34	22	8.5	55	1	5	8	12	13	18	35
35–49	188	9.1	57	1	4	8	11	19	23	38
50–64	352	8.6	71	1	3	7	11	17	24	37
65+	134	7.2	28	1	2	7	10	14	17	25
GRAND TOTAL	709	8.7	62	1	4	7	11	17	24	35

39.2: OTHER SHUNT/VASC BYPASS

Type of Patients	Observed Patients	Avg. Stay	Variance	Percentiles						
				10th	25th	50th	75th	90th	95th	99th
1. SINGLE DX										
0–19 Years	3	4.0	3	3	3	3	6	6	6	6
20–34	2	2.0	2	1	1	3	3	3	3	3
35–49	10	3.4	6	1	2	3	4	9	9	9
50–64	29	2.9	2	1	2	3	4	5	6	7
65+	28	3.1	6	1	2	3	3	4	6	14
2. MULTIPLE DX										
0–19 Years	278	9.6	124	3	4	7	10	23	32	>99
20–34	359	7.7	55	1	3	6	11	17	22	35
35–49	1,077	7.5	60	1	3	5	10	15	21	42
50–64	4,021	7.0	54	1	3	5	9	15	20	40
65+	6,898	7.2	48	2	3	5	9	15	20	32
TOTAL SINGLE DX	72	3.1	4	1	2	3	4	5	6	14
TOTAL MULTIPLE DX	12,633	7.3	55	2	3	5	9	15	21	39
TOTAL										
0–19 Years	281	9.6	123	3	4	7	10	21	32	>99
20–34	361	7.7	55	1	3	6	11	17	22	35
35–49	1,087	7.5	60	1	3	5	9	15	21	42
50–64	4,050	7.0	54	1	3	5	9	15	20	40
65+	6,926	7.2	48	2	3	5	9	15	20	32
GRAND TOTAL	12,705	7.3	55	2	3	5	9	15	20	39

39.21: CAVAL-PA ANASTOMOSIS

Type of Patients	Observed Patients	Avg. Stay	Variance	Percentiles						
				10th	25th	50th	75th	90th	95th	99th
1. SINGLE DX										
0–19 Years	0									
20–34	0									
35–49	0									
50–64	0									
65+	0									
2. MULTIPLE DX										
0–19 Years	187	10.8	144	4	5	7	12	23	38	>99
20–34	1	4.0	0	4	4	4	4	4	4	4
35–49	1	7.0	0	7	7	7	7	7	7	7
50–64	1	11.0	0	11	11	11	11	11	11	11
65+	0									
TOTAL SINGLE DX	0									
TOTAL MULTIPLE DX	190	10.8	144	4	5	7	12	23	38	>99
TOTAL										
0–19 Years	187	10.8	144	4	5	7	12	23	38	>99
20–34	1	4.0	0	4	4	4	4	4	4	4
35–49	1	7.0	0	7	7	7	7	7	7	7
50–64	1	11.0	0	11	11	11	11	11	11	11
65+	0									
GRAND TOTAL	190	10.8	144	4	5	7	12	23	38	>99

LOS by Diagnosis and Operation, Western Region, 45th Edition

Western Region, October 2007–September 2008 Data, by Operation

39.22: AORTA-SCL-CAROTID BYPASS

Type of Patients	Observed Patients	Avg. Stay	Variance	Percentiles						
				10th	25th	50th	75th	90th	95th	99th
1. SINGLE DX										
0–19 Years	0									
20–34	0									
35–49	1									
50–64	2	1.0	0	1	1	1	1	1	1	1
65+	1	2.0	0	2	2	2	2	2	2	2
2. MULTIPLE DX										
0–19 Years	2	22.4	106	4	27	27	27	27	27	27
20–34	2	18.7	537	2	2	35	35	35	35	35
35–49	10	4.4	16	1	2	3	8	13	13	13
50–64	74	4.2	38	1	2	2	4	8	12	45
65+	114	4.9	36	1	2	3	6	11	14	24
TOTAL SINGLE DX	**2**	**1.5**	**<1**	**1**	**1**	**2**	**2**	**2**	**2**	**2**
TOTAL MULTIPLE DX	**202**	**5.2**	**48**	**1**	**2**	**3**	**6**	**11**	**22**	**35**
TOTAL										
0–19 Years	2	22.4	106	4	27	27	27	27	27	27
20–34	2	18.7	537	2	2	35	35	35	35	35
35–49	10	4.4	16	1	2	3	8	13	13	13
50–64	75	4.2	38	1	1	2	4	8	12	45
65+	115	4.9	35	1	2	3	6	11	14	24
GRAND TOTAL	**204**	**5.2**	**48**	**1**	**2**	**2**	**6**	**11**	**22**	**35**

39.25: AORTA-ILIAC-FEMORAL BYP

Type of Patients	Observed Patients	Avg. Stay	Variance	Percentiles						
				10th	25th	50th	75th	90th	95th	99th
1. SINGLE DX										
0–19 Years	0									
20–34	0									
35–49	1	1.0	0	1	1	1	1	1	1	1
50–64	2	4.0	2	3	3	5	5	5	5	5
65+	1	4.0	0	4	4	4	4	4	4	4
2. MULTIPLE DX										
0–19 Years	0									
20–34	6	7.3	34	3	3	3	12	17	17	17
35–49	93	7.4	30	3	4	6	9	13	20	40
50–64	591	7.6	31	3	5	6	8	13	18	33
65+	681	8.6	42	3	5	7	10	16	21	32
TOTAL SINGLE DX	**4**	**3.2**	**3**	**1**	**1**	**3**	**5**	**5**	**5**	**5**
TOTAL MULTIPLE DX	**1,371**	**8.1**	**36**	**3**	**5**	**6**	**9**	**15**	**20**	**32**
TOTAL										
0–19 Years	0									
20–34	6	7.3	34	3	3	3	12	17	17	17
35–49	94	7.3	30	3	4	6	9	13	20	40
50–64	593	7.6	31	3	5	6	8	13	18	33
65+	682	8.6	42	3	5	7	10	16	21	32
GRAND TOTAL	**1,375**	**8.1**	**36**	**3**	**5**	**6**	**9**	**15**	**20**	**32**

39.26: INTRA-ABD VASC SHUNT NEC

Type of Patients	Observed Patients	Avg. Stay	Variance	Percentiles						
				10th	25th	50th	75th	90th	95th	99th
1. SINGLE DX										
0–19 Years	0									
20–34	0									
35–49	0									
50–64	0									
65+	0									
2. MULTIPLE DX										
0–19 Years	0									
20–34	3	8.0	21	3	3	9	12	12	12	12
35–49	5	6.2	6	3	5	6	8	10	10	10
50–64	27	10.2	65	4	5	8	12	19	26	40
65+	36	10.0	81	2	4	7	15	22	29	44
TOTAL SINGLE DX	**0**									
TOTAL MULTIPLE DX	**71**	**9.7**	**66**	**3**	**5**	**7**	**12**	**19**	**26**	**44**
TOTAL										
0–19 Years	0									
20–34	3	8.0	21	3	3	9	12	12	12	12
35–49	5	6.2	6	3	5	6	8	10	10	10
50–64	27	10.2	65	4	5	8	12	19	26	40
65+	36	10.0	81	2	4	7	15	22	29	44
GRAND TOTAL	**71**	**9.7**	**66**	**3**	**5**	**7**	**12**	**19**	**26**	**44**

39.27: ARTERIOVENOSTOMY FOR RD

Type of Patients	Observed Patients	Avg. Stay	Variance	Percentiles						
				10th	25th	50th	75th	90th	95th	99th
1. SINGLE DX										
0–19 Years	0									
20–34	1	1.0	0	1	1	1	1	1	1	1
35–49	2	1.5	<1	1	1	2	2	2	2	2
50–64	3	1.0	0	1	1	1	1	1	1	1
65+	3	1.0	0	1	1	1	1	1	1	1
2. MULTIPLE DX										
0–19 Years	30	6.8	63	1	2	3	9	19	29	29
20–34	277	7.9	52	1	3	6	11	17	20	34
35–49	703	7.9	73	1	3	6	10	17	22	43
50–64	1,586	8.1	84	1	2	6	10	18	24	56
65+	1,981	8.0	75	1	2	6	10	17	22	41
TOTAL SINGLE DX	**9**	**1.1**	**<1**	**1**	**1**	**1**	**1**	**2**	**2**	**2**
TOTAL MULTIPLE DX	**4,577**	**8.0**	**77**	**1**	**2**	**6**	**10**	**17**	**23**	**46**
TOTAL										
0–19 Years	30	6.8	63	1	2	3	9	19	29	29
20–34	278	7.8	52	1	3	6	11	17	20	34
35–49	705	7.9	73	1	3	6	10	17	22	43
50–64	1,589	8.1	84	1	2	6	10	18	24	56
65+	1,984	8.0	75	1	2	6	10	17	22	41
GRAND TOTAL	**4,586**	**8.0**	**77**	**1**	**2**	**6**	**10**	**17**	**23**	**46**

LOS by Diagnosis and Operation, Western Region, 45th Edition

Western Region, October 2007–September 2008 Data, by Operation

39.28: EC-IC VASCULAR BYPASS

Type of Patients	Observed Patients	Avg. Stay	Variance	Percentiles						
				10th	25th	50th	75th	90th	95th	99th
1. SINGLE DX										
0–19 Years	3	4.0	3	3	3	3	6	6	6	6
20–34	0									
35–49	1	3.0	0	3	3	3	3	3	3	3
50–64	0									
65+	0									
2. MULTIPLE DX										
0–19 Years	38	3.2	2	2	2	3	4	4	7	11
20–34	25	5.8	35	3	3	4	5	9	19	29
35–49	42	5.9	15	3	3	4	7	11	12	19
50–64	51	5.7	25	3	3	4	6	10	15	31
65+	16	7.7	83	1	3	5	11	16	38	38
TOTAL SINGLE DX	4	3.8	2	3	3	3	6	6	6	6
TOTAL MULTIPLE DX	172	5.1	23	2	3	3	5	10	12	31
TOTAL										
0–19 Years	41	3.3	3	2	2	3	4	4	7	11
20–34	25	5.8	35	3	3	4	5	9	19	29
35–49	43	5.8	15	3	3	4	7	11	12	19
50–64	51	5.7	25	3	3	4	6	10	15	31
65+	16	7.7	83	1	3	5	11	16	38	38
GRAND TOTAL	176	5.1	23	2	3	3	5	10	11	29

39.3: SUTURE OF VESSEL

Type of Patients	Observed Patients	Avg. Stay	Variance	Percentiles						
				10th	25th	50th	75th	90th	95th	99th
1. SINGLE DX										
0–19 Years	5	1.2	<1	1	1	1	1	2	2	2
20–34	9	1.3	<1	1	1	1	1	3	3	3
35–49	6	2.0	1	1	1	2	2	4	4	4
50–64	3	1.0	0	1	1	1	1	1	1	1
65+	0									
2. MULTIPLE DX										
0–19 Years	88	6.5	123	1	1	3	6	12	26	55
20–34	265	4.4	46	1	1	2	5	9	14	42
35–49	174	5.2	80	1	1	2	5	10	17	57
50–64	194	7.0	88	2	2	4	8	19	30	>99
65+	208	7.8	66	1	3	5	10	18	28	46
TOTAL SINGLE DX	23	1.4	<1	1	1	1	2	2	3	4
TOTAL MULTIPLE DX	929	6.0	75	1	1	3	7	14	24	55
TOTAL										
0–19 Years	93	6.2	118	1	1	3	6	11	20	55
20–34	274	4.3	45	1	1	2	5	9	14	42
35–49	180	5.1	78	1	1	2	7	10	17	57
50–64	197	6.9	87	1	2	4	8	19	30	>99
65+	208	7.8	66	1	3	5	10	18	28	46
GRAND TOTAL	952	5.9	74	1	1	3	6	14	24	55

39.29: VASC SHUNT & BYPASS NEC

Type of Patients	Observed Patients	Avg. Stay	Variance	Percentiles						
				10th	25th	50th	75th	90th	95th	99th
1. SINGLE DX										
0–19 Years	0									
20–34	1	3.0	0	3	3	3	3	3	3	3
35–49	6	4.5	6	2	2	3	3	5	9	9
50–64	23	3.1	2	2	2	3	4	5	6	7
65+	23	3.4	6	2	2	3	4	4	6	14
2. MULTIPLE DX										
0–19 Years	15	6.2	24	2	3	4	9	14	18	18
20–34	42	7.8	81	1	2	4	9	24	29	35
35–49	217	6.7	42	2	2	5	8	15	20	34
50–64	1,686	6.0	32	2	2	4	8	13	17	29
65+	4,053	6.7	34	2	3	5	8	14	18	27
TOTAL SINGLE DX	53	3.4	4	2	2	3	4	5	7	14
TOTAL MULTIPLE DX	6,013	6.5	34	2	3	5	8	14	18	29
TOTAL										
0–19 Years	15	6.2	24	2	3	4	9	14	18	18
20–34	43	7.6	79	1	2	4	9	24	29	35
35–49	223	6.7	41	2	3	5	8	15	20	34
50–64	1,709	5.9	32	2	2	4	7	13	17	29
65+	4,076	6.6	34	2	3	5	8	14	18	27
GRAND TOTAL	6,066	6.5	34	2	3	5	8	13	18	29

39.31: SUTURE OF ARTERY

Type of Patients	Observed Patients	Avg. Stay	Variance	Percentiles						
				10th	25th	50th	75th	90th	95th	99th
1. SINGLE DX										
0–19 Years	5	1.2	<1	1	1	1	1	2	2	2
20–34	7	1.3	<1	1	1	1	1	3	3	3
35–49	5	2.0	1	1	1	2	2	4	4	4
50–64	3	1.0	0	1	1	1	1	1	1	1
65+	0									
2. MULTIPLE DX										
0–19 Years	68	6.5	148	1	1	3	6	10	55	55
20–34	198	4.0	25	1	1	2	5	8	13	26
35–49	119	4.5	61	1	2	3	8	7	16	52
50–64	143	6.9	91	1	3	5	10	19	30	>99
65+	167	7.8	65	1	3	5	10	18	27	46
TOTAL SINGLE DX	20	1.4	<1	1	1	1	1	2	3	4
TOTAL MULTIPLE DX	695	5.9	69	1	1	3	7	14	21	55
TOTAL										
0–19 Years	73	6.2	140	1	1	2	5	10	55	55
20–34	205	3.9	25	1	1	2	5	8	12	22
35–49	124	4.4	59	1	1	3	5	7	15	52
50–64	146	6.8	90	1	2	4	8	19	30	>99
65+	167	7.8	65	1	3	5	10	18	27	46
GRAND TOTAL	715	5.7	68	1	1	3	6	14	20	55

LOS by Diagnosis and Operation, Western Region, 45th Edition

Western Region, October 2007–September 2008 Data, by Operation

39.32: SUTURE OF VEIN

Type of Patients	Observed Patients	Avg. Stay	Variance	10th	25th	50th	75th	90th	95th	99th
1. SINGLE DX										
0–19 Years	0									
20–34	1	1.0	0	1	1	1	1	1	1	1
35–49	1	2.0	0	2	2	2	2	2	2	2
50–64	0									
65+	0									
2. MULTIPLE DX										
0–19 Years	16	7.3	48	1	2	4	10	20	26	26
20–34	57	6.3	123	1	1	3	5	14	32	65
35–49	46	6.2	126	1	1	3	6	15	21	72
50–64	40	6.3	59	1	2	4	6	16	29	30
65+	30	8.9	91	2	3	5	13	23	39	>99
TOTAL SINGLE DX	2	1.5	<1	1	1	2	2	2	2	2
TOTAL MULTIPLE DX	189	6.8	97	1	2	4	7	15	29	72
TOTAL										
0–19 Years	16	7.3	48	1	2	4	10	20	26	26
20–34	58	6.2	121	1	1	3	5	14	32	65
35–49	47	6.1	124	1	1	3	6	15	21	72
50–64	40	6.3	59	1	2	4	6	16	29	30
65+	30	8.9	91	2	3	5	13	23	39	>99
GRAND TOTAL	191	6.7	96	1	2	4	7	15	29	72

39.4: VASCULAR PX REVISION

Type of Patients	Observed Patients	Avg. Stay	Variance	10th	25th	50th	75th	90th	95th	99th
1. SINGLE DX										
0–19 Years	1	2.0	0	2	2	2	2	2	2	2
20–34	0									
35–49	2	1.5	<1	1	1	1	2	2	2	3
50–64	4	1.7	<1	1	1	1	2	3	3	3
65+	11	1.5	<1	1	1	1	2	3	3	3
2. MULTIPLE DX										
0–19 Years	35	12.1	226	1	2	6	20	57	>99	>99
20–34	209	5.8	52	1	2	3	7	13	19	40
35–49	665	5.7	35	1	2	4	8	13	17	31
50–64	1,775	5.8	35	1	2	4	8	13	18	28
65+	2,644	5.9	42	2	2	5	7	13	17	33
TOTAL SINGLE DX	18	1.6	<1	1	1	1	2	3	3	3
TOTAL MULTIPLE DX	5,328	5.9	42	1	2	4	7	13	18	32
TOTAL										
0–19 Years	36	12.0	224	1	2	6	20	57	>99	>99
20–34	209	5.8	52	1	2	3	7	13	19	40
35–49	667	5.7	35	1	2	4	7	13	17	31
50–64	1,779	5.8	34	1	2	4	7	13	18	28
65+	2,655	5.9	42	2	2	5	7	13	17	33
GRAND TOTAL	5,346	5.9	42	1	2	4	7	13	18	32

39.42: REV AV SHUNT FOR RD

Type of Patients	Observed Patients	Avg. Stay	Variance	10th	25th	50th	75th	90th	95th	99th
1. SINGLE DX										
0–19 Years	0									
20–34	0									
35–49	0									
50–64	0									
65+	1	1.0	0	1	1	1	1	1	1	1
2. MULTIPLE DX										
0–19 Years	9	3.6	7	1	1	3	4	8	8	8
20–34	91	5.5	46	1	2	3	6	11	19	49
35–49	268	5.4	40	1	2	3	6	14	18	38
50–64	630	4.9	25	1	1	3	6	11	15	23
65+	762	4.8	36	1	3	3	6	10	14	26
TOTAL SINGLE DX	1	1.0	0	1	1	1	1	1	1	1
TOTAL MULTIPLE DX	1,760	5.0	33	1	1	3	6	11	15	25
TOTAL										
0–19 Years	9	3.6	7	1	1	3	4	8	8	8
20–34	91	5.5	46	1	2	3	6	11	19	49
35–49	268	5.4	40	1	2	3	6	14	18	38
50–64	630	4.9	25	1	1	3	6	11	15	23
65+	763	4.8	36	1	1	3	6	10	14	26
GRAND TOTAL	1,761	5.0	33	1	1	3	6	11	15	25

39.43: RMVL AV SHUNT FOR RD

Type of Patients	Observed Patients	Avg. Stay	Variance	10th	25th	50th	75th	90th	95th	99th
1. SINGLE DX										
0–19 Years	0									
20–34	0									
35–49	0									
50–64	1	1.0	0	1	1	1	1	1	1	1
65+	0									
2. MULTIPLE DX										
0–19 Years	2	27.7	355	7	7	39	39	39	39	39
20–34	23	6.4	37	1	2	5	10	11	15	28
35–49	74	6.3	26	2	3	5	9	13	16	28
50–64	147	8.4	59	2	3	6	12	21	24	31
65+	183	8.6	43	2	4	7	12	17	21	32
TOTAL SINGLE DX	1	1.0	0	1	1	1	1	1	1	1
TOTAL MULTIPLE DX	429	8.2	50	2	3	6	11	17	24	32
TOTAL										
0–19 Years	2	27.7	355	7	7	39	39	39	39	39
20–34	23	6.4	37	1	3	5	10	11	15	28
35–49	74	6.3	26	2	3	5	9	13	16	28
50–64	148	8.4	59	2	3	6	12	21	24	31
65+	183	8.6	43	2	4	7	12	17	21	32
GRAND TOTAL	430	8.1	50	2	3	6	11	17	24	32

LOS by Diagnosis and Operation, Western Region, 45th Edition

Western Region, October 2007–September 2008 Data, by Operation

39.49: VASCULAR PX REVISION NEC

Type of Patients	Observed Patients	Avg. Stay	Variance	10th	25th	50th	75th	90th	95th	99th
1. SINGLE DX										
0–19 Years	1	2.0	0	2	2	2	2	2	2	2
20–34	0									
35–49	2	1.5	<1	1	1	2	2	2	2	2
50–64	3	2.0	1	1	1	2	3	3	3	3
65+	10	1.5	<1	1	1	1	2	3	3	3
2. MULTIPLE DX										
0–19 Years	24	15.6	276	2	4	15	24	57	>99	>99
20–34	95	6.0	61	1	2	3	6	15	19	53
35–49	319	5.8	34	1	2	4	8	13	17	31
50–64	995	5.9	36	1	2	4	8	13	18	28
65+	1,692	6.1	43	1	2	4	8	13	17	36
TOTAL SINGLE DX	16	1.6	<1	1	1	1	2	3	3	3
TOTAL MULTIPLE DX	3,125	6.1	45	1	2	4	8	13	18	36
TOTAL										
0–19 Years	25	15.2	273	2	4	14	24	57	>99	>99
20–34	95	6.0	61	1	2	3	6	15	19	53
35–49	321	5.8	34	1	2	4	8	13	17	31
50–64	998	5.9	36	1	2	4	8	13	18	28
65+	1,702	6.0	43	1	2	4	8	13	17	36
GRAND TOTAL	3,141	6.1	44	1	2	4	8	13	18	36

39.50: PTA/ATHERECT OTH VESSEL

Type of Patients	Observed Patients	Avg. Stay	Variance	10th	25th	50th	75th	90th	95th	99th
1. SINGLE DX										
0–19 Years	23	1.7	5	1	1	1	1	7	7	11
20–34	11	1.8	2	1	1	1	2	4	5	5
35–49	17	1.8	3	1	1	1	2	3	8	8
50–64	51	1.3	<1	1	1	1	1	2	3	5
65+	125	1.3	<1	1	1	1	1	2	2	5
2. MULTIPLE DX										
0–19 Years	314	4.4	86	1	1	4	4	10	19	45
20–34	281	5.7	43	1	2	4	7	12	16	37
35–49	967	5.9	45	1	2	4	7	13	18	38
50–64	3,811	4.8	46	1	1	2	6	12	16	33
65+	9,688	4.2	32	1	1	2	5	10	15	26
TOTAL SINGLE DX	227	1.4	2	1	1	1	1	2	4	7
TOTAL MULTIPLE DX	15,061	4.5	40	1	1	2	6	11	16	30
TOTAL										
0–19 Years	337	4.2	82	1	1	4	3	10	18	45
20–34	292	5.5	42	1	2	4	7	11	16	36
35–49	984	5.8	45	1	1	4	7	13	18	38
50–64	3,862	4.8	46	1	1	2	6	12	16	33
65+	9,813	4.2	32	1	1	2	5	10	15	26
GRAND TOTAL	15,288	4.5	39	1	1	2	6	11	16	29

39.5: OTHER VESSEL REPAIR

Type of Patients	Observed Patients	Avg. Stay	Variance	10th	25th	50th	75th	90th	95th	99th
1. SINGLE DX										
0–19 Years	30	2.4	5	1	1	1	4	5	7	11
20–34	26	3.5	12	1	1	2	4	9	12	16
35–49	39	3.9	16	1	1	2	5	13	15	15
50–64	73	2.2	6	1	1	1	3	4	7	13
65+	135	1.4	1	1	1	1	1	2	4	7
2. MULTIPLE DX										
0–19 Years	421	5.2	89	1	1	1	5	13	23	43
20–34	468	7.3	70	1	2	5	9	16	22	44
35–49	1,344	7.2	65	1	2	4	7	16	24	46
50–64	4,739	5.9	61	1	1	3	7	14	21	40
65+	10,738	4.6	38	1	1	2	6	11	16	29
TOTAL SINGLE DX	303	2.2	6	1	1	1	3	5	7	13
TOTAL MULTIPLE DX	17,710	5.2	51	1	1	3	7	13	18	35
TOTAL										
0–19 Years	451	5.1	85	1	1	1	5	12	22	43
20–34	494	7.0	67	1	2	4	9	16	22	42
35–49	1,383	7.1	64	1	2	4	9	16	24	46
50–64	4,812	5.8	61	1	1	3	7	14	21	40
65+	10,873	4.6	38	1	1	2	6	11	16	28
GRAND TOTAL	18,013	5.2	50	1	1	3	7	13	18	34

39.51: CLIPPING OF ANEURYSM

Type of Patients	Observed Patients	Avg. Stay	Variance	10th	25th	50th	75th	90th	95th	99th
1. SINGLE DX										
0–19 Years	0									
20–34	6	7.8	30	2	3	5	12	16	16	16
35–49	16	5.8	18	2	3	4	8	13	15	15
50–64	15	5.4	13	2	3	4	7	12	13	13
65+	1	3.0	0	3	3	3	3	3	3	3
2. MULTIPLE DX										
0–19 Years	8	21.7	268	11	13	19	22	35	72	72
20–34	64	14.2	153	4	6	11	18	29	35	68
35–49	229	12.6	109	3	4	10	18	27	34	59
50–64	514	12.5	112	3	5	10	18	26	32	59
65+	205	12.5	138	3	5	8	16	28	32	70
TOTAL SINGLE DX	38	5.9	17	2	3	4	8	13	15	16
TOTAL MULTIPLE DX	1,020	12.8	122	3	4	10	18	26	33	70
TOTAL										
0–19 Years	8	21.7	268	11	13	19	22	35	72	72
20–34	70	13.7	145	3	5	11	17	26	35	68
35–49	245	12.1	106	3	4	10	16	27	30	59
50–64	529	12.3	110	3	4	10	17	26	32	59
65+	206	12.4	138	3	4	8	16	28	32	70
GRAND TOTAL	1,058	12.5	120	3	4	10	17	26	32	70

LOS by Diagnosis and Operation, Western Region, 45th Edition

Western Region, October 2007–September 2008 Data, by Operation

39.52: ANEURYSM REPAIR NEC

Type of Patients	Observed Patients	Avg. Stay	Vari-ance	10th	25th	50th	75th	90th	95th	99th
1. SINGLE DX										
0–19 Years	1	5.0	0	5	5	5	5	5	5	5
20–34	0									
35–49	1	1.0	0	1	1	1	1	1	1	1
50–64	2	2.0	2	1	1	2	3	3	3	3
65+	8	3.5	7	1	1	2	7	7	7	7
2. MULTIPLE DX										
0–19 Years	5	4.9	13	2	2	5	5	13	13	13
20–34	21	10.8	140	2	3	6	14	31	37	42
35–49	46	6.7	20	2	4	6	8	12	15	22
50–64	224	7.7	89	2	3	5	9	17	24	53
65+	579	8.1	64	2	3	6	9	17	22	44
TOTAL SINGLE DX	12	3.6	5	1	1	4	5	7	7	7
TOTAL MULTIPLE DX	875	8.0	69	2	3	6	9	16	23	48
TOTAL										
0–19 Years	6	4.9	8	2	2	5	5	5	13	13
20–34	21	10.8	140	2	2	6	14	31	37	42
35–49	47	6.6	20	2	4	6	8	12	15	22
50–64	226	7.7	88	1	3	5	9	17	24	53
65+	587	8.1	63	2	3	6	9	16	22	44
GRAND TOTAL	887	7.9	68	2	3	6	9	16	23	48

39.53: AV FISTULA REPAIR

Type of Patients	Observed Patients	Avg. Stay	Vari-ance	10th	25th	50th	75th	90th	95th	99th
1. SINGLE DX										
0–19 Years	1	1.0	0	1	1	1	1	1	1	1
20–34	2	2.5	4	1	1	4	4	4	4	4
35–49	1	15.0	0	15	15	15	15	15	15	15
50–64	3	3.3	6	1	1	6	6	6	6	6
65+	1	1.0	0	1	1	1	1	1	1	1
2. MULTIPLE DX										
0–19 Years	5	11.7	187	1	1	3	20	20	43	43
20–34	11	5.2	20	1	2	3	9	11	13	13
35–49	26	6.6	47	1	2	4	9	13	15	34
50–64	82	5.9	34	1	1	4	9	14	18	27
65+	111	5.3	43	1	1	3	7	11	20	34
TOTAL SINGLE DX	8	4.0	23	1	1	3	6	15	15	15
TOTAL MULTIPLE DX	235	6.0	47	1	1	4	7	14	20	34
TOTAL										
0–19 Years	6	10.9	180	1	1	1	20	20	43	43
20–34	13	4.8	18	1	2	3	9	11	13	13
35–49	27	6.9	48	1	2	5	9	15	15	34
50–64	85	5.8	33	1	1	4	9	14	18	27
65+	112	5.3	43	1	1	3	7	11	20	34
GRAND TOTAL	243	5.9	46	1	1	3	7	14	20	34

39.56: REP VESS W TISS PATCH

Type of Patients	Observed Patients	Avg. Stay	Vari-ance	10th	25th	50th	75th	90th	95th	99th
1. SINGLE DX										
0–19 Years	3	3.7	<1	2	4	4	4	4	4	4
20–34	6	3.8	2	2	3	4	5	6	6	6
35–49	3	2.3	5	1	1	1	5	5	5	5
50–64	0									
65+	0									
2. MULTIPLE DX										
0–19 Years	59	7.5	60	2	3	4	8	20	25	28
20–34	50	5.5	39	1	2	4	6	11	18	33
35–49	35	6.7	57	2	3	5	8	11	15	46
50–64	42	7.3	117	1	2	5	8	12	17	53
65+	42	7.0	46	1	2	5	9	17	20	31
TOTAL SINGLE DX	12	3.5	2	1	2	4	4	5	6	6
TOTAL MULTIPLE DX	228	6.9	62	1	3	4	8	17	25	46
TOTAL										
0–19 Years	62	7.3	58	2	3	4	7	20	25	28
20–34	56	5.3	35	1	2	4	6	8	18	33
35–49	38	6.3	54	1	2	4	8	11	15	46
50–64	42	7.3	117	1	2	5	8	12	17	53
65+	42	7.0	46	1	2	5	9	17	20	31
GRAND TOTAL	240	6.8	60	1	3	4	7	17	25	39

39.57: REP VESS W SYNTH PATCH

Type of Patients	Observed Patients	Avg. Stay	Vari-ance	10th	25th	50th	75th	90th	95th	99th
1. SINGLE DX										
0–19 Years	0									
20–34	1	2.0	0	2	2	2	2	2	2	2
35–49	1	6.0	0	6	6	6	6	6	6	6
50–64	2	1.0	0	1	1	1	1	1	1	1
65+	0									
2. MULTIPLE DX										
0–19 Years	18	8.3	62	3	4	4	8	27	27	27
20–34	27	10.5	61	2	3	10	17	20	28	29
35–49	12	17.6	377	2	6	6	44	48	52	52
50–64	34	5.8	32	2	2	4	7	11	22	27
65+	57	6.3	58	1	2	4	7	15	24	40
TOTAL SINGLE DX	4	2.5	6	1	1	2	6	6	6	6
TOTAL MULTIPLE DX	148	8.1	84	2	2	5	10	20	27	48
TOTAL										
0–19 Years	18	8.3	62	3	4	4	8	27	27	27
20–34	28	10.2	61	2	3	10	12	20	28	29
35–49	13	16.7	356	2	5	6	22	48	52	52
50–64	36	5.6	31	1	2	4	8	11	22	27
65+	57	6.3	58	1	2	4	7	15	24	40
GRAND TOTAL	152	8.0	83	1	2	5	10	20	27	48

Percentiles

LOS by Diagnosis and Operation, Western Region, 45th Edition

Western Region, October 2007–September 2008 Data, by Operation

39.59: REPAIR OF VESSEL NEC

Type of Patients	Observed Patients	Avg. Stay	Variance	Percentiles						
				10th	25th	50th	75th	90th	95th	99th
1. SINGLE DX										
0–19 Years	2	4.0	0	4	4	4	4	4	4	4
20–34	0									
35–49	0									
50–64	0									
65+	0									
2. MULTIPLE DX										
0–19 Years	12	6.7	40	2	3	5	7	12	14	35
20–34	11	3.9	10	1	2	3	5	7	12	12
35–49	21	5.2	25	1	2	3	7	12	16	19
50–64	28	6.0	42	1	2	4	7	11	18	33
65+	39	5.6	53	1	1	3	6	15	31	33
TOTAL SINGLE DX	2	4.0	0	4	4	4	4	4	4	4
TOTAL MULTIPLE DX	111	5.7	39	1	2	4	7	12	17	33
TOTAL										
0–19 Years	14	6.1	33	2	3	5	7	12	14	35
20–34	11	3.9	10	1	2	3	5	7	12	12
35–49	21	5.2	25	1	2	3	7	12	16	19
50–64	28	6.0	42	1	2	4	7	11	18	33
65+	39	5.6	53	1	1	3	6	15	31	33
GRAND TOTAL	113	5.6	37	1	2	4	7	12	17	33

39.6: OPEN HEART AUXILIARY PX

Type of Patients	Observed Patients	Avg. Stay	Variance	Percentiles						
				10th	25th	50th	75th	90th	95th	99th
1. SINGLE DX										
0–19 Years	0									
20–34	0									
35–49	0									
50–64	0									
65+	0									
2. MULTIPLE DX										
0–19 Years	34	34.9	566	6	23	34	55	97	>99	>99
20–34	3	33.3	531	12	12	30	58	58	58	58
35–49	4	25.0	405	1	17	35	35	47	47	47
50–64	10	16.6	243	3	6	15	19	29	55	55
65+	7	8.0	35	2	3	7	14	18	18	18
TOTAL SINGLE DX	0									
TOTAL MULTIPLE DX	58	31.3	552	3	12	34	52	97	>99	>99
TOTAL										
0–19 Years	34	34.9	566	6	23	34	55	97	>99	>99
20–34	3	33.3	531	12	12	30	58	58	58	58
35–49	4	25.0	405	1	17	35	35	47	47	47
50–64	10	16.6	243	3	6	15	19	29	55	55
65+	7	8.0	35	2	3	7	14	18	18	18
GRAND TOTAL	58	31.3	552	3	12	34	52	97	>99	>99

39.7: ENDOVASCULAR VESSEL REP

Type of Patients	Observed Patients	Avg. Stay	Variance	Percentiles						
				10th	25th	50th	75th	90th	95th	99th
1. SINGLE DX										
0–19 Years	44	2.2	6	1	1	1	3	5	7	18
20–34	36	2.3	6	1	1	1	2	7	8	9
35–49	63	2.3	16	1	1	1	2	3	12	23
50–64	77	1.6	2	1	1	1	2	3	4	10
65+	66	1.3	<1	1	1	1	1	2	2	4
2. MULTIPLE DX										
0–19 Years	209	8.1	250	1	1	3	8	19	28	95
20–34	343	7.7	77	1	2	5	10	17	22	43
35–49	775	6.5	63	1	1	4	8	16	22	42
50–64	1,828	6.1	77	1	1	3	7	15	22	44
65+	5,020	4.3	37	1	1	2	5	10	15	31
TOTAL SINGLE DX	286	1.9	6	1	1	1	2	4	6	15
TOTAL MULTIPLE DX	8,175	5.2	61	1	1	2	6	13	19	41
TOTAL										
0–19 Years	253	7.0	210	1	1	2	7	16	25	92
20–34	379	7.1	73	1	2	4	9	17	22	43
35–49	838	6.2	61	1	1	3	8	16	22	39
50–64	1,905	6.0	75	1	1	2	7	15	21	44
65+	5,086	4.3	37	1	1	2	5	10	15	31
GRAND TOTAL	8,461	5.1	59	1	1	2	6	12	19	40

39.71: ENDOVASCULAR GRAFT-AAA

Type of Patients	Observed Patients	Avg. Stay	Variance	Percentiles						
				10th	25th	50th	75th	90th	95th	99th
1. SINGLE DX										
0–19 Years	0									
20–34	0									
35–49	0									
50–64	9	1.4	<1	1	1	1	1	3	3	3
65+	39	1.4	<1	1	1	1	2	2	3	4
2. MULTIPLE DX										
0–19 Years	1	2.0	0	2	2	2	2	2	2	2
20–34	0									
35–49	16	3.7	6	1	1	4	6	7	8	8
50–64	476	2.9	13	1	1	2	3	6	9	22
65+	3,256	3.3	23	1	1	2	3	7	10	26
TOTAL SINGLE DX	48	1.4	<1	1	1	1	2	3	3	4
TOTAL MULTIPLE DX	3,749	3.2	21	1	1	2	3	7	10	25
TOTAL										
0–19 Years	1	2.0	0	2	2	2	2	2	2	2
20–34	0									
35–49	16	3.7	6	1	1	4	6	7	8	8
50–64	485	2.9	13	1	1	2	3	6	8	22
65+	3,295	3.3	23	1	1	2	3	7	10	25
GRAND TOTAL	3,797	3.2	21	1	1	2	3	7	10	25

LOS by Diagnosis and Operation, Western Region, 45th Edition

Western Region, October 2007–September 2008 Data, by Operation

39.72: ENDOV REP HN VESSEL

Type of Patients	Observed Patients	Avg. Stay	Vari-ance	Percentiles						
				10th	25th	50th	75th	90th	95th	99th
1. SINGLE DX										
0–19 Years	28	2.3	8	1	1	1	3	4	7	18
20–34	29	2.4	6	1	1	1	2	8	8	9
35–49	34	3.4	27	1	1	1	2	12	16	23
50–64	47	1.5	2	1	1	1	2	2	3	10
65+	15	1.1	<1	1	1	1	1	1	2	2
2. MULTIPLE DX										
0–19 Years	76	9.9	391	1	1	2	8	21	64	92
20–34	133	6.8	84	1	1	3	10	17	24	42
35–49	340	5.6	59	1	1	2	7	16	22	36
50–64	689	6.8	93	1	1	2	9	18	24	46
65+	487	6.4	101	1	1	2	7	19	26	55
TOTAL SINGLE DX	153	2.2	9	1	1	1	2	5	8	18
TOTAL MULTIPLE DX	1,725	6.7	110	1	1	2	8	18	25	54
TOTAL										
0–19 Years	104	7.7	291	1	1	2	5	18	52	92
20–34	162	6.0	73	1	1	2	8	15	22	42
35–49	374	5.4	57	1	1	2	7	16	21	36
50–64	736	6.5	88	1	1	2	9	18	23	44
65+	502	6.2	98	1	1	2	7	18	26	50
GRAND TOTAL	1,878	6.3	102	1	1	2	7	17	24	52

39.73: ENDOV GRAFT THOR AORTA

Type of Patients	Observed Patients	Avg. Stay	Vari-ance	Percentiles						
				10th	25th	50th	75th	90th	95th	99th
1. SINGLE DX										
0–19 Years	1	1.0	0	1	1	1	1	1		1
20–34	0									
35–49	1	1.0	0	1	1	1	1	1	1	1
50–64	2	2.5	4	1	1	3	4	4	4	4
65+	0									
2. MULTIPLE DX										
0–19 Years	5	8.2	32	1	6	6	13	15	15	15
20–34	9	13.7	97	2	5	11	20	31	31	31
35–49	26	9.6	46	2	2	8	15	19	22	26
50–64	74	9.6	183	2	2	5	9	27	42	80
65+	205	7.0	42	2	3	5	9	14	20	31
TOTAL SINGLE DX	4	1.8	2	1	1	1	4	4	4	4
TOTAL MULTIPLE DX	319	8.0	78	2	3	5	10	17	24	44
TOTAL										
0–19 Years	6	7.0	35	1	1	6	13	15	15	15
20–34	9	13.7	97	2	5	11	20	31	31	31
35–49	27	9.2	47	1	5	7	15	19	22	26
50–64	76	9.4	179	2	2	5	8	27	42	80
65+	205	7.0	42	2	3	5	9	14	20	31
GRAND TOTAL	323	7.9	77	2	3	5	10	17	24	44

39.74: ENDOV RMVL HN VESS OBSTR

Type of Patients	Observed Patients	Avg. Stay	Vari-ance	Percentiles						
				10th	25th	50th	75th	90th	95th	99th
1. SINGLE DX										
0–19 Years	0									
20–34	0									
35–49	0									
50–64	0									
65+										
2. MULTIPLE DX										
0–19 Years	2	11.6	17	7	7	14	14	14	14	14
20–34	7	5.7	14	3	3	4	7	13	13	13
35–49	26	8.5	39	3	4	6	12	17	20	26
50–64	52	10.5	92	3	6	8	12	19	22	66
65+	87	8.9	41	3	4	7	11	18	22	32
TOTAL SINGLE DX	0									
TOTAL MULTIPLE DX	174	9.3	55	3	4	7	12	18	22	32
TOTAL										
0–19 Years	2	11.6	17	7	7	14	14	14	14	14
20–34	7	5.7	14	3	3	4	7	13	13	13
35–49	26	8.5	39	3	4	6	12	17	20	26
50–64	52	10.5	92	3	6	8	12	19	22	66
65+	87	8.9	41	3	4	7	11	18	22	32
GRAND TOTAL	174	9.3	55	3	4	7	12	18	22	32

39.79: ENDOV REP VESSELS NEC

Type of Patients	Observed Patients	Avg. Stay	Vari-ance	Percentiles						
				10th	25th	50th	75th	90th	95th	99th
1. SINGLE DX										
0–19 Years	15	1.9	2	1	1	1	4	5	5	5
20–34	7	2.3	5	1	1	2	2	7	7	7
35–49	28	1.2	<1	1	1	1	1	2	2	3
50–64	19	1.7	2	1	1	1	2	4	6	6
65+	12	1.1	<1	1	1	1	1	1	2	2
2. MULTIPLE DX										
0–19 Years	125	7.1	183	1	1	3	8	16	24	95
20–34	194	8.0	73	1	3	6	10	17	21	47
35–49	367	7.1	71	1	2	5	9	15	24	42
50–64	537	7.3	85	1	2	4	9	16	22	45
65+	985	5.9	40	1	2	4	8	13	18	35
TOTAL SINGLE DX	81	1.6	2	1	1	1	1	4	5	6
TOTAL MULTIPLE DX	2,208	6.7	73	1	2	4	8	15	20	42
TOTAL										
0–19 Years	140	6.5	163	1	1	5	7	14	24	95
20–34	201	7.8	71	1	3	5	9	16	20	43
35–49	395	6.6	68	1	1	4	8	15	23	42
50–64	556	7.1	83	1	2	4	9	16	22	45
65+	997	5.8	40	1	2	4	7	13	18	32
GRAND TOTAL	2,289	6.5	71	1	1	4	8	15	20	42

LOS by Diagnosis and Operation, Western Region, 45th Edition

158

Western Region, October 2007–September 2008 Data, by Operation

39.90: NON-DRUG PERIPH STENT

Type of Patients	Observed Patients	Avg. Stay	Variance	Percentiles						
				10th	25th	50th	75th	90th	95th	99th
1. SINGLE DX										
0–19 Years	0									
20–34	0									
35–49	0									
50–64	0									
65+	2	1.5	<1	1	1	2	2	2	2	2
2. MULTIPLE DX										
0–19 Years	3	1.0	0	1	1	1	1	1	1	1
20–34	1	1.0	0	1	1	1	1	1	1	1
35–49	7	4.0	11	1	1	3	7	9	9	9
50–64	18	5.2	30	1	1	4	8	8	24	24
65+	30	3.7	32	1	1	1	3	14	18	25
TOTAL SINGLE DX	2	1.5	<1	1	1	2	2	2	2	2
TOTAL MULTIPLE DX	59	3.5	24	1	1	1	4	8	14	25
TOTAL										
0–19 Years	3	1.0	0	1	1	1	1	1	1	1
20–34	1	1.0	0	1	1	1	1	1	1	1
35–49	7	4.0	11	1	1	3	7	9	9	9
50–64	18	5.2	30	1	1	4	8	8	24	24
65+	32	3.6	30	1	1	1	3	7	18	25
GRAND TOTAL	61	3.5	23	1	1	1	4	8	14	25

39.93: INSERT VESS-VESS CANNULA

Type of Patients	Observed Patients	Avg. Stay	Variance	Percentiles						
				10th	25th	50th	75th	90th	95th	99th
1. SINGLE DX										
0–19 Years	0									
20–34	0									
35–49	0									
50–64	0									
65+	0									
2. MULTIPLE DX										
0–19 Years	3	5.7	16	1	1	8	8	8	8	8
20–34	14	6.4	27	1	2	6	9	13	19	19
35–49	30	11.7	144	2	4	6	10	32	47	47
50–64	58	8.0	61	1	2	6	10	19	39	39
65+	71	7.7	32	2	3	6	11	15	18	27
TOTAL SINGLE DX	0									
TOTAL MULTIPLE DX	176	8.3	61	1	3	6	10	18	23	47
TOTAL										
0–19 Years	3	5.7	16	1	1	8	8	8	8	8
20–34	14	6.4	27	1	2	6	9	13	19	19
35–49	30	11.7	144	2	4	6	10	32	47	47
50–64	58	8.0	61	1	2	6	10	19	25	39
65+	71	7.7	32	2	3	6	11	15	18	27
GRAND TOTAL	176	8.3	61	1	3	6	10	18	23	47

39.8: VASCULAR BODY OPERATIONS

Type of Patients	Observed Patients	Avg. Stay	Variance	Percentiles						
				10th	25th	50th	75th	90th	95th	99th
1. SINGLE DX										
0–19 Years	0									
20–34	4	1.3	<1	1	1	1	1	2	2	2
35–49	3	2.0	<1	1	1	2	3	3	3	3
50–64	3	1.3	<1	1	1	1	2	2	2	2
65+	0									
2. MULTIPLE DX										
0–19 Years	1	6.0	0	6	6	6	6	6	6	6
20–34	2	5.5	24	2	2	9	9	9	9	9
35–49	19	3.6	40	1	1	2	3	4	29	29
50–64	39	2.7	7	1	1	2	3	6	10	13
65+	37	2.8	17	1	1	2	3	5	7	25
TOTAL SINGLE DX	10	1.5	<1	1	1	1	2	2	3	3
TOTAL MULTIPLE DX	98	3.0	17	1	1	2	3	6	9	29
TOTAL										
0–19 Years	1	6.0	0	6	6	6	6	6	6	6
20–34	6	2.7	10	1	1	2	2	9	9	9
35–49	22	3.3	34	1	1	2	3	4	4	29
50–64	42	2.6	7	1	1	2	3	6	7	13
65+	37	2.8	17	1	1	2	3	5	7	25
GRAND TOTAL	108	2.9	15	1	1	2	3	6	7	25

39.9: OTHER VESSEL OPERATIONS

Type of Patients	Observed Patients	Avg. Stay	Variance	Percentiles						
				10th	25th	50th	75th	90th	95th	99th
1. SINGLE DX										
0–19 Years	20	1.1	<1	1	1	1	1	1	2	3
20–34	17	1.7	2	1	1	1	2	5	6	6
35–49	17	2.1	6	1	1	1	2	4	11	11
50–64	4	1.0	0	1	1	1	1	1	1	1
65+	6	1.5	<1	1	1	1	2	3	3	3
2. MULTIPLE DX										
0–19 Years	363	5.9	67	1	2	3	7	15	22	58
20–34	3,517	4.0	24	1	2	3	5	8	11	24
35–49	7,986	4.1	19	1	2	3	5	8	11	23
50–64	16,033	4.5	23	1	2	3	5	9	13	23
65+	21,888	4.9	21	1	2	4	6	10	13	23
TOTAL SINGLE DX	64	1.4	2	1	1	1	1	2	3	6
TOTAL MULTIPLE DX	49,787	4.6	22	1	2	3	6	9	13	23
TOTAL										
0–19 Years	383	5.5	63	1	1	3	6	14	20	58
20–34	3,534	4.0	24	1	2	3	5	8	11	24
35–49	8,003	4.1	19	1	2	3	5	8	11	23
50–64	16,037	4.5	23	1	2	3	5	9	13	23
65+	21,894	4.9	21	1	2	4	6	10	13	23
GRAND TOTAL	49,851	4.6	22	1	2	3	6	9	13	23

LOS by Diagnosis and Operation, Western Region, 45th Edition

Western Region, October 2007–September 2008 Data, by Operation

39.95: HEMODIALYSIS

Type of Patients	Observed Patients	Avg. Stay	Vari-ance	Percentiles						
				10th	25th	50th	75th	90th	95th	99th
1. SINGLE DX										
0–19 Years	1	1.0	0	1	1	1	1	1	1	1
20–34	1	6.0	0	6	6	6	6	6	6	6
35–49	4	4.0	22	1	1	1	3	11	11	11
50–64	1	1.0	0	1	1	1	1	1	1	1
65+	4	1.5	1	1	1	1	3	3	3	3
2. MULTIPLE DX										
0–19 Years	287	5.8	43	1	2	3	7	15	22	54
20–34	3,401	4.0	22	1	2	3	5	8	11	23
35–49	7,803	4.0	18	1	2	3	5	8	11	21
50–64	15,747	4.5	22	1	2	3	5	9	12	23
65+	21,558	4.9	20	1	2	4	6	9	13	23
TOTAL SINGLE DX	11	2.7	10	1	1	1	3	6	11	11
TOTAL MULTIPLE DX	48,796	4.6	21	1	2	3	6	9	12	23
TOTAL										
0–19 Years	288	5.8	43	1	2	3	7	15	22	54
20–34	3,402	4.0	22	1	2	3	5	8	11	23
35–49	7,807	4.0	18	1	2	3	5	8	11	21
50–64	15,748	4.5	22	1	2	3	5	9	12	23
65+	21,562	4.9	20	1	2	4	6	9	13	23
GRAND TOTAL	48,807	4.6	21	1	2	3	6	9	12	23

39.99: VESSEL OPERATION NEC

Type of Patients	Observed Patients	Avg. Stay	Vari-ance	Percentiles						
				10th	25th	50th	75th	90th	95th	99th
1. SINGLE DX										
0–19 Years	2	2.2	<1	2	2	2	2	3	3	3
20–34	1	1.0	0	1	1	1	1	1	1	1
35–49	0									
50–64	1	1.0	0	1	1	1	1	1	1	1
65+	0									
2. MULTIPLE DX										
0–19 Years	12	9.3	259	2	2	3	8	26	45	72
20–34	16	11.5	59	2	5	9	16	20	33	33
35–49	24	9.8	61	2	5	7	11	23	27	28
50–64	31	11.1	163	1	3	4	15	27	34	56
65+	25	8.7	63	2	3	7	10	18	28	32
TOTAL SINGLE DX	4	1.9	<1	1	1	2	2	3	3	3
TOTAL MULTIPLE DX	108	10.1	124	2	3	7	14	26	32	56
TOTAL										
0–19 Years	14	8.1	221	2	2	2	8	14	45	72
20–34	17	11.0	61	2	5	9	16	20	33	33
35–49	24	9.8	61	2	5	7	11	23	27	28
50–64	32	10.8	161	1	2	4	15	27	34	56
65+	25	8.7	63	2	3	7	10	18	28	32
GRAND TOTAL	112	9.6	121	2	2	6	14	23	32	56

39.98: HEMORRHAGE CONTROL NOS

Type of Patients	Observed Patients	Avg. Stay	Vari-ance	Percentiles						
				10th	25th	50th	75th	90th	95th	99th
1. SINGLE DX										
0–19 Years	15	1.0	<1	1	1	1	1	1	1	3
20–34	14	1.4	1	1	1	1	1	2	5	5
35–49	12	1.5	<1	1	2	2	2	2	4	4
50–64	0									
65+	0									
2. MULTIPLE DX										
0–19 Years	49	7.2	181	1	1	2	5	18	58	58
20–34	76	3.8	20	1	1	3	4	7	20	>99
35–49	107	5.6	85	1	2	4	6	13	20	53
50–64	157	7.3	77	1	2	4	9	20	31	39
65+	188	6.6	75	1	2	3	8	14	22	51
TOTAL SINGLE DX	41	1.2	<1	1	1	1	1	1	2	5
TOTAL MULTIPLE DX	577	6.3	83	1	2	3	7	16	24	58
TOTAL										
0–19 Years	64	4.5	111	1	1	1	2	9	18	58
20–34	90	3.4	18	1	1	2	4	6	19	>99
35–49	119	5.2	78	1	1	2	5	12	20	53
50–64	157	7.3	77	1	2	4	9	20	31	39
65+	188	6.6	75	1	2	3	8	14	22	51
GRAND TOTAL	618	5.7	76	1	1	3	6	14	22	58

40.0: INC LYMPHATIC STRUCTURE

Type of Patients	Observed Patients	Avg. Stay	Vari-ance	Percentiles						
				10th	25th	50th	75th	90th	95th	99th
1. SINGLE DX										
0–19 Years	16	3.0	3	2	2	3	3	4	7	8
20–34	1	1.0	0	1	1	1	1	1	1	1
35–49	0									
50–64	0									
65+	0									
2. MULTIPLE DX										
0–19 Years	51	5.2	23	2	2	4	7	10	13	24
20–34	2	2.0	0	2	2	2	2	2	2	2
35–49	3	7.6	30	4	4	5	14	14	14	14
50–64	3	7.7	30	7	7	7	9	9	9	9
65+	14	5.7	56	1	2	4	6	9	31	31
TOTAL SINGLE DX	17	3.0	3	2	2	3	3	4	7	8
TOTAL MULTIPLE DX	73	5.4	26	2	2	4	7	10	14	24
TOTAL										
0–19 Years	67	4.8	20	2	2	3	5	9	13	24
20–34	3	1.7	<1	1	1	1	2	2	2	2
35–49	3	7.6	30	4	4	5	14	14	14	14
50–64	3	7.7	30	7	7	7	9	9	9	9
65+	14	5.7	56	1	2	4	6	9	31	31
GRAND TOTAL	90	5.0	23	2	2	4	6	9	13	24

LOS by Diagnosis and Operation, Western Region, 45th Edition

Western Region, October 2007–September 2008 Data, by Operation

40.1: LYMPHATIC DXTIC PX

Type of Patients	Observed Patients	Avg. Stay	Variance	Percentiles 10th	25th	50th	75th	90th	95th	99th
1. SINGLE DX										
0–19 Years	30	5.7	42	1	2	4	5	12	23	30
20–34	19	1.8	<1	1	1	2	2	4	4	4
35–49	56	1.6	<1	1	1	1	2	3	3	4
50–64	81	1.5	2	1	1	1	2	2	3	10
65+	44	1.5	1	1	1	1	2	3	3	7
2. MULTIPLE DX										
0–19 Years	176	9.4	89	1	3	7	12	21	24	59
20–34	315	8.1	88	1	3	6	10	17	22	49
35–49	735	6.1	51	1	2	4	8	14	21	34
50–64	1,287	6.2	59	1	2	4	8	15	20	43
65+	1,587	6.2	41	1	2	4	9	14	18	29
TOTAL SINGLE DX	230	2.4	12	1	1	1	2	5	7	23
TOTAL MULTIPLE DX	4,100	6.6	57	1	2	4	9	15	21	37
TOTAL										
0–19 Years	206	8.9	84	1	3	7	11	21	24	48
20–34	334	7.8	85	1	3	5	9	16	20	49
35–49	791	5.8	49	1	2	3	7	14	20	34
50–64	1,368	5.9	57	1	1	3	8	14	19	41
65+	1,631	6.1	40	1	1	4	9	14	18	28
GRAND TOTAL	4,330	6.4	55	1	2	4	8	15	20	36

40.11: LYMPHATIC STRUCT BIOPSY

Type of Patients	Observed Patients	Avg. Stay	Variance	Percentiles 10th	25th	50th	75th	90th	95th	99th
1. SINGLE DX										
0–19 Years	30	5.7	42	1	2	4	5	12	23	30
20–34	17	1.8	<1	1	1	2	2	4	4	4
35–49	54	1.6	<1	1	1	1	2	3	3	4
50–64	78	1.5	2	1	1	1	2	2	3	10
65+	44	1.5	1	1	1	1	2	3	3	7
2. MULTIPLE DX										
0–19 Years	173	9.4	90	1	3	7	12	21	24	59
20–34	314	8.1	88	1	3	6	10	17	22	49
35–49	708	6.2	52	1	2	4	8	14	21	34
50–64	1,239	6.4	60	1	2	4	8	15	21	43
65+	1,533	6.3	42	1	2	4	9	14	19	29
TOTAL SINGLE DX	223	2.4	13	1	1	1	2	5	7	23
TOTAL MULTIPLE DX	3,967	6.7	58	1	2	4	9	15	21	38
TOTAL										
0–19 Years	203	9.0	85	1	3	7	11	21	24	48
20–34	331	7.8	86	1	3	5	9	16	20	49
35–49	762	5.9	50	1	2	3	8	14	20	34
50–64	1,317	6.1	58	1	1	3	8	14	20	41
65+	1,577	6.2	41	1	2	4	9	14	18	29
GRAND TOTAL	4,190	6.5	56	1	2	4	9	15	21	36

40.2: SMP EXC LYMPHATIC STRUCT

Type of Patients	Observed Patients	Avg. Stay	Variance	Percentiles 10th	25th	50th	75th	90th	95th	99th
1. SINGLE DX										
0–19 Years	45	2.0	3	1	1	1	3	4	5	13
20–34	27	1.9	2	1	1	1	3	4	5	5
35–49	120	1.7	1	1	1	1	2	3	5	6
50–64	112	1.5	<1	1	1	1	2	2	4	5
65+	64	1.5	<1	1	1	1	2	2	3	4
2. MULTIPLE DX										
0–19 Years	58	7.9	78	1	2	5	11	15	22	49
20–34	155	5.1	43	1	1	3	6	12	18	39
35–49	619	2.9	11	1	1	2	3	6	9	18
50–64	1,173	2.5	18	1	1	1	2	5	8	21
65+	1,304	2.7	18	1	1	1	2	5	9	20
TOTAL SINGLE DX	368	1.7	2	1	1	1	2	3	4	6
TOTAL MULTIPLE DX	3,309	2.9	21	1	1	1	3	6	10	22
TOTAL										
0–19 Years	103	5.4	54	1	1	2	6	14	18	48
20–34	182	4.6	38	1	1	3	5	11	14	39
35–49	739	2.7	9	1	1	2	3	5	8	17
50–64	1,285	2.4	17	1	1	1	2	5	7	20
65+	1,368	2.6	17	1	1	1	2	5	8	20
GRAND TOTAL	3,677	2.8	19	1	1	1	3	6	9	21

40.21: EXC DEEP CERVICAL NODE

Type of Patients	Observed Patients	Avg. Stay	Variance	Percentiles 10th	25th	50th	75th	90th	95th	99th
1. SINGLE DX										
0–19 Years	9	1.9	<1	1	1	2	3	3	3	3
20–34	7	1.7	2	1	1	1	2	5	5	5
35–49	3	2.7	8	1	1	1	6	6	6	6
50–64	2	1.5	<1	1	1	1	2	2	2	2
65+	0									
2. MULTIPLE DX										
0–19 Years	18	5.8	17	1	2	5	8	10	15	15
20–34	25	5.1	21	1	1	4	7	10	12	20
35–49	33	5.3	44	1	1	3	8	16	22	24
50–64	46	5.0	53	1	1	3	5	11	22	40
65+	69	4.9	20	1	1	3	7	12	15	17
TOTAL SINGLE DX	21	1.9	2	1	1	2	2	3	5	6
TOTAL MULTIPLE DX	191	5.2	30	1	1	3	7	11	16	23
TOTAL										
0–19 Years	27	4.8	16	1	2	4	6	10	15	15
20–34	32	4.4	19	1	1	3	7	10	12	20
35–49	36	5.1	42	1	1	3	8	16	22	24
50–64	48	4.9	51	1	1	2	5	11	22	40
65+	69	4.9	20	1	1	3	7	12	15	17
GRAND TOTAL	212	4.8	28	1	1	3	7	11	15	23

LOS by Diagnosis and Operation, Western Region, 45th Edition

Western Region, October 2007–September 2008 Data, by Operation

40.29: SMP EXC LYMPHATIC NEC

Type of Patients	Observed Patients	Avg. Stay	Vari-ance	10th	25th	50th	75th	90th	95th	99th
1. SINGLE DX										
0–19 Years	32	2.0	4	1	1	1	2	5	5	13
20–34	6	2.7	2	1	1	3	3	5	5	5
35–49	13	2.3	3	1	1	1	3	5	6	6
50–64	12	1.6	<1	1	1	1	2	3	4	4
65+	12	1.6	<1	1	1	1	2	3	4	4
2. MULTIPLE DX										
0–19 Years	31	9.7	105	1	1	6	14	22	22	49
20–34	53	5.5	46	1	2	4	6	12	19	39
35–49	74	4.9	23	1	2	4	6	11	17	23
50–64	159	4.6	68	1	2	3	5	8	14	22
65+	140	4.8	35	1	2	3	6	10	15	31
TOTAL SINGLE DX	75	2.0	3	1	1	1	2	5	5	6
TOTAL MULTIPLE DX	457	5.4	55	1	2	3	6	12	18	39
TOTAL										
0–19 Years	63	5.4	62	1	1	2	5	15	22	49
20–34	59	5.2	42	1	2	4	5	12	19	39
35–49	87	4.5	21	1	1	3	5	11	17	23
50–64	171	4.4	64	1	1	3	5	8	12	22
65+	152	4.6	33	1	2	3	5	10	14	31
GRAND TOTAL	532	4.7	47	1	1	3	5	11	15	28

40.3: REGIONAL LYMPH NODE EXC

Type of Patients	Observed Patients	Avg. Stay	Vari-ance	10th	25th	50th	75th	90th	95th	99th
1. SINGLE DX										
0–19 Years	4	1.0	0	1	1	1	1	1	1	1
20–34	12	2.7	2	1	2	2	4	4	5	5
35–49	25	1.6	2	1	1	1	2	3	3	7
50–64	20	1.3	<1	1	1	1	1	2	4	4
65+	18	1.3	1	1	1	1	1	2	6	6
2. MULTIPLE DX										
0–19 Years	11	7.1	20	1	5	5	13	13	14	14
20–34	75	3.6	6	1	1	4	5	7	9	12
35–49	189	2.5	14	1	1	1	2	5	8	19
50–64	438	2.9	29	1	1	1	3	5	9	34
65+	393	2.5	7	1	1	1	3	6	8	16
TOTAL SINGLE DX	79	1.6	1	1	1	1	2	3	4	7
TOTAL MULTIPLE DX	1,106	2.8	18	1	1	1	3	6	8	16
TOTAL										
0–19 Years	15	5.8	22	1	1	5	8	13	13	14
20–34	87	3.5	5	1	1	3	5	7	7	12
35–49	214	2.4	12	1	1	1	2	5	7	12
50–64	458	2.9	28	1	1	1	3	5	8	34
65+	411	2.4	7	1	1	1	3	6	7	15
GRAND TOTAL	1,185	2.7	17	1	1	1	3	6	8	16

40.23: EXC AXILLARY LYMPH NODE

Type of Patients	Observed Patients	Avg. Stay	Vari-ance	10th	25th	50th	75th	90th	95th	99th
1. SINGLE DX										
0–19 Years	0									
20–34	11	1.4	<1	1	1	1	1	2	4	4
35–49	101	1.6	<1	1	1	1	2	3	3	5
50–64	95	1.5	<1	1	1	1	2	2	4	5
65+	50	1.4	<1	1	1	1	2	2	3	3
2. MULTIPLE DX										
0–19 Years	4	11.1	264	4	4	4	7	48	48	48
20–34	58	3.8	28	1	1	2	4	11	13	31
35–49	459	2.1	4	1	1	1	2	4	6	13
50–64	897	2.0	7	1	1	1	2	3	5	15
65+	1,009	2.0	9	1	1	1	2	3	5	15
TOTAL SINGLE DX	257	1.5	<1	1	1	1	2	3	3	5
TOTAL MULTIPLE DX	2,427	2.1	9	1	1	1	2	4	5	15
TOTAL										
0–19 Years	4	11.1	264	4	4	4	7	48	48	48
20–34	69	3.4	24	1	1	2	3	11	12	31
35–49	560	2.0	3	1	1	1	2	4	5	9
50–64	992	1.9	6	1	1	1	2	3	5	10
65+	1,059	2.0	9	1	1	1	2	3	5	15
GRAND TOTAL	2,684	2.0	8	1	1	1	2	3	5	14

40.24: EXC INGUINAL LYMPH NODE

Type of Patients	Observed Patients	Avg. Stay	Vari-ance	10th	25th	50th	75th	90th	95th	99th
1. SINGLE DX										
0–19 Years	4	2.7	4	1	1	1	4	5	5	5
20–34	2	2.5	4	1	1	2	4	4	4	4
35–49	3	3.0	1	3	3	3	3	3	3	3
50–64	1	3.0	0	3	3	3	3	3	3	3
65+	2	1.5	<1	1	1	1	2	2	2	2
2. MULTIPLE DX										
0–19 Years	5	5.5	54	1	2	2	2	22	22	22
20–34	19	7.6	105	1	1	5	10	16	45	45
35–49	50	5.0	16	2	1	4	6	11	14	18
50–64	60	3.8	14	1	1	2	4	10	12	16
65+	76	5.7	85	1	1	3	7	12	20	57
TOTAL SINGLE DX	12	2.3	2	1	1	2	3	4	5	5
TOTAL MULTIPLE DX	210	5.2	49	1	2	3	6	12	15	45
TOTAL										
0–19 Years	9	4.6	38	1	1	2	4	11	22	22
20–34	21	7.1	97	1	1	4	8	14	16	45
35–49	53	4.9	16	1	2	4	5	11	14	18
50–64	61	3.8	14	1	1	3	4	10	12	16
65+	78	5.6	83	1	1	3	6	12	20	57
GRAND TOTAL	222	5.0	47	1	2	3	6	11	14	45

LOS by Diagnosis and Operation, Western Region, 45th Edition

Western Region, October 2007–September 2008 Data, by Operation

40.4: RAD EXC CERV LYMPH NODE

Type of Patients	Observed Patients	Avg. Stay	Vari-ance	Percentiles						
				10th	25th	50th	75th	90th	95th	99th
1. SINGLE DX										
0–19 Years	5	2.1	<1	2	2	2	2	2	4	4
20–34	17	2.0	1	1	1	2	3	4	4	4
35–49	15	2.8	4	1	1	2	4	6	8	8
50–64	34	2.5	2	1	1	2	4	4	5	6
65+	19	2.1	3	1	1	1	2	5	8	8
2. MULTIPLE DX										
0–19 Years	28	4.4	13	1	2	3	7	9	13	13
20–34	104	2.6	3	1	1	3	3	5	7	8
35–49	267	3.2	25	1	1	3	3	6	7	22
50–64	719	3.2	9	1	1	3	4	7	9	17
65+	752	3.7	19	1	2	3	4	7	9	26
TOTAL SINGLE DX	90	2.3	2	1	1	2	3	4	5	8
TOTAL MULTIPLE DX	1,870	3.4	15	1	1	2	4	7	9	19
TOTAL										
0–19 Years	33	4.0	12	1	2	2	5	9	13	13
20–34	121	2.5	3	1	1	2	3	5	6	8
35–49	282	3.2	24	1	1	2	3	6	7	22
50–64	753	3.2	9	1	1	2	4	6	9	17
65+	771	3.6	19	1	2	3	4	7	9	26
GRAND TOTAL	1,960	3.3	15	1	1	2	4	6	9	19

40.41: UNILAT RAD NECK DISSECT

Type of Patients	Observed Patients	Avg. Stay	Vari-ance	Percentiles						
				10th	25th	50th	75th	90th	95th	99th
1. SINGLE DX										
0–19 Years	5	2.1	<1	2	2	2	2	2	4	4
20–34	16	2.0	1	1	1	2	3	4	4	4
35–49	13	2.4	3	1	1	2	3	4	6	6
50–64	29	2.5	2	1	1	2	3	4	5	6
65+	16	2.1	4	1	1	1	3	5	8	8
2. MULTIPLE DX										
0–19 Years	20	4.5	14	1	2	3	5	13	13	13
20–34	84	2.5	3	1	1	2	3	5	7	9
35–49	233	2.8	8	1	1	2	3	5	7	19
50–64	655	3.1	9	1	1	2	4	6	9	16
65+	685	3.5	16	1	2	3	4	6	9	25
TOTAL SINGLE DX	79	2.3	2	1	1	2	3	4	5	8
TOTAL MULTIPLE DX	1,677	3.2	12	1	1	2	4	6	9	18
TOTAL										
0–19 Years	25	4.0	13	1	1	2	4	9	13	13
20–34	100	2.4	3	1	1	2	3	5	7	9
35–49	246	2.8	8	1	1	2	3	5	7	19
50–64	684	3.1	8	1	1	2	4	6	9	16
65+	701	3.5	16	1	2	3	4	6	9	23
GRAND TOTAL	1,756	3.2	11	1	1	2	4	6	9	18

40.42: BILAT RAD NECK DISSECT

Type of Patients	Observed Patients	Avg. Stay	Vari-ance	Percentiles						
				10th	25th	50th	75th	90th	95th	99th
1. SINGLE DX										
0–19 Years	0									
20–34	1	2.0	0	2	2	2	2	2	2	2
35–49	1	3.0	0	3	3	3	3	3	3	3
50–64	0									
65+	2	2.0	0	2	2	2	2	2	2	2
2. MULTIPLE DX										
0–19 Years	6	4.2	8	1	1	4	7	7	7	7
20–34	18	3.1	2	1	2	3	4	5	6	6
35–49	25	4.4	22	2	2	3	4	7	13	24
50–64	48	4.3	21	1	2	4	4	10	16	24
65+	46	4.4	19	1	2	4	5	8	11	28
TOTAL SINGLE DX	4	2.3	<1	2	2	2	3	3	3	3
TOTAL MULTIPLE DX	143	4.2	17	1	2	3	5	7	11	24
TOTAL										
0–19 Years	6	4.2	8	1	1	4	7	7	7	7
20–34	19	3.0	2	1	2	3	4	5	6	6
35–49	26	4.3	22	2	2	3	4	7	13	24
50–64	48	4.3	21	1	2	4	4	10	16	24
65+	48	4.3	19	1	2	4	5	8	11	28
GRAND TOTAL	147	4.1	17	1	2	3	5	7	11	24

40.5: OTH RAD NODE DISSECTION

Type of Patients	Observed Patients	Avg. Stay	Vari-ance	Percentiles						
				10th	25th	50th	75th	90th	95th	99th
1. SINGLE DX										
0–19 Years	7	2.6	14	1	1	1	3	5	15	15
20–34	4	4.0	6	1	1	3	6	6	6	6
35–49	16	3.4	2	1	3	3	4	6	6	6
50–64	20	2.9	2	1	1	3	4	4	6	6
65+	8	2.3	1	1	1	2	3	4	4	4
2. MULTIPLE DX										
0–19 Years	15	7.7	44	3	4	5	7	21	21	21
20–34	75	4.8	8	2	3	4	6	8	9	17
35–49	176	4.0	8	1	2	3	5	7	9	16
50–64	338	4.3	22	1	1	3	5	8	10	18
65+	246	4.8	33	1	1	3	5	11	15	28
TOTAL SINGLE DX	55	3.0	5	1	1	3	4	5	6	15
TOTAL MULTIPLE DX	850	4.5	22	1	2	3	5	8	12	21
TOTAL										
0–19 Years	22	5.9	39	1	1	4	6	21	21	21
20–34	79	4.7	8	2	3	3	6	8	9	17
35–49	192	4.0	7	1	2	3	5	7	9	16
50–64	358	4.2	21	1	2	3	5	8	10	18
65+	254	4.7	32	1	1	3	5	11	15	28
GRAND TOTAL	905	4.4	21	1	2	3	5	8	12	21

LOS by Diagnosis and Operation, Western Region, 45th Edition

163

Western Region, October 2007–September 2008 Data, by Operation

40.51: RAD EXC AXILLARY NODES

Type of Patients	Observed Patients	Avg. Stay	Vari-ance	Percentiles						
				10th	25th	50th	75th	90th	95th	99th
1. SINGLE DX										
0–19 Years	0									
20–34	0									
35–49	2	1.5	<1	1	1	1	2	2	2	2
50–64	1	2.0	0	2	2	2	2	2	2	2
65+	4	1.8	<1	1	1	1	2	3	3	3
2. MULTIPLE DX										
0–19 Years	3	12.1	73	1	6	6	21	21	21	21
20–34	6	1.2	<1	1	1	1	1	2	2	2
35–49	23	1.4	<1	1	1	1	2	2	2	2
50–64	38	1.7	7	1	1	1	2	2	2	4
65+	53	2.2	9	1	1	2	2	4	8	18
TOTAL SINGLE DX	7	1.7	<1	1	1	2	2	3	3	3
TOTAL MULTIPLE DX	123	2.6	18	1	1	2	2	6	9	21
TOTAL										
0–19 Years	3	12.1	73	1	6	6	21	21	21	21
20–34	6	1.2	<1	1	1	1	1	2	2	2
35–49	25	1.4	<1	1	1	1	2	2	2	2
50–64	39	1.7	7	1	1	1	2	2	2	4
65+	57	2.1	9	1	1	2	2	4	8	18
GRAND TOTAL	130	2.5	17	1	1	1	2	4	9	21

40.52: RAD EXC PERIAORTIC NODES

Type of Patients	Observed Patients	Avg. Stay	Vari-ance	Percentiles						
				10th	25th	50th	75th	90th	95th	99th
1. SINGLE DX										
0–19 Years	0									
20–34	0									
35–49	3	4.0	<1	3	3	4	5	5	5	5
50–64	6	3.0	<1	2	2	3	4	4	4	4
65+	0									
2. MULTIPLE DX										
0–19 Years	2	4.0	2	3	3	3	5	5	5	5
20–34	16	5.4	5	3	4	5	8	9	10	10
35–49	34	4.4	4	2	3	4	5	7	8	11
50–64	87	4.7	7	2	3	4	5	8	11	15
65+	52	6.1	45	2	3	4	6	13	15	45
TOTAL SINGLE DX	9	3.3	1	2	3	3	4	5	5	5
TOTAL MULTIPLE DX	191	5.1	17	2	3	4	6	8	12	19
TOTAL										
0–19 Years	2	4.0	2	3	3	3	5	5	5	5
20–34	16	5.4	5	3	4	5	8	9	10	10
35–49	37	4.4	4	2	3	4	5	7	8	11
50–64	93	4.6	7	2	3	4	5	8	11	15
65+	52	6.1	45	2	3	4	6	13	15	45
GRAND TOTAL	200	5.0	16	2	3	4	6	8	12	19

40.53: RAD EXC ILIAC LYMPH NODE

Type of Patients	Observed Patients	Avg. Stay	Vari-ance	Percentiles						
				10th	25th	50th	75th	90th	95th	99th
1. SINGLE DX										
0–19 Years	0									
20–34	0									
35–49	0									
50–64	1	2.0	0	2	2	2	2	2	2	2
65+	2	2.0	2	1	1	3	3	3	3	3
2. MULTIPLE DX										
0–19 Years	1	4.0	0	4	4	4	4	4	4	4
20–34	5	4.4	5	3	3	3	5	8	8	8
35–49	30	3.9	9	1	3	3	4	6	7	17
50–64	63	5.2	67	1	2	3	5	9	11	63
65+	38	5.2	36	1	2	3	6	11	24	28
TOTAL SINGLE DX	3	2.0	<1	1	1	2	3	3	3	3
TOTAL MULTIPLE DX	137	4.9	43	1	2	3	5	8	13	28
TOTAL										
0–19 Years	1	4.0	0	4	4	4	4	4	4	4
20–34	5	4.4	5	3	3	3	5	8	8	8
35–49	30	3.9	9	1	2	3	4	6	7	17
50–64	64	5.1	66	1	2	3	5	9	11	63
65+	40	5.0	34	1	1	3	6	8	17	28
GRAND TOTAL	140	4.8	42	1	2	3	5	8	11	28

40.59: RAD EXC LYMPH NODE NEC

Type of Patients	Observed Patients	Avg. Stay	Vari-ance	Percentiles						
				10th	25th	50th	75th	90th	95th	99th
1. SINGLE DX										
0–19 Years	7	2.6	14	1	1	1	3	5	15	15
20–34	4	4.0	6	1	1	3	6	6	6	6
35–49	9	3.4	2	1	2	3	4	6	6	6
50–64	11	3.0	2	1	3	3	4	4	6	6
65+	1	3.0	0	3	3	3	3	3	3	3
2. MULTIPLE DX										
0–19 Years	8	5.3	16	3	3	4	5	8	17	17
20–34	45	5.1	9	3	3	5	6	7	9	17
35–49	70	4.8	10	2	3	4	5	9	14	16
50–64	115	4.6	15	2	3	4	5	8	9	15
65+	69	6.2	45	1	2	3	9	12	19	43
TOTAL SINGLE DX	32	3.1	7	1	1	3	4	6	6	15
TOTAL MULTIPLE DX	307	5.1	20	2	3	4	6	9	14	20
TOTAL										
0–19 Years	15	3.9	16	1	1	3	4	8	15	17
20–34	49	5.0	9	1	3	5	6	7	9	17
35–49	79	4.5	9	2	3	4	5	9	14	16
50–64	126	4.5	14	2	3	4	5	8	8	15
65+	70	6.1	44	1	2	3	9	12	19	43
GRAND TOTAL	339	4.9	19	2	3	4	5	9	13	20

Western Region, October 2007–September 2008 Data, by Operation

40.6: THORACIC DUCT OPERATIONS

Type of Patients	Observed Patients	Avg. Stay	Variance	Percentiles						
				10th	25th	50th	75th	90th	95th	99th
1. SINGLE DX										
0–19 Years	0									
20–34	0									
35–49	0									
50–64	0									
65+	0									
2. MULTIPLE DX										
0–19 Years	9	28.7	553	4	8	23	49	66	75	75
20–34	1	14.0	0	14	14	14	14	14	14	14
35–49	3	14.6	111	5	5	13	26	26	26	26
50–64	12	15.0	289	1	2	10	23	45	50	50
65+	8	18.9	496	3	11	12	17	73	73	73
TOTAL SINGLE DX	0									
TOTAL MULTIPLE DX	33	22.2	453	3	8	14	29	50	73	75
TOTAL										
0–19 Years	9	28.7	553	4	8	23	49	66	75	75
20–34	1	14.0	0	14	14	14	14	14	14	14
35–49	3	14.6	111	5	5	13	26	26	26	26
50–64	12	15.0	289	1	2	10	23	45	50	50
65+	8	18.9	496	3	11	12	17	73	73	73
GRAND TOTAL	33	22.2	453	3	8	14	29	50	73	75

41.0: BONE MARROW TRANSPLANT

Type of Patients	Observed Patients	Avg. Stay	Variance	Percentiles						
				10th	25th	50th	75th	90th	95th	99th
1. SINGLE DX										
0–19 Years	5	7.0	115	1	1	2	5	26	26	26
20–34	2	19.5	<1	19	19	20	20	20	20	20
35–49	3	7.0	107	1	1	1	1	19	19	19
50–64	6	1.2	<1	1	1	1	1	2	2	2
65+	5	4.4	57	1	1	1	1	18	18	18
2. MULTIPLE DX										
0–19 Years	296	38.1	356	18	27	36	54	76	>99	>99
20–34	216	26.8	186	17	19	23	31	46	59	>99
35–49	286	22.3	100	11	17	21	27	35	40	65
50–64	581	21.2	123	7	16	20	25	32	40	66
65+	203	19.9	114	8	15	20	23	26	41	64
TOTAL SINGLE DX	21	5.9	72	1	1	1	5	19	20	26
TOTAL MULTIPLE DX	1,582	28.2	275	14	19	25	36	57	76	>99
TOTAL										
0–19 Years	301	37.9	361	18	27	36	53	76	>99	>99
20–34	218	26.8	185	17	19	23	29	46	59	>99
35–49	289	22.1	102	10	17	21	27	35	40	65
50–64	587	21.0	126	7	16	20	25	32	40	66
65+	208	19.5	118	3	15	20	23	26	41	64
GRAND TOTAL	1,603	28.0	278	14	18	24	36	57	75	>99

40.9: LYMPHATIC STRUCT OPS NEC

Type of Patients	Observed Patients	Avg. Stay	Variance	Percentiles						
				10th	25th	50th	75th	90th	95th	99th
1. SINGLE DX										
0–19 Years	8	2.3	3	1	1	1	3	5	5	5
20–34	0									
35–49	0									
50–64	0									
65+	1	1.0	0	1	1	1	1	1	1	1
2. MULTIPLE DX										
0–19 Years	4	7.2	80	3	3	4	>99	>99	>99	>99
20–34	3	6.1	61	1	1	2	15	15	15	15
35–49	7	4.9	18	2	2	3	5	14	14	14
50–64	13	3.9	9	1	2	3	5	8	11	11
65+	20	6.0	39	1	2	3	8	20	21	21
TOTAL SINGLE DX	9	2.2	3	1	1	1	3	5	5	5
TOTAL MULTIPLE DX	47	5.6	37	1	2	3	8	26	>99	>99
TOTAL										
0–19 Years	12	4.2	37	1	1	3	5	>99	>99	>99
20–34	3	6.1	61	1	1	2	15	15	15	15
35–49	7	4.9	18	2	2	4	5	14	14	14
50–64	13	3.9	9	1	2	3	5	8	11	11
65+	21	5.8	38	1	2	3	8	15	20	21
GRAND TOTAL	56	4.7	30	1	2	3	5	20	>99	>99

41.03: ALLO MARROW TRANSPL NEC

Type of Patients	Observed Patients	Avg. Stay	Variance	Percentiles						
				10th	25th	50th	75th	90th	95th	99th
1. SINGLE DX										
0–19 Years	2	1.5	<1	1	1	2	2	2	2	2
20–34	0									
35–49	0									
50–64	0									
65+	1	1.0	0	1	1	1	1	1	1	1
2. MULTIPLE DX										
0–19 Years	66	46.4	252	31	36	49	58	>99	>99	>99
20–34	15	29.9	122	20	22	33	36	37	57	57
35–49	12	31.3	61	24	25	31	40	41	47	47
50–64	21	27.5	177	10	21	27	36	46	47	52
65+	6	24.7	182	1	22	26	30	42	42	42
TOTAL SINGLE DX	3	1.3	<1	1	1	1	2	2	2	2
TOTAL MULTIPLE DX	120	42.6	278	25	33	44	57	84	>99	>99
TOTAL										
0–19 Years	68	46.0	268	31	36	49	58	>99	>99	>99
20–34	15	29.9	122	20	22	33	36	37	57	57
35–49	12	31.3	61	24	25	31	40	41	47	47
50–64	21	27.5	177	10	21	27	36	46	47	52
65+	7	21.3	232	1	1	26	30	42	42	42
GRAND TOTAL	123	42.2	294	25	32	44	57	84	>99	>99

LOS by Diagnosis and Operation, Western Region, 45th Edition

Western Region, October 2007–September 2008 Data, by Operation

41.04: AUTLOG STEM CELL TRANSPL

Type of Patients	Observed Patients	Avg. Stay	Variance	Percentiles						
				10th	25th	50th	75th	90th	95th	99th
1. SINGLE DX										
0–19 Years	2	3.0	8	1	1	5	5	5	5	5
20–34	2	19.5	<1	19	19	20	20	20	20	20
35–49	1	19.0	0	19	19	19	19	19	19	19
50–64	1	1.0	0	1	1	1	1	1	1	1
65+	1	18.0	0	18	18	18	18	18	18	18
2. MULTIPLE DX										
0–19 Years	114	28.3	253	13	20	27	33	43	72	>99
20–34	94	20.7	20	17	18	20	23	26	26	40
35–49	148	18.5	52	8	15	18	21	26	33	37
50–64	350	19.8	57	14	16	19	22	28	32	49
65+	141	20.5	101	14	16	19	22	26	34	67
TOTAL SINGLE DX	7	11.9	81	1	1	18	19	20	20	20
TOTAL MULTIPLE DX	847	22.3	131	14	17	20	26	33	42	75
TOTAL										
0–19 Years	116	28.2	255	10	20	27	33	43	72	>99
20–34	96	20.6	20	17	18	20	23	26	26	40
35–49	149	18.5	52	12	15	18	21	26	33	37
50–64	351	19.7	58	14	16	19	22	28	32	49
65+	142	20.4	101	14	16	19	22	26	34	67
GRAND TOTAL	854	22.2	131	14	17	20	26	33	42	75

41.05: ALLO STEM CELL TRANSPL

Type of Patients	Observed Patients	Avg. Stay	Variance	Percentiles						
				10th	25th	50th	75th	90th	95th	99th
1. SINGLE DX										
0–19 Years	1	26.0	0	26	26	26	26	26	26	26
20–34	0									
35–49	2	1.0	0	1	1	1	1	1	1	1
50–64	5	1.2	<1	1	1	1	1	2	2	2
65+	3	1.0	0	1	1	1	1	1	1	1
2. MULTIPLE DX										
0–19 Years	61	40.7	412	19	31	38	50	81	86	>99
20–34	89	29.4	269	18	22	26	33	47	83	>99
35–49	101	26.2	119	18	22	25	32	40	47	>99
50–64	180	23.4	228	1	16	24	28	36	46	91
65+	40	18.7	186	1	2	22	25	34	54	55
TOTAL SINGLE DX	11	3.4	57	1	1	1	1	2	26	26
TOTAL MULTIPLE DX	471	28.6	303	5	21	26	36	51	81	>99
TOTAL										
0–19 Years	62	40.6	411	19	30	38	50	81	86	>99
20–34	89	29.4	269	18	22	26	33	47	83	>99
35–49	103	25.7	129	12	22	25	31	40	47	>99
50–64	185	22.8	235	1	15	24	28	36	46	91
65+	43	17.4	193	1	1	22	25	29	42	55
GRAND TOTAL	482	28.1	310	3	21	26	36	50	81	>99

41.1: PUNCTURE OF SPLEEN

Type of Patients	Observed Patients	Avg. Stay	Variance	Percentiles						
				10th	25th	50th	75th	90th	95th	99th
1. SINGLE DX										
0–19 Years	2	2.5	<1	2	2	3	3	3	3	3
20–34	1	3.0	0	3	3	3	3	3	3	3
35–49	0									
50–64	1	3.0	0	3	3	3	3	3	3	3
65+	0									
2. MULTIPLE DX										
0–19 Years	2	3.5	<1	3	3	3	4	4	4	4
20–34	5	11.8	118	5	6	7	10	31	31	31
35–49	2	9.6	111	2	2	17	17	17	17	17
50–64	4	5.5	8	2	5	6	6	9	9	9
65+	4	9.7	7	6	6	11	12	12	12	12
TOTAL SINGLE DX	4	2.8	<1	2	3	3	3	3	3	3
TOTAL MULTIPLE DX	17	8.6	49	2	5	6	10	17	31	31
TOTAL										
0–19 Years	4	3.0	<1	2	3	3	3	4	4	4
20–34	6	10.3	107	3	5	7	10	31	31	31
35–49	2	9.6	111	2	2	17	17	17	17	17
50–64	5	5.0	7	2	3	5	6	9	9	9
65+	4	9.7	7	6	6	11	12	12	12	12
GRAND TOTAL	21	7.5	45	2	3	6	10	12	17	31

41.2: SPLENOTOMY

Type of Patients	Observed Patients	Avg. Stay	Variance	Percentiles						
				10th	25th	50th	75th	90th	95th	99th
1. SINGLE DX										
0–19 Years	0									
20–34	0									
35–49	0									
50–64	0									
65+	0									
2. MULTIPLE DX										
0–19 Years	0									
20–34	2	7.5	40	3	3	8	12	12	12	12
35–49	1	8.0	0	8	8	8	8	8	8	8
50–64	2	15.0	383	1	1	15	29	29	29	29
65+	1	17.0	0	17	17	17	17	17	17	17
TOTAL SINGLE DX	0									
TOTAL MULTIPLE DX	6	11.7	106	1	3	8	17	29	29	29
TOTAL										
0–19 Years	0									
20–34	2	7.5	40	3	3	8	12	12	12	12
35–49	1	8.0	0	8	8	8	8	8	8	8
50–64	2	15.0	383	1	1	15	29	29	29	29
65+	1	17.0	0	17	17	17	17	17	17	17
GRAND TOTAL	6	11.7	106	1	3	8	17	29	29	29

LOS by Diagnosis and Operation, Western Region, 45th Edition

Western Region, October 2007–September 2008 Data, by Operation

41.3: MARROW & SPLEEN DXTIC PX

Type of Patients	Observed Patients	Avg. Stay	Variance	10th	25th	50th	75th	90th	95th	99th
1. SINGLE DX										
0–19 Years	86	4.6	10	1	2	4	6	9	11	16
20–34	17	6.0	104	1	2	3	6	7	45	45
35–49	12	3.9	28	1	1	3	5	5	20	20
50–64	10	3.2	4	1	2	3	4	7	7	7
65+	11	3.5	13	1	1	1	6	10	10	10
2. MULTIPLE DX										
0–19 Years	775	11.6	147	2	4	8	13	30	36	64
20–34	451	13.5	167	2	4	8	20	32	37	63
35–49	726	10.9	131	2	4	7	13	28	36	58
50–64	1,303	10.4	116	2	4	7	12	26	33	54
65+	2,653	8.7	64	3	4	6	10	17	24	43
TOTAL SINGLE DX	136	4.5	18	1	2	3	6	9	11	16
TOTAL MULTIPLE DX	5,908	10.3	111	2	4	7	12	24	33	51
TOTAL										
0–19 Years	861	11.0	139	2	4	7	13	27	36	64
20–34	468	13.2	166	2	4	8	19	32	37	63
35–49	738	10.8	130	2	4	7	13	28	36	58
50–64	1,313	10.3	115	2	4	7	12	26	33	54
65+	2,664	8.6	64	3	4	6	10	17	24	43
GRAND TOTAL	6,044	10.1	109	2	4	7	12	24	33	51

41.31: BONE MARROW BIOPSY

Type of Patients	Observed Patients	Avg. Stay	Variance	10th	25th	50th	75th	90th	95th	99th
1. SINGLE DX										
0–19 Years	86	4.6	10	1	2	4	6	9	11	16
20–34	17	6.0	104	1	2	3	6	7	45	45
35–49	12	3.9	28	1	1	3	5	5	20	20
50–64	10	3.2	4	1	2	3	4	7	7	7
65+	11	3.5	13	1	1	1	6	10	10	10
2. MULTIPLE DX										
0–19 Years	774	11.6	147	2	4	8	13	30	36	64
20–34	451	13.5	167	2	4	8	20	32	37	63
35–49	722	11.0	131	2	4	7	13	28	36	58
50–64	1,295	10.4	116	2	4	7	12	26	33	54
65+	2,648	8.7	64	3	4	6	10	17	24	43
TOTAL SINGLE DX	136	4.5	18	1	2	3	6	9	11	16
TOTAL MULTIPLE DX	5,890	10.3	112	2	4	7	12	24	33	51
TOTAL										
0–19 Years	860	11.0	139	2	4	7	13	27	36	64
20–34	468	13.2	166	2	4	8	19	32	37	63
35–49	734	11.0	131	2	4	7	13	28	36	58
50–64	1,305	10.4	116	2	4	7	12	26	33	54
65+	2,659	8.6	64	3	4	6	10	17	24	43
GRAND TOTAL	6,026	10.1	110	2	4	7	12	24	33	51

41.4: EXC/DESTR SPLENIC TISSUE

Type of Patients	Observed Patients	Avg. Stay	Variance	10th	25th	50th	75th	90th	95th	99th
1. SINGLE DX										
0–19 Years	8	2.0	<1	1	1	2	3	3	3	3
20–34	3	2.3		1	1	3	3	3	3	3
35–49	2	1.5	<1	1	1	2	2	2	2	2
50–64	0									
65+	0									
2. MULTIPLE DX										
0–19 Years	9	10.0	52	2	5	8	20	20	20	20
20–34	16	4.7	14	2	4	4	6	8	16	16
35–49	7	5.4	54	1	1	3	4	22	22	22
50–64	2	1.0	0	1	1	1	1	1	1	1
65+	6	5.9	41	1	1	3	14	14	14	14
TOTAL SINGLE DX	13	2.0	<1	1	1	2	3	3	3	3
TOTAL MULTIPLE DX	40	6.4	39	1	2	4	8	20	20	22
TOTAL										
0–19 Years	17	5.0	34	1	2	3	5	20	20	20
20–34	19	4.3	12	1	2	3	5	8	16	16
35–49	9	4.5	44	1	1	3	4	22	22	22
50–64	2	1.0	0	1	1	1	1	1	1	1
65+	6	5.9	41	1	1	3	14	14	14	14
GRAND TOTAL	53	4.7	28	1	1	3	5	14	20	22

41.5: TOTAL SPLENECTOMY

Type of Patients	Observed Patients	Avg. Stay	Variance	10th	25th	50th	75th	90th	95th	99th
1. SINGLE DX										
0–19 Years	44	2.3	3	1	1	2	3	4	6	7
20–34	27	2.6	4	1	1	2	3	5	6	10
35–49	23	2.5	2	1	2	3	3	4	5	5
50–64	12	3.6	5	1	2	3	6	7	7	7
65+	6	2.8	3	1	1	3	3	6	6	6
2. MULTIPLE DX										
0–19 Years	201	5.9	45	1	2	4	7	13	18	39
20–34	373	8.5	88	2	4	6	9	17	22	59
35–49	358	8.8	77	2	4	6	10	19	25	42
50–64	558	9.0	102	2	4	6	11	19	25	59
65+	476	9.8	93	2	4	7	12	20	28	53
TOTAL SINGLE DX	112	2.5	3	1	1	2	3	5	6	10
TOTAL MULTIPLE DX	1,966	8.6	85	2	3	6	10	18	24	52
TOTAL										
0–19 Years	245	5.1	38	1	2	3	5	11	18	34
20–34	400	8.1	84	2	3	6	9	15	22	59
35–49	381	8.4	74	2	3	6	10	19	25	42
50–64	570	8.9	101	2	3	6	11	19	24	59
65+	482	9.7	93	2	4	7	12	20	27	53
GRAND TOTAL	2,078	8.1	82	2	3	5	9	17	23	51

LOS by Diagnosis and Operation, Western Region, 45th Edition

Western Region, October 2007–September 2008 Data, by Operation

41.9: OTH SPLEEN & MARROW OPS

Type of Patients	Observed Patients	Avg. Stay	Vari-ance	Percentiles						
				10th	25th	50th	75th	90th	95th	99th
1. SINGLE DX										
0–19 Years	14	1.1	<1	1	1	1	1	1	1	4
20–34	6	1.3	1	1	1	1	1	1	5	5
35–49	1	1.0	0	1	1	1	1	1	1	1
50–64	4	1.0	0	1	1	1	1	1	1	1
65+	0									
2. MULTIPLE DX										
0–19 Years	50	4.3	33	1	1	2	5	10	18	25
20–34	38	6.5	40	1	3	5	8	15	19	32
35–49	25	6.6	36	2	4	5	8	10	12	32
50–64	16	9.5	60	2	4	5	14	23	23	23
65+	6	18.6	301	4	6	13	29	49	49	49
TOTAL SINGLE DX	25	1.1	<1	1	1	1	1	1	1	5
TOTAL MULTIPLE DX	135	6.0	51	1	1	4	7	15	23	32
TOTAL										
0–19 Years	64	3.5	26	1	1	1	4	7	18	25
20–34	44	5.2	35	1	1	3	6	15	19	32
35–49	26	6.4	36	1	1	5	8	10	12	32
50–64	20	7.8	60	1	1	4	10	22	23	23
65+	6	18.6	301	4	6	13	29	49	49	49
GRAND TOTAL	160	4.9	44	1	1	2	6	12	19	32

42.0: ESOPHAGOTOMY

Type of Patients	Observed Patients	Avg. Stay	Vari-ance	Percentiles						
				10th	25th	50th	75th	90th	95th	99th
1. SINGLE DX										
0–19 Years	2	2.5	4	1	1	1	4	4	4	4
20–34	0									
35–49	0									
50–64	0									
65+										
2. MULTIPLE DX										
0–19 Years	1	7.0	0	7	7	7	7	7	7	7
20–34	1	21.0	0	21	21	21	21	21	21	21
35–49	4	11.0	88	3	5	9	14	23	23	23
50–64	9	9.5	51	3	5	8	10	27	27	27
65+	2	9.6	143	1	1	18	18	18	18	18
TOTAL SINGLE DX	2	2.5	4	1	1	1	4	4	4	4
TOTAL MULTIPLE DX	17	10.4	60	3	5	8	14	23	27	27
TOTAL										
0–19 Years	3	4.0	9	1	1	4	7	7	7	7
20–34	1	21.0	0	21	21	21	21	21	21	21
35–49	4	11.0	88	3	4	9	14	23	23	23
50–64	9	9.5	51	3	5	8	10	27	27	27
65+	2	9.6	143	1	1	18	18	18	18	18
GRAND TOTAL	19	9.6	59	1	4	7	14	23	27	27

42.1: ESOPHAGOSTOMY

Type of Patients	Observed Patients	Avg. Stay	Vari-ance	Percentiles						
				10th	25th	50th	75th	90th	95th	99th
1. SINGLE DX										
0–19 Years	0									
20–34	0									
35–49	0									
50–64	0									
65+	0									
2. MULTIPLE DX										
0–19 Years	2	40.0	>999			70	70	70	70	70
20–34	0									
35–49	1	40.0	0	40	40	40	40	40	40	40
50–64	2	24.0	195	14	14	14	34	34	34	34
65+	2	18.0	280	6	6	18	30	30	30	30
TOTAL SINGLE DX	0									
TOTAL MULTIPLE DX	7	29.1	496	9	9	30	40	70	70	70
TOTAL										
0–19 Years	2	40.0	>999			70	70	70	70	70
20–34	0									
35–49	1	40.0	0	40	40	40	40	40	40	40
50–64	2	24.0	195	14	14	14	34	34	34	34
65+	2	18.0	280	6	6	18	30	30	30	30
GRAND TOTAL	7	29.1	496	9	9	30	40	70	70	70

42.2: ESOPHAGEAL DXTIC PX

Type of Patients	Observed Patients	Avg. Stay	Vari-ance	Percentiles						
				10th	25th	50th	75th	90th	95th	99th
1. SINGLE DX										
0–19 Years	124	1.2	<1	1	1	1	1	2	2	3
20–34	1	1.0	0	1	1	1	1	1	1	1
35–49	3	1.3	<1	1	1	1	2	2	3	3
50–64	3	1.7	<1	1	1	1	3	3	3	3
65+	4	1.0	0	1	1	1	1	1	1	1
2. MULTIPLE DX										
0–19 Years	109	4.3	26	1	1	2	5	11	17	23
20–34	24	4.2	31	1	1	3	5	8	13	29
35–49	61	5.7	66	1	2	3	6	10	15	55
50–64	119	5.7	36	1	2	4	7	11	18	29
65+	195	6.1	25	1	3	5	8	14	16	24
TOTAL SINGLE DX	135	1.2	<1	1	1	1	1	2	2	3
TOTAL MULTIPLE DX	508	5.2	32	1	1	4	7	12	16	28
TOTAL										
0–19 Years	233	2.7	15	1	1	2	2	6	11	20
20–34	25	4.1	30	1	1	3	4	8	13	29
35–49	64	5.5	64	1	2	3	6	10	15	55
50–64	122	5.6	36	1	2	4	7	10	17	29
65+	199	6.0	25	1	2	5	8	13	16	23
GRAND TOTAL	643	4.0	26	1	1	2	5	10	15	24

LOS by Diagnosis and Operation, Western Region, 45th Edition

Western Region, October 2007–September 2008 Data, by Operation

42.23: ESOPHAGOSCOPY NEC

Type of Patients	Observed Patients	Avg. Stay	Vari-ance	10th	25th	50th	75th	90th	95th	99th
1. SINGLE DX										
0–19 Years	120	1.2	<1	1	1	1	1	2	2	3
20–34	1	1.0	0	1	1	1	1	1	1	1
35–49	3	1.3	<1	1	1	1	2	2	2	2
50–64	2	2.0	2	1	1	1	3	3	3	3
65+	4	1.0	0	1	1	1	1	1	1	1
2. MULTIPLE DX										
0–19 Years	99	3.9	25	1	1	2	5	10	17	23
20–34	20	4.6	36	1	1	3	5	8	13	29
35–49	45	5.9	84	1	2	3	6	10	19	55
50–64	86	4.9	21	1	2	4	7	9	14	29
65+	158	6.2	25	1	3	5	8	14	16	23
TOTAL SINGLE DX	130	1.2	<1	1	1	1	1	2	2	3
TOTAL MULTIPLE DX	408	4.9	30	1	1	3	6	11	16	24
TOTAL										
0–19 Years	219	2.4	13	1	1	1	2	5	9	23
20–34	21	4.4	35	1	1	3	5	8	13	29
35–49	48	5.6	80	1	2	3	6	10	19	55
50–64	88	4.8	21	1	2	4	7	9	14	29
65+	162	6.0	25	1	2	5	8	13	16	23
GRAND TOTAL	538	3.7	23	1	1	2	5	9	14	23

42.24: CLOSED ESOPHAGEAL BIOPSY

Type of Patients	Observed Patients	Avg. Stay	Vari-ance	10th	25th	50th	75th	90th	95th	99th
1. SINGLE DX										
0–19 Years	0									
20–34	0									
35–49	0									
50–64	0									
65+										
2. MULTIPLE DX										
0–19 Years	7	8.7	29	2	2	8	12	16	16	16
20–34	3	2.3	2	1	1	2	4	4	4	4
35–49	14	4.5	13	1	3	4	5	8	15	15
50–64	26	7.1	48	1	3	6	7	16	20	34
65+	34	5.7	30	1	2	4	8	14	15	27
TOTAL SINGLE DX	0									
TOTAL MULTIPLE DX	84	6.4	33	1	2	5	8	15	16	34
TOTAL										
0–19 Years	7	8.7	29	2	2	8	12	16	16	16
20–34	3	2.3	2	1	1	2	4	4	4	4
35–49	14	4.5	13	1	2	4	5	8	15	15
50–64	26	7.1	48	1	3	6	7	16	20	34
65+	34	5.7	30	1	2	4	8	14	15	27
GRAND TOTAL	84	6.4	33	1	2	5	8	15	16	34

42.3: EXC/DESTR ESOPH LES/TISS

Type of Patients	Observed Patients	Avg. Stay	Vari-ance	10th	25th	50th	75th	90th	95th	99th
1. SINGLE DX										
0–19 Years	6	1.9	<1	1	1	2	3	3	3	3
20–34	1	1.0	0	1	1	1	1	1	1	1
35–49	3	4.7	5	2	2	6	6	6	6	6
50–64	7	2.0	<1	1	1	2	3	3	3	3
65+	5	1.6	<1	1	1	1	2	3	3	3
2. MULTIPLE DX										
0–19 Years	44	6.7	121	1	2	2	6	15	44	49
20–34	239	4.4	30	1	2	3	5	8	11	18
35–49	1,566	4.6	16	2	3	4	5	8	11	22
50–64	2,416	4.8	17	2	3	4	5	8	12	22
65+	1,312	5.1	21	2	3	4	6	9	12	20
TOTAL SINGLE DX	22	2.2	2	1	1	2	3	3	6	6
TOTAL MULTIPLE DX	5,577	4.8	21	2	3	4	5	8	12	23
TOTAL										
0–19 Years	50	6.2	112	1	2	2	6	11	44	49
20–34	240	4.4	30	1	2	3	5	8	11	18
35–49	1,569	4.6	16	2	3	4	5	8	11	22
50–64	2,423	4.8	17	2	3	4	5	8	12	22
65+	1,317	5.0	21	2	3	4	6	9	12	20
GRAND TOTAL	5,599	4.8	21	2	3	4	5	8	12	23

42.33: ENDO EXC/DESTR ESOPH LES

Type of Patients	Observed Patients	Avg. Stay	Vari-ance	10th	25th	50th	75th	90th	95th	99th
1. SINGLE DX										
0–19 Years	2	1.2	<1	1	1	1	1	2	2	2
20–34	1	1.0	0	1	1	1	1	1	1	1
35–49	2	4.0	8	2	2	4	6	6	6	6
50–64	4	1.8	<1	1	1	1	2	3	3	3
65+	4	1.8	<1	1	1	1	2	3	3	3
2. MULTIPLE DX										
0–19 Years	38	6.6	127	1	2	2	6	15	44	49
20–34	235	4.3	29	1	2	3	5	7	11	17
35–49	1,551	4.6	16	2	3	4	5	8	11	22
50–64	2,382	4.8	17	2	3	4	5	8	12	22
65+	1,250	4.8	12	2	3	4	6	9	11	18
TOTAL SINGLE DX	13	1.8	2	1	1	1	2	3	6	6
TOTAL MULTIPLE DX	5,456	4.8	19	2	3	4	5	8	11	22
TOTAL										
0–19 Years	40	6.4	123	1	2	2	6	11	44	49
20–34	236	4.3	29	1	2	3	5	7	11	17
35–49	1,553	4.6	16	2	3	4	5	8	11	22
50–64	2,386	4.8	17	2	3	4	5	8	12	22
65+	1,254	4.8	12	2	3	4	6	9	11	18
GRAND TOTAL	5,469	4.8	19	2	3	4	5	8	11	22

LOS by Diagnosis and Operation, Western Region, 45th Edition

Western Region, October 2007–September 2008 Data, by Operation

42.4: EXCISION OF ESOPHAGUS

Type of Patients	Observed Patients	Avg. Stay	Variance	Percentiles						
				10th	25th	50th	75th	90th	95th	99th
1. SINGLE DX										
0–19 Years	1	7.0	0	7	7	7	7	7	7	7
20–34	0									
35–49	1	8.0	0	8	8	8	8	8	8	8
50–64	1	5.0	0	5	5	5	5	5	5	5
65+	0									
2. MULTIPLE DX										
0–19 Years	9	13.3	34	8	8	13	18	18	23	30
20–34	6	9.7	5	6	9	9	11	12	12	12
35–49	38	12.4	44	7	8	10	16	21	26	35
50–64	230	13.6	89	7	8	11	15	24	29	45
65+	215	16.9	185	7	9	12	19	30	47	70
TOTAL SINGLE DX	**3**	**6.7**	**2**	**5**	**5**	**7**	**8**	**8**	**8**	**8**
TOTAL MULTIPLE DX	**498**	**14.9**	**126**	**7**	**9**	**11**	**16**	**27**	**35**	**63**
TOTAL										
0–19 Years	10	13.0	34	8	8	11	18	18	23	30
20–34	6	9.7	5	6	9	9	11	12	12	12
35–49	39	12.3	44	7	8	10	16	21	26	35
50–64	231	13.6	89	7	8	11	15	24	29	45
65+	215	16.9	185	7	9	12	19	30	47	70
GRAND TOTAL	**501**	**14.8**	**125**	**7**	**9**	**11**	**16**	**27**	**35**	**63**

42.42: TOTAL ESOPHAGECTOMY

Type of Patients	Observed Patients	Avg. Stay	Variance	Percentiles						
				10th	25th	50th	75th	90th	95th	99th
1. SINGLE DX										
0–19 Years	0									
20–34	0									
35–49	0									
50–64	0									
65+	0									
2. MULTIPLE DX										
0–19 Years	1	11.0	0	11	11	11	11	11	11	11
20–34	2	11.5	<1	11	11	12	12	12	12	12
35–49	14	14.4	41	7	9	14	21	21	26	26
50–64	69	13.0	42	8	8	11	16	24	29	33
65+	76	16.4	158	8	10	12	18	30	42	70
TOTAL SINGLE DX	**0**									
TOTAL MULTIPLE DX	**162**	**14.7**	**96**	**8**	**9**	**11**	**16**	**28**	**31**	**63**
TOTAL										
0–19 Years	1	11.0	0	11	11	11	11	11	11	11
20–34	2	11.5	<1	11	11	12	12	12	12	12
35–49	14	14.4	41	7	9	14	21	21	26	26
50–64	69	13.0	42	8	8	11	16	24	29	33
65+	76	16.4	158	8	10	12	18	30	42	70
GRAND TOTAL	**162**	**14.7**	**96**	**8**	**9**	**11**	**16**	**28**	**31**	**63**

42.41: PARTIAL ESOPHAGECTOMY

Type of Patients	Observed Patients	Avg. Stay	Variance	Percentiles						
				10th	25th	50th	75th	90th	95th	99th
1. SINGLE DX										
0–19 Years	1	7.0	0	7	7	7	7	7	7	7
20–34	0									
35–49	1	8.0	0	8	8	8	8	8	8	8
50–64	1	5.0	0	5	5	5	5	5	5	5
65+	0									
2. MULTIPLE DX										
0–19 Years	8	13.8	41	8	8	13	18	23	30	30
20–34	4	8.8	4	6	9	9	11	11	11	11
35–49	24	11.3	44	7	8	8	11	16	26	35
50–64	147	14.3	117	7	8	11	16	26	33	55
65+	132	17.4	209	7	10	12	20	32	53	72
TOTAL SINGLE DX	**3**	**6.7**	**2**	**5**	**5**	**7**	**8**	**8**	**8**	**8**
TOTAL MULTIPLE DX	**315**	**15.3**	**147**	**7**	**9**	**11**	**17**	**28**	**39**	**66**
TOTAL										
0–19 Years	9	13.4	41	7	8	13	18	23	30	30
20–34	4	8.8	4	6	9	9	11	11	11	11
35–49	25	11.1	43	7	8	8	11	16	26	35
50–64	148	14.2	117	7	8	11	16	26	33	55
65+	132	17.4	209	7	10	12	20	32	53	72
GRAND TOTAL	**318**	**15.2**	**146**	**7**	**9**	**11**	**17**	**28**	**39**	**66**

42.5: INTRATHOR ESOPH ANAST

Type of Patients	Observed Patients	Avg. Stay	Variance	Percentiles						
				10th	25th	50th	75th	90th	95th	99th
1. SINGLE DX										
0–19 Years	0									
20–34	0									
35–49	0									
50–64	0									
65+	0									
2. MULTIPLE DX										
0–19 Years	5	15.7	211	5	7	17	22	>99	>99	>99
20–34	1	37.0	0	37	37	37	37	37	37	37
35–49	8	22.7	355	3	11	13	41	60	60	60
50–64	15	18.4	323	8	9	12	20	27	80	80
65+	13	14.6	57	8	10	13	17	21	35	35
TOTAL SINGLE DX	**0**									
TOTAL MULTIPLE DX	**42**	**17.6**	**224**	**7**	**8**	**14**	**22**	**60**	**>99**	**>99**
TOTAL										
0–19 Years	5	15.7	211	5	7	17	22	>99	>99	>99
20–34	1	37.0	0	37	37	37	37	37	37	37
35–49	8	22.7	355	3	11	13	41	60	60	60
50–64	15	18.4	323	8	9	12	20	27	80	80
65+	13	14.6	57	8	10	13	17	21	35	35
GRAND TOTAL	**42**	**17.6**	**224**	**7**	**8**	**14**	**22**	**60**	**>99**	**>99**

LOS by Diagnosis and Operation, Western Region, 45th Edition

Western Region, October 2007–September 2008 Data, by Operation

42.8: OTHER ESOPHAGEAL REPAIR

Type of Patients	Observed Patients	Avg. Stay	Vari- ance	10th	25th	50th	75th	90th	95th	99th
1. SINGLE DX										
0–19 Years	0									
20–34	0									
35–49	1	3.0	0	3	3	3	3	3	3	3
50–64	1	2.0	0	2	2	2	2	2	2	2
65+	0									
2. MULTIPLE DX										
0–19 Years	23	22.1	413	4	12	16	50	95	>99	>99
20–34	15	20.4	545	3	5	7	38	67	68	68
35–49	34	12.0	123	2	4	8	18	27	35	46
50–64	90	10.0	87	2	3	8	14	26	33	>99
65+	129	10.6	99	1	4	7	15	20	30	44
TOTAL SINGLE DX	2	2.5	<1	2	2	3	3	3	3	3
TOTAL MULTIPLE DX	291	12.4	171	2	4	9	16	30	47	>99
TOTAL										
0–19 Years	23	22.1	413	4	12	16	50	95	>99	>99
20–34	15	20.4	545	3	5	7	38	67	68	68
35–49	35	11.8	122	2	4	7	18	27	35	46
50–64	91	9.9	87	2	4	7	14	26	33	>99
65+	129	10.6	99	1	4	7	15	20	30	44
GRAND TOTAL	293	12.4	171	2	4	9	16	29	47	>99

42.81: INSERT PERM TUBE ESOPH

Type of Patients	Observed Patients	Avg. Stay	Vari- ance	10th	25th	50th	75th	90th	95th	99th
1. SINGLE DX										
0–19 Years	0									
20–34	0									
35–49	0									
50–64	0									
65+	0									
2. MULTIPLE DX										
0–19 Years	3	5.8	24	3	4	4	4	16	16	16
20–34	2	2.0	2	1	1	1	3	3	3	3
35–49	16	10.3	97	1	4	7	17	27	35	35
50–64	47	6.1	33	2	2	4	9	14	15	28
65+	73	7.8	47	2	4	6	11	15	17	44
TOTAL SINGLE DX	0									
TOTAL MULTIPLE DX	141	7.4	48	1	3	5	9	15	18	35
TOTAL										
0–19 Years	3	5.8	24	3	4	4	4	16	16	16
20–34	2	2.0	2	1	1	1	3	3	3	3
35–49	16	10.3	97	1	4	7	17	27	35	35
50–64	47	6.1	33	2	2	4	9	14	15	28
65+	73	7.8	47	2	4	6	11	15	17	44
GRAND TOTAL	141	7.4	48	1	3	5	9	15	18	35

42.6: ANTESTERNAL ESOPH ANAST

Type of Patients	Observed Patients	Avg. Stay	Vari- ance	10th	25th	50th	75th	90th	95th	99th
1. SINGLE DX										
0–19 Years	0									
20–34	0									
35–49	0									
50–64	0									
65+	0									
2. MULTIPLE DX										
0–19 Years	3	14.5	<1	13	14	15	15	15	15	15
20–34	0									
35–49	1	42.0	0	42	42	42	42	42	42	42
50–64	0									
65+	2	12.0	8	10	10	12	14	14	14	14
TOTAL SINGLE DX	0									
TOTAL MULTIPLE DX	6	17.0	89	10	14	15	15	42	42	42
TOTAL										
0–19 Years	3	14.5	<1	13	14	15	15	15	15	15
20–34	0									
35–49	1	42.0	0	42	42	42	42	42	42	42
50–64	0									
65+	2	12.0	8	10	10	12	14	14	14	14
GRAND TOTAL	6	17.0	89	10	14	15	15	42	42	42

42.7: ESOPHAGOMYOTOMY

Type of Patients	Observed Patients	Avg. Stay	Vari- ance	10th	25th	50th	75th	90th	95th	99th
1. SINGLE DX										
0–19 Years	7	2.2	2	1	1	2	4	4	4	4
20–34	12	2.8	4	1	1	3	4	4	8	8
35–49	13	2.9	7	1	2	2	2	6	10	10
50–64	11	2.3	3	1	2	2	2	2	7	7
65+	1	3.0	0	3	3	3	3	3	3	3
2. MULTIPLE DX										
0–19 Years	19	2.9	3	2	2	2	4	7	7	>99
20–34	47	4.1	24	1	1	2	5	10	11	27
35–49	84	4.3	88	1	1	2	3	8	12	84
50–64	121	2.9	5	1	1	2	4	6	7	11
65+	94	5.0	33	2	2	3	6	11	14	35
TOTAL SINGLE DX	44	2.6	4	1	1	2	3	4	7	10
TOTAL MULTIPLE DX	365	3.9	34	1	2	2	4	7	11	28
TOTAL										
0–19 Years	26	2.7	2	1	2	2	4	4	7	>99
20–34	59	3.8	20	1	1	2	4	8	11	27
35–49	97	4.1	78	1	1	2	3	8	12	84
50–64	132	2.8	5	1	2	2	4	6	7	11
65+	95	5.0	33	1	2	3	6	11	14	35
GRAND TOTAL	409	3.7	30	1	2	2	4	7	11	27

LOS by Diagnosis and Operation, Western Region, 45th Edition

Western Region, October 2007–September 2008 Data, by Operation

42.9: OTHER ESOPHAGEAL OPS

Type of Patients	Observed Patients	Avg. Stay	Vari-ance	10th	25th	50th	75th	90th	95th	99th
1. SINGLE DX										
0–19 Years	10	1.9	3	1	1	1	3	3	7	7
20–34	1	1.0	0	1	1	1	1	1	1	1
35–49	1	1.0	0	1	1	1	1	1	1	1
50–64	2	1.0	0	1	1	1	1	1	1	1
65+	1	1.0		1	1	1	1	1	1	1
2. MULTIPLE DX										
0–19 Years	71	3.3	15	1	1	2	4	8	13	19
20–34	55	5.1	32	1	2	3	5	10	22	29
35–49	141	4.4	11	1	2	3	5	10	12	14
50–64	375	5.3	28	1	2	4	7	10	14	27
65+	1,073	5.2	20	1	2	4	7	10	14	22
TOTAL SINGLE DX	15	1.7	2	1	1	1	2	3	3	7
TOTAL MULTIPLE DX	1,715	5.0	21	1	2	4	6	10	13	22
TOTAL										
0–19 Years	81	3.2	14	1	1	2	4	7	13	19
20–34	56	5.0	32	1	2	3	5	10	22	29
35–49	142	4.4	11	1	2	5	5	10	12	14
50–64	377	5.2	28	1	2	4	7	10	14	27
65+	1,074	5.2	20	1	2	4	7	10	14	22
GRAND TOTAL	1,730	4.9	21	1	2	4	6	10	13	22

42.92: ESOPHAGEAL DILATION

Type of Patients	Observed Patients	Avg. Stay	Vari-ance	10th	25th	50th	75th	90th	95th	99th
1. SINGLE DX										
0–19 Years	10	1.9	3	1	1	1	3	3	7	7
20–34	1	1.0	0	1	1	1	1	1	1	1
35–49	1	1.0	0	1	1	1	1	1	1	1
50–64	2	1.0	0	1	1	1	1	1	1	1
65+	0									
2. MULTIPLE DX										
0–19 Years	71	3.3	15	1	1	2	4	8	13	19
20–34	55	5.1	32	1	2	3	5	10	22	29
35–49	135	4.4	12	1	2	3	5	10	12	14
50–64	362	5.3	29	1	2	4	7	10	14	27
65+	1,067	5.3	20	1	2	4	7	10	14	22
TOTAL SINGLE DX	14	1.8	2	1	1	1	2	3	3	7
TOTAL MULTIPLE DX	1,690	5.0	22	1	2	4	6	10	13	22
TOTAL										
0–19 Years	81	3.2	14	1	1	2	4	7	13	19
20–34	56	5.0	32	1	2	3	5	10	22	29
35–49	136	4.4	12	1	2	3	5	10	13	14
50–64	364	5.3	28	1	2	4	7	10	14	27
65+	1,067	5.3	20	1	2	4	7	10	14	22
GRAND TOTAL	1,704	5.0	21	1	2	4	6	10	13	22

43.0: GASTROTOMY

Type of Patients	Observed Patients	Avg. Stay	Vari-ance	10th	25th	50th	75th	90th	95th	99th
1. SINGLE DX										
0–19 Years	1	4.0	0	4	4	4	4	4	4	4
20–34	1	4.0	0	4	4	4	4	4	4	4
35–49	0									
50–64	1	2.0	0	2	2	2	2	2	2	2
65+	0									
2. MULTIPLE DX										
0–19 Years	16	18.1	559	4	5	9	14	34	84	84
20–34	15	10.3	54	4	5	7	10	23	23	23
35–49	29	9.6	93	2	4	6	11	23	36	42
50–64	32	9.8	61	2	4	7	13	21	23	33
65+	29	14.3	176	4	8	10	16	27	34	72
TOTAL SINGLE DX	3	3.7	<1	2	4	4	4	4	4	4
TOTAL MULTIPLE DX	121	13.0	235	3	5	9	14	23	34	84
TOTAL										
0–19 Years	17	16.8	524	4	4	9	14	34	84	84
20–34	16	10.0	53	4	5	7	10	23	23	23
35–49	29	9.6	93	2	4	6	11	23	36	42
50–64	33	9.6	61	2	4	7	13	21	23	33
65+	29	14.3	176	4	8	10	16	27	34	72
GRAND TOTAL	124	12.6	229	3	4	8	14	23	34	84

43.1: GASTROSTOMY

Type of Patients	Observed Patients	Avg. Stay	Vari-ance	10th	25th	50th	75th	90th	95th	99th
1. SINGLE DX										
0–19 Years	22	2.4	13	1	1	2	2	4	7	23
20–34	1	13.0	0	13	13	13	13	13	13	13
35–49	4	1.8	<1	1	1	1	2	3	2	2
50–64	15	2.7	23	1	1	1	1	3	20	20
65+	8	1.6	2	1	1	1	1	5	5	5
2. MULTIPLE DX										
0–19 Years	703	8.3	154	1	2	3	10	22	32	88
20–34	143	12.2	159	2	4	9	15	29	35	53
35–49	447	11.3	122	2	4	8	14	25	33	51
50–64	1,376	10.7	112	2	4	8	13	22	32	60
65+	7,310	10.5	53	4	6	9	13	19	24	36
TOTAL SINGLE DX	50	2.5	14	1	1	2	2	4	7	23
TOTAL MULTIPLE DX	9,979	10.2	81	2	5	8	13	20	26	46
TOTAL										
0–19 Years	725	8.2	151	1	2	3	10	22	32	84
20–34	144	12.2	158	2	4	9	15	29	35	53
35–49	451	11.3	122	2	4	8	14	25	33	51
50–64	1,391	10.6	112	2	4	8	13	22	32	60
65+	7,318	10.5	53	4	6	9	13	19	24	36
GRAND TOTAL	10,029	10.2	81	2	5	8	13	20	26	46

172

Western Region, October 2007–September 2008 Data, by Operation

43.11: PEG

Type of Patients	Observed Patients	Avg. Stay	Variance	10th	25th	50th	75th	90th	95th	99th
1. SINGLE DX										
0–19 Years	14	1.6	<1	1	1	2	2	2	2	2
20–34	1	13.0	0	13	13	13	13	13	13	13
35–49	2	2.0	0	2	2	2	2	2	2	2
50–64	13	2.9	27	1	1	1	2	3	20	20
65+	7	1.1	<1	1	1	1	1	2	2	2
2. MULTIPLE DX										
0–19 Years	434	7.6	132	1	1	3	10	20	29	89
20–34	124	12.1	171	2	4	9	14	33	37	53
35–49	393	11.5	126	2	4	8	15	25	34	77
50–64	1,269	10.7	113	2	4	8	13	23	32	60
65+	7,100	10.5	53	4	6	9	13	19	24	37
TOTAL SINGLE DX	37	2.1	10	1	1	2	2	2	3	20
TOTAL MULTIPLE DX	9,320	10.3	75	2	5	8	13	20	26	43
TOTAL										
0–19 Years	448	7.5	130	1	1	3	10	20	29	89
20–34	125	12.1	170	2	4	9	14	33	37	53
35–49	395	11.5	126	2	4	8	14	25	34	77
50–64	1,282	10.7	112	2	4	8	13	22	32	60
65+	7,107	10.5	53	4	6	9	13	19	24	37
GRAND TOTAL	9,357	10.2	75	2	5	8	13	20	26	43

43.19: GASTROSTOMY NEC

Type of Patients	Observed Patients	Avg. Stay	Variance	10th	25th	50th	75th	90th	95th	99th
1. SINGLE DX										
0–19 Years	8	4.0	39	1	1	2	4	7	23	23
20–34	0									
35–49	2	1.5	<1	1	1	1	2	2	2	2
50–64	2	1.5	<1	1	1	1	2	2	2	2
65+	1	5.0	0	5	5	5	5	5	5	5
2. MULTIPLE DX										
0–19 Years	269	9.6	189	1	2	3	12	29	47	73
20–34	19	12.3	74	1	6	10	19	26	32	32
35–49	54	10.2	94	1	3	8	13	20	28	50
50–64	107	10.0	109	2	3	7	13	19	32	41
65+	210	9.3	42	2	5	8	13	18	21	27
TOTAL SINGLE DX	13	3.5	28	1	1	2	4	7	23	23
TOTAL MULTIPLE DX	659	9.6	142	1	2	6	13	22	32	69
TOTAL										
0–19 Years	277	9.4	187	1	2	3	12	29	47	73
20–34	19	12.3	74	1	6	10	19	26	32	32
35–49	56	9.9	93	1	3	8	13	20	28	50
50–64	109	9.8	108	2	3	7	12	19	32	41
65+	211	9.3	42	2	5	8	13	18	21	27
GRAND TOTAL	672	9.5	141	1	2	5	13	22	32	69

43.3: PYLOROMYOTOMY

Type of Patients	Observed Patients	Avg. Stay	Variance	10th	25th	50th	75th	90th	95th	99th
1. SINGLE DX										
0–19 Years	866	2.0	<1	1	1	2	2	3	4	5
20–34	0									
35–49	0									
50–64	0									
65+	0									
2. MULTIPLE DX										
0–19 Years	778	3.4	19	1	2	2	4	6	8	21
20–34										
35–49	1	1.0	0	1	1	1	1	1	1	1
50–64	4	13.0	145	5	8	8	8	31	31	31
65+	2	22.5	4	21	21	24	24	24	24	24
TOTAL SINGLE DX	866	2.0	<1	1	1	2	2	3	4	5
TOTAL MULTIPLE DX	785	3.4	20	1	2	2	4	6	9	28
TOTAL										
0–19 Years	1,644	2.6	10	1	2	2	3	4	6	13
20–34	0									
35–49	1	1.0	0	1	1	1	1	1	1	1
50–64	4	13.0	145	5	8	8	8	31	31	31
65+	2	22.5	4	21	21	24	24	24	24	24
GRAND TOTAL	1,651	2.7	10	1	2	2	3	4	6	16

43.4: LOC EXC GASTRIC LES

Type of Patients	Observed Patients	Avg. Stay	Variance	10th	25th	50th	75th	90th	95th	99th
1. SINGLE DX										
0–19 Years	5	2.0	1	1	1	1	3	4	4	4
20–34	3	3.7	1	3	3	3	5	5	5	5
35–49	0									
50–64	13	3.3	3	2	2	3	4	5	7	7
65+	7	3.3	3	1	2	4	5	5	5	5
2. MULTIPLE DX										
0–19 Years	7	5.8	143	1	2	2	4	50	>99	>99
20–34	54	5.1	20	1	2	4	6	14	15	20
35–49	169	5.8	23	2	3	5	7	11	14	31
50–64	398	5.4	23	2	3	4	7	11	13	23
65+	881	5.5	23	2	3	4	7	10	14	24
TOTAL SINGLE DX	28	3.0	2	1	2	3	4	5	5	7
TOTAL MULTIPLE DX	1,509	5.5	24	2	3	4	7	11	14	24
TOTAL										
0–19 Years	12	4.6	97	1	1	2	4	8	50	>99
20–34	57	5.0	19	1	2	4	6	14	15	20
35–49	169	5.8	23	2	3	5	7	11	14	31
50–64	411	5.3	22	2	2	4	6	11	13	23
65+	888	5.4	23	2	3	4	7	10	14	24
GRAND TOTAL	1,537	5.4	24	2	3	4	7	11	14	24

LOS by Diagnosis and Operation, Western Region, 45th Edition

Western Region, October 2007–September 2008 Data, by Operation

43.41: ENDO EXC GASTRIC LES

Type of Patients	Observed Patients	Avg. Stay	Vari-ance	Percentiles 10th	25th	50th	75th	90th	95th	99th
1. SINGLE DX										
0–19 Years	1	2.0	0	2	2	2	2	2	2	2
20–34	1	5.0	0	5	5	5	5	5	5	5
35–49	0									
50–64	1	2.0	0	2	2	2	2	2	2	2
65+	0									
2. MULTIPLE DX										
0–19 Years	4	3.0	5	1	1	2	4	4	8	8
20–34	36	4.0	15	1	2	3	5	7	15	20
35–49	113	4.9	13	2	3	4	6	10	13	17
50–64	289	4.5	13	2	2	4	5	9	12	20
65+	693	4.7	12	2	2	4	6	9	12	17
TOTAL SINGLE DX	3	3.0	3	2	2	2	5	5	5	5
TOTAL MULTIPLE DX	1,135	4.6	12	2	2	4	6	9	12	17
TOTAL										
0–19 Years	5	2.9	5	1	1	2	4	4	8	8
20–34	37	4.0	14	1	2	3	5	7	15	20
35–49	113	4.9	13	2	3	4	6	10	13	17
50–64	290	4.5	13	2	2	4	5	9	12	20
65+	693	4.7	12	2	2	4	6	9	12	17
GRAND TOTAL	1,138	4.6	12	2	2	4	6	9	12	17

43.42: LOC GASTRIC LES EXC NEC

Type of Patients	Observed Patients	Avg. Stay	Vari-ance	Percentiles 10th	25th	50th	75th	90th	95th	99th
1. SINGLE DX										
0–19 Years	2	3.0	0	3	3	3	3	3	3	3
20–34	2	3.0	0	3	3	3	3	3	3	3
35–49	0									
50–64	12	3.4	3	2	2	3	5	5	7	7
65+	7	3.3	3	1	2	4	5	5	5	5
2. MULTIPLE DX										
0–19 Years	3	10.6	379	2	2	2	50	>99	>99	>99
20–34	17	7.6	23	2	5	6	9	15	17	17
35–49	55	7.7	38	3	5	8	10	13	21	35
50–64	106	7.8	44	2	4	6	10	13	16	34
65+	181	8.5	58	3	4	7	10	15	19	41
TOTAL SINGLE DX	23	3.3	2	2	2	3	4	5	5	7
TOTAL MULTIPLE DX	362	8.1	53	3	4	6	10	15	19	48
TOTAL										
0–19 Years	5	8.7	283	2	2	3	5	>99	>99	>99
20–34	19	7.1	22	2	4	6	8	15	17	17
35–49	55	7.7	38	3	5	6	8	13	21	35
50–64	118	7.3	41	2	4	6	9	13	16	34
65+	188	8.3	57	3	4	7	10	15	19	41
GRAND TOTAL	385	7.8	52	2	4	6	9	14	19	48

43.5: PROXIMAL GASTRECTOMY

Type of Patients	Observed Patients	Avg. Stay	Vari-ance	Percentiles 10th	25th	50th	75th	90th	95th	99th
1. SINGLE DX										
0–19 Years	0									
20–34	1	4.0	0	4	4	4	4	4	4	4
35–49	1	3.0	0	3	3	3	3	3	3	3
50–64	0									
65+	1	4.0	0	4	4	4	4	4	4	4
2. MULTIPLE DX										
0–19 Years	0									
20–34	4	16.0	17	11	15	17	21	21	21	21
35–49	16	16.5	178	5	6	11	24	41	48	48
50–64	51	14.5	236	5	6	9	16	41	54	65
65+	82	12.4	74	6	7	10	16	25	31	47
TOTAL SINGLE DX	3	3.7	<1	3	3	4	4	4	4	4
TOTAL MULTIPLE DX	153	13.6	137	5	7	10	16	27	41	63
TOTAL										
0–19 Years	0									
20–34	5	13.6	42	4	11	15	17	21	21	21
35–49	17	15.7	177	5	6	11	24	41	48	48
50–64	51	14.5	236	5	6	9	16	41	54	65
65+	83	12.3	74	6	7	10	16	25	31	47
GRAND TOTAL	156	13.4	136	5	6	10	16	27	41	63

43.6: DISTAL GASTRECTOMY

Type of Patients	Observed Patients	Avg. Stay	Vari-ance	Percentiles 10th	25th	50th	75th	90th	95th	99th
1. SINGLE DX										
0–19 Years	1	9.0	0	9	9	9	9	9	9	9
20–34	1	6.0	0	6	6	6	6	6	6	6
35–49	2	4.0	2	3	3	5	5	5	5	5
50–64	4	6.5	9	3	5	9	9	9	9	9
65+	0									
2. MULTIPLE DX										
0–19 Years	1	8.0	0	8	8	8	8	8	8	8
20–34	9	13.1	83	4	7	10	15	28	28	28
35–49	26	13.9	192	5	6	7	14	39	40	64
50–64	91	11.2	121	4	5	7	12	24	30	81
65+	134	10.6	69	4	6	8	12	18	29	45
TOTAL SINGLE DX	8	6.1	7	3	5	6	9	9	9	9
TOTAL MULTIPLE DX	261	11.2	98	4	6	8	12	21	30	51
TOTAL										
0–19 Years	2	8.2	<1	8	8	8	9	9	9	9
20–34	10	12.4	79	6	6	9	15	28	28	28
35–49	28	13.2	185	5	6	7	14	39	40	64
50–64	95	11.0	117	4	5	7	11	24	30	81
65+	134	10.6	69	4	6	8	12	18	29	45
GRAND TOTAL	269	11.0	96	4	6	8	12	21	30	51

LOS by Diagnosis and Operation, Western Region, 45th Edition

Western Region, October 2007–September 2008 Data, by Operation

43.7: PART GASTRECTOMY W ANAST

Type of Patients	Observed Patients	Avg. Stay	Vari-ance	10th	25th	50th	75th	90th	95th	99th
1. SINGLE DX										
0–19 Years	0									
20–34	1	5.0	0	5	5	5	5	5	5	5
35–49	4									
50–64	0	6.3	<1	5	5	6	7	7	7	7
65+	1	10.0	0	10	10	10	10	10	10	10
2. MULTIPLE DX										
0–19 Years	2	24.5	4	23	23	25	26	26	26	26
20–34	32	11.7	90	2	6	9	17	23	35	35
35–49	140	12.4	130	4	6	8	14	29	38	57
50–64	365	13.0	106	5	7	9	16	25	34	49
65+	534	13.6	93	6	7	11	17	25	32	48
TOTAL SINGLE DX	6	6.7	3	5	5	7	7	10	10	10
TOTAL MULTIPLE DX	1,073	13.2	102	5	7	10	16	26	34	49
TOTAL										
0–19 Years	2	24.5	4	23	23	25	26	26	26	26
20–34	33	11.5	88	4	6	8	16	23	35	35
35–49	140	12.4	130	4	6	9	14	29	38	57
50–64	369	12.9	105	5	7	9	16	25	34	49
65+	535	13.6	93	6	7	11	17	25	32	48
GRAND TOTAL	1,079	13.1	102	5	7	10	16	26	34	49

43.8: OTH PARTIAL GASTRECTOMY

Type of Patients	Observed Patients	Avg. Stay	Vari-ance	10th	25th	50th	75th	90th	95th	99th
1. SINGLE DX										
0–19 Years	1	13.0	0	13	13	13	13	13	13	13
20–34	5	4.0	6	1	3	4	6	7	7	7
35–49	8	4.6	9	3	3	4	7	10	10	10
50–64	8	6.7	84	1	1	4	6	29	29	29
65+	2	4.5	<1	4	4	5	5	5	5	5
2. MULTIPLE DX										
0–19 Years	4	7.4	32	1	1	2	5	12	12	12
20–34	66	4.4	20	1	2	2	5	12	14	22
35–49	215	6.2	95	1	2	2	6	15	22	50
50–64	375	5.5	62	1	2	3	6	12	20	54
65+	248	9.8	57	3	5	8	13	20	25	49
TOTAL SINGLE DX	24	5.5	33	1	2	4	7	10	13	29
TOTAL MULTIPLE DX	908	6.8	69	1	2	4	9	15	22	49
TOTAL										
0–19 Years	5	8.1	32	1	2	12	12	13	13	13
20–34	71	4.3	19	1	2	2	5	9	14	22
35–49	223	6.1	92	1	2	2	6	15	22	50
50–64	383	5.6	62	1	2	3	6	12	20	54
65+	250	9.8	57	3	5	8	13	19	25	49
GRAND TOTAL	932	6.8	68	1	2	4	8	15	22	49

43.89: PARTIAL GASTRECTOMY NEC

Type of Patients	Observed Patients	Avg. Stay	Vari-ance	10th	25th	50th	75th	90th	95th	99th
1. SINGLE DX										
0–19 Years	1	13.0	0	13	13	13	13	13	13	13
20–34	5	4.0	6	1	3	3	6	7	7	7
35–49	8	4.6	9	1	3	4	7	10	10	10
50–64	8	6.7	84	1	1	4	6	29	29	29
65+	2	4.5	<1	4	4	5	5	5	5	5
2. MULTIPLE DX										
0–19 Years	4	7.4	32	1	1	2	5	12	12	12
20–34	66	4.4	20	1	2	2	5	12	14	22
35–49	215	6.2	95	1	2	2	6	15	22	50
50–64	374	5.5	62	1	2	3	6	12	20	54
65+	246	9.8	56	3	5	8	13	19	24	49
TOTAL SINGLE DX	24	5.5	33	1	2	4	7	10	13	29
TOTAL MULTIPLE DX	905	6.8	68	1	2	4	8	15	22	49
TOTAL										
0–19 Years	5	8.1	32	1	2	12	12	13	13	13
20–34	71	4.3	19	1	2	2	5	9	14	22
35–49	223	6.1	92	1	2	2	6	15	22	50
50–64	382	5.6	62	1	2	3	6	12	20	54
65+	248	9.7	56	3	5	8	12	19	24	49
GRAND TOTAL	929	6.7	68	1	2	4	8	15	22	49

43.9: TOTAL GASTRECTOMY

Type of Patients	Observed Patients	Avg. Stay	Vari-ance	10th	25th	50th	75th	90th	95th	99th
1. SINGLE DX										
0–19 Years	0									
20–34	0									
35–49	4	11.0	<1	10	10	11	11	12	12	12
50–64	5	7.6	3	5	7	8	8	10	10	10
65+	0									
2. MULTIPLE DX										
0–19 Years	2	19.0	31	15	15	19	23	23	23	23
20–34	10	13.1	150	6	7	11	11	20	46	46
35–49	51	14.0	74	7	8	11	17	27	32	50
50–64	187	15.3	123	7	9	12	18	28	39	70
65+	279	16.8	134	8	9	13	21	31	41	70
TOTAL SINGLE DX	9	9.1	5	5	8	10	11	12	12	12
TOTAL MULTIPLE DX	529	16.0	125	7	9	12	19	29	40	65
TOTAL										
0–19 Years	2	19.0	31	15	15	19	23	23	23	23
20–34	10	13.1	150	6	7	9	11	20	46	46
35–49	55	13.8	70	7	8	11	17	27	32	50
50–64	192	15.1	122	7	9	12	17	28	39	70
65+	279	16.8	134	8	9	13	21	31	41	70
GRAND TOTAL	538	15.9	123	7	9	12	19	29	40	65

LOS by Diagnosis and Operation, Western Region, 45th Edition

Western Region, October 2007–September 2008 Data, by Operation

43.99: TOTAL GASTRECTOMY NEC

Type of Patients	Observed Patients	Avg. Stay	Vari- ance	10th	25th	50th	75th	90th	95th	99th
1. SINGLE DX										
0–19 Years	0									
20–34	0									
35–49	4	11.0	<1	10	10	11	11	12	12	12
50–64	5	7.6	3	5	7	8	8	10	10	10
65+	0									
2. MULTIPLE DX										
0–19 Years	2	19.0	31	15	15	19	23	23	23	23
20–34	10	13.1	150	6	7	9	11	20	46	46
35–49	51	14.0	74	7	8	11	17	27	32	50
50–64	182	15.3	126	7	9	12	17	28	39	70
65+	275	16.9	135	8	9	13	21	31	41	70
TOTAL SINGLE DX	9	9.1	5	5	8	10	11	12	12	12
TOTAL MULTIPLE DX	520	16.0	126	7	9	12	19	30	40	65
TOTAL										
0–19 Years	2	19.0	31	15	15	19	23	23	23	23
20–34	10	13.1	150	6	7	9	11	20	46	46
35–49	55	13.8	70	7	7	11	17	27	32	50
50–64	187	15.1	124	7	9	12	17	28	39	70
65+	275	16.9	135	8	9	13	21	31	41	70
GRAND TOTAL	529	15.9	125	7	9	12	19	29	40	65

44.1: GASTRIC DXTIC PX

Type of Patients	Observed Patients	Avg. Stay	Vari- ance	10th	25th	50th	75th	90th	95th	99th
1. SINGLE DX										
0–19 Years	4	1.0	0	1	1	1	1	1	1	1
20–34	0									
35–49	1	1.0	0	1	1	1	1	1	1	1
50–64	0									
65+	0									
2. MULTIPLE DX										
0–19 Years	27	13.8	325	2	4	6	14	35	68	68
20–34	36	4.0	7	1	2	3	5	9	11	11
35–49	78	4.7	16	1	2	3	6	10	14	21
50–64	112	6.9	40	2	3	5	8	13	21	31
65+	194	6.6	42	2	3	5	9	12	17	43
TOTAL SINGLE DX	5	1.0	0	1	1	1	1	1	1	1
TOTAL MULTIPLE DX	447	7.1	77	2	3	4	8	13	21	61
TOTAL										
0–19 Years	31	12.9	312	1	2	6	14	35	68	68
20–34	36	4.0	7	1	2	3	5	9	11	11
35–49	79	4.7	16	1	2	3	6	10	14	21
50–64	112	6.9	40	2	3	5	8	13	21	31
65+	194	6.6	42	2	3	5	9	12	17	43
GRAND TOTAL	452	7.0	76	1	3	4	8	13	21	61

44.13: GASTROSCOPY NEC

Type of Patients	Observed Patients	Avg. Stay	Vari- ance	10th	25th	50th	75th	90th	95th	99th
1. SINGLE DX										
0–19 Years	4	1.0	0	1	1	1	1	1	1	1
20–34	0									
35–49	0									
50–64	0									
65+	0									
2. MULTIPLE DX										
0–19 Years	18	5.6	15	2	2	4	7	11	14	14
20–34	26	3.9	6	1	2	3	5	7	9	11
35–49	45	4.5	14	1	2	3	5	10	14	16
50–64	54	5.6	19	1	3	5	7	13	14	23
65+	82	5.8	31	2	2	4	8	11	12	43
TOTAL SINGLE DX	4	1.0	0	1	1	1	1	1	1	1
TOTAL MULTIPLE DX	225	5.3	20	1	2	4	7	11	14	21
TOTAL										
0–19 Years	22	5.1	15	1	2	3	7	11	14	14
20–34	26	3.9	6	1	2	3	5	7	9	11
35–49	45	4.5	14	1	2	3	5	10	14	16
50–64	54	5.6	19	2	3	5	7	13	14	23
65+	82	5.8	31	2	2	4	8	11	12	43
GRAND TOTAL	229	5.2	20	1	2	4	7	11	14	21

44.0: VAGOTOMY

Type of Patients	Observed Patients	Avg. Stay	Vari- ance	10th	25th	50th	75th	90th	95th	99th
1. SINGLE DX										
0–19 Years	0									
20–34	0									
35–49	0									
50–64	1	6.0	0	6	6	6	6	6	6	6
65+	0									
2. MULTIPLE DX										
0–19 Years	2	3.0	8	1	1	3	5	5	5	5
20–34	4	7.5	1	6	6	8	8	8	8	8
35–49	16	10.4	33	4	5	10	17	19	19	19
50–64	30	10.5	55	4	6	8	14	18	22	39
65+	24	13.9	119	7	7	12	15	18	31	58
TOTAL SINGLE DX	1	6.0	0	6	6	6	6	6	6	6
TOTAL MULTIPLE DX	76	11.2	70	4	6	9	14	18	22	58
TOTAL										
0–19 Years	2	3.0	8	1	1	3	5	5	5	5
20–34	4	7.5	1	6	6	8	8	8	8	8
35–49	16	10.4	33	4	5	10	17	19	19	19
50–64	31	10.3	54	4	6	8	14	18	22	39
65+	24	13.9	119	7	7	12	15	18	31	58
GRAND TOTAL	77	11.1	69	4	6	8	14	18	22	58

LOS by Diagnosis and Operation, Western Region, 45th Edition

Western Region, October 2007–September 2008 Data, by Operation

44.14: CLOSED GASTRIC BIOPSY

Type of Patients	Observed Patients	Avg. Stay	Variance	10th	25th	50th	75th	90th	95th	99th
1. SINGLE DX										
0–19 Years	0									
20–34	0									
35–49	1	1.0	0	1	1	1	1	1	1	1
50–64	0									
65+	0									
2. MULTIPLE DX										
0–19 Years	6	39.1	623	7	35	35	68	68	68	68
20–34	7	4.6	15	2	2	2	9	11	11	11
35–49	20	3.1	5	1	1	3	4	7	7	9
50–64	38	4.9	18	2	3	4	7	9	10	25
65+	85	5.8	18	2	3	4	7	13	14	18
TOTAL SINGLE DX	1	1.0	0	1	1	1	1	1	1	1
TOTAL MULTIPLE DX	156	7.7	137	2	3	4	7	13	35	68
TOTAL										
0–19 Years	6	39.1	623	7	35	35	68	68	68	68
20–34	7	4.6	15	2	2	2	9	11	11	11
35–49	21	3.0	5	1	1	3	4	6	7	9
50–64	38	4.9	18	2	3	4	7	9	10	25
65+	85	5.8	18	2	3	4	7	13	14	18
GRAND TOTAL	157	7.6	137	2	2	4	7	13	35	68

44.22: ENDO DILATION PYLORUS

Type of Patients	Observed Patients	Avg. Stay	Variance	10th	25th	50th	75th	90th	95th	99th
1. SINGLE DX										
0–19 Years	0									
20–34	1	3.0	0	3	3	3	3	3	3	3
35–49	1	1.0	0	1	1	1	1	1	1	1
50–64	1	4.0	0	4	4	4	4	4	4	4
65+	0									
2. MULTIPLE DX										
0–19 Years	8	4.6	12	2	2	3	8	8	12	12
20–34	53	3.1	3	1	2	3	4	5	7	8
35–49	80	4.8	78	1	2	3	5	9	16	74
50–64	126	5.0	19	1	2	3	6	10	14	22
65+	109	6.4	30	2	3	5	8	13	17	26
TOTAL SINGLE DX	3	2.7	2	1	1	3	4	4	4	4
TOTAL MULTIPLE DX	376	5.1	33	1	2	3	6	10	14	25
TOTAL										
0–19 Years	8	4.6	12	2	2	3	8	8	12	12
20–34	54	3.1	3	1	2	3	4	5	7	8
35–49	81	4.8	77	1	2	3	5	7	13	74
50–64	127	5.0	18	1	2	3	6	10	14	22
65+	109	6.4	30	2	3	5	8	13	17	26
GRAND TOTAL	379	5.1	32	1	2	3	6	10	14	25

44.2: PYLOROPLASTY

Type of Patients	Observed Patients	Avg. Stay	Variance	10th	25th	50th	75th	90th	95th	99th
1. SINGLE DX										
0–19 Years	7	3.3	3	2	2	3	4	6	7	7
20–34	1	3.0	0	3	3	3	3	3	3	3
35–49	2	3.5	12	1	3	3	3	4	6	6
50–64	1	4.0	0	4	4	4	4	4	4	4
65+	0									
2. MULTIPLE DX										
0–19 Years	41	9.1	75	3	3	5	13	21	28	45
20–34	66	4.0	9	1	2	3	5	8	11	17
35–49	133	6.4	63	2	3	4	8	14	18	25
50–64	210	8.0	91	2	3	5	9	15	22	57
65+	224	9.6	90	3	4	7	12	17	26	52
TOTAL SINGLE DX	11	3.3	3	2	2	3	4	6	7	7
TOTAL MULTIPLE DX	674	7.9	78	2	3	5	9	16	22	45
TOTAL										
0–19 Years	48	8.3	70	2	3	4	8	21	25	45
20–34	67	4.0	9	1	2	3	5	8	11	17
35–49	135	6.4	62	1	2	4	8	14	18	25
50–64	211	8.0	90	2	3	5	9	15	22	57
65+	224	9.6	90	3	4	7	12	17	26	52
GRAND TOTAL	685	7.9	77	2	3	5	9	16	22	45

44.29: OTHER PYLOROPLASTY

Type of Patients	Observed Patients	Avg. Stay	Variance	10th	25th	50th	75th	90th	95th	99th
1. SINGLE DX										
0–19 Years	7	3.3	3	2	2	3	4	6	7	7
20–34	0									
35–49	1	6.0	0	6	6	6	6	6	6	6
50–64	0									
65+	0									
2. MULTIPLE DX										
0–19 Years	33	10.1	85	3	4	6	15	22	29	45
20–34	13	7.8	15	5	5	6	11	11	17	17
35–49	53	8.8	32	2	4	8	12	17	21	25
50–64	82	12.5	170	4	6	8	13	25	44	71
65+	115	12.7	127	4	6	9	14	24	36	55
TOTAL SINGLE DX	8	3.5	3	2	2	3	4	6	7	7
TOTAL MULTIPLE DX	296	11.4	112	3	5	8	13	21	35	57
TOTAL										
0–19 Years	40	9.0	78	3	3	5	15	22	28	45
20–34	13	7.8	15	5	5	6	11	11	17	17
35–49	54	8.8	32	2	4	8	12	17	21	25
50–64	82	12.5	170	4	6	8	13	25	44	71
65+	115	12.7	127	4	6	9	14	24	36	55
GRAND TOTAL	304	11.1	110	3	5	8	13	21	35	57

LOS by Diagnosis and Operation, Western Region, 45th Edition

Western Region, October 2007–September 2008 Data, by Operation

44.32: PERC GASTROJEJUNOSTOMY

Type of Patients	Observed Patients	Avg. Stay	Vari-ance	Percentiles						
				10th	25th	50th	75th	90th	95th	99th
1. SINGLE DX										
0–19 Years	0									
20–34	0									
35–49	0									
50–64	0									
65+	0									
2. MULTIPLE DX										
0–19 Years	88	13.6	232	1	2	7	22	37	41	73
20–34	41	18.3	427	3	6	14	19	38	59	98
35–49	71	15.8	268	3	5	11	20	36	47	95
50–64	138	18.5	228	4	8	15	25	40	54	>99
65+	348	14.7	124	4	7	12	20	30	37	48
TOTAL SINGLE DX	0									
TOTAL MULTIPLE DX	686	15.3	200	2	5	11	21	34	43	77
TOTAL										
0–19 Years	88	13.6	232	1	2	7	22	37	41	73
20–34	41	18.3	427	3	6	14	19	38	59	98
35–49	71	15.8	268	3	5	11	20	36	47	95
50–64	138	18.5	228	4	8	15	25	40	54	>99
65+	348	14.7	124	4	7	12	20	30	37	48
GRAND TOTAL	686	15.3	200	2	5	11	21	34	43	77

44.38: LAPSCP GASTROENTEROSTOMY

Type of Patients	Observed Patients	Avg. Stay	Vari-ance	Percentiles						
				10th	25th	50th	75th	90th	95th	99th
1. SINGLE DX										
0–19 Years	6	2.5	<1	2	2	3	3	3	3	3
20–34	29	2.2	<1	1	2	2	2	3	4	4
35–49	21	2.6	2	1	2	2	3	5	5	7
50–64	17	2.5	2	2	2	2	3	4	7	7
65+	1	2.0	0	2	2	2	2	2	2	2
2. MULTIPLE DX										
0–19 Years	46	3.9	27	1	1	2	4	13	14	30
20–34	2,157	2.2	2	1	2	2	2	3	4	7
35–49	3,763	2.3	4	1	2	2	3	3	4	9
50–64	4,716	2.4	6	1	2	2	3	4	4	9
65+	338	3.7	20	1	2	2	3	7	13	23
TOTAL SINGLE DX	74	2.4	1	2	2	2	3	3	5	7
TOTAL MULTIPLE DX	11,020	2.4	5	1	2	2	3	3	4	9
TOTAL										
0–19 Years	52	3.7	24	1	2	2	3	8	14	30
20–34	2,186	2.2	2	1	2	2	3	3	4	7
35–49	3,784	2.3	4	1	2	2	3	3	4	7
50–64	4,733	2.4	6	1	2	2	3	4	4	9
65+	339	3.7	20	1	2	2	3	7	13	23
GRAND TOTAL	11,094	2.4	5	1	2	2	3	3	4	9

44.3: GASTROENTEROSTOMY

Type of Patients	Observed Patients	Avg. Stay	Vari-ance	Percentiles						
				10th	25th	50th	75th	90th	95th	99th
1. SINGLE DX										
0–19 Years	7	1.9	<1	1	1	2	3	3	3	3
20–34	32	2.2	<1	1	2	2	2	3	4	4
35–49	24	2.5	2	1	2	2	3	5	5	7
50–64	18	2.5	2	2	2	2	3	4	7	7
65+	1	2.0	0	2	2	2	2	2	2	2
2. MULTIPLE DX										
0–19 Years	162	14.1	307	1	2	5	22	37	58	75
20–34	2,364	2.7	20	1	2	2	3	3	5	19
35–49	4,237	2.9	18	1	2	2	3	4	6	21
50–64	5,398	3.4	31	1	2	2	3	5	9	31
65+	994	11.1	114	2	3	8	15	25	32	47
TOTAL SINGLE DX	82	2.3	1	1	2	2	3	3	4	7
TOTAL MULTIPLE DX	13,155	4.0	44	1	2	2	3	7	14	37
TOTAL										
0–19 Years	169	13.7	302	1	2	5	22	37	58	75
20–34	2,396	2.7	20	1	2	2	3	3	5	19
35–49	4,261	2.9	18	1	2	2	3	4	6	21
50–64	5,416	3.4	31	1	2	2	3	5	9	31
65+	995	11.1	114	2	3	8	15	25	32	47
GRAND TOTAL	13,237	3.9	44	1	2	2	3	7	14	37

44.31: HIGH GASTRIC BYPASS

Type of Patients	Observed Patients	Avg. Stay	Vari-ance	Percentiles						
				10th	25th	50th	75th	90th	95th	99th
1. SINGLE DX										
0–19 Years	0									
20–34	0									
35–49	0									
50–64	0									
65+										
2. MULTIPLE DX										
0–19 Years	0									
20–34	5	1.6	<1	1	1	1	2	3	3	3
35–49	22	1.5	3	1	1	1	1	2	2	9
50–64	13	1.2	<1	1	1	1	1	1	4	4
65+	1	1.0	0	1	1	1	1	1	1	1
TOTAL SINGLE DX	0									
TOTAL MULTIPLE DX	41	1.4	2	1	1	1	1	2	3	9
TOTAL										
0–19 Years	0									
20–34	5	1.6	<1	1	1	1	2	3	3	3
35–49	22	1.5	3	1	1	1	1	2	2	9
50–64	13	1.2	<1	1	1	1	1	1	4	4
65+	1	1.0	0	1	1	1	1	1	1	1
GRAND TOTAL	41	1.4	2	1	1	1	1	2	3	9

LOS by Diagnosis and Operation, Western Region, 45th Edition

Western Region, October 2007–September 2008 Data, by Operation

44.41: SUT GASTRIC ULCER SITE

Type of Patients	Observed Patients	Avg. Stay	Vari-ance	10th	25th	50th	75th	90th	95th	99th
1. SINGLE DX										
0–19 Years	0									
20–34	4	5.8	<1	5	5	5	6	7	7	7
35–49	3	5.4	4	3	3	6	7	7	7	7
50–64	6	5.2	3	3	4	7	8	8	8	8
65+	3	7.0	1	6	6	7	8	8	8	8
2. MULTIPLE DX										
0–19 Years	8	4.5	11	1	1	6	7	7	10	10
20–34	54	7.4	27	4	5	6	8	10	18	34
35–49	102	9.3	101	4	5	7	9	15	24	45
50–64	204	10.7	107	4	6	8	12	20	34	57
65+	207	11.7	70	6	7	9	14	21	28	48
TOTAL SINGLE DX	16	5.7	2	3	5	6	7	8	8	8
TOTAL MULTIPLE DX	575	10.4	85	4	6	8	11	19	28	54
TOTAL										
0–19 Years	8	4.5	11	1	1	6	7	7	10	10
20–34	58	7.3	25	4	5	6	7	10	18	34
35–49	105	9.2	99	4	5	7	9	15	24	45
50–64	210	10.6	104	4	5	8	11	19	34	57
65+	210	11.7	69	6	7	9	14	21	28	48
GRAND TOTAL	591	10.3	83	4	6	8	11	18	27	54

44.42: SUT DUODENAL ULCER SITE

Type of Patients	Observed Patients	Avg. Stay	Vari-ance	10th	25th	50th	75th	90th	95th	99th
1. SINGLE DX										
0–19 Years	4	5.5	<1	5	5	5	5	7	7	7
20–34	8	4.6	2	3	4	5	5	7	7	7
35–49	7	5.6	1	4	5	6	7	7	7	7
50–64	10	6.2	2	6	6	6	8	8	8	8
65+	1	6.0	0	6	6	6	6	6	6	6
2. MULTIPLE DX										
0–19 Years	19	8.2	26	4	5	6	13	18	18	18
20–34	81	7.2	72	3	5	6	7	10	12	77
35–49	189	8.8	57	4	5	8	9	16	23	49
50–64	273	12.2	138	6	6	8	14	24	40	58
65+	415	13.5	94	6	7	10	17	25	33	55
TOTAL SINGLE DX	30	5.5	2	4	5	5	7	8	8	8
TOTAL MULTIPLE DX	977	11.6	100	4	6	8	14	22	31	55
TOTAL										
0–19 Years	23	7.9	23	4	5	5	9	18	18	18
20–34	89	7.0	67	3	5	7	7	8	12	77
35–49	196	8.7	55	4	5	7	9	16	23	49
50–64	283	12.0	135	6	6	7	14	24	38	58
65+	416	13.4	94	6	7	10	17	25	33	55
GRAND TOTAL	1,007	11.4	98	4	6	8	14	22	29	55

44.39: GASTROENTEROSTOMY NEC

Type of Patients	Observed Patients	Avg. Stay	Vari-ance	10th	25th	50th	75th	90th	95th	99th
1. SINGLE DX										
0–19 Years	1	1.0	0	1	1	1	1	1	1	1
20–34	3	2.3	2	1	1	2	4	4	4	4
35–49	3	1.7	<1	1	1	2	2	2	2	2
50–64	1	2.0	0	2	2	2	2	2	2	2
65+	0									
2. MULTIPLE DX										
0–19 Years	28	25.1	638	2	3	20	38	63	75	93
20–34	161	5.3	83	2	2	3	4	7	20	55
35–49	381	6.4	65	2	2	3	7	16	24	48
50–64	531	8.3	107	2	3	4	9	21	30	57
65+	307	15.2	115	4	8	13	20	29	36	52
TOTAL SINGLE DX	8	1.6	<1	1	1	1	2	2	4	4
TOTAL MULTIPLE DX	1,408	9.6	136	2	3	4	13	24	32	58
TOTAL										
0–19 Years	29	23.4	631	1	3	13	37	63	75	93
20–34	164	5.3	81	2	2	3	4	7	20	55
35–49	384	6.3	65	2	2	3	7	15	23	48
50–64	532	8.3	107	2	3	4	9	21	30	57
65+	307	15.2	115	4	8	13	20	29	36	52
GRAND TOTAL	1,416	9.5	135	2	3	4	12	24	32	58

44.4: CNTRL PEPTIC ULCER HEMOR

Type of Patients	Observed Patients	Avg. Stay	Vari-ance	10th	25th	50th	75th	90th	95th	99th
1. SINGLE DX										
0–19 Years	6	4.6	2	2	4	5	5	7	7	7
20–34	16	4.1	4	1	3	5	5	7	7	7
35–49	15	4.4	4	2	3	5	6	7	7	7
50–64	24	4.5	6	1	3	5	6	8	8	8
65+	5	6.0	3	3	6	6	7	8	8	8
2. MULTIPLE DX										
0–19 Years	56	5.8	17	2	3	5	7	11	13	18
20–34	433	4.6	28	1	2	3	5	8	11	25
35–49	1,112	5.4	39	2	2	4	6	10	15	34
50–64	2,516	5.5	41	2	2	4	6	10	15	38
65+	5,377	5.8	33	2	3	4	7	11	16	29
TOTAL SINGLE DX	66	4.5	4	1	3	5	6	7	8	8
TOTAL MULTIPLE DX	9,494	5.6	35	2	3	4	6	11	15	31
TOTAL										
0–19 Years	62	5.7	16	2	3	5	7	11	13	18
20–34	449	4.6	27	1	2	3	5	8	10	25
35–49	1,127	5.4	39	2	2	4	6	10	14	34
50–64	2,540	5.5	41	2	2	4	6	10	15	38
65+	5,382	5.8	33	2	3	4	7	11	16	29
GRAND TOTAL	9,560	5.6	35	2	3	4	6	11	15	31

LOS by Diagnosis and Operation, Western Region, 45th Edition

44.43: ENDO CNTRL GASTRIC BLEED

Type of Patients	Observed Patients	Avg. Stay	Vari-ance	Percentiles						
				10th	25th	50th	75th	90th	95th	99th
1. SINGLE DX										
0–19 Years	2	3.3	1	2	2	4	4	4	4	4
20–34	4	1.3	<1	1	1	1	1	2	2	2
35–49	5	2.2	<1	1	2	2	3	3	3	3
50–64	8	1.9	<1	1	1	2	2	3	3	3
65+	1	3.0	0	3	3	3	3	3	3	3
2. MULTIPLE DX										
0–19 Years	29	4.5	8	2	2	4	6	8	11	11
20–34	295	3.3	11	1	2	3	4	5	8	20
35–49	804	4.0	16	2	2	3	4	7	10	22
50–64	2,009	4.1	11	2	2	3	5	7	10	18
65+	4,712	4.8	18	2	3	4	6	9	12	21
TOTAL SINGLE DX	**20**	**2.1**	**<1**	**1**	**1**	**2**	**3**	**3**	**4**	**4**
TOTAL MULTIPLE DX	**7,849**	**4.5**	**16**	**2**	**2**	**3**	**5**	**8**	**11**	**20**
TOTAL										
0–19 Years	31	4.4	8	2	2	4	6	8	11	11
20–34	299	3.3	11	1	2	3	4	5	8	20
35–49	809	4.0	16	2	2	3	4	7	10	22
50–64	2,017	4.1	11	2	2	3	5	7	10	18
65+	4,713	4.8	18	2	3	4	6	9	12	21
GRAND TOTAL	**7,869**	**4.5**	**16**	**2**	**2**	**3**	**5**	**8**	**11**	**20**

44.5: REVISION GASTRIC ANAST

Type of Patients	Observed Patients	Avg. Stay	Vari-ance	Percentiles						
				10th	25th	50th	75th	90th	95th	99th
1. SINGLE DX										
0–19 Years	0									
20–34	0									
35–49	0									
50–64	0									
65+	0									
2. MULTIPLE DX										
0–19 Years	4	34.5	163	17	23	36	36	58	58	58
20–34	53	7.5	42	2	3	6	9	16	20	32
35–49	110	8.7	110	2	3	6	10	16	35	71
50–64	136	9.8	111	2	4	6	12	23	33	51
65+	49	12.6	79	3	7	11	15	28	30	41
TOTAL SINGLE DX	**0**									
TOTAL MULTIPLE DX	**352**	**10.0**	**110**	**2**	**4**	**7**	**12**	**23**	**36**	**60**
TOTAL										
0–19 Years	4	34.5	163	17	23	36	36	58	58	58
20–34	53	7.5	42	2	3	6	9	16	20	32
35–49	110	8.7	110	2	3	6	10	16	35	71
50–64	136	9.8	111	2	4	6	12	23	33	51
65+	49	12.6	79	3	7	11	15	28	30	41
GRAND TOTAL	**352**	**10.0**	**110**	**2**	**4**	**7**	**12**	**23**	**36**	**60**

44.6: OTHER GASTRIC REPAIR

Type of Patients	Observed Patients	Avg. Stay	Vari-ance	Percentiles						
				10th	25th	50th	75th	90th	95th	99th
1. SINGLE DX										
0–19 Years	74	2.0	2	1	1	2	2	4	5	6
20–34	42	1.8	2	1	1	1	2	4	5	6
35–49	44	1.8	1	1	1	2	2	3	3	5
50–64	51	1.9	2	1	1	1	2	4	4	7
65+	12	3.1	6	1	1	2	4	5	10	10
2. MULTIPLE DX										
0–19 Years	956	10.7	237	1	2	5	13	29	49	>99
20–34	510	4.1	28	1	1	2	5	9	14	28
35–49	1,098	3.4	27	1	1	2	4	7	11	25
50–64	1,854	3.6	31	1	1	2	3	7	11	29
65+	1,342	5.2	40	1	2	3	6	11	17	35
TOTAL SINGLE DX	**223**	**2.0**	**2**	**1**	**1**	**2**	**2**	**4**	**5**	**7**
TOTAL MULTIPLE DX	**5,760**	**5.9**	**99**	**1**	**1**	**3**	**6**	**14**	**25**	**72**
TOTAL										
0–19 Years	1,030	10.1	225	1	2	4	12	28	48	>99
20–34	552	4.0	26	1	1	2	5	9	13	28
35–49	1,142	3.4	26	1	1	2	3	7	10	24
50–64	1,905	3.5	30	1	1	2	3	7	11	29
65+	1,354	5.2	40	1	2	3	6	11	17	35
GRAND TOTAL	**5,983**	**5.8**	**96**	**1**	**1**	**2**	**6**	**14**	**25**	**67**

44.61: SUTURE GASTRIC LAC

Type of Patients	Observed Patients	Avg. Stay	Vari-ance	Percentiles						
				10th	25th	50th	75th	90th	95th	99th
1. SINGLE DX										
0–19 Years	3	4.3	4	2	2	5	6	6	6	6
20–34	3	4.0	3	3	3	3	6	6	6	6
35–49	0									
50–64	0									
65+	0									
2. MULTIPLE DX										
0–19 Years	42	8.6	78	3	4	6	10	12	20	55
20–34	89	8.8	43	4	5	6	11	17	21	42
35–49	48	12.1	218	4	5	7	12	24	55	78
50–64	31	10.7	83	2	4	8	13	27	32	34
65+	36	12.5	59	5	7	11	15	28	30	>99
TOTAL SINGLE DX	**6**	**4.2**	**3**	**2**	**3**	**3**	**6**	**6**	**6**	**6**
TOTAL MULTIPLE DX	**246**	**10.1**	**91**	**3**	**5**	**7**	**12**	**19**	**29**	**56**
TOTAL										
0–19 Years	45	8.3	75	3	4	6	10	12	20	55
20–34	92	8.6	42	3	5	6	11	16	21	42
35–49	48	12.1	218	4	5	7	12	24	55	78
50–64	31	10.7	83	2	4	8	13	27	32	34
65+	36	12.5	59	5	7	11	15	28	30	>99
GRAND TOTAL	**252**	**10.0**	**90**	**3**	**5**	**7**	**12**	**19**	**28**	**56**

Western Region, October 2007–September 2008 Data, by Operation

44.63: CLOSE STOM FISTULA NEC

Type of Patients	Observed Patients	Avg. Stay	Vari-ance	10th	25th	50th	75th	90th	95th	99th
1. SINGLE DX										
0–19 Years	8	1.0	0	1	1	1	1	1	1	1
20–34	0									
35–49	2	3.0	0	3	3	3	3	3	3	3
50–64	1	4.0	0	4	4	4	4	4	4	4
65+	0									
2. MULTIPLE DX										
0–19 Years	60	8.5	311	1	1	1	9	21	27	86
20–34	12	8.3	41	1	4	7	11	14	24	24
35–49	22	8.7	125	1	2	5	9	26	26	48
50–64	36	11.0	111	3	4	7	13	32	37	43
65+	57	11.3	132	1	4	8	14	25	28	75
TOTAL SINGLE DX	11	1.5	1	1	1	1	1	3	4	4
TOTAL MULTIPLE DX	187	9.6	202	1	1	5	12	24	28	86
TOTAL										
0–19 Years	68	7.8	285	1	1	1	6	21	27	86
20–34	12	8.3	41	1	4	7	11	14	24	24
35–49	24	8.2	117	1	2	5	9	26	26	48
50–64	37	10.9	110	3	4	7	13	32	37	43
65+	57	11.3	132	1	4	8	14	25	28	75
GRAND TOTAL	198	9.1	194	1	1	4	11	24	27	86

44.66: CREAT EG SPHINCT COMPET

Type of Patients	Observed Patients	Avg. Stay	Vari-ance	10th	25th	50th	75th	90th	95th	99th
1. SINGLE DX										
0–19 Years	3	4.2	2	2	3	5	5	5	5	5
20–34	2	1.0	0	1	1	1	1	1	1	1
35–49	2	1.0	0	1	1	1	1	1	1	1
50–64	2	4.5	<1	4	4	5	5	5	5	5
65+	1	5.0	0	5	5	5	5	5	5	5
2. MULTIPLE DX										
0–19 Years	221	16.9	311	3	5	10	23	56	83	>99
20–34	42	4.8	16	1	2	3	6	10	14	20
35–49	106	5.0	13	1	2	4	7	10	13	15
50–64	227	6.4	38	1	3	5	7	12	18	38
65+	222	8.6	61	3	4	6	10	15	24	47
TOTAL SINGLE DX	10	3.3	3	1	1	4	5	5	5	5
TOTAL MULTIPLE DX	818	10.9	175	2	4	6	12	27	49	>99
TOTAL										
0–19 Years	224	16.8	309	3	5	10	23	56	82	>99
20–34	44	4.6	16	1	2	3	6	10	14	20
35–49	108	4.9	13	1	2	4	7	10	13	15
50–64	229	6.3	38	1	3	5	7	12	18	38
65+	223	8.6	61	3	4	6	10	15	24	47
GRAND TOTAL	828	10.8	173	2	4	6	12	27	48	>99

44.67: LAPSCP PX EGS COMPET

Type of Patients	Observed Patients	Avg. Stay	Vari-ance	10th	25th	50th	75th	90th	95th	99th
1. SINGLE DX										
0–19 Years	48	2.1	2	1	1	2	2	3	4	14
20–34	33	1.4	<1	1	1	1	2	2	2	4
35–49	38	1.6	<1	1	1	2	2	3	3	4
50–64	47	1.7	1	1	1	2	2	3	4	7
65+	11	2.9	7	1	2	4	4	4	10	10
2. MULTIPLE DX										
0–19 Years	538	9.7	224	1	2	4	10	28	44	98
20–34	264	2.2	7	1	1	2	2	3	5	12
35–49	706	2.2	4	1	1	2	2	4	5	12
50–64	1,221	2.2	4	1	1	2	2	3	5	11
65+	905	3.2	11	2	2	2	3	6	9	15
TOTAL SINGLE DX	177	1.9	2	1	1	2	2	3	4	7
TOTAL MULTIPLE DX	3,634	4.4	75	1	1	2	3	8	18	49
TOTAL										
0–19 Years	586	9.2	212	1	2	3	9	26	42	98
20–34	297	2.1	6	1	1	2	2	3	5	11
35–49	744	2.2	4	1	1	2	2	3	5	12
50–64	1,268	2.2	4	1	1	2	2	3	5	11
65+	916	3.2	11	2	2	2	3	6	9	15
GRAND TOTAL	3,811	4.3	71	1	1	2	3	7	17	48

44.68: LAPSCP GASTROPLASTY

Type of Patients	Observed Patients	Avg. Stay	Vari-ance	10th	25th	50th	75th	90th	95th	99th
1. SINGLE DX										
0–19 Years	0									
20–34	1	1.0	0	1	1	1	1	1	1	1
35–49	1	5.0	0	5	5	5	5	5	5	5
50–64	1	2.0	0	2	2	2	2	2	2	2
65+	0									
2. MULTIPLE DX										
0–19 Years	3	4.7	5	1	3	6	6	6	6	6
20–34	54	3.8	73	1	1	1	1	7	34	34
35–49	96	1.9	5	1	1	1	1	4	7	14
50–64	156	1.6	7	1	1	1	1	2	3	19
65+	18	4.2	39	1	1	2	3	19	21	21
TOTAL SINGLE DX	3	2.7	4	1	1	2	5	5	5	5
TOTAL MULTIPLE DX	327	2.3	20	1	1	1	2	3	7	34
TOTAL										
0–19 Years	3	4.7	5	1	3	6	6	6	6	6
20–34	55	3.8	72	1	1	1	1	7	34	34
35–49	97	2.0	5	1	1	1	1	4	7	14
50–64	157	1.6	7	1	1	1	1	2	3	19
65+	18	4.2	39	1	1	2	3	19	21	21
GRAND TOTAL	330	2.3	20	1	1	1	2	3	7	34

LOS by Diagnosis and Operation, Western Region, 45th Edition

Western Region, October 2007–September 2008 Data, by Operation

44.69: GASTRIC REPAIR NEC

Type of Patients	Observed Patients	Avg. Stay	Vari-ance	Percentiles						
				10th	25th	50th	75th	90th	95th	99th
1. SINGLE DX										
0–19 Years	0									
20–34	3	4.7	<1	4	4	5	5	5	5	5
35–49	1	5.0	0	5	5	5	5	5	5	5
50–64	0									
65+	0									
2. MULTIPLE DX										
0–19 Years	29	10.8	129	2	3	6	17	28	39	39
20–34	45	4.9	9	1	3	5	6	9	11	12
35–49	116	6.0	41	2	2	4	7	13	19	45
50–64	158	7.5	129	2	2	4	7	16	25	62
65+	63	10.6	88	3	5	7	15	26	45	>99
TOTAL SINGLE DX	4	4.8	<1	4	5	5	5	5	5	5
TOTAL MULTIPLE DX	411	7.7	91	2	3	5	8	17	26	62
TOTAL										
0–19 Years	29	10.8	129	2	3	6	17	28	39	39
20–34	48	4.9	8	1	3	5	6	9	11	12
35–49	117	6.0	41	2	2	4	7	13	19	45
50–64	158	7.5	129	2	2	4	7	16	25	62
65+	63	10.6	88	3	5	7	15	26	45	>99
GRAND TOTAL	415	7.7	90	2	3	5	8	17	26	62

44.95: LAPSCP GASTRIC REST PX

Type of Patients	Observed Patients	Avg. Stay	Vari-ance	Percentiles						
				10th	25th	50th	75th	90th	95th	99th
1. SINGLE DX										
0–19 Years	2	1.0	0							
20–34	15	1.0	<1	1	1	1	1	1	1	1
35–49	14	1.0	0	1	1	1	1	1	1	1
50–64	13	1.0	0	1	1	1	1	1	1	1
65+	1	1.0	0	1	1	1	1	1	1	1
2. MULTIPLE DX										
0–19 Years	32	1.1	<1	1	1	1	1	1	2	2
20–34	641	1.1	<1	1	1	1	1	1	2	2
35–49	1,360	1.1	<1	1	1	1	1	1	2	3
50–64	1,792	1.2	<1	1	1	1	1	2	2	4
65+	449	1.2	<1	1	1	1	1	2	2	3
TOTAL SINGLE DX	45	1.0	<1	1	1	1	1	1	1	2
TOTAL MULTIPLE DX	4,274	1.1	<1	1	1	1	1	1	2	3
TOTAL										
0–19 Years	34	1.1	<1	1	1	1	1	1	2	2
20–34	656	1.1	<1	1	1	1	1	1	2	2
35–49	1,374	1.1	<1	1	1	1	1	1	2	3
50–64	1,805	1.2	<1	1	1	1	1	2	2	4
65+	450	1.2	<1	1	1	1	2	2	2	3
GRAND TOTAL	4,319	1.1	<1	1	1	1	1	1	2	3

44.9: OTHER STOMACH OPERATIONS

Type of Patients	Observed Patients	Avg. Stay	Vari-ance	Percentiles						
				10th	25th	50th	75th	90th	95th	99th
1. SINGLE DX										
0–19 Years	8	1.7	<1	1	1	1	2	3	3	3
20–34	15	1.1	<1	1	1	1	1	1	2	2
35–49	18	1.2	<1	1	1	1	1	2	3	3
50–64	16	1.1	<1	1	1	1	1	1	2	2
65+	1	1.0	0	1	1	1	1	1	1	1
2. MULTIPLE DX										
0–19 Years	45	1.5	1	1	1	1	2	2	3	7
20–34	732	1.5	13	1	1	1	1	2	4	8
35–49	1,524	1.4	3	1	1	1	1	2	3	7
50–64	1,967	1.4	3	1	1	1	1	2	3	9
65+	515	1.9	11	1	1	1	1	3	7	15
TOTAL SINGLE DX	58	1.3	<1	1	1	1	1	2	3	3
TOTAL MULTIPLE DX	4,783	1.5	5	1	1	1	1	2	3	10
TOTAL										
0–19 Years	53	1.5	<1	1	1	1	2	3	3	7
20–34	747	1.5	13	1	1	1	1	2	4	8
35–49	1,542	1.4	3	1	1	1	1	2	3	7
50–64	1,983	1.4	3	1	1	1	1	2	3	9
65+	516	1.9	11	1	1	1	1	3	7	15
GRAND TOTAL	4,841	1.5	5	1	1	1	1	2	3	10

44.96: LAPSCP REV GAST REST PX

Type of Patients	Observed Patients	Avg. Stay	Vari-ance	Percentiles						
				10th	25th	50th	75th	90th	95th	99th
1. SINGLE DX										
0–19 Years	0									
20–34	0									
35–49	2	2.0	2	1	1	3	3	3	3	3
50–64	0									
65+	0									
2. MULTIPLE DX										
0–19 Years	3	1.7	<1	1	1	2	2	2	2	2
20–34	32	2.3	5	1	1	1	3	4	8	10
35–49	48	1.8	2	1	1	1	2	3	5	8
50–64	52	2.1	1	1	1	2	3	4	4	5
65+	10	7.5	219	1	1	2	7	8	49	49
TOTAL SINGLE DX	2	2.0	2	1	1	3	3	3	3	3
TOTAL MULTIPLE DX	145	2.4	18	1	1	1	3	4	6	10
TOTAL										
0–19 Years	3	1.7	<1	1	1	2	2	2	2	2
20–34	32	2.3	5	1	1	1	3	4	8	10
35–49	50	1.8	2	1	1	1	2	3	5	8
50–64	52	2.1	1	1	1	2	3	4	4	5
65+	10	7.5	219	1	1	2	7	8	49	49
GRAND TOTAL	147	2.4	18	1	1	1	3	4	6	10

LOS by Diagnosis and Operation, Western Region, 45th Edition

45.0: ENTEROTOMY

Type of Patients	Observed Patients	Avg. Stay	Vari-ance	Percentiles						
				10th	25th	50th	75th	90th	95th	99th
1. SINGLE DX										
0–19 Years	1	5.0	0	5	5	5	5	5	5	5
20–34	3	4.3	10	2	2	3	8	8	8	8
35–49	4	5.0	<1	4	5	5	6	6	6	6
50–64	3	3.3	2	2	2	3	6	5	5	5
65+	1	6.0	0	6	6	6	6	6	6	6
2. MULTIPLE DX										
0–19 Years	27	21.4	549	4	5	14	31	77	>99	>99
20–34	30	7.0	23	3	4	6	8	16	20	20
35–49	43	9.3	56	3	5	6	12	21	26	35
50–64	69	10.7	79	3	5	7	12	25	30	38
65+	111	11.2	82	4	5	8	14	22	29	40
TOTAL SINGLE DX	12	4.6	3	2	3	5	5	6	8	8
TOTAL MULTIPLE DX	280	12.0	163	3	5	8	14	26	38	94
TOTAL										
0–19 Years	28	20.1	525	4	5	14	31	77	>99	>99
20–34	33	6.8	22	3	4	6	8	15	20	20
35–49	47	8.9	53	3	5	6	11	21	26	35
50–64	72	10.4	78	3	5	7	12	25	30	38
65+	112	11.1	82	4	5	8	14	22	29	40
GRAND TOTAL	292	11.7	158	3	5	7	14	26	38	94

45.02: SM INTEST INCISION NEC

Type of Patients	Observed Patients	Avg. Stay	Vari-ance	Percentiles						
				10th	25th	50th	75th	90th	95th	99th
1. SINGLE DX										
0–19 Years	1	5.0	0	5	5	5	5	5	5	5
20–34	0									
35–49	1	6.0	0	6	6	6	6	6	6	6
50–64	1	5.0	0	5	5	6	6	6	6	6
65+	0									
2. MULTIPLE DX										
0–19 Years	13	32.2	963	4	5	31	75	>99	>99	>99
20–34	16	7.4	21	4	5	6	9	15	20	20
35–49	22	9.3	52	3	5	7	11	23	26	27
50–64	40	10.3	82	3	5	7	11	25	38	38
65+	75	10.1	55	4	5	7	13	18	25	40
TOTAL SINGLE DX	3	5.2	<1	5	5	5	5	6	6	6
TOTAL MULTIPLE DX	166	12.6	222	4	5	7	15	31	40	>99
TOTAL										
0–19 Years	14	28.0	908	4	5	31	75	94	>99	>99
20–34	16	7.4	21	4	5	6	9	15	20	20
35–49	23	9.1	50	4	5	6	11	23	26	27
50–64	41	10.2	81	3	5	7	10	24	25	38
65+	75	10.1	55	4	5	7	13	18	25	40
GRAND TOTAL	169	12.3	216	4	5	7	13	31	40	>99

44.97: LAPSCP RMV GAST REST DEV

Type of Patients	Observed Patients	Avg. Stay	Vari-ance	Percentiles						
				10th	25th	50th	75th	90th	95th	99th
1. SINGLE DX										
0–19 Years	1	1.0	0	1	1	1	1	1	1	1
20–34	0									
35–49	1	2.0	0	2	2	2	2	2	2	2
50–64	2	1.0	0	1	1	1	1	1	1	1
65+	0									
2. MULTIPLE DX										
0–19 Years	2	4.0	2	3	3	4	5	5	5	5
20–34	36	3.9	8	1	2	2	6	8	9	12
35–49	69	3.6	9	1	1	2	5	8	10	16
50–64	65	3.5	15	1	1	2	4	9	13	18
65+	11	3.5	13	1	1	2	4	7	13	13
TOTAL SINGLE DX	4	1.3	<1	1	1	1	2	2	2	2
TOTAL MULTIPLE DX	183	3.6	11	1	1	2	5	8	11	16
TOTAL										
0–19 Years	3	3.0	4	1	1	3	5	5	5	5
20–34	36	3.9	8	1	2	2	6	8	9	12
35–49	70	3.6	9	1	1	2	5	8	10	16
50–64	67	3.5	14	1	1	2	4	9	13	18
65+	11	3.5	13	1	1	2	4	7	13	13
GRAND TOTAL	187	3.6	11	1	1	2	5	8	11	16

44.99: GASTRIC OPERATION NEC

Type of Patients	Observed Patients	Avg. Stay	Vari-ance	Percentiles						
				10th	25th	50th	75th	90th	95th	99th
1. SINGLE DX										
0–19 Years	4	1.4	<1	1	1	1	2	2	2	2
20–34	0									
35–49	0									
50–64	0									
65+	0									
2. MULTIPLE DX										
0–19 Years	7	2.1	2	1	1	2	2	3	7	7
20–34	16	4.3	11	1	2	3	6	10	12	12
35–49	27	6.4	81	1	3	4	6	10	21	47
50–64	38	7.2	55	1	2	4	10	18	25	33
65+	14	6.1	26	1	2	5	12	13	16	16
TOTAL SINGLE DX	4	1.4	<1	1	1	1	2	2	2	2
TOTAL MULTIPLE DX	102	5.7	46	1	2	3	6	12	18	33
TOTAL										
0–19 Years	11	1.8	1	1	1	2	2	2	3	7
20–34	16	4.3	11	1	2	3	6	10	12	12
35–49	27	6.4	81	1	3	4	6	10	21	47
50–64	38	7.2	55	1	2	4	10	18	25	33
65+	14	6.1	26	1	2	5	12	13	16	16
GRAND TOTAL	106	5.2	42	1	2	3	6	12	17	33

LOS by Diagnosis and Operation, Western Region, 45th Edition

Western Region, October 2007–September 2008 Data, by Operation

45.1: SMALL INTEST DXTIC PX

Type of Patients	Observed Patients	Avg. Stay	Variance	10th	25th	50th	75th	90th	95th	99th
1. SINGLE DX										
0–19 Years	215	1.8	3	1	1	1	2	4	5	9
20–34	78	2.8	8	1	1	2	3	6	7	22
35–49	59	2.6	4	1	1	2	4	5	7	12
50–64	42	2.8	5	1	1	2	4	6	6	11
65+	15	3.6	12	1	1	2	5	7	14	14
2. MULTIPLE DX										
0–19 Years	2,500	6.1	55	1	2	4	7	13	19	39
20–34	6,943	4.1	17	1	2	3	5	8	11	20
35–49	15,453	4.3	17	1	2	3	5	8	11	20
50–64	23,893	4.7	20	1	2	3	6	9	12	22
65+	45,445	5.0	17	2	2	4	6	10	13	21
TOTAL SINGLE DX	409	2.1	4	1	1	1	2	5	6	9
TOTAL MULTIPLE DX	94,234	4.8	20	1	2	4	6	9	12	23
TOTAL										
0–19 Years	2,715	5.8	53	1	2	4	7	13	18	38
20–34	7,021	4.1	17	1	2	3	5	8	10	20
35–49	15,512	4.3	17	1	2	3	5	8	11	20
50–64	23,935	4.7	20	1	2	3	6	9	12	22
65+	45,460	5.0	17	2	2	4	6	10	13	21
GRAND TOTAL	94,643	4.8	20	2	2	4	6	9	12	23

45.12: ENDO S-INTEST THRU STOMA

Type of Patients	Observed Patients	Avg. Stay	Variance	10th	25th	50th	75th	90th	95th	99th
1. SINGLE DX										
0–19 Years	3	1.0	0	1	1	1	1	1	1	1
20–34	1	1.0	0	1	1	1	1	1	1	1
35–49	0									
50–64	0									
65+	0									
2. MULTIPLE DX										
0–19 Years	6	7.7	138	1	1	1	13	13	38	38
20–34	13	7.1	86	1	2	4	8	26	31	31
35–49	16	4.7	16	1	2	3	6	12	15	15
50–64	29	4.6	42	1	2	3	4	8	11	36
65+	37	5.1	34	1	2	3	5	12	24	28
TOTAL SINGLE DX	4	1.0	0	1	1	1	1	1	1	1
TOTAL MULTIPLE DX	101	5.4	49	1	2	3	6	13	24	36
TOTAL										
0–19 Years	9	5.9	106	1	1	2	9	13	38	38
20–34	14	6.7	83	1	1	4	8	26	31	31
35–49	16	4.7	16	1	2	4	6	12	15	15
50–64	29	4.6	42	1	2	3	4	8	11	36
65+	37	5.1	34	1	2	3	5	12	24	28
GRAND TOTAL	105	5.2	48	1	1	3	6	12	24	36

45.13: SM INTEST ENDOSCOPY NEC

Type of Patients	Observed Patients	Avg. Stay	Variance	10th	25th	50th	75th	90th	95th	99th
1. SINGLE DX										
0–19 Years	116	1.3	1	1	1	1	1	2	3	5
20–34	31	2.6	4	1	1	2	3	5	7	9
35–49	26	3.2	8	1	1	2	5	7	7	12
50–64	25	2.8	3	1	2	2	4	5	6	6
65+	8	3.7	19	1	1	3	3	14	14	14
2. MULTIPLE DX										
0–19 Years	465	5.3	40	1	1	3	7	13	20	38
20–34	2,449	4.1	17	1	2	3	5	8	11	21
35–49	5,835	4.4	21	1	2	3	5	9	12	23
50–64	8,693	4.9	24	2	2	4	6	10	13	24
65+	16,310	5.1	18	2	2	4	6	10	13	23
TOTAL SINGLE DX	206	1.8	3	1	1	1	2	4	5	9
TOTAL MULTIPLE DX	33,752	4.8	21	1	2	4	6	9	13	23
TOTAL										
0–19 Years	581	4.4	34	1	1	2	5	12	16	35
20–34	2,480	4.1	17	1	2	3	5	8	11	21
35–49	5,861	4.4	21	1	2	3	5	9	12	23
50–64	8,718	4.9	24	1	2	3	6	10	13	24
65+	16,318	5.1	18	2	2	4	6	10	13	23
GRAND TOTAL	33,958	4.8	21	1	2	4	6	9	13	23

45.14: CLOSED SMALL INTEST BX

Type of Patients	Observed Patients	Avg. Stay	Variance	10th	25th	50th	75th	90th	95th	99th
1. SINGLE DX										
0–19 Years	1	1.0	0	1	1	1	1	1	1	1
20–34	1	2.0	0	2	2	2	2	2	2	2
35–49	0									
50–64	0									
65+	0									
2. MULTIPLE DX										
0–19 Years	31	7.3	64	2	2	5	9	15	29	36
20–34	55	4.3	7	1	3	3	6	7	11	13
35–49	66	4.7	11	2	3	3	6	9	12	17
50–64	103	5.4	20	2	3	4	6	10	15	21
65+	154	5.3	18	2	2	4	7	9	14	24
TOTAL SINGLE DX	2	1.2	<1	1	1	1	1	2	2	2
TOTAL MULTIPLE DX	409	5.4	25	2	3	4	6	11	15	29
TOTAL										
0–19 Years	32	7.0	62	1	2	4	9	15	29	36
20–34	56	4.3	7	1	3	3	6	7	11	13
35–49	66	4.7	11	2	3	3	6	9	12	17
50–64	103	5.4	20	2	3	4	6	10	15	21
65+	154	5.3	18	2	2	4	7	9	14	24
GRAND TOTAL	411	5.4	24	2	2	4	6	10	15	29

LOS by Diagnosis and Operation, Western Region, 45th Edition

Western Region, October 2007–September 2008 Data, by Operation

45.16: EGD W CLOSED BIOPSY

Type of Patients	Observed Patients	Avg. Stay	Vari-ance	Percentiles						
				10th	25th	50th	75th	90th	95th	99th
1. SINGLE DX										
0–19 Years	95	2.4	4	1	1	2	3	5	7	9
20–34	45	3.0	11	1	2	2	3	6	6	22
35–49	33	2.2	2	1	1	2	3	4	5	5
50–64	17	2.8	9	1	1	2	3	9	11	11
65+	7	3.4	6	1	1	2	6	7	7	7
2. MULTIPLE DX										
0–19 Years	1,988	6.2	55	1	2	4	7	13	18	39
20–34	4,422	4.1	17	1	2	3	5	8	10	20
35–49	9,518	4.2	15	1	2	3	5	8	11	20
50–64	15,043	4.6	17	1	2	3	5	9	12	21
65+	28,913	5.0	17	2	2	4	6	9	12	21
TOTAL SINGLE DX	197	2.5	5	1	1	2	3	5	7	9
TOTAL MULTIPLE DX	59,884	4.8	19	2	2	4	6	9	12	22
TOTAL										
0–19 Years	2,083	6.0	54	1	2	4	7	13	18	39
20–34	4,467	4.1	17	1	2	3	5	8	10	20
35–49	9,551	4.2	15	1	2	3	5	8	11	20
50–64	15,060	4.6	17	1	2	3	5	9	12	21
65+	28,920	5.0	17	2	2	4	6	9	12	21
GRAND TOTAL	60,081	4.8	19	2	2	4	6	9	12	22

45.22: ENDO L-INTEST THRU STOMA

Type of Patients	Observed Patients	Avg. Stay	Vari-ance	Percentiles						
				10th	25th	50th	75th	90th	95th	99th
1. SINGLE DX										
0–19 Years	0									
20–34	0									
35–49	0									
50–64	0									
65+	0									
2. MULTIPLE DX										
0–19 Years	2	8.5	59	3	3	14	14	14	14	14
20–34	5	3.8	4	2	3	3	4	7	7	7
35–49	25	4.6	17	2	3	3	5	7	9	22
50–64	31	4.9	26	1	3	4	5	9	13	28
65+	84	5.2	24	2	2	4	6	10	14	37
TOTAL SINGLE DX	0									
TOTAL MULTIPLE DX	147	5.0	23	2	2	4	6	10	14	28
TOTAL										
0–19 Years	2	8.5	59	3	3	14	14	14	14	14
20–34	5	3.8	4	2	3	3	4	7	7	7
35–49	25	4.6	17	2	3	3	5	7	9	22
50–64	31	4.9	26	1	3	4	5	9	13	28
65+	84	5.2	24	2	2	4	6	10	14	37
GRAND TOTAL	147	5.0	23	2	2	4	6	10	14	28

45.2: LG INTESTINE DXTIC PX

Type of Patients	Observed Patients	Avg. Stay	Vari-ance	Percentiles						
				10th	25th	50th	75th	90th	95th	99th
1. SINGLE DX										
0–19 Years	69	2.7	5	1	1	2	3	6	6	10
20–34	126	3.1	5	1	2	3	4	6	8	10
35–49	75	3.2	5	1	2	3	4	6	8	14
50–64	53	2.9	4	1	2	3	4	5	6	13
65+	23	2.8	3	1	2	2	4	5	5	8
2. MULTIPLE DX										
0–19 Years	611	6.6	60	1	2	4	8	15	20	35
20–34	2,743	4.6	17	2	2	3	5	9	11	22
35–49	4,649	4.6	16	2	2	4	6	9	12	19
50–64	7,633	4.8	21	2	2	4	6	9	13	22
65+	17,545	5.1	19	2	2	4	6	10	13	22
TOTAL SINGLE DX	346	3.0	5	1	2	2	4	6	7	13
TOTAL MULTIPLE DX	33,181	5.0	20	2	2	4	6	9	13	22
TOTAL										
0–19 Years	680	6.2	56	1	2	4	7	14	20	34
20–34	2,869	4.5	16	2	2	3	5	9	11	22
35–49	4,724	4.6	16	2	2	4	6	9	11	19
50–64	7,686	4.8	21	2	2	4	6	9	13	22
65+	17,568	5.1	19	2	2	4	6	10	13	22
GRAND TOTAL	33,527	4.9	20	2	2	4	6	9	13	22

45.23: COLONOSCOPY

Type of Patients	Observed Patients	Avg. Stay	Vari-ance	Percentiles						
				10th	25th	50th	75th	90th	95th	99th
1. SINGLE DX										
0–19 Years	12	2.4	2	1	1	2	3	4	5	5
20–34	29	2.5	5	1	1	2	3	5	8	10
35–49	20	2.0	1	1	1	2	2	4	4	5
50–64	25	2.9	3	1	2	2	3	6	6	7
65+	17	2.8	4	1	2	2	3	5	8	8
2. MULTIPLE DX										
0–19 Years	87	5.7	63	1	1	3	5	16	27	35
20–34	694	4.4	15	1	2	3	5	8	11	22
35–49	1,700	4.2	12	1	2	3	5	8	10	16
50–64	3,188	4.4	19	1	2	3	5	8	11	22
65+	8,468	4.6	14	2	2	4	6	8	11	19
TOTAL SINGLE DX	103	2.5	3	1	1	2	3	5	6	8
TOTAL MULTIPLE DX	14,137	4.5	15	1	2	3	5	8	11	20
TOTAL										
0–19 Years	99	5.3	57	1	1	3	4	16	27	35
20–34	723	4.3	14	1	2	3	5	8	11	21
35–49	1,720	4.1	11	1	2	3	5	8	10	16
50–64	3,213	4.4	19	1	2	3	5	8	11	22
65+	8,485	4.6	14	2	2	4	6	8	11	19
GRAND TOTAL	14,240	4.5	15	1	2	3	5	8	11	20

LOS by Diagnosis and Operation, Western Region, 45th Edition

Western Region, October 2007–September 2008 Data, by Operation

45.24: FLEXIBLE SIGMOIDOSCOPY

Type of Patients	Observed Patients	Avg. Stay	Vari-ance	Percentiles						
				10th	25th	50th	75th	90th	95th	99th
1. SINGLE DX										
0–19 Years	4	5.6	52	2	2	2	3	18	18	18
20–34	3	6.4	14	2	2	8	9	9	9	9
35–49	1	4.0	0	4	4	4	4	4	4	4
50–64	3	2.3	2	1	1	2	4	4	4	4
65+	0									
2. MULTIPLE DX										
0–19 Years	27	4.6	35	1	1	3	4	11	12	34
20–34	160	4.7	28	1	2	3	5	10	11	29
35–49	216	4.7	15	1	2	4	6	9	13	17
50–64	364	5.2	26	1	2	4	6	11	15	28
65+	1,147	5.9	34	2	3	4	7	12	15	29
TOTAL SINGLE DX	11	4.8	24	2	2	3	8	9	18	18
TOTAL MULTIPLE DX	1,914	5.5	30	1	2	4	7	11	15	28
TOTAL										
0–19 Years	31	4.7	36	1	2	2	4	11	18	34
20–34	163	4.7	28	1	2	3	5	10	11	29
35–49	217	4.7	15	1	2	4	6	9	13	17
50–64	367	5.2	26	1	2	4	6	11	15	28
65+	1,147	5.9	34	2	3	4	7	12	15	29
GRAND TOTAL	1,925	5.5	30	1	2	4	7	11	15	28

45.25: CLOSED LG INTEST BIOPSY

Type of Patients	Observed Patients	Avg. Stay	Vari-ance	Percentiles						
				10th	25th	50th	75th	90th	95th	99th
1. SINGLE DX										
0–19 Years	53	2.5	3	1	1	2	3	6	6	10
20–34	94	3.2	5	1	2	3	4	6	8	16
35–49	54	3.6	6	1	2	3	4	7	8	14
50–64	25	3.0	6	1	2	2	4	5	6	13
65+	6	2.8	2	1	2	3	4	5	5	5
2. MULTIPLE DX										
0–19 Years	489	6.5	43	2	3	4	8	14	20	31
20–34	1,883	4.7	16	2	2	4	6	9	12	22
35–49	2,702	4.9	19	2	2	4	6	9	12	23
50–64	4,043	5.1	22	2	3	4	6	10	13	23
65+	7,827	5.5	21	2	3	4	7	10	14	23
TOTAL SINGLE DX	232	3.1	5	1	2	3	4	6	7	13
TOTAL MULTIPLE DX	16,944	5.3	22	2	3	4	6	10	14	23
TOTAL										
0–19 Years	542	6.1	41	1	2	4	7	13	19	31
20–34	1,977	4.6	16	2	2	4	6	9	12	21
35–49	2,756	4.9	19	2	2	4	6	9	12	22
50–64	4,068	5.1	22	2	3	4	6	10	13	23
65+	7,833	5.5	21	2	3	4	7	10	14	23
GRAND TOTAL	17,176	5.3	21	2	3	4	6	10	13	23

45.3: LOC EXC/DESTR SMB LES

Type of Patients	Observed Patients	Avg. Stay	Vari-ance	Percentiles						
				10th	25th	50th	75th	90th	95th	99th
1. SINGLE DX										
0–19 Years	14	4.5	6	2	2	4	6	8	10	10
20–34	8	5.3	16	1	2	5	9	12	12	12
35–49	4	3.8	8	1	1	2	7	7	7	7
50–64	3	4.0	13	1	1	3	8	8	8	8
65+	1	7.0	0	7	7	7	7	7	7	7
2. MULTIPLE DX										
0–19 Years	81	5.8	31	3	3	5	6	10	12	34
20–34	39	4.7	6	3	3	4	6	8	9	15
35–49	70	6.4	46	2	2	4	8	12	16	41
50–64	149	6.2	37	2	3	4	7	12	17	34
65+	295	6.1	23	2	3	5	8	12	14	26
TOTAL SINGLE DX	30	4.6	7	2	2	4	6	9	10	12
TOTAL MULTIPLE DX	634	6.0	29	2	3	4	7	11	14	31
TOTAL										
0–19 Years	95	5.5	26	2	3	4	6	10	10	30
20–34	47	4.8	8	2	3	4	6	8	9	15
35–49	74	6.2	44	2	2	4	8	12	16	41
50–64	152	6.2	36	2	3	4	8	12	17	34
65+	296	6.1	23	2	3	5	8	12	14	26
GRAND TOTAL	664	5.9	27	2	3	4	7	11	14	31

45.30: ENDO EXC/DESTR DUOD LES

Type of Patients	Observed Patients	Avg. Stay	Vari-ance	Percentiles						
				10th	25th	50th	75th	90th	95th	99th
1. SINGLE DX										
0–19 Years	0									
20–34	0									
35–49	0									
50–64	0									
65+	0									
2. MULTIPLE DX										
0–19 Years	1	5.0	0	5	5	5	5	5	5	5
20–34	6	6.4	21	2	3	6	6	15	15	15
35–49	12	3.9	12	1	2	2	7	9	12	12
50–64	57	5.0	26	2	2	3	6	14	17	27
65+	157	4.7	10	2	2	4	6	10	12	14
TOTAL SINGLE DX	0									
TOTAL MULTIPLE DX	233	4.8	14	2	2	4	6	10	14	17
TOTAL										
0–19 Years	1	5.0	0	5	5	5	5	5	5	5
20–34	6	6.4	21	2	3	6	6	15	15	15
35–49	12	3.9	12	1	2	2	7	9	12	12
50–64	57	5.0	26	2	2	3	6	14	17	27
65+	157	4.7	10	2	2	4	6	10	12	14
GRAND TOTAL	233	4.8	14	2	2	4	6	10	14	17

LOS by Diagnosis and Operation, Western Region, 45th Edition

Western Region, October 2007–September 2008 Data, by Operation

45.31: LOC EXC DUOD LES NEC

Type of Patients	Observed Patients	Avg. Stay	Variance	Percentiles						
				10th	25th	50th	75th	90th	95th	99th
1. SINGLE DX										
0–19 Years	2	5.0	1			6	6	6	6	6
20–34	1	8.0	0			8	8	8	8	8
35–49	1	7.0	0			7	7	7	7	7
50–64	0									
65+	1	7.0	0			7	7	7	7	7
2. MULTIPLE DX										
0–19 Years	6	6.1	19	4	4	5	6	12	22	22
20–34	2	4.0	0	4	4	4	4	4	4	4
35–49	20	8.3	18	3	5	8	10	13	16	19
50–64	31	8.5	51	4	5	7	8	10	29	34
65+	56	9.5	35	4	6	7	12	17	23	31
TOTAL SINGLE DX	5	5.6	2	4	4	6	7	7	8	8
TOTAL MULTIPLE DX	115	8.5	34	4	5	7	10	15	22	31
TOTAL										
0–19 Years	8	5.8	14	4	4	5	6	6	12	22
20–34	3	5.3	5	4	4	4	8	8	8	8
35–49	21	8.2	17	4	5	8	10	13	16	19
50–64	31	8.5	51	4	5	7	8	10	29	34
65+	57	9.4	35	4	6	7	12	17	23	31
GRAND TOTAL	120	8.2	32	4	5	7	9	14	22	31

45.33: LOC EXC S-INTEST LES NEC

Type of Patients	Observed Patients	Avg. Stay	Variance	Percentiles						
				10th	25th	50th	75th	90th	95th	99th
1. SINGLE DX										
0–19 Years	12	4.4	7	2	2	4	6	10	10	10
20–34	7	4.9	17	1	2	3	9	12	12	12
35–49	2	1.5	<1	1	1	2	2	2	2	2
50–64	3	4.0	13	1	1	3	8	8	8	8
65+	0									
2. MULTIPLE DX										
0–19 Years	70	5.8	33	2	3	4	6	10	10	34
20–34	30	4.5	4	2	3	4	6	8	8	9
35–49	34	6.4	76	2	3	4	7	12	36	41
50–64	46	5.7	20	2	3	4	7	12	16	20
65+	49	7.3	38	2	4	6	10	13	14	41
TOTAL SINGLE DX	24	4.3	9	2	2	4	6	10	10	12
TOTAL MULTIPLE DX	229	6.0	34	2	3	4	7	10	12	36
TOTAL										
0–19 Years	82	5.5	28	2	3	4	6	10	10	34
20–34	37	4.6	6	2	3	4	6	8	9	12
35–49	36	6.1	73	2	3	3	6	12	36	41
50–64	49	5.6	20	2	3	4	7	12	16	20
65+	49	7.3	38	2	4	6	10	13	14	41
GRAND TOTAL	253	5.7	31	2	3	4	6	10	12	36

45.4: LOC DESTR LG INTEST LES

Type of Patients	Observed Patients	Avg. Stay	Variance	Percentiles						
				10th	25th	50th	75th	90th	95th	99th
1. SINGLE DX										
0–19 Years	3	2.9	1	2	2	2	4	4	4	4
20–34	1	1.0	0	2	2	1	1	1	1	1
35–49	3	3.3	5	2	2	2	6	6	6	6
50–64	13	2.4	5	1	1	2	2	6	8	8
65+	14	4.2	5	1	2	4	6	7	8	8
2. MULTIPLE DX										
0–19 Years	27	4.6	35	1	2	2	4	13	21	21
20–34	131	3.4	5	1	2	3	4	7	8	11
35–49	648	3.8	11	1	2	3	5	7	9	16
50–64	2,098	4.0	18	1	2	3	5	8	10	19
65+	5,923	4.5	13	2	2	3	6	8	11	19
TOTAL SINGLE DX	34	3.2	4	1	2	2	4	6	7	8
TOTAL MULTIPLE DX	8,827	4.3	14	1	2	3	5	8	11	19
TOTAL										
0–19 Years	30	4.3	29	1	2	2	4	13	21	21
20–34	132	3.4	5	1	2	3	4	7	8	11
35–49	651	3.8	11	1	2	3	5	7	9	16
50–64	2,111	4.0	18	1	2	3	5	8	10	19
65+	5,937	4.5	13	2	2	3	6	8	11	19
GRAND TOTAL	8,861	4.3	14	1	2	3	5	8	11	19

45.41: EXC LG INTEST LESION

Type of Patients	Observed Patients	Avg. Stay	Variance	Percentiles						
				10th	25th	50th	75th	90th	95th	99th
1. SINGLE DX										
0–19 Years	2	3.0	1	2	2	2	4	4	4	4
20–34	0									
35–49	1	6.0	0	6	6	6	6	6	6	6
50–64	1	4.5	25	1	1	5	8	8	8	8
65+	6	5.2	3	3	4	4	7	7	7	7
2. MULTIPLE DX										
0–19 Years	2	3.5	4	2	2	2	5	5	5	5
20–34	8	3.7	6	1	2	2	6	7	7	7
35–49	14	4.2	8	1	3	4	6	9	10	10
50–64	46	5.4	13	2	3	4	7	11	11	17
65+	58	6.2	43	2	3	4	7	17	21	34
TOTAL SINGLE DX	11	4.1	4	2	2	4	6	7	8	8
TOTAL MULTIPLE DX	128	5.5	26	2	3	4	7	11	17	28
TOTAL										
0–19 Years	4	3.1	1	2	2	2	4	4	5	5
20–34	7	3.7	6	1	2	2	6	7	7	7
35–49	15	4.3	8	1	3	3	6	9	10	10
50–64	48	5.3	13	2	3	4	7	11	11	17
65+	64	6.1	39	2	3	4	7	14	19	34
GRAND TOTAL	139	5.3	23	2	3	4	7	10	14	28

LOS by Diagnosis and Operation, Western Region, 45th Edition

Western Region, October 2007–September 2008 Data, by Operation

45.42: ENDO COLON POLYPECTOMY

Type of Patients	Observed Patients	Avg. Stay	Vari-ance	Percentiles						
				10th	25th	50th	75th	90th	95th	99th
1. SINGLE DX										
0–19 Years	1	2.0	0	2	2	2	2	2	2	2
20–34	0									
35–49	0									
50–64	2	4.0	8	2	2	6	6	6	6	6
65+	5	4.2	10	1	1	5	6	8	8	8
2. MULTIPLE DX										
0–19 Years	19	5.5	46	1	2	3	4	21	21	21
20–34	94	3.4	5	1	2	3	4	6	8	11
35–49	528	3.8	9	1	2	3	5	7	9	13
50–64	1,502	4.3	20	1	2	3	5	8	10	19
65+	4,367	4.7	14	2	2	4	6	9	12	19
TOTAL SINGLE DX	8	3.9	7	1	1	5	6	8	8	8
TOTAL MULTIPLE DX	6,510	4.5	15	1	2	3	6	9	11	19
TOTAL										
0–19 Years	20	5.4	44	1	2	2	4	21	21	21
20–34	94	3.4	5	1	2	3	4	6	8	11
35–49	528	3.8	9	1	2	3	5	7	9	13
50–64	1,504	4.3	20	1	2	3	5	8	10	19
65+	4,372	4.7	14	2	2	4	6	9	12	19
GRAND TOTAL	6,518	4.5	15	1	2	3	6	9	11	19

45.5: INTESTINAL SEG ISOLATION

Type of Patients	Observed Patients	Avg. Stay	Vari-ance	Percentiles						
				10th	25th	50th	75th	90th	95th	99th
1. SINGLE DX										
0–19 Years	0									
20–34	0									
35–49	0									
50–64	0									
65+	0									
2. MULTIPLE DX										
0–19 Years	3	7.4	5	4	7	9	9	9	9	9
20–34	4	15.5	209	6	6	11	37	37	37	37
35–49	5	6.2	2	4	6	6	7	8	8	8
50–64	10	6.5	7	3	5	6	9	9	11	11
65+	14	12.0	93	3	6	10	14	29	36	36
TOTAL SINGLE DX	0									
TOTAL MULTIPLE DX	36	9.4	59	4	6	8	10	14	29	37
TOTAL										
0–19 Years	3	7.4	5	4	7	9	9	9	9	9
20–34	4	15.5	209	6	6	11	37	37	37	37
35–49	5	6.2	2	4	6	6	7	8	8	8
50–64	10	6.5	7	3	5	6	9	9	11	11
65+	14	12.0	93	3	6	10	14	29	36	36
GRAND TOTAL	36	9.4	59	4	6	8	10	14	29	37

45.43: ENDO DESTR COLON LES NEC

Type of Patients	Observed Patients	Avg. Stay	Vari-ance	Percentiles						
				10th	25th	50th	75th	90th	95th	99th
1. SINGLE DX										
0–19 Years	0									
20–34	1	1.0	0	1	1	1	1	1	1	1
35–49	2	2.0	6	2	1	2	2	2	2	2
50–64	9	1.6	<1	1	1	2	2	2	2	2
65+	3	2.3	<1	2	2	2	3	3	3	3
2. MULTIPLE DX										
0–19 Years	6	2.0	7	1	1	2	2	5	5	5
20–34	27	3.1	7	1	2	3	4	5	10	12
35–49	106	3.5	21	1	1	2	4	6	8	19
50–64	549	3.1	13	1	1	2	4	6	8	20
65+	1,490	3.9	10	1	2	3	5	7	9	17
TOTAL SINGLE DX	15	1.7	<1	1	1	2	2	2	3	3
TOTAL MULTIPLE DX	2,178	3.6	11	1	2	3	4	7	9	18
TOTAL										
0–19 Years	6	2.0	1	1	1	2	2	5	5	5
20–34	28	3.0	6	1	2	3	4	5	10	12
35–49	108	3.5	21	1	2	2	4	6	8	19
50–64	558	3.1	13	1	1	2	4	6	8	20
65+	1,493	3.8	10	1	2	3	5	7	9	17
GRAND TOTAL	2,193	3.6	11	1	2	3	4	7	9	18

45.6: SM INTEST EXCISION NEC

Type of Patients	Observed Patients	Avg. Stay	Vari-ance	Percentiles						
				10th	25th	50th	75th	90th	95th	99th
1. SINGLE DX										
0–19 Years	26	6.5	11	3	4	7	8	8	16	16
20–34	19	4.9	2	3	4	5	6	7	7	7
35–49	38	4.7	6	2	3	5	6	8	9	11
50–64	30	4.4	6	2	3	5	5	6	8	14
65+	9	3.9	2	2	3	3	5	6	6	6
2. MULTIPLE DX										
0–19 Years	423	16.5	424	5	6	9	23	91	>99	>99
20–34	633	9.9	87	4	5	7	11	19	28	68
35–49	1,263	10.3	81	4	5	8	12	21	27	52
50–64	2,366	11.4	113	4	5	8	13	23	33	64
65+	4,035	12.6	84	5	7	10	15	23	30	52
TOTAL SINGLE DX	122	5.3	8	3	3	5	7	8	8	16
TOTAL MULTIPLE DX	8,720	12.1	120	4	6	9	14	24	34	96
TOTAL										
0–19 Years	449	15.8	401	4	6	8	21	86	>99	>99
20–34	652	9.7	85	4	5	7	11	19	27	68
35–49	1,301	10.1	80	3	5	7	12	21	27	51
50–64	2,396	11.4	112	4	5	8	13	23	33	64
65+	4,044	12.5	84	5	7	10	15	23	30	52
GRAND TOTAL	8,842	11.9	119	4	6	9	14	24	33	95

Western Region, October 2007–September 2008 Data, by Operation

45.61: MULT SEG S-INTEST RESECT

Type of Patients	Observed Patients	Avg. Stay	Vari- ance	Percentiles						
				10th	25th	50th	75th	90th	95th	99th
1. SINGLE DX										
0–19 Years	2	5.5	4	4	4	7	7	7	7	7
20–34	0									
35–49	1	7.0	0	7	7	7	7	7	7	7
50–64	0									
65+	1	2.0	0	2	2	2	2	2	2	2
2. MULTIPLE DX										
0–19 Years	20	13.8	173	5	6	12	54	>99	>99	>99
20–34	37	11.6	72	5	6	9	17	25	44	>99
35–49	63	14.0	110	4	6	12	20	27	34	55
50–64	122	16.1	219	5	7	11	18	35	44	77
65+	210	16.1	145	6	9	13	19	28	37	63
TOTAL SINGLE DX	4	5.0	6	2	2	7	7	7	7	7
TOTAL MULTIPLE DX	452	15.3	156	5	7	12	19	32	44	>99
TOTAL										
0–19 Years	22	13.1	163	5	6	10	54	>99	>99	>99
20–34	37	11.6	72	5	6	9	17	25	44	>99
35–49	64	13.9	109	4	6	12	19	27	34	55
50–64	122	16.1	219	5	7	11	18	35	44	77
65+	211	16.0	145	6	8	13	19	28	37	63
GRAND TOTAL	456	15.3	156	5	7	12	19	32	44	>99

45.62: PART S-INTEST RESECT NEC

Type of Patients	Observed Patients	Avg. Stay	Vari- ance	Percentiles						
				10th	25th	50th	75th	90th	95th	99th
1. SINGLE DX										
0–19 Years	24	6.5	11	3	4	7	8	8	16	16
20–34	19	4.9	2	3	4	5	6	7	7	7
35–49	37	4.6	6	2	3	4	6	8	9	11
50–64	30	4.4	6	2	3	5	5	6	8	14
65+	8	4.1	2	3	3	3	5	6	6	6
2. MULTIPLE DX										
0–19 Years	399	16.4	428	5	6	9	21	86	>99	>99
20–34	592	9.8	88	4	5	7	11	19	27	68
35–49	1,193	10.1	79	4	5	8	12	21	26	52
50–64	2,238	11.2	106	5	5	8	13	23	32	62
65+	3,807	12.3	80	5	7	10	15	23	29	49
TOTAL SINGLE DX	118	5.3	8	3	3	5	7	8	8	16
TOTAL MULTIPLE DX	8,229	11.9	117	4	6	9	14	23	33	92
TOTAL										
0–19 Years	423	15.7	404	4	6	8	19	80	>99	>99
20–34	611	9.6	86	4	5	7	10	18	26	64
35–49	1,230	9.9	78	3	5	7	11	20	26	51
50–64	2,268	11.1	105	4	5	8	13	23	31	62
65+	3,815	12.3	80	5	7	10	15	23	29	49
GRAND TOTAL	8,347	11.7	116	4	6	8	14	23	33	92

45.7: PART LG INTEST EXCISION

Type of Patients	Observed Patients	Avg. Stay	Vari- ance	Percentiles						
				10th	25th	50th	75th	90th	95th	99th
1. SINGLE DX										
0–19 Years	43	5.0	3	3	3	5	6	7	8	12
20–34	124	4.8	3	3	3	4	6	8	8	11
35–49	270	4.7	5	3	3	4	6	7	8	12
50–64	464	4.1	3	2	3	4	5	6	7	9
65+	197	4.4	3	2	3	4	5	6	7	10
2. MULTIPLE DX										
0–19 Years	383	13.7	312	4	5	7	14	39	80	>99
20–34	1,384	9.0	62	4	5	7	10	16	23	42
35–49	4,223	8.3	49	3	4	6	10	15	20	39
50–64	10,619	8.3	54	3	4	6	9	15	21	42
65+	17,416	9.5	59	4	5	7	11	18	23	40
TOTAL SINGLE DX	1,098	4.5	4	3	3	4	5	7	8	10
TOTAL MULTIPLE DX	34,025	9.0	61	3	5	7	11	17	23	42
TOTAL										
0–19 Years	426	12.7	284	4	5	7	13	36	74	>99
20–34	1,508	8.6	59	3	5	6	10	16	22	42
35–49	4,493	8.1	47	3	4	6	9	15	20	39
50–64	11,083	8.1	53	3	4	6	9	15	21	41
65+	17,613	9.5	59	4	5	7	11	18	23	40
GRAND TOTAL	35,123	8.9	60	3	5	7	10	17	22	42

45.71: MULT SEG L-INTEST RESECT

Type of Patients	Observed Patients	Avg. Stay	Vari- ance	Percentiles						
				10th	25th	50th	75th	90th	95th	99th
1. SINGLE DX										
0–19 Years	1	8.0	0	8	8	8	8	8	8	8
20–34	0									
35–49	1	6.0	0	6	6	6	6	6	6	6
50–64	1	4.0	0	4	4	4	4	4	4	4
65+	0									
2. MULTIPLE DX										
0–19 Years	3	8.0	0	8	8	8	8	8	8	8
20–34	6	10.4	65	3	5	8	16	24	24	24
35–49	13	15.8	208	4	6	9	22	31	53	53
50–64	49	9.6	48	5	6	7	12	18	24	39
65+	62	10.8	62	5	6	7	13	23	26	43
TOTAL SINGLE DX	3	6.4	4	4	4	6	8	8	8	8
TOTAL MULTIPLE DX	133	10.8	70	4	6	7	12	23	28	43
TOTAL										
0–19 Years	4	8.0	0	8	8	8	8	8	8	8
20–34	6	10.4	65	3	5	7	16	24	24	24
35–49	14	15.1	199	4	6	7	22	31	53	53
50–64	50	9.5	48	4	5	7	12	18	24	39
65+	62	10.8	62	5	6	7	13	23	26	43
GRAND TOTAL	136	10.6	69	4	6	7	12	23	28	43

LOS by Diagnosis and Operation, Western Region, 45th Edition

Western Region, October 2007–September 2008 Data, by Operation

45.72: CECECTOMY

Type of Patients	Observed Patients	Avg. Stay	Vari-ance	Percentiles						
				10th	25th	50th	75th	90th	95th	99th
1. SINGLE DX										
0–19 Years	16	5.5	5	2	4	5	7	8	12	12
20–34	25	4.3	5	2	3	4	5	8	8	10
35–49	22	4.4	4	2	3	4	6	7	8	8
50–64	21	3.9	5	1	2	4	6	6	8	9
65+	8	3.4	4	1	2	2	5	7	7	7
2. MULTIPLE DX										
0–19 Years	89	13.5	269	4	5	8	14	38	65	>99
20–34	236	8.1	37	3	4	6	9	15	21	31
35–49	264	8.7	92	3	4	6	10	17	25	47
50–64	421	8.6	83	3	4	6	10	17	26	52
65+	576	8.5	45	3	4	7	11	16	22	35
TOTAL SINGLE DX	92	4.4	5	2	3	4	6	7	8	12
TOTAL MULTIPLE DX	1,586	8.9	81	3	4	6	10	17	26	51
TOTAL										
0–19 Years	105	12.5	243	4	5	7	11	36	65	>99
20–34	261	7.8	35	3	4	6	9	14	21	31
35–49	286	8.4	86	3	4	6	9	16	24	47
50–64	442	8.4	80	2	4	6	10	16	25	52
65+	584	8.4	45	2	4	7	11	16	22	35
GRAND TOTAL	1,678	8.7	78	3	4	6	10	17	25	49

45.73: RIGHT HEMICOLECTOMY

Type of Patients	Observed Patients	Avg. Stay	Vari-ance	Percentiles						
				10th	25th	50th	75th	90th	95th	99th
1. SINGLE DX										
0–19 Years	11	4.1	1	3	3	4	5	5	5	6
20–34	24	5.0	4	3	3	5	6	8	8	11
35–49	48	4.6	4	3	3	5	5	6	7	14
50–64	146	4.0	2	2	3	4	5	6	6	8
65+	103	4.1	2	2	3	4	5	6	6	7
2. MULTIPLE DX										
0–19 Years	126	12.8	362	4	5	7	11	44	99	>99
20–34	397	9.2	76	4	5	7	10	16	23	51
35–49	970	8.7	57	4	5	7	10	16	21	45
50–64	3,388	8.0	58	3	4	6	9	15	21	42
65+	8,008	9.0	52	4	5	7	11	17	21	38
TOTAL SINGLE DX	332	4.2	2	3	3	4	5	6	6	9
TOTAL MULTIPLE DX	12,889	8.8	59	3	5	6	10	16	22	42
TOTAL										
0–19 Years	137	11.8	329	3	5	6	9	36	98	>99
20–34	421	8.9	73	4	5	6	10	15	22	42
35–49	1,018	8.5	55	3	5	6	10	16	21	45
50–64	3,534	7.9	56	3	4	6	9	14	20	42
65+	8,111	8.9	51	4	5	7	11	17	21	38
GRAND TOTAL	13,221	8.6	58	3	4	6	10	16	21	42

45.74: TRANSVERSE COLON RESECT

Type of Patients	Observed Patients	Avg. Stay	Vari-ance	Percentiles						
				10th	25th	50th	75th	90th	95th	99th
1. SINGLE DX										
0–19 Years	2	6.2	<1	6	6	6	6	7	7	7
20–34	3	4.3	5	3	3	3	7	7	7	7
35–49	3	4.0	<1	3	3	4	5	5	5	5
50–64	20	4.1	3	2	3	4	4	6	10	10
65+	9	4.8	2	3	4	5	5	7	7	7
2. MULTIPLE DX										
0–19 Years	32	25.0	715	5	8	13	31	76	91	93
20–34	44	9.1	35	4	5	8	10	16	17	32
35–49	134	9.1	73	3	5	7	10	18	26	39
50–64	475	8.9	74	4	5	6	10	18	24	54
65+	910	9.8	64	4	5	7	12	20	24	39
TOTAL SINGLE DX	37	4.5	3	3	3	4	6	6	7	10
TOTAL MULTIPLE DX	1,595	9.8	87	4	5	7	11	19	26	54
TOTAL										
0–19 Years	34	22.7	665	5	6	13	29	75	81	93
20–34	47	8.8	34	4	5	7	10	16	17	32
35–49	137	9.0	72	3	5	7	10	18	26	39
50–64	495	8.8	72	3	4	6	10	18	24	54
65+	919	9.8	64	4	5	7	12	20	24	39
GRAND TOTAL	1,632	9.7	86	4	5	7	11	19	26	54

45.75: LEFT HEMICOLECTOMY

Type of Patients	Observed Patients	Avg. Stay	Vari-ance	Percentiles						
				10th	25th	50th	75th	90th	95th	99th
1. SINGLE DX										
0–19 Years	1	6.0	0	6	6	6	6	6	6	6
20–34	14	5.4	8	3	4	4	5	9	13	13
35–49	23	5.0	3	3	4	4	6	7	7	10
50–64	31	4.3	3	2	3	4	6	7	7	8
65+	17	4.5	2	3	4	5	5	6	7	7
2. MULTIPLE DX										
0–19 Years	33	15.5	309	5	5	7	16	47	74	>99
20–34	126	10.9	66	4	6	8	13	19	24	44
35–49	430	9.4	57	4	5	7	11	17	21	38
50–64	1,177	9.4	59	4	5	7	11	17	23	42
65+	1,830	11.1	82	4	6	8	14	20	26	47
TOTAL SINGLE DX	86	4.7	4	3	3	4	6	7	8	13
TOTAL MULTIPLE DX	3,596	10.4	76	4	5	8	12	19	26	47
TOTAL										
0–19 Years	34	15.3	305	5	5	7	16	47	74	>99
20–34	140	10.3	63	4	5	8	13	19	24	44
35–49	453	9.2	56	4	5	7	11	16	20	38
50–64	1,208	9.3	59	4	5	7	11	17	23	42
65+	1,847	11.0	81	4	6	8	14	20	26	47
GRAND TOTAL	3,682	10.3	75	4	5	8	12	19	26	47

LOS by Diagnosis and Operation, Western Region, 45th Edition

Western Region, October 2007–September 2008 Data, by Operation

45.76: SIGMOIDECTOMY

Type of Patients	Observed Patients	Avg. Stay	Vari-ance	10th	25th	50th	75th	90th	95th	99th
1. SINGLE DX										
0–19 Years	6	6.3	2	5	5	6	7	8	10	10
20–34	41	4.9	3	3	4	5	6	7	8	10
35–49	147	4.7	6	3	3	4	6	7	8	12
50–64	192	4.3	2	3	3	4	5	6	7	9
65+	49	4.9	4	3	4	5	6	7	9	11
2. MULTIPLE DX										
0–19 Years	42	14.3	286	3	5	9	14	39	62	81
20–34	438	8.6	60	4	5	7	10	15	21	42
35–49	1,970	7.7	32	3	4	6	9	14	18	30
50–64	4,153	8.0	42	3	4	6	9	15	19	36
65+	4,677	10.0	59	4	5	8	12	19	24	41
TOTAL SINGLE DX	435	4.6	4	3	3	4	5	7	8	10
TOTAL MULTIPLE DX	11,280	8.8	50	3	5	7	11	16	21	37
TOTAL										
0–19 Years	48	12.6	235	4	5	7	13	26	50	81
20–34	479	8.3	56	3	4	6	9	15	21	42
35–49	2,117	7.5	31	3	4	6	9	14	18	29
50–64	4,345	7.8	41	3	4	6	9	14	18	36
65+	4,726	9.9	58	4	5	8	12	19	24	39
GRAND TOTAL	11,715	8.7	49	3	5	7	10	16	21	37

45.79: PART LG INTEST EXC NEC

Type of Patients	Observed Patients	Avg. Stay	Vari-ance	10th	25th	50th	75th	90th	95th	99th
1. SINGLE DX										
0–19 Years	6	3.4	<1	3	3	3	3	4	6	6
20–34	17	5.1	3	3	4	5	6	7	9	9
35–49	26	5.0	5	3	4	4	6	7	10	11
50–64	53	3.9	3	2	3	4	5	6	7	11
65+	11	4.6	3	3	3	4	6	7	8	8
2. MULTIPLE DX										
0–19 Years	58	10.9	130	3	5	7	15	21	43	>99
20–34	137	9.1	74	3	4	6	10	19	28	46
35–49	442	8.5	56	3	4	6	10	15	20	44
50–64	956	8.4	63	3	4	6	10	17	24	47
65+	1,353	9.4	70	3	4	7	11	20	25	43
TOTAL SINGLE DX	113	4.3	4	2	3	4	5	7	8	11
TOTAL MULTIPLE DX	2,946	9.0	68	3	4	6	10	18	24	46
TOTAL										
0–19 Years	64	10.2	122	3	4	7	14	21	39	>99
20–34	154	8.7	67	3	4	6	9	17	28	46
35–49	468	8.3	54	3	4	6	9	15	20	44
50–64	1,009	8.2	60	3	4	6	9	16	23	46
65+	1,364	9.4	69	3	4	7	11	20	25	43
GRAND TOTAL	3,059	8.8	66	3	4	6	10	18	24	46

45.8: TOT INTRA-ABD COLECTOMY

Type of Patients	Observed Patients	Avg. Stay	Vari-ance	10th	25th	50th	75th	90th	95th	99th
1. SINGLE DX										
0–19 Years	9	5.8	3	4	4	6	7	7	9	9
20–34	14	4.3	3	3	3	4	5	7	8	8
35–49	11	6.9	6	4	5	7	9	9	11	11
50–64	11	5.9	12	3	3	6	7	8	15	15
65+	2	5.5	<1	5	5	6	6	6	6	6
2. MULTIPLE DX										
0–19 Years	56	16.2	209	5	7	9	20	46	49	53
20–34	161	12.2	134	4	6	8	14	26	36	70
35–49	243	12.4	132	4	6	9	14	26	34	59
50–64	362	13.2	128	5	6	9	17	26	34	78
65+	432	16.8	151	6	8	14	22	33	40	73
TOTAL SINGLE DX	47	5.6	6	3	4	5	7	9	9	15
TOTAL MULTIPLE DX	1,254	14.4	148	5	7	10	18	29	42	68
TOTAL										
0–19 Years	65	15.2	199	5	7	9	17	42	49	53
20–34	175	11.6	128	4	5	7	13	26	36	70
35–49	254	12.2	128	4	6	9	14	24	34	59
50–64	373	13.0	126	5	6	9	17	26	34	78
65+	434	16.7	150	6	8	14	22	33	40	73
GRAND TOTAL	1,301	14.1	145	5	6	10	18	29	40	68

45.9: INTESTINAL ANASTOMOSIS

Type of Patients	Observed Patients	Avg. Stay	Vari-ance	10th	25th	50th	75th	90th	95th	99th
1. SINGLE DX										
0–19 Years	6	7.8	21	4	4	6	10	16	16	16
20–34	2	6.0	0	6	6	6	6	6	6	6
35–49	13	5.0	4	3	4	5	6	8	9	9
50–64	17	5.4	4	4	4	5	6	8	11	11
65+	9	6.3	6	3	5	6	7	10	10	10
2. MULTIPLE DX										
0–19 Years	102	12.3	99	4	6	8	16	30	37	>99
20–34	94	8.5	130	3	4	6	8	15	20	99
35–49	229	8.7	44	3	4	6	11	17	21	36
50–64	440	9.1	69	3	4	6	11	17	25	39
65+	457	11.2	68	4	6	9	14	20	27	48
TOTAL SINGLE DX	47	5.8	7	3	4	5	7	10	10	16
TOTAL MULTIPLE DX	1,322	10.1	74	4	5	7	12	19	28	44
TOTAL										
0–19 Years	108	12.1	97	4	6	8	15	30	37	>99
20–34	96	8.4	128	3	4	6	8	15	20	99
35–49	242	8.5	43	3	4	6	10	17	20	36
50–64	457	9.0	67	3	4	6	10	17	24	39
65+	466	11.1	67	4	6	9	14	20	26	48
GRAND TOTAL	1,369	10.0	73	3	5	7	12	19	27	44

LOS by Diagnosis and Operation, Western Region, 45th Edition

45.91: SM-TO-SM INTEST ANAST

Type of Patients	Observed Patients	Avg. Stay	Variance	10th	25th	50th	75th	90th	95th	99th
1. SINGLE DX										
0–19 Years	4	8.9	25	4	4	10	10	16	16	16
20–34	0									
35–49	2	8.5	<1	8	8	8	9	9	9	9
50–64	2	7.5	24	4	8	8	11	11	11	11
65+	1	10.0	0	10	10	10	10	10	10	10
2. MULTIPLE DX										
0–19 Years	50	18.7	132	6	9	17	30	34	41	>99
20–34	37	9.7	296	2	3	5	8	17	47	99
35–49	78	8.3	60	3	3	6	11	18	24	43
50–64	123	7.9	67	3	3	5	9	16	19	38
65+	119	13.0	85	5	7	10	15	24	36	48
TOTAL SINGLE DX	9	8.7	14	4	4	10	10	16	16	16
TOTAL MULTIPLE DX	407	11.4	115	3	4	8	15	25	34	55
TOTAL										
0–19 Years	54	18.0	130	5	8	17	30	34	41	>99
20–34	37	9.7	296	2	3	5	8	17	47	99
35–49	80	8.4	58	3	3	6	11	18	24	43
50–64	125	7.9	66	3	3	5	9	16	19	38
65+	120	12.9	84	5	7	10	15	24	36	48
GRAND TOTAL	416	11.3	113	3	4	8	14	25	33	55

45.93: SM-LG INTEST ANAST NEC

Type of Patients	Observed Patients	Avg. Stay	Variance	10th	25th	50th	75th	90th	95th	99th
1. SINGLE DX										
0–19 Years	0									
20–34	0									
35–49	2	2.5	<1	2	2	3	3	3	3	3
50–64	1	3.0	0	3	3	3	3	3	3	3
65+	1	6.0	0	6	6	6	6	6	6	6
2. MULTIPLE DX										
0–19 Years	19	9.7	73	4	5	8	11	17	44	>99
20–34	18	9.2	58	3	4	6	12	26	27	27
35–49	44	11.3	78	4	6	7	16	21	36	37
50–64	104	12.8	92	4	7	9	16	25	30	39
65+	122	13.7	69	6	8	12	18	23	27	43
TOTAL SINGLE DX	4	3.5	3	2	3	3	6	6	6	6
TOTAL MULTIPLE DX	307	12.4	79	4	6	10	16	24	30	44
TOTAL										
0–19 Years	19	9.7	73	4	5	8	11	17	44	>99
20–34	18	9.2	58	3	4	6	12	26	27	27
35–49	46	11.0	78	4	5	7	16	21	36	37
50–64	105	12.7	92	4	6	9	16	25	30	39
65+	123	13.7	69	6	8	12	18	23	27	43
GRAND TOTAL	311	12.3	79	4	6	10	16	23	30	44

45.94: LG-TO-LG INTEST ANAST

Type of Patients	Observed Patients	Avg. Stay	Variance	10th	25th	50th	75th	90th	95th	99th
1. SINGLE DX										
0–19 Years	0									
20–34	0									
35–49	3	4.7	<1	4	4	5	5	5	5	5
50–64	8	4.9	2	3	4	6	5	7	7	8
65+	6	6.3	4	5	5	6	7	10	10	10
2. MULTIPLE DX										
0–19 Years	11	7.4	23	4	4	7	10	10	12	26
20–34	11	6.3	3	4	5	6	8	8	8	8
35–49	55	7.6	15	4	5	6	10	12	17	19
50–64	144	7.5	49	3	5	6	8	13	15	39
65+	164	9.1	54	4	5	7	10	15	18	52
TOTAL SINGLE DX	17	5.4	3	4	5	5	6	7	10	10
TOTAL MULTIPLE DX	385	8.1	44	4	5	6	10	14	17	39
TOTAL										
0–19 Years	11	7.4	23	4	4	7	10	10	12	26
20–34	11	6.3	3	4	5	6	8	8	8	8
35–49	58	7.5	15	4	5	6	10	12	17	19
50–64	152	7.3	46	3	4	6	8	13	15	39
65+	170	9.0	53	4	5	7	10	15	18	52
GRAND TOTAL	402	8.0	43	4	5	6	9	13	17	39

45.95: ANASTOMOSIS TO ANUS

Type of Patients	Observed Patients	Avg. Stay	Variance	10th	25th	50th	75th	90th	95th	99th
1. SINGLE DX										
0–19 Years	2	5.0	2	4	4	5	6	6	6	6
20–34	2	6.0	0	6	6	6	6	6	6	6
35–49	5	5.2	2	4	4	5	6	7	7	7
50–64	3	6.0	4	4	4	6	8	8	8	8
65+	0									
2. MULTIPLE DX										
0–19 Years	19	7.1	11	4	5	7	7	11	11	23
20–34	28	7.2	11	4	5	6	10	13	13	16
35–49	41	8.0	17	5	5	7	10	13	14	23
50–64	55	8.4	31	5	5	6	8	16	24	30
65+	35	7.8	25	3	5	6	9	14	16	28
TOTAL SINGLE DX	12	5.5	2	4	4	6	6	7	8	8
TOTAL MULTIPLE DX	178	7.8	20	4	5	6	9	13	16	24
TOTAL										
0–19 Years	21	7.0	11	4	5	6	7	11	11	23
20–34	30	7.1	10	4	5	6	9	13	13	16
35–49	46	7.7	16	4	5	6	10	13	14	23
50–64	58	8.2	29	5	5	6	8	16	24	30
65+	35	7.8	25	3	5	6	9	14	16	28
GRAND TOTAL	190	7.6	19	4	5	6	9	13	16	24

LOS by Diagnosis and Operation, Western Region, 45th Edition

Western Region, October 2007–September 2008 Data, by Operation

46.0: INTEST EXTERIORIZATION

Type of Patients	Observed Patients	Avg. Stay	Variance	10th	25th	50th	75th	90th	95th	99th
1. SINGLE DX										
0–19 Years	6	6.4	2	5	6	6	8	8	8	8
20–34	3	5.0	4	3	3	5	7	7	7	7
35–49	13	4.6	4	3	4	5	5	6	10	10
50–64	13	4.1	2	2	3	4	5	5	6	6
65+	4	5.0	5	3	3	4	8	8	8	8
2. MULTIPLE DX										
0–19 Years	22	19.7	416	4	7	13	57	>99	>99	>99
20–34	89	11.8	119	3	5	9	14	26	33	70
35–49	270	10.9	100	3	5	8	12	21	30	69
50–64	572	10.7	84	3	5	8	13	22	26	50
65+	672	11.3	71	4	6	9	14	21	27	46
TOTAL SINGLE DX	39	5.0	4	3	4	5	6	8	8	10
TOTAL MULTIPLE DX	1,625	11.2	88	4	5	8	13	22	29	56
TOTAL										
0–19 Years	28	15.0	306	4	6	8	25	>99	>99	>99
20–34	92	11.6	116	3	5	9	14	23	33	70
35–49	283	10.6	97	3	5	8	12	21	30	69
50–64	585	10.5	83	3	5	8	13	21	26	50
65+	676	11.3	71	4	6	9	14	21	27	46
GRAND TOTAL	1,664	11.0	87	4	5	8	13	22	28	56

46.01: S-INTEST EXTERIORIZATION

Type of Patients	Observed Patients	Avg. Stay	Variance	10th	25th	50th	75th	90th	95th	99th
1. SINGLE DX										
0–19 Years	1	3.0	0	3	3	3	3	3	3	3
20–34	2	4.0	2	3	3	3	5	5	5	5
35–49	11	5.0	4	3	4	5	5	6	10	10
50–64	10	4.4	1	2	4	5	5	5	6	6
65+	2	4.5	<1	4	4	4	5	5	5	5
2. MULTIPLE DX										
0–19 Years	8	23.2	583	2	10	25	>99	>99	>99	>99
20–34	58	11.3	135	3	4	9	13	23	30	70
35–49	142	9.6	71	4	5	7	11	19	23	41
50–64	292	10.2	77	3	5	7	12	21	26	50
65+	278	11.9	84	4	6	9	15	22	30	49
TOTAL SINGLE DX	26	4.6	2	3	4	5	5	6	6	10
TOTAL MULTIPLE DX	778	10.9	89	4	5	8	13	22	29	56
TOTAL										
0–19 Years	9	21.0	556	2	10	25	>99	>99	>99	>99
20–34	60	11.1	132	3	4	8	11	23	30	70
35–49	153	9.3	67	3	5	7	11	17	23	41
50–64	302	10.0	76	4	5	7	12	20	25	49
65+	280	11.9	83	4	6	9	15	22	29	49
GRAND TOTAL	804	10.7	88	4	5	8	13	21	28	55

46.03: L-INTEST EXTERIORIZATION

Type of Patients	Observed Patients	Avg. Stay	Variance	10th	25th	50th	75th	90th	95th	99th
1. SINGLE DX										
0–19 Years	5	6.7	1	6	6	6	8	8	8	8
20–34	1	7.0	0	7	7	7	7	7	7	7
35–49	1	1.0	0	1	1	1	1	1	1	1
50–64	3	3.0	<1	2	2	3	4	4	4	4
65+	2	5.5	12	3	3	8	8	8	8	8
2. MULTIPLE DX										
0–19 Years	14	17.7	346	6	7	10	25	61	>99	>99
20–34	27	12.5	103	4	5	9	14	33	33	39
35–49	117	12.2	133	3	6	9	15	28	32	78
50–64	270	11.3	91	3	5	9	14	23	27	53
65+	365	11.0	64	4	6	9	13	21	26	44
TOTAL SINGLE DX	12	5.7	5	2	4	6	8	8	8	8
TOTAL MULTIPLE DX	793	11.5	90	4	6	9	14	23	29	57
TOTAL										
0–19 Years	19	12.8	218	6	6	8	13	57	61	>99
20–34	28	12.3	101	4	5	9	14	33	33	39
35–49	118	12.2	133	3	6	9	15	28	32	78
50–64	273	11.2	91	4	6	9	14	23	27	53
65+	367	11.0	64	4	6	9	13	21	26	44
GRAND TOTAL	805	11.3	89	3	6	9	14	22	28	57

46.1: COLOSTOMY

Type of Patients	Observed Patients	Avg. Stay	Variance	10th	25th	50th	75th	90th	95th	99th
1. SINGLE DX										
0–19 Years	6	2.7	<1	2	2	3	3	3	4	4
20–34	1	5.0	0	5	5	5	5	5	5	5
35–49	2	5.5	4	4	4	7	7	7	7	7
50–64	7	4.7	13	1	1	4	7	11	11	11
65+	2	1.5	<1	1	1	1	2	2	2	2
2. MULTIPLE DX										
0–19 Years	138	12.0	171	2	4	7	16	25	46	70
20–34	53	10.1	87	2	4	8	12	26	31	>99
35–49	155	13.0	137	3	6	10	17	30	48	56
50–64	413	13.0	139	3	6	10	16	26	39	77
65+	570	12.5	110	4	6	9	15	25	33	63
TOTAL SINGLE DX	18	3.4	5	1	2	3	4	7	7	11
TOTAL MULTIPLE DX	1,329	12.6	130	3	6	9	15	25	35	70
TOTAL										
0–19 Years	144	11.4	165	2	3	6	15	25	35	70
20–34	54	10.0	86	2	4	7	12	23	31	>99
35–49	157	12.9	136	3	6	10	16	30	48	56
50–64	420	12.9	138	4	6	10	16	26	37	77
65+	572	12.5	110	4	6	9	15	25	33	63
GRAND TOTAL	1,347	12.4	130	3	6	9	15	25	35	70

LOS by Diagnosis and Operation, Western Region, 45th Edition

Western Region, October 2007–September 2008 Data, by Operation

46.10: COLOSTOMY NOS

Type of Patients	Observed Patients	Avg. Stay	Variance	Percentiles						
				10th	25th	50th	75th	90th	95th	99th
1. SINGLE DX										
0–19 Years	4	2.6	<1	2	2	3	3	3	4	4
20–34	1	5.0	0	5	5	5	5	5	5	5
35–49	1	4.0	0	4	4	4	4	4	4	4
50–64	5	5.2	18	1	1	6	7	11	11	11
65+	1	2.0	0	2	2	2	2	2	2	2
2. MULTIPLE DX										
0–19 Years	82	10.1	112	2	3	6	16	24	25	50
20–34	28	10.8	90	5	6	10	12	26	48	>99
35–49	89	13.6	142	4	6	9	16	33	41	56
50–64	237	13.4	147	4	6	10	17	28	43	83
65+	334	12.7	113	4	6	10	15	23	32	51
TOTAL SINGLE DX	12	3.5	6	1	2	3	4	7	11	11
TOTAL MULTIPLE DX	770	12.5	126	3	6	9	16	25	34	66
TOTAL										
0–19 Years	86	9.6	108	2	3	5	14	24	25	50
20–34	29	10.6	88	3	5	8	12	22	48	>99
35–49	90	13.5	141	4	6	9	16	33	41	56
50–64	242	13.2	146	4	6	10	17	27	42	83
65+	335	12.6	113	4	6	10	15	23	32	51
GRAND TOTAL	782	12.3	125	3	5	9	15	25	34	66

46.13: PERMANENT COLOSTOMY

Type of Patients	Observed Patients	Avg. Stay	Variance	Percentiles						
				10th	25th	50th	75th	90th	95th	99th
1. SINGLE DX										
0–19 Years	1	3.0	0	3	3	3	3	3	3	3
20–34	0									
35–49	0									
50–64	1	4.0	0	4	4	4	4	4	4	4
65+	0									
2. MULTIPLE DX										
0–19 Years	8	6.6	8	3	6	6	7	10	14	14
20–34	7	4.2	24	1	1	2	6	7	17	17
35–49	34	11.9	162	3	6	7	15	30	56	>99
50–64	88	12.0	156	3	5	8	13	26	49	66
65+	119	10.6	58	4	6	8	13	22	28	36
TOTAL SINGLE DX	2	3.5	<1	3	3	3	4	4	4	4
TOTAL MULTIPLE DX	256	10.8	102	3	5	8	13	24	28	61
TOTAL										
0–19 Years	9	6.3	8	3	6	6	7	10	14	14
20–34	7	4.2	24	1	1	2	6	7	17	17
35–49	34	11.9	162	3	6	7	15	30	56	>99
50–64	89	12.0	155	3	5	8	13	26	49	66
65+	119	10.6	58	4	6	8	13	22	28	36
GRAND TOTAL	258	10.7	102	3	5	7	13	24	28	61

46.11: TEMPORARY COLOSTOMY

Type of Patients	Observed Patients	Avg. Stay	Variance	Percentiles						
				10th	25th	50th	75th	90th	95th	99th
1. SINGLE DX										
0–19 Years	1	3.0	0	3	3	3	3	3	3	3
20–34	0									
35–49	1	7.0	0	7	7	7	7	7	7	7
50–64	1	3.0	0	3	3	3	3	3	3	3
65+	1	1.0	0	1	1	1	1	1	1	1
2. MULTIPLE DX										
0–19 Years	48	16.3	274	4	6	10	23	49	59	50
20–34	18	12.2	101	2	5	9	18	31	31	>99
35–49	32	12.7	105	3	6	9	18	23	32	50
50–64	88	13.1	103	4	6	12	16	23	28	77
65+	117	14.2	150	4	6	12	18	32	47	>99
TOTAL SINGLE DX	4	3.3	3	1	3	3	3	7	7	7
TOTAL MULTIPLE DX	303	14.1	160	4	6	11	18	30	46	81
TOTAL										
0–19 Years	49	15.6	268	3	6	8	19	49	59	50
20–34	18	12.2	101	5	5	9	18	31	31	>99
35–49	33	12.6	103	3	6	10	18	23	32	50
50–64	89	12.9	103	4	6	12	16	23	28	77
65+	118	14.1	150	4	6	12	18	32	47	>99
GRAND TOTAL	307	13.9	160	4	6	10	17	30	46	81

46.2: ILEOSTOMY

Type of Patients	Observed Patients	Avg. Stay	Variance	Percentiles						
				10th	25th	50th	75th	90th	95th	99th
1. SINGLE DX										
0–19 Years	3	6.7	10	3	3	8	9	9	9	9
20–34	1	6.0	0	6	6	6	6	6	6	6
35–49	4	5.5	3	4	4	4	5	7	7	7
50–64	4	4.3	<1	4	4	4	5	5	5	5
65+	2	3.0	2	2	2	4	4	4	4	4
2. MULTIPLE DX										
0–19 Years	20	19.2	533	5	7	12	29	>99	>99	>99
20–34	24	10.4	109	3	5	8	12	19	23	52
35–49	64	10.8	93	4	5	7	15	21	26	55
50–64	157	10.5	75	4	5	7	12	21	26	52
65+	147	11.8	105	4	6	8	14	23	32	95
TOTAL SINGLE DX	14	5.1	4	3	4	4	7	8	9	9
TOTAL MULTIPLE DX	412	11.9	146	4	6	8	14	25	38	>99
TOTAL										
0–19 Years	23	18.5	511	5	6	10	29	>99	>99	>99
20–34	25	10.2	105	3	5	7	12	19	23	52
35–49	68	10.5	89	3	5	7	15	21	26	55
50–64	161	10.3	74	4	5	7	12	21	25	52
65+	149	11.6	104	4	6	8	14	23	32	95
GRAND TOTAL	426	11.7	143	4	5	8	14	25	38	>99

Western Region, October 2007–September 2008 Data, by Operation

46.20: ILEOSTOMY NOS

Type of Patients	Observed Patients	Avg. Stay	Variance	Percentiles						
				10th	25th	50th	75th	90th	95th	99th
1. SINGLE DX										
0–19 Years	2	6.0	18	3	3	9	9	9	9	9
20–34	0									
35–49	1	7.0	0	7	7	7	7	7	7	7
50–64	4	4.3	<1	4	4	4	5	5	5	5
65+	1	2.0	0	2	2	2	2	2	2	2
2. MULTIPLE DX										
0–19 Years	4	17.4	461	3	12	12	>99	>99	>99	>99
20–34	8	16.5	241	3	8	12	23	52	52	52
35–49	27	13.6	150	4	5	10	16	31	42	55
50–64	72	10.5	79	4	5	7	11	22	25	55
65+	67	12.8	157	5	6	9	16	22	29	95
TOTAL SINGLE DX	8	4.8	5	2	4	4	7	9	9	9
TOTAL MULTIPLE DX	178	12.3	138	4	6	8	15	25	42	>99
TOTAL										
0–19 Years	6	14.8	373	3	5	12	65	>99	>99	>99
20–34	8	16.5	241	3	8	12	23	52	52	52
35–49	28	13.4	146	4	5	10	16	31	42	55
50–64	76	10.1	77	4	5	7	11	22	25	55
65+	68	12.7	156	5	6	9	16	22	29	95
GRAND TOTAL	186	12.0	135	4	6	8	14	24	42	>99

46.23: PERMANENT ILEOSTOMY NEC

Type of Patients	Observed Patients	Avg. Stay	Variance	Percentiles						
				10th	25th	50th	75th	90th	95th	99th
1. SINGLE DX										
0–19 Years	1	8.0	0	8	8	8	8	8	8	8
20–34	0									
35–49	3	5.0	3	4	4	4	7	7	7	7
50–64	0									
65+	0									
2. MULTIPLE DX										
0–19 Years	7	12.8	81	5	6	7	17	29	29	29
20–34	10	8.7	33	3	4	7	10	19	19	19
35–49	20	9.1	54	4	5	5	10	23	26	26
50–64	47	10.7	82	4	5	8	13	21	29	52
65+	41	11.9	78	4	6	8	14	24	32	39
TOTAL SINGLE DX	4	5.7	4	4	4	4	8	8	8	8
TOTAL MULTIPLE DX	125	11.0	73	4	5	8	14	23	29	39
TOTAL										
0–19 Years	8	12.6	78	5	6	7	17	29	29	29
20–34	10	8.7	33	3	4	7	10	19	19	19
35–49	23	8.6	49	4	4	5	10	20	23	26
50–64	47	10.7	82	4	5	8	13	21	29	52
65+	41	11.9	78	4	6	8	14	24	32	39
GRAND TOTAL	129	10.9	72	4	5	8	14	23	29	39

46.3: OTHER ENTEROSTOMY

Type of Patients	Observed Patients	Avg. Stay	Variance	Percentiles						
				10th	25th	50th	75th	90th	95th	99th
1. SINGLE DX										
0–19 Years	1	2.0	0	2	2	2	2	2	2	2
20–34	1	1.0	0	1	1	1	1	1	1	1
35–49	2	1.5	<1	1	1	1	2	2	2	2
50–64	0									
65+	1	1.0	0	1	1	1	1	1	1	1
2. MULTIPLE DX										
0–19 Years	23	12.3	182	2	2	7	14	27	49	56
20–34	38	10.0	75	2	4	8	12	22	29	42
35–49	89	10.7	105	2	4	7	15	27	32	55
50–64	155	12.1	188	2	5	8	14	22	39	78
65+	289	10.3	93	2	4	7	13	22	29	48
TOTAL SINGLE DX	5	1.6	<1	1	1	2	2	2	2	2
TOTAL MULTIPLE DX	594	10.9	122	2	4	8	14	22	32	55
TOTAL										
0–19 Years	24	11.1	172	2	2	6	14	27	49	56
20–34	39	9.8	75	2	4	8	12	22	25	42
35–49	91	10.5	104	2	4	7	15	22	32	55
50–64	155	12.1	188	2	5	8	14	22	39	78
65+	290	10.3	93	2	4	7	13	22	29	48
GRAND TOTAL	599	10.8	122	2	4	8	13	22	32	55

46.32: PEJ

Type of Patients	Observed Patients	Avg. Stay	Variance	Percentiles						
				10th	25th	50th	75th	90th	95th	99th
1. SINGLE DX										
0–19 Years	0									
20–34	0									
35–49	1	2.0	0	2	2	2	2	2	2	2
50–64	0									
65+	0									
2. MULTIPLE DX										
0–19 Years	11	13.7	91	6	6	11	14	27	39	39
20–34	13	10.5	55	3	4	10	11	22	25	25
35–49	32	10.9	90	2	4	8	16	27	32	34
50–64	34	12.2	142	2	4	10	14	32	41	53
65+	121	8.4	42	2	5	7	10	16	23	29
TOTAL SINGLE DX	1	2.0	0	2	2	2	2	2	2	2
TOTAL MULTIPLE DX	211	9.9	71	2	4	8	13	22	28	39
TOTAL										
0–19 Years	11	13.7	91	6	6	11	14	27	39	39
20–34	13	10.5	55	3	4	10	11	22	25	25
35–49	33	10.7	90	2	4	8	15	27	32	34
50–64	34	12.2	142	2	4	10	14	32	41	53
65+	121	8.4	42	2	5	7	10	16	23	29
GRAND TOTAL	212	9.8	71	2	4	8	13	22	28	39

LOS by Diagnosis and Operation, Western Region, 45th Edition

Western Region, October 2007–September 2008 Data, by Operation

46.41: SM INTEST STOMA REVISION

Type of Patients	Observed Patients	Avg. Stay	Variance	10th	25th	50th	75th	90th	95th	99th
1. SINGLE DX										
0–19 Years	0									
20–34	1	3.0	0	3	3	3	3	3	3	3
35–49	2	1.5	<1	1	1	1	2	2	2	2
50–64	6	3.5	6	1	2	3	6	7	7	7
65+	1	2.0	0	2	2	2	2	2	2	2
2. MULTIPLE DX										
0–19 Years	20	10.0	77	2	2	6	21	22	22	30
20–34	14	8.7	15	4	5	8	11	14	16	16
35–49	45	7.9	55	2	3	5	9	17	20	37
50–64	83	8.5	82	2	3	5	11	19	23	47
65+	105	9.1	109	2	3	5	10	22	32	42
TOTAL SINGLE DX	10	2.9	4	1	2	2	3	7	7	7
TOTAL MULTIPLE DX	267	8.8	83	2	3	5	11	21	25	44
TOTAL										
0–19 Years	20	10.0	77	2	2	6	21	22	22	30
20–34	15	8.3	16	4	4	8	11	14	16	16
35–49	47	7.6	54	2	3	5	9	17	20	37
50–64	89	8.1	78	2	3	5	10	19	23	47
65+	106	9.0	109	2	3	5	10	22	32	42
GRAND TOTAL	277	8.6	82	2	3	5	11	21	25	44

46.42: PERICOLOSTOMY HERNIA REP

Type of Patients	Observed Patients	Avg. Stay	Variance	10th	25th	50th	75th	90th	95th	99th
1. SINGLE DX										
0–19 Years	0									
20–34	0									
35–49	1	2.0	0	2	2	2	2	2	2	2
50–64	0									
65+	4	2.3	4	1	1	1	5	5	5	5
2. MULTIPLE DX										
0–19 Years	0									
20–34	3	8.3	4	6	6	9	10	10	10	10
35–49	25	6.1	30	4	3	4	6	13	17	27
50–64	78	5.0	16	1	2	4	7	10	13	23
65+	147	7.9	111	1	2	5	9	14	30	61
TOTAL SINGLE DX	5	2.2	3	1	1	2	2	5	5	5
TOTAL MULTIPLE DX	253	6.8	74	1	2	5	8	11	18	56
TOTAL										
0–19 Years	0									
20–34	3	8.3	4	6	6	9	10	10	10	10
35–49	26	5.9	30	2	3	4	6	13	17	27
50–64	78	5.0	16	1	2	4	7	10	13	23
65+	151	7.7	109	1	2	5	9	12	30	61
GRAND TOTAL	258	6.7	73	1	2	5	8	11	18	56

46.39: ENTEROSTOMY NEC

Type of Patients	Observed Patients	Avg. Stay	Variance	10th	25th	50th	75th	90th	95th	99th
1. SINGLE DX										
0–19 Years	1	2.0	0	2	2	2	2	2	2	2
20–34	1	1.0	0	1	1	1	1	1	1	1
35–49	1	1.0	0	1	1	1	1	1	1	1
50–64	0									
65+	1	1.0	0	1	1	1	1	1	1	1
2. MULTIPLE DX										
0–19 Years	12	11.2	260	2	2	3	15	49	56	56
20–34	25	9.7	89	2	4	7	12	20	29	42
35–49	57	10.5	115	2	4	7	11	21	37	55
50–64	121	12.0	203	3	5	8	14	21	36	78
65+	168	11.7	125	2	4	8	16	25	35	50
TOTAL SINGLE DX	4	1.6	<1	1	1	2	2	2	2	2
TOTAL MULTIPLE DX	383	11.5	150	2	4	8	15	23	37	63
TOTAL										
0–19 Years	13	9.5	223	2	2	2	9	22	49	56
20–34	26	9.4	88	2	4	7	12	20	29	42
35–49	58	10.4	114	2	4	7	11	21	37	55
50–64	121	12.0	203	3	5	8	14	21	36	78
65+	169	11.7	125	2	4	8	16	25	35	50
GRAND TOTAL	387	11.3	149	2	4	7	15	22	37	63

46.4: INTESTINAL STOMA REV

Type of Patients	Observed Patients	Avg. Stay	Variance	10th	25th	50th	75th	90th	95th	99th
1. SINGLE DX										
0–19 Years	1	2.0	0	2	2	2	2	2	2	2
20–34	1	3.0	0	3	3	3	3	3	3	3
35–49	4	2.8	5	2	3	2	6	6	6	6
50–64	7	3.6	5	1	1	3	6	7	7	7
65+	8	3.1	3	1	1	4	5	5	5	5
2. MULTIPLE DX										
0–19 Years	26	12.5	110	2	4	8	22	30	30	30
20–34	24	7.8	12	4	5	8	9	13	14	16
35–49	102	6.9	38	1	3	5	9	15	17	29
50–64	233	6.4	53	1	2	4	8	16	20	40
65+	329	7.8	90	1	2	5	9	16	26	56
TOTAL SINGLE DX	21	3.2	4	1	2	2	5	6	6	7
TOTAL MULTIPLE DX	714	7.6	72	1	2	5	9	17	24	40
TOTAL										
0–19 Years	27	12.3	110	2	4	8	22	30	30	30
20–34	25	7.6	12	4	5	8	9	13	14	16
35–49	106	6.8	37	1	3	5	8	15	17	29
50–64	240	6.3	52	1	2	4	8	16	19	40
65+	337	7.7	89	1	2	5	9	16	26	56
GRAND TOTAL	735	7.5	71	1	2	5	9	17	23	40

LOS by Diagnosis and Operation, Western Region, 45th Edition

46.43: LG INTEST STOMA REV NEC

Type of Patients	Observed Patients	Avg. Stay	Vari-ance	10th	25th	50th	75th	90th	95th	99th
1. SINGLE DX										
0–19 Years	1	2.0	0	2	2	2	2	2	2	2
20–34	0									
35–49	1	6.0	0	6	6	6	6	6	6	6
50–64	0									
65+	2	5.0	0	5	5	5	5	5	5	5
2. MULTIPLE DX										
0–19 Years	6	19.0	146	4	8	30	30	30	30	30
20–34	5	5.6	5	2	5	6	7	8	8	8
35–49	24	5.9	18	1	2	5	9	12	13	14
50–64	64	5.4	41	1	1	3	7	14	20	32
65+	68	6.0	22	1	2	5	8	13	14	21
TOTAL SINGLE DX	4	4.5	3	2	5	5	6	6	6	6
TOTAL MULTIPLE DX	167	6.9	51	1	2	5	8	14	30	30
TOTAL										
0–19 Years	7	18.0	154	2	8	10	30	30	30	30
20–34	5	5.6	5	2	5	6	7	8	8	8
35–49	25	5.9	17	1	2	5	8	12	13	14
50–64	64	5.4	41	1	1	3	7	14	20	32
65+	70	6.0	21	1	2	5	8	13	14	21
GRAND TOTAL	171	6.8	50	1	2	5	8	14	28	30

46.5: INTESTINAL STOMA CLOSURE

Type of Patients	Observed Patients	Avg. Stay	Vari-ance	10th	25th	50th	75th	90th	95th	99th
1. SINGLE DX										
0–19 Years	59	4.7	3	3	3	4	6	7	8	9
20–34	61	4.4	2	3	3	4	5	6	7	8
35–49	87	4.4	2	2	3	4	5	7	7	9
50–64	78	4.5	5	2	3	4	6	7	7	9
65+	19	4.8	4	2	3	5	7	8	8	16
2. MULTIPLE DX										
0–19 Years	216	6.7	56	3	4	5	7	9	18	31
20–34	285	5.7	14	3	3	5	7	9	13	17
35–49	664	6.0	25	3	4	5	7	10	14	23
50–64	1,286	6.1	26	3	4	5	7	10	14	28
65+	1,182	6.9	28	3	4	6	8	12	15	28
TOTAL SINGLE DX	304	4.5	3	3	3	4	6	7	8	9
TOTAL MULTIPLE DX	3,633	6.4	29	3	4	5	7	11	15	28
TOTAL										
0–19 Years	275	6.3	46	3	4	5	7	9	15	31
20–34	346	5.5	12	3	3	5	6	9	12	17
35–49	751	5.8	23	3	4	5	7	9	13	23
50–64	1,364	6.0	25	3	3	5	7	10	14	28
65+	1,201	6.8	28	3	4	6	8	12	15	28
GRAND TOTAL	3,937	6.2	28	3	4	5	7	10	14	28

46.51: SM INTEST STOMA CLOSURE

Type of Patients	Observed Patients	Avg. Stay	Vari-ance	10th	25th	50th	75th	90th	95th	99th
1. SINGLE DX										
0–19 Years	20	4.7	2	3	3	5	5	7	7	9
20–34	23	3.8	3	3	3	4	5	5	7	8
35–49	40	3.5	2	2	3	3	4	6	7	7
50–64	30	3.8	2	2	3	4	4	6	6	7
65+	6	4.3	5	2	2	4	7	7	7	7
2. MULTIPLE DX										
0–19 Years	92	8.5	126	3	3	6	9	18	30	89
20–34	160	5.1	10	2	3	4	6	9	12	17
35–49	293	5.8	30	2	3	4	6	12	14	23
50–64	625	5.8	32	2	3	4	6	11	14	31
65+	496	7.1	49	2	3	5	8	15	20	46
TOTAL SINGLE DX	119	4.0	3	2	3	4	5	7	7	9
TOTAL MULTIPLE DX	1,666	6.4	45	2	3	4	7	12	17	31
TOTAL										
0–19 Years	112	7.8	105	3	3	5	7	15	24	31
20–34	183	4.9	9	2	3	4	6	9	12	17
35–49	333	5.5	27	2	3	4	6	11	14	23
50–64	655	5.7	30	2	3	4	6	11	14	31
65+	502	7.0	48	2	3	5	8	15	20	39
GRAND TOTAL	1,785	6.2	42	2	3	4	7	12	17	31

46.52: LG INTEST STOMA CLOSURE

Type of Patients	Observed Patients	Avg. Stay	Vari-ance	10th	25th	50th	75th	90th	95th	99th
1. SINGLE DX										
0–19 Years	39	4.7	3	3	3	4	6	8	8	9
20–34	38	4.7	2	3	4	4	6	7	7	8
35–49	47	5.1	2	4	4	4	6	7	8	9
50–64	48	4.9	7	2	3	4	6	7	10	16
65+	13	5.1	4	3	3	5	6	8	8	8
2. MULTIPLE DX										
0–19 Years	123	5.4	7	3	4	5	6	8	9	18
20–34	125	6.5	18	3	4	6	7	11	14	24
35–49	371	6.2	21	3	4	5	7	9	12	25
50–64	660	6.4	21	3	4	5	7	10	12	28
65+	685	6.8	13	3	5	6	8	11	14	21
TOTAL SINGLE DX	185	4.9	4	3	4	5	6	7	8	10
TOTAL MULTIPLE DX	1,964	6.4	17	3	4	5	7	10	12	23
TOTAL										
0–19 Years	162	5.3	6	3	4	5	6	8	9	14
20–34	163	6.1	15	3	4	5	7	9	12	24
35–49	418	6.1	19	3	4	5	7	9	11	20
50–64	708	6.3	20	3	4	5	7	10	12	28
65+	698	6.7	13	3	5	6	8	11	14	21
GRAND TOTAL	2,149	6.2	16	3	4	5	7	9	12	22

Western Region, October 2007–September 2008 Data, by Operation

46.6: FIXATION OF INTESTINE

Type of Patients	Observed Patients	Avg. Stay	Vari-ance	Percentiles						
				10th	25th	50th	75th	90th	95th	99th
1. SINGLE DX										
0–19 Years	0									
20–34	0									
35–49	2	2.0	0	2	2	2	2	2	2	2
50–64	2	2.0	2	1	1	3	3	3	3	3
65+	0									
2. MULTIPLE DX										
0–19 Years	1	16.0	0	16	16	16	16	16	16	16
20–34	2	2.0	2	1	1	1	3	3	3	3
35–49	10	4.2	11	1	2	3	4	9	11	11
50–64	6	9.3	89	1	1	5	17	25	25	25
65+	7	9.3	65	1	5	7	12	26	26	26
TOTAL SINGLE DX	4	2.0	<1	1	1	2	3	3	3	3
TOTAL MULTIPLE DX	26	7.0	48	1	3	4	9	17	25	26
TOTAL										
0–19 Years	1	16.0	0	16	16	16	16	16	16	16
20–34	2	2.0	2	1	1	3	3	3	3	3
35–49	12	3.8	10	1	2	3	4	9	11	11
50–64	8	7.5	75	1	1	5	5	25	25	25
65+	7	9.3	65	1	5	7	12	26	26	26
GRAND TOTAL	30	6.4	45	1	2	4	8	16	25	26

46.71: DUODENAL LAC SUTURE

Type of Patients	Observed Patients	Avg. Stay	Vari-ance	Percentiles						
				10th	25th	50th	75th	90th	95th	99th
1. SINGLE DX										
0–19 Years	2	8.4	2	6	9	9	9	9	9	9
20–34	1	9.0	0	9	9	9	9	9	9	9
35–49	0									
50–64	0									
65+	0									
2. MULTIPLE DX										
0–19 Years	11	10.6	163	5	5	5	8	33	53	53
20–34	21	10.8	25	6	7	10	14	18	20	20
35–49	20	12.6	149	3	4	9	18	30	50	50
50–64	15	24.5	481	5	8	9	51	56	63	63
65+	30	12.3	48	5	8	10	15	24	27	31
TOTAL SINGLE DX	3	8.5	1	6	9	9	9	9	9	9
TOTAL MULTIPLE DX	97	13.5	159	4	6	9	15	28	50	56
TOTAL										
0–19 Years	13	10.1	125	5	5	6	9	13	33	53
20–34	22	10.7	24	6	7	10	14	18	20	20
35–49	20	12.6	149	3	4	9	18	30	50	50
50–64	15	24.5	481	5	8	9	51	56	63	63
65+	30	12.3	48	5	8	10	15	24	27	31
GRAND TOTAL	100	13.3	152	4	6	9	14	28	50	56

46.7: OTHER INTESTINAL REPAIR

Type of Patients	Observed Patients	Avg. Stay	Vari-ance	Percentiles						
				10th	25th	50th	75th	90th	95th	99th
1. SINGLE DX										
0–19 Years	17	5.6	7	2	4	6	9	9	9	9
20–34	16	5.8	13	3	4	5	6	9	17	17
35–49	2	5.5	4	2	4	6	7	7	7	7
50–64	7	5.0	11	2	3	4	8	11	11	11
65+	2	9.0	18	6	6	12	12	12	12	12
2. MULTIPLE DX										
0–19 Years	200	12.9	285	3	5	6	14	41	61	>99
20–34	417	9.3	88	3	4	6	11	21	28	62
35–49	501	10.7	106	3	5	7	13	24	31	56
50–64	734	11.3	131	3	5	8	13	23	37	92
65+	935	11.6	111	4	5	8	14	23	30	58
TOTAL SINGLE DX	44	5.7	10	2	4	4	8	9	11	17
TOTAL MULTIPLE DX	2,787	11.2	129	3	5	7	13	23	32	79
TOTAL										
0–19 Years	217	12.4	269	3	5	6	13	31	58	>99
20–34	433	9.2	86	3	4	6	10	20	28	62
35–49	503	10.7	106	3	5	7	13	24	31	56
50–64	741	11.3	130	3	5	8	13	23	34	92
65+	937	11.6	110	4	5	8	14	23	30	58
GRAND TOTAL	2,831	11.1	128	3	5	7	13	23	32	77

46.73: SMALL INTEST SUTURE NEC

Type of Patients	Observed Patients	Avg. Stay	Vari-ance	Percentiles						
				10th	25th	50th	75th	90th	95th	99th
1. SINGLE DX										
0–19 Years	12	4.6	4	2	4	4	6	7	9	9
20–34	7	4.0	1	3	3	4	5	6	6	6
35–49	2	5.5	13	4	6	6	7	7	7	7
50–64	5	5.8	13	3	3	4	8	11	11	11
65+	1	12.0	0	12	12	12	12	12	12	12
2. MULTIPLE DX										
0–19 Years	83	8.6	77	3	4	6	11	19	29	>99
20–34	200	8.3	77	3	4	6	9	18	26	76
35–49	234	10.4	108	4	5	7	12	22	33	53
50–64	308	10.3	61	4	5	8	13	20	25	46
65+	401	11.0	78	3	6	9	14	22	27	40
TOTAL SINGLE DX	27	5.0	7	3	3	4	6	9	11	12
TOTAL MULTIPLE DX	1,226	10.1	80	3	5	7	12	20	27	57
TOTAL										
0–19 Years	95	8.2	71	3	4	6	10	19	29	>99
20–34	207	8.2	75	3	4	6	9	18	26	76
35–49	236	10.4	107	3	5	7	12	22	33	53
50–64	313	10.2	60	3	5	8	13	20	25	46
65+	402	11.0	78	3	6	9	14	22	27	40
GRAND TOTAL	1,253	10.0	79	3	5	7	12	20	27	57

Western Region, October 2007–September 2008 Data, by Operation

46.74: CLOSURE SMB FISTULA NEC

Type of Patients	Observed Patients	Avg. Stay	Variance	Percentiles						
				10th	25th	50th	75th	90th	95th	99th
1. SINGLE DX										
0–19 Years	0									
20–34	0									
35–49	0									
50–64	0									
65+	0									
2. MULTIPLE DX										
0–19 Years	11	28.4	821	2	5	16	41	84	84	84
20–34	32	15.2	197	5	6	10	21	26	42	74
35–49	50	17.5	232	4	6	14	25	42	61	>99
50–64	104	17.2	398	4	6	11	19	50	74	>99
65+	123	17.3	303	4	6	10	22	45	59	82
TOTAL SINGLE DX	0									
TOTAL MULTIPLE DX	320	17.9	355	4	6	11	23	46	70	>99
TOTAL										
0–19 Years	11	28.4	821	2	5	16	41	84	84	84
20–34	32	15.2	197	5	6	10	21	26	42	74
35–49	50	17.5	232	4	6	14	25	42	61	>99
50–64	104	17.2	398	4	6	11	19	50	74	>99
65+	123	17.3	303	4	6	10	22	45	59	82
GRAND TOTAL	320	17.9	355	4	6	11	23	46	70	>99

46.75: LARGE INTESTINE SUTURE

Type of Patients	Observed Patients	Avg. Stay	Variance	Percentiles						
				10th	25th	50th	75th	90th	95th	99th
1. SINGLE DX										
0–19 Years	1	8.0	0	8	8	8	8	8	8	8
20–34	5	8.6	25	4	6	7	9	17	17	17
35–49	0									
50–64	2	3.0	2	2	2	3	4	4	4	4
65+	1	6.0	0	6	6	6	6	6	6	6
2. MULTIPLE DX										
0–19 Years	59	10.6	252	2	5	6	9	21	23	99
20–34	127	8.4	67	3	4	5	9	21	29	38
35–49	116	8.4	54	3	4	6	9	16	22	43
50–64	153	8.8	55	3	4	7	10	18	26	43
65+	204	9.0	54	3	5	7	10	19	24	32
TOTAL SINGLE DX	9	7.0	19	2	4	6	8	17	17	17
TOTAL MULTIPLE DX	659	8.9	80	3	4	6	10	19	25	44
TOTAL										
0–19 Years	60	10.6	249	2	5	6	9	21	23	99
20–34	132	8.4	65	3	4	5	9	20	29	38
35–49	116	8.4	54	3	4	6	9	16	22	43
50–64	155	8.7	55	3	4	7	10	18	26	43
65+	205	9.0	54	3	5	7	10	19	24	32
GRAND TOTAL	668	8.9	79	3	4	6	10	19	25	43

46.79: REPAIR OF INTESTINE NEC

Type of Patients	Observed Patients	Avg. Stay	Variance	Percentiles						
				10th	25th	50th	75th	90th	95th	99th
1. SINGLE DX										
0–19 Years	2	3.0	2	2	2	4	4	4	4	4
20–34	3	4.0	4	2	2	4	6	6	6	6
35–49	0									
50–64	0									
65+	0									
2. MULTIPLE DX										
0–19 Years	34	19.6	370	5	6	11	26	55	73	>99
20–34	29	9.9	125	3	4	6	9	36	39	45
35–49	64	8.6	39	2	4	6	13	18	19	31
50–64	125	9.4	58	3	5	8	12	16	27	49
65+	148	11.6	105	4	6	9	14	22	29	38
TOTAL SINGLE DX	5	3.6	3	2	2	4	4	6	6	6
TOTAL MULTIPLE DX	400	11.2	119	3	5	8	14	22	32	73
TOTAL										
0–19 Years	36	18.9	366	3	6	11	25	55	73	>99
20–34	32	9.4	116	3	4	5	9	19	39	45
35–49	64	8.6	39	2	4	6	13	18	19	31
50–64	125	9.4	58	3	5	8	12	16	27	49
65+	148	11.6	105	4	6	9	14	22	29	38
GRAND TOTAL	405	11.1	119	3	5	8	13	22	31	73

46.8: BOWEL DILATION & MANIP

Type of Patients	Observed Patients	Avg. Stay	Variance	Percentiles						
				10th	25th	50th	75th	90th	95th	99th
1. SINGLE DX										
0–19 Years	81	2.7	2	1	2	3	3	4	5	7
20–34	3	2.0	<1	1	1	2	3	3	3	3
35–49	2	4.5	12	3	3	3	7	7	7	7
50–64	3	3.7	1	3	3	3	5	5	5	5
65+	1	3.0	0	3	3	3	3	3	3	3
2. MULTIPLE DX										
0–19 Years	193	7.0	86	2	3	4	7	13	19	57
20–34	82	5.7	23	1	3	4	7	12	15	27
35–49	134	6.0	23	2	3	5	9	12	15	26
50–64	220	7.0	31	2	3	6	9	14	18	23
65+	510	7.7	47	2	3	6	10	14	20	32
TOTAL SINGLE DX	90	2.7	2	1	2	3	3	4	5	7
TOTAL MULTIPLE DX	1,139	7.1	53	2	3	5	9	14	19	38
TOTAL										
0–19 Years	274	5.7	63	2	2	4	5	11	14	51
20–34	85	5.5	23	1	3	4	7	12	15	27
35–49	136	6.0	23	2	3	5	9	12	15	26
50–64	223	6.9	31	2	3	6	9	14	18	23
65+	511	7.7	47	2	3	6	10	14	20	32
GRAND TOTAL	1,229	6.5	49	2	3	4	8	13	18	36

LOS by Diagnosis and Operation, Western Region, 45th Edition

Western Region, October 2007–September 2008 Data, by Operation

46.81: INTRA-ABD S-INTEST MANIP

Type of Patients	Observed Patients	Avg. Stay	Variance	Percentiles						
				10th	25th	50th	75th	90th	95th	99th
1. SINGLE DX										
0–19 Years	38	2.9	3	1	2	3	3	5	7	11
20–34	2	2.0	2	1	1	1	3	3	3	3
35–49	0									
50–64	2	4.0	2	3	3	4	5	5	5	5
65+	0									
2. MULTIPLE DX										
0–19 Years	102	7.7	119	2	3	5	7	12	32	57
20–34	41	6.0	22	1	3	5	7	13	15	20
35–49	51	6.8	16	2	4	6	8	12	14	20
50–64	61	7.5	29	2	4	6	12	15	18	22
65+	99	10.1	32	4	6	9	13	17	20	31
TOTAL SINGLE DX	42	2.9	3	1	2	3	3	5	7	11
TOTAL MULTIPLE DX	354	7.9	73	2	4	5	9	14	20	57
TOTAL										
0–19 Years	140	6.4	91	2	3	4	6	11	15	57
20–34	43	5.8	21	1	3	4	7	13	15	20
35–49	51	6.8	16	2	4	6	8	12	14	20
50–64	63	7.4	28	2	4	6	12	15	18	22
65+	99	10.1	32	4	6	9	13	17	20	31
GRAND TOTAL	396	7.1	65	2	3	5	8	14	18	55

46.82: INTRA-ABD L-INTEST MANIP

Type of Patients	Observed Patients	Avg. Stay	Variance	Percentiles						
				10th	25th	50th	75th	90th	95th	99th
1. SINGLE DX										
0–19 Years	30	2.6	1	1	2	3	3	4	5	5
20–34	0									
35–49	1	7.0	0	7	7	7	7	7	7	7
50–64	0									
65+	0									
2. MULTIPLE DX										
0–19 Years	58	5.5	24	2	3	4	7	13	16	18
20–34	6	8.7	86	1	5	5	7	27	27	27
35–49	10	4.3	3	3	3	5	5	7	7	7
50–64	19	6.7	8	3	5	6	9	11	12	12
65+	38	9.7	45	4	5	7	12	20	24	32
TOTAL SINGLE DX	31	2.7	1	1	2	3	3	4	5	7
TOTAL MULTIPLE DX	131	6.4	30	2	3	5	7	13	18	32
TOTAL										
0–19 Years	88	4.4	17	2	2	3	4	7	13	18
20–34	6	8.7	86	5	5	5	7	27	27	27
35–49	11	4.5	3	3	3	5	6	7	7	7
50–64	19	6.7	8	3	5	6	9	11	12	12
65+	38	9.7	45	4	5	7	12	20	24	32
GRAND TOTAL	162	5.4	24	2	2	4	6	11	17	27

46.85: DILATION OF INTESTINE

Type of Patients	Observed Patients	Avg. Stay	Variance	Percentiles						
				10th	25th	50th	75th	90th	95th	99th
1. SINGLE DX										
0–19 Years	3	1.7	3	1	1	1	1	5	5	5
20–34	1	2.0	0	2	2	2	2	2	2	2
35–49	1	2.0	0	2	2	2	2	2	2	2
50–64	0									
65+	1	3.0	0	3	3	3	3	3	3	3
2. MULTIPLE DX										
0–19 Years	15	10.8	173	2	2	3	25	35	35	35
20–34	32	4.8	15	1	2	4	6	11	12	16
35–49	67	5.5	31	1	2	3	6	13	16	31
50–64	135	6.9	36	2	3	6	9	13	18	26
65+	367	6.9	49	2	3	5	9	14	20	36
TOTAL SINGLE DX	6	1.9	2	1	1	1	2	5	5	5
TOTAL MULTIPLE DX	616	6.8	48	2	3	5	8	14	20	35
TOTAL										
0–19 Years	18	9.0	152	1	2	3	9	35	35	35
20–34	33	4.7	15	1	2	4	6	11	12	16
35–49	68	5.4	31	1	2	3	6	13	16	31
50–64	135	6.9	36	2	3	6	9	13	18	26
65+	368	6.9	49	2	3	5	9	14	20	36
GRAND TOTAL	622	6.7	48	2	3	5	8	14	20	35

46.9: OTHER INTESTINAL OPS

Type of Patients	Observed Patients	Avg. Stay	Variance	Percentiles						
				10th	25th	50th	75th	90th	95th	99th
1. SINGLE DX										
0–19 Years	2	3.4	6	2	2	2	6	6	6	6
20–34	0									
35–49	0									
50–64	0									
65+	0									
2. MULTIPLE DX										
0–19 Years	17	22.4	468	3	8	13	25	66	66	68
20–34	22	9.1	66	3	5	7	10	32	33	>99
35–49	39	9.9	131	3	6	9	12	21	34	63
50–64	66	11.9	91	3	5	9	17	24	30	49
65+	71	14.5	191	4	7	12	17	25	40	79
TOTAL SINGLE DX	2	3.4	6	2	2	2	6	6	6	6
TOTAL MULTIPLE DX	215	13.7	196	3	5	10	16	27	49	76
TOTAL										
0–19 Years	19	21.0	458	3	7	12	25	66	66	68
20–34	22	9.1	66	3	5	6	10	32	33	>99
35–49	39	9.9	131	2	3	6	12	21	34	63
50–64	66	11.9	91	3	5	9	17	24	30	49
65+	71	14.5	191	4	7	12	17	25	40	79
GRAND TOTAL	217	13.5	195	3	5	9	16	27	49	76

LOS by Diagnosis and Operation, Western Region, 45th Edition

Western Region, October 2007–September 2008 Data, by Operation

46.93: REVISION SM INTEST ANAST

Type of Patients	Observed Patients	Avg. Stay	Vari- ance	Percentiles						
				10th	25th	50th	75th	90th	95th	99th
1. SINGLE DX										
0–19 Years	1	6.0	0	6	6	6	6	6	6	6
20–34	0									
35–49	0									
50–64	0									
65+	0									
2. MULTIPLE DX										
0–19 Years	6	12.7	43	7	8	8	21	21	21	21
20–34	15	5.7	5	3	4	5	8	8	9	9
35–49	22	7.4	49	2	3	5	11	15	15	32
50–64	29	11.9	124	2	8	8	15	27	34	49
65+	18	18.1	297	4	8	14	23	30	79	79
TOTAL SINGLE DX	1	6.0	0	6	6	6	6	6	6	6
TOTAL MULTIPLE DX	90	11.2	124	2	4	8	15	23	30	79
TOTAL										
0–19 Years	7	12.2	43	6	8	8	21	21	21	21
20–34	15	5.7	5	3	4	5	8	8	9	9
35–49	22	7.4	49	2	3	5	11	15	15	32
50–64	29	11.9	124	2	8	8	15	27	34	49
65+	18	18.1	297	4	8	14	23	30	79	79
GRAND TOTAL	91	11.1	123	2	4	8	15	23	30	79

47.0: APPENDECTOMY

Type of Patients	Observed Patients	Avg. Stay	Vari- ance	Percentiles						
				10th	25th	50th	75th	90th	95th	99th
1. SINGLE DX										
0–19 Years	13,003	2.4	4	1	1	2	3	5	6	9
20–34	8,735	1.6	1	1	1	1	2	3	4	6
35–49	4,016	1.7	1	1	1	1	2	3	4	6
50–64	1,598	1.8	1	1	1	1	2	3	4	6
65+	175	1.8	1	1	1	1	2	3	4	5
2. MULTIPLE DX										
0–19 Years	8,388	3.8	13	1	1	3	5	7	10	18
20–34	9,514	2.4	6	1	1	2	3	5	6	12
35–49	7,972	2.7	8	1	1	2	3	5	8	13
50–64	7,020	3.2	11	1	2	2	4	7	9	16
65+	3,797	4.5	22	1	2	3	6	9	12	22
TOTAL SINGLE DX	27,527	2.1	3	1	1	1	2	4	6	8
TOTAL MULTIPLE DX	36,691	3.2	12	1	1	2	4	7	9	16
TOTAL										
0–19 Years	21,391	2.9	8	1	1	2	4	6	8	13
20–34	18,249	2.0	4	1	1	1	2	4	5	10
35–49	11,988	2.3	6	1	1	2	3	5	7	12
50–64	8,618	2.9	10	1	2	2	4	6	8	15
65+	3,972	4.3	22	1	2	3	5	9	12	22
GRAND TOTAL	64,218	2.7	8	1	1	2	3	6	7	13

47.01: LAPSCP APPENDECTOMY

Type of Patients	Observed Patients	Avg. Stay	Vari- ance	Percentiles						
				10th	25th	50th	75th	90th	95th	99th
1. SINGLE DX										
0–19 Years	8,843	2.4	4	1	1	2	3	5	6	9
20–34	6,456	1.5	<1	1	1	1	2	2	3	5
35–49	3,026	1.6	1	1	1	1	2	3	3	5
50–64	1,211	1.7	1	1	1	1	2	3	4	6
65+	133	1.7	<1	1	1	1	2	3	4	5
2. MULTIPLE DX										
0–19 Years	5,470	3.4	11	1	1	2	5	7	9	15
20–34	6,938	2.1	4	1	1	1	2	4	6	10
35–49	5,860	2.3	6	1	1	1	3	4	6	11
50–64	4,902	2.6	7	1	1	2	3	5	7	13
65+	2,480	3.7	18	1	1	2	4	8	10	18
TOTAL SINGLE DX	19,669	2.0	3	1	1	1	2	5	6	8
TOTAL MULTIPLE DX	25,650	2.7	9	1	1	2	3	6	8	13
TOTAL										
0–19 Years	14,313	2.8	7	1	1	2	4	6	7	12
20–34	13,394	1.8	3	1	1	1	2	3	4	8
35–49	8,886	2.0	4	1	1	1	2	4	5	10
50–64	6,113	2.4	6	1	1	2	3	5	6	11
65+	2,613	3.6	17	1	1	2	4	7	10	17
GRAND TOTAL	45,319	2.4	6	1	1	2	3	5	6	11

47.09: OTHER APPENDECTOMY

Type of Patients	Observed Patients	Avg. Stay	Vari- ance	Percentiles						
				10th	25th	50th	75th	90th	95th	99th
1. SINGLE DX										
0–19 Years	4,160	2.5	4	1	1	2	3	5	6	9
20–34	2,279	2.0	2	1	1	2	2	4	4	7
35–49	990	2.1	2	1	1	2	3	4	5	7
50–64	387	2.3	2	1	1	2	3	4	5	8
65+	42	2.1	1	1	1	2	3	3	4	5
2. MULTIPLE DX										
0–19 Years	2,918	4.5	17	1	2	3	6	9	12	21
20–34	2,576	3.3	12	1	1	2	4	6	9	16
35–49	2,112	3.8	12	1	2	3	5	8	10	16
50–64	2,118	4.6	19	1	2	3	6	9	12	21
65+	1,317	5.9	28	2	3	5	7	11	15	27
TOTAL SINGLE DX	7,858	2.3	3	1	1	2	3	4	6	9
TOTAL MULTIPLE DX	11,041	4.3	17	1	2	3	5	8	11	20
TOTAL										
0–19 Years	7,078	3.4	11	1	1	2	4	7	9	16
20–34	4,855	2.7	8	1	1	2	3	5	7	13
35–49	3,102	3.3	9	1	1	3	4	7	9	15
50–64	2,505	4.2	17	1	2	3	5	8	11	20
65+	1,359	5.8	28	1	3	5	7	11	15	27
GRAND TOTAL	18,899	3.5	12	1	1	2	4	7	9	17

LOS by Diagnosis and Operation, Western Region, 45th Edition

Western Region, October 2007–September 2008 Data, by Operation

47.2: DRAIN APPENDICEAL ABSC

Type of Patients	Observed Patients	Avg. Stay	Variance	10th	25th	50th	75th	90th	95th	99th
1. SINGLE DX										
0–19 Years	46	6.8	12	3	4	6	9	14	14	15
20–34	16	5.5	7	2	3	5	7	8	12	12
35–49	17	4.0	4	2	3	4	5	6	9	9
50–64	7	3.7	6	1	2	3	4	9	9	9
65+	1	2.0	0	2	2	2	2	2	2	2
2. MULTIPLE DX										
0–19 Years	60	8.8	25	4	5	7	11	16	19	22
20–34	28	4.3	5	2	3	4	5	9	10	10
35–49	43	6.6	31	2	3	6	8	11	12	35
50–64	68	6.5	29	3	3	5	7	12	14	40
65+	42	5.6	12	2	3	4	7	11	12	17
TOTAL SINGLE DX	87	6.2	11	3	4	6	8	12	14	15
TOTAL MULTIPLE DX	241	7.2	25	3	4	6	9	14	16	22
TOTAL										
0–19 Years	106	7.8	20	3	5	6	10	15	16	22
20–34	44	4.7	6	2	3	4	5	8	10	12
35–49	60	5.9	24	2	3	5	7	11	12	35
50–64	75	6.3	27	3	3	5	7	11	14	40
65+	43	5.5	12	2	3	4	7	11	12	17
GRAND TOTAL	328	6.9	21	3	4	6	9	13	15	22

47.9: OTHER APPENDICEAL OPS

Type of Patients	Observed Patients	Avg. Stay	Variance	10th	25th	50th	75th	90th	95th	99th
1. SINGLE DX										
0–19 Years	0									
20–34	1	4.0	0	4	4	4	4	4	4	4
35–49	0									
50–64	1	4.0	0	4	4	4	4	4	4	4
65+	0									
2. MULTIPLE DX										
0–19 Years	33	4.5	16	1	3	3	5	8	12	30
20–34	1	8.0	0	8	8	8	8	8	8	8
35–49	3	3.4	6	1	1	3	6	6	6	6
50–64	4	14.9	309	3	3	5	11	41	41	41
65+	4	4.3	7	2	3	4	8	8	8	8
TOTAL SINGLE DX	2	4.0	0	4	4	4	4	4	4	4
TOTAL MULTIPLE DX	45	4.9	29	1	3	3	6	8	12	41
TOTAL										
0–19 Years	33	4.5	16	1	3	3	5	8	12	30
20–34	3	6.0	8	4	4	3	8	8	8	8
35–49	3	3.4	6	1	1	3	6	6	6	6
50–64	5	12.7	256	3	4	5	11	41	41	41
65+	4	4.3	7	2	3	4	8	8	8	8
GRAND TOTAL	47	4.9	28	1	3	3	5	8	12	41

47.1: INCIDENTAL APPENDECTOMY

Type of Patients	Observed Patients	Avg. Stay	Variance	10th	25th	50th	75th	90th	95th	99th
1. SINGLE DX										
0–19 Years	22	1.8	<1	1	1	2	2	3	3	4
20–34	17	1.4	<1	1	1	1	2	2	3	3
35–49	2	4.5	12	2	2	5	7	7	7	7
50–64	0									
65+	0									
2. MULTIPLE DX										
0–19 Years	43	5.0	153	1	1	2	4	7	22	91
20–34	71	3.3	10	1	2	3	4	6	8	23
35–49	38	3.3	12	1	2	2	4	6	16	17
50–64	20	11.8	194	1	4	6	13	40	41	41
65+	15	10.2	104	2	4	6	11	28	36	36
TOTAL SINGLE DX	41	1.8	1	1	1	1	2	3	3	7
TOTAL MULTIPLE DX	187	5.2	83	1	2	3	5	9	21	40
TOTAL										
0–19 Years	65	4.1	109	1	1	2	3	5	7	91
20–34	88	2.9	9	1	2	2	3	6	8	23
35–49	40	3.4	12	1	2	2	4	6	16	17
50–64	20	11.8	194	1	4	6	13	40	41	41
65+	15	10.2	104	2	4	6	11	28	36	36
GRAND TOTAL	228	4.5	70	1	1	2	4	8	16	40

47.11: LAPSCP INCIDENTAL APPY

Type of Patients	Observed Patients	Avg. Stay	Variance	10th	25th	50th	75th	90th	95th	99th
1. SINGLE DX										
0–19 Years	22	1.8	<1	1	1	2	2	3	3	4
20–34	15	1.4	<1	1	1	1	2	2	3	3
35–49	2	4.5	12	2	2	5	7	7	7	7
50–64	0									
65+	0									
2. MULTIPLE DX										
0–19 Years	36	2.6	4	1	1	2	3	5	7	12
20–34	63	3.1	4	1	2	3	4	6	7	10
35–49	31	2.5	2	1	2	3	3	4	5	8
50–64	16	8.8	123	1	3	4	8	31	40	40
65+	8	6.3	41	1	4	4	9	21	21	21
TOTAL SINGLE DX	39	1.8	1	1	1	2	2	3	3	7
TOTAL MULTIPLE DX	154	3.5	20	1	2	2	4	7	9	31
TOTAL										
0–19 Years	58	2.3	3	1	1	2	3	4	6	12
20–34	78	2.7	4	1	2	2	3	5	7	10
35–49	33	2.6	3	1	2	2	3	5	7	10
50–64	16	8.8	123	1	3	4	8	31	40	40
65+	8	6.3	41	1	4	4	9	21	21	21
GRAND TOTAL	193	3.2	17	1	1	2	3	6	8	21

Western Region, October 2007–September 2008 Data, by Operation

48.0: PROCTOTOMY

Type of Patients	Observed Patients	Avg. Stay	Variance	10th	25th	50th	75th	90th	95th	99th
1. SINGLE DX										
0–19 Years	1	3.0	0	3	3	3	3	3	3	3
20–34	4	1.3	<1	1	1	1	1	2	2	2
35–49	12	2.1	2	1	1	1	3	4	6	6
50–64	3	1.7	<1	1	1	2	2	2	2	2
65+	0									
2. MULTIPLE DX										
0–19 Years	7	7.7	70	2	4	7	7	10	32	32
20–34	24	4.7	51	1	1	2	6	8	11	36
35–49	55	4.3	29	1	1	2	5	9	15	30
50–64	40	4.6	33	1	2	3	6	9	18	32
65+	35	6.8	69	1	2	5	7	10	31	41
TOTAL SINGLE DX	20	2.1	2	1	1	2	3	3	4	6
TOTAL MULTIPLE DX	161	5.2	45	1	2	3	6	9	18	36
TOTAL										
0–19 Years	8	6.4	54	2	3	4	7	10	32	32
20–34	28	4.2	45	1	1	2	5	8	11	36
35–49	67	3.9	25	1	1	2	4	8	11	30
50–64	43	4.4	31	1	2	3	5	9	14	32
65+	35	6.8	69	1	2	5	7	10	31	41
GRAND TOTAL	181	4.8	40	1	1	3	6	9	15	36

48.2: RECTAL/PERIRECT DXTIC PX

Type of Patients	Observed Patients	Avg. Stay	Variance	10th	25th	50th	75th	90th	95th	99th
1. SINGLE DX										
0–19 Years	28	2.8	2	1	2	2	3	4	7	7
20–34	15	3.4	9	1	1	2	5	7	12	12
35–49	17	2.4	6	1	1	1	3	7	9	9
50–64	8	1.8	2	1	1	1	2	5	5	5
65+	3	2.3	2	1	1	2	4	4	4	4
2. MULTIPLE DX										
0–19 Years	213	7.7	99	1	3	5	9	14	25	73
20–34	191	4.4	17	1	2	3	5	10	13	21
35–49	323	5.0	39	1	2	4	6	9	12	32
50–64	460	5.2	19	1	2	4	7	11	14	21
65+	1,018	6.1	31	2	3	5	7	12	16	26
TOTAL SINGLE DX	71	2.7	4	1	1	2	3	6	7	12
TOTAL MULTIPLE DX	2,205	5.9	41	1	2	4	7	12	16	32
TOTAL										
0–19 Years	241	7.2	91	1	3	4	8	13	24	73
20–34	206	4.3	17	1	2	3	5	10	13	20
35–49	340	4.8	37	1	2	4	6	9	12	32
50–64	468	5.2	19	1	2	4	7	11	14	21
65+	1,021	6.1	31	2	3	5	7	12	16	26
GRAND TOTAL	2,276	5.8	40	1	2	4	7	12	16	31

48.1: PROCTOSTOMY

Type of Patients	Observed Patients	Avg. Stay	Variance	10th	25th	50th	75th	90th	95th	99th
1. SINGLE DX										
0–19 Years	0									
20–34	0									
35–49	0									
50–64	0									
65+	0									
2. MULTIPLE DX										
0–19 Years	0									
20–34	0									
35–49	1	11.0	0	11	11	11	11	11	11	11
50–64	1	7.0	0	7	7	7	7	7	7	7
65+										
TOTAL SINGLE DX	0									
TOTAL MULTIPLE DX	2	9.0	8	7	7	9	11	11	11	11
TOTAL										
0–19 Years	0									
20–34	0									
35–49	1	11.0	0	11	11	11	11	11	11	11
50–64	1	7.0	0	7	7	7	7	7	7	7
65+										
GRAND TOTAL	2	9.0	8	7	7	9	11	11	11	11

48.23: RIG PROCTOSIGMOIDOSCOPY

Type of Patients	Observed Patients	Avg. Stay	Variance	10th	25th	50th	75th	90th	95th	99th
1. SINGLE DX										
0–19 Years	5	1.6	<1	1	1	1	2	3	3	3
20–34	9	2.0		1	1	2	2	5	5	5
35–49	9	1.0	0	1	1	1	1	1	1	1
50–64		1.0	0	1	1	1	1	1	1	1
65+	3	2.3	2	1	1	2	4	4	4	4
2. MULTIPLE DX										
0–19 Years	15	5.1	12	1	2	5	8	10	10	11
20–34	48	3.3	19	1	1	2	4	6	7	29
35–49	72	3.5	12	1	1	3	5	7	10	22
50–64	94	3.5	9	1	1	3	4	7	11	14
65+	165	5.8	40	1	2	4	6	11	15	34
TOTAL SINGLE DX	30	1.5	1	1	1	1	2	3	4	5
TOTAL MULTIPLE DX	394	4.5	24	1	2	3	5	10	12	22
TOTAL										
0–19 Years	20	4.5	11	1	2	3	8	10	10	11
20–34	57	3.1	17	1	1	2	4	6	7	29
35–49	81	3.2	11	1	1	2	4	7	9	22
50–64	98	3.4	9	1	2	3	4	6	11	14
65+	168	5.7	39	1	2	4	6	11	15	34
GRAND TOTAL	424	4.3	23	1	1	3	5	9	12	22

LOS by Diagnosis and Operation, Western Region, 45th Edition

Western Region, October 2007–September 2008 Data, by Operation

48.24: CLOSED RECTAL BIOPSY

Type of Patients	Observed Patients	Avg. Stay	Variance	10th	25th	50th	75th	90th	95th	99th
1. SINGLE DX										
0–19 Years	14	2.8	<1	2	2	3	3	4	4	4
20–34	6	5.5	14	2	3	3	7	12	12	12
35–49	8	3.9	8	1	2	4	7	9	9	9
50–64	3	2.7	4	1	1	2	5	5	5	5
65+	0									
2. MULTIPLE DX										
0–19 Years	154	6.5	56	1	2	4	8	12	22	42
20–34	137	4.7	15	1	2	4	5	11	13	19
35–49	244	5.3	46	1	2	4	6	9	13	43
50–64	351	5.6	20	1	2	4	7	12	14	21
65+	827	6.1	28	2	3	5	8	12	16	26
TOTAL SINGLE DX	31	3.4	5	1	2	3	4	6	7	12
TOTAL MULTIPLE DX	1,713	5.9	33	2	3	4	7	12	15	30
TOTAL										
0–19 Years	168	6.2	53	1	2	4	8	11	21	41
20–34	143	4.7	15	1	2	4	6	11	13	19
35–49	252	5.3	45	1	2	4	6	9	13	43
50–64	354	5.6	20	1	2	4	7	12	14	21
65+	827	6.1	28	2	3	5	8	12	16	26
GRAND TOTAL	1,744	5.8	32	2	3	4	7	12	15	30

48.35: LOC EXC RECTAL LES/TISS

Type of Patients	Observed Patients	Avg. Stay	Variance	10th	25th	50th	75th	90th	95th	99th
1. SINGLE DX										
0–19 Years	2	2.5	<1	2	2	3	3	3	3	3
20–34	3	1.3	<1	1	1	3	2	2	2	2
35–49	1	1.0	0	1	1	1	1	1	1	1
50–64	18	1.9	2	1	1	1	2	5	5	5
65+	14	1.2	<1	1	1	1	1	2	3	3
2. MULTIPLE DX										
0–19 Years	3	4.8	1	3	4	4	6	6	6	6
20–34	4	5.3	4	4	4	5	8	8	8	8
35–49	23	3.2	9	1	1	2	5	6	9	13
50–64	104	2.7	10	1	1	1	3	6	10	16
65+	217	3.2	17	1	1	2	4	7	9	19
TOTAL SINGLE DX	38	1.7	1	1	1	1	2	3	5	5
TOTAL MULTIPLE DX	351	3.1	14	1	1	2	4	6	9	17
TOTAL										
0–19 Years	5	3.7	2	2	3	3	4	6	6	6
20–34	7	3.6	6	1	1	4	5	8	8	8
35–49	24	3.1	9	1	1	1	3	6	9	13
50–64	122	2.6	9	1	1	1	3	5	8	16
65+	231	3.1	16	1	1	2	4	6	9	19
GRAND TOTAL	389	2.9	13	1	1	2	4	6	9	16

48.3: LOC DESTR RECTAL LESION

Type of Patients	Observed Patients	Avg. Stay	Variance	10th	25th	50th	75th	90th	95th	99th
1. SINGLE DX										
0–19 Years	4	2.0	<1	1	1	3	3	3	3	3
20–34	3	1.3	<1	1	1	3	2	2	2	2
35–49	1	1.0	0	1	1	1	1	1	1	1
50–64	20	1.9	2	1	1	1	2	5	5	5
65+	20	1.2	<1	1	1	1	1	2	2	3
2. MULTIPLE DX										
0–19 Years	17	3.6	11	1	1	3	4	6	7	18
20–34	30	3.4	6	1	2	3	4	9	9	10
35–49	147	3.7	10	1	2	3	5	8	9	17
50–64	320	3.6	11	1	1	3	5	7	9	20
65+	730	3.9	16	2	2	3	5	8	11	19
TOTAL SINGLE DX	48	1.6	1	1	1	1	2	3	5	5
TOTAL MULTIPLE DX	1,244	3.8	14	1	1	3	5	8	10	19
TOTAL										
0–19 Years	21	3.1	8	1	1	3	4	6	6	18
20–34	33	3.2	6	1	2	3	4	8	9	10
35–49	148	3.7	10	1	2	3	5	8	9	17
50–64	340	3.5	11	1	1	2	5	7	9	20
65+	750	3.9	16	2	2	3	5	8	11	19
GRAND TOTAL	1,292	3.7	13	1	1	3	5	7	10	19

48.36: ENDO RECTAL POLYPECTOMY

Type of Patients	Observed Patients	Avg. Stay	Variance	10th	25th	50th	75th	90th	95th	99th
1. SINGLE DX										
0–19 Years	2	1.2	<1	1	1	1	1	2	2	2
20–34	0									
35–49	2	1.5	<1	1	1	2	2	2	2	2
50–64	6	1.2	<1	1	1	1	1	2	2	2
65+										
2. MULTIPLE DX										
0–19 Years	13	3.1	16	1	1	2	3	7	18	18
20–34	25	2.9	4	1	2	3	4	4	9	9
35–49	122	3.8	11	1	2	3	4	8	9	17
50–64	205	4.1	12	1	2	3	5	8	9	20
65+	476	4.3	15	1	2	3	5	8	11	19
TOTAL SINGLE DX	10	1.2	<1	1	1	1	1	2	2	2
TOTAL MULTIPLE DX	841	4.1	13	1	2	3	5	8	11	20
TOTAL										
0–19 Years	15	2.7	13	1	1	1	3	4	7	18
20–34	25	2.9	4	1	2	3	3	4	9	9
35–49	122	3.8	11	1	2	3	4	8	9	17
50–64	207	4.1	12	1	2	3	5	8	9	20
65+	482	4.3	15	1	2	3	5	8	11	19
GRAND TOTAL	851	4.1	13	1	2	3	5	8	11	20

LOS by Diagnosis and Operation, Western Region, 45th Edition

Western Region, October 2007–September 2008 Data, by Operation

48.4: PULL-THRU RECT RESECTION

Type of Patients	Observed Patients	Avg. Stay	Vari-ance	10th	25th	50th	75th	90th	95th	99th
1. SINGLE DX										
0–19 Years	57	4.0	11	1	3	3	5	6	6	20
20–34	1	10.0	0	10	10	10	10	10	10	10
35–49	0									
50–64	3	4.0	1	3	3	4	5	5	5	5
65+	3	2.0	<1	1	1	2	3	3	3	3
2. MULTIPLE DX										
0–19 Years	167	6.2	115	2	2	4	6	9	18	78
20–34	4	6.0	17	2	2	9	10	10	10	10
35–49	8	4.9	2	3	4	5	5	8	8	8
50–64	28	4.4	12	1	2	3	6	9	13	15
65+	159	3.8	15	1	2	3	5	7	8	24
TOTAL SINGLE DX	64	4.0	11	1	3	3	5	6	6	20
TOTAL MULTIPLE DX	366	5.4	80	1	2	3	5	9	13	63
TOTAL										
0–19 Years	224	5.6	90	2	2	3	5	9	18	63
20–34	5	6.8	16	2	3	9	10	10	10	10
35–49	8	4.9	2	3	4	5	5	8	8	8
50–64	31	4.4	11	1	2	3	6	8	13	15
65+	162	3.8	15	1	2	3	5	7	8	24
GRAND TOTAL	430	5.1	67	1	2	3	5	8	13	63

48.49: PULL-THRU RECT RESECT

Type of Patients	Observed Patients	Avg. Stay	Vari-ance	10th	25th	50th	75th	90th	95th	99th
1. SINGLE DX										
0–19 Years	40	3.4	3	1	2	3	4	6	6	7
20–34	0									
35–49	0									
50–64	3	4.0	1	3	3	4	5	5	5	5
65+	3	2.0	<1	1	1	2	3	3	3	3
2. MULTIPLE DX										
0–19 Years	133	5.8	128	2	2	3	5	9	13	78
20–34	4	6.0	17	2	2	9	10	10	10	10
35–49	8	4.9	2	3	4	5	5	8	8	8
50–64	28	4.4	12	1	2	3	6	9	13	15
65+	158	3.8	15	1	2	3	5	7	10	24
TOTAL SINGLE DX	46	3.4	2	1	2	3	4	6	6	7
TOTAL MULTIPLE DX	331	5.1	83	1	2	3	5	8	12	63
TOTAL										
0–19 Years	173	5.2	100	2	2	3	5	8	12	78
20–34	4	6.0	17	2	2	9	10	10	10	10
35–49	8	4.9	2	3	4	5	5	8	8	8
50–64	31	4.4	11	1	2	3	6	8	13	15
65+	161	3.8	15	1	2	3	5	7	8	24
GRAND TOTAL	377	4.8	70	1	2	3	5	8	10	63

48.5: ABD-PERINEAL RECT RESECT

Type of Patients	Observed Patients	Avg. Stay	Vari-ance	10th	25th	50th	75th	90th	95th	99th
1. SINGLE DX										
0–19 Years	0									
20–34	4	8.3	38	4	4	4	17	17	17	17
35–49	5	7.4	7	3	7	8	9	10	10	10
50–64	13	7.2	9	5	5	6	8	12	14	14
65+	7	5.6	5	2	4	5	8	8	8	8
2. MULTIPLE DX										
0–19 Years	2	12.5	110	5	5	20	20	20	20	20
20–34	26	8.7	29	4	5	7	10	17	18	25
35–49	129	9.3	69	5	6	7	9	16	22	44
50–64	333	8.9	36	5	6	8	10	15	21	39
65+	499	9.9	47	5	6	8	11	17	22	41
TOTAL SINGLE DX	29	7.0	11	4	5	6	8	12	14	17
TOTAL MULTIPLE DX	989	9.5	45	5	6	8	11	16	22	43
TOTAL										
0–19 Years	2	12.5	110	5	5	20	20	20	20	20
20–34	30	8.6	29	4	4	7	10	17	18	25
35–49	134	9.3	66	5	6	7	9	16	22	44
50–64	346	8.8	35	5	6	8	10	15	21	39
65+	506	9.8	46	5	6	8	11	17	22	41
GRAND TOTAL	1,018	9.4	45	5	6	8	10	16	22	41

48.6: OTHER RECTAL RESECTION

Type of Patients	Observed Patients	Avg. Stay	Vari-ance	10th	25th	50th	75th	90th	95th	99th
1. SINGLE DX										
0–19 Years	5	4.5	6	1	2	5	5	9	9	9
20–34	12	4.2	3	1	3	5	5	6	7	7
35–49	47	4.5	2	3	3	4	5	7	8	9
50–64	97	4.8	4	3	3	4	6	7	8	15
65+	30	4.5	5	2	3	4	5	8	10	11
2. MULTIPLE DX										
0–19 Years	16	6.1	12	1	4	6	8	10	11	14
20–34	70	6.7	17	3	4	5	8	12	15	24
35–49	426	6.8	28	3	4	6	8	11	14	23
50–64	1,308	6.8	25	3	4	6	8	11	15	25
65+	1,897	8.0	38	3	5	6	9	14	19	33
TOTAL SINGLE DX	191	4.6	4	3	3	4	5	7	8	14
TOTAL MULTIPLE DX	3,717	7.4	32	3	4	6	8	13	17	29
TOTAL										
0–19 Years	21	5.7	10	1	4	6	8	9	11	14
20–34	82	6.3	16	1	4	5	7	10	15	24
35–49	473	6.6	26	3	4	5	7	11	14	23
50–64	1,405	6.7	24	3	4	5	7	11	14	25
65+	1,927	8.0	38	3	5	6	9	14	18	32
GRAND TOTAL	3,908	7.3	31	3	4	6	8	13	17	29

Western Region, October 2007–September 2008 Data, by Operation

48.62: ANT RECT RESECT W COLOST

Type of Patients	Observed Patients	Avg. Stay	Variance	10th	25th	50th	75th	90th	95th	99th
1. SINGLE DX										
0–19 Years	0									
20–34	0									
35–49	5	6.2	<1	5	6	6	7	7	7	7
50–64	6	6.8	4	4	6	6	8	10	10	10
65+	4	4.3	2	3	3	3	5	6	6	6
2. MULTIPLE DX										
0–19 Years	0									
20–34	8	11.3	42	5	7	10	16	24	24	24
35–49	35	10.3	118	4	6	8	12	15	19	69
50–64	123	9.1	25	5	6	8	11	16	21	24
65+	261	11.6	72	5	7	9	14	21	29	60
TOTAL SINGLE DX	15	5.9	3	3	5	6	7	8	10	10
TOTAL MULTIPLE DX	427	10.8	62	5	6	8	13	19	24	51
TOTAL										
0–19 Years	0									
20–34	8	11.3	42	5	7	10	16	24	24	24
35–49	40	9.8	105	4	6	7	11	14	19	69
50–64	129	9.0	24	5	6	8	10	16	21	24
65+	265	11.5	71	5	6	9	14	21	29	60
GRAND TOTAL	442	10.6	61	5	6	8	12	18	24	51

48.63: ANTERIOR RECT RESECT NEC

Type of Patients	Observed Patients	Avg. Stay	Variance	10th	25th	50th	75th	90th	95th	99th
1. SINGLE DX										
0–19 Years	0									
20–34	7	4.9	1	3	4	5	5	7	7	7
35–49	39	4.3	2	3	4	4	5	6	8	9
50–64	77	4.8	4	3	4	4	5	7	7	15
65+	20	4.9	6	3	3	4	6	10	11	11
2. MULTIPLE DX										
0–19 Years	1	10.0	0	10	10	10	10	10	10	10
20–34	40	5.6	7	3	4	5	7	9	10	15
35–49	327	6.3	10	3	4	5	7	10	13	18
50–64	988	6.6	22	3	4	5	7	11	14	24
65+	1,255	7.7	24	4	5	6	9	14	17	28
TOTAL SINGLE DX	143	4.7	4	3	3	4	5	7	8	14
TOTAL MULTIPLE DX	2,611	7.1	21	4	5	6	8	12	15	24
TOTAL										
0–19 Years	1	10.0	0	10	10	10	10	10	10	10
20–34	47	5.5	6	3	4	5	7	9	10	15
35–49	366	6.0	10	3	4	5	7	10	13	18
50–64	1,065	6.5	21	3	4	5	7	10	14	24
65+	1,275	7.6	24	4	5	6	9	14	17	28
GRAND TOTAL	2,754	6.9	21	3	4	6	8	12	15	24

48.69: RECTAL RESECTION NEC

Type of Patients	Observed Patients	Avg. Stay	Variance	10th	25th	50th	75th	90th	95th	99th
1. SINGLE DX										
0–19 Years	1	4.0	0	4	4	4	4	4	4	4
20–34	2	3.0	8	1	1	1	5	5	5	5
35–49	3	4.7	2	3	3	5	6	6	6	6
50–64	14	3.7	3	1	2	4	5	6	6	6
65+	6	3.3	1	2	3	3	4	5	5	5
2. MULTIPLE DX										
0–19 Years	5	3.8	16	1	1	1	4	11	11	11
20–34	21	7.2	21	3	4	6	8	12	15	21
35–49	62	7.7	66	3	4	6	7	12	19	48
50–64	194	6.5	39	2	3	5	7	10	14	43
65+	373	6.8	54	2	3	5	8	13	17	40
TOTAL SINGLE DX	26	3.7	3	1	3	4	5	6	6	6
TOTAL MULTIPLE DX	655	6.8	49	2	3	5	8	12	17	43
TOTAL										
0–19 Years	6	3.8	14	1	1	3	4	11	11	11
20–34	23	6.8	21	2	4	6	8	12	15	21
35–49	65	7.5	64	3	4	6	7	12	19	48
50–64	208	6.3	37	2	4	5	7	9	13	37
65+	379	6.7	54	2	3	5	8	13	17	40
GRAND TOTAL	681	6.7	48	2	3	5	8	12	15	43

48.7: REPAIR OF RECTUM

Type of Patients	Observed Patients	Avg. Stay	Variance	10th	25th	50th	75th	90th	95th	99th
1. SINGLE DX										
0–19 Years	7	1.3	<1	1	1	1	2	3	3	3
20–34	5	4.8	5	2	4	4	7	7	7	7
35–49	10	2.6	2	1	1	3	4	5	5	5
50–64	16	2.7	3	1	1	3	3	5	7	7
65+	8	2.9	2	1	2	3	4	5	5	5
2. MULTIPLE DX										
0–19 Years	21	6.0	10	3	3	6	7	11	11	19
20–34	52	4.6	13	2	3	3	6	8	12	21
35–49	113	4.9	33	2	3	3	6	9	12	17
50–64	200	5.7	33	2	2	4	6	12	19	35
65+	351	5.1	26	1	2	4	6	10	13	26
TOTAL SINGLE DX	46	2.6	3	1	1	2	4	5	7	7
TOTAL MULTIPLE DX	737	5.2	27	1	2	4	6	10	14	27
TOTAL										
0–19 Years	28	5.1	12	1	3	5	7	9	11	19
20–34	57	4.6	12	2	2	3	6	8	12	21
35–49	123	4.7	31	1	2	3	6	9	11	17
50–64	216	5.5	31	1	2	4	6	12	18	27
65+	359	5.0	25	1	2	4	6	10	13	26
GRAND TOTAL	783	5.1	26	1	2	4	6	10	13	26

LOS by Diagnosis and Operation, Western Region, 45th Edition

Western Region, October 2007–September 2008 Data, by Operation

48.75: ABDOMINAL PROCTOPEXY

Type of Patients	Observed Patients	Avg. Stay	Vari-ance	10th	25th	50th	75th	90th	95th	99th
1. SINGLE DX										
0–19 Years	2	1.0	0	1	1	1		1	1	1
20–34	0									
35–49	4	3.3	<1	2	3	4	4	4	4	4
50–64	8	3.5	3	1	3	3	5	7	7	7
65+	3	3.7	2	2	2	4	5	5	5	5
2. MULTIPLE DX										
0–19 Years	5	3.4	2	2	3	3	3	6	6	6
20–34	18	4.0	3	2	3	3	5	7	8	8
35–49	50	5.7	61	3	3	4	6	9	13	56
50–64	85	5.9	32	3	3	5	6	9	14	36
65+	108	6.5	23	3	3	5	8	12	16	27
TOTAL SINGLE DX	17	2.9	3	1	1	3	4	5	7	7
TOTAL MULTIPLE DX	266	5.9	32	3	3	4	6	10	14	35
TOTAL										
0–19 Years	7	2.2	3	1	1	1	3	6	6	6
20–34	18	4.0	3	2	3	3	5	7	8	8
35–49	54	5.5	57	3	3	4	6	8	13	56
50–64	93	5.7	30	3	3	4	6	8	14	36
65+	111	6.4	23	3	3	5	8	12	16	27
GRAND TOTAL	283	5.7	30	2	3	4	6	10	14	35

48.76: PROCTOPEXY NEC

Type of Patients	Observed Patients	Avg. Stay	Vari-ance	10th	25th	50th	75th	90th	95th	99th
1. SINGLE DX										
0–19 Years	2	1.5	<1	1	1	1	2	2	2	2
20–34	3	5.0	3	4	4	4	7	7	7	7
35–49	3	1.7	1	1	1	1	3	3	3	3
50–64	4	2.3	<1	1	1	2	3	3	3	3
65+	5	2.4	1	1	2	2	3	4	4	4
2. MULTIPLE DX										
0–19 Years	4	5.6	4	2	6	6	7	7	7	7
20–34	14	3.4	2	2	3	3	4	6	7	7
35–49	31	3.5	9	1	2	3	4	7	9	15
50–64	65	5.3	31	1	2	4	6	12	18	27
65+	176	3.9	11	1	2	3	5	9	12	16
TOTAL SINGLE DX	17	2.6	3	1	1	2	3	4	7	7
TOTAL MULTIPLE DX	290	4.2	15	1	2	3	5	9	12	20
TOTAL										
0–19 Years	6	4.9	6	2	2	6	7	7	7	7
20–34	17	3.7	3	2	3	3	4	7	7	7
35–49	34	3.4	8	1	1	3	4	7	9	15
50–64	69	5.2	30	1	2	3	6	12	18	27
65+	181	3.8	11	1	2	3	5	8	12	16
GRAND TOTAL	307	4.1	14	1	2	3	5	8	12	19

48.8: PERIRECT TISS INC/EXC

Type of Patients	Observed Patients	Avg. Stay	Vari-ance	10th	25th	50th	75th	90th	95th	99th
1. SINGLE DX										
0–19 Years	49	2.3	4	1	1	2	3	4	5	11
20–34	121	1.8	1	1	1	1	2	3	4	5
35–49	128	1.8	1	1	1	1	2	3	4	6
50–64	38	1.9	1	1	1	2	2	3	4	7
65+	4	3.0	3				5	5	5	5
2. MULTIPLE DX										
0–19 Years	124	4.9	18	1	2	3	6	11	13	20
20–34	415	2.8	7	1	1	2	3	6	8	14
35–49	694	3.5	21	1	1	2	4	7	9	23
50–64	630	4.2	24	1	2	3	5	8	12	25
65+	382	5.5	29	1	2	4	7	12	15	27
TOTAL SINGLE DX	340	2.0	2	1	1	2	2	4	4	11
TOTAL MULTIPLE DX	2,245	4.0	21	1	2	3	5	8	12	23
TOTAL										
0–19 Years	173	4.0	15	1	2	3	5	10	12	20
20–34	536	2.6	6	1	1	2	3	5	7	13
35–49	822	3.2	18	1	1	2	4	6	9	18
50–64	668	4.1	23	1	2	3	5	8	11	25
65+	386	5.4	29	1	2	4	7	12	15	27
GRAND TOTAL	2,585	3.7	19	1	1	2	4	8	11	22

48.81: PERIRECTAL INCISION

Type of Patients	Observed Patients	Avg. Stay	Vari-ance	10th	25th	50th	75th	90th	95th	99th
1. SINGLE DX										
0–19 Years	49	2.3	4	1	1	2	3	4	5	11
20–34	120	1.8	1	1	1	1	3	3	4	5
35–49	126	1.8	1	1	1	1	2	3	4	6
50–64	38	1.9	1	1	1	2	2	3	4	7
65+	4	3.0	3				5	5	5	5
2. MULTIPLE DX										
0–19 Years	122	4.9	18	1	2	3	6	11	13	20
20–34	410	2.8	7	1	1	2	3	6	8	14
35–49	683	3.5	21	1	1	2	4	7	9	23
50–64	612	4.2	24	1	2	3	5	8	12	25
65+	362	5.5	30	1	2	4	7	12	16	27
TOTAL SINGLE DX	337	2.0	2	1	1	2	2	4	4	11
TOTAL MULTIPLE DX	2,189	4.0	21	1	2	3	5	8	12	23
TOTAL										
0–19 Years	171	4.0	15	1	2	3	5	10	12	20
20–34	530	2.6	6	1	1	2	3	5	7	13
35–49	809	3.2	18	1	1	2	4	6	9	18
50–64	650	4.1	23	1	2	3	5	8	11	25
65+	366	5.5	30	1	2	4	7	12	16	27
GRAND TOTAL	2,526	3.7	19	1	1	2	4	8	11	22

LOS by Diagnosis and Operation, Western Region, 45th Edition

Western Region, October 2007–September 2008 Data, by Operation

48.9: OTH RECTAL/PERIRECT OP

Type of Patients	Observed Patients	Avg. Stay	Variance	Percentiles						
				10th	25th	50th	75th	90th	95th	99th
1. SINGLE DX										
0–19 Years	3	1.7	<1	1	1	2	2	2	2	2
20–34	1	1.0	0	1	1	1	1	1	1	1
35–49	1	1.0	0	1	1	1	1	1	1	1
50–64	0									
65+	0									
2. MULTIPLE DX										
0–19 Years	5	9.0	77	1	1	4	18	18	27	27
20–34	8	4.5	30	1	1	2	7	17	17	17
35–49	14	3.8	12	1	1	2	5	9	12	12
50–64	15	3.2	4	1	1	3	5	6	7	7
65+	10	3.9	12	1	1	2	7	8	10	10
TOTAL SINGLE DX	5	1.5	<1	1	1	2	2	2	2	2
TOTAL MULTIPLE DX	52	5.0	31	1	1	3	6	12	18	27
TOTAL										
0–19 Years	8	6.8	64	1	1	2	9	18	18	27
20–34	9	4.1	28	1	1	2	5	17	17	17
35–49	15	3.6	12	1	1	2	5	9	12	12
50–64	15	3.2	4	1	1	3	5	6	7	7
65+	10	3.9	12	1	1	2	7	8	10	10
GRAND TOTAL	57	4.6	29	1	1	2	5	12	18	27

49.0: PERIANAL TISS INC/EXC

Type of Patients	Observed Patients	Avg. Stay	Variance	Percentiles						
				10th	25th	50th	75th	90th	95th	99th
1. SINGLE DX										
0–19 Years	43	2.1	1	1	1	2	2	4	4	5
20–34	55	1.8	1	1	1	1	2	3	4	6
35–49	62	1.8	1	1	1	2	2	3	4	6
50–64	18	1.7	<1	1	1	2	2	3	3	3
65+	4	2.0	<1	1	2	2	3	3	3	3
2. MULTIPLE DX										
0–19 Years	63	3.8	25	1	1	3	4	7	13	27
20–34	194	3.4	16	1	1	2	4	6	9	24
35–49	337	4.3	30	1	1	3	5	8	13	27
50–64	282	4.3	44	1	2	3	5	8	11	23
65+	154	5.8	29	1	2	4	7	12	16	31
TOTAL SINGLE DX	182	1.9	1	1	1	2	2	3	4	6
TOTAL MULTIPLE DX	1,030	4.3	31	1	2	3	5	8	13	27
TOTAL										
0–19 Years	106	3.2	16	1	1	2	3	5	7	27
20–34	249	3.1	13	1	1	2	3	6	8	23
35–49	399	3.9	26	1	1	2	4	8	12	22
50–64	300	4.2	42	1	2	3	5	8	11	22
65+	158	5.7	29	1	2	4	7	12	16	31
GRAND TOTAL	1,212	3.9	27	1	1	3	4	8	11	27

49.01: INC PERIANAL ABSCESS

Type of Patients	Observed Patients	Avg. Stay	Variance	Percentiles						
				10th	25th	50th	75th	90th	95th	99th
1. SINGLE DX										
0–19 Years	40	2.1	1	1	1	2	2	4	4	5
20–34	52	1.8	1	1	1	1	2	3	4	6
35–49	58	1.8	1	1	1	2	2	3	5	6
50–64	18	1.7	<1	1	1	1	2	3	3	3
65+	3	2.0	<1	1	1	2	3	3	3	3
2. MULTIPLE DX										
0–19 Years	56	3.8	29	1	1	3	4	7	14	27
20–34	168	3.4	15	1	1	2	4	6	9	24
35–49	311	4.2	31	1	2	3	5	8	13	27
50–64	258	4.4	46	1	2	3	5	8	11	23
65+	142	5.9	31	1	2	4	8	12	16	31
TOTAL SINGLE DX	171	1.9	1	1	1	2	2	3	4	6
TOTAL MULTIPLE DX	935	4.3	32	1	2	3	5	9	13	27
TOTAL										
0–19 Years	96	3.1	18	1	1	2	3	4	7	27
20–34	220	3.0	12	1	1	2	3	6	8	20
35–49	369	3.9	27	1	2	3	4	8	12	27
50–64	276	4.3	43	1	2	3	5	8	11	23
65+	145	5.8	30	1	2	4	7	12	16	31
GRAND TOTAL	1,106	3.9	28	1	1	2	4	8	12	27

49.1: INC/EXC OF ANAL FISTULA

Type of Patients	Observed Patients	Avg. Stay	Variance	Percentiles						
				10th	25th	50th	75th	90th	95th	99th
1. SINGLE DX										
0–19 Years	3	2.8	<1	2	3	3	3	3	3	3
20–34	5	1.6	<1	1	1	1	2	3	3	3
35–49	9	2.0	2	1	1	1	3	5	5	5
50–64	1	4.0	0	4	4	4	4	4	4	4
65+	0									
2. MULTIPLE DX										
0–19 Years	11	1.8	1	1	1	2	2	3	5	5
20–34	45	3.7	22	1	1	2	4	9	10	29
35–49	57	3.5	42	1	1	2	3	7	14	44
50–64	60	3.0	9	1	2	2	4	6	7	16
65+	36	4.9	22	1	2	3	6	11	14	24
TOTAL SINGLE DX	18	2.2	1	1	1	2	3	3	4	5
TOTAL MULTIPLE DX	209	3.5	22	1	1	2	4	7	11	24
TOTAL										
0–19 Years	14	2.1	1	1	1	2	3	3	3	5
20–34	50	3.5	20	1	1	2	4	9	10	29
35–49	66	3.3	37	1	1	1	3	7	8	44
50–64	61	3.0	9	1	1	2	4	6	7	16
65+	36	4.9	22	1	2	3	6	11	14	24
GRAND TOTAL	227	3.4	21	1	1	2	4	7	10	24

Western Region, October 2007–September 2008 Data, by Operation

49.11: ANAL FISTULOTOMY

Type of Patients	Observed Patients	Avg. Stay	Variance	Percentiles						
				10th	25th	50th	75th	90th	95th	99th
1. SINGLE DX										
0–19 Years	1	3.0	0	3	3	3	3	3	3	3
20–34	2	1.0	0	1	1	1	1	1	1	1
35–49	4	1.8	<1	1	1	2	2	3	3	3
50–64	1	4.0	0	4	4	4	4	4	4	4
65+	0									
2. MULTIPLE DX										
0–19 Years	6	2.0	2	1	1	2	2	5	5	5
20–34	27	3.8	30	1	1	2	4	7	9	29
35–49	31	3.4	63	1	1	1	3	4	14	44
50–64	29	3.2	10	1	1	2	4	7	7	16
65+	24	4.6	15	1	2	3	8	11	12	14
TOTAL SINGLE DX	8	2.0	1	1	1	2	3	4	4	4
TOTAL MULTIPLE DX	117	3.6	29	1	1	2	4	7	12	29
TOTAL										
0–19 Years	7	2.1	2	1	1	2	2	5	5	5
20–34	29	3.6	28	1	1	2	4	7	9	29
35–49	35	3.2	56	1	1	2	3	4	14	44
50–64	30	3.2	10	1	1	2	4	6	7	16
65+	24	4.6	15	1	2	3	8	11	12	14
GRAND TOTAL	125	3.5	27	1	1	2	4	7	11	29

49.12: ANAL FISTULECTOMY

Type of Patients	Observed Patients	Avg. Stay	Variance	Percentiles						
				10th	25th	50th	75th	90th	95th	99th
1. SINGLE DX										
0–19 Years	2	2.8	<1	2	3	3	3	3	3	3
20–34	3	2.0	<1	1	1	2	3	3	3	3
35–49	5	2.2	3	1	1	1	3	5	5	5
50–64	0									
65+	0									
2. MULTIPLE DX										
0–19 Years	5	1.6	<1	1	1	1	2	3	3	3
20–34	18	3.6	12	1	1	2	5	10	12	12
35–49	26	2.9	19	1	1	2	3	8	8	22
50–64	31	3.2	8	1	1	2	4	6	8	15
65+	12	5.5	38	2	2	3	5	9	24	24
TOTAL SINGLE DX	10	2.4	1	1	1	3	3	3	5	5
TOTAL MULTIPLE DX	92	3.4	15	1	1	2	4	8	10	24
TOTAL										
0–19 Years	7	2.0	<1	1	1	2	3	3	3	3
20–34	21	3.3	10	1	1	2	3	9	10	12
35–49	31	3.3	17	1	1	2	3	7	8	22
50–64	31	2.9	8	1	1	2	4	6	8	15
65+	12	5.5	38	2	2	3	5	9	24	24
GRAND TOTAL	102	3.3	14	1	1	2	3	7	9	22

49.2: ANAL & PERIANAL DXTIC PX

Type of Patients	Observed Patients	Avg. Stay	Variance	Percentiles						
				10th	25th	50th	75th	90th	95th	99th
1. SINGLE DX										
0–19 Years	2	1.0	0	1	1	1	1	1	1	1
20–34	2	2.0	2	3	3	3	3	3	3	3
35–49	1	1.0	0	1	1	1	1	1	1	1
50–64	1	20.0	0	20	20	20	20	20	20	20
65+	1	4.0	0	4	4	4	4	4	4	4
2. MULTIPLE DX										
0–19 Years	7	2.6	4	1	1	1	5	5	5	5
20–34	29	4.4	26	1	1	2	4	16	16	16
35–49	56	2.5	5	1	1	2	3	6	8	12
50–64	55	5.2	169	1	1	2	4	6	12	76
65+	135	3.7	7	1	2	3	5	7	10	13
TOTAL SINGLE DX	7	4.4	48	1	1	1	4	20	20	20
TOTAL MULTIPLE DX	282	3.8	40	1	1	2	4	7	10	16
TOTAL										
0–19 Years	9	2.4	4	1	1	1	5	5	5	5
20–34	31	4.3	25	1	1	2	4	16	16	16
35–49	57	2.5	5	1	1	2	3	6	8	12
50–64	56	5.5	170	1	1	2	4	10	20	76
65+	136	3.7	7	1	2	3	5	7	10	13
GRAND TOTAL	289	3.8	40	1	1	2	4	7	10	20

49.21: ANOSCOPY

Type of Patients	Observed Patients	Avg. Stay	Variance	Percentiles						
				10th	25th	50th	75th	90th	95th	99th
1. SINGLE DX										
0–19 Years	1	1.0	0	1	1	1	1	1	1	1
20–34	2	2.0	2	3	3	3	3	3	3	3
35–49	1	1.0	0	1	1	1	1	1	1	1
50–64	1	20.0	0	20	20	20	20	20	20	20
65+	1	4.0	0	4	4	4	4	4	4	4
2. MULTIPLE DX										
0–19 Years	6	2.8	4	1	1	2	5	5	5	5
20–34	25	2.8	7	1	1	2	3	6	8	13
35–49	45	2.2	2	1	1	2	3	4	4	7
50–64	41	5.9	222	1	1	2	4	6	10	76
65+	130	3.6	7	1	2	3	5	7	9	11
TOTAL SINGLE DX	6	5.0	55	1	1	3	4	20	20	20
TOTAL MULTIPLE DX	247	3.6	42	1	1	2	4	7	8	14
TOTAL										
0–19 Years	7	2.6	4	1	1	1	5	5	5	5
20–34	27	2.8	7	1	1	2	3	6	8	13
35–49	46	2.2	2	1	1	2	3	4	4	7
50–64	42	6.2	222	1	1	2	4	6	10	76
65+	131	3.6	7	1	2	3	5	7	9	11
GRAND TOTAL	253	3.6	42	1	1	2	4	7	9	20

LOS by Diagnosis and Operation, Western Region, 45th Edition

Western Region, October 2007–September 2008 Data, by Operation

49.3: LOC DESTR ANAL LES NEC

Type of Patients	Observed Patients	Avg. Stay	Vari-ance	Percentiles						
				10th	25th	50th	75th	90th	95th	99th
1. SINGLE DX										
0–19 Years	1	1.0	0	1	1	1	1	1	1	1
20–34	3	1.0	0	1	1	1	1	1	1	1
35–49	6	2.7	6	1	1	2	4	7	7	7
50–64	8	1.1	<1	1	1	1	1	2	2	2
65+	3	2.0	3	1	1	1	4	4	4	4
2. MULTIPLE DX										
0–19 Years	4	3.3	15	1	1	3	3	3	14	14
20–34	22	2.9	9	1	1	2	3	5	6	15
35–49	49	4.1	47	1	1	2	4	6	19	40
50–64	59	4.5	65	1	1	3	4	7	17	60
65+	75	4.5	46	1	1	2	5	8	14	52
TOTAL SINGLE DX	21	1.7	2	1	1	1	1	4	4	7
TOTAL MULTIPLE DX	209	4.2	46	1	1	2	4	7	14	40
TOTAL										
0–19 Years	5	3.1	14	1	1	3	3	3	14	14
20–34	25	2.6	8	1	1	2	3	5	6	15
35–49	55	3.9	42	1	1	2	4	6	19	40
50–64	67	4.1	59	1	1	2	4	7	11	60
65+	78	4.4	44	1	1	2	5	8	14	52
GRAND TOTAL	230	3.9	42	1	1	2	4	7	14	40

49.39: OTH LOC DESTR ANAL LES

Type of Patients	Observed Patients	Avg. Stay	Vari-ance	Percentiles						
				10th	25th	50th	75th	90th	95th	99th
1. SINGLE DX										
0–19 Years	1	1.0	0	1	1	1	1	1	1	1
20–34	3	1.0	0	1	1	1	1	1	1	1
35–49	6	2.7	6	1	1	2	4	7	7	7
50–64	8	1.1	<1	1	1	1	1	2	2	2
65+	2	2.5	4	1	1	3	4	4	4	4
2. MULTIPLE DX										
0–19 Years	4	3.3	15	1	1	3	3	3	14	14
20–34	19	3.0	10	1	1	2	3	6	15	15
35–49	47	4.2	48	1	1	2	4	6	19	40
50–64	53	4.4	69	1	1	3	4	7	11	60
65+	64	4.8	52	1	1	2	6	12	14	52
TOTAL SINGLE DX	20	1.7	2	1	1	1	2	4	7	7
TOTAL MULTIPLE DX	187	4.3	49	1	1	2	4	7	14	52
TOTAL										
0–19 Years	5	3.1	14	1	1	3	3	3	14	14
20–34	22	2.8	9	1	1	2	3	5	6	15
35–49	53	4.0	44	1	1	2	4	6	19	40
50–64	61	3.9	61	1	1	2	4	6	8	60
65+	66	4.8	51	1	1	2	5	12	14	52
GRAND TOTAL	207	4.0	46	1	1	2	4	7	14	40

49.4: HEMORRHOID PROCEDURES

Type of Patients	Observed Patients	Avg. Stay	Vari-ance	Percentiles						
				10th	25th	50th	75th	90th	95th	99th
1. SINGLE DX										
0–19 Years	0									
20–34	9	1.9	1	1	1	2	2	4	4	4
35–49	30	1.7	1	1	1	1	2	3	4	6
50–64	21	1.3	<1	1	1	1	2	2	2	3
65+	1	1.0	0	1	1	1	1	1	1	1
2. MULTIPLE DX										
0–19 Years	7	4.0	55	1	1	1	2	6	25	25
20–34	141	2.8	12	1	1	2	3	5	6	24
35–49	380	3.0	7	1	1	2	4	7	8	14
50–64	376	3.5	12	1	1	3	5	7	10	21
65+	408	4.3	17	2	2	3	5	8	12	23
TOTAL SINGLE DX	61	1.6	<1	1	1	1	2	3	3	6
TOTAL MULTIPLE DX	1,312	3.6	13	1	1	2	5	7	9	19
TOTAL										
0–19 Years	7	4.0	55	1	1	1	2	6	25	25
20–34	150	2.7	11	1	1	2	3	5	6	24
35–49	410	2.9	6	1	1	2	4	6	8	12
50–64	397	3.4	12	1	1	2	4	7	10	21
65+	409	4.3	17	2	2	3	5	8	12	23
GRAND TOTAL	1,373	3.5	12	1	1	2	4	7	9	19

49.45: HEMORRHOID LIGATION

Type of Patients	Observed Patients	Avg. Stay	Vari-ance	Percentiles						
				10th	25th	50th	75th	90th	95th	99th
1. SINGLE DX										
0–19 Years	0									
20–34	0									
35–49	1	1.0	0	1	1	1	1	1	1	1
50–64	0									
65+	1	1.0	0	1	1	1	1	1	1	1
2. MULTIPLE DX										
0–19 Years	2	13.3	261	2	2	2	25	25	25	25
20–34	16	2.9	2	1	2	3	4	5	6	6
35–49	43	3.2	9	1	1	3	3	6	6	19
50–64	55	4.3	15	1	2	3	6	10	15	>99
65+	107	4.6	15	1	2	3	5	9	12	21
TOTAL SINGLE DX	2	1.0	0	1	1	1	1	1	1	1
TOTAL MULTIPLE DX	223	4.2	15	1	2	3	5	9	12	23
TOTAL										
0–19 Years	2	13.3	261	2	2	2	25	25	25	25
20–34	16	2.9	2	1	2	3	4	5	6	6
35–49	44	3.2	9	1	1	3	3	6	6	19
50–64	55	4.3	15	1	2	3	6	10	15	>99
65+	108	4.5	15	1	2	3	5	9	12	21
GRAND TOTAL	225	4.2	15	1	2	3	5	9	12	23

LOS by Diagnosis and Operation, Western Region, 45th Edition

Western Region, October 2007–September 2008 Data, by Operation

49.46: EXC OF HEMORRHOIDS

Type of Patients	Observed Patients	Avg. Stay	Vari-ance	Percentiles						
				10th	25th	50th	75th	90th	95th	99th
1. SINGLE DX										
0–19 Years	0									
20–34	8	2.0	1	1	1	2	3	4	4	4
35–49	28	1.8	1	1	1	1	2	3	4	6
50–64	19	1.4	<1	1	1	1	2	2	3	3
65+	0									
2. MULTIPLE DX										
0–19 Years	2	1.5	<1	1	1	2	2	2	2	2
20–34	105	2.7	7	1	1	2	3	5	6	7
35–49	283	3.1	7	1	1	2	4	7	8	14
50–64	282	3.4	12	1	1	2	4	7	9	17
65+	254	4.2	16	1	2	3	5	8	10	24
TOTAL SINGLE DX	55	1.7	<1	1	1	1	2	3	4	6
TOTAL MULTIPLE DX	926	3.4	11	1	1	2	4	7	9	16
TOTAL										
0–19 Years	2	1.5	<1	1	1	2	2	2	2	2
20–34	113	2.6	6	1	1	2	3	5	6	7
35–49	311	3.0	6	1	1	2	4	7	8	12
50–64	301	3.2	11	1	1	2	4	7	9	17
65+	254	4.2	16	2	2	3	5	8	10	24
GRAND TOTAL	981	3.3	11	1	1	2	4	7	9	16

49.5: ANAL SPHINCTER DIVISION

Type of Patients	Observed Patients	Avg. Stay	Vari-ance	Percentiles						
				10th	25th	50th	75th	90th	95th	99th
1. SINGLE DX										
0–19 Years	0									
20–34	2	1.0	0	1	1	1	1	1	1	1
35–49	3	3.4	16	1	1	1	8	8	8	8
50–64	1	2.0	0	2	2	2	2	2	2	2
65+	0									
2. MULTIPLE DX										
0–19 Years	0									
20–34	10	2.3	5	1	1	1	3	6	7	7
35–49	15	1.7	<1	1	1	1	2	3	4	4
50–64	21	5.4	73	1	1	1	4	14	20	35
65+	22	4.9	36	1	1	3	5	13	18	24
TOTAL SINGLE DX	6	2.3	8	1	1	1	2	8	8	8
TOTAL MULTIPLE DX	68	4.0	37	1	1	2	4	12	18	35
TOTAL										
0–19 Years	0									
20–34	12	2.1	5	1	1	1	3	6	7	7
35–49	18	2.0	3	1	1	1	2	4	8	8
50–64	22	5.3	70	1	1	2	4	14	20	35
65+	22	4.9	36	1	1	3	5	13	18	24
GRAND TOTAL	74	3.8	34	1	1	2	3	8	18	35

49.6: EXCISION OF ANUS

Type of Patients	Observed Patients	Avg. Stay	Vari-ance	Percentiles						
				10th	25th	50th	75th	90th	95th	99th
1. SINGLE DX										
0–19 Years	0									
20–34	0									
35–49	0									
50–64	0									
65+	0									
2. MULTIPLE DX										
0–19 Years	0									
20–34	0									
35–49	1	3.0	0	3	3	3	3	3	3	3
50–64	2	10.0	125	18	18	18	18	18	18	18
65+	1	1.0	0	1	1	1	1	1	1	1
TOTAL SINGLE DX	0									
TOTAL MULTIPLE DX	4	6.0	64	1	2	3	18	18	18	18
TOTAL										
0–19 Years	0									
20–34	0									
35–49	1	3.0	0	3	3	3	3	3	3	3
50–64	2	10.0	125	18	18	18	18	18	18	18
65+	1	1.0	0	1	1	1	1	1	1	1
GRAND TOTAL	4	6.0	64	1	2	3	18	18	18	18

49.7: REPAIR OF ANUS

Type of Patients	Observed Patients	Avg. Stay	Vari-ance	Percentiles						
				10th	25th	50th	75th	90th	95th	99th
1. SINGLE DX										
0–19 Years	10	2.7	3	1	1	2	4	5	6	6
20–34	5	1.8	2	1	1	1	2	4	4	4
35–49	16	1.8	<1	1	1	2	2	3	4	4
50–64	14	2.6	3	1	1	2	4	5	5	5
65+	3	2.3	1	1	1	3	3	3	3	3
2. MULTIPLE DX										
0–19 Years	61	4.3	15	1	2	4	5	8	9	22
20–34	53	3.5	11	1	1	3	4	8	11	18
35–49	89	2.6	6	1	1	2	3	5	8	14
50–64	102	2.7	7	1	1	2	3	4	6	13
65+	60	3.0	6	1	1	2	4	6	9	13
TOTAL SINGLE DX	48	2.4	2	1	1	2	3	5	5	6
TOTAL MULTIPLE DX	365	3.2	10	1	1	2	4	6	9	18
TOTAL										
0–19 Years	71	4.0	13	1	2	3	5	7	8	22
20–34	58	3.3	11	1	1	2	4	8	11	18
35–49	105	2.4	5	1	1	2	3	4	6	12
50–64	116	2.7	7	1	1	2	3	5	6	13
65+	63	3.0	6	1	1	2	4	6	8	13
GRAND TOTAL	413	3.1	9	1	1	2	4	6	8	18

LOS by Diagnosis and Operation, Western Region, 45th Edition

Western Region, October 2007–September 2008 Data, by Operation

49.73: CLOSURE OF ANAL FISTULA

Type of Patients	Observed Patients	Avg. Stay	Vari- ance	Percentiles						
				10th	25th	50th	75th	90th	95th	99th
1. SINGLE DX										
0–19 Years	1	4.0	0	4	4	4	4	4	4	4
20–34	1	1.0	0	1	1	1	1	1	1	1
35–49	6	1.5	<1	1	1	1	2	3	3	3
50–64	3	2.3	5	1	1	1	5	5	5	5
65+	0									
2. MULTIPLE DX										
0–19 Years	3	1.3	<1	1	1	1	2	2	2	2
20–34	13	4.5	29	1	1	1	8	11	18	18
35–49	31	3.0	12	1	1	1	3	8	12	14
50–64	22	4.3	24	1	1	3	4	11	13	21
65+	12	4.2	15	1	1	2	8	9	13	13
TOTAL SINGLE DX	11	1.9	2	1	1	1	3	4	5	5
TOTAL MULTIPLE DX	81	3.7	18	1	1	2	4	11	13	21
TOTAL										
0–19 Years	4	1.8	2	1	1	1	2	4	4	4
20–34	14	4.3	28	1	1	1	8	11	18	18
35–49	37	2.8	11	1	1	1	3	8	12	14
50–64	25	4.0	22	1	1	2	4	11	13	21
65+	12	4.2	15	1	1	2	8	9	13	13
GRAND TOTAL	92	3.5	16	1	1	2	4	9	13	21

49.79: ANAL SPHINCTER REP NEC

Type of Patients	Observed Patients	Avg. Stay	Vari- ance	Percentiles						
				10th	25th	50th	75th	90th	95th	99th
1. SINGLE DX										
0–19 Years	8	2.6	2	1	1	2	4	6	6	6
20–34	4	2.0	2	1	1	1	4	4	4	4
35–49	8	1.8	<1	1	1	2	2	3	3	3
50–64	8	3.0	3	1	2	3	4	5	5	5
65+	2	3.0	0	3	3	3	3	3	3	3
2. MULTIPLE DX										
0–19 Years	52	4.7	16	1	3	4	5	8	10	29
20–34	35	2.7	3	1	2	2	3	4	6	9
35–49	52	2.4	3	1	1	2	3	4	5	10
50–64	69	2.2	1	1	1	2	3	4	4	6
65+	41	2.5	2	1	1	2	3	5	5	6
TOTAL SINGLE DX	30	2.5	2	1	1	2	3	4	6	6
TOTAL MULTIPLE DX	249	3.2	8	1	2	3	4	6	7	18
TOTAL										
0–19 Years	60	4.2	14	1	2	4	5	7	8	22
20–34	39	2.6	3	1	1	2	3	4	6	9
35–49	60	2.3	3	1	1	2	3	4	5	10
50–64	77	2.3	2	1	1	2	3	4	5	6
65+	43	2.5	2	1	1	2	3	5	5	6
GRAND TOTAL	279	3.1	7	1	2	3	4	5	7	11

49.9: OTH OPERATIONS ON ANUS

Type of Patients	Observed Patients	Avg. Stay	Vari- ance	Percentiles						
				10th	25th	50th	75th	90th	95th	99th
1. SINGLE DX										
0–19 Years	0									
20–34	2	1.5	<1	1	1	2	2	2	2	2
35–49	2	1.5	<1	1	1	2	2	2	2	2
50–64	6	1.7	1	1	1	1	2	4	4	4
65+	3	1.3	<1	1	1	1	2	2	2	2
2. MULTIPLE DX										
0–19 Years	6	2.6	3	1	2	2	3	6	6	6
20–34	16	2.4	3	1	1	2	3	6	6	6
35–49	40	3.0	8	1	1	2	4	7	11	14
50–64	33	4.2	25	1	2	3	5	8	16	25
65+	39	4.1	10	1	2	3	5	9	13	14
TOTAL SINGLE DX	13	1.5	<1	1	1	1	2	2	4	4
TOTAL MULTIPLE DX	134	3.5	12	1	1	2	4	7	11	16
TOTAL										
0–19 Years	6	2.6	3	1	2	2	3	6	6	6
20–34	18	2.3	2	1	1	2	3	6	6	6
35–49	42	2.9	8	1	1	2	3	7	7	14
50–64	39	3.8	22	1	2	2	4	8	16	25
65+	42	3.9	10	1	2	3	5	7	11	14
GRAND TOTAL	147	3.3	11	1	1	2	4	6	11	16

50.0: HEPATOTOMY

Type of Patients	Observed Patients	Avg. Stay	Vari- ance	Percentiles						
				10th	25th	50th	75th	90th	95th	99th
1. SINGLE DX										
0–19 Years	0									
20–34	0									
35–49	2	5.0	2	4	4	4	6	6	6	6
50–64	0									
65+	1	6.0	0	6	6	6	6	6	6	6
2. MULTIPLE DX										
0–19 Years	3	20.1	226	6	6	18	36	36	36	36
20–34	5	12.0	52	2	7	15	17	19	19	19
35–49	14	10.5	52	3	4	10	18	23	>99	>99
50–64	39	12.2	229	2	5	7	16	29	36	87
65+	43	12.6	111	2	5	10	18	23	35	49
TOTAL SINGLE DX	3	5.3	1	4	4	6	6	6	6	6
TOTAL MULTIPLE DX	104	12.3	145	2	5	8	17	25	36	87
TOTAL										
0–19 Years	3	20.1	226	6	6	18	36	36	36	36
20–34	5	12.0	52	2	7	15	17	19	19	19
35–49	16	9.8	49	3	4	7	18	23	>99	>99
50–64	39	12.2	229	2	5	7	16	29	36	87
65+	44	12.4	109	2	5	10	18	23	35	49
GRAND TOTAL	107	12.1	142	2	5	8	17	25	36	87

LOS by Diagnosis and Operation, Western Region, 45th Edition

Western Region, October 2007–September 2008 Data, by Operation

50.1: HEPATIC DXTIC PX

Type of Patients	Observed Patients	Avg. Stay	Vari-ance	Percentiles						
				10th	25th	50th	75th	90th	95th	99th
1. SINGLE DX										
0–19 Years	57	2.5	24	1	1	1	2	4	11	30
20–34	6	7.9	26	1	4	8	12	15	15	15
35–49	12	2.5	2	1	1	3	3	4	5	5
50–64	8	1.4	<1	1	1	1	1	3	3	3
65+	2	2.5	4	1	1	1	4	4	4	4
2. MULTIPLE DX										
0–19 Years	372	8.6	128	1	1	5	10	23	35	58
20–34	244	6.9	46	1	3	5	9	13	17	39
35–49	588	7.2	34	2	3	6	9	14	18	27
50–64	1,464	6.6	34	1	3	5	9	13	17	30
65+	1,891	6.8	26	2	3	6	9	12	15	26
TOTAL SINGLE DX	85	2.6	22	1	1	1	2	6	11	30
TOTAL MULTIPLE DX	4,559	7.1	50	1	3	5	9	14	19	39
TOTAL										
0–19 Years	429	7.8	118	1	1	4	9	21	35	58
20–34	250	7.0	46	1	3	5	9	13	16	39
35–49	600	7.1	34	2	3	6	9	14	18	27
50–64	1,472	6.6	34	1	3	5	8	13	17	30
65+	1,893	6.8	26	2	3	6	9	12	15	26
GRAND TOTAL	4,644	7.0	50	1	3	5	9	14	19	39

50.11: CLOSED LIVER BIOPSY

Type of Patients	Observed Patients	Avg. Stay	Vari-ance	Percentiles						
				10th	25th	50th	75th	90th	95th	99th
1. SINGLE DX										
0–19 Years	50	1.6	2	1	1	1	1	3	6	6
20–34	5	7.9	33	1	4	7	12	15	15	15
35–49	9	2.7	2	1	2	3	3	5	5	5
50–64	6	1.2	<1	1	1	1	1	2	2	2
65+	2	2.5	4	1	1	1	4	4	4	4
2. MULTIPLE DX										
0–19 Years	290	7.4	104	1	1	4	8	19	33	58
20–34	197	6.7	40	1	3	5	9	13	16	31
35–49	465	7.0	31	1	3	5	8	13	16	27
50–64	1,162	6.5	30	2	3	5	8	13	16	27
65+	1,675	6.6	23	2	4	6	9	12	14	25
TOTAL SINGLE DX	72	1.8	4	1	1	1	2	4	6	12
TOTAL MULTIPLE DX	3,789	6.8	41	1	3	5	9	13	17	35
TOTAL										
0–19 Years	340	6.5	93	1	1	3	7	16	29	58
20–34	202	6.8	40	1	3	5	9	13	16	31
35–49	474	6.9	31	1	3	5	9	13	16	27
50–64	1,168	6.5	30	2	3	5	8	13	16	27
65+	1,677	6.6	23	2	4	6	9	12	14	25
GRAND TOTAL	3,861	6.6	41	1	3	5	8	13	17	35

50.12: OPEN BIOPSY OF LIVER

Type of Patients	Observed Patients	Avg. Stay	Vari-ance	Percentiles						
				10th	25th	50th	75th	90th	95th	99th
1. SINGLE DX										
0–19 Years	5	3.3	19	1	1	1	1	11	11	11
20–34	0									
35–49	1	1.0	0	1	1	1	1	1	1	1
50–64	0									
65+	0									
2. MULTIPLE DX										
0–19 Years	55	14.3	216	2	5	9	15	40	50	61
20–34	4	5.5	18	2	2	4	7	12	12	12
35–49	25	8.6	47	2	5	6	13	21	22	25
50–64	70	8.3	54	2	4	6	10	22	26	34
65+	83	8.4	39	3	4	6	12	18	21	31
TOTAL SINGLE DX	6	3.2	18	1	1	1	1	11	11	11
TOTAL MULTIPLE DX	237	10.8	125	2	4	7	13	23	39	50
TOTAL										
0–19 Years	60	13.0	206	1	5	8	15	40	50	61
20–34	4	5.5	18	2	2	4	7	12	12	12
35–49	26	8.3	48	2	4	5	13	21	22	25
50–64	70	8.3	54	2	4	6	10	22	26	34
65+	83	8.4	39	3	4	6	12	18	21	31
GRAND TOTAL	243	10.4	122	2	4	7	13	23	34	50

50.13: TRANSJUGULAR LIVER BX

Type of Patients	Observed Patients	Avg. Stay	Vari-ance	Percentiles						
				10th	25th	50th	75th	90th	95th	99th
1. SINGLE DX										
0–19 Years	1	30.0	0	30	30	30	30	30	30	30
20–34	0									
35–49	1	4.0	0	4	4	4	4	4	4	4
50–64	1	3.0	0	3	3	3	3	3	3	3
65+	0									
2. MULTIPLE DX										
0–19 Years	10	10.8	170	2	3	4	9	39	39	39
20–34	30	9.0	100	2	3	6	11	14	21	56
35–49	58	7.9	44	1	3	5	12	19	21	24
50–64	128	7.6	55	2	5	5	10	16	23	35
65+	33	8.3	32	2	5	7	10	14	17	29
TOTAL SINGLE DX	3	21.3	185	3	4	30	30	30	30	30
TOTAL MULTIPLE DX	259	8.2	65	2	3	6	10	17	23	39
TOTAL										
0–19 Years	11	13.4	191	2	3	8	30	39	39	39
20–34	30	9.0	100	2	3	5	11	14	21	56
35–49	59	7.8	43	1	3	5	12	19	21	24
50–64	129	7.6	55	2	3	5	10	16	23	35
65+	33	8.3	32	2	5	7	10	14	17	29
GRAND TOTAL	262	8.5	71	2	3	6	11	19	29	39

LOS by Diagnosis and Operation, Western Region, 45th Edition

Western Region, October 2007–September 2008 Data, by Operation

50.22: PARTIAL HEPATECTOMY

Type of Patients	Observed Patients	Avg. Stay	Vari-ance	10th	25th	50th	75th	90th	95th	99th
1. SINGLE DX										
0–19 Years	2	8.0	0	8	8	8	8	8	8	8
20–34	5	4.4	3	3	3	4	5	7	7	7
35–49	9	4.8	5	2	3	5	6	8	8	8
50–64	1	3.0	0	3	3	3	3	3	3	3
65+	1	3.0	0	3	3	3	3	3	3	3
2. MULTIPLE DX										
0–19 Years	20	9.0	90	3	4	6	8	33	33	43
20–34	41	6.7	30	3	4	5	7	10	14	35
35–49	131	6.8	45	3	4	6	7	11	14	25
50–64	385	6.9	20	4	4	6	8	12	17	27
65+	309	7.7	41	4	5	6	8	12	18	31
TOTAL SINGLE DX	18	4.8	4	2	3	4	7	8	8	8
TOTAL MULTIPLE DX	886	7.3	35	4	4	6	8	12	17	33
TOTAL										
0–19 Years	22	9.0	86	4	4	6	8	33	33	43
20–34	46	6.4	27	3	4	5	7	10	14	35
35–49	140	6.7	43	3	4	6	7	10	13	25
50–64	386	6.9	20	4	4	6	8	12	17	27
65+	310	7.7	41	4	5	6	8	12	18	31
GRAND TOTAL	904	7.2	34	3	4	6	8	12	17	33

50.23: OPEN ABLAT LIVER LESION

Type of Patients	Observed Patients	Avg. Stay	Vari-ance	10th	25th	50th	75th	90th	95th	99th
1. SINGLE DX										
0–19 Years	0									
20–34	0									
35–49	1	2.0	0	2	2	2	2	2	2	2
50–64	0									
65+	0									
2. MULTIPLE DX										
0–19 Years	0									
20–34	2	4.0	2	3	3	5	5	5	5	5
35–49	18	5.8	12	3	4	4	6	12	16	16
50–64	58	5.7	9	3	4	5	7	9	11	21
65+	51	6.1	9	3	4	6	8	10	12	17
TOTAL SINGLE DX	1	2.0	0	2	2	2	2	2	2	2
TOTAL MULTIPLE DX	129	5.8	9	3	4	5	7	9	12	17
TOTAL										
0–19 Years	0									
20–34	2	4.0	2	3	3	4	5	5	5	5
35–49	19	5.6	12	3	4	4	6	9	11	16
50–64	58	5.7	9	3	4	5	7	10	12	21
65+	51	6.1	9	3	4	6	8	10	12	17
GRAND TOTAL	130	5.8	9	3	4	5	7	9	12	17

50.14: LAPAROSCOPIC LIVER BX

Type of Patients	Observed Patients	Avg. Stay	Vari-ance	10th	25th	50th	75th	90th	95th	99th
1. SINGLE DX										
0–19 Years	1	1.0	0	1	1	1	1	1	1	1
20–34	1	8.0	0	8	8	8	8	8	8	8
35–49	1	1.0	0	1	1	1	1	1	1	1
50–64	1	1.0	0	1	1	1	1	1	1	1
65+	0									
2. MULTIPLE DX										
0–19 Years	17	11.6	143	1	5	8	15	24	24	72
20–34	13	5.9	30	1	2	4	9	14	18	18
35–49	40	7.6	48	1	2	5	11	18	18	32
50–64	104	5.6	41	1	1	2	8	15	19	24
65+	99	7.1	64	1	2	4	9	17	25	54
TOTAL SINGLE DX	4	2.7	12	1	1	1	1	8	8	8
TOTAL MULTIPLE DX	273	7.2	67	1	1	5	11	18	23	34
TOTAL										
0–19 Years	18	11.4	142	1	5	8	15	24	24	72
20–34	14	6.1	28	1	2	4	9	14	18	18
35–49	41	7.4	48	1	2	5	11	17	18	32
50–64	105	5.6	41	1	1	2	8	15	19	24
65+	99	7.1	64	1	2	4	9	17	25	54
GRAND TOTAL	277	7.2	66	1	1	5	11	17	22	32

50.2: LOC EXC/DESTR LIVER LES

Type of Patients	Observed Patients	Avg. Stay	Vari-ance	10th	25th	50th	75th	90th	95th	99th
1. SINGLE DX										
0–19 Years	6	3.5	15	1	1	1	8	10	10	10
20–34	9	4.9	5	1	3	5	7	8	8	8
35–49	15	4.0	5	2	2	4	6	7	8	8
50–64	7	1.6	<1	1	1	1	2	3	3	3
65+	6	2.8	7	1	1	1	3	8	8	8
2. MULTIPLE DX										
0–19 Years	31	10.2	87	3	4	6	10	24	33	43
20–34	67	6.9	37	2	4	5	8	14	19	35
35–49	221	5.9	33	2	3	5	7	10	13	21
50–64	718	5.7	22	1	3	5	7	10	15	26
65+	628	6.0	31	1	3	5	7	11	15	28
TOTAL SINGLE DX	43	3.6	7	1	1	3	6	8	8	10
TOTAL MULTIPLE DX	1,665	6.0	30	1	3	5	7	11	16	28
TOTAL										
0–19 Years	37	9.4	83	1	4	6	9	21	33	43
20–34	76	6.7	33	2	3	5	8	13	19	35
35–49	236	5.8	31	2	3	5	7	10	13	21
50–64	725	5.6	22	1	3	5	7	10	15	26
65+	634	5.9	31	1	3	5	7	11	15	28
GRAND TOTAL	1,708	6.0	30	1	3	5	7	11	16	28

LOS by Diagnosis and Operation, Western Region, 45th Edition

214

Western Region, October 2007–September 2008 Data, by Operation

50.24: PERC ABLAT LIVER LESION

Type of Patients	Observed Patients	Avg. Stay	Variance	10th	25th	50th	75th	90th	95th	99th
1. SINGLE DX										
0–19 Years	0									
20–34	0									
35–49	0									
50–64	0									
65+	1	1.0	0			1			1	1
2. MULTIPLE DX										
0–19 Years	0									
20–34	3	1.3	<1	1	1	1	2	2	2	2
35–49	14	2.0	4	1	1	1	3	3	8	8
50–64	54	2.7	21	1	1	1	2	5	7	26
65+	80	2.4	13	1	1	1	2	4	7	26
TOTAL SINGLE DX	1	1.0	0	1	1	1	1	1	1	1
TOTAL MULTIPLE DX	151	2.4	15	1	1	1	2	4	7	26
TOTAL										
0–19 Years	0									
20–34	3	1.3	<1	1	1	1	2	2	2	2
35–49	14	2.0	4	1	1	1	3	3	8	8
50–64	54	2.7	21	1	1	1	2	5	7	26
65+	81	2.4	13	1	1	1	2	4	7	26
GRAND TOTAL	152	2.4	15	1	1	1	2	4	7	26

50.25: LAPSCP ABLAT LIVER LES

Type of Patients	Observed Patients	Avg. Stay	Variance	10th	25th	50th	75th	90th	95th	99th
1. SINGLE DX										
0–19 Years	2	1.0	0	1	1	1	1	1	1	1
20–34	1	1.0	0	1	1	1	1	1	1	1
35–49	1	5.0	0	5	5	5	5	5	5	5
50–64	0									
65+	0									
2. MULTIPLE DX										
0–19 Years	0									
20–34	2	12.5	83	6	6	13	19	19	19	19
35–49	14	3.5	20	1	1	2	4	7	18	18
50–64	84	3.4	16	1	1	2	4	6	14	21
65+	71	3.6	12	1	1	2	5	8	11	16
TOTAL SINGLE DX	4	1.6	2	1	1	1	1	5	5	5
TOTAL MULTIPLE DX	171	3.6	16	1	1	2	4	7	14	21
TOTAL										
0–19 Years	2	1.0	0	1	1	1	1	1	1	1
20–34	3	8.7	85	1	1	6	19	19	19	19
35–49	15	3.6	19	1	1	2	4	7	18	18
50–64	84	3.4	16	1	1	2	4	6	14	21
65+	71	3.6	12	1	1	2	5	8	11	16
GRAND TOTAL	175	3.5	15	1	1	2	4	7	14	21

50.29: HEPATIC LESION DESTR NEC

Type of Patients	Observed Patients	Avg. Stay	Variance	10th	25th	50th	75th	90th	95th	99th
1. SINGLE DX										
0–19 Years	2	5.5	40	1	1	10	10	10	10	10
20–34	2	7.0	2	6	6	7	8	8	8	8
35–49	2	1.5	<1	1	1	2	2	2	2	2
50–64	4	1.5	<1	1	1	2	2	2	2	2
65+	3	4.0	13	1	1	3	8	8	8	8
2. MULTIPLE DX										
0–19 Years	10	14.4	62	2	9	16	21	24	25	25
20–34	18	8.4	53	1	3	8	11	22	26	26
35–49	36	5.4	9	2	4	5	7	10	11	15
50–64	99	4.7	19	1	2	4	6	9	12	27
65+	79	5.5	16	2	3	5	7	11	14	25
TOTAL SINGLE DX	13	3.5	11	1	1	2	6	8	10	10
TOTAL MULTIPLE DX	242	6.0	27	1	2	4	7	12	18	26
TOTAL										
0–19 Years	12	13.4	65	1	8	16	21	24	25	25
20–34	20	8.3	48	1	4	8	11	22	26	26
35–49	38	5.2	9	2	4	5	7	10	11	15
50–64	103	4.6	19	2	3	4	6	9	12	27
65+	82	5.4	16	2	3	5	7	10	12	25
GRAND TOTAL	255	5.8	27	1	2	4	7	11	16	26

50.3: HEPATIC LOBECTOMY

Type of Patients	Observed Patients	Avg. Stay	Variance	10th	25th	50th	75th	90th	95th	99th
1. SINGLE DX										
0–19 Years	1	4.0	0	4	4	4	4	4	4	4
20–34	5	6.0	<1	5	6	6	6	7	7	7
35–49	4	9.8	57	5	7	7	21	21	21	21
50–64	2	7.0	7	7	7	7	7	7	7	7
65+	1	3.0	0	3	3	3	3	3	3	3
2. MULTIPLE DX										
0–19 Years	24	18.3	262	6	7	13	15	52	57	57
20–34	29	8.0	37	3	5	6	9	14	14	34
35–49	73	8.3	100	4	5	6	8	12	15	88
50–64	154	8.3	35	4	5	6	9	14	21	35
65+	118	10.2	89	4	5	7	11	21	23	48
TOTAL SINGLE DX	13	6.9	19	4	5	6	7	7	21	21
TOTAL MULTIPLE DX	398	10.3	106	4	5	7	11	19	33	57
TOTAL										
0–19 Years	25	18.1	261	6	7	13	15	52	57	57
20–34	34	7.7	32	4	5	6	8	14	14	34
35–49	77	8.4	97	4	5	6	8	12	16	88
50–64	156	8.3	34	4	5	6	9	14	21	35
65+	119	10.2	89	4	5	7	11	21	23	48
GRAND TOTAL	411	10.2	104	4	5	7	11	19	32	57

LOS by Diagnosis and Operation, Western Region, 45th Edition

Western Region, October 2007–September 2008 Data, by Operation

50.4: TOTAL HEPATECTOMY

Type of Patients	Observed Patients	Avg. Stay	Variance	Percentiles						
				10th	25th	50th	75th	90th	95th	99th
1. SINGLE DX										
0–19 Years	0									
20–34	1	4.0	0	4	4		4	4	4	4
35–49	0									
50–64	0									
65+	0									
2. MULTIPLE DX										
0–19 Years	0									
20–34	1	1.0	0	1	1	1	1	1	1	1
35–49	2	5.0	2	4	4	6	6	6	6	6
50–64	7	16.5	590	4	4	9	12	71	71	71
65+	1	3.0	0	3	3	3	3	3	3	3
TOTAL SINGLE DX	1	4.0	0	4	4		4	4	4	4
TOTAL MULTIPLE DX	11	11.8	398	3	4	5	10	12	71	71
TOTAL										
0–19 Years	0									
20–34	2	2.5	4	1	1	1	6	6	6	6
35–49	2	5.0	2	4	4	6	6	6	6	6
50–64	7	16.5	590	4	4	9	12	71	71	71
65+	1	3.0	0	3	3	3	3	3	3	3
GRAND TOTAL	12	11.1	367	3	4	5	10	12	71	71

50.59: LIVER TRANSPLANT NEC

Type of Patients	Observed Patients	Avg. Stay	Variance	Percentiles						
				10th	25th	50th	75th	90th	95th	99th
1. SINGLE DX										
0–19 Years	1	14.0	0	14	14	14	14	14	14	14
20–34	0									
35–49	1	8.0	0	8	8	8	8	8	8	8
50–64	1	11.0	0	11	11	11	11	11	11	11
65+	0									
2. MULTIPLE DX										
0–19 Years	61	26.6	357	11	13	21	32	72	79	>99
20–34	22	13.7	171	6	8	9	15	23	24	71
35–49	109	14.0	77	6	7	11	18	28	38	>99
50–64	426	15.9	242	6	7	11	18	38	56	89
65+	64	16.5	238	6	7	11	20	48	57	>99
TOTAL SINGLE DX	3	11.0	9	8	8	11	14	14	14	14
TOTAL MULTIPLE DX	682	17.7	258	6	7	11	21	41	63	>99
TOTAL										
0–19 Years	62	26.5	356	11	13	21	32	72	79	>99
20–34	22	13.7	171	6	8	9	15	23	24	71
35–49	110	14.0	77	6	7	11	18	28	38	>99
50–64	427	15.9	242	6	7	11	18	38	56	89
65+	64	16.5	238	6	7	11	20	48	57	>99
GRAND TOTAL	685	17.7	257	6	8	11	21	40	63	>99

50.5: LIVER TRANSPLANT

Type of Patients	Observed Patients	Avg. Stay	Variance	Percentiles						
				10th	25th	50th	75th	90th	95th	99th
1. SINGLE DX										
0–19 Years	1	14.0	0	14	14	14	14	14	14	14
20–34	0									
35–49	1	8.0	0	8	8	8	8	8	8	8
50–64	1	11.0	0	11	11	11	11	11	11	11
65+	0									
2. MULTIPLE DX										
0–19 Years	62	27.3	368	11	13	21	33	72	79	>99
20–34	22	13.7	171	6	8	9	15	23	24	71
35–49	110	14.0	77	6	7	11	18	28	38	>99
50–64	433	16.0	242	6	7	9	19	39	57	93
65+	64	16.5	238	6	7	11	20	48	57	>99
TOTAL SINGLE DX	3	11.0	9	8	8	11	14	14	14	14
TOTAL MULTIPLE DX	691	17.9	263	6	8	12	22	42	63	>99
TOTAL										
0–19 Years	63	27.2	367	11	13	21	33	72	79	>99
20–34	22	13.7	171	6	8	9	15	23	24	71
35–49	111	13.9	76	6	8	11	18	28	38	>99
50–64	434	15.9	242	6	7	9	19	39	57	93
65+	64	16.5	238	6	7	11	20	48	57	>99
GRAND TOTAL	694	17.9	262	6	8	11	22	42	63	>99

50.6: REPAIR OF LIVER

Type of Patients	Observed Patients	Avg. Stay	Variance	Percentiles						
				10th	25th	50th	75th	90th	95th	99th
1. SINGLE DX										
0–19 Years	2	5.5	<1	5	5	5	6	6	6	6
20–34	5	4.0	3	2	3	4	5	6	6	6
35–49	0									
50–64	1	10.0	0	10	10	10	10	10	10	10
65+	0									
2. MULTIPLE DX										
0–19 Years	39	9.2	145	4	5	6	11	12	15	86
20–34	125	9.7	122	3	4	6	12	20	25	49
35–49	63	10.0	187	2	4	6	12	19	28	92
50–64	42	14.7	298	2	4	7	14	38	58	62
65+	34	10.2	61	3	4	7	14	18	27	37
TOTAL SINGLE DX	8	5.1	6	2	4	5	6	10	10	10
TOTAL MULTIPLE DX	303	10.4	157	3	4	6	12	21	34	62
TOTAL										
0–19 Years	41	9.0	140	4	5	6	11	12	15	86
20–34	130	9.5	119	2	3	6	11	19	25	49
35–49	63	10.0	187	2	3	6	12	19	28	92
50–64	43	14.6	292	2	4	8	14	38	58	62
65+	34	10.2	61	3	4	7	14	18	27	37
GRAND TOTAL	311	10.3	154	3	4	6	12	20	34	62

LOS by Diagnosis and Operation, Western Region, 45th Edition

Western Region, October 2007–September 2008 Data, by Operation

50.61: CLOSURE OF LIVER LAC

Type of Patients	Observed Patients	Avg. Stay	Variance	10th	25th	50th	75th	90th	95th	99th
1. SINGLE DX										
0–19 Years	2	5.5	<1	5	5	5	6	6	6	6
20–34	5	4.0	3	2	3	4	5	6	6	6
35–49	0									
50–64	0									
65+	0									
2. MULTIPLE DX										
0–19 Years	37	9.2	152	4	5	6	11	12	15	86
20–34	121	9.5	124	3	4	6	10	19	25	49
35–49	56	9.6	201	2	3	5	11	19	32	92
50–64	37	15.2	328	2	4	8	14	57	60	62
65+	24	9.2	46	2	4	6	14	18	21	27
TOTAL SINGLE DX	7	4.4	2	2	3	5	6	6	6	6
TOTAL MULTIPLE DX	275	10.2	165	2	4	6	12	19	34	86
TOTAL										
0–19 Years	39	9.0	146	4	5	6	11	12	15	86
20–34	126	9.2	120	2	4	6	9	19	25	49
35–49	56	9.6	201	2	4	5	11	19	32	92
50–64	37	15.2	328	2	4	8	14	57	60	62
65+	24	9.2	46	2	4	6	14	18	21	27
GRAND TOTAL	282	10.0	162	2	4	6	12	19	34	86

50.91: PERC LIVER ASPIRATION

Type of Patients	Observed Patients	Avg. Stay	Variance	10th	25th	50th	75th	90th	95th	99th
1. SINGLE DX										
0–19 Years	2	3.5	12	1	1	6	6	6	6	6
20–34	4	6.5	7	3	3	6	9	9	9	9
35–49	5	3.6	10	1	2	3	3	9	9	9
50–64	3	4.3	5	3	3	3	7	7	7	7
65+	0									
2. MULTIPLE DX										
0–19 Years	21	9.9	53	2	5	9	12	18	30	30
20–34	66	7.6	20	2	4	7	10	13	17	21
35–49	133	8.9	36	3	5	7	12	19	20	25
50–64	261	8.5	42	3	4	8	10	15	19	40
65+	297	9.7	41	3	5	8	13	17	21	41
TOTAL SINGLE DX	14	4.6	8	1	3	3	7	9	9	9
TOTAL MULTIPLE DX	778	9.0	40	3	5	8	11	17	20	30
TOTAL										
0–19 Years	23	9.7	53	2	5	9	12	16	30	30
20–34	70	7.6	19	3	4	7	10	13	17	21
35–49	138	8.7	36	3	4	7	12	19	20	25
50–64	264	8.4	42	3	5	7	10	15	19	40
65+	297	9.7	41	3	5	8	13	17	21	41
GRAND TOTAL	792	8.9	40	3	5	7	11	17	20	30

50.9: OTHER LIVER OPERATIONS

Type of Patients	Observed Patients	Avg. Stay	Variance	10th	25th	50th	75th	90th	95th	99th
1. SINGLE DX										
0–19 Years	2	3.5	12	1	1	6	6	6	6	6
20–34	4	6.5	7	3	3	6	9	9	9	9
35–49	5	3.6	10	1	2	3	3	9	9	9
50–64	3	4.3	5	3	3	3	7	7	7	7
65+	1	1.0	0	1	1	1	1	1	1	1
2. MULTIPLE DX										
0–19 Years	23	12.1	73	2	5	10	16	25	30	30
20–34	68	7.5	20	2	4	7	10	13	17	21
35–49	149	8.4	36	2	4	7	9	19	20	25
50–64	324	7.4	45	1	3	6	9	14	18	40
65+	359	8.5	43	1	4	7	12	16	20	31
TOTAL SINGLE DX	15	4.3	8	1	2	3	7	9	9	9
TOTAL MULTIPLE DX	923	8.2	44	2	4	7	10	16	20	30
TOTAL										
0–19 Years	25	11.8	74	2	5	9	16	25	30	30
20–34	72	7.4	20	3	4	6	10	12	17	21
35–49	154	8.3	36	2	4	7	11	18	20	25
50–64	327	7.4	45	1	3	6	9	14	18	40
65+	360	8.4	43	1	4	7	12	16	20	31
GRAND TOTAL	938	8.2	44	2	4	7	10	16	20	30

50.94: HEPATIC INJECTION NEC

Type of Patients	Observed Patients	Avg. Stay	Variance	10th	25th	50th	75th	90th	95th	99th
1. SINGLE DX										
0–19 Years	0									
20–34	0									
35–49	0									
50–64	0									
65+	1	1.0	0	1	1	1	1	1	1	1
2. MULTIPLE DX										
0–19 Years	0									
20–34	1	1.0	0	1	1	1	1	1	1	1
35–49	15	4.3	17	1	2	3	5	6	18	18
50–64	56	3.0	40	1	1	1	3	5	11	46
65+	56	2.7	10	1	1	1	3	5	13	15
TOTAL SINGLE DX	1	1.0	0	1	1	1	1	1	1	1
TOTAL MULTIPLE DX	128	3.0	24	1	1	2	3	5	11	18
TOTAL										
0–19 Years	0									
20–34	1	1.0	0	1	1	3	5	6	1	1
35–49	15	4.3	17	1	2	3	5	6	18	18
50–64	56	3.0	40	1	1	1	3	5	11	46
65+	57	2.7	10	1	1	1	3	5	13	15
GRAND TOTAL	129	3.0	24	1	1	1	3	5	11	18

LOS by Diagnosis and Operation, Western Region, 45th Edition

Western Region, October 2007–September 2008 Data, by Operation

51.0: GB INC & CHOLECYSTOSTOMY

Type of Patients	Observed Patients	Avg. Stay	Variance	Percentiles 10th	25th	50th	75th	90th	95th	99th
1. SINGLE DX										
0–19 Years	2	3.5	<1	3	3	4	4	4	4	4
20–34	2	1.0	0	1	1	1	1	1	1	1
35–49	4	2.8	<1	2	2	3	3	3	3	3
50–64	1	4.0	0	4	4	4	4	4	4	4
65+	3	5.7	2	4	4	6	7	7	7	7
2. MULTIPLE DX										
0–19 Years	6	2.7	2	1	2	2	3	5	5	5
20–34	31	13.1	334	2	2	5	18	42	56	75
35–49	84	8.3	66	2	4	5	10	15	21	51
50–64	167	10.2	87	3	4	7	13	20	26	62
65+	556	9.4	56	3	5	7	11	17	23	43
TOTAL SINGLE DX	12	3.4	3	1	2	3	4	6	7	7
TOTAL MULTIPLE DX	844	9.5	73	3	4	7	11	17	24	48
TOTAL										
0–19 Years	8	2.8	2	2	2	2	4	5	5	5
20–34	33	12.4	322	1	2	5	14	42	56	75
35–49	88	8.0	65	2	4	5	9	15	21	51
50–64	168	10.2	87	3	4	7	13	20	26	62
65+	559	9.4	56	3	5	7	11	17	23	43
GRAND TOTAL	856	9.4	73	3	4	7	11	17	24	48

51.01: PERC ASPIRATION OF GB

Type of Patients	Observed Patients	Avg. Stay	Variance	Percentiles 10th	25th	50th	75th	90th	95th	99th
1. SINGLE DX										
0–19 Years	1	4.0	0	4	4	4	4	4	4	4
20–34	2	1.0	0	1	1	1	1	1	1	1
35–49	2	2.5	<1	2	2	2	3	3	3	3
50–64	1	4.0	0	4	4	4	4	4	4	4
65+	2	6.5	<1	6	6	7	7	7	7	7
2. MULTIPLE DX										
0–19 Years	2	4.0	2	3	3	3	5	5	5	5
20–34	10	8.3	142	2	4	4	7	9	42	42
35–49	45	8.2	59	2	4	7	10	14	16	51
50–64	95	8.8	87	2	4	6	11	15	20	65
65+	355	8.9	46	3	5	7	11	16	20	41
TOTAL SINGLE DX	8	3.5	5	1	1	3	4	7	7	7
TOTAL MULTIPLE DX	507	8.8	56	3	4	7	11	15	20	43
TOTAL										
0–19 Years	3	4.0	1	3	3	4	4	5	5	5
20–34	12	7.1	124	1	2	4	5	9	42	42
35–49	47	7.9	58	2	4	6	10	14	16	51
50–64	96	8.8	87	3	4	6	11	15	20	65
65+	357	8.9	46	3	5	7	11	16	20	41
GRAND TOTAL	515	8.7	56	3	4	7	11	15	20	43

51.03: CHOLECYSTOSTOMY NEC

Type of Patients	Observed Patients	Avg. Stay	Variance	Percentiles 10th	25th	50th	75th	90th	95th	99th
1. SINGLE DX										
0–19 Years	1	3.0	0	3	3	3	3	3	3	3
20–34	0									
35–49	1	3.0	0	3	3	3	3	3	3	3
50–64	0									
65+	1	4.0	0	4	4	4	4	4	4	4
2. MULTIPLE DX										
0–19 Years	2	2.6	2	2	2	2	2	5	5	5
20–34	13	14.0	234	2	3	11	19	28	56	56
35–49	24	9.4	107	2	4	5	11	22	32	43
50–64	46	12.4	65	4	6	11	17	24	31	36
65+	133	10.5	58	4	6	8	13	19	26	41
TOTAL SINGLE DX	3	3.3	<1	3	3	3	4	4	4	4
TOTAL MULTIPLE DX	218	10.8	75	3	5	8	14	20	30	43
TOTAL										
0–19 Years	3	2.7	1	2	2	2	3	5	5	5
20–34	13	14.0	234	2	3	11	19	28	56	56
35–49	25	9.2	105	2	4	5	11	22	32	43
50–64	46	12.4	65	4	6	11	17	24	31	36
65+	134	10.5	58	4	6	8	13	19	26	41
GRAND TOTAL	221	10.7	75	3	5	8	14	20	30	43

51.04: CHOLECYSTOTOMY NEC

Type of Patients	Observed Patients	Avg. Stay	Variance	Percentiles 10th	25th	50th	75th	90th	95th	99th
1. SINGLE DX										
0–19 Years	0									
20–34	0									
35–49	0									
50–64	0									
65+	0									
2. MULTIPLE DX										
0–19 Years	1	1.0	0	1	1	1	1	1	1	1
20–34	6	22.4	992	1	2	5	48	75	75	75
35–49	12	5.2	8	3	3	4	5	9	11	11
50–64	17	11.6	79	3	4	10	15	26	34	34
65+	50	11.3	129	2	5	8	15	21	23	64
TOTAL SINGLE DX	0									
TOTAL MULTIPLE DX	86	11.2	164	2	3	8	15	21	34	75
TOTAL										
0–19 Years	1	1.0	0	1	1	1	1	1	1	1
20–34	6	22.4	992	1	3	5	48	75	75	75
35–49	12	5.2	8	1	3	4	5	9	11	11
50–64	17	11.6	79	2	4	10	15	26	34	34
65+	50	11.3	129	2	5	8	15	21	23	64
GRAND TOTAL	86	11.2	164	2	3	8	15	21	34	75

218

LOS by Diagnosis and Operation, Western Region, 45th Edition

Western Region, October 2007–September 2008 Data, by Operation

51.1: BILIARY TRACT DXTIC PX

Type of Patients	Observed Patients	Avg. Stay	Variance	10th	25th	50th	75th	90th	95th	99th
1. SINGLE DX										
0–19 Years	6	5.5	9	1	3	7	8	8	8	8
20–34	24	2.6	2	1	2	2	3	4	5	7
35–49	16	4.4	20	1	2	3	5	7	20	20
50–64	9	2.9	2	1	2	3	4	5	5	5
65+	1	6.0	0	6	6	6	6	6	6	6
2. MULTIPLE DX										
0–19 Years	56	5.0	12	1	2	4	8	10	11	14
20–34	239	5.1	22	2	3	4	6	9	13	22
35–49	434	5.8	31	2	3	4	7	11	15	23
50–64	759	5.8	23	2	3	5	7	12	15	27
65+	1,331	6.0	20	2	3	5	8	11	14	22
TOTAL SINGLE DX	56	3.6	9	1	2	3	4	7	8	20
TOTAL MULTIPLE DX	2,819	5.8	23	2	3	4	7	11	14	23
TOTAL										
0–19 Years	62	5.1	11	1	2	4	8	10	11	14
20–34	263	4.9	20	2	3	4	6	8	13	22
35–49	450	5.8	30	2	3	4	7	11	15	23
50–64	768	5.8	23	2	3	4	7	12	15	27
65+	1,332	6.0	20	2	3	5	8	11	14	22
GRAND TOTAL	2,875	5.8	22	2	3	4	7	11	14	23

51.10: ERCP

Type of Patients	Observed Patients	Avg. Stay	Variance	10th	25th	50th	75th	90th	95th	99th
1. SINGLE DX										
0–19 Years	6	5.5	9	1	3	7	8	8	8	8
20–34	20	2.7	2	1	2	3	3	5	7	7
35–49	14	4.7	22	1	2	4	5	7	20	20
50–64	8	2.9	3	1	1	2	4	5	5	5
65+	1	6.0	0	6	6	6	6	6	6	6
2. MULTIPLE DX										
0–19 Years	53	5.0	12	1	2	4	7	10	11	14
20–34	221	4.9	20	2	3	4	5	8	13	21
35–49	365	5.9	30	2	3	4	7	12	15	22
50–64	619	5.9	23	2	3	4	7	12	15	25
65+	1,032	6.0	21	2	3	5	8	11	14	23
TOTAL SINGLE DX	49	3.8	10	1	2	3	5	7	8	20
TOTAL MULTIPLE DX	2,290	5.8	23	2	3	4	7	11	14	22
TOTAL										
0–19 Years	59	5.1	11	1	2	4	8	10	11	14
20–34	241	4.7	19	2	3	4	5	8	13	21
35–49	379	5.8	29	2	3	4	7	12	15	22
50–64	627	5.8	23	2	3	4	7	12	15	25
65+	1,033	6.0	21	2	3	5	8	11	14	23
GRAND TOTAL	2,339	5.8	23	2	3	4	7	11	14	22

51.14: CLSD BD/SPHINCT ODDI BX

Type of Patients	Observed Patients	Avg. Stay	Variance	10th	25th	50th	75th	90th	95th	99th
1. SINGLE DX										
0–19 Years	0									
20–34	3	2.7	1	2	2	2	4	4	4	4
35–49	2	2.0	2	1	1	1	3	3	3	3
50–64	1	3.0	0	3	3	3	3	3	3	3
65+	0									
2. MULTIPLE DX										
0–19 Years	1	4.0	0	4	4	4	4	4	4	4
20–34	9	7.1	6	4	6	6	8	13	13	13
35–49	50	5.8	44	1	2	5	7	10	11	39
50–64	116	5.3	21	2	2	4	7	11	12	25
65+	243	5.7	18	2	3	5	7	10	14	21
TOTAL SINGLE DX	6	2.5	1	1	2	2	3	4	4	4
TOTAL MULTIPLE DX	419	5.6	22	2	3	5	7	10	14	29
TOTAL										
0–19 Years	1	4.0	0	4	4	4	4	4	4	4
20–34	12	6.0	9	2	4	6	7	8	13	13
35–49	52	5.6	43	1	2	4	7	9	11	39
50–64	117	5.3	21	2	3	4	7	11	12	25
65+	243	5.7	18	2	3	5	7	10	14	21
GRAND TOTAL	425	5.6	22	2	3	4	7	10	13	29

51.2: CHOLECYSTECTOMY

Type of Patients	Observed Patients	Avg. Stay	Variance	10th	25th	50th	75th	90th	95th	99th
1. SINGLE DX										
0–19 Years	756	2.2	3	1	1	2	3	4	6	9
20–34	3,469	2.1	2	1	1	2	3	4	5	7
35–49	2,047	2.1	2	1	1	2	3	4	5	7
50–64	928	2.1	2	1	1	2	3	4	5	8
65+	248	1.8	1	1	1	1	2	3	4	6
2. MULTIPLE DX										
0–19 Years	2,135	4.2	27	1	2	3	5	8	13	28
20–34	13,780	3.2	8	1	2	3	4	6	8	14
35–49	14,222	3.5	14	1	2	3	4	7	9	17
50–64	15,860	4.1	18	1	2	3	5	8	11	21
65+	18,306	5.7	28	1	2	4	7	11	15	27
TOTAL SINGLE DX	7,448	2.1	2	1	1	2	3	4	5	7
TOTAL MULTIPLE DX	64,303	4.2	19	1	2	3	5	8	11	22
TOTAL										
0–19 Years	2,891	3.6	21	1	1	2	4	7	10	25
20–34	17,249	3.0	7	1	1	2	4	5	7	13
35–49	16,269	3.3	12	1	1	3	4	6	8	16
50–64	16,788	4.0	17	1	2	3	5	8	10	20
65+	18,554	5.7	28	1	2	4	7	11	15	27
GRAND TOTAL	71,751	4.0	18	1	2	3	5	8	11	21

LOS by Diagnosis and Operation, Western Region, 45th Edition

Western Region, October 2007–September 2008 Data, by Operation

51.22: CHOLECYSTECTOMY NOS

Type of Patients	Observed Patients	Avg. Stay	Vari-ance	Percentiles						
				10th	25th	50th	75th	90th	95th	99th
1. SINGLE DX										
0–19 Years	20	2.5	4	1	1	2	3	6	6	10
20–34	31	3.5	10	1	1	3	4	7	8	16
35–49	29	3.4	7	1	2	2	5	9	9	9
50–64	21	4.7	6	2	3	4	6	8	9	10
65+	8	3.8	6	1	1	4	5	8	8	8
2. MULTIPLE DX										
0–19 Years	124	8.5	148	1	3	5	9	19	29	69
20–34	810	5.6	23	2	3	5	7	9	13	29
35–49	1,255	6.4	44	2	3	5	7	11	16	36
50–64	2,226	6.9	42	2	4	5	8	12	17	36
65+	3,171	8.8	47	3	5	7	11	16	22	37
TOTAL SINGLE DX	109	3.2	7	1	1	2	3	6	8	10
TOTAL MULTIPLE DX	7,586	7.5	47	3	4	6	9	14	19	37
TOTAL										
0–19 Years	144	7.1	121	1	2	4	7	16	25	69
20–34	841	5.5	23	2	3	5	7	9	13	29
35–49	1,284	6.3	44	2	3	5	7	11	16	36
50–64	2,247	6.9	41	2	4	5	8	12	17	36
65+	3,179	8.8	47	3	5	7	11	16	22	37
GRAND TOTAL	7,695	7.4	46	2	4	6	9	14	19	36

51.23: LAPSCP CHOLECYSTECTOMY

Type of Patients	Observed Patients	Avg. Stay	Vari-ance	Percentiles						
				10th	25th	50th	75th	90th	95th	99th
1. SINGLE DX										
0–19 Years	733	2.2	3	1	1	2	3	4	5	9
20–34	3,431	2.1	2	1	1	2	3	4	5	7
35–49	2,015	2.0	2	1	1	2	3	4	5	7
50–64	902	2.0	2	1	1	2	3	4	4	7
65+	239	1.7	1	1	1	1	2	3	4	6
2. MULTIPLE DX										
0–19 Years	2,006	3.8	15	1	2	3	4	7	10	24
20–34	12,946	3.1	7	1	2	2	4	6	7	13
35–49	12,938	3.2	9	1	2	2	4	6	8	15
50–64	13,586	3.7	13	1	2	3	5	7	9	18
65+	15,058	5.0	22	2	3	4	6	10	13	23
TOTAL SINGLE DX	7,320	2.0	2	1	1	2	3	4	5	7
TOTAL MULTIPLE DX	56,534	3.8	14	1	2	3	5	7	10	19
TOTAL										
0–19 Years	2,739	3.3	12	1	1	2	4	6	9	20
20–34	16,377	2.9	6	1	1	2	4	5	7	11
35–49	14,953	3.1	9	1	1	2	4	6	8	14
50–64	14,488	3.6	12	1	2	3	4	7	9	17
65+	15,297	5.0	21	2	2	4	6	10	13	23
GRAND TOTAL	63,854	3.6	13	1	2	3	4	7	9	18

51.3: BILIARY TRACT ANAST

Type of Patients	Observed Patients	Avg. Stay	Vari-ance	Percentiles						
				10th	25th	50th	75th	90th	95th	99th
1. SINGLE DX										
0–19 Years	10	7.5	9	4	5	7	11	12	12	12
20–34		11.0	31	7	7	15	15	15	15	15
35–49	2	6.0	2	5	5	7	7	7	7	7
50–64	2	5.0	2	4	4	5	6	6	6	6
65+	2	8.0	18	5	5	8	11	11	11	11
2. MULTIPLE DX										
0–19 Years	57	11.4	46	5	7	9	15	21	25	27
20–34	37	12.2	149	4	6	8	15	23	41	67
35–49	78	11.8	75	5	6	9	14	24	35	43
50–64	213	11.1	60	5	6	9	14	20	26	41
65+	281	11.6	71	5	7	9	14	20	25	57
TOTAL SINGLE DX	18	7.5	10	4	5	7	11	12	12	15
TOTAL MULTIPLE DX	666	11.5	67	5	7	9	14	21	26	45
TOTAL										
0–19 Years	67	11.0	43	5	6	9	15	21	25	27
20–34	39	12.2	142	4	6	8	15	23	41	67
35–49	80	11.7	74	5	6	9	14	24	35	43
50–64	215	11.1	60	5	6	9	14	20	26	41
65+	283	11.6	70	5	7	9	14	20	25	57
GRAND TOTAL	684	11.4	65	5	6	9	14	21	26	45

51.36: CHOLEDOCHOENTEROSTOMY

Type of Patients	Observed Patients	Avg. Stay	Vari-ance	Percentiles						
				10th	25th	50th	75th	90th	95th	99th
1. SINGLE DX										
0–19 Years	3	6.3	<1	6	6	6	7	7	7	7
20–34	0									
35–49	1	7.0	0	7	7	7	7	7	7	7
50–64	1	6.0	0	6	6	6	6	6	6	6
65+	1	11.0	0	11	11	11	11	11	11	11
2. MULTIPLE DX										
0–19 Years	4	13.5	104	5	5	7	26	26	26	26
20–34	21	10.3	51	4	6	7	13	19	23	31
35–49	41	12.6	81	5	6	9	14	27	28	42
50–64	108	11.4	63	5	7	9	15	21	30	41
65+	168	11.6	69	5	7	9	14	20	27	46
TOTAL SINGLE DX	6	6.9	3	6	6	6	7	11	11	11
TOTAL MULTIPLE DX	342	11.6	68	5	7	9	14	22	28	41
TOTAL										
0–19 Years	7	10.9	77	5	6	7	7	26	26	26
20–34	21	10.3	51	4	6	7	13	19	23	31
35–49	42	12.5	80	5	7	9	14	27	28	42
50–64	109	11.3	63	5	6	9	14	21	30	41
65+	169	11.6	68	5	7	9	14	20	27	46
GRAND TOTAL	348	11.5	67	5	6	9	14	22	28	41

LOS by Diagnosis and Operation, Western Region, 45th Edition

Western Region, October 2007–September 2008 Data, by Operation

51.37: HEPATIC DUCT-GI ANAST

Type of Patients	Observed Patients	Avg. Stay	Variance	Percentiles						
				10th	25th	50th	75th	90th	95th	99th
1. SINGLE DX										
0–19 Years	7	8.0	12	4	4	8	11	12	12	12
20–34	1	7.0	0	7	7	7	7	7	7	7
35–49	1	5.0	0	5	5	5	5	5	5	5
50–64	1	4.0	0	4	4	4	4	4	4	4
65+	1	5.0	0	5	5	5	5	5	5	5
2. MULTIPLE DX										
0–19 Years	48	11.4	40	5	7	9	15	21	21	25
20–34	14	15.7	309	5	6	9	15	41	67	67
35–49	31	9.9	57	4	5	8	11	17	20	43
50–64	81	10.2	45	5	6	8	11	17	21	48
65+	77	11.7	95	6	7	9	13	20	34	62
TOTAL SINGLE DX	11	7.4	11	4	4	7	11	12	12	12
TOTAL MULTIPLE DX	251	11.2	67	5	6	9	14	20	22	48
TOTAL										
0–19 Years	55	11.1	39	5	7	9	15	21	21	25
20–34	15	15.1	292	5	6	8	15	41	67	67
35–49	32	9.7	56	4	5	8	11	17	20	43
50–64	82	10.1	149	5	6	8	11	17	21	48
65+	78	11.7	94	5	7	9	13	20	34	62
GRAND TOTAL	262	11.0	65	5	6	9	13	18	22	48

51.43: INSERT CBD-HEP TUBE

Type of Patients	Observed Patients	Avg. Stay	Variance	Percentiles						
				10th	25th	50th	75th	90th	95th	99th
1. SINGLE DX										
0–19 Years	0									
20–34	0									
35–49	0									
50–64	1	4.0	0	4	4	4	4	4	4	4
65+	0									
2. MULTIPLE DX										
0–19 Years	1	3.0	0	3	3	3	3	3	3	3
20–34	10	8.2	35	3	4	7	9	20	20	20
35–49	19	10.5	66	3	5	9	13	29	33	33
50–64	36	11.4	98	2	4	6	16	29	34	35
65+	81	10.7	76	4	5	9	12	21	32	45
TOTAL SINGLE DX	1	4.0	0	4	4	4	4	4	4	4
TOTAL MULTIPLE DX	147	10.5	76	3	4	8	13	21	32	43
TOTAL										
0–19 Years	1	3.0	0	3	3	3	3	3	3	3
20–34	10	8.2	35	3	4	7	9	20	20	20
35–49	19	10.5	66	3	5	9	13	29	33	33
50–64	37	11.2	96	2	4	6	15	29	34	35
65+	81	10.7	76	4	5	9	12	21	32	45
GRAND TOTAL	148	10.4	76	3	4	7	13	21	32	43

51.4: INC BILE DUCT OBSTR

Type of Patients	Observed Patients	Avg. Stay	Variance	Percentiles						
				10th	25th	50th	75th	90th	95th	99th
1. SINGLE DX										
0–19 Years	0									
20–34	1	4.0	0	4	4	4	4	4	4	4
35–49	1	5.0	0	5	5	5	5	5	5	5
50–64	2	5.0	2	4	4	6	6	6	6	6
65+	0									
2. MULTIPLE DX										
0–19 Years	3	3.8	3	3	3	3	4	7	7	7
20–34	25	7.8	25	2	4	7	9	17	17	20
35–49	31	11.5	162	2	5	7	13	14	33	70
50–64	58	12.2	149	2	4	8	16	31	35	63
65+	137	10.0	57	4	5	8	11	19	28	43
TOTAL SINGLE DX	4	4.8	<1	4	4	5	5	6	6	6
TOTAL MULTIPLE DX	254	10.3	87	3	5	8	12	20	31	46
TOTAL										
0–19 Years	3	3.8	3	3	3	3	4	7	7	7
20–34	26	7.6	25	4	4	7	9	17	17	20
35–49	32	11.2	158	3	5	7	12	14	33	70
50–64	60	12.0	145	2	4	7	16	31	35	63
65+	137	10.0	57	4	5	8	11	19	28	43
GRAND TOTAL	258	10.2	86	3	5	7	12	20	29	46

51.5: OTHER BILE DUCT INCISION

Type of Patients	Observed Patients	Avg. Stay	Variance	Percentiles						
				10th	25th	50th	75th	90th	95th	99th
1. SINGLE DX										
0–19 Years	0									
20–34	3	4.7	5	2	2	6	6	6	6	6
35–49	0									
50–64	1	2.0	0	2	2	2	2	2	2	2
65+	0									
2. MULTIPLE DX										
0–19 Years	7	6.5	72	1	1	2	15	22	22	22
20–34	15	3.5	13	1	2	2	5	6	15	15
35–49	10	9.8	46	2	7	9	13	24	24	24
50–64	36	5.6	20	1	3	4	7	11	16	22
65+	39	8.9	42	3	4	7	14	18	23	28
TOTAL SINGLE DX	4	4.0	5	2	2	2	6	6	6	6
TOTAL MULTIPLE DX	107	6.9	38	1	3	4	10	16	22	24
TOTAL										
0–19 Years	7	6.5	72	1	1	2	15	22	22	22
20–34	18	3.7	11	1	2	2	6	6	15	15
35–49	10	9.8	46	2	7	9	13	24	24	24
50–64	37	5.5	19	1	3	4	7	11	16	22
65+	39	8.9	42	3	4	7	14	18	23	28
GRAND TOTAL	111	6.8	37	1	2	4	9	16	22	24

LOS by Diagnosis and Operation, Western Region, 45th Edition

Western Region, October 2007–September 2008 Data, by Operation

51.6: LOC EXC BD & S OF O LES

Type of Patients	Observed Patients	Avg. Stay	Variance	10th	25th	50th	75th	90th	95th	99th
1. SINGLE DX										
0–19 Years	4	7.4	4	5	5	9	9	9	9	9
20–34	0									
35–49	1	8.0	0	8	8	8	8	8	8	8
50–64	2	4.0	18	1	1	4	7	7	7	7
65+	0									
2. MULTIPLE DX										
0–19 Years	22	11.0	59	5	6	7	13	24	24	30
20–34	20	11.4	154	4	6	7	12	15	23	61
35–49	17	7.7	17	2	6	7	9	15	18	18
50–64	34	8.3	33	3	6	7	8	14	22	32
65+	60	8.2	18	3	6	7	10	14	17	21
TOTAL SINGLE DX	7	6.8	7	5	5	8	9	9	9	9
TOTAL MULTIPLE DX	153	9.3	48	4	6	7	10	17	23	32
TOTAL										
0–19 Years	26	10.5	53	5	6	8	13	24	24	30
20–34	20	11.4	154	4	6	7	12	15	23	61
35–49	18	7.7	16	2	6	8	9	15	18	18
50–64	36	8.0	33	3	6	7	8	14	22	32
65+	60	8.2	18	3	6	7	10	14	17	21
GRAND TOTAL	160	9.2	46	4	6	7	10	17	23	32

51.8: SPHINCTER OF ODDI OP NEC

Type of Patients	Observed Patients	Avg. Stay	Variance	10th	25th	50th	75th	90th	95th	99th
1. SINGLE DX										
0–19 Years	38	3.0	3	1	2	3	4	5	6	9
20–34	167	2.9	3	1	2	2	4	5	7	7
35–49	92	2.7	2	1	1	2	4	5	5	5
50–64	59	2.6	5	1	1	2	3	5	6	8
65+	24	3.2	11	1	1	3	3	6	9	16
2. MULTIPLE DX										
0–19 Years	175	4.6	26	1	2	3	5	8	15	29
20–34	1,288	4.5	33	1	2	3	5	8	11	25
35–49	1,596	4.7	20	2	2	4	6	8	12	20
50–64	2,493	5.1	24	2	2	4	6	10	13	23
65+	4,967	5.5	17	2	3	4	7	10	13	21
TOTAL SINGLE DX	380	2.8	4	1	2	2	4	5	6	9
TOTAL MULTIPLE DX	10,519	5.1	21	2	3	4	6	10	13	22
TOTAL										
0–19 Years	213	4.3	22	1	2	3	5	8	11	26
20–34	1,455	4.3	30	1	2	3	5	8	10	23
35–49	1,688	4.6	19	2	2	3	6	8	12	20
50–64	2,552	5.1	24	2	2	4	6	10	13	22
65+	4,991	5.4	17	2	3	4	7	10	13	21
GRAND TOTAL	10,899	5.1	21	2	2	4	6	10	13	22

51.7: REPAIR OF BILE DUCTS

Type of Patients	Observed Patients	Avg. Stay	Variance	10th	25th	50th	75th	90th	95th	99th
1. SINGLE DX										
0–19 Years	0									
20–34	0									
35–49	0									
50–64	0									
65+	0									
2. MULTIPLE DX										
0–19 Years	4	8.3	111	2	3	4	24	24	24	24
20–34	32	6.7	23	3	4	5	8	11	16	27
35–49	32	4.9	9	2	3	4	6	7	11	16
50–64	73	7.7	48	3	4	6	8	17	23	42
65+	51	12.1	104	4	6	9	15	20	45	49
TOTAL SINGLE DX	0									
TOTAL MULTIPLE DX	192	8.2	59	3	4	6	9	17	22	47
TOTAL										
0–19 Years	4	8.3	111	2	3	4	24	24	24	24
20–34	32	6.7	23	3	4	5	8	11	16	27
35–49	32	4.9	9	2	3	4	6	7	11	16
50–64	73	7.7	48	3	4	6	8	17	23	42
65+	51	12.1	104	4	6	9	15	20	45	49
GRAND TOTAL	192	8.2	59	3	4	6	9	17	22	47

51.84: ENDO AMPULLA & BD DILAT

Type of Patients	Observed Patients	Avg. Stay	Variance	10th	25th	50th	75th	90th	95th	99th
1. SINGLE DX										
0–19 Years	3	4.7	2	3	3	5	6	6	6	6
20–34	2	3.5	4	2	2	2	5	5	5	5
35–49	1	2.0		2	2	2	2	2	2	2
50–64	2	10.4	60	5	5	5	16	16	16	16
65+	1	1.0		1	1	1	1	1	1	1
2. MULTIPLE DX										
0–19 Years	5	13.4	154	1	2	2	6	26	26	26
20–34	28	3.7	5	2	2	3	5	6	8	12
35–49	52	4.7	21	2	2	3	7	8	13	30
50–64	130	5.3	22	1	2	3	7	12	14	20
65+	170	5.5	23	2	3	4	7	11	14	19
TOTAL SINGLE DX	9	5.0	20	1	2	5	5	16	16	16
TOTAL MULTIPLE DX	385	5.4	25	2	2	4	6	11	14	26
TOTAL										
0–19 Years	8	11.2	128	1	3	6	26	26	26	26
20–34	30	3.7	5	2	2	3	5	5	8	12
35–49	53	4.6	21	1	2	3	6	8	13	30
50–64	132	5.4	23	2	2	4	7	12	16	20
65+	171	5.4	23	2	3	4	7	11	14	19
GRAND TOTAL	394	5.4	25	2	2	4	6	11	14	26

LOS by Diagnosis and Operation, Western Region, 45th Edition

Western Region, October 2007–September 2008 Data, by Operation

51.85: ENDO SPHINCTOT/PAPILLOT

Type of Patients	Observed Patients	Avg. Stay	Vari-ance	10th	25th	50th	75th	90th	95th	99th
1. SINGLE DX										
0–19 Years	17	2.7	2	1	1	2	4	5	6	6
20–34	83	2.8	3	1	2	2	4	5	7	9
35–49	44	2.6	2	1	2	2	3	4	5	6
50–64	27	1.9	<1	1	1	2	2	3	4	4
65+	10	3.3	6	1	2	3	3	6	9	9
2. MULTIPLE DX										
0–19 Years	101	3.3	4	1	2	3	4	6	7	9
20–34	763	4.4	30	1	2	3	5	8	10	22
35–49	908	4.9	20	2	2	4	6	9	13	22
50–64	1,292	4.9	19	2	2	4	6	9	12	22
65+	2,480	5.4	16	2	3	4	7	10	13	20
TOTAL SINGLE DX	181	2.6	3	1	2	2	3	5	6	9
TOTAL MULTIPLE DX	5,544	5.0	19	2	3	4	6	9	12	21
TOTAL										
0–19 Years	118	3.2	4	1	2	2	4	6	7	9
20–34	846	4.2	27	1	2	3	5	8	10	21
35–49	952	4.8	20	2	2	4	6	9	12	22
50–64	1,319	4.9	19	2	2	4	6	9	12	22
65+	2,490	5.4	16	2	3	4	7	10	13	20
GRAND TOTAL	5,725	4.9	19	2	2	4	6	9	12	21

51.87: ENDO INSERT BD STENT

Type of Patients	Observed Patients	Avg. Stay	Vari-ance	10th	25th	50th	75th	90th	95th	99th
1. SINGLE DX										
0–19 Years	4	3.3	<1	2	2	4	4	4	4	4
20–34	10	4.2	4	3	3	3	7	7	7	7
35–49	13	2.8	2	1	2	2	4	5	6	6
50–64	10	2.0	<1	1	1	2	3	3	3	3
65+	2	8.5	110	1	1	16	16	16	16	16
2. MULTIPLE DX										
0–19 Years	22	7.4	58	1	2	4	9	16	29	29
20–34	173	5.3	29	2	3	4	6	9	13	30
35–49	277	5.0	27	2	3	4	6	9	12	17
50–64	588	6.0	41	2	3	4	7	11	16	28
65+	1,049	5.7	17	2	3	5	7	11	13	20
TOTAL SINGLE DX	39	3.3	7	1	2	3	4	7	7	16
TOTAL MULTIPLE DX	2,109	5.6	26	2	3	4	7	11	14	22
TOTAL										
0–19 Years	26	6.8	51	1	2	4	8	16	29	29
20–34	183	5.2	28	3	3	4	6	9	12	30
35–49	290	4.9	26	2	2	4	6	9	12	17
50–64	598	5.9	41	2	3	4	7	11	16	28
65+	1,051	5.7	17	2	3	5	7	11	14	20
GRAND TOTAL	2,148	5.6	26	2	3	4	7	11	14	22

51.88: ENDO RMVL BILIARY STONE

Type of Patients	Observed Patients	Avg. Stay	Vari-ance	10th	25th	50th	75th	90th	95th	99th
1. SINGLE DX										
0–19 Years	14	3.2	4	1	2	2	4	5	9	9
20–34	70	2.8	3	1	2	3	4	5	6	7
35–49	34	2.8	3	1	2	3	4	5	6	8
50–64	18	3.1	4	1	1	3	4	7	7	7
65+	11	2.3	1	1	1	2	3	3	4	4
2. MULTIPLE DX										
0–19 Years	45	4.1	10	1	2	3	5	6	12	15
20–34	313	4.2	43	1	2	3	4	6	10	27
35–49	333	4.0	11	2	2	3	5	7	8	15
50–64	450	4.4	14	2	3	4	6	8	12	18
65+	1,223	5.2	18	2	3	4	6	10	13	22
TOTAL SINGLE DX	147	2.8	3	1	1	3	4	5	6	8
TOTAL MULTIPLE DX	2,364	4.7	20	2	2	4	6	9	12	22
TOTAL										
0–19 Years	59	3.9	9	1	2	3	5	6	11	15
20–34	383	4.0	36	1	2	3	4	6	9	27
35–49	367	3.9	10	1	2	3	5	7	8	15
50–64	468	4.4	14	1	2	3	5	8	11	18
65+	1,234	5.2	18	2	3	4	6	10	13	22
GRAND TOTAL	2,511	4.6	19	2	2	4	5	8	12	21

51.9: OTHER BILIARY TRACT OPS

Type of Patients	Observed Patients	Avg. Stay	Vari-ance	10th	25th	50th	75th	90th	95th	99th
1. SINGLE DX										
0–19 Years	0	0								
20–34	0	0								
35–49	3	5.0	19	2	2	3	10	10	10	10
50–64	3	2.5	4	1	1	1	4	4	4	4
65+	1	1.0	0	1	1	1	1	1	1	1
2. MULTIPLE DX										
0–19 Years	31	6.0	37	1	2	3	9	15	15	36
20–34	35	6.8	43	1	2	5	8	18	22	27
35–49	77	9.8	109	2	4	7	11	21	34	61
50–64	214	6.4	32	1	3	5	8	12	18	30
65+	328	7.0	25	2	3	6	10	14	17	24
TOTAL SINGLE DX	6	3.5	11	1	1	2	4	10	10	10
TOTAL MULTIPLE DX	685	7.0	39	2	3	5	9	14	18	32
TOTAL										
0–19 Years	31	6.0	37	1	2	3	9	15	15	36
20–34	35	6.8	43	1	2	5	8	18	22	27
35–49	80	9.6	107	2	4	6	10	21	33	61
50–64	216	6.3	31	1	3	5	8	12	18	30
65+	329	7.0	26	2	3	6	10	14	17	24
GRAND TOTAL	691	7.0	39	2	3	5	9	14	18	32

LOS by Diagnosis and Operation, Western Region, 45th Edition

Western Region, October 2007–September 2008 Data, by Operation

51.98: PERC OP ON BIL TRACT NEC

Type of Patients	Observed Patients	Avg. Stay	Vari-ance	10th	25th	50th	75th	90th	95th	99th
1. SINGLE DX										
0–19 Years	0									
20–34	0									
35–49	3	5.0	19	2	2	3	10	10	10	10
50–64	2	2.5	4	1	1	1	1	4	4	4
65+	1	1.0	0	1	1	1	1	1	1	1
2. MULTIPLE DX										
0–19 Years	28	5.2	20	1	2	3	8	11	15	15
20–34	24	7.3	50	1	3	5	8	18	22	27
35–49	62	9.9	129	2	4	6	11	21	34	61
50–64	172	5.9	26	1	3	5	8	12	14	30
65+	270	6.7	23	2	3	5	9	13	16	22
TOTAL SINGLE DX	6	3.5	11	1	1	2	4	10	10	10
TOTAL MULTIPLE DX	556	6.7	37	2	3	5	9	13	17	32
TOTAL										
0–19 Years	28	5.2	20	1	2	3	8	11	15	15
20–34	24	7.3	50	1	3	5	8	18	22	27
35–49	65	9.7	125	2	4	6	11	21	34	61
50–64	174	5.9	26	1	3	5	8	12	14	30
65+	271	6.7	23	2	3	5	9	13	16	22
GRAND TOTAL	562	6.7	37	2	3	5	9	13	17	32

52.01: DRAIN PANC CYST BY CATH

Type of Patients	Observed Patients	Avg. Stay	Vari-ance	10th	25th	50th	75th	90th	95th	99th
1. SINGLE DX										
0–19 Years	1	3.0	0	3	3	3	3	3	3	3
20–34	0									
35–49	1	2.0	0	2	2	2	2	2	2	2
50–64	2	4.5	12	2	2	7	7	7	7	7
65+	0									
2. MULTIPLE DX										
0–19 Years	7	23.3	151	8	13	24	31	44	44	44
20–34	28	15.2	264	4	5	9	23	34	51	73
35–49	72	12.7	201	3	5	9	14	30	48	>99
50–64	86	15.8	203	2	6	11	20	40	45	69
65+	44	15.9	142	2	6	13	23	41	46	>99
TOTAL SINGLE DX	4	3.5	6	2	2	3	7	7	7	7
TOTAL MULTIPLE DX	237	15.0	198	3	5	10	20	38	46	86
TOTAL										
0–19 Years	8	20.8	181	3	8	24	31	44	44	44
20–34	28	15.2	264	4	5	9	23	34	51	73
35–49	73	12.6	200	3	5	8	14	30	48	>99
50–64	88	15.5	201	2	6	11	20	40	45	69
65+	44	15.9	142	2	6	13	23	41	46	>99
GRAND TOTAL	241	14.8	196	3	5	10	20	37	46	86

52.0: PANCREATOMY

Type of Patients	Observed Patients	Avg. Stay	Vari-ance	10th	25th	50th	75th	90th	95th	99th
1. SINGLE DX										
0–19 Years	1	3.0	0	3	3	3	3	3	3	3
20–34	1	6.0	0	6	6	6	6	6	6	6
35–49	1	2.0	0	2	2	2	2	2	2	2
50–64	2	4.5	12	2	2	7	7	7	7	7
65+	1	8.0	0	8	8	8	8	8	8	8
2. MULTIPLE DX										
0–19 Years	10	22.1	85	8	20	24	26	31	44	44
20–34	37	18.6	419	4	5	10	23	56	73	79
35–49	94	13.5	231	3	6	9	16	37	52	>99
50–64	121	17.7	256	3	6	11	23	41	51	69
65+	57	16.8	196	3	9	14	23	41	48	>99
TOTAL SINGLE DX	6	4.7	7	2	2	6	7	8	8	8
TOTAL MULTIPLE DX	319	16.6	251	3	6	11	22	41	51	82
TOTAL										
0–19 Years	11	20.9	100	5	16	20	26	31	44	44
20–34	38	18.3	412	4	5	10	23	56	73	79
35–49	95	13.4	230	3	5	9	16	37	52	>99
50–64	123	17.4	255	3	6	11	23	41	51	69
65+	58	16.6	194	3	8	13	23	41	48	>99
GRAND TOTAL	325	16.4	249	3	6	11	21	41	51	82

52.1: PANCREATIC DXTIC PX

Type of Patients	Observed Patients	Avg. Stay	Vari-ance	10th	25th	50th	75th	90th	95th	99th
1. SINGLE DX										
0–19 Years	0									
20–34	0									
35–49	2	3.0	2	2	2	2	4	4	4	4
50–64	4	5.3	<1	5	5	5	6	6	6	6
65+	0									
2. MULTIPLE DX										
0–19 Years	0									
20–34	26	7.8	81	2	3	4	8	29	29	36
35–49	76	7.0	25	2	3	5	10	14	17	24
50–64	202	7.1	41	2	3	5	9	14	18	34
65+	351	7.0	32	2	3	6	9	13	18	27
TOTAL SINGLE DX	6	4.5	2	2	4	5	5	6	6	6
TOTAL MULTIPLE DX	655	7.0	36	2	3	5	9	14	18	34
TOTAL										
0–19 Years	0									
20–34	26	7.8	81	2	3	4	8	29	29	36
35–49	78	6.9	25	2	3	5	9	14	17	24
50–64	206	7.0	40	2	3	5	9	14	18	34
65+	351	7.0	32	2	3	6	9	13	18	27
GRAND TOTAL	661	7.0	35	2	3	5	9	14	18	34

LOS by Diagnosis and Operation, Western Region, 45th Edition

Western Region, October 2007–September 2008 Data, by Operation

52.11: PANCREAS ASPIRATION BX

Type of Patients	Observed Patients	Avg. Stay	Vari-ance	Percentiles						
				10th	25th	50th	75th	90th	95th	99th
1. SINGLE DX										
0–19 Years	0									
20–34	0									
35–49	1	4.0	0	4	4	4	4	4	4	4
50–64	0									
65+	0									
2. MULTIPLE DX										
0–19 Years	0									
20–34	17	7.8	71	2	3	5	8	29	29	29
35–49	56	7.2	28	2	3	6	10	15	18	24
50–64	150	6.6	35	2	3	5	9	12	15	34
65+	266	6.6	26	2	3	5	8	13	16	27
TOTAL SINGLE DX	1	4.0	0	4	4	4	4	4	4	4
TOTAL MULTIPLE DX	489	6.7	31	2	3	5	9	13	17	29
TOTAL										
0–19 Years	0									
20–34	17	7.8	71	2	3	5	8	29	29	29
35–49	57	7.2	28	2	4	5	10	15	18	24
50–64	150	6.6	35	2	3	5	9	12	15	34
65+	266	6.6	26	2	3	5	8	13	16	27
GRAND TOTAL	490	6.7	31	2	3	5	9	13	17	29

52.22: PANC DUCT LES DESTR NEC

Type of Patients	Observed Patients	Avg. Stay	Vari-ance	Percentiles						
				10th	25th	50th	75th	90th	95th	99th
1. SINGLE DX										
0–19 Years	1	12.0	0	12	12	12	12	12	12	12
20–34	0									
35–49	1	3.0	0	3	3	3	3	3	3	3
50–64	0									
65+	1	5.0	0	5	5	5	5	5	5	5
2. MULTIPLE DX										
0–19 Years	5	6.9	2	4	7	8	8	8	8	8
20–34	25	17.1	281	3	5	12	21	40	53	68
35–49	38	19.3	328	4	7	13	24	48	52	87
50–64	73	15.8	229	3	5	11	22	45	58	>99
65+	43	16.8	308	3	4	8	26	49	54	62
TOTAL SINGLE DX	3	6.7	22	3	3	5	12	12	12	12
TOTAL MULTIPLE DX	184	16.5	266	3	5	10	22	47	54	>99
TOTAL										
0–19 Years	6	7.4	5	4	7	8	8	12	12	12
20–34	25	17.1	281	3	5	12	21	40	53	68
35–49	39	18.9	326	4	6	12	24	48	52	87
50–64	73	15.8	229	3	5	11	22	45	58	>99
65+	44	16.5	304	3	4	7	26	49	54	62
GRAND TOTAL	187	16.4	263	3	5	10	22	45	54	>99

52.2: PANC/PANC DUCT LES DESTR

Type of Patients	Observed Patients	Avg. Stay	Vari-ance	Percentiles						
				10th	25th	50th	75th	90th	95th	99th
1. SINGLE DX										
0–19 Years	1	12.0	0	12	12	12	12	12	12	12
20–34	0									
35–49	1	3.0	0	3	3	3	3	3	3	3
50–64	0									
65+	1	5.0	0	5	5	5	5	5	5	5
2. MULTIPLE DX										
0–19 Years	5	6.9	2	4	7	8	8	8	8	8
20–34	25	17.1	281	3	5	12	21	40	53	68
35–49	40	18.5	325	4	6	12	24	48	52	87
50–64	74	15.7	226	3	6	11	22	45	58	>99
65+	45	16.4	298	3	4	8	23	49	54	62
TOTAL SINGLE DX	3	6.7	22	3	3	5	12	12	12	12
TOTAL MULTIPLE DX	189	16.3	262	3	5	10	22	45	54	>99
TOTAL										
0–19 Years	6	7.4	5	4	7	8	8	12	12	12
20–34	25	17.1	281	3	5	12	21	40	53	68
35–49	41	18.1	323	4	6	12	22	47	48	87
50–64	74	15.7	226	3	6	11	22	45	58	>99
65+	46	16.2	294	3	4	7	23	49	54	62
GRAND TOTAL	192	16.1	259	3	5	10	22	45	54	>99

52.3: PANCREATIC CYST MARSUP

Type of Patients	Observed Patients	Avg. Stay	Vari-ance	Percentiles						
				10th	25th	50th	75th	90th	95th	99th
1. SINGLE DX										
0–19 Years	0									
20–34	0									
35–49	0									
50–64	0									
65+	0									
2. MULTIPLE DX										
0–19 Years	0									
20–34	4	19.7	196	8	8	11	39	39	39	39
35–49	3	26.7	562	5	5	23	52	52	52	52
50–64	4	6.5	4	5	6	7	9	9	9	9
65+	1	5.0	0	5	5	5	5	5	5	5
TOTAL SINGLE DX	0									
TOTAL MULTIPLE DX	12	15.8	238	5	6	8	21	39	52	52
TOTAL										
0–19 Years	0									
20–34	4	19.7	196	8	8	11	39	39	39	39
35–49	3	26.7	562	5	5	23	52	52	52	52
50–64	4	6.5	4	5	6	7	9	9	9	9
65+	1	5.0	0	5	5	5	5	5	5	5
GRAND TOTAL	12	15.8	238	5	6	8	21	39	52	52

LOS by Diagnosis and Operation, Western Region, 45th Edition

Western Region, October 2007–September 2008 Data, by Operation

52.52: DISTAL PANCREATECTOMY

Type of Patients	Observed Patients	Avg. Stay	Vari- ance	Percentiles						
				10th	25th	50th	75th	90th	95th	99th
1. SINGLE DX										
0–19 Years	2	3.5	<1	3	3	4	4	4	4	4
20–34	6	7.2	10	5	5	7	8	13	13	13
35–49	4	5.0	3	3	3	4	7	7	7	7
50–64	8	5.4	1	4	4	5	6	7	7	7
65+	1	7.0	0	7	7	7	7	7	7	7
2. MULTIPLE DX										
0–19 Years	20	13.8	77	6	9	12	14	19	39	48
20–34	49	12.1	179	4	5	8	13	30	59	>99
35–49	86	10.7	165	4	5	7	10	17	30	93
50–64	194	8.9	54	4	6	7	9	15	23	59
65+	203	8.7	25	4	6	7	10	15	19	25
TOTAL SINGLE DX	21	5.7	5	4	4	6	7	7	8	13
TOTAL MULTIPLE DX	552	9.7	74	4	6	7	11	16	24	59
TOTAL										
0–19 Years	22	13.2	78	6	9	12	14	16	36	48
20–34	55	11.5	163	4	5	7	13	28	59	>99
35–49	90	10.5	159	4	5	7	10	17	30	93
50–64	202	8.8	52	4	5	7	9	15	22	51
65+	204	8.7	25	4	6	7	10	15	19	25
GRAND TOTAL	573	9.6	72	4	6	7	10	16	24	59

52.59: PART PANCREATECTOMY NEC

Type of Patients	Observed Patients	Avg. Stay	Vari- ance	Percentiles						
				10th	25th	50th	75th	90th	95th	99th
1. SINGLE DX										
0–19 Years	1	5.0	0	5	5	5	5	5	5	5
20–34	2	6.0	2	5	5	6	7	7	7	7
35–49	1	6.0	0	6	6	6	6	6	6	6
50–64	0									
65+	0									
2. MULTIPLE DX										
0–19 Years	1	12.0	0	12	12	12	12	12	12	12
20–34	5	14.9	412	5	5	6	7	51	51	51
35–49	16	11.9	214	3	6	8	10	28	62	62
50–64	29	17.1	437	5	6	8	17	46	68	97
65+	33	10.6	90	4	6	8	11	19	33	52
TOTAL SINGLE DX	4	5.8	<1	5	5	5	7	7	7	7
TOTAL MULTIPLE DX	84	13.4	249	5	6	8	12	28	51	97
TOTAL										
0–19 Years	2	8.5	24	5	5	5	12	12	12	12
20–34	7	12.3	293	5	6	6	10	51	51	51
35–49	17	11.5	203	3	6	6	10	28	62	62
50–64	29	17.1	437	5	6	8	17	46	68	97
65+	33	10.6	90	4	6	8	11	19	33	52
GRAND TOTAL	88	13.0	240	5	6	8	12	28	51	97

52.4: INT DRAIN PANC CYST

Type of Patients	Observed Patients	Avg. Stay	Vari- ance	Percentiles						
				10th	25th	50th	75th	90th	95th	99th
1. SINGLE DX										
0–19 Years	0									
20–34	0									
35–49	2	6.0	2	5	5	6	7	7	7	7
50–64	0									
65+	0									
2. MULTIPLE DX										
0–19 Years	2	42.8	134	22	48	48	48	48	48	48
20–34	19	10.3	79	4	5	8	13	21	41	41
35–49	42	13.6	226	3	5	11	14	28	42	81
50–64	39	11.0	88	4	5	8	15	23	30	49
65+	17	14.1	262	4	5	9	16	25	72	72
TOTAL SINGLE DX	2	6.0	2	5	5	6	7	7	7	7
TOTAL MULTIPLE DX	119	13.5	194	3	5	9	15	28	48	72
TOTAL										
0–19 Years	2	42.8	134	22	48	48	48	48	48	48
20–34	19	10.3	79	4	5	8	13	21	41	41
35–49	44	13.2	218	3	5	11	14	28	42	81
50–64	39	11.0	88	4	5	8	15	23	30	49
65+	17	14.1	262	4	5	9	16	25	72	72
GRAND TOTAL	121	13.4	192	3	5	9	15	28	48	72

52.5: PARTIAL PANCREATECTOMY

Type of Patients	Observed Patients	Avg. Stay	Vari- ance	Percentiles						
				10th	25th	50th	75th	90th	95th	99th
1. SINGLE DX										
0–19 Years	3	4.0	<1	3	3	4	5	5	5	5
20–34	8	6.9	8	4	5	7	8	13	13	13
35–49	5	5.2	3	3	5	6	6	7	7	7
50–64	8	5.4	1	4	4	5	6	7	7	7
65+	1	7.0	0	7	7	7	7	7	7	7
2. MULTIPLE DX										
0–19 Years	23	14.0	77	7	9	12	14	19	36	48
20–34	56	13.0	226	4	5	7	13	34	59	>99
35–49	112	11.1	172	4	5	7	10	17	31	69
50–64	245	10.1	104	4	6	7	11	17	27	68
65+	269	9.3	36	5	6	8	11	15	20	35
TOTAL SINGLE DX	25	5.7	4	4	4	6	7	7	8	13
TOTAL MULTIPLE DX	705	10.4	98	4	6	8	11	17	28	62
TOTAL										
0–19 Years	26	13.3	78	6	9	12	14	19	36	48
20–34	64	12.2	202	4	5	7	13	30	58	>99
35–49	117	10.8	166	4	6	7	10	17	31	69
50–64	253	9.9	102	4	6	7	10	17	27	68
65+	270	9.3	36	5	6	8	11	15	20	35
GRAND TOTAL	730	10.2	96	4	6	7	11	17	28	62

Western Region, October 2007–September 2008 Data, by Operation

52.6: TOTAL PANCREATECTOMY

Type of Patients	Observed Patients	Avg. Stay	Vari-ance	10th	25th	50th	75th	90th	95th	99th
1. SINGLE DX										
0–19 Years	0									
20–34	0									
35–49	0									
50–64	0									
65+	0									
2. MULTIPLE DX										
0–19 Years	0									
20–34	4	34.1	871	5	19	29	73	73	73	73
35–49	11	9.3	34	5	5	7	15	19	20	20
50–64	31	13.9	122	5	7	10	17	27	41	50
65+	31	16.4	128	7	8	13	23	29	47	50
TOTAL SINGLE DX	0									
TOTAL MULTIPLE DX	77	15.3	162	5	7	11	19	34	47	73
TOTAL										
0–19 Years	0									
20–34	4	34.1	871	5	19	29	73	73	73	73
35–49	11	9.3	34	5	5	7	15	19	20	20
50–64	31	13.9	122	5	7	10	17	27	41	50
65+	31	16.4	128	7	8	13	23	29	47	50
GRAND TOTAL	77	15.3	162	5	7	11	19	34	47	73

52.7: RAD PANC/DUODENECTOMY

Type of Patients	Observed Patients	Avg. Stay	Vari-ance	10th	25th	50th	75th	90th	95th	99th
1. SINGLE DX										
0–19 Years	0									
20–34	2	10.0	8	8	8	8	12	12	12	12
35–49	1	13.0	0	13	13	13	13	13	13	13
50–64	4	8.2	28	4	6	7	7	16	16	16
65+	2	9.0	2	8	8	8	10	10	10	10
2. MULTIPLE DX										
0–19 Years	0									
20–34	16	18.1	151	7	12	14	19	39	52	52
35–49	111	16.4	104	8	9	13	20	30	36	53
50–64	440	15.2	99	7	9	12	18	27	35	52
65+	611	15.3	100	7	9	12	18	27	34	57
TOTAL SINGLE DX	9	9.3	14	4	7	8	12	16	16	16
TOTAL MULTIPLE DX	1,178	15.4	100	7	9	12	19	28	35	57
TOTAL										
0–19 Years	0									
20–34	18	17.2	141	7	9	14	19	39	52	52
35–49	112	16.4	104	8	9	13	20	30	36	53
50–64	444	15.2	99	7	9	12	18	27	35	52
65+	613	15.3	99	7	9	12	18	27	34	57
GRAND TOTAL	1,187	15.4	100	7	9	12	18	28	35	57

52.8: TRANSPLANT OF PANCREAS

Type of Patients	Observed Patients	Avg. Stay	Vari-ance	10th	25th	50th	75th	90th	95th	99th
1. SINGLE DX										
0–19 Years	0									
20–34	0									
35–49	0									
50–64	0									
65+	0									
2. MULTIPLE DX										
0–19 Years	1	18.0	0	18	18	18	18	18	18	18
20–34	12	11.0	29	7	7	9	9	20	23	23
35–49	22	10.6	78	5	6	9	9	18	28	43
50–64	24	10.4	27	5	6	8	13	18	20	23
65+	1	16.0	0	16	16	16	16	16	16	16
TOTAL SINGLE DX	0									
TOTAL MULTIPLE DX	60	10.8	45	5	7	9	13	18	23	43
TOTAL										
0–19 Years	1	18.0	0	18	18	18	18	18	18	18
20–34	12	11.0	29	7	7	9	9	20	23	23
35–49	22	10.6	78	5	6	9	9	18	28	43
50–64	24	10.4	27	5	6	8	13	18	20	23
65+	1	16.0	0	16	16	16	16	16	16	16
GRAND TOTAL	60	10.8	45	5	7	9	13	18	23	43

52.9: OTHER OPS ON PANCREAS

Type of Patients	Observed Patients	Avg. Stay	Vari-ance	10th	25th	50th	75th	90th	95th	99th
1. SINGLE DX										
0–19 Years	0									
20–34	2	4.0	2	3	3	5	5	5	5	5
35–49	2	4.0	2	3	3	3	5	5	5	5
50–64	3	4.4	10	2	2	3	5	8	8	8
65+	1	6.0	0	6	6	6	6	6	6	6
2. MULTIPLE DX										
0–19 Years	32	15.5	173	1	6	11	20	33	51	51
20–34	71	7.3	27	2	3	6	10	14	19	26
35–49	117	6.6	42	1	3	5	9	12	16	30
50–64	168	7.4	89	1	3	5	9	15	21	41
65+	143	7.7	78	2	3	6	8	14	26	41
TOTAL SINGLE DX	8	4.4	4	2	3	5	6	8	8	8
TOTAL MULTIPLE DX	531	8.2	84	2	3	6	10	17	26	51
TOTAL										
0–19 Years	32	15.5	173	1	6	11	20	33	51	51
20–34	73	7.2	27	2	3	6	10	14	19	26
35–49	119	6.6	41	1	3	5	9	12	16	30
50–64	171	7.4	88	2	3	5	9	15	21	41
65+	144	7.7	78	2	3	6	8	14	26	41
GRAND TOTAL	539	8.2	83	2	3	6	10	17	25	51

LOS by Diagnosis and Operation, Western Region, 45th Edition

Western Region, October 2007–September 2008 Data, by Operation

53.0: UNILAT IH REPAIR

Type of Patients	Observed Patients	Avg. Stay	Variance	Percentiles						
				10th	25th	50th	75th	90th	95th	99th
1. SINGLE DX										
0–19 Years	130	1.3	<1	1	1	1	1	2	3	4
20–34	145	1.5	<1	1	1	1	1	2	3	5
35–49	115	1.6	<1	1	1	1	2	3	3	4
50–64	116	1.6	1	1	1	1	2	3	4	6
65+	67	1.5	<1	1	1	1	2	3	3	5
2. MULTIPLE DX										
0–19 Years	262	5.9	262	1	1	1	2	9	64	>99
20–34	209	1.9	2	1	1	1	2	3	4	7
35–49	458	2.8	14	1	1	2	3	6	9	14
50–64	848	2.9	14	1	1	2	3	6	8	20
65+	2,086	3.5	13	2	1	2	4	8	10	19
TOTAL SINGLE DX	573	1.5	<1	1	1	1	2	2	3	5
TOTAL MULTIPLE DX	3,863	3.5	47	1	1	2	4	7	10	44
TOTAL										
0–19 Years	392	4.6	189	1	1	1	2	5	41	>99
20–34	354	1.8	2	1	1	1	2	3	4	7
35–49	573	2.5	11	1	1	2	3	5	8	13
50–64	964	2.8	12	1	1	2	3	6	8	18
65+	2,153	3.4	13	2	1	2	4	7	10	19
GRAND TOTAL	4,436	3.2	41	1	1	2	3	6	9	35

53.00: UNILAT IH REPAIR NOS

Type of Patients	Observed Patients	Avg. Stay	Variance	Percentiles						
				10th	25th	50th	75th	90th	95th	99th
1. SINGLE DX										
0–19 Years	62	1.4	<1	1	1	1	1	2	3	4
20–34	9	1.5	<1	1	1	1	2	3	3	3
35–49	10	1.7	<1	1	1	1	2	3	3	3
50–64	7	1.4	<1	1	1	1	2	2	2	2
65+	5	1.2	<1	1	1	1	1	2	2	2
2. MULTIPLE DX										
0–19 Years	129	7.6	339	1	1	1	3	35	73	>99
20–34	19	2.0	2	1	2	1	3	4	5	5
35–49	21	3.0	3	1	1	2	4	5	6	7
50–64	42	3.0	7	1	2	2	4	5	9	13
65+	137	4.2	12	1	2	3	5	9	11	17
TOTAL SINGLE DX	93	1.4	<1	1	1	1	2	2	3	4
TOTAL MULTIPLE DX	348	5.7	184	1	1	2	4	10	40	>99
TOTAL										
0–19 Years	191	5.7	242	1	1	1	2	9	52	>99
20–34	28	1.8	1	1	1	1	3	4	4	5
35–49	31	2.5	3	1	1	2	3	5	6	7
50–64	49	2.8	6	1	1	2	4	5	9	13
65+	142	4.1	12	1	1	3	5	9	11	17
GRAND TOTAL	441	4.7	145	1	1	1	3	8	24	96

52.93: ENDO INSERT PANC STENT

Type of Patients	Observed Patients	Avg. Stay	Variance	Percentiles						
				10th	25th	50th	75th	90th	95th	99th
1. SINGLE DX										
0–19 Years	0									
20–34	2	4.0	2	3	3	5	5	5	5	5
35–49	2	4.0	2	3	3	3	5	5	5	5
50–64	0									
65+	0									
2. MULTIPLE DX										
0–19 Years	17	13.8	130	1	3	10	27	33	33	33
20–34	33	6.6	23	2	3	4	9	13	15	19
35–49	60	5.8	48	2	3	4	7	11	15	50
50–64	83	5.6	17	1	3	4	8	12	14	21
65+	107	6.5	32	2	3	5	8	11	16	26
TOTAL SINGLE DX	4	4.0	1	3	3	5	5	5	5	5
TOTAL MULTIPLE DX	300	6.9	45	1	3	5	9	14	20	33
TOTAL										
0–19 Years	17	13.8	130	1	3	10	27	33	33	33
20–34	35	6.4	22	2	3	4	9	13	15	19
35–49	62	5.8	46	2	3	4	7	11	15	50
50–64	83	5.6	17	1	3	4	8	12	14	21
65+	107	6.5	32	2	3	5	8	11	16	26
GRAND TOTAL	304	6.8	45	1	3	5	8	14	20	33

52.96: PANCREATIC ANASTOMOSIS

Type of Patients	Observed Patients	Avg. Stay	Variance	Percentiles						
				10th	25th	50th	75th	90th	95th	99th
1. SINGLE DX										
0–19 Years	0									
20–34	0									
35–49	0									
50–64	2	5.5	12	3	3	8	8	8	8	8
65+	1	6.0	0	6	6	6	6	6	6	6
2. MULTIPLE DX										
0–19 Years	6	22.8	332	4	10	17	51	51	51	51
20–34	18	9.0	24	5	6	7	12	19	19	19
35–49	31	9.8	40	5	6	7	11	16	29	30
50–64	30	16.1	317	5	7	10	17	25	41	98
65+	14	13.3	88	6	7	9	17	33	33	33
TOTAL SINGLE DX	3	5.7	6	3	3	6	8	8	8	8
TOTAL MULTIPLE DX	99	13.7	177	5	7	10	16	29	41	51
TOTAL										
0–19 Years	6	22.8	332	4	10	17	51	51	51	51
20–34	18	9.0	24	5	6	7	12	19	19	19
35–49	31	9.8	40	5	6	7	11	16	29	30
50–64	32	15.5	304	5	7	10	16	25	41	98
65+	15	12.8	85	6	7	9	17	33	33	33
GRAND TOTAL	102	13.5	174	5	6	10	16	25	41	51

LOS by Diagnosis and Operation, Western Region, 45th Edition

Western Region, October 2007–September 2008 Data, by Operation

53.01: UNILAT REP DIRECT IH

Type of Patients	Observed Patients	Avg. Stay	Variance	Percentiles						
				10th	25th	50th	75th	90th	95th	99th
1. SINGLE DX										
0–19 Years	6	1.0	0	1	1	1	1	1	1	1
20–34	3	1.0	0	1	1	1	1	1	1	1
35–49	5	1.6	2	1	1	1	2	4	4	4
50–64	3	1.3	<1	1	1	1	2	2	2	2
65+	5	2.4	3	1	1	2	3	5	5	5
2. MULTIPLE DX										
0–19 Years	16	1.4	<1	1	1	1	1	2	4	4
20–34	4	1.8	<1	1	1	1	3	3	3	3
35–49	16	2.7	8	1	1	1	3	8	11	11
50–64	27	5.5	49	1	1	3	7	10	17	35
65+	78	4.7	23	1	2	3	5	11	17	27
TOTAL SINGLE DX	22	1.4	1	1	1	1	1	3	4	5
TOTAL MULTIPLE DX	141	3.7	22	1	1	2	4	8	11	27
TOTAL										
0–19 Years	22	1.3	<1	1	1	1	1	2	4	4
20–34	7	1.4	<1	1	1	1	2	3	3	3
35–49	21	2.4	7	1	1	1	3	4	8	11
50–64	30	5.1	46	1	1	3	7	10	17	35
65+	83	4.6	22	1	1	3	5	11	15	27
GRAND TOTAL	163	3.4	19	1	1	2	4	7	11	27

53.02: UNILAT REP INDIRECT IH

Type of Patients	Observed Patients	Avg. Stay	Variance	Percentiles						
				10th	25th	50th	75th	90th	95th	99th
1. SINGLE DX										
0–19 Years	54	1.1	<1	1	1	1	1	2	2	2
20–34	6	1.7	<1	1	1	2	2	2	2	2
35–49	3	1.0	0	1	1	1	2	2	1	1
50–64	4	1.3	<1	1	1	1	2	2	2	2
65+	5	1.8	<1	1	1	2	2	3	3	3
2. MULTIPLE DX										
0–19 Years	103	5.1	235	1	1	2	2	5	64	>99
20–34	14	1.6	<1	1	1	2	2	3	4	4
35–49	13	3.2	9	1	2	2	3	9	10	10
50–64	36	2.9	6	1	1	2	4	7	8	11
65+	85	4.0	16	1	1	3	5	9	13	24
TOTAL SINGLE DX	72	1.2	<1	1	1	1	1	2	2	2
TOTAL MULTIPLE DX	251	4.5	154	1	1	3	3	7	14	89
TOTAL										
0–19 Years	157	3.9	169	1	1	1	2	3	14	>99
20–34	20	1.7	<1	1	1	2	2	3	4	4
35–49	16	2.8	8	1	1	2	3	9	10	10
50–64	40	2.7	6	1	1	2	4	7	8	11
65+	90	3.9	15	1	1	3	5	8	13	24
GRAND TOTAL	323	3.7	119	1	1	2	2	6	11	89

53.03: UNILAT REP DIR IH/GRAFT

Type of Patients	Observed Patients	Avg. Stay	Variance	Percentiles						
				10th	25th	50th	75th	90th	95th	99th
1. SINGLE DX										
0–19 Years	0									
20–34	21	1.4	<1	1	1	1	2	2	2	3
35–49	20	1.6	<1	1	1	1	2	3	3	4
50–64	29	1.6	<1	1	1	1	2	3	4	4
65+	14	1.7	1	1	1	1	2	2	5	5
2. MULTIPLE DX										
0–19 Years	1	2.0	0	2	2	2	2	2	2	2
20–34	41	2.2	3	1	1	2	2	5	6	9
35–49	108	2.3	5	1	1	1	3	5	7	9
50–64	198	2.4	11	1	1	2	3	5	6	15
65+	569	2.9	7	1	1	2	4	6	8	13
TOTAL SINGLE DX	84	1.6	<1	1	1	1	2	2	3	5
TOTAL MULTIPLE DX	917	2.7	7	1	1	2	3	5	8	13
TOTAL										
0–19 Years	1	2.0	0	2	2	2	2	2	2	2
20–34	62	2.0	2	1	1	2	2	3	5	9
35–49	128	2.2	4	1	1	1	3	5	7	9
50–64	227	2.3	9	1	1	2	4	5	6	15
65+	583	2.8	7	1	1	2	4	6	8	13
GRAND TOTAL	1,001	2.6	7	1	1	2	3	5	7	13

53.04: UNILAT INDIRECT IH/GRAFT

Type of Patients	Observed Patients	Avg. Stay	Variance	Percentiles						
				10th	25th	50th	75th	90th	95th	99th
1. SINGLE DX										
0–19 Years	5	2.6	3	1	1	2	4	5	5	5
20–34	52	1.4	<1	1	1	1	2	2	3	4
35–49	41	1.5	<1	1	1	1	2	3	3	4
50–64	34	1.5	<1	1	1	1	2	2	3	6
65+	20	1.2	<1	1	1	1	1	2	2	2
2. MULTIPLE DX										
0–19 Years	8	2.5	7	1	1	1	2	7	7	7
20–34	70	1.8	3	1	1	1	2	3	4	14
35–49	143	2.7	10	1	1	1	3	5	10	14
50–64	269	2.8	12	1	1	2	3	6	8	27
65+	637	3.2	11	1	1	2	4	7	10	19
TOTAL SINGLE DX	152	1.4	<1	1	1	1	2	2	3	5
TOTAL MULTIPLE DX	1,127	3.0	11	1	1	2	3	7	9	19
TOTAL										
0–19 Years	13	2.5	6	1	1	1	4	7	7	7
20–34	122	1.6	2	1	1	1	2	3	4	6
35–49	184	2.4	8	1	1	1	3	4	9	14
50–64	303	2.7	11	1	1	2	3	6	8	23
65+	657	3.2	11	1	1	2	4	7	10	19
GRAND TOTAL	1,279	2.8	10	1	1	2	3	6	9	19

LOS by Diagnosis and Operation, Western Region, 45th Edition

Western Region, October 2007–September 2008 Data, by Operation

53.05: UNILAT REP IH/GRAFT NOS

Type of Patients	Observed Patients	Avg. Stay	Variance	10th	25th	50th	75th	90th	95th	99th
1. SINGLE DX										
0–19 Years	3	2.3	5	1	1	1	5	5	5	5
20–34	54	1.8	2	1	1	1	2	3	5	7
35–49	36	1.8	<1	1	1	1	2	3	3	5
50–64	39	1.8	2	1	1	1	2	4	5	7
65+	18	1.5	<1	1	1	1	2	3	3	3
2. MULTIPLE DX										
0–19 Years	5	18.0	692	1	1	1	26	61	61	61
20–34	61	1.8	<1	1	1	1	2	3	4	4
35–49	157	3.1	25	1	1	2	3	6	10	38
50–64	276	3.1	15	1	1	2	4	6	9	20
65+	580	3.9	19	1	1	2	5	8	13	23
TOTAL SINGLE DX	150	1.8	1	1	1	1	2	3	4	7
TOTAL MULTIPLE DX	1,079	3.5	22	1	1	2	4	7	11	23
TOTAL										
0–19 Years	8	12.2	465	1	1	1	26	61	61	61
20–34	115	1.8	1	1	1	1	2	3	4	5
35–49	193	2.8	21	1	1	2	3	5	8	38
50–64	315	3.0	14	1	1	2	3	6	8	18
65+	598	3.9	19	1	1	2	5	8	13	23
GRAND TOTAL	1,229	3.3	20	1	1	2	4	7	10	21

53.1: BILAT IH REPAIR

Type of Patients	Observed Patients	Avg. Stay	Variance	10th	25th	50th	75th	90th	95th	99th
1. SINGLE DX										
0–19 Years	95	1.1	<1	1	1	1	1	1	2	2
20–34	5	1.8	<1	1	1	2	2	3	3	3
35–49	7	1.1	<1	1	1	1	1	2	2	2
50–64	13	1.3	<1	1	1	1	2	2	2	2
65+	13	1.8	2	1	1	1	3	4	4	4
2. MULTIPLE DX										
0–19 Years	337	9.5	513	1	1	1	2	71	91	>99
20–34	14	1.7	1	1	1	1	2	3	5	5
35–49	49	2.1	3	1	1	1	2	6	6	8
50–64	130	2.4	7	1	1	2	3	5	6	13
65+	292	3.0	13	1	1	2	3	6	12	21
TOTAL SINGLE DX	133	1.2	<1	1	1	1	1	2	2	3
TOTAL MULTIPLE DX	822	6.8	319	1	1	2	3	15	74	>99
TOTAL										
0–19 Years	432	7.9	424	1	1	2	2	52	85	>99
20–34	19	1.7	1	1	1	1	2	3	5	5
35–49	56	2.0	3	1	1	1	2	5	6	8
50–64	143	2.3	7	1	1	2	3	4	6	13
65+	305	2.9	12	1	1	2	3	5	9	18
GRAND TOTAL	955	5.9	275	1	1	2	2	9	71	>99

53.10: BILAT IH REPAIR NOS

Type of Patients	Observed Patients	Avg. Stay	Variance	10th	25th	50th	75th	90th	95th	99th
1. SINGLE DX										
0–19 Years	54	1.0	<1	1	1	1	1	1	1	3
20–34	0									
35–49	0									
50–64	1	1.0	0	1	1	1	1	1	1	1
65+	0									
2. MULTIPLE DX										
0–19 Years	184	13.3	702	1	1	1	5	75	98	>99
20–34	1	2.0	0	2	2	2	2	3	2	2
35–49	1	8.0	0	8	8	8	8	8	8	8
50–64	3	1.3	<1	1	1	1	2	2	2	2
65+	5	3.8	6	2	2	2	6	7	7	7
TOTAL SINGLE DX	55	1.0	<1	1	1	1	1	1	1	3
TOTAL MULTIPLE DX	194	13.0	685	1	1	1	5	75	97	>99
TOTAL										
0–19 Years	238	10.6	575	1	1	1	2	71	89	>99
20–34	1	2.0	0	2	2	2	2	3	2	2
35–49	1	8.0	0	8	8	8	8	8	8	8
50–64	4	1.3	<1	1	1	1	1	2	2	2
65+	5	3.8	6	2	2	2	6	7	7	7
GRAND TOTAL	249	10.4	562	1	1	1	2	71	89	>99

53.12: BILAT INDIRECT IH REPAIR

Type of Patients	Observed Patients	Avg. Stay	Variance	10th	25th	50th	75th	90th	95th	99th
1. SINGLE DX										
0–19 Years	34	1.1	<1	1	1	1	1	2	2	2
20–34	0									
35–49	0									
50–64	0									
65+	0									
2. MULTIPLE DX										
0–19 Years	139	5.7	289	1	1	1	1	10	73	>99
20–34	0									
35–49	0									
50–64	2	1.0	0	1	1	1	1	1	1	1
65+	6	1.3	<1	1	1	1	2	2	2	2
TOTAL SINGLE DX	34	1.1	<1	1	1	1	1	2	2	2
TOTAL MULTIPLE DX	147	5.6	282	1	1	1	1	9	73	>99
TOTAL										
0–19 Years	173	5.0	246	1	1	1	1	3	67	>99
20–34	0									
35–49	0									
50–64	2	1.0	0	1	1	1	1	1	1	1
65+	6	1.3	<1	1	1	1	2	2	2	2
GRAND TOTAL	181	4.9	241	1	1	1	1	3	62	>99

LOS by Diagnosis and Operation, Western Region, 45th Edition

Western Region, October 2007–September 2008 Data, by Operation

53.14: BILAT DIRECT IH REP-GRFT

Type of Patients	Observed Patients	Avg. Stay	Variance	10th	25th	50th	75th	90th	95th	99th
1. SINGLE DX										
0–19 Years	0									
20–34	2	1.0	0	1	1	1	1	1	2	1
35–49	2	1.5	<1	1	1	2	2	2	2	2
50–64	4	1.0	0	1	1	1	1	1	1	1
65+	3	1.7	1	1	1	1	3	3	3	3
2. MULTIPLE DX										
0–19 Years	0									
20–34	3	2.0	<1	1	1	2	3	3	3	3
35–49	14	1.6	2	1	1	1	2	2	6	6
50–64	55	2.2	4	1	1	2	3	5	6	10
65+	80	2.9	13	1	1	2	3	5	12	18
TOTAL SINGLE DX	11	1.3	<1	1	1	1	1	2	3	3
TOTAL MULTIPLE DX	152	2.5	8	1	1	2	3	5	6	18
TOTAL										
0–19 Years	0									
20–34	5	1.6	<1	1	1	1	2	3	3	3
35–49	16	1.6	2	1	1	1	2	2	6	6
50–64	59	2.1	4	1	1	2	3	5	6	10
65+	83	2.9	12	1	1	2	3	5	12	18
GRAND TOTAL	163	2.4	8	1	1	1	3	5	6	18

53.15: BILAT INDIRECT IH-GRAFT

Type of Patients	Observed Patients	Avg. Stay	Variance	10th	25th	50th	75th	90th	95th	99th
1. SINGLE DX										
0–19 Years	1	1.0	0	1	1	1	1	1	1	1
20–34	2	2.5	<1	2	2	3	3	3	3	3
35–49	0									
50–64	3	1.3	0	1	1	1	2	2	2	2
65+	2	1.0	0	1	1	1	1	1	1	1
2. MULTIPLE DX										
0–19 Years	1	1.0	0	1	1	1	1	1	1	1
20–34	5	1.8	3	1	1	1	1	5	5	5
35–49	12	1.5	<1	1	1	1	2	2	4	4
50–64	21	1.9	2	1	1	2	3	3	4	4
65+	68	2.3	5	1	1	2	3	5	6	15
TOTAL SINGLE DX	8	1.5	<1	1	1	1	2	3	3	3
TOTAL MULTIPLE DX	107	2.1	4	1	1	2	3	4	5	9
TOTAL										
0–19 Years	2	1.0	0	1	1	1	1	1	1	1
20–34	7	2.0	2	1	1	1	3	5	5	5
35–49	12	1.5	<1	1	1	1	2	2	4	4
50–64	24	1.8	2	1	1	2	3	3	4	4
65+	70	2.3	5	1	1	2	3	4	6	15
GRAND TOTAL	115	2.1	4	1	1	1	3	4	5	9

53.16: DIRECT/INDIRECT IH-GRAFT

Type of Patients	Observed Patients	Avg. Stay	Variance	10th	25th	50th	75th	90th	95th	99th
1. SINGLE DX										
0–19 Years	0									
20–34	1	2.0	0	2	2	2	2	2	2	2
35–49	4	1.0	0	1	1	1	1	1	1	1
50–64	3	1.7	<1	1	1	2	2	2	2	2
65+	3	2.0	3	1	1	1	4	4	4	4
2. MULTIPLE DX										
0–19 Years	2	1.4	<1	1	1	1	1	3	3	3
20–34	2	2.0	2	1	1	2	3	3	3	3
35–49	8	2.3	3	1	1	2	3	6	6	6
50–64	19	2.6	8	1	1	2	3	5	13	13
65+	63	2.6	10	1	1	2	3	4	6	21
TOTAL SINGLE DX	11	1.5	<1	1	1	2	2	2	4	4
TOTAL MULTIPLE DX	94	2.5	8	1	1	2	3	4	6	21
TOTAL										
0–19 Years	2	1.4	<1	1	1	1	1	3	3	3
20–34	3	2.0	<1	1	1	2	3	3	3	3
35–49	12	1.8	2	1	1	2	3	4	6	6
50–64	22	2.5	7	1	1	2	3	4	5	13
65+	66	2.6	9	1	1	2	3	4	6	21
GRAND TOTAL	105	2.4	7	1	1	2	3	4	6	13

53.17: BILAT IH REP-GRAFT NOS

Type of Patients	Observed Patients	Avg. Stay	Variance	10th	25th	50th	75th	90th	95th	99th
1. SINGLE DX										
0–19 Years	1	1.0	0	1	1	1	1	1	1	1
20–34	0									
35–49	2	1.0	0	1	1	1	1	1	1	1
50–64	2	1.5	<1	1	1	1	2	2	2	2
65+	5	2.0	2	1	1	1	3	4	4	4
2. MULTIPLE DX										
0–19 Years	1	1.0	0	1	1	1	1	1	1	1
20–34	3	1.0	0	1	1	1	1	1	1	1
35–49	12	3.0	5	1	1	2	4	6	8	8
50–64	30	3.2	17	1	1	2	3	6	13	21
65+	64	3.7	16	1	1	3	4	7	12	22
TOTAL SINGLE DX	9	1.7	1	1	1	1	2	4	4	4
TOTAL MULTIPLE DX	110	3.4	15	1	1	2	4	6	12	21
TOTAL										
0–19 Years	2	1.0	0	1	1	1	1	1	1	1
20–34	3	1.0	0	1	1	1	1	1	1	1
35–49	13	2.8	5	1	1	2	4	6	8	8
50–64	32	3.1	16	1	1	2	3	6	13	21
65+	69	3.6	15	1	1	3	4	7	12	22
GRAND TOTAL	119	3.3	14	1	1	2	4	6	12	21

LOS by Diagnosis and Operation, Western Region, 45th Edition

Western Region, October 2007–September 2008 Data, by Operation

53.2: UNILAT FH REPAIR

Type of Patients	Observed Patients	Avg. Stay	Variance	10th	25th	50th	75th	90th	95th	99th
1. SINGLE DX										
0–19 Years	1	1.0	0	1	1	1	1	1	1	1
20–34	2	1.0	0	1	1	1	1	1	1	1
35–49	13	1.5	1	1	1	1	2	2	5	5
50–64	8	1.0	0	1	1	1	1	1	1	1
65+	8	2.0	2	1	1	2	2	5	5	5
2. MULTIPLE DX										
0–19 Years	0									
20–34	5	3.2	4	1	2	3	4	6	6	6
35–49	37	2.3	11	1	1	1	2	4	9	19
50–64	68	2.9	9	1	1	2	4	7	8	16
65+	379	4.4	19	1	2	3	5	9	12	21
TOTAL SINGLE DX	32	1.5	1	1	1	1	2	2	5	5
TOTAL MULTIPLE DX	489	4.1	17	1	1	3	5	9	11	19
TOTAL										
0–19 Years	1	1.0	0	1	1	1	1	1	1	1
20–34	7	2.6	4	1	1	2	4	6	6	6
35–49	50	2.1	8	1	1	1	2	4	7	19
50–64	76	2.7	8	1	1	2	4	6	8	16
65+	387	4.4	19	1	2	3	5	9	12	21
GRAND TOTAL	521	3.9	17	1	1	3	5	8	11	19

53.29: UNILAT FH REP NEC

Type of Patients	Observed Patients	Avg. Stay	Variance	10th	25th	50th	75th	90th	95th	99th
1. SINGLE DX										
0–19 Years	0									
20–34	1	1.0	0	1	1	1	1	1	1	1
35–49	4	2.3	4	1	1	2	2	5	5	5
50–64	1	1.0	0	1	1	1	1	1	1	1
65+	1	2.0	0	2	2	2	2	2	2	2
2. MULTIPLE DX										
0–19 Years	0									
20–34	2	4.0	8	2	2	6	6	6	6	6
35–49	10	3.9	32	1	1	1	4	4	9	19
50–64	17	2.9	4	1	1	2	4	6	7	7
65+	121	4.5	15	1	2	4	6	8	11	21
TOTAL SINGLE DX	7	1.9	2	1	1	1	2	5	5	5
TOTAL MULTIPLE DX	150	4.3	15	1	2	3	5	8	11	21
TOTAL										
0–19 Years	0									
20–34	3	3.0	7	1	1	2	4	6	6	6
35–49	14	3.4	23	1	1	1	4	7	19	19
50–64	18	2.8	4	1	1	2	4	6	7	7
65+	122	4.5	15	1	2	4	6	8	11	21
GRAND TOTAL	157	4.2	15	1	2	3	5	8	11	21

53.21: UNILAT FH REP W GRAFT

Type of Patients	Observed Patients	Avg. Stay	Variance	10th	25th	50th	75th	90th	95th	99th
1. SINGLE DX										
0–19 Years	1	1.0	0	1	1	1	1	1	1	1
20–34	1	1.0	0	1	1	1	1	1	1	1
35–49	9	1.2	<1	1	1	1	1	2	2	2
50–64	7	1.0	0	1	1	1	1	1	1	1
65+	7	2.0	2	1	1	2	2	5	5	5
2. MULTIPLE DX										
0–19 Years	0									
20–34	3	2.7	2	1	1	3	4	4	4	4
35–49	27	1.6	3	1	1	1	2	2	4	9
50–64	51	2.9	10	1	2	2	3	7	9	16
65+	258	4.4	21	1	2	3	5	9	13	19
TOTAL SINGLE DX	25	1.4	<1	1	1	1	1	2	2	5
TOTAL MULTIPLE DX	339	4.0	18	1	1	3	5	9	12	18
TOTAL										
0–19 Years	1	1.0	0	1	1	1	1	1	1	1
20–34	4	2.2	2	1	1	1	3	4	4	4
35–49	36	1.5	2	1	1	1	2	2	4	9
50–64	58	2.7	10	1	1	2	3	7	9	16
65+	265	4.4	21	1	2	3	5	9	12	19
GRAND TOTAL	364	3.8	18	1	1	2	5	9	11	18

53.3: BILAT FH REPAIR

Type of Patients	Observed Patients	Avg. Stay	Variance	10th	25th	50th	75th	90th	95th	99th
1. SINGLE DX										
0–19 Years	0									
20–34	0									
35–49	0									
50–64	0									
65+	0									
2. MULTIPLE DX										
0–19 Years	0									
20–34	2	2.0	2	1	1	1	3	3	3	3
35–49	2	2.5	<1	2	2	2	3	3	3	3
65+	2	8.0	2	7	7	7	9	9	9	9
TOTAL SINGLE DX	0									
TOTAL MULTIPLE DX	6	4.2	10	1	2	3	7	9	9	9
TOTAL										
0–19 Years	0									
20–34	2	2.0	2	1	1	1	3	3	3	3
35–49	2	2.5	<1	2	2	2	3	3	3	3
65+	2	8.0	2	7	7	7	9	9	9	9
GRAND TOTAL	6	4.2	10	1	2	3	7	9	9	9

Western Region, October 2007–September 2008 Data, by Operation

53.4: UMBILICAL HERNIA REPAIR

Type of Patients	Observed Patients	Avg. Stay	Variance	10th	25th	50th	75th	90th	95th	99th
1. SINGLE DX										
0–19 Years	13	1.5	<1	1	1	1	2	3	4	4
20–34	29	1.5	<1	1	1	1	2	3	4	4
35–49	80	1.4	<1	1	1	1	2	2	3	4
50–64	43	1.5	<1	1	1	1	2	3	3	3
65+	5	1.4	<1	1	1	1	1	3	3	3
2. MULTIPLE DX										
0–19 Years	98	9.7	290	1	1	3	10	33	62	>99
20–34	171	2.7	16	1	1	2	3	3	7	28
35–49	541	2.7	10	1	1	2	3	5	7	15
50–64	720	3.3	12	1	1	2	4	7	10	18
65+	505	3.9	16	1	1	3	5	8	12	22
TOTAL SINGLE DX	170	1.5	<1	1	1	1	2	3	3	4
TOTAL MULTIPLE DX	2,035	3.8	40	1	1	2	4	7	12	33
TOTAL										
0–19 Years	111	8.4	251	1	1	3	6	28	58	>99
20–34	200	2.5	14	1	1	2	3	4	6	17
35–49	621	2.5	9	1	1	2	3	5	6	14
50–64	763	3.2	12	1	1	2	4	7	9	18
65+	510	3.9	16	1	1	3	5	8	12	22
GRAND TOTAL	2,205	3.6	37	1	1	2	4	7	11	32

53.49: UMB HERNIA REPAIR NEC

Type of Patients	Observed Patients	Avg. Stay	Variance	10th	25th	50th	75th	90th	95th	99th
1. SINGLE DX										
0–19 Years	13	1.5	<1	1	1	1	2	3	4	4
20–34	11	1.4	<1	1	1	1	2	2	3	3
35–49	39	1.4	<1	1	1	1	2	3	3	3
50–64	18	1.6	<1	1	1	1	2	3	3	3
65+	4	1.5	<1	1	1	1	1	3	3	3
2. MULTIPLE DX										
0–19 Years	91	9.5	303	1	1	3	9	33	62	>99
20–34	95	2.8	14	1	1	2	3	5	7	28
35–49	260	3.2	16	1	1	2	4	6	8	24
50–64	337	3.8	17	1	1	2	4	8	13	21
65+	220	4.4	21	1	2	3	5	9	14	24
TOTAL SINGLE DX	85	1.5	<1	1	1	1	2	3	3	4
TOTAL MULTIPLE DX	1,003	4.5	65	1	1	2	4	9	14	58
TOTAL										
0–19 Years	104	8.1	258	1	1	2	5	26	58	97
20–34	106	2.7	13	1	1	2	3	5	7	17
35–49	299	2.9	15	1	1	2	3	6	8	24
50–64	355	3.6	16	1	1	2	4	8	12	21
65+	224	4.4	21	1	2	3	5	9	14	24
GRAND TOTAL	1,088	4.3	60	1	1	2	4	8	14	51

53.5: REP OTH ABD WALL HERNIA

Type of Patients	Observed Patients	Avg. Stay	Variance	10th	25th	50th	75th	90th	95th	99th
1. SINGLE DX										
0–19 Years	10	1.3	<1	1	1	1	1	2	2	2
20–34	10	1.7	4	1	1	1	1	7	7	7
35–49	39	2.0	2	1	1	1	2	4	5	7
50–64	25	2.1	2	1	1	2	3	4	4	6
65+	9	1.5	<1	1	1	1	2	3	3	3
2. MULTIPLE DX										
0–19 Years	38	3.6	8	1	1	2	6	8	9	9
20–34	113	3.0	5	1	1	3	4	5	8	9
35–49	369	3.5	12	1	2	3	5	7	10	24
50–64	564	4.6	35	1	2	3	5	10	13	36
65+	564	5.4	32	1	2	4	7	11	17	24
TOTAL SINGLE DX	93	1.8	2	1	1	1	2	4	5	7
TOTAL MULTIPLE DX	1,648	4.5	26	1	2	3	5	9	13	27
TOTAL										
0–19 Years	48	3.2	7	1	1	2	4	8	9	9
20–34	123	2.9	5	1	1	2	4	5	7	9
35–49	408	3.4	11	1	1	2	4	6	9	21
50–64	589	4.5	34	1	2	3	5	9	13	36
65+	573	5.3	32	1	2	4	7	11	17	24
GRAND TOTAL	1,741	4.3	25	1	2	3	5	9	12	26

53.41: UH REP-GRAFT/PROSTH

Type of Patients	Observed Patients	Avg. Stay	Variance	10th	25th	50th	75th	90th	95th	99th
1. SINGLE DX										
0–19 Years	0									
20–34	18	1.6	1	1	1	1	2	4	4	4
35–49	41	1.3	<1	1	1	1	1	2	2	3
50–64	25	1.4	<1	1	1	1	2	3	3	3
65+	1	1.0	0	1	1	1	1	1	1	1
2. MULTIPLE DX										
0–19 Years	7	11.7	168	1	2	5	24	42	>99	>99
20–34	76	2.5	19	1	1	2	3	4	5	38
35–49	281	2.3	3	1	1	2	4	4	6	10
50–64	383	2.9	8	1	1	2	4	6	8	15
65+	285	3.6	13	1	1	2	4	7	10	22
TOTAL SINGLE DX	85	1.4	<1	1	1	1	2	2	3	4
TOTAL MULTIPLE DX	1,032	3.0	13	1	1	2	4	6	9	22
TOTAL										
0–19 Years	7	11.7	168	1	2	5	24	42	>99	>99
20–34	94	2.3	15	1	1	2	3	4	4	38
35–49	322	2.2	3	1	1	2	3	4	5	9
50–64	408	2.8	8	1	1	2	4	6	8	14
65+	286	3.6	13	1	1	2	4	7	10	22
GRAND TOTAL	1,117	2.9	12	1	1	2	3	6	8	22

LOS by Diagnosis and Operation, Western Region, 45th Edition

Western Region, October 2007–September 2008 Data, by Operation

53.51: INCISIONAL HERNIA REPAIR

Type of Patients	Observed Patients	Avg. Stay	Vari-ance	Percentiles						
				10th	25th	50th	75th	90th	95th	99th
1. SINGLE DX										
0–19 Years	5	1.3	<1	1	1	1	1	2	2	2
20–34	5	2.4	7	1	1	1	2	7	7	7
35–49	17	2.6	3	1	1	2	4	5	7	7
50–64	11	1.8	<1	1	1	2	3	3	3	3
65+	6	1.3	<1	1	1	1	1	3	3	3
2. MULTIPLE DX										
0–19 Years	27	4.1	9	1	1	3	7	8	9	9
20–34	64	3.3	6	1	2	3	4	5	8	16
35–49	216	3.6	13	1	2	3	4	7	9	21
50–64	338	4.7	36	1	2	3	5	10	13	36
65+	331	5.2	29	1	2	4	7	10	15	23
TOTAL SINGLE DX	44	2.0	2	1	1	1	3	4	5	7
TOTAL MULTIPLE DX	976	4.5	25	1	2	3	5	9	12	26
TOTAL										
0–19 Years	32	3.7	9	1	1	2	7	8	9	9
20–34	69	3.3	6	1	1	3	4	7	8	16
35–49	233	3.5	12	1	2	3	4	7	9	21
50–64	349	4.6	35	1	2	3	5	10	13	36
65+	337	5.1	28	1	2	3	6	10	15	23
GRAND TOTAL	1,020	4.4	25	1	2	3	5	9	12	26

53.59: ABD WALL HERNIA REP NEC

Type of Patients	Observed Patients	Avg. Stay	Vari-ance	Percentiles						
				10th	25th	50th	75th	90th	95th	99th
1. SINGLE DX										
0–19 Years	5	1.2	<1	1	1	1	1	2	2	2
20–34	5	1.0	0	1	1	1	1	1	1	1
35–49	22	1.5	<1	1	1	1	2	2	2	5
50–64	14	2.4	2	1	1	2	3	4	6	6
65+	3	1.7	<1	1	1	2	2	2	2	2
2. MULTIPLE DX										
0–19 Years	11	2.2	2	1	1	2	4	4	4	4
20–34	49	2.5	3	1	1	2	5	5	6	9
35–49	153	3.4	10	1	1	2	5	6	10	24
50–64	226	4.5	35	1	2	3	5	9	13	34
65+	233	5.7	37	2	2	4	7	11	18	24
TOTAL SINGLE DX	49	1.6	1	1	1	1	2	3	4	6
TOTAL MULTIPLE DX	672	4.5	28	1	2	3	5	9	13	28
TOTAL										
0–19 Years	16	1.9	1	1	1	2	2	4	4	4
20–34	54	2.4	3	1	1	2	3	5	6	9
35–49	175	3.2	9	1	1	2	4	6	10	24
50–64	240	4.4	33	1	1	3	5	8	13	34
65+	236	5.7	37	1	2	4	7	11	18	24
GRAND TOTAL	721	4.3	27	1	1	3	5	9	13	27

53.6: REP OTH ABD HERNIA-GRAFT

Type of Patients	Observed Patients	Avg. Stay	Vari-ance	Percentiles						
				10th	25th	50th	75th	90th	95th	99th
1. SINGLE DX										
0–19 Years	3	4.0	9	1	1	4	7	7	7	7
20–34	84	2.3	2	1	1	2	3	5	5	6
35–49	230	2.2	3	1	1	2	3	4	5	10
50–64	195	2.1	3	1	1	2	3	4	5	9
65+	104	2.1	1	1	1	2	3	3	4	5
2. MULTIPLE DX										
0–19 Years	19	5.7	39	1	3	3	5	21	21	21
20–34	408	3.6	15	1	1	3	4	7	9	17
35–49	1,903	3.2	10	1	2	3	4	6	7	17
50–64	3,524	3.6	13	1	2	3	4	7	9	16
65+	3,359	4.0	16	1	2	3	5	8	11	20
TOTAL SINGLE DX	616	2.2	3	1	1	2	3	4	5	8
TOTAL MULTIPLE DX	9,213	3.7	14	1	2	3	4	7	9	19
TOTAL										
0–19 Years	22	5.6	36	1	3	3	5	21	21	21
20–34	492	3.3	13	1	1	3	4	6	8	17
35–49	2,133	3.1	10	1	1	3	4	6	7	16
50–64	3,719	3.5	12	1	2	3	4	7	9	16
65+	3,463	4.0	15	1	2	3	5	8	11	20
GRAND TOTAL	9,829	3.6	13	1	2	3	4	7	9	18

53.61: INC HERN REP-GRFT/PROSTH

Type of Patients	Observed Patients	Avg. Stay	Vari-ance	Percentiles						
				10th	25th	50th	75th	90th	95th	99th
1. SINGLE DX										
0–19 Years	3	4.0	9	1	1	4	7	7	7	7
20–34	47	2.7	2	1	2	2	4	5	5	6
35–49	165	2.3	4	1	1	2	3	4	5	11
50–64	140	2.2	3	1	1	2	3	4	6	9
65+	87	2.1	1	1	1	2	3	4	4	5
2. MULTIPLE DX										
0–19 Years	10	8.5	60	1	4	5	21	21	21	21
20–34	305	3.7	15	1	2	3	4	7	10	14
35–49	1,463	3.3	11	1	2	3	4	6	7	16
50–64	2,765	3.6	13	1	2	3	4	7	9	16
65+	2,652	4.0	15	1	2	3	5	8	11	20
TOTAL SINGLE DX	442	2.3	3	1	1	2	3	4	5	9
TOTAL MULTIPLE DX	7,195	3.7	14	1	2	3	5	7	9	18
TOTAL										
0–19 Years	13	7.8	54	1	4	5	9	21	21	21
20–34	352	3.6	13	1	1	3	4	7	9	14
35–49	1,628	3.2	10	1	1	3	4	6	7	16
50–64	2,905	3.5	13	1	2	3	4	7	9	16
65+	2,739	3.9	15	1	2	3	5	8	10	20
GRAND TOTAL	7,637	3.6	13	1	2	3	4	7	9	18

LOS by Diagnosis and Operation, Western Region, 45th Edition

Western Region, October 2007–September 2008 Data, by Operation

53.69: HERN NEC REP-GRFT/PROSTH

Type of Patients	Observed Patients	Avg. Stay	Vari-ance	Percentiles						
				10th	25th	50th	75th	90th	95th	99th
1. SINGLE DX										
0–19 Years	0									
20–34	37	1.7	<1	1	1	1	2	3	3	5
35–49	65	1.7	<1	1	1	1	2	3	4	4
50–64	55	1.9	2	1	1	1	2	4	5	8
65+	17	1.9	<1	1	1	2	2	3	3	3
2. MULTIPLE DX										
0–19 Years	9	2.8	1	1	2	3	3	4	5	5
20–34	103	3.1	14	1	1	2	3	5	7	21
35–49	440	3.0	9	1	1	2	3	6	7	18
50–64	759	3.5	11	1	1	3	4	7	9	17
65+	707	4.1	17	1	2	3	5	8	11	20
TOTAL SINGLE DX	174	1.8	1	1	1	1	2	3	4	5
TOTAL MULTIPLE DX	2,018	3.6	13	1	1	3	4	7	9	20
TOTAL										
0–19 Years	9	2.8	1	1	2	3	3	4	5	5
20–34	140	2.7	11	1	1	2	3	4	6	21
35–49	505	2.8	9	1	1	2	3	5	7	16
50–64	814	3.4	10	1	1	2	4	7	9	15
65+	724	4.1	17	1	2	3	5	8	11	20
GRAND TOTAL	2,192	3.4	12	1	1	2	4	7	9	19

53.7: ABD REP-DIAPH HERNIA

Type of Patients	Observed Patients	Avg. Stay	Vari-ance	Percentiles						
				10th	25th	50th	75th	90th	95th	99th
1. SINGLE DX										
0–19 Years	21	2.8	7	1	1	2	2	9	9	10
20–34	2	1.5	<1	1	1	2	2	2	2	2
35–49	4	2.0	4	1	1	1	1	5	5	5
50–64	7	2.4	4	1	1	2	4	6	6	6
65+	3	1.7	<1	1	1	2	2	3	2	2
2. MULTIPLE DX										
0–19 Years	120	11.2	215	2	3	6	12	26	46	75
20–34	44	5.6	63	1	2	4	6	8	13	51
35–49	137	4.9	44	1	2	3	5	9	14	29
50–64	316	5.4	63	1	2	3	6	11	14	33
65+	500	8.4	74	2	3	6	10	18	25	50
TOTAL SINGLE DX	37	2.6	6	1	1	2	2	6	9	10
TOTAL MULTIPLE DX	1,117	7.7	100	1	2	5	9	15	25	57
TOTAL										
0–19 Years	141	9.9	193	1	2	5	10	24	46	75
20–34	46	5.4	61	1	1	3	6	8	13	51
35–49	141	4.8	43	1	1	3	5	9	14	29
50–64	323	5.3	62	1	2	3	6	11	14	33
65+	503	8.3	74	2	3	6	10	18	25	50
GRAND TOTAL	1,154	7.5	97	1	2	5	8	15	25	57

53.8: REPAIR DH THOR APPR

Type of Patients	Observed Patients	Avg. Stay	Vari-ance	Percentiles						
				10th	25th	50th	75th	90th	95th	99th
1. SINGLE DX										
0–19 Years	8	3.1	3	2	2	2	4	6	6	6
20–34	0									
35–49	0									
50–64	1	7.0	0	7	7	7	7	7	7	7
65+	0									
2. MULTIPLE DX										
0–19 Years	51	13.4	257	2	3	6	18	30	42	98
20–34	15	11.2	271	3	4	6	11	16	69	69
35–49	29	6.7	20	1	4	6	9	13	14	19
50–64	101	6.8	49	2	3	5	8	13	20	36
65+	82	8.2	58	2	4	5	9	16	24	40
TOTAL SINGLE DX	9	3.3	3	2	2	2	4	6	6	7
TOTAL MULTIPLE DX	278	9.4	130	2	4	6	11	21	30	71
TOTAL										
0–19 Years	59	11.7	229	2	3	5	16	30	42	98
20–34	15	11.2	271	3	4	6	11	16	69	69
35–49	29	6.7	20	1	4	6	9	13	14	19
50–64	102	6.8	48	2	4	5	8	13	20	36
65+	82	8.2	58	2	4	5	9	16	24	40
GRAND TOTAL	287	9.0	124	2	3	5	11	21	30	71

53.80: REPAIR DH THOR APPR NOS

Type of Patients	Observed Patients	Avg. Stay	Vari-ance	Percentiles						
				10th	25th	50th	75th	90th	95th	99th
1. SINGLE DX										
0–19 Years	5	2.7	1	2	2	2	4	4	4	4
20–34	0									
35–49	0									
50–64	1	7.0	0	7	7	7	7	7	7	7
65+	0									
2. MULTIPLE DX										
0–19 Years	34	11.5	125	1	3	5	18	29	39	>99
20–34	11	7.8	19	3	4	6	11	13	16	16
35–49	24	6.8	23	2	3	5	8	13	14	19
50–64	75	6.9	40	2	3	5	8	14	21	36
65+	65	8.4	53	3	4	6	11	16	23	40
TOTAL SINGLE DX	6	3.1	2	2	2	2	4	4	7	7
TOTAL MULTIPLE DX	209	8.6	67	2	3	6	12	20	27	41
TOTAL										
0–19 Years	39	10.2	116	1	3	5	18	27	38	>99
20–34	11	7.8	19	3	4	6	11	13	16	16
35–49	24	6.8	23	2	3	5	8	13	14	19
50–64	76	6.9	39	2	3	5	8	14	21	36
65+	65	8.4	53	3	4	6	11	16	23	40
GRAND TOTAL	215	8.4	65	2	3	5	11	20	27	41

LOS by Diagnosis and Operation, Western Region, 45th Edition

Western Region, October 2007–September 2008 Data, by Operation

53.9: OTHER HERNIA REPAIR

Type of Patients	Observed Patients	Avg. Stay	Variance	10th	25th	50th	75th	90th	95th	99th
1. SINGLE DX										
0–19 Years	0									
20–34	3	2.0	3	1	1	1	4	4	4	4
35–49	4	4.5	15	1	3	4	4	10	10	10
50–64	4	5.5	4	1	2	4	6	8	8	8
65+	2	2.0	0	2	2	2	2	2	2	2
2. MULTIPLE DX										
0–19 Years	7	6.4	20	1	3	6	8	9	17	17
20–34	59	3.4	6	1	2	3	5	8	9	10
35–49	116	3.6	12	1	1	2	5	7	10	15
50–64	107	5.4	56	1	2	3	7	11	14	38
65+	89	7.9	60	2	4	6	9	15	20	58
TOTAL SINGLE DX	13	3.8	8	1	2	4	4	8	10	10
TOTAL MULTIPLE DX	378	5.1	38	1	2	3	6	10	14	32
TOTAL										
0–19 Years	7	6.4	20	1	3	6	8	9	17	17
20–34	62	3.3	6	1	2	2	4	8	9	10
35–49	120	3.6	12	1	1	2	5	7	10	15
50–64	111	5.4	54	1	2	3	7	11	14	38
65+	91	7.8	59	2	3	6	9	15	20	58
GRAND TOTAL	391	5.1	37	1	2	3	6	10	14	32

54.1: LAPAROTOMY

Type of Patients	Observed Patients	Avg. Stay	Variance	10th	25th	50th	75th	90th	95th	99th
1. SINGLE DX										
0–19 Years	47	3.4	5	1	2	3	6	7	7	10
20–34	60	3.1	5	1	2	2	4	6	8	14
35–49	42	3.5	18	1	2	2	4	5	6	26
50–64	12	4.0	15	1	1	3	5	6	15	15
65+	1	2.0	0	2	2	3	2	2	2	2
2. MULTIPLE DX										
0–19 Years	280	11.1	217	2	4	7	14	44	96	>99
20–34	673	7.3	73	2	3	5	8	16	24	55
35–49	728	9.2	114	2	3	6	11	21	27	58
50–64	829	11.3	139	3	3	7	14	25	37	73
65+	782	11.6	122	3	5	8	14	24	33	59
TOTAL SINGLE DX	162	3.3	8	1	2	3	4	6	7	15
TOTAL MULTIPLE DX	3,292	10.1	128	2	4	6	12	22	34	90
TOTAL										
0–19 Years	327	10.1	195	2	3	6	12	30	90	>99
20–34	733	6.9	68	2	3	4	8	15	21	48
35–49	770	8.9	111	2	3	6	10	20	27	58
50–64	841	11.2	138	2	4	7	14	25	37	73
65+	783	11.6	122	3	5	8	14	24	33	59
GRAND TOTAL	3,454	9.8	125	2	3	6	12	22	33	90

54.0: ABDOMINAL WALL INCISION

Type of Patients	Observed Patients	Avg. Stay	Variance	10th	25th	50th	75th	90th	95th	99th
1. SINGLE DX										
0–19 Years	27	2.5	2	1	1	3	3	4	6	6
20–34	21	2.3	3	1	1	2	2	4	4	9
35–49	10	2.8	1	2	1	3	3	5	5	5
50–64	9	1.3	<1	1	1	1	2	2	2	2
65+	4	2.5	6	1	1	2	6	6	6	6
2. MULTIPLE DX										
0–19 Years	121	4.4	35	1	2	3	5	8	10	76
20–34	197	5.2	32	1	2	4	6	11	14	31
35–49	337	6.4	49	1	2	4	8	14	19	43
50–64	495	7.5	83	1	3	5	9	15	22	57
65+	405	7.9	85	1	3	5	9	17	22	48
TOTAL SINGLE DX	71	2.4	2	1	1	2	3	4	5	9
TOTAL MULTIPLE DX	1,555	6.7	66	1	3	4	8	14	20	48
TOTAL										
0–19 Years	148	4.1	30	1	2	3	5	7	10	28
20–34	218	4.9	30	1	2	3	6	10	13	31
35–49	347	6.3	48	1	2	4	7	13	18	43
50–64	504	7.4	82	1	3	5	9	15	21	55
65+	409	7.9	85	1	3	5	9	17	22	48
GRAND TOTAL	1,626	6.5	64	1	2	4	7	14	19	46

54.11: EXPLORATORY LAPAROTOMY

Type of Patients	Observed Patients	Avg. Stay	Variance	10th	25th	50th	75th	90th	95th	99th
1. SINGLE DX										
0–19 Years	31	2.9	3	1	1	3	3	4	6	7
20–34	36	3.2	6	1	2	3	4	4	8	14
35–49	29	2.9	7	1	1	2	3	5	6	14
50–64	9	2.4	2	1	1	2	3	6	5	5
65+	0									
2. MULTIPLE DX										
0–19 Years	181	11.1	259	2	3	5	13	28	90	>99
20–34	405	6.6	66	2	3	4	7	14	20	46
35–49	369	8.8	106	2	3	6	10	21	27	58
50–64	446	10.8	134	3	4	7	13	23	35	60
65+	477	10.6	87	3	5	8	13	21	30	49
TOTAL SINGLE DX	105	2.9	5	1	2	2	3	6	6	14
TOTAL MULTIPLE DX	1,878	9.6	122	2	3	6	11	21	30	78
TOTAL										
0–19 Years	212	10.0	233	2	3	5	11	28	78	>99
20–34	441	6.4	62	2	3	4	7	14	19	46
35–49	398	8.4	101	2	3	5	9	19	27	58
50–64	455	10.6	133	2	4	7	13	23	35	60
65+	477	10.6	87	3	5	8	13	21	30	49
GRAND TOTAL	1,983	9.2	118	2	3	6	11	20	28	78

LOS by Diagnosis and Operation, Western Region, 45th Edition

Western Region, October 2007–September 2008 Data, by Operation

54.12: REOPEN RECENT LAP SITE

Type of Patients	Observed Patients	Avg. Stay	Vari-ance	Percentiles						
				10th	25th	50th	75th	90th	95th	99th
1. SINGLE DX										
0–19 Years	2	3.5	<1	3	3	4	4	4	4	4
20–34	8	2.9	3	2	3	3	3	7	7	7
35–49	2	3.5	<1	3	3	3	4	4	4	4
50–64	1	6.0	0	6	6	6	6	6	6	6
65+	0									
2. MULTIPLE DX										
0–19 Years	18	12.6	237	3	4	6	14	38	62	62
20–34	75	9.0	124	2	3	5	10	27	37	>99
35–49	115	9.4	103	2	3	6	12	21	25	60
50–64	106	11.5	168	2	4	8	14	33	52	>99
65+	89	11.5	131	2	4	7	13	29	34	61
TOTAL SINGLE DX	13	3.3	3	2	2	3	4	6	7	7
TOTAL MULTIPLE DX	403	10.5	136	2	4	7	12	26	38	80
TOTAL										
0–19 Years	20	11.6	219	3	3	5	14	38	62	62
20–34	83	8.4	115	2	3	5	8	24	37	>99
35–49	117	9.3	102	2	3	6	12	21	25	60
50–64	107	11.4	167	2	4	8	14	33	52	>99
65+	89	11.5	131	2	4	7	13	29	34	61
GRAND TOTAL	416	10.2	134	2	3	6	12	25	38	80

54.2: ABD REGION DXTIC PX

Type of Patients	Observed Patients	Avg. Stay	Vari-ance	Percentiles						
				10th	25th	50th	75th	90th	95th	99th
1. SINGLE DX										
0–19 Years	55	1.9	3	1	1	1	2	4	4	15
20–34	91	1.8	2	1	1	1	2	4	5	7
35–49	48	1.9	<1	1	1	2	3	3	4	4
50–64	27	4.0	11	1	1	3	7	8	10	12
65+	11	2.3	4	1	1	1	3	4	7	7
2. MULTIPLE DX										
0–19 Years	263	8.8	165	1	2	4	10	23	30	79
20–34	715	3.8	18	1	1	3	4	8	11	20
35–49	631	5.3	39	1	2	3	7	12	17	35
50–64	763	6.4	48	1	2	5	8	14	19	34
65+	984	7.1	47	1	3	5	9	15	19	38
TOTAL SINGLE DX	232	2.1	3	1	1	1	2	4	6	10
TOTAL MULTIPLE DX	3,356	6.2	56	1	2	4	8	14	19	38
TOTAL										
0–19 Years	318	7.6	144	1	1	3	8	19	28	79
20–34	806	3.6	16	1	1	2	4	8	10	19
35–49	679	5.1	37	1	1	3	6	11	17	35
50–64	790	6.3	47	1	2	4	8	14	19	34
65+	995	7.1	47	1	3	5	9	15	19	36
GRAND TOTAL	3,588	5.9	53	1	2	4	7	13	18	37

54.19: LAPAROTOMY NEC

Type of Patients	Observed Patients	Avg. Stay	Vari-ance	Percentiles						
				10th	25th	50th	75th	90th	95th	99th
1. SINGLE DX										
0–19 Years	14	4.3	7	2	2	4	7	7	7	10
20–34	16	2.9	4	1	2	2	3	6	8	8
35–49	11	5.2	49	2	2	3	5	5	26	26
50–64	2	10.0	50	5	5	5	15	15	15	15
65+	1	2.0	0	2	2	2	2	2	2	2
2. MULTIPLE DX										
0–19 Years	81	11.1	129	3	5	8	14	52	>99	>99
20–34	193	7.8	66	2	3	6	9	18	25	57
35–49	244	9.7	133	2	3	6	11	20	28	58
50–64	277	12.2	137	2	5	8	16	26	34	63
65+	216	13.7	191	3	6	10	17	25	41	88
TOTAL SINGLE DX	44	4.2	17	2	2	3	5	7	10	26
TOTAL MULTIPLE DX	1,011	11.0	137	2	4	8	14	24	41	>99
TOTAL										
0–19 Years	95	10.1	117	2	4	8	13	45	>99	>99
20–34	209	7.5	62	2	3	6	9	15	22	55
35–49	255	9.5	130	2	4	6	11	20	28	58
50–64	279	12.2	136	2	5	8	16	26	34	63
65+	217	13.6	191	3	5	10	17	25	41	88
GRAND TOTAL	1,055	10.7	133	2	4	7	13	24	39	>99

54.21: LAPAROSCOPY

Type of Patients	Observed Patients	Avg. Stay	Vari-ance	Percentiles						
				10th	25th	50th	75th	90th	95th	99th
1. SINGLE DX										
0–19 Years	49	1.9	4	1	1	1	2	4	4	15
20–34	88	1.7	2	1	1	1	2	3	5	7
35–49	43	1.8	<1	1	1	2	3	3	3	4
50–64	17	2.8	6	2	2	1	4	7	8	8
65+	2	3.0	2	2	2	2	4	4	4	4
2. MULTIPLE DX										
0–19 Years	224	7.2	165	1	2	3	7	14	34	79
20–34	622	3.4	12	1	1	2	4	7	9	14
35–49	424	4.3	27	1	1	3	5	9	14	28
50–64	351	5.3	44	1	1	3	7	12	17	25
65+	330	6.6	47	2	2	4	9	15	20	30
TOTAL SINGLE DX	199	1.9	2	1	1	1	2	4	5	7
TOTAL MULTIPLE DX	1,951	5.0	52	1	1	3	6	11	15	34
TOTAL										
0–19 Years	273	6.1	137	1	1	2	6	12	25	79
20–34	710	3.2	11	1	1	2	4	6	9	14
35–49	467	4.1	25	1	1	3	5	9	13	28
50–64	368	5.2	43	1	1	3	7	12	16	25
65+	332	6.6	47	2	2	4	9	15	20	30
GRAND TOTAL	2,150	4.7	48	1	1	3	5	10	15	34

LOS by Diagnosis and Operation, Western Region, 45th Edition

Western Region, October 2007–September 2008 Data, by Operation

54.22: ABD WALL OR UMBILICUS BX

Type of Patients	Observed Patients	Avg. Stay	Variance	10th	25th	50th	75th	90th	95th	99th
1. SINGLE DX										
0–19 Years	0									
20–34	0									
35–49	0									
50–64	2	6.6	60	1	1	12	12	12	12	12
65+	1	1.0	0	1	1	1	1	1	1	1
2. MULTIPLE DX										
0–19 Years	1	13.0	0	13	13	13	13	13	13	13
20–34	2	2.5	<1	2	2	2	3	3	3	3
35–49	20	10.3	108	2	4	6	11	31	39	39
50–64	33	9.1	74	2	3	6	9	23	32	34
65+	43	10.0	119	2	3	7	12	19	26	58
TOTAL SINGLE DX	3	4.7	40	1	1	1	12	12	12	12
TOTAL MULTIPLE DX	99	9.7	95	2	3	6	13	21	31	44
TOTAL										
0–19 Years	1	13.0	0	13	13	13	13	13	13	13
20–34	2	2.5	<1	2	2	2	3	3	3	3
35–49	20	10.3	108	2	4	6	11	31	39	39
50–64	35	9.0	72	2	3	6	11	23	32	34
65+	44	9.8	118	2	3	7	12	19	26	58
GRAND TOTAL	102	9.6	94	2	3	6	12	21	31	44

54.24: CLSD INTRA-ABD MASS BX

Type of Patients	Observed Patients	Avg. Stay	Variance	10th	25th	50th	75th	90th	95th	99th
1. SINGLE DX										
0–19 Years	5	2.4	2	1	2	2	2	5	5	5
20–34	1	4.0	0	4	4	4	4	4	4	4
35–49	3	1.7	1	1	1	1	3	3	3	3
50–64	6	7.2	4	4	7	7	8	10	10	10
65+	5	2.6	7	1	1	1	3	7	7	7
2. MULTIPLE DX										
0–19 Years	7	11.1	94	2	3	8	24	24	24	24
20–34	51	6.1	52	2	3	4	7	11	16	48
35–49	107	6.4	43	1	3	4	8	12	17	37
50–64	209	7.3	60	1	3	5	9	16	24	43
65+	417	6.6	28	2	3	6	9	13	16	22
TOTAL SINGLE DX	20	3.9	8	1	1	3	7	8	10	10
TOTAL MULTIPLE DX	791	6.8	41	1	3	5	9	13	17	37
TOTAL										
0–19 Years	12	8.7	83	2	2	3	16	24	24	24
20–34	52	6.1	51	2	3	4	7	11	16	48
35–49	110	6.3	43	1	3	5	8	12	17	37
50–64	215	7.3	58	1	2	5	9	16	24	43
65+	422	6.6	27	2	3	6	9	13	16	22
GRAND TOTAL	811	6.8	40	1	3	5	9	13	17	37

54.23: PERITONEAL BIOPSY

Type of Patients	Observed Patients	Avg. Stay	Variance	10th	25th	50th	75th	90th	95th	99th
1. SINGLE DX										
0–19 Years	0									
20–34	1	1.0	0	1	1	1	1	1	1	1
35–49	2	3.5	<1	3	3	4	4	4	4	4
50–64	2	3.0	2	2	2	3	4	4	4	4
65+	3	1.7	1	1	1	1	3	3	3	3
2. MULTIPLE DX										
0–19 Years	28	15.5	144	4	8	12	20	28	53	53
20–34	29	9.4	51	2	4	8	13	19	26	30
35–49	64	8.5	61	2	4	7	10	17	24	44
50–64	150	6.8	32	1	2	5	10	16	18	21
65+	186	8.5	72	1	3	6	11	18	24	50
TOTAL SINGLE DX	8	2.4	2	1	1	2	3	4	4	4
TOTAL MULTIPLE DX	457	9.1	74	2	3	7	12	19	24	53
TOTAL										
0–19 Years	28	15.5	144	4	8	12	20	28	53	53
20–34	30	9.1	52	2	4	8	13	19	26	30
35–49	66	8.4	60	2	4	7	10	17	24	44
50–64	152	6.8	32	1	2	5	10	16	18	21
65+	189	8.4	71	1	3	6	11	18	24	50
GRAND TOTAL	465	9.0	74	2	3	7	12	19	24	53

54.3: EXC/DESTR ABD WALL LES

Type of Patients	Observed Patients	Avg. Stay	Variance	10th	25th	50th	75th	90th	95th	99th
1. SINGLE DX										
0–19 Years	12	3.6	4	1	2	3	5	5	7	9
20–34	23	2.5	3	1	1	2	3	5	5	7
35–49	19	2.1	1	1	1	2	3	4	4	4
50–64	9	2.7	4	1	1	2	4	6	6	6
65+	1	1.0	0	1	1	1	1	1	1	1
2. MULTIPLE DX										
0–19 Years	36	8.7	57	1	3	7	15	23	24	29
20–34	89	6.0	58	1	2	4	6	13	17	>99
35–49	156	6.1	51	1	2	4	8	13	15	39
50–64	211	7.7	76	1	2	5	9	16	24	43
65+	186	7.2	47	1	2	5	10	16	21	30
TOTAL SINGLE DX	64	2.7	3	1	1	2	4	5	6	9
TOTAL MULTIPLE DX	678	7.1	59	1	2	5	9	15	21	43
TOTAL										
0–19 Years	48	7.5	49	1	3	5	9	20	24	29
20–34	112	5.3	49	1	2	3	6	12	16	51
35–49	175	5.7	47	1	2	4	7	11	15	39
50–64	220	7.4	74	1	2	5	9	16	21	43
65+	187	7.2	47	1	2	5	10	16	21	30
GRAND TOTAL	742	6.7	56	1	2	4	8	15	21	43

Western Region, October 2007–September 2008 Data, by Operation

54.4: EXC/DESTR PERITON TISS

Type of Patients	Observed Patients	Avg. Stay	Vari-ance	Percentiles						
				10th	25th	50th	75th	90th	95th	99th
1. SINGLE DX										
0–19 Years	33	4.5	12	1	2	3	6	9	12	17
20–34	21	2.3	3	1	2	3	3	4	7	7
35–49	12	2.3	1	1	2	2	3	4	4	7
50–64	20	3.4	3	1	2	4	5	5	5	7
65+	5	3.4	<1	2	3	4	4	4	4	4
2. MULTIPLE DX										
0–19 Years	105	10.0	156	2	4	6	10	19	31	72
20–34	147	4.5	13	2	2	4	6	9	11	21
35–49	304	5.8	58	2	3	4	6	10	14	35
50–64	505	7.0	67	2	3	5	8	13	23	41
65+	439	8.1	73	3	4	6	9	16	21	47
TOTAL SINGLE DX	91	3.7	8	1	2	3	5	7	9	12
TOTAL MULTIPLE DX	1,500	7.3	77	2	3	5	8	13	21	52
TOTAL										
0–19 Years	138	8.7	128	2	3	6	9	17	28	72
20–34	168	4.2	12	1	2	3	6	9	10	21
35–49	316	5.7	56	2	3	4	7	9	14	35
50–64	525	6.9	65	2	3	5	8	13	22	41
65+	444	8.1	72	3	4	6	9	15	20	47
GRAND TOTAL	1,591	7.0	73	2	3	5	8	13	20	50

54.51: LAPSCP PERITON ADHESIO

Type of Patients	Observed Patients	Avg. Stay	Vari-ance	Percentiles						
				10th	25th	50th	75th	90th	95th	99th
1. SINGLE DX										
0–19 Years	10	5.5	16	1	2	5	10	10	11	11
20–34	26	3.3	5	1	2	5	5	7	7	7
35–49	31	2.4	4	1	1	2	3	4	6	10
50–64	22	2.4	4	1	1	2	3	5	6	8
65+	6	2.8	5	1	1	2	4	7	7	7
2. MULTIPLE DX										
0–19 Years	212	4.5	16	1	2	4	6	9	11	21
20–34	589	3.7	15	1	1	2	4	8	11	21
35–49	1,004	4.2	17	1	1	3	5	9	11	21
50–64	1,187	4.6	27	1	2	3	5	9	13	27
65+	977	6.9	57	1	3	5	8	13	18	33
TOTAL SINGLE DX	95	3.1	7	1	1	2	4	7	10	11
TOTAL MULTIPLE DX	3,969	4.9	31	1	2	3	6	10	14	26
TOTAL										
0–19 Years	222	4.6	16	1	2	4	6	10	11	21
20–34	615	3.7	15	1	1	3	5	7	11	20
35–49	1,035	4.1	17	1	1	3	5	9	11	21
50–64	1,209	4.6	27	1	2	3	5	9	13	27
65+	983	6.8	57	1	3	5	8	13	18	33
GRAND TOTAL	4,064	4.9	30	1	2	3	6	10	14	26

54.5: PERITONEAL ADHESIOLYSIS

Type of Patients	Observed Patients	Avg. Stay	Vari-ance	Percentiles						
				10th	25th	50th	75th	90th	95th	99th
1. SINGLE DX										
0–19 Years	36	6.4	13	2	4	6	10	10	12	19
20–34	55	4.1	6	1	2	4	6	7	8	11
35–49	61	3.5	7	1	1	3	4	7	9	11
50–64	54	4.4	9	1	2	4	6	8	10	13
65+	16	5.7	11	1	2	6	7	11	11	11
2. MULTIPLE DX										
0–19 Years	598	8.9	101	2	4	6	10	20	24	97
20–34	1,291	5.7	38	1	2	4	7	12	16	32
35–49	2,648	6.1	36	1	3	5	8	12	17	28
50–64	3,764	7.4	56	2	3	5	9	15	21	38
65+	4,559	9.9	61	3	5	8	12	18	23	38
TOTAL SINGLE DX	222	4.6	10	1	2	4	7	10	10	12
TOTAL MULTIPLE DX	12,860	7.9	58	2	3	6	10	16	21	38
TOTAL										
0–19 Years	634	8.7	97	2	4	6	10	20	23	97
20–34	1,346	5.6	37	1	2	4	8	11	16	32
35–49	2,709	6.1	36	1	3	4	8	12	17	27
50–64	3,818	7.3	56	2	3	5	9	14	21	38
65+	4,575	9.9	61	3	5	8	12	18	23	38
GRAND TOTAL	13,082	7.9	58	2	3	6	10	16	21	37

54.59: PERITON ADHESIOLYSIS NEC

Type of Patients	Observed Patients	Avg. Stay	Vari-ance	Percentiles						
				10th	25th	50th	75th	90th	95th	99th
1. SINGLE DX										
0–19 Years	26	6.7	11	3	4	6	9	10	12	19
20–34	29	4.9	6	3	3	5	7	8	8	11
35–49	30	4.6	8	1	3	4	7	9	10	11
50–64	32	5.8	8	3	4	5	8	10	11	13
65+	10	7.5	6	4	6	6	10	11	11	11
2. MULTIPLE DX										
0–19 Years	386	10.9	128	4	5	8	12	23	28	>99
20–34	702	7.4	52	2	3	5	9	14	20	37
35–49	1,644	7.3	44	2	3	6	9	14	19	34
50–64	2,577	8.6	64	3	4	7	10	16	22	44
65+	3,582	10.7	59	4	6	9	13	19	24	38
TOTAL SINGLE DX	127	5.7	9	2	3	5	7	10	11	13
TOTAL MULTIPLE DX	8,891	9.3	65	3	5	7	11	18	23	41
TOTAL										
0–19 Years	412	10.7	123	4	5	8	12	22	28	>99
20–34	731	7.3	50	2	3	5	9	14	20	37
35–49	1,674	7.2	44	2	3	6	9	14	19	34
50–64	2,609	8.6	64	3	4	7	10	16	22	44
65+	3,592	10.7	59	4	6	9	13	19	24	38
GRAND TOTAL	9,018	9.2	64	3	5	7	11	18	23	41

Western Region, October 2007–September 2008 Data, by Operation

54.6: ABD WALL/PERITON SUTURE

Type of Patients	Observed Patients	Avg. Stay	Variance	Percentiles						
				10th	25th	50th	75th	90th	95th	99th
1. SINGLE DX										
0–19 Years	8	1.6	2	1	1	1	1	4	5	5
20–34	15	2.5	2	1	1	2	4	4	6	6
35–49	6	4.0	6	1	3	4	5	8	8	8
50–64	4	2.8	3	1	2	3	5	5	5	5
65+	1	1.0	0	1	1	1	1	1	1	1
2. MULTIPLE DX										
0–19 Years	28	4.0	20	1	1	2	6	17	>99	>99
20–34	90	3.5	7	1	1	3	5	7	7	13
35–49	85	6.7	56	2	3	5	7	13	23	42
50–64	114	7.5	100	1	3	4	7	17	24	48
65+	120	8.0	82	1	3	6	9	17	23	47
TOTAL SINGLE DX	34	2.5	3	1	1	2	4	5	6	8
TOTAL MULTIPLE DX	437	6.4	65	1	2	4	7	14	22	71
TOTAL										
0–19 Years	36	3.3	16	1	1	2	5	16	>99	>99
20–34	105	3.3	7	1	1	3	4	6	9	13
35–49	91	6.6	53	2	3	5	7	13	23	42
50–64	118	7.3	97	1	3	4	7	17	24	48
65+	121	8.0	82	1	3	6	9	16	22	47
GRAND TOTAL	471	6.1	61	1	2	4	7	13	21	71

54.61: RECLOSE POSTOP DISRUPT

Type of Patients	Observed Patients	Avg. Stay	Variance	Percentiles						
				10th	25th	50th	75th	90th	95th	99th
1. SINGLE DX										
0–19 Years	1	1.0	0	1	1	1	1	1	1	1
20–34	3	3.0	0	3	3	3	3	3	3	3
35–49	4	3.3	3	3	3	4	5	5	5	5
50–64	3	2.0	1	1	1	2	3	3	3	3
65+	1	1.0	0	1	1	1	1	1	1	1
2. MULTIPLE DX										
0–19 Years	6	4.0	3	2	2	4	6	>99	>99	>99
20–34	14	3.5	6	1	2	3	5	8	9	9
35–49	46	6.7	41	2	3	5	8	11	23	36
50–64	85	7.1	93	1	2	4	7	17	23	72
65+	103	7.5	50	1	3	6	9	16	20	35
TOTAL SINGLE DX	12	2.5	2	1	1	3	3	4	5	5
TOTAL MULTIPLE DX	254	6.9	59	1	3	5	8	14	23	47
TOTAL										
0–19 Years	7	3.6	4	1	2	4	6	>99	>99	>99
20–34	17	3.4	5	3	3	3	4	8	9	9
35–49	50	6.5	39	2	3	5	8	11	23	36
50–64	88	6.9	91	1	2	4	7	17	23	72
65+	104	7.4	50	1	3	6	9	16	20	35
GRAND TOTAL	266	6.7	58	1	3	4	8	14	22	47

54.63: ABD WALL SUTURE NEC

Type of Patients	Observed Patients	Avg. Stay	Variance	Percentiles						
				10th	25th	50th	75th	90th	95th	99th
1. SINGLE DX										
0–19 Years	5	1.0	0	1	1	1	1	1	1	1
20–34	9	1.8	2	1	1	1	2	4	4	4
35–49	0									
50–64	0									
65+	0									
2. MULTIPLE DX										
0–19 Years	19	3.5	20	1	1	2	5	17	>99	>99
20–34	48	2.7	6	1	1	2	3	6	7	13
35–49	19	5.9	86	1	2	3	6	13	42	42
50–64	13	4.2	4	2	3	4	6	7	7	7
65+	6	10.7	74	1	4	15	16	23	23	23
TOTAL SINGLE DX	14	1.4	1	1	1	1	1	4	4	4
TOTAL MULTIPLE DX	105	4.1	29	1	1	2	5	10	16	>99
TOTAL										
0–19 Years	24	2.8	15	1	1	1	4	14	>99	>99
20–34	57	2.5	5	1	1	3	3	5	7	13
35–49	19	5.9	86	1	2	3	6	13	42	42
50–64	13	4.2	4	2	3	4	6	7	7	7
65+	6	10.7	74	1	4	15	16	23	23	23
GRAND TOTAL	119	3.7	26	1	1	2	4	7	15	>99

54.7: OTH ABD WALL PERITON REP

Type of Patients	Observed Patients	Avg. Stay	Variance	Percentiles						
				10th	25th	50th	75th	90th	95th	99th
1. SINGLE DX										
0–19 Years	0									
20–34	4	4.0	1	3	3	3	5	5	5	5
35–49	2	2.5	<1	2	2	3	3	3	3	3
50–64	3	3.3	6	1	1	3	6	6	6	6
65+	0									
2. MULTIPLE DX										
0–19 Years	243	35.8	432	16	22	32	54	85	>99	>99
20–34	56	5.0	7	2	3	5	6	8	11	13
35–49	47	6.4	57	2	2	4	7	11	15	51
50–64	62	6.4	47	2	2	4	7	16	20	40
65+	28	10.3	193	2	5	8	11	14	30	75
TOTAL SINGLE DX	9	3.4	3	1	3	3	5	6	6	6
TOTAL MULTIPLE DX	436	23.5	487	3	5	20	37	71	98	>99
TOTAL										
0–19 Years	243	35.8	432	16	22	32	54	85	>99	>99
20–34	60	4.9	7	2	3	5	6	8	11	13
35–49	49	5.8	55	1	3	4	6	11	15	51
50–64	65	6.3	46	1	2	4	7	16	20	40
65+	28	10.3	193	2	5	8	11	14	30	75
GRAND TOTAL	445	23.2	485	3	5	20	37	69	98	>99

Western Region, October 2007–September 2008 Data, by Operation

54.71: REPAIR OF GASTROSCHISIS

Type of Patients	Observed Patients	Avg. Stay	Vari-ance	10th	25th	50th	75th	90th	95th	99th
1. SINGLE DX										
0–19 Years	0									
20–34	0									
35–49	0									
50–64	0									
65+	0									
2. MULTIPLE DX										
0–19 Years	230	37.3	402	18	23	34	55	86	>99	>99
20–34	0									
35–49	0									
50–64	0									
65+	0									
TOTAL SINGLE DX	0									
TOTAL MULTIPLE DX	230	37.3	402	18	23	34	55	86	>99	>99
TOTAL										
0–19 Years	230	37.3	402	18	23	34	55	86	>99	>99
20–34	0									
35–49	0									
50–64	0									
65+	0									
GRAND TOTAL	230	37.3	402	18	23	34	55	86	>99	>99

54.72: ABDOMEN WALL REPAIR NEC

Type of Patients	Observed Patients	Avg. Stay	Vari-ance	10th	25th	50th	75th	90th	95th	99th
1. SINGLE DX										
0–19 Years	0									
20–34	1	3.0	0	3	3	3	3	3	3	3
35–49	1	2.0	0	2	2	2	2	2	2	2
50–64	2	4.5	4	3	3	6	6	6	6	6
65+	0									
2. MULTIPLE DX										
0–19 Years	1	10.0	0	10	10	10	10	10	10	10
20–34	21	4.2	4	2	3	4	5	7	7	8
35–49	20	4.3	13	2	2	4	7	8	8	16
50–64	44	5.3	22	2	2	4	7	9	16	25
65+	17	10.3	296	1	2	6	10	14	75	75
TOTAL SINGLE DX	4	3.5	3	2	2	3	6	6	6	6
TOTAL MULTIPLE DX	103	5.8	63	1	2	4	7	10	14	25
TOTAL										
0–19 Years	1	10.0	0	10	10	10	10	10	10	10
20–34	22	4.1	3	2	2	4	5	7	7	8
35–49	21	4.2	13	1	2	3	5	8	8	16
50–64	46	5.3	21	2	2	4	7	9	16	25
65+	17	10.3	296	1	2	6	10	14	75	75
GRAND TOTAL	107	5.7	61	1	2	4	7	10	14	25

54.9: OTHER ABD REGION OPS

Type of Patients	Observed Patients	Avg. Stay	Vari-ance	10th	25th	50th	75th	90th	95th	99th
1. SINGLE DX										
0–19 Years	119	5.6	8	2	4	5	7	9	10	15
20–34	105	3.6	5	1	2	3	5	7	8	10
35–49	76	3.2	5	1	2	3	4	6	7	14
50–64	37	3.4	5	1	2	3	5	7	9	9
65+	17	2.9	3	1	2	3	3	5	7	7
2. MULTIPLE DX										
0–19 Years	1,015	8.1	118	1	2	5	9	17	28	72
20–34	1,775	5.9	31	2	3	4	7	12	16	31
35–49	5,329	5.8	37	1	2	4	7	12	16	28
50–64	9,536	5.9	36	1	3	4	7	12	16	29
65+	6,805	6.3	29	2	3	5	8	12	16	26
TOTAL SINGLE DX	354	4.5	8	1	2	4	6	8	9	15
TOTAL MULTIPLE DX	24,460	6.2	41	2	3	4	7	12	17	31
TOTAL										
0–19 Years	1,134	7.9	108	1	3	5	9	16	27	59
20–34	1,880	5.7	29	2	3	4	7	11	16	30
35–49	5,405	5.8	37	1	2	4	7	11	16	28
50–64	9,573	5.9	36	1	2	4	7	12	16	29
65+	6,822	6.3	29	2	3	5	8	12	16	26
GRAND TOTAL	24,814	6.1	41	2	3	4	7	12	17	31

54.91: PERC ABD DRAINAGE

Type of Patients	Observed Patients	Avg. Stay	Vari-ance	10th	25th	50th	75th	90th	95th	99th
1. SINGLE DX										
0–19 Years	104	5.7	8	2	4	5	7	9	10	15
20–34	91	3.8	5	1	2	3	5	7	8	11
35–49	69	3.4	5	1	2	3	4	6	7	14
50–64	35	3.5	5	1	2	3	5	7	9	9
65+	13	3.4	2	2	3	3	3	5	7	7
2. MULTIPLE DX										
0–19 Years	449	8.2	57	3	4	6	10	16	21	43
20–34	1,207	6.0	31	2	3	5	7	12	16	30
35–49	4,479	5.8	33	2	2	4	7	12	16	26
50–64	8,250	5.9	34	2	3	4	7	12	16	29
65+	5,749	6.3	27	2	3	5	8	12	16	26
TOTAL SINGLE DX	312	4.6	8	2	3	4	6	8	10	15
TOTAL MULTIPLE DX	20,134	6.1	33	2	3	5	7	12	16	28
TOTAL										
0–19 Years	553	7.7	47	3	4	6	9	14	19	38
20–34	1,298	5.9	29	2	3	4	7	11	15	29
35–49	4,548	5.7	33	2	2	4	7	11	16	26
50–64	8,285	5.9	34	2	3	4	7	12	16	29
65+	5,762	6.3	27	2	3	5	8	12	16	26
GRAND TOTAL	20,446	6.0	32	2	3	4	7	12	16	27

LOS by Diagnosis and Operation, Western Region, 45th Edition

Western Region, October 2007–September 2008 Data, by Operation

54.92: RMVL FB PERITON CAVITY

Type of Patients	Observed Patients	Avg. Stay	Vari-ance	Percentiles						
				10th	25th	50th	75th	90th	95th	99th
1. SINGLE DX										
0–19 Years	1	1.0	0	1	1	1	1	1	1	1
20–34	7	1.9	1	1	1	3	3	4	4	4
35–49	3	2.3	<1	2	2	2	3	3	3	3
50–64	1	2.0	0	2	2	2	2	2	2	2
65+	1	3.0	0	3	3	3	3	3	3	3
2. MULTIPLE DX										
0–19 Years	11	8.1	42	2	4	7	7	15	15	28
20–34	35	4.1	7	2	3	3	5	8	9	14
35–49	52	7.8	72	1	3	5	9	21	31	38
50–64	75	8.1	117	2	3	5	8	18	25	72
65+	56	7.0	72	2	3	5	7	14	19	56
TOTAL SINGLE DX	13	2.0	1	1	1	2	3	3	4	4
TOTAL MULTIPLE DX	229	7.2	75	2	3	4	7	15	24	51
TOTAL										
0–19 Years	12	7.8	43	2	3	7	7	15	15	28
20–34	42	3.7	6	1	2	3	4	7	8	14
35–49	55	7.5	70	2	3	5	9	21	31	38
50–64	76	8.0	116	2	3	5	7	18	25	72
65+	57	7.0	71	2	3	5	7	14	19	56
GRAND TOTAL	242	6.9	72	2	3	4	7	15	23	51

54.93: CREATE CUTANEOPERIT FIST

Type of Patients	Observed Patients	Avg. Stay	Vari-ance	Percentiles						
				10th	25th	50th	75th	90th	95th	99th
1. SINGLE DX										
0–19 Years	1	1.0	0	1	1	1	1	1	1	1
20–34	1	2.0	0	2	2	2	2	2	2	2
35–49	0									
50–64	0									
65+	0									
2. MULTIPLE DX										
0–19 Years	110	12.5	221	1	2	7	16	31	45	74
20–34	81	5.9	22	1	2	5	8	14	16	>99
35–49	128	7.1	43	1	2	6	10	17	21	30
50–64	202	6.1	43	1	2	4	8	12	21	56
65+	139	6.5	52	1	2	4	8	13	20	44
TOTAL SINGLE DX	2	1.5	<1	1	1	2	2	2	2	2
TOTAL MULTIPLE DX	660	8.7	118	1	2	5	11	21	31	74
TOTAL										
0–19 Years	111	12.4	221	1	2	7	16	31	45	74
20–34	82	5.8	22	1	2	5	8	14	16	>99
35–49	128	7.1	43	1	2	6	10	17	21	30
50–64	202	6.1	43	1	2	4	8	12	21	56
65+	139	6.5	52	1	2	4	8	13	20	44
GRAND TOTAL	662	8.7	118	1	2	5	11	21	31	74

54.95: PERITONEAL INCISION

Type of Patients	Observed Patients	Avg. Stay	Vari-ance	Percentiles						
				10th	25th	50th	75th	90th	95th	99th
1. SINGLE DX										
0–19 Years	12	5.1	8	1	3	5	7	9	9	9
20–34	5	2.6	3	1	1	2	4	5	5	5
35–49	3	2.0	3	1	1	1	4	4	4	4
50–64	1	1.0	0	1	1	1	1	1	1	1
65+	1	1.0	0	1	1	1	1	1	1	1
2. MULTIPLE DX										
0–19 Years	256	7.5	155	1	2	4	8	15	25	98
20–34	156	6.8	48	1	2	4	9	14	20	36
35–49	197	8.1	135	1	2	5	10	16	26	79
50–64	236	8.9	93	2	3	6	10	21	28	45
65+	223	9.0	87	2	3	6	11	20	24	46
TOTAL SINGLE DX	22	4.2	8	1	1	5	7	9	9	9
TOTAL MULTIPLE DX	1,068	8.0	119	1	2	5	9	16	25	77
TOTAL										
0–19 Years	268	7.4	149	1	2	5	8	14	20	93
20–34	161	6.7	47	1	2	4	9	14	19	36
35–49	200	8.1	134	1	2	5	10	16	26	79
50–64	237	8.8	93	2	3	6	10	21	28	45
65+	224	8.9	87	2	3	6	11	20	24	46
GRAND TOTAL	1,090	7.9	117	1	2	5	9	16	25	77

54.98: PERITONEAL DIALYSIS

Type of Patients	Observed Patients	Avg. Stay	Vari-ance	Percentiles						
				10th	25th	50th	75th	90th	95th	99th
1. SINGLE DX										
0–19 Years	0									
20–34	0									
35–49	0									
50–64	0									
65+										
2. MULTIPLE DX										
0–19 Years	175	5.4	80	1	2	3	5	11	17	53
20–34	280	4.7	19	2	2	3	6	8	12	23
35–49	455	4.3	12	1	2	3	5	8	11	20
50–64	735	4.6	22	2	2	3	6	8	11	20
65+	587	5.1	16	2	3	4	6	10	14	20
TOTAL SINGLE DX	0									
TOTAL MULTIPLE DX	2,232	4.8	28	1	2	3	6	9	13	23
TOTAL										
0–19 Years	175	5.4	80	1	2	3	5	11	17	53
20–34	280	4.7	19	2	2	3	6	8	12	23
35–49	455	4.3	12	1	2	3	5	8	11	20
50–64	735	4.6	22	2	2	3	6	8	11	20
65+	587	5.1	16	2	3	4	6	10	14	20
GRAND TOTAL	2,232	4.8	28	1	2	3	6	9	13	23

LOS by Diagnosis and Operation, Western Region, 45th Edition

Western Region, October 2007–September 2008 Data, by Operation

55.0: NEPHROTOMY & NEPHROSTOMY

Type of Patients	Observed Patients	Avg. Stay	Vari- ance	10th	25th	50th	75th	90th	95th	99th
1. SINGLE DX										
0–19 Years	9	2.9	2	2	2	2	4	4	4	7
20–34	57	2.4	2	1	1	2	3	4	5	6
35–49	61	2.2	2	1	1	2	3	4	5	6
50–64	64	2.0	1	1	1	2	3	3	5	6
65+	17	2.5	3	1	2	2	3	4	8	8
2. MULTIPLE DX										
0–19 Years	114	5.6	20	2	2	4	8	12	16	21
20–34	602	5.0	32	2	2	4	6	10	12	28
35–49	1,056	5.7	33	1	2	4	7	12	17	28
50–64	1,844	6.2	42	1	2	4	8	14	18	31
65+	2,334	7.8	51	2	3	6	10	16	20	33
TOTAL SINGLE DX	208	2.3	2	1	1	2	3	4	5	6
TOTAL MULTIPLE DX	5,950	6.6	43	1	2	5	8	14	19	31
TOTAL										
0–19 Years	123	5.4	19	2	2	4	7	10	16	21
20–34	659	4.8	30	1	2	3	5	10	12	28
35–49	1,117	5.5	32	1	2	4	7	11	17	28
50–64	1,908	6.0	42	1	2	4	8	14	18	31
65+	2,351	7.8	51	2	3	6	10	16	20	33
GRAND TOTAL	6,158	6.4	42	1	2	4	8	14	18	30

55.02: NEPHROSTOMY

Type of Patients	Observed Patients	Avg. Stay	Vari- ance	10th	25th	50th	75th	90th	95th	99th
1. SINGLE DX										
0–19 Years	0									
20–34	0									
35–49	0									
50–64	3	3.0	3	2	2	2	5	5	5	5
65+	0									
2. MULTIPLE DX										
0–19 Years	13	4.5	9	2	2	3	7	10	10	10
20–34	50	5.7	16	2	3	5	8	11	15	18
35–49	97	7.6	34	2	3	6	10	17	20	28
50–64	195	8.6	82	2	4	6	11	16	21	45
65+	309	9.7	79	3	4	7	12	18	27	53
TOTAL SINGLE DX	3	3.0	3	2	2	2	5	5	5	5
TOTAL MULTIPLE DX	664	8.6	68	2	4	7	10	16	22	45
TOTAL										
0–19 Years	13	4.5	9	2	2	3	7	10	10	10
20–34	50	5.7	16	2	3	5	8	11	15	18
35–49	97	7.6	34	2	3	6	10	17	20	28
50–64	198	8.5	81	2	4	6	11	16	21	45
65+	309	9.7	79	3	4	7	12	18	27	53
GRAND TOTAL	667	8.5	68	2	4	6	10	16	22	45

55.01: NEPHROTOMY

Type of Patients	Observed Patients	Avg. Stay	Vari- ance	10th	25th	50th	75th	90th	95th	99th
1. SINGLE DX										
0–19 Years	1	2.0	0	2	2	2	2	2	2	2
20–34	14	2.2	1	1	1	2	3	4	4	4
35–49	8	3.3	3	1	2	3	3	6	6	6
50–64	16	2.1	2	1	1	2	2	5	5	5
65+	5	2.4	<1	2	2	2	2	4	4	4
2. MULTIPLE DX										
0–19 Years	6	6.1	8	2	5	7	7	11	11	11
20–34	51	4.5	62	1	2	3	4	7	9	59
35–49	92	5.7	69	1	2	3	5	15	25	53
50–64	160	3.9	22	1	2	3	4	7	13	22
65+	106	3.8	12	1	2	3	4	8	10	19
TOTAL SINGLE DX	44	2.4	2	1	1	2	3	5	5	6
TOTAL MULTIPLE DX	415	4.4	35	1	2	3	4	8	13	31
TOTAL										
0–19 Years	7	4.9	9	2	2	5	7	7	11	11
20–34	65	4.1	51	1	2	3	4	6	9	59
35–49	100	5.5	64	1	2	3	5	15	25	53
50–64	176	3.7	20	1	2	3	4	7	11	22
65+	111	3.7	12	1	2	3	4	7	10	19
GRAND TOTAL	459	4.2	32	1	2	3	4	7	12	31

55.03: PERC NEPHROSTOMY S FRAG

Type of Patients	Observed Patients	Avg. Stay	Vari- ance	10th	25th	50th	75th	90th	95th	99th
1. SINGLE DX										
0–19 Years	3	2.3	<1	1	2	2	3	3	3	3
20–34	13	2.8	3	1	2	2	3	6	6	6
35–49	16	1.7	<1	1	1	1	2	3	4	4
50–64	16	1.7	<1	1	1	1	2	3	4	4
65+	8	3.0	5	2	2	2	3	8	8	8
2. MULTIPLE DX										
0–19 Years	77	6.3	25	2	3	4	8	13	16	21
20–34	377	5.5	36	2	2	4	7	10	14	29
35–49	626	6.2	31	2	3	4	8	13	17	28
50–64	1,078	7.3	44	2	3	5	10	15	21	33
65+	1,675	8.4	50	2	4	7	11	16	21	31
TOTAL SINGLE DX	56	2.2	2	1	1	2	3	3	4	8
TOTAL MULTIPLE DX	3,833	7.4	44	2	3	6	10	15	20	31
TOTAL										
0–19 Years	80	6.0	24	2	3	4	8	13	16	21
20–34	390	5.5	35	1	2	4	7	10	14	29
35–49	642	6.1	31	1	2	4	8	13	17	28
50–64	1,094	7.2	44	2	3	5	10	15	21	33
65+	1,683	8.4	50	2	4	7	11	16	21	31
GRAND TOTAL	3,889	7.3	44	2	3	5	9	15	20	31

LOS by Diagnosis and Operation, Western Region, 45th Edition

Western Region, October 2007–September 2008 Data, by Operation

55.04: PERC NEPHROSTOMY W FRAG

Type of Patients	Observed Patients	Avg. Stay	Vari-ance	Percentiles						
				10th	25th	50th	75th	90th	95th	99th
1. SINGLE DX										
0–19 Years	5	3.9	2	2	4	4	4	7	7	7
20–34	30	2.3	1	1	1	2	3	4	4	5
35–49	37	2.3	1	1	2	2	3	4	4	5
50–64	29	1.9	1	1	2	2	2	3	3	6
65+	4	1.8	<1	1	1	2	2	3	3	3
2. MULTIPLE DX										
0–19 Years	18	3.4	6	1	2	2	5	8	8	10
20–34	124	3.3	8	1	2	2	4	6	8	18
35–49	241	3.5	16	1	2	3	4	6	8	26
50–64	411	3.0	9	1	2	2	3	5	8	15
65+	244	3.5	11	1	2	2	4	6	9	18
TOTAL SINGLE DX	105	2.3	1	1	1	2	3	4	4	6
TOTAL MULTIPLE DX	1,038	3.3	11	1	2	2	4	6	8	17
TOTAL										
0–19 Years	23	3.5	5	1	2	3	5	8	8	10
20–34	154	3.1	7	1	1	2	4	5	7	18
35–49	278	3.4	14	1	2	3	4	6	7	26
50–64	440	2.9	8	1	1	2	3	5	8	15
65+	248	3.4	11	1	2	2	4	6	9	18
GRAND TOTAL	1,143	3.2	10	1	2	2	4	6	8	17

55.11: PYELOTOMY

Type of Patients	Observed Patients	Avg. Stay	Vari-ance	Percentiles						
				10th	25th	50th	75th	90th	95th	99th
1. SINGLE DX										
0–19 Years	0									
20–34	1	4.0	0	4	4	4	4	4	4	4
35–49	1	3.0	0	3	3	3	3	3	3	3
50–64	1	2.0	0	2	2	2	2	2	2	2
65+	0									
2. MULTIPLE DX										
0–19 Years	5	2.3	4	1	1	2	2	4	8	8
20–34	11	3.8	5	1	3	3	6	6	8	8
35–49	23	4.3	21	1	2	3	5	9	11	22
50–64	21	4.9	12	1	2	4	6	10	11	12
65+	17	4.0	12	1	1	3	5	9	14	14
TOTAL SINGLE DX	3	3.0	<1	2	2	3	4	4	4	4
TOTAL MULTIPLE DX	77	4.1	13	1	2	3	5	9	11	22
TOTAL										
0–19 Years	5	2.3	4	1	1	2	2	4	8	8
20–34	12	3.8	4	1	3	3	4	6	8	8
35–49	24	4.2	21	1	2	3	5	9	11	22
50–64	22	4.8	12	1	2	4	6	10	11	12
65+	17	4.0	12	1	1	3	5	9	14	14
GRAND TOTAL	80	4.0	12	1	2	3	5	9	11	22

55.2: RENAL DIAGNOSTIC PX

Type of Patients	Observed Patients	Avg. Stay	Vari-ance	Percentiles						
				10th	25th	50th	75th	90th	95th	99th
1. SINGLE DX										
0–19 Years	80	1.5	1	1	1	1	1	4	4	6
20–34	14	2.5	5	1	1	1	4	5	8	8
35–49	14	1.3	<1	1	1	1	1	2	4	4
50–64	4	3.3	11	1	1	3	8	8	8	8
65+	1	1.0	0	1	1	1	1	1	1	1
2. MULTIPLE DX										
0–19 Years	526	4.9	57	1	1	3	6	11	15	41
20–34	574	6.3	42	1	2	5	8	12	17	30
35–49	630	6.5	36	1	2	5	9	13	17	30
50–64	877	7.0	50	1	3	5	9	15	21	29
65+	694	7.3	35	2	3	6	10	15	19	28
TOTAL SINGLE DX	113	1.6	2	1	1	1	1	4	5	7
TOTAL MULTIPLE DX	3,301	6.3	46	1	2	5	8	13	18	30
TOTAL										
0–19 Years	606	4.4	49	1	1	2	5	9	14	30
20–34	588	6.2	42	1	2	5	8	12	17	28
35–49	644	6.4	35	1	2	5	8	13	17	30
50–64	881	7.0	50	1	2	5	9	15	20	29
65+	695	7.3	35	2	3	6	10	15	19	28
GRAND TOTAL	3,414	6.0	45	1	2	4	8	13	18	30

55.1: PYELOTOMY & PYELOSTOMY

Type of Patients	Observed Patients	Avg. Stay	Vari-ance	Percentiles						
				10th	25th	50th	75th	90th	95th	99th
1. SINGLE DX										
0–19 Years	0									
20–34	1	4.0	0	4	4	4	4	4	4	4
35–49	1	3.0	0	3	3	3	3	3	3	3
50–64	1	2.0	0	2	2	2	2	2	2	2
65+	0									
2. MULTIPLE DX										
0–19 Years	14	5.2	29	1	1	3	6	12	12	24
20–34	22	5.1	7	3	3	5	8	8	9	12
35–49	33	6.2	66	1	2	4	6	13	22	43
50–64	31	6.3	26	1	2	5	10	12	15	21
65+	30	5.6	22	1	3	4	7	14	15	20
TOTAL SINGLE DX	3	3.0	<1	2	2	3	4	4	4	4
TOTAL MULTIPLE DX	130	5.7	31	1	2	4	7	12	15	24
TOTAL										
0–19 Years	14	5.2	29	1	1	3	6	12	12	24
20–34	23	5.0	7	3	3	5	6	8	9	12
35–49	34	6.1	64	1	2	4	6	13	22	43
50–64	32	6.2	25	1	2	5	10	12	15	21
65+	30	5.6	22	1	3	4	7	14	15	20
GRAND TOTAL	133	5.7	31	1	2	4	7	12	15	24

LOS by Diagnosis and Operation, Western Region, 45th Edition

Western Region, October 2007–September 2008 Data, by Operation

55.33: PERC ABLAT RENAL LESION

Type of Patients	Observed Patients	Avg. Stay	Vari-ance	10th	25th	50th	75th	90th	95th	99th
1. SINGLE DX										
0–19 Years	0									
20–34	1	1.0	0	1	1	1	1	1	1	1
35–49	1	2.0	0	2	2	2	2	2	2	2
50–64	2	2.5	4	1	1	1	4	4	4	4
65+	3	1.0	0	1	1	1	1	1	1	1
2. MULTIPLE DX										
0–19 Years	1	2.0	0	2	2	2	2	2	2	2
20–34	1	8.0	0	8	8	8	8	8	8	8
35–49	2	4.0	8	2	2	2	2	6	6	8
50–64	24	2.7	18	1	1	1	2	6	10	20
65+	59	2.1	4	1	1	1	2	5	8	10
TOTAL SINGLE DX	7	1.6	1	1	1	1	2	4	4	4
TOTAL MULTIPLE DX	87	2.4	8	1	1	1	2	5	8	20
TOTAL										
0–19 Years	1	2.0	0	2	2	2	2	2	2	2
20–34	2	4.5	24	1	1	8	8	8	8	8
35–49	3	3.3	5	2	2	2	2	6	6	6
50–64	26	2.7	17	1	1	1	2	6	10	20
65+	62	2.1	4	1	1	1	2	5	8	10
GRAND TOTAL	94	2.3	8	1	1	1	2	5	8	20

55.34: LAPSCP ABLAT RENAL LES

Type of Patients	Observed Patients	Avg. Stay	Vari-ance	10th	25th	50th	75th	90th	95th	99th
1. SINGLE DX										
0–19 Years	1	2.0	0	2	2	2	2	2	2	2
20–34	1	1.0	0	1	1	1	1	1	1	1
35–49	1	1.0	0	1	1	1	1	1	1	1
50–64	12	1.5	<1	1	1	1	2	2	2	2
65+	4	1.8	<1	1	1	2	3	3	3	3
2. MULTIPLE DX										
0–19 Years	3	1.6	<1	1	1	1	2	2	>99	>99
20–34	10	1.7	2	1	1	1	2	3	5	5
35–49	23	3.0	5	1	2	2	3	6	9	10
50–64	94	2.5	5	1	1	2	3	5	6	16
65+	212	2.7	5	1	1	2	3	5	6	14
TOTAL SINGLE DX	19	1.5	<1	1	1	1	2	2	3	3
TOTAL MULTIPLE DX	342	2.6	5	1	1	2	3	5	6	14
TOTAL										
0–19 Years	4	1.6	<1	1	1	1	2	2	>99	>99
20–34	11	1.6	2	1	1	1	3	3	5	5
35–49	24	2.9	5	1	2	2	3	5	9	10
50–64	106	2.4	4	1	1	2	3	4	5	8
65+	216	2.7	5	1	1	2	3	5	6	14
GRAND TOTAL	361	2.5	4	1	1	2	3	4	6	14

55.23: CLOSED RENAL BIOPSY

Type of Patients	Observed Patients	Avg. Stay	Vari-ance	10th	25th	50th	75th	90th	95th	99th
1. SINGLE DX										
0–19 Years	78	1.5	1	1	1	1	1	3	4	6
20–34	14	2.5	5	1	1	1	4	5	8	8
35–49	14	1.3	<1	1	1	1	1	2	4	4
50–64	3	3.4	16	1	1	1	8	8	8	8
65+	1	1.0	0	1	1	1	1	1	1	1
2. MULTIPLE DX										
0–19 Years	499	4.4	34	1	1	2	6	9	14	30
20–34	567	6.3	42	1	2	5	8	12	17	30
35–49	616	6.6	36	1	2	5	9	13	17	30
50–64	865	7.0	49	1	2	5	9	15	20	29
65+	677	7.4	34	2	3	6	10	15	19	26
TOTAL SINGLE DX	110	1.5	2	1	1	1	1	4	5	7
TOTAL MULTIPLE DX	3,224	6.2	40	1	2	5	8	13	18	29
TOTAL										
0–19 Years	577	3.9	30	1	1	2	5	9	12	28
20–34	581	6.2	41	1	2	5	8	12	17	30
35–49	630	6.4	36	1	2	5	8	13	17	30
50–64	868	7.0	48	1	2	5	9	15	20	29
65+	678	7.4	34	2	3	6	10	15	19	26
GRAND TOTAL	3,334	5.9	39	1	2	4	8	13	17	28

55.3: LOC EXC/DESTR RENAL LES

Type of Patients	Observed Patients	Avg. Stay	Vari-ance	10th	25th	50th	75th	90th	95th	99th
1. SINGLE DX										
0–19 Years	2	2.5	<1	2	2	3	3	3	3	3
20–34	4	1.0	0	1	1	1	1	1	1	1
35–49	4	1.8	<1	1	1	1	2	2	3	3
50–64	18	1.7	<1	1	1	1	2	4	4	4
65+	16	1.6	<1	1	1	1	3	3	3	3
2. MULTIPLE DX										
0–19 Years	6	1.5	<1	1	1	1	2	2	>99	>99
20–34	18	2.5	4	1	1	2	3	5	8	8
35–49	54	3.8	25	1	2	3	4	6	10	36
50–64	171	2.9	13	1	1	2	4	5	8	20
65+	375	2.8	5	1	1	2	4	5	7	14
TOTAL SINGLE DX	44	1.6	<1	1	1	1	2	3	3	4
TOTAL MULTIPLE DX	624	2.9	9	1	1	2	4	5	8	15
TOTAL										
0–19 Years	8	1.6	<1	1	1	2	2	3	>99	>99
20–34	22	2.2	3	1	1	2	3	4	5	8
35–49	58	3.7	23	1	2	2	4	6	10	36
50–64	189	2.8	12	1	1	2	3	5	8	20
65+	391	2.7	5	1	1	2	4	5	7	14
GRAND TOTAL	668	2.8	9	1	1	2	3	5	7	15

LOS by Diagnosis and Operation, Western Region, 45th Edition

Western Region, October 2007–September 2008 Data, by Operation

55.39: LOC DESTR RENAL LES NEC

Type of Patients	Observed Patients	Avg. Stay	Vari-ance	Percentiles						
				10th	25th	50th	75th	90th	95th	99th
1. SINGLE DX										
0–19 Years	1	3.0	0	3	3	3	3	3	3	3
20–34	2	1.0	0	1	1	1	1	1	1	1
35–49	2	2.0	2	1	1	2	3	3	3	3
50–64	4	2.0	2	1	1	1	2	4	4	4
65+	4	2.0	1	1	1	3	3	3	3	3
2. MULTIPLE DX										
0–19 Years	2	1.2	<1	1	1	1	1	2	2	2
20–34	5	2.6	1	1	2	3	3	4	4	4
35–49	19	3.2	5	1	2	3	4	5	11	11
50–64	38	3.1	6	1	1	2	4	8	10	10
65+	53	3.2	4	1	2	3	4	5	5	12
TOTAL SINGLE DX	13	1.9	1	1	1	1	3	3	4	4
TOTAL MULTIPLE DX	117	3.0	4	1	1	3	4	5	6	11
TOTAL										
0–19 Years	3	1.5	<1	1	1	1	2	3	3	3
20–34	7	2.1	1	1	1	2	3	4	4	4
35–49	21	3.0	5	1	2	2	4	4	5	11
50–64	42	3.0	6	1	1	2	4	6	8	10
65+	57	3.1	3	1	2	3	4	5	5	12
GRAND TOTAL	130	2.9	4	1	1	3	4	5	6	11

55.4: PARTIAL NEPHRECTOMY

Type of Patients	Observed Patients	Avg. Stay	Vari-ance	Percentiles						
				10th	25th	50th	75th	90th	95th	99th
1. SINGLE DX										
0–19 Years	5	4.7	5	3	3	4	8	8	8	8
20–34	13	3.7	<1	3	3	4	4	5	5	5
35–49	29	3.7	2	2	2	4	4	6	6	8
50–64	51	3.1	2	2	2	3	4	5	5	9
65+	9	3.3	3	1	2	4	5	5	5	5
2. MULTIPLE DX										
0–19 Years	63	3.9	23	1	2	3	4	5	9	25
20–34	51	4.7	40	2	3	4	5	6	7	48
35–49	294	4.0	5	2	3	4	5	6	7	15
50–64	681	4.1	10	2	3	4	5	6	8	12
65+	589	4.5	7	2	3	4	5	7	9	16
TOTAL SINGLE DX	107	3.5	3	2	3	3	4	5	8	8
TOTAL MULTIPLE DX	1,678	4.2	10	2	3	4	5	7	9	16
TOTAL										
0–19 Years	68	4.0	21	1	2	3	4	8	9	25
20–34	64	4.5	32	2	3	4	5	6	7	48
35–49	323	4.0	5	2	3	4	5	6	7	13
50–64	732	4.0	9	2	3	4	5	6	8	12
65+	598	4.5	7	2	3	4	5	7	9	16
GRAND TOTAL	1,785	4.2	10	2	3	4	5	7	8	15

55.5: COMPLETE NEPHRECTOMY

Type of Patients	Observed Patients	Avg. Stay	Vari-ance	Percentiles						
				10th	25th	50th	75th	90th	95th	99th
1. SINGLE DX										
0–19 Years	35	3.4	8	1	1	2	6	7	11	11
20–34	191	2.4	<1	1	2	2	3	4	4	5
35–49	227	2.7	1	1	2	3	3	4	5	6
50–64	243	2.7	2	1	2	3	3	4	5	7
65+	47	3.2	2	2	2	3	4	4	6	8
2. MULTIPLE DX										
0–19 Years	260	7.5	159	1	2	4	8	15	29	69
20–34	423	6.0	58	2	3	4	6	13	21	45
35–49	1,073	4.7	27	2	2	3	5	8	11	30
50–64	2,511	4.9	29	2	3	4	5	8	12	28
65+	2,691	5.5	26	2	3	4	6	10	14	28
TOTAL SINGLE DX	743	2.7	2	1	2	3	3	4	5	8
TOTAL MULTIPLE DX	6,958	5.4	40	2	3	4	6	9	14	32
TOTAL										
0–19 Years	295	7.0	143	1	1	4	7	14	27	69
20–34	614	4.9	43	2	2	3	4	9	17	45
35–49	1,300	4.3	23	2	2	4	5	7	10	23
50–64	2,754	4.7	27	2	2	4	5	8	12	26
65+	2,738	5.5	26	2	3	4	6	10	14	27
GRAND TOTAL	7,701	5.1	37	2	2	4	5	9	13	31

55.51: NEPHROURETERECTOMY

Type of Patients	Observed Patients	Avg. Stay	Vari-ance	Percentiles						
				10th	25th	50th	75th	90th	95th	99th
1. SINGLE DX										
0–19 Years	35	3.4	8	1	1	2	6	7	11	11
20–34	191	2.4	<1	1	2	2	3	4	4	5
35–49	227	2.7	1	1	2	3	3	4	5	6
50–64	243	2.7	2	1	2	3	3	4	5	7
65+	47	3.2	2	2	2	3	4	4	6	8
2. MULTIPLE DX										
0–19 Years	233	6.4	127	1	1	3	7	11	19	69
20–34	362	5.4	44	2	3	3	5	10	19	45
35–49	989	4.5	21	2	2	3	5	8	11	24
50–64	2,415	4.7	26	2	3	4	5	8	12	26
65+	2,648	5.5	25	2	3	4	6	10	13	26
TOTAL SINGLE DX	743	2.7	2	1	2	3	3	4	5	8
TOTAL MULTIPLE DX	6,647	5.1	34	2	3	4	6	9	13	30
TOTAL										
0–19 Years	268	6.0	113	1	1	3	7	10	18	69
20–34	553	4.4	31	2	2	3	4	6	13	36
35–49	1,216	4.1	18	2	2	3	4	7	9	23
50–64	2,658	4.6	24	2	3	4	5	7	10	24
65+	2,695	5.4	25	2	3	4	6	9	13	26
GRAND TOTAL	7,390	4.9	31	2	2	4	5	8	12	29

LOS by Diagnosis and Operation, Western Region, 45th Edition

Western Region, October 2007–September 2008 Data, by Operation

55.53: REJECTED KID NEPHRECTOMY

Type of Patients	Observed Patients	Avg. Stay	Vari-ance	Percentiles						
				10th	25th	50th	75th	90th	95th	99th
1. SINGLE DX										
0–19 Years	0									
20–34	0									
35–49	0									
50–64	0									
65+	0									
2. MULTIPLE DX										
0–19 Years	15	7.7	34	3	3	6	14	18	18	21
20–34	53	8.2	56	3	4	5	10	18	22	45
35–49	53	5.6	16	2	3	4	7	11	14	20
50–64	47	8.5	138	2	3	4	10	14	28	72
65+	24	10.5	160	3	3	5	12	28	29	58
TOTAL SINGLE DX	**0**									
TOTAL MULTIPLE DX	**192**	**7.8**	**72**	**2**	**3**	**5**	**10**	**17**	**21**	**45**
TOTAL										
0–19 Years	15	7.7	34	3	3	6	14	18	18	21
20–34	53	8.2	56	3	4	5	10	18	22	45
35–49	53	5.6	16	2	3	4	7	11	14	20
50–64	47	8.5	138	2	3	4	10	14	28	72
65+	24	10.5	160	3	3	5	12	28	29	58
GRAND TOTAL	**192**	**7.8**	**72**	**2**	**3**	**5**	**10**	**17**	**21**	**45**

55.6: KIDNEY TRANSPLANT

Type of Patients	Observed Patients	Avg. Stay	Vari-ance	Percentiles						
				10th	25th	50th	75th	90th	95th	99th
1. SINGLE DX										
0–19 Years	1	4.0	0	4	4	4	4	4	4	4
20–34	0									
35–49	0									
50–64	2	5.0	0	5	5	5	5	5	5	5
65+	0									
2. MULTIPLE DX										
0–19 Years	145	10.1	25	5	7	9	12	15	21	31
20–34	390	6.8	31	3	4	5	7	11	15	31
35–49	738	6.6	18	4	4	6	8	11	15	23
50–64	1,172	7.0	27	4	5	6	8	11	14	26
65+	374	7.6	25	4	5	6	8	13	16	26
TOTAL SINGLE DX	**3**	**4.7**	**<1**	**4**	**4**	**5**	**5**	**5**	**5**	**5**
TOTAL MULTIPLE DX	**2,819**	**7.3**	**26**	**4**	**5**	**6**	**8**	**12**	**16**	**27**
TOTAL										
0–19 Years	146	10.0	25	5	7	9	12	15	21	31
20–34	390	6.8	31	3	4	5	7	11	15	31
35–49	738	6.6	18	4	4	6	8	11	15	23
50–64	1,174	7.0	27	4	5	6	8	11	14	26
65+	374	7.6	25	4	5	6	8	13	16	26
GRAND TOTAL	**2,822**	**7.3**	**26**	**4**	**5**	**6**	**8**	**12**	**16**	**26**

55.54: BILATERAL NEPHRECTOMY

Type of Patients	Observed Patients	Avg. Stay	Vari-ance	Percentiles						
				10th	25th	50th	75th	90th	95th	99th
1. SINGLE DX										
0–19 Years	0									
20–34	0									
35–49	0									
50–64	0									
65+	0									
2. MULTIPLE DX										
0–19 Years	10	21.4	523	5	7	7	27	59	67	67
20–34	7	20.9	629	1	2	10	45	67	67	67
35–49	22	7.3	95	2	3	6	8	10	10	49
50–64	39	8.2	33	4	5	6	10	19	23	24
65+	11	8.3	52	3	4	5	14	14	26	26
TOTAL SINGLE DX	**0**									
TOTAL MULTIPLE DX	**89**	**12.2**	**240**	**3**	**4**	**7**	**10**	**27**	**59**	**67**
TOTAL										
0–19 Years	10	21.4	523	5	7	7	27	59	67	67
20–34	7	20.9	629	1	2	10	45	67	67	67
35–49	22	7.3	95	2	3	6	8	10	10	49
50–64	39	8.2	33	4	5	6	10	19	23	24
65+	11	8.3	52	3	4	5	14	14	26	26
GRAND TOTAL	**89**	**12.2**	**240**	**3**	**4**	**7**	**10**	**27**	**59**	**67**

55.69: KIDNEY TRANSPLANT NEC

Type of Patients	Observed Patients	Avg. Stay	Vari-ance	Percentiles						
				10th	25th	50th	75th	90th	95th	99th
1. SINGLE DX										
0–19 Years	1	4.0	0	4	4	4	4	4	4	4
20–34	0									
35–49	0									
50–64	2	5.0	0	5	5	5	5	5	5	5
65+	0									
2. MULTIPLE DX										
0–19 Years	144	10.1	25	5	7	9	12	15	21	31
20–34	390	6.8	31	3	4	5	7	11	15	31
35–49	736	6.7	18	4	4	6	8	11	15	23
50–64	1,169	7.0	27	4	5	6	8	11	15	26
65+	374	7.6	25	4	5	6	8	13	16	26
TOTAL SINGLE DX	**3**	**4.7**	**<1**	**4**	**4**	**5**	**5**	**5**	**5**	**5**
TOTAL MULTIPLE DX	**2,813**	**7.3**	**26**	**4**	**5**	**6**	**8**	**12**	**16**	**27**
TOTAL										
0–19 Years	145	10.1	25	5	7	9	12	15	21	31
20–34	390	6.8	31	3	4	5	7	11	15	31
35–49	736	6.7	18	4	4	6	8	11	15	23
50–64	1,171	7.0	27	4	5	6	8	11	14	26
65+	374	7.6	25	4	5	6	8	13	16	26
GRAND TOTAL	**2,816**	**7.3**	**26**	**4**	**5**	**6**	**8**	**12**	**16**	**27**

LOS by Diagnosis and Operation, Western Region, 45th Edition

Western Region, October 2007–September 2008 Data, by Operation

55.7: NEPHROPEXY

Type of Patients	Observed Patients	Avg. Stay	Vari- ance	Percentiles						
				10th	25th	50th	75th	90th	95th	99th
1. SINGLE DX										
0–19 Years	0									
20–34	0									
35–49	1	1.0	0	1	1	1	1	1	1	1
50–64	2	1.5	<1	1	1	2	2	2	2	2
65+	0									
2. MULTIPLE DX										
0–19 Years	1	1.0	0	1	1	1	1	1	1	1
20–34	2	2.0	0	2	2	2	2	2	2	2
35–49	5	1.4	<1	1	1	1	2	2	2	2
50–64	1	1.3	<1	1	1	1	1	2	2	2
65+	0	1.3	0	1	1	1	1	2	1	1
TOTAL SINGLE DX	3	1.3	<1	1	1	2	2	2	2	2
TOTAL MULTIPLE DX	9	1.3	<1	1	1	2	2	2	2	2
TOTAL										
0–19 Years	1	1.0	0	1	1	2	1	1	1	1
20–34	2	2.0	0	2	2	2	2	2	2	2
35–49	6	1.3	<1	1	1	1	2	2	2	2
50–64	3	1.3	<1	1	1	1	2	2	2	2
65+	0									
GRAND TOTAL	12	1.3	<1	1	1	2	2	2	2	2

55.8: OTHER KIDNEY REPAIR

Type of Patients	Observed Patients	Avg. Stay	Vari- ance	Percentiles						
				10th	25th	50th	75th	90th	95th	99th
1. SINGLE DX										
0–19 Years	120	2.0	1	1	1	2	2	3	4	6
20–34	27	2.2	1	1	1	2	3	4	4	6
35–49	18	2.4	1	1	2	2	3	4	4	4
50–64	6	2.7	<1	1	2	3	4	4	4	4
65+	2	2.0	0	2	2	2	2	2	2	2
2. MULTIPLE DX										
0–19 Years	363	3.2	19	1	1	2	3	5	9	18
20–34	166	3.2	5	1	2	3	4	5	7	12
35–49	110	3.7	39	1	2	3	4	6	11	16
50–64	119	3.0	<1	1	2	3	4	6	7	12
65+	75	3.3	6	1	2	3	4	6	8	12
TOTAL SINGLE DX	173	2.0	1	1	1	2	3	3	4	6
TOTAL MULTIPLE DX	833	3.2	17	1	2	2	3	5	9	18
TOTAL										
0–19 Years	483	2.9	15	1	1	2	3	5	8	18
20–34	193	3.0	5	1	2	2	4	5	6	12
35–49	128	3.5	33	1	2	2	4	5	9	16
50–64	125	3.0	4	1	2	3	4	5	6	12
65+	77	3.3	6	2	2	2	4	6	8	12
GRAND TOTAL	1,006	3.0	14	1	2	2	3	5	8	17

55.87: CORRECTION OF UPJ

Type of Patients	Observed Patients	Avg. Stay	Vari- ance	Percentiles						
				10th	25th	50th	75th	90th	95th	99th
1. SINGLE DX										
0–19 Years	119	2.0	1	1	1	2	2	3	4	6
20–34	27	2.2	1	1	1	2	3	4	4	6
35–49	18	2.4	<1	1	2	2	3	4	4	4
50–64	6	2.7	1	1	2	3	4	4	4	4
65+	2	2.0	0	2	2	2	2	2	2	2
2. MULTIPLE DX										
0–19 Years	349	3.2	20	1	1	2	3	5	9	18
20–34	154	2.8	2	1	2	3	3	5	5	9
35–49	101	3.6	41	1	2	2	4	5	9	61
50–64	114	2.9	3	1	2	2	4	5	6	8
65+	73	3.3	6	1	2	2	4	6	8	12
TOTAL SINGLE DX	172	2.0	1	1	1	2	3	3	4	6
TOTAL MULTIPLE DX	791	3.1	17	1	2	2	3	5	8	18
TOTAL										
0–19 Years	468	2.9	16	1	1	2	3	4	7	18
20–34	181	2.7	2	1	2	2	3	4	5	9
35–49	119	3.4	35	1	2	2	3	5	9	16
50–64	120	2.9	3	1	2	2	4	5	6	8
65+	75	3.2	6	1	2	2	4	6	8	12
GRAND TOTAL	963	2.9	14	1	1	2	3	5	6	17

55.9: OTHER RENAL OPERATIONS

Type of Patients	Observed Patients	Avg. Stay	Vari- ance	Percentiles						
				10th	25th	50th	75th	90th	95th	99th
1. SINGLE DX										
0–19 Years	2	2.0	0	2	2	2	2	2	2	2
20–34	4	1.3	<1	1	1	1	1	2	2	2
35–49	3	1.3	<1	1	1	1	2	2	2	2
50–64	2	1.5	<1	1	1	1	2	2	2	2
65+	2	1.0	0	1	1	1	1	1	1	1
2. MULTIPLE DX										
0–19 Years	14	3.6	5	2	2	2	6	7	7	7
20–34	102	4.5	11	1	2	4	6	9	10	16
35–49	200	5.3	33	1	2	4	6	11	13	33
50–64	282	5.6	26	1	2	4	7	11	16	29
65+	399	5.0	25	1	2	4	6	9	12	23
TOTAL SINGLE DX	13	1.5	<1	1	1	2	2	2	2	2
TOTAL MULTIPLE DX	997	5.1	25	1	2	4	6	9	13	24
TOTAL										
0–19 Years	16	3.3	4	2	2	2	4	7	7	7
20–34	106	4.4	11	1	2	4	6	9	10	16
35–49	203	5.3	32	1	2	4	6	9	13	33
50–64	284	5.5	26	1	2	4	7	11	16	29
65+	401	5.0	25	1	2	4	6	9	12	23
GRAND TOTAL	1,010	5.1	25	1	2	4	6	9	13	24

LOS by Diagnosis and Operation, Western Region, 45th Edition

Western Region, October 2007–September 2008 Data, by Operation

55.92: PERC RENAL ASPIRATION

Type of Patients	Observed Patients	Avg. Stay	Variance	10th	25th	50th	75th	90th	95th	99th
1. SINGLE DX										
0–19 Years	2	2.0	0	2	2	2	2	2	2	2
20–34	3	1.3	<1	1	1	1	2	2	2	2
35–49	1	2.0	0	2	2	2	2	2	2	2
50–64	0									
65+	0									
2. MULTIPLE DX										
0–19 Years	5	4.1	5	2	2	5	6	7	7	7
20–34	31	5.2	8	2	3	5	8	9	9	13
35–49	41	5.6	5	3	4	5	7	8	9	13
50–64	38	6.3	35	1	3	6	6	15	19	31
65+	51	6.6	26	2	3	6	9	12	16	28
TOTAL SINGLE DX	6	1.8	<1	1	2	2	2	2	2	2
TOTAL MULTIPLE DX	166	5.9	19	2	3	5	7	10	13	28
TOTAL										
0–19 Years	7	3.1	4	2	2	2	5	6	7	7
20–34	34	4.9	9	1	2	4	7	9	9	13
35–49	42	5.5	5	3	4	5	7	8	9	13
50–64	38	6.3	35	1	3	6	6	15	19	31
65+	51	6.6	26	2	3	6	9	12	16	28
GRAND TOTAL	172	5.7	19	2	3	5	7	9	13	28

55.93: REPL NEPHROSTOMY TUBE

Type of Patients	Observed Patients	Avg. Stay	Variance	10th	25th	50th	75th	90th	95th	99th
1. SINGLE DX										
0–19 Years	0									
20–34	1	1.0	0	1	1	1	1	1	1	1
35–49	1	1.0	0	1	1	1	1	1	1	1
50–64	0									
65+	2	1.0	0	1	1	1	1	1	1	1
2. MULTIPLE DX										
0–19 Years	9	3.4	5	2	2	2	4	7	7	7
20–34	69	4.2	11	1	2	4	5	7	12	16
35–49	148	5.4	42	1	2	4	6	10	14	43
50–64	230	5.6	26	1	2	4	7	11	16	24
65+	333	4.9	25	1	2	4	6	9	11	23
TOTAL SINGLE DX	4	1.0	0	1	1	1	1	1	1	1
TOTAL MULTIPLE DX	789	5.1	27	1	2	4	6	10	14	24
TOTAL										
0–19 Years	9	3.4	5	2	2	2	4	7	7	7
20–34	70	4.2	11	1	2	4	5	7	12	16
35–49	149	5.4	42	1	2	4	6	10	14	43
50–64	230	5.6	26	1	2	4	7	11	16	24
65+	335	4.9	25	1	2	4	6	9	11	23
GRAND TOTAL	793	5.1	27	1	2	4	6	10	14	24

56.0: TU RMVL URETERAL OBSTR

Type of Patients	Observed Patients	Avg. Stay	Variance	10th	25th	50th	75th	90th	95th	99th
1. SINGLE DX										
0–19 Years	13	1.9	3	1	1	1	2	4	6	6
20–34	85	1.6	<1	1	1	1	2	2	3	6
35–49	109	1.5	<1	1	1	1	2	3	4	4
50–64	66	1.5	<1	1	1	1	2	2	3	4
65+	16	1.6	1	1	1	1	2	3	5	5
2. MULTIPLE DX										
0–19 Years	126	2.6	5	1	1	2	3	5	8	12
20–34	963	2.3	4	1	1	2	3	4	6	9
35–49	1,404	2.6	6	1	1	2	3	5	7	14
50–64	1,666	2.9	13	1	1	2	3	5	9	17
65+	1,235	4.0	19	1	1	3	5	9	12	23
TOTAL SINGLE DX	289	1.6	<1	1	1	1	2	3	3	5
TOTAL MULTIPLE DX	5,394	3.0	11	1	1	2	3	6	9	17
TOTAL										
0–19 Years	139	2.6	5	1	1	2	3	5	7	12
20–34	1,048	2.3	3	1	1	2	3	4	6	9
35–49	1,513	2.5	6	1	1	2	3	5	7	14
50–64	1,732	2.8	13	1	1	2	3	5	8	17
65+	1,251	4.0	19	1	1	3	5	9	12	23
GRAND TOTAL	5,683	2.9	11	1	1	2	3	6	8	16

56.1: URETERAL MEATOTOMY

Type of Patients	Observed Patients	Avg. Stay	Variance	10th	25th	50th	75th	90th	95th	99th
1. SINGLE DX										
0–19 Years	0									
20–34	0									
35–49	0									
50–64	0									
65+	0									
2. MULTIPLE DX										
0–19 Years	0									
20–34	3	7.7	65	3	3	3	17	17	17	17
35–49	8	2.4	3	1	2	3	5	6	6	6
50–64	7	3.9	9	1	2	3	5	10	10	10
65+	7	2.7	3	1	2	2	4	6	6	6
TOTAL SINGLE DX	0									
TOTAL MULTIPLE DX	25	3.5	12	1	2	2	4	6	10	17
TOTAL										
0–19 Years	0									
20–34	3	7.7	65	3	3	3	17	17	17	17
35–49	8	2.4	3	1	2	3	5	6	6	6
50–64	7	3.9	9	1	2	3	5	10	10	10
65+	7	2.7	3	1	2	2	4	6	6	6
GRAND TOTAL	25	3.5	12	1	2	2	4	6	10	17

LOS by Diagnosis and Operation, Western Region, 45th Edition

Western Region, October 2007–September 2008 Data, by Operation

56.2: URETEROTOMY

Type of Patients	Observed Patients	Avg. Stay	Variance	10th	25th	50th	75th	90th	95th	99th
1. SINGLE DX										
0–19 Years	3	1.2	<1	1	1	1	1	2	2	2
20–34	2	1.5	<1	1	1	1	2	2	2	2
35–49	2	1.0	0	1	1	1	1	1	1	1
50–64	2	1.5	<1	1	1	1	2	2	2	2
65+	1	2.0	0	2	2	2	2	2	2	2
2. MULTIPLE DX										
0–19 Years	23	5.1	82	1	1	2	7	7	10	58
20–34	18	3.1	4	1	1	3	4	6	8	8
35–49	25	3.0	3	1	2	2	4	6	7	7
50–64	45	4.4	81	1	2	2	4	7	9	61
65+	56	5.2	18	2	2	4	7	12	15	20
TOTAL SINGLE DX	10	1.3	<1	1	1	1	2	2	2	2
TOTAL MULTIPLE DX	167	4.5	45	1	1	3	5	8	12	58
TOTAL										
0–19 Years	26	4.6	74	1	1	2	7	7	10	58
20–34	20	2.9	4	1	1	2	4	6	8	8
35–49	27	2.8	3	1	1	2	4	6	7	7
50–64	47	4.3	78	1	1	2	4	7	9	61
65+	57	5.1	18	2	2	4	6	12	15	20
GRAND TOTAL	177	4.3	43	1	1	3	5	7	10	25

56.31: URETEROSCOPY

Type of Patients	Observed Patients	Avg. Stay	Variance	10th	25th	50th	75th	90th	95th	99th
1. SINGLE DX										
0–19 Years	1	2.0	0	2	2	2	2	2	2	2
20–34	6	1.2	<1	1	1	1	1	2	2	2
35–49	4	1.3	<1	1	1	1	2	2	2	2
50–64	8	1.4	<1	1	1	1	2	2	2	2
65+	0									
2. MULTIPLE DX										
0–19 Years	7	1.9	<1	1	1	2	3	3	3	3
20–34	42	2.7	3	1	1	2	3	5	7	9
35–49	53	3.2	9	1	1	2	4	6	11	16
50–64	57	3.1	4	1	2	2	3	6	7	10
65+	59	4.4	12	1	2	3	6	10	11	18
TOTAL SINGLE DX	19	1.3	<1	1	1	1	2	2	2	2
TOTAL MULTIPLE DX	218	3.4	8	1	2	3	4	7	10	13
TOTAL										
0–19 Years	8	1.9	<1	1	1	2	2	3	3	3
20–34	48	2.5	3	1	1	2	3	5	7	9
35–49	57	3.1	9	1	1	2	3	6	11	16
50–64	65	2.9	4	1	2	2	3	6	7	10
65+	59	4.4	12	1	2	3	6	10	11	18
GRAND TOTAL	237	3.2	7	1	1	2	4	7	10	13

56.3: URETERAL DIAGNOSTIC PX

Type of Patients	Observed Patients	Avg. Stay	Variance	10th	25th	50th	75th	90th	95th	99th
1. SINGLE DX										
0–19 Years	1	2.0	0	2	2	2	2	2	2	2
20–34	6	1.2	<1	1	1	1	1	2	2	2
35–49	4	1.3	<1	1	1	1	2	2	1	1
50–64	8	1.4	<1	1	1	2	2	2	2	2
65+	0									
2. MULTIPLE DX										
0–19 Years	8	1.8	<1	1	1	1	2	3	3	3
20–34	43	2.7	3	1	1	2	3	5	7	9
35–49	55	3.3	9	1	1	3	4	6	11	16
50–64	75	3.6	16	1	2	3	4	7	9	33
65+	106	4.6	14	1	2	3	6	11	12	17
TOTAL SINGLE DX	19	1.3	<1	1	1	1	2	2	2	2
TOTAL MULTIPLE DX	287	3.7	12	1	2	3	5	7	11	17
TOTAL										
0–19 Years	9	1.8	<1	1	1	2	2	3	3	3
20–34	49	2.5	3	1	1	2	3	5	7	9
35–49	59	3.1	8	1	1	2	4	6	11	16
50–64	83	3.4	15	1	2	2	4	6	8	33
65+	106	4.6	14	1	2	3	6	11	12	17
GRAND TOTAL	306	3.6	12	1	1	3	4	7	10	16

56.4: URETERECTOMY

Type of Patients	Observed Patients	Avg. Stay	Variance	10th	25th	50th	75th	90th	95th	99th
1. SINGLE DX										
0–19 Years	4	1.4	<1	1	1	1	1	4	4	4
20–34	0									
35–49	4	2.0	2	1	3	3	4	4	4	4
50–64	4	3.3	<1	3	3	3	4	4	4	4
65+	4	3.8	13	1	1	3	9	9	9	9
2. MULTIPLE DX										
0–19 Years	61	2.5	9	1	1	2	2	4	9	15
20–34	13	4.8	18	1	3	3	6	8	17	17
35–49	26	4.0	5	2	2	4	5	7	8	9
50–64	53	4.1	6	2	2	4	5	8	10	11
65+	154	5.1	22	2	2	4	5	10	14	27
TOTAL SINGLE DX	16	2.3	4	1	1	1	3	4	4	9
TOTAL MULTIPLE DX	307	3.9	15	1	2	3	4	8	12	18
TOTAL										
0–19 Years	65	2.5	9	1	1	2	2	4	9	15
20–34	13	4.8	18	1	2	3	6	8	17	17
35–49	30	3.7	5	2	2	3	5	6	8	9
50–64	57	4.0	6	2	2	4	5	8	10	11
65+	158	5.0	22	2	2	4	5	10	14	27
GRAND TOTAL	323	3.8	15	1	1	3	4	8	11	17

LOS by Diagnosis and Operation, Western Region, 45th Edition

Western Region, October 2007–September 2008 Data, by Operation

56.41: PARTIAL URETERECTOMY

Type of Patients	Observed Patients	Avg. Stay	Vari-ance	10th	25th	50th	75th	90th	95th	99th
1. SINGLE DX										
0–19 Years	4	1.4	<1	1	1	1	1	4	4	4
20–34	0									
35–49	4	2.0	2	1	4	2	4	4	4	4
50–64	1	4.0	0	4	4	4	4	4	4	4
65+	2	1.5	<1	1	1	1	2	2	2	2
2. MULTIPLE DX										
0–19 Years	60	2.5	9	1	1	2	2	4	9	15
20–34	12	5.1	18	1	3	3	6	8	17	17
35–49	24	4.1	5	2	2	4	6	7	8	9
50–64	42	3.8	5	1	2	4	5	6	8	11
65+	124	5.0	21	2	2	5	5	9	14	24
TOTAL SINGLE DX	11	1.7	1	1	1	1	2	4	4	4
TOTAL MULTIPLE DX	262	3.7	14	1	1	3	4	8	11	17
TOTAL										
0–19 Years	64	2.5	9	1	1	2	2	4	9	15
20–34	12	5.1	18	1	3	3	6	8	17	17
35–49	28	3.8	5	1	2	4	6	7	8	9
50–64	43	3.8	5	1	2	4	5	6	8	11
65+	126	4.9	21	2	2	4	5	9	14	24
GRAND TOTAL	273	3.6	14	1	1	3	4	8	11	17

56.5: CUTAN URETERO-ILEOSTOMY

Type of Patients	Observed Patients	Avg. Stay	Vari-ance	10th	25th	50th	75th	90th	95th	99th
1. SINGLE DX										
0–19 Years	0									
20–34	0									
35–49	0									
50–64	1	1.0	0	1	1	1	1	1	1	1
65+	1	7.0	0	7	7	7	7	7	7	7
2. MULTIPLE DX										
0–19 Years	8	6.1	20	1	1	6	8	14	14	14
20–34	12	11.5	33	5	7	12	12	16	28	28
35–49	21	13.0	124	6	7	9	18	32	51	>99
50–64	82	9.8	51	4	6	8	12	16	21	48
65+	134	11.7	72	5	7	9	13	20	28	50
TOTAL SINGLE DX	2	4.0	18	1	1	4	7	7	7	7
TOTAL MULTIPLE DX	257	10.7	65	4	6	8	13	19	27	51
TOTAL										
0–19 Years	8	6.1	20	1	1	6	8	14	14	14
20–34	12	11.5	33	5	7	12	12	16	28	28
35–49	21	13.0	124	6	7	9	18	32	51	>99
50–64	83	9.7	51	4	6	8	12	16	21	48
65+	135	11.6	72	5	7	9	13	20	28	50
GRAND TOTAL	259	10.7	65	4	6	8	13	19	27	51

56.51: FORM CUTAN ILEOURETEROST

Type of Patients	Observed Patients	Avg. Stay	Vari-ance	10th	25th	50th	75th	90th	95th	99th
1. SINGLE DX										
0–19 Years	0									
20–34	0									
35–49	0									
50–64	0									
65+	1	7.0	0	7	7	7	7	7	7	7
2. MULTIPLE DX										
0–19 Years	5	9.6	11	7	7	8	14	14	14	14
20–34	11	11.9	32	6	10	12	12	16	28	28
35–49	16	14.9	146	7	8	10	18	32	51	51
50–64	62	10.5	31	6	7	9	12	16	21	35
65+	116	12.3	74	5	7	9	14	22	28	50
TOTAL SINGLE DX	1	7.0	0	7	7	7	7	7	7	7
TOTAL MULTIPLE DX	210	11.8	62	6	7	9	13	20	27	50
TOTAL										
0–19 Years	5	9.6	11	7	7	8	14	14	14	14
20–34	11	11.9	32	6	10	12	12	16	28	28
35–49	16	14.9	146	7	8	10	18	32	51	51
50–64	62	10.5	31	6	7	9	12	16	21	35
65+	117	12.2	74	5	7	9	14	22	28	50
GRAND TOTAL	211	11.8	61	6	7	9	13	20	27	50

56.6: EXT URIN DIVERSION NEC

Type of Patients	Observed Patients	Avg. Stay	Vari-ance	10th	25th	50th	75th	90th	95th	99th
1. SINGLE DX										
0–19 Years	1	1.0	0	1	1	1	1	1	1	1
20–34	0									
35–49	0									
50–64	0									
65+	0									
2. MULTIPLE DX										
0–19 Years	16	5.2	39	1	1	1	7	20	20	20
20–34	3	5.3	10	3	3	4	9	9	9	9
35–49	1	3.0	0	3	2	5	3	3	3	3
50–64	7	5.6	15	2	1	4	8	13	13	13
65+	5	7.5	72	1	1	4	11	21	21	21
TOTAL SINGLE DX	1	1.0	0	1	1	1	1	1	1	1
TOTAL MULTIPLE DX	32	5.4	35	1	1	3	7	20	20	21
TOTAL										
0–19 Years	17	5.1	38	1	1	1	7	20	20	20
20–34	3	5.3	10	3	3	4	9	9	9	9
35–49	1	3.0	0	3	2	5	3	3	3	3
50–64	7	5.6	15	2	1	4	8	13	13	13
65+	5	7.5	72	1	1	4	11	21	21	21
GRAND TOTAL	33	5.4	35	1	1	3	7	20	20	21

LOS by Diagnosis and Operation, Western Region, 45th Edition

Western Region, October 2007–September 2008 Data, by Operation

56.7: OTHER URETERAL ANAST

Type of Patients	Observed Patients	Avg. Stay	Vari-ance	Percentiles						
				10th	25th	50th	75th	90th	95th	99th
1. SINGLE DX										
0–19 Years	218	1.8	<1	1	1	2	2	3	4	5
20–34	4	2.0	<1	1	1	2	2	3	3	3
35–49	2	5.5	12	3	3	8	8	8	8	8
50–64	3	3.0	7	1	1	2	6	6	6	6
65+	0									
2. MULTIPLE DX										
0–19 Years	641	2.6	4	1	1	2	3	5	6	10
20–34	50	4.3	7	2	3	4	5	8	10	14
35–49	105	5.3	19	2	3	4	6	9	12	24
50–64	106	5.6	13	2	3	5	7	10	12	15
65+	53	6.2	21	2	3	5	8	10	16	24
TOTAL SINGLE DX	227	1.8	<1	1	1	2	2	3	4	5
TOTAL MULTIPLE DX	955	3.1	7	1	2	2	3	6	8	14
TOTAL										
0–19 Years	859	2.4	3	1	1	2	3	4	6	9
20–34	54	4.2	7	2	2	3	5	8	10	14
35–49	107	5.3	19	2	2	4	6	9	12	24
50–64	109	5.5	13	2	3	5	7	10	12	15
65+	53	6.2	21	2	3	5	8	10	16	24
GRAND TOTAL	1,182	2.8	6	1	1	2	3	5	7	12

56.8: REPAIR OF URETER

Type of Patients	Observed Patients	Avg. Stay	Vari-ance	Percentiles						
				10th	25th	50th	75th	90th	95th	99th
1. SINGLE DX										
0–19 Years	2	2.0	1	1	1	2	3	3	3	3
20–34	0									
35–49	1	4.0	0	4	4	4	4	4	4	4
50–64	0									
65+	0									
2. MULTIPLE DX										
0–19 Years	21	2.7	3	1	1	2	4	6	6	7
20–34	6	7.7	66	3	4	4	7	24	24	24
35–49	9	5.8	16	3	3	4	6	14	14	14
50–64	11	4.6	12	1	3	4	5	6	14	14
65+	8	3.8	4	1	3	4	6	6	6	6
TOTAL SINGLE DX	3	2.2	1	1	1	3	3	4	4	4
TOTAL MULTIPLE DX	55	3.7	12	1	2	3	4	6	7	24
TOTAL										
0–19 Years	23	2.6	3	1	1	2	4	6	6	7
20–34	6	7.7	66	3	4	4	7	24	24	24
35–49	10	5.6	14	3	3	4	6	11	14	14
50–64	11	4.6	12	1	3	4	5	6	14	14
65+	8	3.8	4	1	3	4	6	6	6	6
GRAND TOTAL	58	3.6	11	1	2	3	4	6	7	24

56.74: URETERONEOCYSTOSTOMY

Type of Patients	Observed Patients	Avg. Stay	Vari-ance	Percentiles						
				10th	25th	50th	75th	90th	95th	99th
1. SINGLE DX										
0–19 Years	218	1.8	<1	1	1	2	2	3	4	5
20–34	3	2.0	<1	1	1	2	2	3	3	3
35–49	2	5.5	12	3	3	8	8	8	8	8
50–64	3	3.0	7	1	1	2	6	6	6	6
65+	0									
2. MULTIPLE DX										
0–19 Years	627	2.6	3	1	1	2	3	5	6	10
20–34	42	4.1	5	2	3	3	5	8	9	11
35–49	91	4.9	14	2	3	4	6	8	12	24
50–64	86	5.3	13	2	3	5	7	9	12	15
65+	40	5.7	17	2	3	5	7	10	16	22
TOTAL SINGLE DX	226	1.8	<1	1	1	2	2	3	4	5
TOTAL MULTIPLE DX	886	2.9	5	1	2	2	3	6	7	12
TOTAL										
0–19 Years	845	2.4	3	1	1	2	3	4	6	9
20–34	45	4.0	5	2	3	3	5	8	9	11
35–49	93	4.9	14	2	3	4	6	8	12	24
50–64	89	5.2	13	2	3	5	7	9	12	15
65+	40	5.7	17	2	3	5	7	10	16	22
GRAND TOTAL	1,112	2.7	4	1	1	2	3	5	7	11

56.9: OTHER URETERAL OPERATION

Type of Patients	Observed Patients	Avg. Stay	Vari-ance	Percentiles						
				10th	25th	50th	75th	90th	95th	99th
1. SINGLE DX										
0–19 Years	0									
20–34	0									
35–49	0									
50–64	0									
65+	0									
2. MULTIPLE DX										
0–19 Years	9	1.3	<1	1	1	1	2	2	2	4
20–34	2	2.0	2	1	1	1	3	3	3	3
35–49	3	6.3	69	1	1	2	16	16	16	16
50–64	6	3.2	5	1	2	2	5	7	7	7
65+	10	5.3	17	1	2	6	7	14	14	14
TOTAL SINGLE DX	0									
TOTAL MULTIPLE DX	30	2.6	9	1	1	1	2	6	9	16
TOTAL										
0–19 Years	9	1.3	<1	1	1	1	2	2	2	4
20–34	2	2.0	2	1	1	1	3	3	3	3
35–49	3	6.3	69	1	1	2	16	16	16	16
50–64	6	3.2	5	1	2	2	5	7	7	7
65+	10	5.3	17	1	2	6	7	14	14	14
GRAND TOTAL	30	2.6	9	1	1	1	2	6	9	16

LOS by Diagnosis and Operation, Western Region, 45th Edition

Western Region, October 2007–September 2008 Data, by Operation

57.0: TU BLADDER CLEARANCE

Type of Patients	Observed Patients	Avg. Stay	Variance	10th	25th	50th	75th	90th	95th	99th
1. SINGLE DX										
0–19 Years	4	1.6	<1	1	1	1	3	3	3	3
20–34	3	1.0	0	1	1	1	1	1	1	1
35–49	4	2.0	<1	1	1	2	3	3	3	3
50–64	8	1.3	<1	1	1	1	2	2	2	2
65+	4	1.0	0	1	1	1	1	1	1	1
2. MULTIPLE DX										
0–19 Years	15	15.0	844	1	1	2	10	87	87	>99
20–34	44	3.7	20	1	1	2	4	11	14	21
35–49	71	4.4	19	1	1	2	7	11	13	17
50–64	207	3.5	12	1	1	2	4	8	11	16
65+	591	4.7	24	1	2	3	6	10	14	25
TOTAL SINGLE DX	23	1.4	<1	1	1	1	2	3	3	3
TOTAL MULTIPLE DX	928	4.7	50	1	1	3	6	10	14	26
TOTAL										
0–19 Years	19	10.9	621	1	1	2	6	87	87	>99
20–34	47	3.6	19	1	1	2	4	11	14	21
35–49	75	4.3	18	1	1	2	7	11	13	17
50–64	215	3.4	12	1	1	2	4	8	11	16
65+	595	4.7	24	1	2	3	6	10	14	25
GRAND TOTAL	951	4.6	48	1	1	3	6	10	13	26

57.17: PERCUTANEOUS CYSTOSTOMY

Type of Patients	Observed Patients	Avg. Stay	Variance	10th	25th	50th	75th	90th	95th	99th
1. SINGLE DX										
0–19 Years	1	1.0	0	1	1	1	1	1	1	1
20–34	0									
35–49	0									
50–64	1	1.0	0	1	1	1	1	1	1	1
65+	0									
2. MULTIPLE DX										
0–19 Years	10	7.6	46	2	2	4	10	21	21	21
20–34	16	4.0	5	1	3	4	6	7	9	9
35–49	37	5.8	35	1	2	4	8	10	20	29
50–64	68	6.9	32	1	2	5	11	14	17	30
65+	219	6.5	39	1	2	5	8	13	17	36
TOTAL SINGLE DX	2	1.0	0	1	1	1	1	1	1	1
TOTAL MULTIPLE DX	350	6.5	36	1	2	5	8	14	17	30
TOTAL										
0–19 Years	11	7.3	46	2	2	4	10	21	21	21
20–34	16	4.0	5	1	3	4	6	7	9	9
35–49	37	5.8	35	1	2	4	8	10	20	29
50–64	69	6.9	32	1	2	5	11	14	17	30
65+	219	6.5	39	1	2	5	8	13	17	36
GRAND TOTAL	352	6.5	36	1	2	5	8	14	17	30

57.1: CYSTOTOMY & CYSTOSTOMY

Type of Patients	Observed Patients	Avg. Stay	Variance	10th	25th	50th	75th	90th	95th	99th
1. SINGLE DX										
0–19 Years	2	1.0	0	1	1	1	1	1	1	1
20–34	5	1.6	<1	1	1	1	2	3	3	3
35–49	5	1.6	<1	1	1	2	2	3	3	3
50–64	10	1.9	<1	1	1	1	2	2	4	4
65+	1	1.0	0	1	1	1	1	1	1	1
2. MULTIPLE DX										
0–19 Years	44	4.6	24	1	2	3	5	14	21	>99
20–34	74	5.3	51	1	2	3	7	10	12	58
35–49	137	5.6	45	1	2	3	6	14	21	29
50–64	252	5.8	40	1	2	4	7	14	17	30
65+	613	5.8	32	1	2	4	8	12	16	26
TOTAL SINGLE DX	23	1.7	<1	1	1	1	2	3	3	4
TOTAL MULTIPLE DX	1,120	5.6	36	1	2	4	7	13	17	29
TOTAL										
0–19 Years	46	4.6	24	1	2	3	5	14	21	>99
20–34	79	5.1	49	1	2	3	7	10	12	58
35–49	142	5.5	44	1	2	3	6	12	20	29
50–64	262	5.7	39	1	2	4	7	13	17	30
65+	614	5.7	32	1	2	4	8	12	16	26
GRAND TOTAL	1,143	5.5	35	1	2	4	7	12	17	27

57.18: S/P CYSTOSTOMY NEC

Type of Patients	Observed Patients	Avg. Stay	Variance	10th	25th	50th	75th	90th	95th	99th
1. SINGLE DX										
0–19 Years	0									
20–34	2	1.0	0	1	1	1	1	1	1	1
35–49	2	1.5	<1	1	1	2	2	2	2	2
50–64	9	2.0	<1	1	2	2	2	4	4	4
65+	0									
2. MULTIPLE DX										
0–19 Years	15	4.4	17	1	1	4	5	14	14	>99
20–34	35	6.7	82	1	2	4	9	10	11	58
35–49	70	5.7	59	1	2	3	5	12	22	49
50–64	134	5.9	52	1	2	4	7	15	20	35
65+	295	5.5	25	1	2	4	7	12	14	25
TOTAL SINGLE DX	13	1.8	<1	1	1	2	2	2	4	4
TOTAL MULTIPLE DX	549	5.7	39	1	2	4	7	12	17	34
TOTAL										
0–19 Years	15	4.4	17	1	1	4	5	14	14	>99
20–34	37	6.4	79	1	2	3	9	10	11	58
35–49	72	5.6	57	1	2	3	5	12	22	49
50–64	143	5.6	50	1	2	3	6	13	18	35
65+	295	5.5	25	1	2	4	7	12	14	25
GRAND TOTAL	562	5.6	38	1	2	4	7	12	17	34

LOS by Diagnosis and Operation, Western Region, 45th Edition

Western Region, October 2007–September 2008 Data, by Operation

57.19: CYSTOTOMY NEC

Type of Patients	Observed Patients	Avg. Stay	Vari-ance	Percentiles						
				10th	25th	50th	75th	90th	95th	99th
1. SINGLE DX										
0–19 Years	1	1.0	0	1	1	1	1	1	1	1
20–34	3	2.0	1	1	1	2	3	3	3	3
35–49	3	1.7	1	1	1	1	3	3	3	3
50–64	0									
65+	1	1.0	0	1	1	1	1	1	1	1
2. MULTIPLE DX										
0–19 Years	18	2.3	2	1	1	2	3	4	5	5
20–34	20	3.6	28	1	1	2	3	11	15	22
35–49	30	5.2	30	1	1	3	6	14	18	19
50–64	48	4.0	15	1	1	2	5	10	13	17
65+	96	4.8	36	1	2	2	5	11	17	38
TOTAL SINGLE DX	8	1.6	<1	1	1	1	3	3	3	3
TOTAL MULTIPLE DX	212	4.2	25	1	1	2	4	10	15	22
TOTAL										
0–19 Years	19	2.3	2	1	1	2	3	4	5	5
20–34	23	3.4	25	1	1	2	3	11	15	22
35–49	33	4.9	28	1	1	3	6	14	18	19
50–64	48	4.0	15	1	1	2	5	10	13	17
65+	97	4.8	36	1	2	2	5	11	17	38
GRAND TOTAL	220	4.1	25	1	1	2	4	10	15	22

57.3: BLADDER DIAGNOSTIC PX

Type of Patients	Observed Patients	Avg. Stay	Vari-ance	Percentiles						
				10th	25th	50th	75th	90th	95th	99th
1. SINGLE DX										
0–19 Years	2	1.0	0	1	1	1	1	1	1	1
20–34	3	1.3	<1	1	1	1	2	2	2	2
35–49	5	1.4	<1	1	1	1	2	2	2	2
50–64	4	1.3	<1	1	1	1	1	2	2	2
65+	8	1.3	<1	1	1	1	1	3	3	3
2. MULTIPLE DX										
0–19 Years	45	5.1	44	1	2	2	5	14	24	27
20–34	124	4.5	17	1	2	3	5	9	13	20
35–49	238	5.3	66	1	2	3	6	10	15	63
50–64	458	5.9	41	1	2	4	8	12	16	35
65+	1,084	6.2	32	1	2	5	8	13	16	32
TOTAL SINGLE DX	22	1.3	<1	1	1	1	1	2	2	3
TOTAL MULTIPLE DX	1,949	5.9	38	1	2	4	8	12	16	33
TOTAL										
0–19 Years	47	5.0	43	1	1	2	5	12	20	27
20–34	127	4.4	17	1	2	3	5	9	13	20
35–49	243	5.2	65	1	2	4	6	10	14	63
50–64	462	5.8	41	1	2	4	7	12	16	35
65+	1,092	6.2	32	1	2	5	8	13	16	32
GRAND TOTAL	1,971	5.8	38	1	2	4	8	12	16	33

57.2: VESICOSTOMY

Type of Patients	Observed Patients	Avg. Stay	Vari-ance	Percentiles						
				10th	25th	50th	75th	90th	95th	99th
1. SINGLE DX										
0–19 Years	1	1.0	0	1	1	1	1	1	1	1
20–34	0									
35–49	0									
50–64	0									
65+	0									
2. MULTIPLE DX										
0–19 Years	61	4.5	63	1	1	2	5	10	19	30
20–34	6	6.8	2	4	7	7	8	8	8	8
35–49	3	3.7	21	1	1	1	9	9	9	9
50–64	3	4.3	6	2	2	5	7	7	7	7
65+	5	9.8	131	3	3	5	8	30	30	30
TOTAL SINGLE DX	1	1.0	0	1	1	1	1	1	1	1
TOTAL MULTIPLE DX	78	4.8	59	1	1	2	6	9	19	30
TOTAL										
0–19 Years	62	4.4	62	1	1	2	4	10	19	30
20–34	6	6.8	2	4	7	7	8	8	8	8
35–49	3	3.7	21	1	1	1	9	9	9	9
50–64	3	4.3	6	2	2	4	7	7	7	7
65+	5	9.8	131	3	3	5	8	30	30	30
GRAND TOTAL	79	4.7	58	1	1	2	6	9	19	30

57.32: CYSTOSCOPY NEC

Type of Patients	Observed Patients	Avg. Stay	Vari-ance	Percentiles						
				10th	25th	50th	75th	90th	95th	99th
1. SINGLE DX										
0–19 Years	1	1.0	0	1	1	1	1	1	1	1
20–34	2	1.5	<1	1	1	2	2	2	2	2
35–49	4	1.3	<1	1	1	1	2	2	2	2
50–64	2	1.5	<1	1	1	1	2	2	2	2
65+	2	1.0	0	1	1	1	1	1	1	1
2. MULTIPLE DX										
0–19 Years	35	5.1	46	1	1	2	5	12	27	27
20–34	103	4.5	18	1	2	3	5	9	15	20
35–49	178	5.5	82	1	2	3	6	11	15	80
50–64	292	5.6	34	1	2	4	7	11	16	35
65+	674	6.2	28	1	2	5	8	13	16	27
TOTAL SINGLE DX	11	1.3	<1	1	1	1	2	2	2	2
TOTAL MULTIPLE DX	1,282	5.8	37	1	2	4	7	12	16	28
TOTAL										
0–19 Years	36	5.1	45	1	1	2	5	12	27	27
20–34	105	4.5	18	1	2	3	5	9	15	20
35–49	182	5.4	81	1	1	3	6	10	14	80
50–64	294	5.6	34	1	2	4	7	11	16	35
65+	676	6.2	28	1	2	5	8	13	16	27
GRAND TOTAL	1,293	5.7	37	1	2	4	7	12	16	28

LOS by Diagnosis and Operation, Western Region, 45th Edition

Western Region, October 2007–September 2008 Data, by Operation

57.49: TU DESTR BLADDER LES NEC

Type of Patients	Observed Patients	Avg. Stay	Variance	10th	25th	50th	75th	90th	95th	99th
1. SINGLE DX										
0–19 Years	0									
20–34	1	1.0	0	1	1	1	1	1	1	1
35–49	4	1.5	<1	1	1	1	2	2	2	2
50–64	25	1.4	<1	1	1	1	1	3	3	4
65+	44	1.8	2	1	1	1	2	3	4	9
2. MULTIPLE DX										
0–19 Years	7	2.7	10	1	1	1	2	9	11	11
20–34	32	3.8	30	1	1	2	4	7	9	32
35–49	147	5.6	108	1	2	3	6	11	16	56
50–64	699	3.7	23	1	1	2	4	9	12	30
65+	3,299	3.9	21	1	1	2	5	9	12	21
TOTAL SINGLE DX	74	1.6	2	1	1	1	2	3	4	9
TOTAL MULTIPLE DX	4,184	3.9	25	1	1	2	5	9	12	23
TOTAL										
0–19 Years	7	2.7	10	1	1	1	2	9	11	11
20–34	33	3.7	29	1	1	2	4	7	9	32
35–49	151	5.5	106	1	2	3	6	11	16	56
50–64	724	3.6	22	1	1	2	4	9	11	25
65+	3,343	3.9	21	1	1	2	5	9	12	21
GRAND TOTAL	4,258	3.9	24	1	1	2	5	9	12	23

57.5: BLADDER LES DESTR NEC

Type of Patients	Observed Patients	Avg. Stay	Variance	10th	25th	50th	75th	90th	95th	99th
1. SINGLE DX										
0–19 Years	11	1.8	<1	1	1	2	2	3	3	4
20–34	9	2.2	3	1	1	2	2	5	5	5
35–49	3	2.7	<1	2	2	3	3	3	3	3
50–64	1	4.0	0	4	4	4	4	4	4	4
65+	0									
2. MULTIPLE DX										
0–19 Years	29	3.9	10	1	1	4	6	10	>99	>99
20–34	10	3.6	13	1	2	3	4	13	13	13
35–49	21	4.9	23	1	2	3	5	9	17	18
50–64	39	3.2	5	1	2	3	4	6	7	13
65+	67	4.7	26	2	3	3	5	9	12	33
TOTAL SINGLE DX	24	2.0	1	1	1	2	3	3	4	5
TOTAL MULTIPLE DX	166	4.1	16	1	2	3	5	9	13	>99
TOTAL										
0–19 Years	40	3.3	8	1	1	2	4	10	12	>99
20–34	19	3.0	8	1	2	3	4	6	13	13
35–49	24	4.6	20	2	2	3	4	9	17	18
50–64	40	3.2	5	1	2	3	4	5	6	13
65+	67	4.7	26	2	3	3	5	9	12	33
GRAND TOTAL	190	3.8	14	1	2	3	4	9	12	>99

57.33: CLOSED BLADDER BIOPSY

Type of Patients	Observed Patients	Avg. Stay	Variance	10th	25th	50th	75th	90th	95th	99th
1. SINGLE DX										
0–19 Years	1	1.0	0	1	1	1	1	1	1	1
20–34	1	1.0	0	1	1	1	1	1	1	1
35–49	1	2.0	0	2	2	2	2	2	2	2
50–64	2	2.0	0	1	1	1	1	1	1	1
65+	6	1.3	<1	1	1	1	1	3	3	3
2. MULTIPLE DX										
0–19 Years	4	2.3	1	1	1	3	3	3	4	4
20–34	18	4.2	10	1	2	3	6	9	13	13
35–49	59	4.7	19	1	1	3	7	11	15	22
50–64	163	6.1	51	1	2	4	8	12	17	47
65+	400	6.3	39	1	2	4	8	13	17	34
TOTAL SINGLE DX	11	1.3	<1	1	1	1	1	2	3	3
TOTAL MULTIPLE DX	644	6.0	39	1	2	4	8	12	16	34
TOTAL										
0–19 Years	5	2.2	1	1	1	3	3	3	4	4
20–34	19	4.1	10	1	2	3	6	9	13	13
35–49	60	4.7	19	1	2	3	7	10	14	22
50–64	165	6.1	51	1	2	4	8	12	17	47
65+	406	6.2	39	1	2	4	8	13	17	33
GRAND TOTAL	655	5.9	39	1	2	4	8	12	16	34

57.4: TU EXC/DESTR BLADDER LES

Type of Patients	Observed Patients	Avg. Stay	Variance	10th	25th	50th	75th	90th	95th	99th
1. SINGLE DX										
0–19 Years	0									
20–34	1	1.0	0	1	1	1	1	1	1	1
35–49	4	1.5	<1	1	1	1	2	2	2	2
50–64	25	1.4	<1	1	1	1	1	3	3	4
65+	44	1.8	2	1	1	1	2	3	4	9
2. MULTIPLE DX										
0–19 Years	7	2.7	10	1	1	1	2	9	11	11
20–34	32	3.8	30	1	1	2	4	7	9	32
35–49	148	5.6	107	1	2	3	6	11	16	56
50–64	699	3.7	23	1	1	2	4	9	12	30
65+	3,299	3.9	21	1	1	2	5	9	12	21
TOTAL SINGLE DX	74	1.6	2	1	1	1	2	3	4	9
TOTAL MULTIPLE DX	4,185	3.9	25	1	1	2	5	9	12	23
TOTAL										
0–19 Years	7	2.7	10	1	1	1	2	9	11	11
20–34	33	3.7	29	1	1	2	4	7	9	32
35–49	152	5.5	105	1	2	3	6	11	16	56
50–64	724	3.6	22	1	1	2	4	9	11	25
65+	3,343	3.9	21	1	1	2	5	9	12	21
GRAND TOTAL	4,259	3.9	24	1	1	2	5	9	12	23

LOS by Diagnosis and Operation, Western Region, 45th Edition

Western Region, October 2007–September 2008 Data, by Operation

57.7: TOTAL CYSTECTOMY

Type of Patients	Observed Patients	Avg. Stay	Variance	Percentiles						
				10th	25th	50th	75th	90th	95th	99th
1. SINGLE DX										
0–19 Years	0									
20–34	1	7.0	0	7	7	7	7	7	7	7
35–49		8.0	0	8	8	8	8	8	8	8
50–64	10	7.3	2	6	6	7	8	8	10	10
65+	7	8.0	2	7	7	7	9	11	11	11
2. MULTIPLE DX										
0–19 Years	3	20.0	74	11	11	24	28	28	28	28
20–34	3	11.3	26	7	7	10	17	17	17	17
35–49	57	10.3	64	5	7	8	10	15	31	55
50–64	380	10.9	81	6	7	8	11	19	26	56
65+	910	11.4	69	6	7	9	13	20	28	50
TOTAL SINGLE DX	19	7.6	2	6	7	7	8	10	11	11
TOTAL MULTIPLE DX	1,353	11.3	73	6	7	9	12	20	28	51
TOTAL										
0–19 Years	3	20.0	74	11	11	24	28	28	28	28
20–34	4	10.3	22	7	7	9	10	17	17	17
35–49	58	10.3	63	5	7	8	10	15	31	55
50–64	390	10.8	79	6	7	8	11	18	26	56
65+	917	11.4	69	6	7	9	13	20	28	50
GRAND TOTAL	1,372	11.2	72	6	7	9	12	20	28	51

57.71: RADICAL CYSTECTOMY

Type of Patients	Observed Patients	Avg. Stay	Variance	Percentiles						
				10th	25th	50th	75th	90th	95th	99th
1. SINGLE DX										
0–19 Years	0									
20–34	1	7.0	0	7	7	7	7	7	7	7
35–49		8.0	0	8	8	8	8	8	8	8
50–64	10	7.3	2	6	6	7	8	8	10	10
65+	7	8.0	2	7	7	7	9	11	11	11
2. MULTIPLE DX										
0–19 Years	2	19.5	82	11	11	20	28	28	28	28
20–34	3	11.3	26	7	7	10	17	17	17	17
35–49	47	10.8	75	5	7	8	11	17	31	55
50–64	355	10.8	75	5	7	8	11	18	26	54
65+	854	11.3	62	6	7	9	13	20	27	48
TOTAL SINGLE DX	19	7.6	2	6	7	7	8	10	11	11
TOTAL MULTIPLE DX	1,261	11.2	66	6	7	9	12	19	27	51
TOTAL										
0–19 Years	2	19.5	82	11	11	20	28	28	28	28
20–34	4	10.3	22	7	7	9	10	17	17	17
35–49	48	10.7	74	5	7	8	11	17	31	55
50–64	365	10.7	73	5	7	8	11	18	25	54
65+	861	11.2	62	6	7	9	12	19	27	48
GRAND TOTAL	1,280	11.1	66	6	7	9	12	19	27	51

57.59: OTH BLADDER LESION DESTR

Type of Patients	Observed Patients	Avg. Stay	Variance	Percentiles						
				10th	25th	50th	75th	90th	95th	99th
1. SINGLE DX										
0–19 Years	1	3.0	0	3	3	3	3	3	3	3
20–34	0									
35–49	0									
50–64	1	4.0	0	4	4	4	4	4	4	4
65+	0									
2. MULTIPLE DX										
0–19 Years	6	3.2	3	2	2	3	4	4	8	8
20–34	2	4.0	8	2	2	6	6	6	6	6
35–49	14	5.2	17	2	3	3	7	9	17	17
50–64	35	3.2	5	2	3	3	4	6	7	13
65+	65	4.7	26	2	3	3	5	9	12	33
TOTAL SINGLE DX	2	3.5	<1	3	3	3	4	4	4	4
TOTAL MULTIPLE DX	122	4.2	17	2	2	3	4	8	10	23
TOTAL										
0–19 Years	7	3.1	3	2	2	3	4	4	8	8
20–34	2	4.0	8	2	2	6	6	6	6	6
35–49	14	5.2	17	2	3	3	7	9	17	17
50–64	36	3.3	5	1	2	3	4	6	7	13
65+	65	4.7	26	2	3	3	5	9	12	33
GRAND TOTAL	124	4.2	17	2	2	3	4	8	10	23

57.6: PARTIAL CYSTECTOMY

Type of Patients	Observed Patients	Avg. Stay	Variance	Percentiles						
				10th	25th	50th	75th	90th	95th	99th
1. SINGLE DX										
0–19 Years	1	3.0	0	3	3	3	3	3	3	3
20–34	3	2.0	0	2	2	2	2	2	2	2
35–49	5	3.4	<1	3	3	3	4	4	4	4
50–64	4	1.8	<1	1	1	1	2	3	3	3
65+	2	3.5	4	2	2	4	5	5	5	5
2. MULTIPLE DX										
0–19 Years	5	4.4	8	2	3	3	7	9	9	9
20–34	9	4.6	12	1	4	6	6	12	12	12
35–49	20	7.7	137	3	4	5	7	16	57	57
50–64	74	6.7	43	2	3	4	7	16	23	32
65+	193	6.1	25	2	3	5	7	12	16	29
TOTAL SINGLE DX	15	2.7	1	1	2	3	3	4	5	5
TOTAL MULTIPLE DX	301	6.2	35	2	3	4	7	12	17	29
TOTAL										
0–19 Years	6	4.3	8	2	3	3	7	9	9	9
20–34	12	4.0	10	2	3	4	6	7	12	12
35–49	25	6.8	111	3	3	4	6	8	9	57
50–64	78	6.5	42	2	3	4	7	16	23	32
65+	195	6.1	25	2	3	5	7	12	16	29
GRAND TOTAL	316	6.1	34	3	3	4	7	12	17	29

Western Region, October 2007–September 2008 Data, by Operation

57.79: TOTAL CYSTECTOMY NEC

Type of Patients	Observed Patients	Avg. Stay	Variance	10th	25th	50th	75th	90th	95th	99th
1. SINGLE DX										
0–19 Years	0									
20–34	0									
35–49	0									
50–64	0									
65+	0									
2. MULTIPLE DX										
0–19 Years	1	24.0	0	24	24	24	24	24	24	24
20–34	0									
35–49	10	8.2	9	5	7	9	10	14	14	14
50–64	25	13.5	169	5	7	9	14	25	30	67
65+	56	13.8	178	5	8	10	13	25	49	82
TOTAL SINGLE DX	0									
TOTAL MULTIPLE DX	92	13.2	158	5	7	9	13	24	35	82
TOTAL										
0–19 Years	1	24.0	0	24	24	24	24	24	24	24
20–34	0									
35–49	10	8.2	9	5	7	9	10	14	14	14
50–64	25	13.5	169	5	7	9	14	25	30	67
65+	56	13.8	178	5	8	10	13	25	49	82
GRAND TOTAL	92	13.2	158	5	7	9	13	24	35	82

57.81: SUTURE BLADDER LAC

Type of Patients	Observed Patients	Avg. Stay	Variance	10th	25th	50th	75th	90th	95th	99th
1. SINGLE DX										
0–19 Years	0									
20–34	3	4.7	2	3	3	5	6	6	6	6
35–49	0									
50–64	2	4.0	0	4	4	4	4	4	4	4
65+	0									
2. MULTIPLE DX										
0–19 Years	10	12.7	66	6	6	6	21	24	24	24
20–34	39	7.0	43	2	3	5	8	17	21	35
35–49	43	6.0	17	2	3	5	8	11	15	19
50–64	33	12.4	364	2	3	5	12	27	57	99
65+	37	8.3	81	2	3	5	11	16	26	49
TOTAL SINGLE DX	5	4.4	1	3	4	4	5	6	6	6
TOTAL MULTIPLE DX	162	8.7	112	2	4	6	10	21	24	57
TOTAL										
0–19 Years	10	12.7	66	6	6	6	21	24	24	24
20–34	42	6.8	40	2	3	5	8	12	21	35
35–49	43	6.0	17	2	3	5	8	11	15	19
50–64	35	11.9	346	2	3	6	12	27	57	99
65+	37	8.3	81	2	3	5	11	16	26	49
GRAND TOTAL	167	8.6	110	2	4	6	10	21	24	57

57.8: OTH URIN BLADDER REPAIR

Type of Patients	Observed Patients	Avg. Stay	Variance	10th	25th	50th	75th	90th	95th	99th
1. SINGLE DX										
0–19 Years	0									
20–34	4	4.3	2	3	3	5	6	6	6	6
35–49	15	2.6	4	1	1	2	3	6	6	8
50–64	9	3.1	5	1	2	3	4	8	8	8
65+	2	2.0	0	2	2	2	2	2	2	2
2. MULTIPLE DX										
0–19 Years	170	9.3	113	2	4	7	9	18	25	49
20–34	105	7.8	51	2	4	6	9	15	21	37
35–49	203	5.6	20	2	3	5	7	10	14	19
50–64	296	7.8	83	2	3	6	9	14	21	57
65+	327	9.8	66	3	5	7	12	20	26	45
TOTAL SINGLE DX	30	2.9	4	1	1	2	4	6	8	8
TOTAL MULTIPLE DX	1,101	8.4	77	2	4	6	9	16	23	49
TOTAL										
0–19 Years	170	9.3	113	2	4	7	9	18	25	49
20–34	109	7.7	49	2	4	6	9	15	21	37
35–49	218	5.4	19	1	2	4	7	10	14	19
50–64	305	7.7	81	2	3	6	8	14	21	48
65+	329	9.8	66	3	5	7	12	19	26	45
GRAND TOTAL	1,131	8.3	76	2	4	6	9	16	23	49

57.83: ENTEROVESICAL FIST REP

Type of Patients	Observed Patients	Avg. Stay	Variance	10th	25th	50th	75th	90th	95th	99th
1. SINGLE DX										
0–19 Years	0									
20–34	0									
35–49	0									
50–64	0									
65+										
2. MULTIPLE DX										
0–19 Years	4	9.2	45	5	5	5	13	23	23	23
20–34	15	8.0	10	4	5	8	10	12	15	15
35–49	46	7.7	34	3	4	7	8	12	14	40
50–64	127	7.5	28	3	4	6	8	13	15	23
65+	194	10.9	55	5	6	8	14	21	26	45
TOTAL SINGLE DX	0									
TOTAL MULTIPLE DX	386	9.3	44	4	5	7	11	17	23	45
TOTAL										
0–19 Years	4	9.2	45	5	5	5	13	23	23	23
20–34	15	8.0	10	4	5	8	10	12	15	15
35–49	46	7.7	34	3	4	7	8	12	14	40
50–64	127	7.5	28	3	4	6	8	13	15	23
65+	194	10.9	55	5	6	8	14	21	26	45
GRAND TOTAL	386	9.3	44	4	5	7	11	17	23	45

LOS by Diagnosis and Operation, Western Region, 45th Edition

Western Region, October 2007–September 2008 Data, by Operation

57.84: REP OTH FISTULA BLADDER

Type of Patients	Observed Patients	Avg. Stay	Vari-ance	Percentiles						
				10th	25th	50th	75th	90th	95th	99th
1. SINGLE DX										
0–19 Years	0									
20–34	1	3.0	0	3	3	3	3	3	3	3
35–49	15	2.6	4	3	3	2	3	6	8	8
50–64	5	2.2	2	1	1	2	3	4	4	4
65+	2	2.0	0	2	2	2	2	2	2	2
2. MULTIPLE DX										
0–19 Years	1	1.0	0	1	1	1	1	1	1	1
20–34	13	3.1	3	1	2	3	4	5	7	7
35–49	71	3.0	4	1	2	3	4	5	7	11
50–64	54	4.8	36	1	2	3	6	10	14	41
65+	21	6.5	61	1	3	5	8	10	12	38
TOTAL SINGLE DX	23	2.5	3	1	1	2	3	4	6	8
TOTAL MULTIPLE DX	160	4.0	23	1	1	3	5	8	10	38
TOTAL										
0–19 Years	1	1.0	0	1	1	1	1	1	1	1
20–34	14	3.1	3	1	2	3	4	5	7	7
35–49	86	3.0	4	1	2	3	4	5	7	11
50–64	59	4.6	34	1	1	3	5	10	11	41
65+	23	6.1	57	1	2	4	8	10	12	38
GRAND TOTAL	183	3.8	21	1	1	3	4	8	10	38

57.89: BLADDER REPAIR NEC

Type of Patients	Observed Patients	Avg. Stay	Vari-ance	Percentiles						
				10th	25th	50th	75th	90th	95th	99th
1. SINGLE DX										
0–19 Years	0									
20–34	0									
35–49	0									
50–64	1	1.0	0	1	1	1	1	1	1	1
65+	0									
2. MULTIPLE DX										
0–19 Years	42	3.4	19	1	2	2	4	10	10	28
20–34	8	5.6	9	3	4	5	8	12	12	12
35–49	15	6.1	23	1	3	5	7	16	17	17
50–64	37	9.8	131	1	3	6	13	24	30	58
65+	36	9.4	104	1	3	7	9	25	39	42
TOTAL SINGLE DX	1	1.0	0	1	1	1	1	1	1	1
TOTAL MULTIPLE DX	138	6.9	75	1	2	4	7	16	25	42
TOTAL										
0–19 Years	42	3.4	19	1	2	2	4	10	10	28
20–34	8	5.6	9	3	4	5	8	12	12	12
35–49	15	6.1	23	1	3	5	7	16	17	17
50–64	38	9.5	129	1	2	6	13	24	30	58
65+	36	9.4	104	1	3	7	9	25	39	42
GRAND TOTAL	139	6.9	75	1	2	4	7	16	25	42

57.87: URINARY BLADDER RECONST

Type of Patients	Observed Patients	Avg. Stay	Vari-ance	Percentiles						
				10th	25th	50th	75th	90th	95th	99th
1. SINGLE DX										
0–19 Years	0									
20–34	0									
35–49	0									
50–64	1	8.0	0	8	8	8	8	8	8	8
65+	0									
2. MULTIPLE DX										
0–19 Years	85	10.1	136	3	5	7	10	17	25	78
20–34	24	10.3	44	5	7	9	10	15	28	37
35–49	21	8.1	17	5	6	8	8	13	17	19
50–64	31	9.0	35	5	6	8	9	15	26	29
65+	22	10.2	89	4	7	8	10	17	20	49
TOTAL SINGLE DX	1	8.0	0	8	8	8	8	8	8	8
TOTAL MULTIPLE DX	183	9.9	108	3	5	7	10	17	25	78
TOTAL										
0–19 Years	85	10.1	136	3	5	7	10	17	25	78
20–34	24	10.3	44	5	7	9	10	15	28	37
35–49	21	8.1	17	5	6	8	8	13	17	19
50–64	32	9.0	34	5	6	8	9	15	26	29
65+	22	10.2	89	4	7	8	10	17	20	49
GRAND TOTAL	184	9.9	108	3	5	7	10	17	25	78

57.9: OTHER BLADDER OPERATIONS

Type of Patients	Observed Patients	Avg. Stay	Vari-ance	Percentiles						
				10th	25th	50th	75th	90th	95th	99th
1. SINGLE DX										
0–19 Years	19	2.5	2	1	1	2	4	4	4	5
20–34	11	1.6	<1	1	1	1	2	2	4	4
35–49	12	1.8	<1	1	1	2	2	3	4	4
50–64	4	2.5	6	1	1	2	6	6	6	6
65+	6	2.3	2	1	1	2	3	5	5	5
2. MULTIPLE DX										
0–19 Years	244	3.3	7	1	2	3	4	6	7	15
20–34	491	3.1	7	1	1	3	4	7	9	14
35–49	804	4.0	21	1	2	3	5	8	11	23
50–64	1,630	4.6	20	1	2	3	6	9	13	23
65+	7,827	4.7	12	2	3	4	6	8	11	18
TOTAL SINGLE DX	52	2.2	2	1	1	2	3	4	5	6
TOTAL MULTIPLE DX	10,996	4.5	14	1	2	4	6	8	11	19
TOTAL										
0–19 Years	263	3.2	7	1	2	3	4	6	7	15
20–34	502	3.0	7	1	1	3	4	6	9	13
35–49	816	4.0	20	1	2	3	5	8	11	23
50–64	1,634	4.6	20	1	2	3	6	9	13	23
65+	7,833	4.7	12	2	3	4	6	8	11	18
GRAND TOTAL	11,048	4.5	14	1	2	4	6	8	11	19

Western Region, October 2007–September 2008 Data, by Operation

57.91: BLADDER SPHINCTEROTOMY

Type of Patients	Observed Patients	Avg. Stay	Variance	10th	25th	50th	75th	90th	95th	99th
1. SINGLE DX										
0–19 Years	0									
20–34	0									
35–49	1	1.0	0	1	1	1	1	1	1	1
50–64	1	1.0	0	1	1	1	1	1	1	1
65+	2	1.0	0	1	1	1	1	1	1	1
2. MULTIPLE DX										
0–19 Years	4	7.7	45			5	15	15	15	15
20–34	1	4.0	0	4	4	4	4	4	4	4
35–49	8	6.4	165	1	1	2	3	38	38	38
50–64	37	1.9	2	1	1	1	3	4	6	6
65+	141	3.1	18	1	1	2	3	7	9	26
TOTAL SINGLE DX	4	1.0	0	1	1	1	1	1	1	1
TOTAL MULTIPLE DX	191	3.2	23	1	1	2	3	7	15	28
TOTAL										
0–19 Years	4	7.7	45			5	15	15	15	15
20–34	1	4.0	0	4	4	4	4	4	4	4
35–49	9	5.8	147	1	1	2	3	38	38	38
50–64	38	1.9	2	1	1	1	3	4	6	6
65+	143	3.0	18	1	1	2	3	7	9	26
GRAND TOTAL	195	3.2	23	1	1	1	3	7	15	28

57.93: CONTROL BLADDER HEMOR

Type of Patients	Observed Patients	Avg. Stay	Variance	10th	25th	50th	75th	90th	95th	99th
1. SINGLE DX										
0–19 Years	0									
20–34	1	1.0	0	1	1	1	1	1	1	1
35–49	0									
50–64	0									
65+	1	2.0	0	2	2	2	2	2	2	2
2. MULTIPLE DX										
0–19 Years	0									
20–34	11	4.0	0	4	4	4	4	4	4	4
35–49	11	5.8	121	1	1	3	4	5	39	39
50–64	47	5.5	60	1	1	3	6	13	14	39
65+	215	5.1	26	1	2	4	6	11	16	24
TOTAL SINGLE DX	3	1.7	<1	1	1	2	2	2	2	2
TOTAL MULTIPLE DX	274	5.2	35	1	2	3	6	11	16	36
TOTAL										
0–19 Years	0									
20–34	2	2.5	4	1	1	3	4	4	4	4
35–49	11	5.8	121	1	1	3	5	5	39	39
50–64	48	5.4	59	1	1	3	6	13	14	39
65+	216	5.1	26	1	2	4	6	11	16	24
GRAND TOTAL	277	5.1	35	2	2	3	6	11	16	36

57.94: INSERT INDWELL URIN CATH

Type of Patients	Observed Patients	Avg. Stay	Variance	10th	25th	50th	75th	90th	95th	99th
1. SINGLE DX										
0–19 Years	19	2.5	2	1	1	2	4	4	4	5
20–34	10	1.6	<1	1	1	1	2	4	4	4
35–49	11	1.8	<1	1	1	2	2	3	4	4
50–64	2	3.5	12	2	6	6	6	6	6	6
65+	3	3.3	2	2	2	3	5	5	5	5
2. MULTIPLE DX										
0–19 Years	238	3.2	6	1	2	3	4	6	7	14
20–34	474	3.1	7	1	1	3	4	7	9	14
35–49	749	3.9	17	1	2	3	5	7	10	21
50–64	1,455	4.6	18	1	2	3	6	9	13	22
65+	7,112	4.7	12	2	3	4	6	8	11	17
TOTAL SINGLE DX	45	2.3	2	1	1	2	3	4	5	6
TOTAL MULTIPLE DX	10,028	4.5	13	1	2	4	6	8	11	18
TOTAL										
0–19 Years	257	3.1	5	1	2	3	4	5	7	14
20–34	484	3.0	7	1	1	2	4	7	9	14
35–49	760	3.9	17	1	2	3	5	7	10	21
50–64	1,457	4.6	18	2	2	3	6	9	13	22
65+	7,115	4.7	12	2	3	4	6	8	11	17
GRAND TOTAL	10,073	4.5	13	1	2	4	6	8	11	18

57.95: REPL INDWELL URIN CATH

Type of Patients	Observed Patients	Avg. Stay	Variance	10th	25th	50th	75th	90th	95th	99th
1. SINGLE DX										
0–19 Years	0									
20–34	0									
35–49	0									
50–64	0									
65+	0									
2. MULTIPLE DX										
0–19 Years	1	1.0	0	1	1	1	1	1	1	1
20–34	13	3.2	2	1	2	3	4	5	6	6
35–49	35	5.0	27	1	1	4	6	9	15	28
50–64	75	4.5	16	1	2	3	6	8	11	28
65+	292	4.6	11	1	2	4	6	9	13	17
TOTAL SINGLE DX	0									
TOTAL MULTIPLE DX	416	4.5	13	1	2	4	6	9	13	17
TOTAL										
0–19 Years	1	1.0	0	1	1	1	1	1	1	1
20–34	13	3.2	2	1	2	3	4	5	6	6
35–49	35	5.0	27	1	1	4	6	9	15	28
50–64	75	4.5	16	2	2	3	6	8	11	28
65+	292	4.6	11	1	2	4	6	9	13	17
GRAND TOTAL	416	4.5	13	1	2	4	6	9	13	17

LOS by Diagnosis and Operation, Western Region, 45th Edition

Western Region, October 2007–September 2008 Data, by Operation

58.0: URETHROTOMY

Type of Patients	Observed Patients	Avg. Stay	Variance	10th	25th	50th	75th	90th	95th	99th
1. SINGLE DX										
0–19 Years	0									
20–34	0									
35–49	1	2.0	0	2	2	2	2	2	2	2
50–64	1	2.0	0	2	2	2	2	2	2	2
65+	0									
2. MULTIPLE DX										
0–19 Years	5	1.5	<1	1	1	1	2	2	2	2
20–34	5	2.6	3	1	1	3	3	5	5	5
35–49	6	1.7	<1	1	1	1	2	3	3	3
50–64	7	8.1	185	2	2	3	4	39	39	39
65+	17	3.7	19	1	1	2	4	7	19	19
TOTAL SINGLE DX	2	2.0	0	2	2	2	2	2	2	2
TOTAL MULTIPLE DX	40	3.6	39	1	1	2	3	5	7	39
TOTAL										
0–19 Years	5	1.5	<1	1	1	1	2	2	2	2
20–34	5	2.6	3	1	1	3	3	5	5	5
35–49	7	1.7	<1	1	1	1	2	3	3	3
50–64	8	7.4	163	2	2	3	4	39	39	39
65+	17	3.7	19	1	1	2	4	7	19	19
GRAND TOTAL	42	3.5	37	1	1	2	3	5	7	39

58.1: URETHRAL MEATOTOMY

Type of Patients	Observed Patients	Avg. Stay	Variance	10th	25th	50th	75th	90th	95th	99th
1. SINGLE DX										
0–19 Years	0									
20–34	0									
35–49	0									
50–64	0									
65+										
2. MULTIPLE DX										
0–19 Years	1	21.0	0	21	21	21	21	21	21	21
20–34	1	1.0	0	1	1	1	1	1	1	1
35–49	4	1.3	<1	1	1	1	2	2	2	2
50–64	1	2.0	0	2	2	2	2	2	2	2
65+	1	3.0	0	3	3	3	3	3	3	3
TOTAL SINGLE DX	0									
TOTAL MULTIPLE DX	8	8.7	97	1	1	2	21	21	21	21
TOTAL										
0–19 Years	1	21.0	0	21	21	21	21	21	21	21
20–34	1	1.0	0	1	1	1	1	1	1	1
35–49	4	1.3	<1	1	1	1	2	2	2	2
50–64	1	2.0	0	2	2	2	2	2	2	2
65+	1	3.0	0	3	3	3	3	3	3	3
GRAND TOTAL	8	8.7	97	1	1	2	21	21	21	21

58.2: URETHRAL DIAGNOSTIC PX

Type of Patients	Observed Patients	Avg. Stay	Variance	10th	25th	50th	75th	90th	95th	99th
1. SINGLE DX										
0–19 Years	0									
20–34	0									
35–49	0									
50–64	0									
65+	0									
2. MULTIPLE DX										
0–19 Years	1	5.0	0	5	5	5	5	5	5	5
20–34	8	3.3	8	1	1	2	4	8	8	8
35–49	12	3.6	9	1	1	3	5	6	11	11
50–64	19	4.8	62	1	2	2	5	7	36	36
65+	31	5.7	21	1	2	4	8	11	15	21
TOTAL SINGLE DX	0									
TOTAL MULTIPLE DX	71	4.8	28	1	2	3	7	9	11	36
TOTAL										
0–19 Years	1	5.0	0	5	5	5	5	5	5	5
20–34	8	3.3	8	1	1	2	4	8	8	8
35–49	12	3.6	9	1	1	3	5	6	11	11
50–64	19	4.8	62	1	2	2	5	7	36	36
65+	31	5.7	21	1	2	4	8	11	15	21
GRAND TOTAL	71	4.8	28	1	2	3	7	9	11	36

58.3: EXC/DESTR URETHRAL LES

Type of Patients	Observed Patients	Avg. Stay	Variance	10th	25th	50th	75th	90th	95th	99th
1. SINGLE DX										
0–19 Years	4	1.0	0	1	1	1	1	1	1	1
20–34	5	1.4	<1	1	1	1	1	3	3	3
35–49	5	1.0	0	1	1	1	1	1	1	1
50–64	1	1.0	0	1	1	1	1	1	1	1
65+	0									
2. MULTIPLE DX										
0–19 Years	26	7.5	33	1	4	6	11	17	19	30
20–34	8	1.3	<1	1	1	1	1	2	2	2
35–49	19	2.1	4	1	1	2	2	4	9	9
50–64	14	3.1	22	1	1	1	2	7	18	18
65+	66	4.0	14	1	1	3	5	10	12	17
TOTAL SINGLE DX	15	1.1	<1	1	1	1	1	1	1	3
TOTAL MULTIPLE DX	133	4.8	23	1	1	3	7	11	15	19
TOTAL										
0–19 Years	30	6.4	33	1	1	5	8	15	17	30
20–34	13	1.3	<1	1	1	1	1	2	3	3
35–49	24	1.9	3	1	1	1	2	3	4	9
50–64	15	2.9	21	1	1	1	2	7	18	18
65+	66	4.0	14	1	1	3	5	10	12	17
GRAND TOTAL	148	4.3	22	1	1	2	6	11	15	19

LOS by Diagnosis and Operation, Western Region, 45th Edition

Western Region, October 2007–September 2008 Data, by Operation

58.31: ENDO URETHRAL LES DESTR

Type of Patients	Observed Patients	Avg. Stay	Variance	10th	25th	50th	75th	90th	95th	99th
1. SINGLE DX										
0–19 Years	3	1.0	0	1	1	1	1	1	1	1
20–34	2	2.0	2	1	1	1	3	3	3	3
35–49	2	1.0	0	1	1	1	1	3	1	1
50–64	0									
65+	0									
2. MULTIPLE DX										
0–19 Years	20	8.3	34	1	5	7	11	17	19	30
20–34	0									
35–49	3	3.7	21	1	1	1	9	9	9	9
50–64	5	6.8	45	1	2	6	7	18	18	18
65+	43	4.8	17	1	2	3	6	11	13	17
TOTAL SINGLE DX	7	1.2	<1	1	1	1	1	1	3	3
TOTAL MULTIPLE DX	71	6.5	28	1	2	5	9	14	17	30
TOTAL										
0–19 Years	23	7.0	35	1	1	6	9	15	19	30
20–34	2	2.0	2	1	1	1	3	3	3	3
35–49	5	2.6	13	1	1	1	1	9	9	9
50–64	5	6.8	45	1	2	6	7	18	18	18
65+	43	4.8	17	1	2	3	6	11	13	17
GRAND TOTAL	78	5.8	28	1	1	4	8	13	17	19

58.45: HYPOSPAD/EPISPADIAS REP

Type of Patients	Observed Patients	Avg. Stay	Variance	10th	25th	50th	75th	90th	95th	99th
1. SINGLE DX										
0–19 Years	56	1.9	2	1	1	1	2	4	4	9
20–34	2	1.0	0	1	1	1	1	1	1	1
35–49	0									
50–64	0									
65+										
2. MULTIPLE DX										
0–19 Years	96	1.8	7	1	1	1	2	3	4	20
20–34	7	1.2	<1	1	1	1	1	2	2	2
35–49	2	2.0	0	2	2	2	2	2	2	2
50–64	0									
65+	1	9.0	0	9	9	9	9	9	9	9
TOTAL SINGLE DX	58	1.9	2	1	1	1	2	4	4	9
TOTAL MULTIPLE DX	106	1.8	7	1	1	1	2	3	4	20
TOTAL										
0–19 Years	152	1.9	5	1	1	1	2	3	4	12
20–34	9	1.2	<1	1	1	1	1	2	2	2
35–49	2	2.0	0	2	2	2	2	2	2	2
50–64	0									
65+	1	9.0	0	9	9	9	9	9	9	9
GRAND TOTAL	164	1.9	5	1	1	1	2	3	4	12

58.4: REPAIR OF URETHRA

Type of Patients	Observed Patients	Avg. Stay	Variance	10th	25th	50th	75th	90th	95th	99th
1. SINGLE DX										
0–19 Years	64	1.8	2	1	1	1	2	3	4	9
20–34	25	1.6	<1	1	1	1	2	2	3	5
35–49	19	1.9	3	1	1	1	2	6	7	7
50–64	15	1.5	<1	1	1	1	2	2	3	3
65+	3	1.7	<1	1	1	2	2	2	2	2
2. MULTIPLE DX										
0–19 Years	135	2.4	18	1	1	1	2	4	6	35
20–34	49	3.1	52	1	1	2	3	5	6	54
35–49	62	2.0	2	1	1	2	2	3	6	7
50–64	89	3.2	10	1	2	2	5	7	8	24
65+	61	2.7	13	1	2	1	3	6	8	25
TOTAL SINGLE DX	126	1.8	2	1	1	1	2	3	4	9
TOTAL MULTIPLE DX	396	2.6	18	1	2	1	3	5	7	24
TOTAL										
0–19 Years	199	2.2	12	1	1	1	2	4	5	20
20–34	74	2.6	36	1	1	1	2	4	6	54
35–49	81	2.0	7	1	1	1	2	3	6	7
50–64	104	3.0	9	1	1	2	4	6	7	9
65+	64	2.7	12	1	1	2	3	6	8	25
GRAND TOTAL	522	2.3	13	1	1	1	2	4	6	20

58.46: URETHRAL RECONST NEC

Type of Patients	Observed Patients	Avg. Stay	Variance	10th	25th	50th	75th	90th	95th	99th
1. SINGLE DX										
0–19 Years	2	1.0	0	1	1	1	1	1	1	1
20–34	7	2.0	2	1	1	1	3	5	5	5
35–49	6	2.2	6	1	1	1	2	6	7	7
50–64	2	1.5	<1	1	1	2	2	2	2	2
65+	1	2.0	0	2	2	2	2	2	2	2
2. MULTIPLE DX										
0–19 Years	9	2.6	3	1	1	1	2	4	5	6
20–34	23	2.6	3	1	1	2	3	5	6	6
35–49	24	2.2	3	1	1	2	3	5	6	7
50–64	40	3.2	4	1	1	2	5	6	7	7
65+	10	2.9	5	1	1	2	4	7	8	7
TOTAL SINGLE DX	18	1.8	2	1	1	1	2	3	5	7
TOTAL MULTIPLE DX	106	2.7	4	1	1	2	5	6	6	7
TOTAL										
0–19 Years	11	2.3	3	1	1	1	3	5	5	6
20–34	30	2.5	3	1	1	2	4	5	6	6
35–49	30	2.2	2	1	1	1	2	5	6	7
50–64	42	3.1	4	1	1	2	5	6	7	7
65+	11	2.8	5	1	1	2	4	6	7	7
GRAND TOTAL	124	2.6	4	1	1	2	4	6	6	7

LOS by Diagnosis and Operation, Western Region, 45th Edition

Western Region, October 2007–September 2008 Data, by Operation

58.49: URETHRAL REPAIR NEC

Type of Patients	Observed Patients	Avg. Stay	Variance	Percentiles						
				10th	25th	50th	75th	90th	95th	99th
1. SINGLE DX										
0–19 Years	4	1.5	<1	1	1	1	2	2	2	2
20–34	13	1.5	<1	1	1	1	2	2	2	2
35–49	11	1.5	<1	1	1	1	2	2	3	2
50–64	8	1.5	<1	1	1	1	2	3	3	3
65+	1	1.0	0	1	1	1	1	1	1	1
2. MULTIPLE DX										
0–19 Years	7	2.3	<1	1	1	2	3	3	4	4
20–34	10	1.6	<1	1	1	2	2	2	3	3
35–49	22	1.9	2	1	1	2	2	3	3	7
50–64	29	2.9	20	1	1	1	2	7	8	24
65+	27	2.0	4	1	1	1	2	3	5	11
TOTAL SINGLE DX	37	1.5	<1	1	1	1	2	2	2	3
TOTAL MULTIPLE DX	95	2.3	7	1	1	2	3	3	5	11
TOTAL										
0–19 Years	11	2.0	<1	1	1	2	3	3	3	4
20–34	23	1.5	<1	1	1	1	2	2	2	3
35–49	33	1.8	1	1	1	1	2	3	3	7
50–64	37	2.6	16	1	1	2	2	5	8	24
65+	28	2.0	4	1	1	1	2	3	5	11
GRAND TOTAL	132	2.0	5	1	1	2	2	3	4	11

58.5: URETHRAL STRICTURE REL

Type of Patients	Observed Patients	Avg. Stay	Variance	Percentiles						
				10th	25th	50th	75th	90th	95th	99th
1. SINGLE DX										
0–19 Years	1	1.0	0	1	1	1	1	1	1	1
20–34	0									
35–49	2	1.0	0	1	1	1	1	1	1	1
50–64	2	1.0	0	1	1	1	1	1	1	1
65+	0									
2. MULTIPLE DX										
0–19 Years	1	4.0	0	4	4	4	4	4	4	4
20–34	19	4.5	22	1	1	2	7	13	16	16
35–49	32	4.8	25	1	1	3	8	11	15	21
50–64	114	4.3	23	1	1	2	6	11	14	21
65+	259	4.2	18	1	1	2	5	10	14	19
TOTAL SINGLE DX	5	1.0	0	1	1	1	1	1	1	1
TOTAL MULTIPLE DX	425	4.3	20	1	1	2	6	10	14	21
TOTAL										
0–19 Years	2	2.5	5	1	1	3	4	4	4	4
20–34	19	4.5	22	1	1	2	7	13	16	16
35–49	34	4.6	24	1	1	2	7	11	15	21
50–64	116	4.3	23	1	1	2	6	11	14	21
65+	259	4.2	18	1	1	2	5	10	14	19
GRAND TOTAL	430	4.3	20	1	1	2	6	10	14	21

58.6: URETHRAL DILATION

Type of Patients	Observed Patients	Avg. Stay	Variance	Percentiles						
				10th	25th	50th	75th	90th	95th	99th
1. SINGLE DX										
0–19 Years	0									
20–34	1	3.0	0	3	3	3	3	3	3	3
35–49	1	1.0	0	1	1	1	1	1	1	1
50–64	2	1.0	0	1	1	1	1	1	1	1
65+	0									
2. MULTIPLE DX										
0–19 Years	11	3.7	9	1	2	3	5	8	8	13
20–34	27	5.3	55	1	2	3	6	10	16	38
35–49	52	5.2	31	1	2	3	6	12	19	28
50–64	116	6.5	56	1	3	5	7	14	17	43
65+	433	5.8	22	1	3	5	7	11	14	21
TOTAL SINGLE DX	4	1.5	1	1	1	1	3	3	3	3
TOTAL MULTIPLE DX	639	5.7	30	1	2	4	7	11	15	29
TOTAL										
0–19 Years	11	3.7	9	1	2	3	5	8	8	13
20–34	28	5.2	53	1	2	3	6	10	16	38
35–49	53	5.1	31	1	2	3	6	12	19	28
50–64	118	6.4	55	1	2	5	7	14	17	43
65+	433	5.8	22	1	3	5	7	11	14	21
GRAND TOTAL	643	5.7	30	1	2	4	7	11	15	29

58.9: OTHER URETHRAL OPS

Type of Patients	Observed Patients	Avg. Stay	Variance	Percentiles						
				10th	25th	50th	75th	90th	95th	99th
1. SINGLE DX										
0–19 Years	1	3.0	0	3	3	3	3	3	3	3
20–34	0									
35–49	2	1.0	0	1	1	1	1	1	1	1
50–64	2	1.0	0	1	1	1	1	1	1	1
65+	4	1.5	<1	1	1	1	2	2	2	2
2. MULTIPLE DX										
0–19 Years	2	8.8	7	4	10	10	10	10	10	10
20–34	12	3.2	8	1	1	2	6	8	8	8
35–49	12	9.2	305	1	1	3	10	13	63	63
50–64	79	1.8	5	1	1	1	2	3	6	18
65+	314	2.3	8	1	1	1	2	5	7	15
TOTAL SINGLE DX	8	1.9	<1	1	1	2	3	3	3	3
TOTAL MULTIPLE DX	416	2.5	17	1	1	1	2	6	9	16
TOTAL										
0–19 Years	3	6.3	13	3	3	4	10	10	10	10
20–34	9	3.2	8	1	1	2	6	8	8	8
35–49	13	8.6	284	1	1	2	8	13	63	63
50–64	81	1.7	5	1	1	1	2	3	6	18
65+	318	2.3	8	1	1	1	2	5	7	15
GRAND TOTAL	424	2.5	17	1	1	1	2	5	9	16

LOS by Diagnosis and Operation, Western Region, 45th Edition

Western Region, October 2007–September 2008 Data, by Operation

58.93: IMPLANTATION OF AUS

Type of Patients	Observed Patients	Avg. Stay	Vari-ance	Percentiles						
				10th	25th	50th	75th	90th	95th	99th
1. SINGLE DX										
0–19 Years	0									
20–34	0									
35–49	0									
50–64	2	1.0	0	1	1	1	1	1	1	1
65+	3	1.3	<1	1	1	1	2	2	2	2
2. MULTIPLE DX										
0–19 Years	0									
20–34	4	2.7	8	1	1	2	2	7	7	7
35–49	6	12.5	616	1	1	1	8	63	63	63
50–64	64	1.3	<1	1	1	1	1	2	2	2
65+	220	1.4	3	1	1	1	1	2	3	4
TOTAL SINGLE DX	5	1.2	<1	1	1	1	1	2	2	2
TOTAL MULTIPLE DX	294	1.6	15	1	1	1	1	2	3	8
TOTAL										
0–19 Years	0									
20–34	4	2.7	8	1	1	2	2	7	7	7
35–49	6	12.5	616	1	1	1	8	63	63	63
50–64	66	1.3	<1	1	1	1	1	2	2	2
65+	223	1.4	3	1	1	1	1	2	3	4
GRAND TOTAL	299	1.6	15	1	1	1	1	2	3	8

59.0: RETROPERITON DISSECTION

Type of Patients	Observed Patients	Avg. Stay	Vari-ance	Percentiles						
				10th	25th	50th	75th	90th	95th	99th
1. SINGLE DX										
0–19 Years	0									
20–34	0									
35–49	3	5.0	7	3	3	4	8	8	8	8
50–64	3	6.0	7	3	3	7	8	8	8	8
65+	0									
2. MULTIPLE DX										
0–19 Years	2	2.5	<1	2	2	3	3	3	3	3
20–34	10	5.8	23	2	2	5	6	17	17	17
35–49	38	6.7	42	3	3	4	9	13	21	36
50–64	42	5.8	23	2	3	4	8	12	15	>99
65+	33	6.4	22	2	3	4	9	14	17	19
TOTAL SINGLE DX	6	5.5	6	3	3	6	8	8	8	8
TOTAL MULTIPLE DX	125	6.2	28	2	3	4	8	13	17	36
TOTAL										
0–19 Years	2	2.5	<1	2	2	3	3	3	3	3
20–34	10	5.8	23	2	2	5	6	17	17	17
35–49	41	6.6	39	3	3	4	8	12	16	36
50–64	45	5.8	22	2	3	4	8	12	15	>99
65+	33	6.4	22	2	3	4	9	14	17	19
GRAND TOTAL	131	6.2	27	2	3	4	8	12	17	36

58.99: PERIURETHRAL OPS NEC

Type of Patients	Observed Patients	Avg. Stay	Vari-ance	Percentiles						
				10th	25th	50th	75th	90th	95th	99th
1. SINGLE DX										
0–19 Years	1	3.0	0	3	3	3	3	3	3	3
20–34	0									
35–49	1	1.0	0	1	1	1	1	1	1	1
50–64	0									
65+	1	2.0	0	2	2	2	2	2	2	2
2. MULTIPLE DX										
0–19 Years	1	4.0	0	4	4	4	4	4	4	4
20–34	4	4.3	11	1	1	2	8	8	8	8
35–49	4	13.0	0	13	13	13	13	13	13	13
50–64	15	3.7	20	1	1	1	3	9	18	18
65+	89	4.2	13	1	1	3	5	10	12	17
TOTAL SINGLE DX	3	2.5	<1	1	2	3	3	3	3	3
TOTAL MULTIPLE DX	110	4.2	14	1	1	3	5	10	12	17
TOTAL										
0–19 Years	2	3.2	<1	3	3	3	3	4	4	4
20–34	4	4.3	11	1	1	1	8	8	8	8
35–49	2	7.0	70	1	1	13	13	13	13	13
50–64	15	3.7	20	1	1	2	3	9	18	18
65+	90	4.2	12	1	1	3	5	10	12	17
GRAND TOTAL	113	4.1	13	1	1	3	5	10	12	17

59.02: PERIRENAL ADHESIO NEC

Type of Patients	Observed Patients	Avg. Stay	Vari-ance	Percentiles						
				10th	25th	50th	75th	90th	95th	99th
1. SINGLE DX										
0–19 Years	0									
20–34	0									
35–49	3	5.0	7	3	3	4	8	8	8	8
50–64	3	6.0	7	3	3	7	8	8	8	8
65+	0									
2. MULTIPLE DX										
0–19 Years	2	2.5	<1	2	2	3	3	3	3	3
20–34	4	9.2	37	3	3	6	11	17	17	17
35–49	25	6.1	21	3	4	5	7	13	16	21
50–64	29	6.6	26	2	3	5	8	12	15	28
65+	19	6.0	18	2	3	4	8	15	17	17
TOTAL SINGLE DX	6	5.5	6	3	3	6	8	8	8	8
TOTAL MULTIPLE DX	79	6.4	22	3	3	5	8	13	17	28
TOTAL										
0–19 Years	2	2.5	<1	2	3	3	3	3	3	3
20–34	4	9.2	37	3	3	6	11	17	17	17
35–49	28	6.0	19	3	3	4	7	13	16	21
50–64	32	6.6	24	3	3	5	8	9	15	28
65+	19	6.0	18	2	3	4	8	15	17	17
GRAND TOTAL	85	6.3	21	3	3	5	8	12	16	28

LOS by Diagnosis and Operation, Western Region, 45th Edition

Western Region, October 2007–September 2008 Data, by Operation

59.1: PERIVESICAL INCISION

Type of Patients	Observed Patients	Avg. Stay	Variance	Percentiles						
				10th	25th	50th	75th	90th	95th	99th
1. SINGLE DX										
0–19 Years	0									
20–34	0									
35–49	0									
50–64	0									
65+	0									
2. MULTIPLE DX										
0–19 Years	0									
20–34	0									
35–49	1	2.0	0	2	2	2	2	2	2	2
50–64	0									
65+	4	7.3	42	4	4	4	17	17	17	17
TOTAL SINGLE DX	0									
TOTAL MULTIPLE DX	5	6.2	37	2	4	4	4	17	17	17
TOTAL										
0–19 Years	0									
20–34	0									
35–49	1	2.0	0	2	2	2	2	2	2	2
50–64	0									
65+	4	7.3	42	4	4	4	17	17	17	17
GRAND TOTAL	5	6.2	37	2	4	4	4	17	17	17

59.2: PERIRENAL DXTIC PX

Type of Patients	Observed Patients	Avg. Stay	Variance	Percentiles						
				10th	25th	50th	75th	90th	95th	99th
1. SINGLE DX										
0–19 Years	0									
20–34	0									
35–49	0									
50–64	0									
65+	0									
2. MULTIPLE DX										
0–19 Years	0									
20–34	0									
35–49	1	8.0	0	8	8	8	8	8	8	8
50–64	1	10.0	0	10	10	10	10	10	10	10
65+	5	6.4	27	2	3	5	7	15	15	15
TOTAL SINGLE DX	0									
TOTAL MULTIPLE DX	7	7.2	20	2	3	7	10	15	15	15
TOTAL										
0–19 Years	0									
20–34	0									
35–49	1	8.0	0	8	8	8	8	8	8	8
50–64	1	10.0	0	10	10	10	10	10	10	10
65+	5	6.4	27	2	3	5	7	15	15	15
GRAND TOTAL	7	7.2	20	2	3	7	10	15	15	15

59.3: URETHROVES JUNCT PLICAT

Type of Patients	Observed Patients	Avg. Stay	Variance	Percentiles						
				10th	25th	50th	75th	90th	95th	99th
1. SINGLE DX										
0–19 Years	0									
20–34	0									
35–49	0									
50–64	0									
65+	0									
2. MULTIPLE DX										
0–19 Years	0									
20–34	0									
35–49	2	1.5	<1	1	1	2	2	2	2	2
50–64	2	2.0	0	2	2	2	2	2	2	2
65+	1	2.0	0	2	2	2	2	2	2	2
TOTAL SINGLE DX	0									
TOTAL MULTIPLE DX	5	1.8	<1	1	2	2	2	2	2	2
TOTAL										
0–19 Years	0									
20–34	0									
35–49	2	1.5	<1	1	2	2	2	2	2	2
50–64	2	2.0	0	2	2	2	2	2	2	2
65+	1	2.0	0	2	2	2	2	2	2	2
GRAND TOTAL	5	1.8	<1	1	2	2	2	2	2	2

59.4: SUPRAPUBIC SLING OP

Type of Patients	Observed Patients	Avg. Stay	Variance	Percentiles						
				10th	25th	50th	75th	90th	95th	99th
1. SINGLE DX										
0–19 Years	0									
20–34	3	1.0	0	1	1	1	1	1	1	1
35–49	13	1.2	<1	1	1	1	1	1	3	3
50–64	14	1.1	<1	1	1	1	1	1	3	3
65+	4	1.0	0	1	1	1	1	1	1	1
2. MULTIPLE DX										
0–19 Years	1	7.0	0	7	7	7	7	7	7	7
20–34	11	1.1	<1	1	1	1	1	1	2	2
35–49	105	1.3	<1	1	1	1	1	2	3	4
50–64	169	1.3	<1	1	1	1	1	2	2	3
65+	153	1.4	<1	1	1	1	2	2	3	8
TOTAL SINGLE DX	34	1.1	<1	1	1	1	1	1	3	3
TOTAL MULTIPLE DX	439	1.4	<1	1	1	1	1	2	3	7
TOTAL										
0–19 Years	1	7.0	0	7	7	7	7	7	7	7
20–34	14	1.1	<1	1	1	1	1	1	2	2
35–49	118	1.3	<1	1	1	1	1	2	3	4
50–64	183	1.3	<1	1	1	1	2	2	2	3
65+	157	1.4	<1	1	1	1	2	2	3	8
GRAND TOTAL	473	1.4	<1	1	1	1	1	2	3	7

Western Region, October 2007–September 2008 Data, by Operation

59.5: RETROPUBIC URETHRAL SUSP

Type of Patients	Observed Patients	Avg. Stay	Variance	10th	25th	50th	75th	90th	95th	99th
1. SINGLE DX										
0–19 Years	0									
20–34	6	1.2	<1	1	1	1	1	2	2	2
35–49	16	1.8	<1	1	1	2	2	3	4	4
50–64	9	1.8	<1	1	1	2	2	3	3	3
65+	6	1.7	<1	1	1	1	2	3	3	3
2. MULTIPLE DX										
0–19 Years	1	2.0	0	2	2	2	2	2	2	2
20–34	8	2.1	<1	2	2	2	3	4	4	4
35–49	94	2.1	1	1	1	2	2	3	5	6
50–64	120	2.1	4	1	1	2	2	3	4	8
65+	95	2.5	7	1	1	2	3	4	5	21
TOTAL SINGLE DX	37	1.7	<1	1	1	2	2	3	3	4
TOTAL MULTIPLE DX	318	2.2	4	1	1	2	3	3	4	8
TOTAL										
0–19 Years	1	2.0	0	2	2	2	2	2	2	2
20–34	14	1.7	<1	1	1	1	2	3	4	4
35–49	110	2.1	1	1	1	2	2	3	4	6
50–64	129	2.1	4	1	1	2	2	3	4	8
65+	101	2.4	6	1	1	2	3	4	5	15
GRAND TOTAL	355	2.2	4	1	1	2	3	3	4	8

59.6: PARAURETHRAL SUSPENSION

Type of Patients	Observed Patients	Avg. Stay	Variance	10th	25th	50th	75th	90th	95th	99th
1. SINGLE DX										
0–19 Years	0									
20–34	0									
35–49	1	2.0	0	2	2	2	2	2	2	2
50–64	0									
65+	0									
2. MULTIPLE DX										
0–19 Years	0									
20–34	1	3.0	0	3	3	3	3	3	3	3
35–49	5	2.2	<1	2	2	2	3	3	3	3
50–64	18	1.5	<1	1	1	1	2	3	3	3
65+	31	1.7	2	1	1	1	2	3	5	7
TOTAL SINGLE DX	1	2.0	0	2	2	2	2	2	2	2
TOTAL MULTIPLE DX	55	1.7	1	1	1	1	2	3	4	7
TOTAL										
0–19 Years	0									
20–34	1	3.0	0	3	3	3	3	3	3	3
35–49	6	2.2	<1	2	2	2	3	3	3	3
50–64	18	1.5	<1	1	1	1	2	3	3	3
65+	31	1.7	2	1	1	1	2	3	5	7
GRAND TOTAL	56	1.7	1	1	1	1	2	3	4	7

59.7: OTH URINARY INCONT REP

Type of Patients	Observed Patients	Avg. Stay	Variance	10th	25th	50th	75th	90th	95th	99th
1. SINGLE DX										
0–19 Years	0									
20–34	19	1.1	<1	1	1	1	1	1	2	2
35–49	92	1.1	<1	1	1	1	1	2	2	3
50–64	89	1.2	<1	1	1	1	1	2	2	3
65+	26	1.2	<1	1	1	1	1	2	2	3
2. MULTIPLE DX										
0–19 Years	8	1.7	<1	1	1	2	2	3	3	3
20–34	70	1.5	2	1	1	1	1	2	4	9
35–49	708	1.4	<1	1	1	1	1	2	3	4
50–64	1,071	1.4	<1	1	1	1	2	2	3	4
65+	955	1.5	1	1	1	1	2	2	3	6
TOTAL SINGLE DX	226	1.1	<1	1	1	1	1	2	2	3
TOTAL MULTIPLE DX	2,812	1.4	<1	1	1	1	2	2	3	5
TOTAL										
0–19 Years	8	1.7	<1	1	1	2	2	3	3	3
20–34	89	1.4	2	1	1	1	1	2	4	9
35–49	800	1.3	<1	1	1	1	1	2	3	4
50–64	1,160	1.3	<1	1	1	1	2	2	3	4
65+	981	1.5	1	1	1	1	2	2	3	6
GRAND TOTAL	3,038	1.4	<1	1	1	1	2	2	3	5

59.79: URIN INCONT REPAIR NEC

Type of Patients	Observed Patients	Avg. Stay	Variance	10th	25th	50th	75th	90th	95th	99th
1. SINGLE DX										
0–19 Years	0									
20–34	19	1.1	<1	1	1	1	1	1	2	2
35–49	91	1.1	<1	1	1	1	1	2	2	3
50–64	89	1.2	<1	1	1	1	1	2	2	3
65+	26	1.2	<1	1	1	1	1	2	2	3
2. MULTIPLE DX										
0–19 Years	3	1.7	<1	1	1	2	2	3	3	3
20–34	70	1.5	2	1	1	1	1	2	4	9
35–49	704	1.4	<1	1	1	1	1	2	3	4
50–64	1,053	1.4	<1	1	1	1	2	2	3	4
65+	941	1.5	1	1	1	1	2	2	3	6
TOTAL SINGLE DX	225	1.1	<1	1	1	1	1	2	2	3
TOTAL MULTIPLE DX	2,771	1.4	<1	1	1	1	2	2	3	5
TOTAL										
0–19 Years	3	1.7	<1	1	1	2	2	3	3	3
20–34	89	1.4	2	1	1	1	1	2	4	9
35–49	795	1.3	<1	1	1	1	1	2	3	4
50–64	1,142	1.3	<1	1	1	1	2	2	3	4
65+	967	1.5	1	1	1	1	2	2	3	6
GRAND TOTAL	2,996	1.4	<1	1	1	1	2	2	3	5

LOS by Diagnosis and Operation, Western Region, 45th Edition

Western Region, October 2007–September 2008 Data, by Operation

59.8: URETERAL CATHETERIZATION

Type of Patients	Observed Patients	Avg. Stay	Variance	10th	25th	50th	75th	90th	95th	99th
1. SINGLE DX										
0–19 Years	11	3.8	10	1	1	4	8	8	11	11
20–34	53	1.4	<1	1	1	1	2	2	3	4
35–49	56	1.6	1	1	1	1	2	3	4	7
50–64	46	1.5	<1	1	1	1	2	2	3	4
65+	6	2.8	11	1	1	1	4	9	9	9
2. MULTIPLE DX										
0–19 Years	175	3.5	12	1	1	2	4	7	9	18
20–34	1,163	3.0	7	1	1	2	4	6	8	13
35–49	1,556	3.0	10	1	1	2	4	6	8	14
50–64	1,986	3.6	16	1	1	2	4	7	11	17
65+	2,223	4.8	17	1	2	4	6	10	13	19
TOTAL SINGLE DX	172	1.8	3	1	1	1	2	4	4	9
TOTAL MULTIPLE DX	7,103	3.7	14	1	1	3	5	8	11	18
TOTAL										
0–19 Years	186	3.5	12	1	1	2	4	7	9	18
20–34	1,216	2.9	7	1	1	2	4	6	8	13
35–49	1,612	3.0	10	1	1	2	4	6	8	14
50–64	2,032	3.5	15	1	1	2	4	7	11	17
65+	2,229	4.8	17	1	2	4	6	10	13	19
GRAND TOTAL	7,275	3.7	14	1	1	3	5	8	10	18

59.9: OTHER URINARY SYSTEM OPS

Type of Patients	Observed Patients	Avg. Stay	Variance	10th	25th	50th	75th	90th	95th	99th
1. SINGLE DX										
0–19 Years	1	1.0	0	1	1	1	1	1	1	1
20–34	3	2.3	<1	2	2	2	3	3	3	3
35–49	2	1.0	0	1	1	1	1	1	1	1
50–64	1	2.0	0	2	2	2	2	2	2	2
65+	0									
2. MULTIPLE DX										
0–19 Years	5	7.1	27	2	4	4	10	10	19	19
20–34	33	5.7	49	1	2	3	6	12	22	36
35–49	60	3.2	4	1	1	3	5	6	8	9
50–64	89	5.0	13	1	3	4	6	10	13	17
65+	147	5.7	28	2	2	4	7	12	15	30
TOTAL SINGLE DX	7	1.7	<1	1	1	2	2	3	3	3
TOTAL MULTIPLE DX	334	5.1	23	1	2	4	6	10	14	26
TOTAL										
0–19 Years	6	6.6	28	1	4	10	10	10	19	19
20–34	36	5.4	46	2	2	3	6	12	22	36
35–49	62	3.1	4	1	1	3	5	6	7	9
50–64	90	5.0	13	1	3	4	6	10	13	17
65+	147	5.7	28	2	2	4	7	12	15	30
GRAND TOTAL	341	5.0	23	1	2	4	6	10	14	26

59.94: REPL CYSTOSTOMY TUBE

Type of Patients	Observed Patients	Avg. Stay	Variance	10th	25th	50th	75th	90th	95th	99th
1. SINGLE DX										
0–19 Years	0									
20–34	0									
35–49	0									
50–64	0									
65+	0									
2. MULTIPLE DX										
0–19 Years	3	10.0	32	1	10	10	10	19	19	19
20–34	18	8.3	74	1	3	5	9	22	36	36
35–49	34	4.2	4	1	3	4	5	7	8	9
50–64	60	5.9	14	3	3	5	7	13	15	17
65+	119	6.0	31	2	3	4	7	12	17	30
TOTAL SINGLE DX	0									
TOTAL MULTIPLE DX	234	6.0	27	2	3	5	7	12	15	30
TOTAL										
0–19 Years	3	10.0	32	1	10	10	10	19	19	19
20–34	18	8.3	74	1	3	5	9	22	36	36
35–49	34	4.2	4	1	3	4	5	7	8	9
50–64	60	5.9	14	3	3	5	7	13	15	17
65+	119	6.0	31	2	3	4	7	12	17	30
GRAND TOTAL	234	6.0	27	2	3	5	7	12	15	30

60.0: INCISION OF PROSTATE

Type of Patients	Observed Patients	Avg. Stay	Variance	10th	25th	50th	75th	90th	95th	99th
1. SINGLE DX										
0–19 Years	0									
20–34	0									
35–49	0									
50–64	0									
65+	1	1.0	0	1	1	1	1	1	1	1
2. MULTIPLE DX										
0–19 Years	0									
20–34	2	1.0	0	1	1	1	1	1	1	1
35–49	10	5.0	18	1	1	5	8	12	12	12
50–64	36	4.6	41	1	1	1	5	18	22	22
65+	41	3.0	12	1	1	1	4	6	11	16
TOTAL SINGLE DX	1	1.0	0	1	1	1	1	1	1	1
TOTAL MULTIPLE DX	89	3.8	25	1	1	1	5	11	16	22
TOTAL										
0–19 Years	0									
20–34	2	1.0	0	1	1	1	1	1	1	1
35–49	10	5.0	18	1	1	5	8	12	12	12
50–64	36	4.6	41	1	1	1	5	18	22	22
65+	42	3.0	12	1	1	1	4	6	11	16
GRAND TOTAL	90	3.8	24	1	1	1	5	11	16	22

Western Region, October 2007–September 2008 Data, by Operation

60.1: PROS/SEM VESICL DXTIC PX

Type of Patients	Observed Patients	Avg. Stay	Variance	10th	25th	50th	75th	90th	95th	99th
						Percentiles				
1. SINGLE DX										
0–19 Years	0									
20–34	0									
35–49	0									
50–64	1	1.0	0	1	1	1	1	1	1	1
65+	0									
2. MULTIPLE DX										
0–19 Years	1	21.0	0	21	21	21	21	21	21	21
20–34	0									
35–49	2	7.5	4	6	6	6	6	9	9	9
50–64	39	6.4	42	1	2	5	8	16	25	31
65+	106	5.8	15	2	3	5	7	11	13	17
TOTAL SINGLE DX	1	1.0	0	1	1	1	1	1	1	1
TOTAL MULTIPLE DX	148	6.1	23	1	3	5	8	11	16	25
TOTAL										
0–19 Years	1	21.0	0	21	21	21	21	21	21	21
20–34	0									
35–49	2	7.5	4	6	6	6	6	9	9	9
50–64	40	6.3	41	1	2	5	8	16	25	31
65+	106	5.8	15	2	3	5	7	11	13	17
GRAND TOTAL	149	6.1	23	1	3	5	8	11	16	25

60.11: CLSD PROSTATIC BX

Type of Patients	Observed Patients	Avg. Stay	Variance	10th	25th	50th	75th	90th	95th	99th
						Percentiles				
1. SINGLE DX										
0–19 Years	0									
20–34	0									
35–49	0									
50–64	1	1.0	0	1	1	1	1	1	1	1
65+	0									
2. MULTIPLE DX										
0–19 Years	1	21.0	0	21	21	21	21	21	21	21
20–34	0									
35–49	2	7.5	4	6	6	6	6	9	9	9
50–64	39	6.4	42	1	2	5	8	16	25	31
65+	105	5.8	15	2	3	5	7	11	13	17
TOTAL SINGLE DX	1	1.0	0	1	1	1	1	1	1	1
TOTAL MULTIPLE DX	147	6.1	23	1	3	5	8	11	16	25
TOTAL										
0–19 Years	1	21.0	0	21	21	21	21	21	21	21
20–34	0									
35–49	2	7.5	4	6	6	6	6	9	9	9
50–64	40	6.3	41	1	2	5	8	16	25	31
65+	105	5.8	15	2	3	5	7	11	13	17
GRAND TOTAL	148	6.0	23	1	3	5	8	11	16	25

60.2: TU PROSTATECTOMY

Type of Patients	Observed Patients	Avg. Stay	Variance	10th	25th	50th	75th	90th	95th	99th
						Percentiles				
1. SINGLE DX										
0–19 Years	0									
20–34	0									
35–49	8	1.0	0	1	1	1	1	1	1	1
50–64	107	1.4	<1	1	1	1	2	2	2	5
65+	195	1.4	<1	1	1	1	2	2	2	4
2. MULTIPLE DX										
0–19 Years	1	7.0	0	7	7	7	7	7	7	7
20–34	2	13.0	72	7	7	13	19	19	19	19
35–49	111	2.4	7	1	1	1	2	4	8	14
50–64	2,362	2.1	10	1	1	1	2	3	6	15
65+	9,865	2.5	10	1	1	2	2	5	8	17
TOTAL SINGLE DX	310	1.4	<1	1	1	1	2	2	2	4
TOTAL MULTIPLE DX	12,341	2.4	10	1	1	1	2	5	8	16
TOTAL										
0–19 Years	1	7.0	0	7	7	7	7	7	7	7
20–34	2	13.0	72	7	7	13	19	19	19	19
35–49	119	2.3	7	1	1	1	2	4	8	14
50–64	2,469	2.1	10	1	1	1	2	3	6	15
65+	10,060	2.5	10	1	1	2	2	5	8	17
GRAND TOTAL	12,651	2.4	10	1	1	1	2	4	7	16

60.21: TULIP PROCEDURE

Type of Patients	Observed Patients	Avg. Stay	Variance	10th	25th	50th	75th	90th	95th	99th
						Percentiles				
1. SINGLE DX										
0–19 Years	0									
20–34	0									
35–49	0									
50–64	17	1.1	<1	1	1	1	1	2	2	2
65+	39	1.2	<1	1	1	1	1	2	2	4
2. MULTIPLE DX										
0–19 Years	1	7.0	0	7	7	7	7	7	7	7
20–34	0									
35–49	15	1.8	2	1	1	1	2	4	6	6
50–64	286	1.9	7	1	1	1	2	3	6	16
65+	1,339	2.5	14	1	1	1	2	5	10	20
TOTAL SINGLE DX	56	1.1	<1	1	1	1	1	2	2	4
TOTAL MULTIPLE DX	1,641	2.4	13	1	1	1	2	5	9	19
TOTAL										
0–19 Years	1	7.0	0	7	7	7	7	7	7	7
20–34	0									
35–49	15	1.8	2	1	1	1	2	4	6	6
50–64	303	1.9	7	1	1	1	2	3	6	16
65+	1,378	2.5	13	1	1	1	2	5	10	20
GRAND TOTAL	1,697	2.4	12	1	1	1	2	5	9	19

LOS by Diagnosis and Operation, Western Region, 45th Edition

Western Region, October 2007–September 2008 Data, by Operation

60.29: TU PROSTATECTOMY NEC

Type of Patients	Observed Patients	Avg. Stay	Variance	Percentiles						
				10th	25th	50th	75th	90th	95th	99th
1. SINGLE DX										
0–19 Years	0									
20–34	0									
35–49	8	1.0	0	1	1	1	1	1	1	1
50–64	90	1.5	<1	1	1	1	2	2	3	6
65+	156	1.5	<1	1	1	1	2	2	2	3
2. MULTIPLE DX										
0–19 Years	0									
20–34	2	13.0	72	7	7	13	19	19	19	19
35–49	96	2.5	8	1	1	2	2	5	11	17
50–64	2,076	2.1	10	1	1	1	2	3	6	15
65+	8,526	2.5	9	1	1	2	2	5	8	16
TOTAL SINGLE DX	254	1.5	<1	1	1	1	2	2	2	4
TOTAL MULTIPLE DX	10,700	2.4	10	1	1	2	2	5	7	15
TOTAL										
0–19 Years	0									
20–34	2	13.0	72	7	7	13	19	19	19	19
35–49	104	2.3	8	1	1	1	2	4	8	15
50–64	2,166	2.1	10	1	1	1	2	3	5	15
65+	8,682	2.5	9	1	1	2	2	5	8	16
GRAND TOTAL	10,954	2.4	9	1	1	2	2	4	7	15

60.4: RETROPUBIC PROSTATECTOMY

Type of Patients	Observed Patients	Avg. Stay	Variance	Percentiles						
				10th	25th	50th	75th	90th	95th	99th
1. SINGLE DX										
0–19 Years	0									
20–34	0									
35–49	0									
50–64	14	2.2	<1	1	2	2	3	3	4	4
65+	2	3.5	4	2	2	2	5	5	5	5
2. MULTIPLE DX										
0–19 Years	0									
20–34	0									
35–49	5	1.6	<1	1	2	1	2	3	3	3
50–64	93	2.8	3	1	2	2	3	4	5	10
65+	277	3.7	7	2	2	3	4	6	8	14
TOTAL SINGLE DX	16	2.4	1	2	2	2	3	4	5	5
TOTAL MULTIPLE DX	375	3.5	6	2	2	3	4	6	8	13
TOTAL										
0–19 Years	0									
20–34	0									
35–49	5	1.6	<1	1	2	1	2	3	3	3
50–64	107	2.7	2	1	2	2	3	4	5	9
65+	279	3.7	7	2	2	3	4	6	8	14
GRAND TOTAL	391	3.4	6	2	2	3	4	6	8	13

60.3: SUPRAPUBIC PROSTATECTOMY

Type of Patients	Observed Patients	Avg. Stay	Variance	Percentiles						
				10th	25th	50th	75th	90th	95th	99th
1. SINGLE DX										
0–19 Years	0									
20–34	0									
35–49	0									
50–64	4	4.2	3	2	2	4	5	6	6	6
65+	9	3.3	<1	2	3	3	4	4	4	4
2. MULTIPLE DX										
0–19 Years	0									
20–34	0									
35–49	0									
50–64	71	4.2	5	2	3	4	5	7	7	14
65+	278	5.1	26	2	3	4	6	8	10	18
TOTAL SINGLE DX	13	3.6	1	2	3	4	4	5	6	6
TOTAL MULTIPLE DX	349	4.9	21	2	3	4	6	8	10	15
TOTAL										
0–19 Years	0									
20–34	0									
35–49	0									
50–64	75	4.2	5	2	3	4	5	7	7	14
65+	287	5.0	25	2	3	4	6	8	10	18
GRAND TOTAL	362	4.9	21	2	3	4	6	8	10	15

60.5: RADICAL PROSTATECTOMY

Type of Patients	Observed Patients	Avg. Stay	Variance	Percentiles						
				10th	25th	50th	75th	90th	95th	99th
1. SINGLE DX										
0–19 Years	0									
20–34	0									
35–49	93	1.8	<1	1	1	2	2	3	3	3
50–64	934	1.9	<1	1	1	2	2	3	3	4
65+	377	2.0	<1	1	1	2	2	3	4	5
2. MULTIPLE DX										
0–19 Years	0									
20–34	2	2.5	<1	2	2	3	3	3	3	3
35–49	358	2.2	2	1	1	2	3	4	5	8
50–64	5,895	2.2	2	1	1	2	3	4	4	8
65+	4,282	2.4	3	1	1	2	3	4	5	9
TOTAL SINGLE DX	1,404	1.9	<1	1	1	2	2	3	3	4
TOTAL MULTIPLE DX	10,537	2.3	3	1	1	2	3	4	5	8
TOTAL										
0–19 Years	0									
20–34	2	2.5	<1	2	2	3	3	3	3	3
35–49	451	2.1	2	1	1	2	3	4	5	8
50–64	6,829	2.2	3	1	1	2	3	4	4	8
65+	4,659	2.4	3	1	1	2	3	4	5	8
GRAND TOTAL	11,941	2.2	3	1	1	2	3	4	5	8

Western Region, October 2007–September 2008 Data, by Operation

60.6: OTHER PROSTATECTOMY

Type of Patients	Observed Patients	Avg. Stay	Vari-ance	Percentiles						
				10th	25th	50th	75th	90th	95th	99th
1. SINGLE DX										
0–19 Years	0									
20–34	0									
35–49	1	1.0	0							
50–64	34	1.5	1	1	1	1	2	3	4	6
65+	47	1.3	<1	1	1	1	2	2	2	3
2. MULTIPLE DX										
0–19 Years	0									
20–34	0									
35–49	9	1.7	4	1	1	1	2	4	4	4
50–64	226	1.9	4	1	1	1	2	3	4	13
65+	569	1.8	5	1	1	1	2	3	5	9
TOTAL SINGLE DX	82	1.4	<1	1	1	1	2	2	3	6
TOTAL MULTIPLE DX	804	1.8	5	1	1	1	2	3	5	11
TOTAL										
0–19 Years	0									
20–34	0									
35–49	10	1.6	<1	1	1	1	2	4	4	4
50–64	260	1.8	3	1	1	1	2	3	4	13
65+	616	1.7	5	1	1	1	2	3	4	9
GRAND TOTAL	886	1.8	4	1	1	1	2	3	4	11

60.62: PERINEAL PROSTATECTOMY

Type of Patients	Observed Patients	Avg. Stay	Vari-ance	Percentiles						
				10th	25th	50th	75th	90th	95th	99th
1. SINGLE DX										
0–19 Years	0									
20–34	0									
35–49	0									
50–64	5	1.0	0	1	1	1	1	1	1	1
65+	33	1.2	<1	1	1	1	1	2	2	3
2. MULTIPLE DX										
0–19 Years	0									
20–34	0									
35–49	1	2.0	0	2	2	2	2	2	2	2
50–64	60	1.4	<1	1	1	1	1	2	3	6
65+	388	1.4	3	1	1	1	1	2	3	8
TOTAL SINGLE DX	38	1.2	<1	1	1	1	1	2	2	3
TOTAL MULTIPLE DX	449	1.4	3	1	1	1	1	2	3	7
TOTAL										
0–19 Years	0									
20–34	0									
35–49	1	2.0	0	2	2	2	2	2	2	2
50–64	65	1.4	<1	1	1	1	1	2	3	6
65+	421	1.4	3	1	1	1	1	2	3	7
GRAND TOTAL	487	1.4	2	1	1	1	2	2	3	7

60.69: PROSTATECTOMY NEC

Type of Patients	Observed Patients	Avg. Stay	Vari-ance	Percentiles						
				10th	25th	50th	75th	90th	95th	99th
1. SINGLE DX										
0–19 Years	0									
20–34	0									
35–49	1	1.0	0	1	1	1	1	1	1	1
50–64	29	1.6	1	1	1	1	2	3	4	6
65+	14	1.7	<1	1	1	2	2	2	3	3
2. MULTIPLE DX										
0–19 Years	0									
20–34	0									
35–49	8	1.6	1	1	1	1	2	4	4	4
50–64	152	2.0	4	1	1	1	2	3	5	13
65+	131	2.6	11	1	1	2	3	5	7	22
TOTAL SINGLE DX	44	1.6	<1	1	1	2	2	3	3	6
TOTAL MULTIPLE DX	291	2.3	7	1	1	2	2	4	6	16
TOTAL										
0–19 Years	0									
20–34	0									
35–49	9	1.6	1	1	1	1	2	4	4	4
50–64	181	1.9	4	1	1	1	2	3	5	13
65+	145	2.5	10	1	1	2	3	5	7	22
GRAND TOTAL	335	2.2	6	1	1	1	2	4	6	13

60.7: SEMINAL VESICLE OPS

Type of Patients	Observed Patients	Avg. Stay	Vari-ance	Percentiles						
				10th	25th	50th	75th	90th	95th	99th
1. SINGLE DX										
0–19 Years	1	2.0	0	2	2	2	2	2	2	2
20–34	0									
35–49	0									
50–64	0									
65+	1	3.0	0	3	3	3	3	3	3	3
2. MULTIPLE DX										
0–19 Years	0									
20–34	0									
35–49	1	4.0	0	4	4	4	4	4	4	4
50–64	1	2.0	0	2	2	2	2	2	2	2
65+	3	4.0	13	1	1	3	8	8	8	8
TOTAL SINGLE DX	2	2.2	<1	2	2	2	2	3	3	3
TOTAL MULTIPLE DX	5	3.6	7	1	2	3	4	8	8	8
TOTAL										
0–19 Years	1	2.0	0	2	2	2	2	2	2	2
20–34	0									
35–49	1	4.0	0	4	4	4	4	4	4	4
50–64	1	2.0	0	2	2	2	2	2	2	2
65+	4	3.8	9	1	3	3	8	8	8	8
GRAND TOTAL	7	2.9	4	2	2	2	3	8	8	8

LOS by Diagnosis and Operation, Western Region, 45th Edition

Western Region, October 2007–September 2008 Data, by Operation

60.8: PERIPROSTATIC INC OR EXC

Type of Patients	Observed Patients	Avg. Stay	Vari-ance	10th	25th	50th	75th	90th	95th	99th
1. SINGLE DX										
0–19 Years	0									
20–34	0									
35–49	0									
50–64	0									
65+	0									
2. MULTIPLE DX										
0–19 Years	0									
20–34	0									
35–49	0									
50–64	1	4.0	0	4	4	4	4	4	4	4
65+	1	20.0	0	20	20	20	20	20	20	20
TOTAL SINGLE DX	**0**									
TOTAL MULTIPLE DX	**2**	**12.0**	**124**	**4**	**4**	**12**	**20**	**20**	**20**	**20**
TOTAL										
0–19 Years	0									
20–34	0									
35–49	0									
50–64	1	4.0	0	4	4	4	4	4	4	4
65+	1	20.0	0	20	20	20	20	20	20	20
GRAND TOTAL	**2**	**12.0**	**124**	**4**	**4**	**12**	**20**	**20**	**20**	**20**

60.94: CNTRL POSTOP PROS HEMOR

Type of Patients	Observed Patients	Avg. Stay	Vari-ance	10th	25th	50th	75th	90th	95th	99th
1. SINGLE DX										
0–19 Years	0									
20–34	0									
35–49	0									
50–64	0									
65+	2	2.0	2	1	1	2	3	3	3	3
2. MULTIPLE DX										
0–19 Years	0									
20–34	0									
35–49	3	2.3	<1	2	2	2	3	3	3	3
50–64	41	3.4	8	1	2	2	4	8	10	12
65+	164	4.7	21	1	2	3	5	10	15	24
TOTAL SINGLE DX	**2**	**2.0**	**2**	**1**	**1**	**2**	**3**	**3**	**3**	**3**
TOTAL MULTIPLE DX	**208**	**4.4**	**18**	**1**	**2**	**3**	**5**	**10**	**13**	**21**
TOTAL										
0–19 Years	0									
20–34	0									
35–49	3	2.3	<1	2	2	2	3	3	3	3
50–64	41	3.4	8	1	2	2	4	8	10	12
65+	166	4.6	21	1	2	3	5	10	15	24
GRAND TOTAL	**210**	**4.4**	**18**	**1**	**2**	**3**	**5**	**10**	**13**	**21**

60.9: OTHER PROSTATIC OPS

Type of Patients	Observed Patients	Avg. Stay	Vari-ance	10th	25th	50th	75th	90th	95th	99th
1. SINGLE DX										
0–19 Years	0									
20–34	1	6.0	0	6	6	6	6	6	6	6
35–49	0									
50–64	0									
65+	4	1.8	<1	1	1	1	3	3	3	3
2. MULTIPLE DX										
0–19 Years	1	6.0	0	6	6	6	6	6	6	6
20–34	5	3.0	0	3	3	3	3	3	3	3
35–49	5	3.4	3	2	2	2	4	6	6	6
50–64	62	3.3	10	1	1	2	4	8	10	17
65+	229	4.7	23	1	2	3	6	10	15	24
TOTAL SINGLE DX	**5**	**2.6**	**4**	**1**	**1**	**2**	**3**	**6**	**6**	**6**
TOTAL MULTIPLE DX	**298**	**4.4**	**20**	**1**	**2**	**3**	**5**	**9**	**15**	**24**
TOTAL										
0–19 Years	1	6.0	0	6	6	6	6	6	6	6
20–34	2	4.5	4	3	3	3	6	6	6	6
35–49	5	3.4	3	2	2	3	4	6	6	6
50–64	62	3.3	10	1	1	2	4	8	10	17
65+	233	4.7	23	1	2	3	6	10	15	24
GRAND TOTAL	**303**	**4.4**	**20**	**1**	**2**	**3**	**5**	**9**	**14**	**23**

61.0: SCROTUM & TUNICA VAG I&D

Type of Patients	Observed Patients	Avg. Stay	Vari-ance	10th	25th	50th	75th	90th	95th	99th
1. SINGLE DX										
0–19 Years	6	1.2	<1	1	1	1	1	3	3	3
20–34	18	1.8	1	1	1	2	2	4	5	5
35–49	17	2.1	1	1	1	1	3	4	4	4
50–64	10	1.8	1	1	1	1	3	4	4	4
65+	3	3.3	5	2	2	2	6	6	6	6
2. MULTIPLE DX										
0–19 Years	33	4.4	32	1	1	2	5	9	23	23
20–34	134	4.4	10	1	2	3	6	10	11	14
35–49	264	4.7	24	1	2	4	7	10	12	19
50–64	217	5.3	33	1	2	4	7	10	13	19
65+	107	4.8	11	1	2	4	6	9	11	17
TOTAL SINGLE DX	**54**	**1.9**	**1**	**1**	**1**	**1**	**2**	**4**	**4**	**6**
TOTAL MULTIPLE DX	**755**	**4.8**	**23**	**1**	**2**	**4**	**6**	**9**	**12**	**22**
TOTAL										
0–19 Years	39	3.9	28	1	1	2	5	8	23	23
20–34	152	4.1	10	1	2	3	6	9	10	14
35–49	281	4.5	23	1	2	3	5	9	12	19
50–64	227	5.2	32	1	2	4	7	9	13	19
65+	110	4.7	11	1	2	4	6	9	11	17
GRAND TOTAL	**809**	**4.6**	**22**	**1**	**2**	**3**	**6**	**9**	**12**	**20**

LOS by Diagnosis and Operation, Western Region, 45th Edition

TOOLS TO GROW YOUR BUSINESS

FROM BENCHMARKING TOOLS FOR INDUSTRY-WIDE INFORMATION TO CUSTOMIZED HOSPITAL-SPECIFIC REPORTS, CHOOSE FROM A VARIETY OF PUBLICATIONS TO MEET YOUR NEEDS. AVAILABLE IN SOFTBOUND, PDF, AND DATA FILE FORMATS.

Hospital Benchmarking Tools and Guides

The Sourcebook — Hospital data by comparison group
The gold standard for measuring hospital operations and financial performance — with five years of proprietary comparative and historical data on nearly 60 key performance measures for 150+ hospital comparison groups. This guide gives true apples-to-apples comparisons.

Profiles of U.S. Hospitals — Individual data on 6,000+ hospitals
Current and in-depth data available on the financial, operational, and clinical performance of nearly every hospital in the United States. The perfect resource for hospital CEOs and CFOs, industry consultants and suppliers, investment bankers, and more.

The MS-DRG Handbook — Six pages of data for each MS-DRG
Detailed clinical, financial, and statistical data on 100 of the most significant diagnosis-related groups (MS-DRGs) for both all-payer and Medicare patient groups.

Length of Stay Series — Data-based LOS norms trusted for more than 40 years
On-target length of stay (LOS) and benchmark information for every ICD-9-CM code. Compiled from an all-payer database representing approximately 20 million discharges.

Thomson Reuters 100 Top Hospitals® Benchmarks Reports

100 Top Hospitals Study Benchmarks Reports
An attractive printed document that lists award winners; describes the program, including database details, criteria, and methodologies; and outlines exciting findings on how the 100 Top Hospitals are setting performance benchmarks.

100 Top Hospitals: National Benchmarks Reports
These new reports are an affordable way to view a snapshot of a hospital's performance — individually, in relation to its peers, and in comparison to the 100 Top Hospitals winners. Reports help to assess current performance and five-year direction and speed of change against the latest benchmarks and peers, and to identify strengths and weaknesses to set performance targets.

100 Top Hospitals: Cardiovascular Benchmarks Reports
Performance measure scores and graphical analysis help you assess your performance against the latest 100 Top Hospitals cardiovascular benchmarks. Performance is evaluated in four key cardiovascular treatment areas for Medicare patients: heart failure, heart attack, angioplasty, and bypass surgery.

100 Top Hospitals Unlimited Access
Includes unlimited access to the most recent 100 Top Hospitals National and Cardiovascular Results Reports, 10 Performance Improvement Leaders Reports, all other 100 Top Hospitals study results released within 12 months, and free PDFs of study publications.

FOR MORE INFORMATION Visit http://www.techstreet.com/trhgate.html

To place an order with our Sales Department, please complete the information on the back and submit via:

- Fax +1 866 314 9717
- Ph +1 616 248 4645
- Email healthcare.pubs@thomsonreuters.com
- Invoice will be mailed separately from shipment.

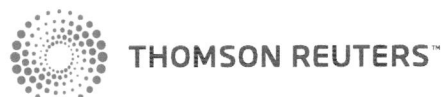
THOMSON REUTERS™

<table>
<tr><th colspan="2">SHIP-TO INFORMATION</th><th colspan="2">BILL-TO INFORMATION (IF DIFFERENT FROM SHIP-TO)</th></tr>
<tr><td colspan="2">Name:</td><td colspan="2">Name:</td></tr>
<tr><td colspan="2">Title:</td><td colspan="2">Title:</td></tr>
<tr><td colspan="2">Organization:</td><td colspan="2">Organization:</td></tr>
<tr><td colspan="2">Address:</td><td colspan="2">Address:</td></tr>
<tr><td colspan="2">City:</td><td colspan="2">City:</td></tr>
<tr><td colspan="2">State:</td><td colspan="2">State:</td></tr>
<tr><td colspan="2">ZIP Code:</td><td colspan="2">ZIP Code:</td></tr>
<tr><td colspan="2">Phone:</td><td colspan="2">Phone:</td></tr>
<tr><td colspan="2">Fax:</td><td colspan="2">Fax:</td></tr>
<tr><td colspan="2">Email:</td><td colspan="2">Email:</td></tr>
</table>

SHIPPING (PLEASE CHECK ONE)

If you have a FedEx or UPS account that you prefer to use, please indicate here:

☐ Ground: $8.95 (covers up to 5 books to one location)

☐ Priority: $18.25 (covers one book or one CD, $4.00 for each additional book)

☐ Standard: $17.25 (covers one book or one CD, $4.00 for each additional book)

☐ 2-Day: $9.25 (covers one book or one CD, $4.00 for each additional book)

SOURCEBOOK

Format	Price	Quantity
Softbound Book	$799	
PDF CD-ROM (1-2 users)	$849	
PDF CD-ROM (3-5 users)	$1,200	
PDF CD-ROM (6 or more users)	$3,000	
ASCII Data File CD (1 user)	$1,399	
Each additional user ASCII	$300	
	Subtotal*	

LENGTH OF STAY

Format	Version	Regular Price	Quantity
Softbound	United States	$599	
	Western Region	$599	
	Southern Region	$599	
	North Central Region	$599	
	Northeastern Region	$599	
	Pediatric	$599	
	Complete Set (includes all versions above)	$1,549	
CD-ROM (PDF file)	1-2 users	$535	
	3-5 users	$1,035	
	6 or more users	$3,000	
		Subtotal*	

PAYMENT METHOD (PLEASE CHECK ONE)

☐ If you have a purchase order #, please indicate here: _____

☐ Invoice me now (payment due in 30 days)

	SUBTOTAL
Sourcebook	
Length of Stay	
MS-DRG Handbook	
Profiles of U.S. Hospitals	
100 Top Hospitals	
Shipping Subtotal	
TOTAL	

MS-DRG HANDBOOK

100 Top MS-DRGs	Price	Quantity
Softbound Book	$649	
PDF CD-ROM (1-2 users)	$657	
PDF CD-ROM (3-5 users)	$1,255	
PDF CD-ROM (6 or more users)	$3,000	
Prices for All MS-DRGs (543)	**Price**	**Quantity**
ASCII Data File All MS-DRGs (1 user)	$1,464	
Each additional user	$315	
	Subtotal*	

PROFILES OF U.S. HOSPITALS

Format	Price	Quantity
Softbound Book	$559	
PDF (1-2 users)	$549	
PDF (3-5 users)	$950	
PDF (6 or more users)	$3,000	
ASCII Data File (1 user)	$1,399	
Each additional user	$300	
	Subtotal*	

To place an order with our Sales Department, please complete this form and submit via:

- Fax +1 866 314 9717
- Ph +1 616 248 4645
- Email healthcare.pubs@ thomsonreuters.com

THOMSON REUTERS 100 TOP HOSPITALS® REPORTS

Please Indicate Hospital Name, City/State, and Type (National or Cardiovascular)

	Type	Price	Quantity
1) Hospital Name, City/State, Type:	National	$1,700	
2) Hospital Name, City/State, Type:			
3) Hospital Name, City/State, Type:	Cardiovascular	$1,195	
4) Unlimited Access			
		Subtotal*	

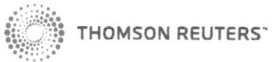

Western Region, October 2007–September 2008 Data, by Operation

61.1: SCROTUM/TUNICA DXTIC PX

Type of Patients	Observed Patients	Avg. Stay	Vari-ance	10th	25th	50th	75th	90th	95th	99th
1. SINGLE DX										
0–19 Years	0									
20–34	0									
35–49	0									
50–64	0									
65+	0									
2. MULTIPLE DX										
0–19 Years	2	6.0	2	5	5	5	7	7	7	7
20–34	2	3.0	8	1	1	5	5	5	5	5
35–49	2	8.0	2	7	7	7	9	9	9	9
50–64	0									
65+	3	3.4	6	1	1	3	6	6	6	6
TOTAL SINGLE DX	0									
TOTAL MULTIPLE DX	9	4.9	8	1	3	5	7	9	9	9
TOTAL										
0–19 Years	2	6.0	2	5	5	5	7	7	7	7
20–34	2	3.0	8	1	1	5	5	5	5	5
35–49	2	8.0	2	7	7	7	9	9	9	9
50–64	0									
65+	3	3.4	6	1	1	3	6	6	6	6
GRAND TOTAL	9	4.9	8	1	3	5	7	9	9	9

61.2: EXCISION OF HYDROCELE

Type of Patients	Observed Patients	Avg. Stay	Vari-ance	10th	25th	50th	75th	90th	95th	99th
1. SINGLE DX										
0–19 Years	1	1.0	0	1	1	1	1	1	1	1
20–34	0									
35–49	2	1.0	0	1	1	1	1	1	1	1
50–64	3	2.3	1	1	1	3	3	3	3	3
65+	0									
2. MULTIPLE DX										
0–19 Years	6	8.6	664	1	1	1	1	2	90	90
20–34	2	30.0	>999	5	5	5	55	55	55	55
35–49	11	2.4	3	1	1	2	3	4	6	6
50–64	16	5.3	124	1	1	2	3	9	46	46
65+	28	3.1	10	1	1	1	3	9	11	11
TOTAL SINGLE DX	6	1.7	1	1	1	1	3	3	3	3
TOTAL MULTIPLE DX	63	5.2	181	1	1	1	3	9	11	90
TOTAL										
0–19 Years	7	8.0	613	1	1	1	1	2	90	90
20–34	2	30.0	>999	5	5	5	55	55	55	55
35–49	13	2.2	2	1	1	1	1	4	6	6
50–64	19	4.9	105	1	1	2	3	9	46	46
65+	28	3.1	10	1	1	1	3	9	11	11
GRAND TOTAL	69	4.9	167	1	1	1	3	7	11	90

61.3: SCROTAL LES EXC/DESTR

Type of Patients	Observed Patients	Avg. Stay	Vari-ance	10th	25th	50th	75th	90th	95th	99th
1. SINGLE DX										
0–19 Years	3	2.0	1	1	1	2	3	3	3	3
20–34	2	3.0	8	1	1	7	5	5	5	5
35–49	1	7.0	0	7	7	7	7	7	7	7
50–64	1	1.0	0	1	1	1	1	1	1	1
65+	0									
2. MULTIPLE DX										
0–19 Years	5	9.6	48	2	2	12	18	18	18	18
20–34	14	7.9	89	2	2	5	8	25	33	33
35–49	55	6.4	14	3	3	6	8	12	14	19
50–64	39	6.7	45	1	3	5	8	16	20	37
65+	31	9.8	102	2	4	7	12	20	32	49
TOTAL SINGLE DX	7	2.8	5	1	1	2	5	7	7	7
TOTAL MULTIPLE DX	144	7.6	50	2	3	6	9	16	20	37
TOTAL										
0–19 Years	8	8.3	48	1	2	5	12	18	18	18
20–34	16	7.3	81	1	2	4	8	25	33	33
35–49	56	6.4	14	3	3	6	8	12	14	19
50–64	40	6.6	45	2	3	5	7	12	19	37
65+	31	9.8	102	2	4	7	12	20	32	49
GRAND TOTAL	151	7.4	49	2	3	6	9	16	19	37

61.4: SCROTUM & TUNICA VAG REP

Type of Patients	Observed Patients	Avg. Stay	Vari-ance	10th	25th	50th	75th	90th	95th	99th
1. SINGLE DX										
0–19 Years	6	1.0	0	1	1	1	1	1	1	1
20–34	1	1.0	0	1	1	1	1	1	1	1
35–49	2	4.0	18	1	1	4	7	7	7	7
50–64	0									
65+	1	2.0	0	2	2	2	2	2	2	2
2. MULTIPLE DX										
0–19 Years	11	1.2	<1	1	1	1	1	1	2	4
20–34	18	6.5	68	1	1	4	6	24	29	29
35–49	22	11.6	165	1	3	7	22	28	38	41
50–64	17	11.2	201	2	3	5	13	24	59	59
65+	6	4.5	3		3	5	5	7	7	7
TOTAL SINGLE DX	10	1.5	3	1	1	1	1	2	7	7
TOTAL MULTIPLE DX	74	7.0	109	1	1	2	7	24	28	59
TOTAL										
0–19 Years	17	1.1	<1	1	1	1	1	1	2	4
20–34	19	6.2	66	1	1	4	6	24	29	29
35–49	24	11.0	156	1	2	7	22	28	38	41
50–64	17	11.2	201	2	3	7	13	24	59	59
65+	7	4.2	3	2	2	5	5	7	7	7
GRAND TOTAL	84	6.3	98	1	1	2	6	21	24	41

LOS by Diagnosis and Operation, Western Region, 45th Edition

Western Region, October 2007–September 2008 Data, by Operation

61.9: OTH SCROT/TUNICA VAG OPS

Type of Patients	Observed Patients	Avg. Stay	Variance	Percentiles						
				10th	25th	50th	75th	90th	95th	99th
1. SINGLE DX										
0–19 Years	0									
20–34	0									
35–49	0									
50–64	0									
65+	0									
2. MULTIPLE DX										
0–19 Years	0									
20–34	2	5.5	4	4	4	4	7	7	7	7
35–49	3	9.3	119	3	3	3	22	22	22	22
50–64	5	12.6	37	5	7	16	17	18	18	18
65+	6	3.2	5	1	1	2	5	6	6	6
TOTAL SINGLE DX	0									
TOTAL MULTIPLE DX	16	7.5	45	1	3	5	7	18	22	22
TOTAL										
0–19 Years	0									
20–34	2	5.5	4	4	4	4	7	7	7	7
35–49	3	9.3	119	3	3	3	22	22	22	22
50–64	5	12.6	37	5	7	16	17	18	18	18
65+	6	3.2	5	1	1	2	5	6	6	6
GRAND TOTAL	16	7.5	45	1	3	5	7	18	22	22

62.1: TESTES DXTIC PX

Type of Patients	Observed Patients	Avg. Stay	Variance	Percentiles						
				10th	25th	50th	75th	90th	95th	99th
1. SINGLE DX										
0–19 Years	2	4.0	0	4	4	4	4	4	4	4
20–34	0									
35–49	0									
50–64	0									
65+	0									
2. MULTIPLE DX										
0–19 Years	6	7.6	63	1	1	4	11	23	23	23
20–34	0									
35–49	2	6.5	59	1	1	7	12	12	12	12
50–64	0									
65+	0									
TOTAL SINGLE DX	2	4.0	0	4	4	4	4	4	4	4
TOTAL MULTIPLE DX	8	7.4	59	1	1	4	11	23	23	23
TOTAL										
0–19 Years	8	6.6	47	1	1	4	11	23	23	23
20–34	0									
35–49	2	6.5	59	1	1	7	12	12	12	12
50–64	0									
65+	0									
GRAND TOTAL	10	6.6	46	1	1	4	11	12	23	23

62.0: INCISION OF TESTIS

Type of Patients	Observed Patients	Avg. Stay	Variance	Percentiles						
				10th	25th	50th	75th	90th	95th	99th
1. SINGLE DX										
0–19 Years	2	1.0	0	1	1	1	1	1	1	1
20–34	1	7.0	0	7	7	7	7	7	7	7
35–49	2	1.0	0	1	1	1	1	1	1	1
50–64	0									
65+	0									
2. MULTIPLE DX										
0–19 Years	3	1.0	0	1	1	1	1	1	1	1
20–34	5	1.6	2	1	1	1	1	4	4	4
35–49	4	6.3	27	2	3	3	5	14	14	14
50–64	3	3.0	<1	2	2	3	4	4	4	4
65+	2	7.5	40	3	3	8	12	12	12	12
TOTAL SINGLE DX	5	2.2	7	1	1	1	1	7	7	7
TOTAL MULTIPLE DX	17	3.2	13	1	1	2	4	12	14	14
TOTAL										
0–19 Years	5	1.0	0	1	1	1	1	1	1	1
20–34	6	2.5	6	1	1	1	4	7	7	7
35–49	6	4.5	24	1	1	3	5	14	14	14
50–64	3	3.0	<1	2	2	3	4	4	4	4
65+	2	7.5	40	3	3	8	12	12	12	12
GRAND TOTAL	22	3.0	12	1	1	1	3	7	12	14

62.2: TESTICULAR LES EXC/DESTR

Type of Patients	Observed Patients	Avg. Stay	Variance	Percentiles						
				10th	25th	50th	75th	90th	95th	99th
1. SINGLE DX										
0–19 Years	6	1.0	0	1	1	1	1	1	1	1
20–34	0									
35–49	1	4.0	0	4	4	4	4	4	4	4
50–64	0									
65+	0									
2. MULTIPLE DX										
0–19 Years	7	1.2	<1	1	1	1	1	2	3	3
20–34	1	3.0	0	3	3	3	3	3	3	3
35–49	1	7.0	0	7	7	7	7	7	7	7
50–64	2	19.5	258	8	8	8	31	31	31	31
65+	0									
TOTAL SINGLE DX	7	1.3	<1	1	1	1	1	1	4	4
TOTAL MULTIPLE DX	11	3.8	53	1	1	3	3	8	31	31
TOTAL										
0–19 Years	13	1.1	<1	1	1	1	1	1	2	3
20–34	1	3.0	0	3	3	3	3	3	3	3
35–49	2	5.5	4	4	4	4	7	7	7	7
50–64	2	19.5	258	8	8	8	31	31	31	31
65+	0									
GRAND TOTAL	18	2.8	33	1	1	1	1	7	8	31

Western Region, October 2007–September 2008 Data, by Operation

62.3: UNILATERAL ORCHIECTOMY

Type of Patients	Observed Patients	Avg. Stay	Variance	10th	25th	50th	75th	90th	95th	99th
1. SINGLE DX										
0–19 Years	54	1.3	<1	1	1	1	1	2	2	4
20–34	41	2.0	7	1	1	1	2	4	4	17
35–49	29	2.1	4	1	1	1	2	6	6	10
50–64	5	1.4	<1	1	1	1	2	2	2	2
65+	2	1.5	<1	1	1	1	2	2	2	2
2. MULTIPLE DX										
0–19 Years	116	2.8	20	1	1	1	3	7	10	12
20–34	141	4.9	79	1	1	2	6	9	16	43
35–49	79	5.7	64	1	1	3	6	14	19	44
50–64	100	4.3	32	1	1	2	5	12	15	42
65+	85	6.8	64	1	2	4	8	15	27	42
TOTAL SINGLE DX	**131**	**1.6**	**3**	**1**	**1**	**1**	**2**	**2**	**4**	**10**
TOTAL MULTIPLE DX	**521**	**4.5**	**49**	**1**	**1**	**2**	**5**	**10**	**14**	**41**
TOTAL										
0–19 Years	170	2.4	15	1	1	1	2	6	10	12
20–34	182	4.3	64	1	1	2	5	8	12	43
35–49	108	4.7	50	1	1	2	6	11	14	41
50–64	105	4.1	31	1	1	2	5	11	13	20
65+	87	6.7	63	1	2	4	8	15	27	42
GRAND TOTAL	**652**	**3.9**	**41**	**1**	**1**	**2**	**4**	**9**	**12**	**35**

62.4: BILATERAL ORCHIECTOMY

Type of Patients	Observed Patients	Avg. Stay	Variance	10th	25th	50th	75th	90th	95th	99th
1. SINGLE DX										
0–19 Years	1	1.0	0	1	1	1	1	1	1	1
20–34	1	1.0	0	1	1	1	1	1	1	1
35–49	1	2.0	0	2	2	2	2	2	2	2
50–64	0									
65+	0									
2. MULTIPLE DX										
0–19 Years	5	1.3	<1	1	1	1	2	2	2	2
20–34	3	7.3	25	2	2	8	12	12	12	12
35–49	8	2.4	7	1	2	2	2	9	9	9
50–64	15	11.7	131	4	4	9	11	31	44	44
65+	78	5.5	31	1	2	3	7	15	19	28
TOTAL SINGLE DX	**3**	**1.3**	**<1**	**1**	**1**	**1**	**2**	**2**	**2**	**2**
TOTAL MULTIPLE DX	**109**	**5.8**	**46**	**1**	**2**	**3**	**8**	**12**	**19**	**31**
TOTAL										
0–19 Years	6	1.3	<1	1	1	1	2	2	2	2
20–34	4	5.7	27	1	2	2	8	12	12	12
35–49	9	2.3	7	1	2	2	2	9	9	9
50–64	15	11.7	131	4	4	9	11	31	44	44
65+	78	5.5	31	1	2	3	7	15	19	28
GRAND TOTAL	**112**	**5.7**	**45**	**1**	**2**	**3**	**8**	**12**	**19**	**31**

62.41: RMVL BOTH TESTES

Type of Patients	Observed Patients	Avg. Stay	Variance	10th	25th	50th	75th	90th	95th	99th
1. SINGLE DX										
0–19 Years	1	1.0	0	1	1	1	1	1	1	1
20–34	1	1.0	0	1	1	1	1	1	1	1
35–49	0									
50–64	0									
65+	0									
2. MULTIPLE DX										
0–19 Years	4	1.4	<1	1	1	1	2	2	2	2
20–34	0									
35–49	3	4.0	19	1	5	2	9	9	9	9
50–64	14	12.3	135	4	5	9	11	31	44	44
65+	78	5.5	31	1	2	3	7	15	19	28
TOTAL SINGLE DX	**2**	**1.0**	**0**	**1**	**1**	**1**	**1**	**1**	**1**	**1**
TOTAL MULTIPLE DX	**99**	**6.1**	**48**	**1**	**2**	**4**	**9**	**15**	**19**	**31**
TOTAL										
0–19 Years	5	1.3	<1	1	1	1	2	2	2	2
20–34	1	1.0	0	1	1	1	1	1	1	1
35–49	3	4.0	19	1	1	9	9	9	9	9
50–64	14	12.3	135	4	5	9	11	31	44	44
65+	78	5.5	31	1	2	3	7	15	19	28
GRAND TOTAL	**101**	**6.0**	**48**	**1**	**2**	**4**	**9**	**15**	**19**	**31**

62.5: ORCHIOPEXY

Type of Patients	Observed Patients	Avg. Stay	Variance	10th	25th	50th	75th	90th	95th	99th
1. SINGLE DX										
0–19 Years	115	1.1	<1	1	1	1	1	2	2	3
20–34	30	1.0	0	1	1	1	1	1	1	1
35–49	6	1.0	0	1	1	1	1	1	1	1
50–64	0									
65+	0									
2. MULTIPLE DX										
0–19 Years	165	1.8	27	1	1	1	1	2	4	9
20–34	26	2.1	5	1	1	1	2	4	5	12
35–49	13	1.8	3	1	1	1	2	3	7	7
50–64	5	4.2	51	1	1	1	1	17	17	17
65+	1	1.0	0	1	1	1	1	1	1	1
TOTAL SINGLE DX	**151**	**1.1**	**<1**	**1**	**1**	**1**	**1**	**2**	**2**	**3**
TOTAL MULTIPLE DX	**210**	**1.8**	**24**	**1**	**1**	**1**	**1**	**2**	**4**	**14**
TOTAL										
0–19 Years	280	1.6	18	1	1	1	1	2	3	6
20–34	56	1.5	3	1	1	1	1	2	4	12
35–49	19	1.5	2	1	1	1	1	3	7	9
50–64	5	4.2	51	1	1	1	1	17	17	17
65+	1	1.0	0	1	1	1	1	1	1	1
GRAND TOTAL	**361**	**1.6**	**16**	**1**	**1**	**1**	**1**	**2**	**3**	**9**

LOS by Diagnosis and Operation, Western Region, 45th Edition

Western Region, October 2007–September 2008 Data, by Operation

62.6: TESTES REPAIR

Type of Patients	Observed Patients	Avg. Stay	Vari-ance	Percentiles						
				10th	25th	50th	75th	90th	95th	99th
1. SINGLE DX										
0–19 Years	1	1.0	0	1	1	1	1	1	1	1
20–34	3	1.3	<1	1	1	1	2	2	2	2
35–49	1	2.0	0	2	2	2	2	2	2	2
50–64	1	3.0	0	3	3	3	3	3	3	3
65+	0									
2. MULTIPLE DX										
0–19 Years	9	2.2	3	1	1	1	3	6	6	6
20–34	12	2.0	3	1	1	1	3	4	6	6
35–49	4	1.5	<1	1	1	1	2	2	2	2
50–64	1	9.0	0	9	9	9	9	9	9	9
65+	0									
TOTAL SINGLE DX	6	1.7	<1	1	1	1	2	3	3	3
TOTAL MULTIPLE DX	26	2.3	4	1	1	1	3	6	6	9
TOTAL										
0–19 Years	10	2.1	3	1	1	1	3	6	6	6
20–34	15	1.9	2	1	1	1	2	4	6	6
35–49	5	1.6	<1	1	1	1	2	2	2	2
50–64	2	6.0	18	3	3	9	9	9	9	9
65+	0									
GRAND TOTAL	32	2.2	4	1	1	1	2	4	6	9

62.7: INSERT TESTICULAR PROSTH

Type of Patients	Observed Patients	Avg. Stay	Vari-ance	Percentiles						
				10th	25th	50th	75th	90th	95th	99th
1. SINGLE DX										
0–19 Years	0									
20–34	1	6.0	0	6	6	6	6	6	6	6
35–49	0									
50–64	0									
65+	0									
2. MULTIPLE DX										
0–19 Years	1	2.0	0	2	2	2	2	2	2	2
20–34	0									
35–49	1	1.0	0	1	1	1	1	1	1	1
50–64	0									
65+	0									
TOTAL SINGLE DX	1	6.0	0	6	6	6	6	6	6	6
TOTAL MULTIPLE DX	2	1.7	<1	1	1	2	2	2	2	2
TOTAL										
0–19 Years	1	2.0	0	2	2	2	2	2	2	2
20–34	1	6.0	0	6	6	6	6	6	6	6
35–49	1	1.0	0	1	1	1	1	1	1	1
50–64	0									
65+	0									
GRAND TOTAL	3	2.8	5	1	1	2	2	4	6	6

62.9: OTHER TESTICULAR OPS

Type of Patients	Observed Patients	Avg. Stay	Vari-ance	Percentiles						
				10th	25th	50th	75th	90th	95th	99th
1. SINGLE DX										
0–19 Years	0									
20–34	0									
35–49	0									
50–64	1	1.0	0	1	1	1	1	1	1	1
65+	0									
2. MULTIPLE DX										
0–19 Years	0									
20–34	0									
35–49	2	7.6	84	1	1	14	14	14	14	14
50–64	0									
65+	3	6.0	16	2	2	6	10	10	10	10
TOTAL SINGLE DX	1	1.0	0	1	1	1	1	1	1	1
TOTAL MULTIPLE DX	5	6.6	30	1	2	6	10	14	14	14
TOTAL										
0–19 Years	0									
20–34	0									
35–49	2	7.6	84	1	1	14	14	14	14	14
50–64	1	1.0	0	1	1	1	1	1	1	1
65+	3	6.0	16	2	2	6	10	10	10	10
GRAND TOTAL	6	5.7	29	1	1	2	10	14	14	14

63.0: SPERMATIC CORD DXTIC PX

Type of Patients	Observed Patients	Avg. Stay	Vari-ance	Percentiles						
				10th	25th	50th	75th	90th	95th	99th
1. SINGLE DX										
0–19 Years	0									
20–34	0									
35–49	0									
50–64	0									
65+	0									
2. MULTIPLE DX										
0–19 Years	0									
20–34	0									
35–49	0									
50–64	0									
65+	0									
TOTAL SINGLE DX	0									
TOTAL MULTIPLE DX	0									
TOTAL										
0–19 Years	0									
20–34	0									
35–49	0									
50–64	0									
65+	0									
GRAND TOTAL	0									

LOS by Diagnosis and Operation, Western Region, 45th Edition

Western Region, October 2007–September 2008 Data, by Operation

63.1: EXC SPERMATIC VARICOCELE

Type of Patients	Observed Patients	Avg. Stay	Vari-ance	Percentiles						
				10th	25th	50th	75th	90th	95th	99th
1. SINGLE DX										
0–19 Years	6	1.5	<1	1	1	1	2	3	3	3
20–34	0									
35–49	2	1.5	<1	1	1	1	2	2	2	2
50–64	0									
65+	0									
2. MULTIPLE DX										
0–19 Years	8	5.1	289	1	1	1	1	1	71	71
20–34	7	2.4	4	1	1	2	2	7	7	7
35–49	8	1.3	<1	1	1	1	2	2	2	2
50–64	13	2.9	20	1	1	1	3	5	17	17
65+	14	3.4	7	2	2	2	4	8	10	10
TOTAL SINGLE DX	8	1.5	<1	1	1	1	2	3	3	3
TOTAL MULTIPLE DX	48	3.5	91	1	1	1	2	5	10	71
TOTAL										
0–19 Years	14	3.8	183	1	1	1	1	3	3	71
20–34	7	2.4	4	1	1	1	2	7	7	7
35–49	8	1.4	<1	1	1	1	2	2	2	2
50–64	13	2.9	20	1	1	1	3	5	17	17
65+	14	3.4	7	1	2	2	4	8	10	10
GRAND TOTAL	56	3.1	76	1	1	1	2	5	8	71

63.2: EXC EPIDIDYMIS CYST

Type of Patients	Observed Patients	Avg. Stay	Vari-ance	Percentiles						
				10th	25th	50th	75th	90th	95th	99th
1. SINGLE DX										
0–19 Years	0									
20–34	0									
35–49	1	1.0	0	1	1	1	1	1	1	1
50–64	1	1.0	0	1	1	1	1	1	1	1
65+	1	1.0	0	1	1	1	1	1	1	1
2. MULTIPLE DX										
0–19 Years	0									
20–34	1	4.0	0	4	4	4	4	4	4	4
35–49	1	1.0	0	1	1	1	1	1	1	1
50–64	7	1.1	<1	1	1	1	1	2	2	2
65+	4	2.5	6	1	2	2	2	6	6	6
TOTAL SINGLE DX	3	1.0	0	1	1	1	1	1	1	1
TOTAL MULTIPLE DX	13	1.8	2	1	1	1	2	4	6	6
TOTAL										
0–19 Years	0									
20–34	1	4.0	0	4	4	4	4	4	4	4
35–49	2	1.0	0	1	1	1	1	1	1	1
50–64	8	1.1	<1	1	1	1	2	2	2	2
65+	5	2.2	5	1	1	1	2	6	6	6
GRAND TOTAL	16	1.6	2	1	1	1	1	4	6	6

63.3: EXC SPERM CORD LES NEC

Type of Patients	Observed Patients	Avg. Stay	Vari-ance	Percentiles						
				10th	25th	50th	75th	90th	95th	99th
1. SINGLE DX										
0–19 Years	1	2.0	0	2	2	2	2	2	2	2
20–34	0									
35–49	0									
50–64	1	6.0	0	6	6	6	6	6	6	6
65+	0									
2. MULTIPLE DX										
0–19 Years	1	1.0	0	1	1	1	1	1	1	1
20–34	5	7.6	47	1	1	8	11	17	17	17
35–49	4	2.0	0	2	2	2	2	2	2	2
50–64	4	4.2	5	1	1	5	6	6	6	6
65+	4	3.0	6	1	1	1	4	6	6	6
TOTAL SINGLE DX	2	4.0	8	2	2	4	6	6	6	6
TOTAL MULTIPLE DX	15	4.7	21	1	1	4	6	11	17	17
TOTAL										
0–19 Years	2	1.5	<1	1	1	2	2	2	2	2
20–34	5	7.6	47	1	1	8	11	17	17	17
35–49	5	2.0	0	2	2	2	2	2	2	2
50–64	5	4.6	4	1	5	5	6	6	6	6
65+	4	3.0	6	1	1	1	4	6	6	6
GRAND TOTAL	17	4.6	19	1	1	4	6	11	17	17

63.4: EPIDIDYMECTOMY

Type of Patients	Observed Patients	Avg. Stay	Vari-ance	Percentiles						
				10th	25th	50th	75th	90th	95th	99th
1. SINGLE DX										
0–19 Years	0									
20–34	0									
35–49	0									
50–64	1	1.0	0	1	1	1	1	1	1	1
65+	0									
2. MULTIPLE DX										
0–19 Years	0									
20–34	2	5.5	<1	5	5	6	6	6	6	6
35–49	2	3.5	<1	3	3	4	4	4	4	4
50–64	3	3.7	6	1	1	4	5	6	6	6
65+	6	3.3	4	1	1	3	5	6	6	6
TOTAL SINGLE DX	1	1.0	0	1	1	1	1	1	1	1
TOTAL MULTIPLE DX	13	3.8	4	1	3	4	5	6	6	6
TOTAL										
0–19 Years	0									
20–34	2	5.5	<1	5	5	6	6	6	6	6
35–49	2	3.5	<1	3	3	4	4	4	4	4
50–64	4	3.0	6	1	1	4	5	6	6	6
65+	6	3.3	4	1	1	3	5	6	6	6
GRAND TOTAL	14	3.6	4	1	1	4	5	6	6	6

LOS by Diagnosis and Operation, Western Region, 45th Edition

Western Region, October 2007–September 2008 Data, by Operation

63.5: SPERM CORD/EPID REPAIR

Type of Patients	Observed Patients	Avg. Stay	Vari-ance	Percentiles						
				10th	25th	50th	75th	90th	95th	99th
1. SINGLE DX										
0–19 Years	4	1.0	0	1	1	1	1	1	1	1
20–34	4	1.0	0	1	1	1	1	1	1	1
35–49	1	1.0	0	1	1	1	1	1	1	1
50–64	0									
65+	0									
2. MULTIPLE DX										
0–19 Years	2	1.0	0	1	1	1	1	1	1	1
20–34	0									
35–49	1	1.0	0	1	1	1	1	1	1	1
50–64	2	7.5	82	1	1	14	14	14	14	14
65+	0									
TOTAL SINGLE DX	9	1.0	0	1	1	1	1	1	1	1
TOTAL MULTIPLE DX	5	2.6	21	1	1	1	1	14	14	14
TOTAL										
0–19 Years	6	1.0	0	1	1	1	1	1	1	1
20–34	4	1.0	0	1	1	1	1	1	1	1
35–49	2	1.0	0	1	1	1	1	1	1	1
50–64	2	7.5	82	1	1	14	14	14	14	14
65+	0									
GRAND TOTAL	14	1.8	10	1	1	1	1	1	14	14

63.6: VASOTOMY

Type of Patients	Observed Patients	Avg. Stay	Vari-ance	Percentiles						
				10th	25th	50th	75th	90th	95th	99th
1. SINGLE DX										
0–19 Years	0									
20–34	0									
35–49	0									
50–64	0									
65+	0									
2. MULTIPLE DX										
0–19 Years	0									
20–34	0									
35–49	0									
50–64	0									
65+	0									
TOTAL SINGLE DX	0									
TOTAL MULTIPLE DX	0									
TOTAL										
0–19 Years	0									
20–34	0									
35–49	0									
50–64	0									
65+	0									
GRAND TOTAL	0									

63.7: VASECTOMY & VAS DEF LIG

Type of Patients	Observed Patients	Avg. Stay	Vari-ance	Percentiles						
				10th	25th	50th	75th	90th	95th	99th
1. SINGLE DX										
0–19 Years	0									
20–34	0									
35–49	0									
50–64	0									
65+	0									
2. MULTIPLE DX										
0–19 Years	0									
20–34	0									
35–49	0									
50–64	1	1.0	0	1	1	1	1	1	1	1
65+	1	12.0	0	12	12	12	12	12	12	12
TOTAL SINGLE DX	0									
TOTAL MULTIPLE DX	2	6.5	59	1	1	1	12	12	12	12
TOTAL										
0–19 Years	0									
20–34	0									
35–49	0									
50–64	1	1.0	0	1	1	1	1	1	1	1
65+	1	12.0	0	12	12	12	12	12	12	12
GRAND TOTAL	2	6.5	59	1	1	1	12	12	12	12

63.8: VAS DEF & EPID REPAIR

Type of Patients	Observed Patients	Avg. Stay	Vari-ance	Percentiles						
				10th	25th	50th	75th	90th	95th	99th
1. SINGLE DX										
0–19 Years	0									
20–34	0									
35–49	0									
50–64	0									
65+	0									
2. MULTIPLE DX										
0–19 Years	0									
20–34	0									
35–49	0									
50–64	0									
65+	0									
TOTAL SINGLE DX	0									
TOTAL MULTIPLE DX	0									
TOTAL										
0–19 Years	0									
20–34	0									
35–49	0									
50–64	0									
65+	0									
GRAND TOTAL	0									

LOS by Diagnosis and Operation, Western Region, 45th Edition

Western Region, October 2007–September 2008 Data, by Operation

63.9: OTH SPERM CORD/EPID OPS

Type of Patients	Observed Patients	Avg. Stay	Variance	Percentiles						
				10th	25th	50th	75th	90th	95th	99th
1. SINGLE DX										
0–19 Years	0									
20–34	1	3.0	0	3	3	3	3	3	3	3
35–49	1									
50–64	0									
65+	0									
2. MULTIPLE DX										
0–19 Years	2	2.6	2	2	2	2	2	5	5	5
20–34	0									
35–49	3	4.0	<1	3	3	4	5	5	5	5
50–64	3	5.7	21	3	3	3	11	11	11	11
65+	2	5.0	8	3	3	3	7	7	7	7
TOTAL SINGLE DX	1	3.0	0	3	3	3	3	3	3	3
TOTAL MULTIPLE DX	10	4.0	7	2	2	3	5	7	11	11
TOTAL										
0–19 Years	2	2.6	2	2	2	2	2	5	5	5
20–34	1	3.0	0	3	3	3	3	3	3	3
35–49	3	4.0	<1	3	3	4	5	5	5	5
50–64	3	5.7	21	3	3	3	11	11	11	11
65+	2	5.0	8	3	3	3	7	7	7	7
GRAND TOTAL	11	3.9	6	2	2	3	5	7	11	11

64.0: CIRCUMCISION

Type of Patients	Observed Patients	Avg. Stay	Variance	Percentiles						
				10th	25th	50th	75th	90th	95th	99th
1. SINGLE DX										
0–19 Years	31,436	2.0	<1	1	1	2	2	3	4	4
20–34	4	1.0	0	1	1	1	1	1	1	1
35–49	1	1.0	0							
50–64	0									
65+	1	1.0	0	1	1	1	1	1	1	1
2. MULTIPLE DX										
0–19 Years	75,298	2.6	11	1	2	2	3	4	4	16
20–34	10	3.3	9	1	1	2	5	6	10	10
35–49	10	2.9	4	1	1	3	4	7	7	7
50–64	9	3.3	15	1	1	1	4	13	13	13
65+	27	5.6	29	2	2	4	7	12	18	24
TOTAL SINGLE DX	31,442	2.0	<1	1	1	2	2	3	4	4
TOTAL MULTIPLE DX	75,354	2.6	11	1	2	2	3	4	4	16
TOTAL										
0–19 Years	106,734	2.4	8	1	2	2	3	4	4	13
20–34	14	2.6	7	1	3	3	3	6	10	10
35–49	11	2.7	4	1	1	3	4	5	7	7
50–64	9	3.3	15	1	1	4	4	13	13	13
65+	28	5.4	29	2	2	4	7	12	18	24
GRAND TOTAL	106,796	2.4	8	1	2	2	3	4	4	13

64.1: PENILE DIAGNOSTIC PX

Type of Patients	Observed Patients	Avg. Stay	Variance	Percentiles						
				10th	25th	50th	75th	90th	95th	99th
1. SINGLE DX										
0–19 Years	0									
20–34	1	2.0	0	2	2	2	2	2	2	2
35–49	0									
50–64	0									
65+	0									
2. MULTIPLE DX										
0–19 Years	0									
20–34	0									
35–49	1	8.0	0	8	8	8	8	8	8	8
50–64	4	9.5	39	2	2	7	13	16	16	16
65+	13	8.2	36	1	2	7	11	18	19	19
TOTAL SINGLE DX	1	2.0	0	2	2	2	2	2	2	2
TOTAL MULTIPLE DX	18	8.4	33	1	2	8	13	18	19	19
TOTAL										
0–19 Years	0									
20–34	1	2.0	0	2	2	2	2	2	2	2
35–49	1	8.0	0	8	8	8	8	8	8	8
50–64	4	9.5	39	2	2	7	13	16	16	16
65+	13	8.2	36	1	2	7	11	18	19	19
GRAND TOTAL	19	8.1	33	1	2	7	13	18	19	19

64.2: LOC EXC/DESTR PENILE LES

Type of Patients	Observed Patients	Avg. Stay	Variance	Percentiles						
				10th	25th	50th	75th	90th	95th	99th
1. SINGLE DX										
0–19 Years	0									
20–34	1	1.0	0	1	1	1	1	1	1	1
35–49	1	3.0	0	3	3	3	3	3	3	3
50–64	3	2.3	5	1	1	1	5	5	5	5
65+	1	1.0	0	1	1	1	1	1	1	1
2. MULTIPLE DX										
0–19 Years	14	5.4	237	1	1	2	3	3	14	80
20–34	11	8.5	87	2	4	5	12	18	32	32
35–49	21	8.3	67	3	4	5	10	12	14	40
50–64	37	8.9	101	2	4	5	14	21	32	49
65+	22	7.8	65	2	2	5	9	20	23	33
TOTAL SINGLE DX	6	2.0	3	1	1	1	3	5	5	5
TOTAL MULTIPLE DX	105	7.8	115	1	2	4	9	17	32	49
TOTAL										
0–19 Years	14	5.4	237	1	1	2	3	3	14	80
20–34	12	7.9	83	1	3	5	12	18	32	32
35–49	22	8.1	66	1	2	5	10	12	14	40
50–64	40	8.4	97	1	2	5	9	17	32	49
65+	23	7.5	64	2	2	5	9	20	23	33
GRAND TOTAL	111	7.5	111	1	2	4	9	16	24	49

LOS by Diagnosis and Operation, Western Region, 45th Edition

Western Region, October 2007–September 2008 Data, by Operation

64.3: AMPUTATION OF PENIS

Type of Patients	Observed Patients	Avg. Stay	Variance	Percentiles						
				10th	25th	50th	75th	90th	95th	99th
1. SINGLE DX										
0–19 Years	0									
20–34	0									
35–49	4	2.0	2	1	1	2	4	4	4	4
50–64	6	2.5	2	1	2	2	3	5	5	5
65+	3	1.0	0	1	1	1	1	1	1	1
2. MULTIPLE DX										
0–19 Years	0									
20–34	1	3.0	0	3	3	3	3	3	3	3
35–49	5	5.0	23	1	2	3	6	13	13	13
50–64	29	3.9	15	1	1	3	4	13	13	15
65+	49	5.7	67	1	1	2	7	16	27	37
TOTAL SINGLE DX	13	2.0	2	1	1	2	2	4	5	5
TOTAL MULTIPLE DX	84	5.0	46	1	1	2	5	13	16	37
TOTAL										
0–19 Years	0									
20–34	1	3.0	0	3	3	3	3	3	3	3
35–49	9	3.7	15	1	1	2	4	13	13	13
50–64	35	3.7	13	1	1	3	4	9	13	15
65+	52	5.5	65	1	1	2	7	11	27	37
GRAND TOTAL	97	4.6	41	1	1	2	5	11	16	37

64.4: PENILE REP/PLASTIC OPS

Type of Patients	Observed Patients	Avg. Stay	Variance	Percentiles						
				10th	25th	50th	75th	90th	95th	99th
1. SINGLE DX										
0–19 Years	14	1.1	<1	1	1	1	1	2	2	3
20–34	17	1.2	<1	1	1	1	1	1	4	4
35–49	15	1.1	<1	1	1	1	1	2	2	2
50–64	4	1.3	<1	1	1	1	2	2	2	2
65+	0									
2. MULTIPLE DX										
0–19 Years	58	2.9	8	1	1	2	4	7	12	12
20–34	32	2.0	4	1	1	1	2	4	5	11
35–49	50	3.7	27	1	1	1	4	8	13	26
50–64	35	3.7	29	1	1	1	4	6	22	24
65+	9	3.8	11	1	1	2	6	10	10	10
TOTAL SINGLE DX	50	1.2	<1	1	1	1	1	2	2	4
TOTAL MULTIPLE DX	184	3.1	16	1	1	2	4	7	12	24
TOTAL										
0–19 Years	72	2.4	6	1	1	1	3	5	7	12
20–34	49	1.7	3	1	1	1	2	4	4	11
35–49	65	3.1	22	1	1	1	2	7	13	26
50–64	39	3.4	26	1	1	2	4	6	22	24
65+	9	3.8	11	1	1	2	6	10	10	10
GRAND TOTAL	234	2.7	13	1	1	1	3	6	8	24

64.49: PENILE REPAIR NEC

Type of Patients	Observed Patients	Avg. Stay	Variance	Percentiles						
				10th	25th	50th	75th	90th	95th	99th
1. SINGLE DX										
0–19 Years	8	1.3	<1	1	1	1	1	2	3	3
20–34	16	1.2	<1	1	1	1	1	1	4	4
35–49	14	1.1	<1	1	1	1	1	2	2	2
50–64	4	1.3	<1	1	1	1	2	2	2	2
65+	0									
2. MULTIPLE DX										
0–19 Years	22	4.1	16	1	1	3	4	12	12	12
20–34	19	1.5	1	1	1	1	2	3	5	5
35–49	34	3.7	35	1	1	2	3	8	24	26
50–64	23	2.3	6	1	1	1	2	5	6	12
65+	6	3.3	13	1	1	2	5	10	10	10
TOTAL SINGLE DX	42	1.2	<1	1	1	1	1	2	2	4
TOTAL MULTIPLE DX	104	3.1	18	1	1	1	3	7	12	24
TOTAL										
0–19 Years	30	3.1	12	1	1	2	3	12	12	12
20–34	35	1.4	<1	1	1	1	1	2	4	5
35–49	48	3.0	26	1	1	1	2	6	13	26
50–64	27	2.1	6	1	1	1	2	5	6	12
65+	6	3.3	13	1	1	2	5	10	10	10
GRAND TOTAL	146	2.5	13	1	1	1	2	5	12	24

64.5: SEX TRANSFORMATION NEC

Type of Patients	Observed Patients	Avg. Stay	Variance	Percentiles						
				10th	25th	50th	75th	90th	95th	99th
1. SINGLE DX										
0–19 Years	0									
20–34	0									
35–49	0									
50–64	0									
65+	0									
2. MULTIPLE DX										
0–19 Years	0									
20–34	0									
35–49	0									
50–64	0									
65+	0									
TOTAL SINGLE DX	0									
TOTAL MULTIPLE DX	0									
TOTAL										
0–19 Years	0									
20–34	0									
35–49	0									
50–64	0									
65+	0									
GRAND TOTAL	0									

LOS by Diagnosis and Operation, Western Region, 45th Edition

Western Region, October 2007–September 2008 Data, by Operation

64.9: OTHER MALE GENITAL OPS

Type of Patients	Observed Patients	Avg. Stay	Variance	10th	25th	50th	75th	90th	95th	99th
1. SINGLE DX										
0–19 Years	7	1.1	<1	1	1	1	1	1	2	2
20–34	9	2.3	5	1	1	1	4	7	7	7
35–49	16	2.1	3	1	1	1	2	5	6	6
50–64	20	1.3	<1	1	1	1	1	2	3	3
65+	23	1.2	<1	1	1	1	1	2	2	2
2. MULTIPLE DX										
0–19 Years	78	5.6	302	1	1	2	3	4	7	91
20–34	61	3.5	26	1	1	2	4	5	7	40
35–49	133	3.6	36	1	1	1	4	7	9	27
50–64	286	2.5	16	1	1	1	2	6	10	20
65+	539	2.2	8	1	1	1	2	5	8	14
TOTAL SINGLE DX	75	1.5	1	1	1	1	1	3	5	7
TOTAL MULTIPLE DX	1,097	2.8	42	1	1	1	2	6	8	20
TOTAL										
0–19 Years	85	5.2	275	1	1	2	2	4	7	91
20–34	70	3.4	23	1	1	2	4	5	7	40
35–49	149	3.5	33	1	1	1	4	7	9	27
50–64	306	2.4	15	1	1	1	2	6	10	19
65+	562	2.2	7	1	1	1	2	5	8	14
GRAND TOTAL	1,172	2.8	39	1	1	1	2	5	8	20

64.92: PENILE INCISION

Type of Patients	Observed Patients	Avg. Stay	Variance	10th	25th	50th	75th	90th	95th	99th
1. SINGLE DX										
0–19 Years	2	1.0	0	1	1	1	1	1	1	1
20–34	3	1.0	0	1	1	1	1	1	1	1
35–49	8	2.1	3	1	1	1	2	5	5	5
50–64	0									
65+	0									
2. MULTIPLE DX										
0–19 Years	28	2.6	3	1	1	2	3	4	7	8
20–34	19	5.2	74	1	2	3	5	6	40	40
35–49	24	5.0	26	1	2	4	6	8	13	25
50–64	19	6.9	45	1	1	5	8	20	22	22
65+	12	4.4	13	1	1	3	4	11	11	11
TOTAL SINGLE DX	13	1.7	2	1	1	1	1	5	5	5
TOTAL MULTIPLE DX	102	4.6	31	1	2	3	5	8	13	25
TOTAL										
0–19 Years	30	2.5	3	1	1	2	3	4	7	8
20–34	22	4.6	65	1	1	3	5	6	6	40
35–49	32	4.3	22	1	1	4	5	8	13	25
50–64	19	6.9	45	1	1	5	8	20	22	22
65+	12	4.4	13	1	1	3	4	11	11	11
GRAND TOTAL	115	4.3	29	1	1	3	5	8	13	25

64.96: RMVL INT PENILE PROSTH

Type of Patients	Observed Patients	Avg. Stay	Variance	10th	25th	50th	75th	90th	95th	99th
1. SINGLE DX										
0–19 Years	0									
20–34	0									
35–49	0									
50–64	2	1.5	<1	1	1	1	2	2	2	2
65+	0									
2. MULTIPLE DX										
0–19 Years	1	2.0	0	2	2	2	2	2	2	2
20–34	0									
35–49	4	5.3	11	2	3	7	9	9	9	9
50–64	24	6.8	65	1	2	6	10	12	13	40
65+	79	4.9	16	1	2	4	7	11	14	20
TOTAL SINGLE DX	2	1.5	<1	1	1	1	2	2	2	2
TOTAL MULTIPLE DX	108	5.3	26	1	2	4	7	11	13	20
TOTAL										
0–19 Years	1	2.0	0	2	2	2	2	2	2	2
20–34	0									
35–49	4	5.3	11	2	3	7	9	9	9	9
50–64	26	6.4	61	1	2	4	7	12	13	40
65+	79	4.9	16	1	2	4	7	11	14	20
GRAND TOTAL	110	5.2	26	1	2	4	7	11	13	20

64.97: INSERT OR REPL IPP

Type of Patients	Observed Patients	Avg. Stay	Variance	10th	25th	50th	75th	90th	95th	99th
1. SINGLE DX										
0–19 Years	0									
20–34	0									
35–49	1	1.0	0	1	1	1	1	1	1	1
50–64	12	1.3	<1	1	1	1	1	2	3	3
65+	18	1.2	<1	1	1	1	1	2	2	2
2. MULTIPLE DX										
0–19 Years	0									
20–34	3	1.0	0	1	1	1	1	1	1	1
35–49	39	1.6	4	1	1	1	1	2	9	10
50–64	191	1.3	<1	1	1	1	1	2	2	4
65+	374	1.4	2	1	1	1	1	2	3	5
TOTAL SINGLE DX	31	1.2	<1	1	1	1	1	2	2	3
TOTAL MULTIPLE DX	607	1.3	1	1	1	1	1	2	3	5
TOTAL										
0–19 Years	0									
20–34	3	1.0	0	1	1	1	1	1	1	1
35–49	40	1.6	4	1	1	1	1	2	9	10
50–64	203	1.3	<1	1	1	1	1	2	2	4
65+	392	1.3	2	1	1	1	1	2	3	5
GRAND TOTAL	638	1.3	1	1	1	1	1	2	3	5

LOS by Diagnosis and Operation, Western Region, 45th Edition

279

Western Region, October 2007–September 2008 Data, by Operation

64.98: PENILE OPERATION NEC

Type of Patients	Observed Patients	Avg. Stay	Vari-ance	10th	25th	50th	75th	90th	95th	99th
1. SINGLE DX										
0–19 Years	2	1.0	0	1	1	1	1	1	1	1
20–34	6	3.0	6	1	1	1	4	7	7	7
35–49	6	2.5	3	1	1	2	3	6	6	6
50–64	2	2.0	2	1	1	2	3	3	3	3
65+	1	2.0	0	2	2	2	2	2	2	2
2. MULTIPLE DX										
0–19 Years	7	20.2	>999	1	1	2	2	91	91	91
20–34	34	3.0	5	1	1	2	3	5	10	11
35–49	58	4.0	56	1	1	2	4	7	8	56
50–64	23	3.1	9	1	1	2	4	7	10	11
65+	7	3.0	8	1	1	1	6	8	8	8
TOTAL SINGLE DX	17	2.1	3	1	1	1	3	4	6	7
TOTAL MULTIPLE DX	129	5.7	237	1	1	2	4	7	11	91
TOTAL										
0–19 Years	9	15.7	>999	1	1	2	2	91	91	91
20–34	40	3.0	5	1	1	2	4	5	7	11
35–49	64	3.9	51	1	1	2	4	7	8	56
50–64	25	3.0	8	1	1	2	3	7	10	11
65+	8	2.9	7	1	2	2	3	8	8	8
GRAND TOTAL	146	5.3	209	1	1	2	4	7	10	91

65.0: OOPHOROTOMY

Type of Patients	Observed Patients	Avg. Stay	Vari-ance	10th	25th	50th	75th	90th	95th	99th
1. SINGLE DX										
0–19 Years	2	1.0	0	1	1	1	1	1	1	1
20–34	15	1.4	<1	1	1	1	2	3	3	3
35–49	2	3.5	<1	3	3	3	4	4	4	4
50–64	0									
65+	0									
2. MULTIPLE DX										
0–19 Years	26	2.3	4	1	1	2	3	6	6	9
20–34	88	2.6	4	1	1	2	3	5	6	14
35–49	64	3.1	7	1	2	2	4	6	7	17
50–64	8	2.9	5	1	1	2	6	7	7	7
65+	2	2.0	2	1	1	2	3	3	3	3
TOTAL SINGLE DX	19	1.6	<1	1	1	1	2	3	4	4
TOTAL MULTIPLE DX	188	2.8	5	1	1	2	3	6	7	14
TOTAL										
0–19 Years	28	2.2	4	1	1	1	3	6	6	9
20–34	103	2.5	4	1	1	2	3	5	5	8
35–49	66	3.1	7	1	2	2	3	6	7	17
50–64	8	2.9	5	1	1	2	6	7	7	7
65+	2	2.0	2	1	1	2	3	3	3	3
GRAND TOTAL	207	2.6	5	1	1	2	3	5	6	10

65.01: LAPSCP OOPHOROTOMY

Type of Patients	Observed Patients	Avg. Stay	Vari-ance	10th	25th	50th	75th	90th	95th	99th
1. SINGLE DX										
0–19 Years	2	1.0	0	1	1	1	1	1	1	1
20–34	13	1.4	<1	1	1	1	1	3	3	3
35–49	0									
50–64	0									
65+	0									
2. MULTIPLE DX										
0–19 Years	24	2.1	3	1	1	1	3	6	6	6
20–34	53	2.0	2	1	1	2	3	4	5	6
35–49	38	2.8	4	1	1	2	4	6	7	10
50–64	5	3.4	8	1	1	2	6	7	7	7
65+	1	1.0	0	1	1	1	1	1	1	1
TOTAL SINGLE DX	15	1.3	<1	1	1	1	1	3	3	3
TOTAL MULTIPLE DX	121	2.3	3	1	1	2	3	5	6	7
TOTAL										
0–19 Years	26	2.0	3	1	1	1	2	6	6	6
20–34	66	1.9	1	1	1	1	3	3	4	6
35–49	38	2.8	4	1	1	2	4	6	7	10
50–64	5	3.4	8	1	1	2	6	7	7	7
65+	1	1.0	0	1	1	1	1	1	1	1
GRAND TOTAL	136	2.2	3	1	1	2	3	5	6	7

65.1: DXTIC PX ON OVARIES

Type of Patients	Observed Patients	Avg. Stay	Vari-ance	10th	25th	50th	75th	90th	95th	99th
1. SINGLE DX										
0–19 Years	1	1.0	0	1	1	1	1	1	1	1
20–34	3	2.0	0	2	2	2	2	2	2	2
35–49	0									
50–64	0									
65+	0									
2. MULTIPLE DX										
0–19 Years	11	2.9	2	1	2	3	4	4	5	5
20–34	27	2.9	13	1	1	2	3	4	7	20
35–49	24	3.3	15	1	2	3	5	9	10	17
50–64	10	4.4	13	1	1	3	5	9	12	12
65+	14	8.4	76	1	1	6	12	14	33	33
TOTAL SINGLE DX	4	1.8	<1	1	2	2	2	2	2	2
TOTAL MULTIPLE DX	86	4.0	24	1	1	3	4	11	14	33
TOTAL										
0–19 Years	12	2.8	2	1	1	3	4	4	5	5
20–34	30	2.8	12	1	1	2	3	4	7	20
35–49	24	3.3	15	1	1	2	3	9	10	17
50–64	10	4.4	13	1	2	3	5	9	12	12
65+	14	8.4	76	1	1	6	12	14	33	33
GRAND TOTAL	90	3.9	24	1	1	3	4	10	14	33

LOS by Diagnosis and Operation, Western Region, 45th Edition

Western Region, October 2007–September 2008 Data, by Operation

65.2: LOC EXC/DESTR OVARY LES

Type of Patients	Observed Patients	Avg. Stay	Vari-ance	Percentiles						
				10th	25th	50th	75th	90th	95th	99th
1. SINGLE DX										
0–19 Years	169	2.1	1	1	1	2	3	4	4	6
20–34	365	1.8	<1	1	1	2	2	3	3	4
35–49	86	1.8	<1	1	1	2	2	3	3	4
50–64	12	1.6	<1	1	1	2	2	3	3	5
65+	1	3.0	0	3	3	3	3	3	3	3
2. MULTIPLE DX										
0–19 Years	344	2.9	8	1	1	2	3	5	7	14
20–34	1,664	2.2	2	1	1	2	3	4	4	7
35–49	838	2.5	5	1	1	2	3	4	5	11
50–64	191	2.9	7	1	2	2	3	5	7	14
65+	66	6.7	43	1	3	4	9	15	23	33
TOTAL SINGLE DX	633	1.9	<1	1	1	2	2	3	4	5
TOTAL MULTIPLE DX	3,103	2.5	5	1	1	2	3	4	5	13
TOTAL										
0–19 Years	513	2.6	6	1	1	2	3	4	6	14
20–34	2,029	2.1	2	1	1	2	3	3	4	6
35–49	924	2.4	5	1	1	2	3	4	5	10
50–64	203	2.8	6	1	1	2	3	5	7	10
65+	67	6.6	43	3	3	4	9	15	23	33
GRAND TOTAL	3,736	2.4	4	1	1	2	3	4	5	11

65.25: LAPSCP OV LES EXC NEC

Type of Patients	Observed Patients	Avg. Stay	Vari-ance	Percentiles						
				10th	25th	50th	75th	90th	95th	99th
1. SINGLE DX										
0–19 Years	58	1.8	1	1	1	1	2	3	4	6
20–34	112	1.4	<1	1	1	1	2	2	3	3
35–49	33	1.5	<1	1	1	1	2	2	3	3
50–64	5	1.0	0	1	1	1	1	1	1	1
65+	0									
2. MULTIPLE DX										
0–19 Years	140	2.3	6	1	1	1	3	4	7	14
20–34	567	1.8	1	1	1	1	2	3	4	6
35–49	274	1.9	3	1	1	1	2	4	5	10
50–64	48	1.9	3	1	1	1	3	4	5	10
65+	12	3.2	7	1	1	2	5	5	10	10
TOTAL SINGLE DX	208	1.5	<1	1	1	1	2	3	3	5
TOTAL MULTIPLE DX	1,041	1.9	3	1	1	1	2	4	4	9
TOTAL										
0–19 Years	198	2.1	4	1	1	1	2	4	5	14
20–34	679	1.7	1	1	1	1	2	3	4	6
35–49	307	1.8	3	1	1	1	2	3	4	9
50–64	53	1.9	3	1	1	1	2	4	5	10
65+	12	3.2	7	1	1	2	5	5	10	10
GRAND TOTAL	1,249	1.8	2	1	1	1	2	3	4	8

65.29: LOC EXC/DESTR OV LES NEC

Type of Patients	Observed Patients	Avg. Stay	Vari-ance	Percentiles						
				10th	25th	50th	75th	90th	95th	99th
1. SINGLE DX										
0–19 Years	109	2.3	1	1	2	2	3	4	4	5
20–34	247	1.9	<1	1	1	2	2	3	3	4
35–49	52	2.1	<1	1	2	2	2	3	4	5
50–64	7	2.0	<1	1	1	2	3	3	3	3
65+	1	3.0	0	3	3	3	3	3	3	3
2. MULTIPLE DX										
0–19 Years	196	3.3	10	1	2	2	4	5	7	20
20–34	1,069	2.5	2	1	2	2	3	4	5	7
35–49	555	2.8	6	1	2	2	3	4	5	13
50–64	143	3.2	8	1	2	3	4	5	7	14
65+	53	7.1	43	2	3	4	9	15	23	33
TOTAL SINGLE DX	416	2.1	<1	1	1	2	2	3	4	5
TOTAL MULTIPLE DX	2,016	2.8	6	1	2	2	3	4	6	14
TOTAL										
0–19 Years	305	2.9	7	1	2	2	3	4	6	20
20–34	1,316	2.4	2	1	2	2	3	4	4	7
35–49	607	2.7	6	1	2	2	3	4	5	11
50–64	150	3.2	7	1	2	2	3	5	7	14
65+	54	7.0	42	2	3	4	9	15	23	33
GRAND TOTAL	2,432	2.7	5	1	2	2	3	4	5	13

65.3: UNILATERAL OOPHORECTOMY

Type of Patients	Observed Patients	Avg. Stay	Vari-ance	Percentiles						
				10th	25th	50th	75th	90th	95th	99th
1. SINGLE DX										
0–19 Years	42	3.1	2	1	2	3	4	5	5	6
20–34	64	2.1	2	1	1	2	2	3	3	13
35–49	40	2.2	1	1	1	2	3	4	4	6
50–64	9	1.8	<1	1	1	2	2	3	3	3
65+	1	2.0	0	2	2	2	2	2	2	2
2. MULTIPLE DX										
0–19 Years	84	4.5	32	1	2	3	5	8	10	31
20–34	312	2.5	2	1	2	2	3	4	5	8
35–49	286	2.7	3	1	2	2	3	4	5	13
50–64	118	3.1	6	1	2	2	4	6	8	12
65+	65	4.0	11	1	2	3	6	9	11	15
TOTAL SINGLE DX	156	2.5	2	1	2	2	3	4	5	6
TOTAL MULTIPLE DX	865	3.0	8	1	2	2	3	5	7	13
TOTAL										
0–19 Years	126	3.9	20	1	2	3	5	7	8	31
20–34	376	2.4	2	1	2	2	3	4	5	10
35–49	326	2.7	3	1	2	2	3	4	5	10
50–64	127	3.0	5	1	2	2	4	6	8	12
65+	66	4.0	11	2	2	3	6	9	11	15
GRAND TOTAL	1,021	2.9	7	1	2	2	3	5	7	13

LOS by Diagnosis and Operation, Western Region, 45th Edition

Western Region, October 2007–September 2008 Data, by Operation

65.31: LAPSCP UNILAT OOPHORECT

Type of Patients	Observed Patients	Avg. Stay	Variance	Percentiles						
				10th	25th	50th	75th	90th	95th	99th
1. SINGLE DX										
0–19 Years	10	1.9	<1	1	1	2	2	3	4	4
20–34	17	1.5	<1	1	1	2	2	3	3	3
35–49	9	2.3	3	1	1	2	3	6	6	6
50–64	2	2.0	2	1	1	2	3	3	3	3
65+	0									
2. MULTIPLE DX										
0–19 Years	18	2.9	7	1	1	2	3	6	10	10
20–34	66	2.1	2	1	1	2	3	4	5	6
35–49	61	2.1	4	1	1	1	2	3	5	14
50–64	29	2.1	6	1	1	1	2	5	7	12
65+	18	2.2	2	1	1	3	3	4	6	6
TOTAL SINGLE DX	38	1.8	1	1	1	2	2	3	4	6
TOTAL MULTIPLE DX	192	2.2	4	1	1	2	3	4	6	12
TOTAL										
0–19 Years	28	2.5	5	1	1	2	3	5	10	10
20–34	83	1.9	1	1	1	1	3	4	4	6
35–49	70	2.1	4	1	1	1	2	4	5	14
50–64	31	2.1	6	1	1	1	2	5	7	12
65+	18	2.2	2	1	1	3	3	4	6	6
GRAND TOTAL	230	2.1	3	1	1	2	3	4	5	10

65.4: UNILATERAL S-O

Type of Patients	Observed Patients	Avg. Stay	Variance	Percentiles						
				10th	25th	50th	75th	90th	95th	99th
1. SINGLE DX										
0–19 Years	77	2.4	1	1	2	2	3	3	4	6
20–34	200	2.1	<1	1	2	2	2	3	3	4
35–49	162	2.0	<1	1	1	2	2	3	4	5
50–64	44	2.1	2	1	1	2	2	3	4	10
65+	5	1.2	<1	1	1	1	1	2	2	2
2. MULTIPLE DX										
0–19 Years	260	3.2	6	1	2	3	4	5	7	17
20–34	1,253	2.7	4	1	2	2	3	4	6	11
35–49	1,744	2.8	5	1	2	2	3	5	7	11
50–64	653	3.1	10	1	2	2	3	6	8	17
65+	306	4.2	21	1	2	3	5	9	12	28
TOTAL SINGLE DX	488	2.1	1	1	1	2	3	3	4	5
TOTAL MULTIPLE DX	4,216	3.0	7	1	2	2	3	5	7	14
TOTAL										
0–19 Years	337	3.0	5	1	2	3	4	5	7	16
20–34	1,453	2.6	4	1	2	2	3	4	5	11
35–49	1,906	2.7	4	1	2	2	3	5	6	11
50–64	697	3.0	10	1	2	2	3	5	7	16
65+	311	4.2	21	1	2	3	5	9	12	28
GRAND TOTAL	4,704	2.9	6	1	2	2	3	5	7	13

65.39: UNILAT OOPHORECTOMY NEC

Type of Patients	Observed Patients	Avg. Stay	Variance	Percentiles						
				10th	25th	50th	75th	90th	95th	99th
1. SINGLE DX										
0–19 Years	32	3.3	2	2	2	4	4	5	5	6
20–34	47	2.3	3	1	2	2	2	3	4	13
35–49	31	2.2	<1	1	2	2	3	3	4	4
50–64	7	1.7	<1	1	1	2	2	3	3	3
65+	1	2.0	0	2	2	2	2	2	2	2
2. MULTIPLE DX										
0–19 Years	66	4.9	38	1	2	3	5	8	11	31
20–34	246	2.6	2	1	2	2	3	4	5	10
35–49	225	2.9	3	1	2	3	3	4	6	10
50–64	89	3.4	5	2	2	3	4	7	8	13
65+	47	4.8	12	2	2	3	7	10	13	15
TOTAL SINGLE DX	118	2.7	2	1	2	2	4	5	5	6
TOTAL MULTIPLE DX	673	3.2	9	1	2	3	3	6	7	14
TOTAL										
0–19 Years	98	4.2	23	1	2	3	5	7	8	31
20–34	293	2.6	3	1	2	2	3	4	5	12
35–49	256	2.8	3	1	2	3	3	4	5	10
50–64	96	3.3	5	2	2	3	4	6	8	13
65+	48	4.7	12	2	2	3	7	10	13	15
GRAND TOTAL	791	3.1	8	1	2	3	3	5	7	13

65.41: LAPSCP UNILATERAL S-O

Type of Patients	Observed Patients	Avg. Stay	Variance	Percentiles						
				10th	25th	50th	75th	90th	95th	99th
1. SINGLE DX										
0–19 Years	17	1.9	2	1	1	1	3	3	4	6
20–34	35	1.5	<1	1	1	1	2	2	3	3
35–49	40	1.4	<1	1	1	1	1	2	3	5
50–64	13	1.4	1	1	1	1	1	2	5	5
65+	4	1.0	0	1	1	1	1	1	1	1
2. MULTIPLE DX										
0–19 Years	60	2.3	3	1	1	2	3	4	5	13
20–34	292	2.0	3	1	1	2	2	3	4	7
35–49	443	2.1	4	1	1	1	2	4	6	11
50–64	168	2.1	4	1	1	1	2	4	5	13
65+	78	2.0	2	1	1	2	3	4	6	6
TOTAL SINGLE DX	109	1.5	<1	1	1	1	2	3	3	5
TOTAL MULTIPLE DX	1,041	2.1	3	1	1	1	2	4	5	11
TOTAL										
0–19 Years	77	2.2	3	1	1	2	3	4	5	8
20–34	327	1.9	3	1	1	1	2	3	4	7
35–49	483	2.0	3	1	1	1	2	4	5	11
50–64	181	2.0	4	1	1	1	2	4	5	13
65+	82	1.9	2	1	1	1	3	4	5	6
GRAND TOTAL	1,150	2.0	3	1	1	1	2	4	5	11

Western Region, October 2007–September 2008 Data, by Operation

65.49: UNILATERAL S-O NEC

Type of Patients	Observed Patients	Avg. Stay	Vari-ance	10th	25th	50th	75th	90th	95th	99th
1. SINGLE DX										
0–19 Years	60	2.5	<1	1	2	2	3	3	4	7
20–34	165	2.2	<1	1	2	2	3	3	4	5
35–49	122	2.1	<1	1	2	2	2	3	4	5
50–64	31	2.4	2	1	2	2	3	3	4	10
65+	1	2.0	0	2	2	2	2	2	2	2
2. MULTIPLE DX										
0–19 Years	200	3.5	7	2	2	3	4	6	8	17
20–34	961	2.9	5	1	2	2	3	5	6	14
35–49	1,301	3.1	5	1	2	3	3	5	7	11
50–64	485	3.4	12	1	2	3	4	6	8	18
65+	228	5.0	25	2	2	3	5	10	14	28
TOTAL SINGLE DX	379	2.3	1	1	2	2	3	3	4	5
TOTAL MULTIPLE DX	3,175	3.2	8	1	2	3	4	5	8	16
TOTAL										
0–19 Years	260	3.3	6	2	2	3	4	5	7	17
20–34	1,126	2.8	4	1	2	2	3	4	6	11
35–49	1,423	3.0	5	1	2	2	3	5	7	11
50–64	516	3.3	11	1	2	2	3	6	8	17
65+	229	5.0	25	2	2	3	5	10	14	28
GRAND TOTAL	3,554	3.1	7	1	2	2	3	5	7	15

65.51: RMVL BOTH OVARIES NEC

Type of Patients	Observed Patients	Avg. Stay	Vari-ance	10th	25th	50th	75th	90th	95th	99th
1. SINGLE DX										
0–19 Years	0									
20–34	0									
35–49	0									
50–64	1	4.0	0	4	4	4	4	4	4	4
65+	1	2.0	0	2	2	2	2	2	2	2
2. MULTIPLE DX										
0–19 Years	1	1.0	0	1	1	1	1	1	1	1
20–34	7	5.4	31	1	2	2	13	14	14	14
35–49	24	2.7	2	2	2	2	3	4	5	7
50–64	34	4.0	11	1	3	3	5	7	10	18
65+	29	4.9	11	2	3	4	6	9	10	17
TOTAL SINGLE DX	2	3.0	2	2	2	4	4	4	4	4
TOTAL MULTIPLE DX	95	4.0	10	1	2	3	5	7	10	18
TOTAL										
0–19 Years	1	1.0	0	1	1	1	1	1	1	1
20–34	7	5.4	31	1	2	2	13	14	14	14
35–49	24	2.7	2	2	2	3	3	4	5	7
50–64	35	4.0	11	1	3	3	5	7	10	18
65+	30	4.8	11	2	3	4	6	9	10	17
GRAND TOTAL	97	3.9	10	1	2	3	5	7	10	18

65.5: BILATERAL OOPHORECTOMY

Type of Patients	Observed Patients	Avg. Stay	Vari-ance	10th	25th	50th	75th	90th	95th	99th
1. SINGLE DX										
0–19 Years	2	2.0	1	1	1	2	3	3	3	3
20–34	1	1.0	0	1	1	1	1	1	1	1
35–49	1	1.0	0	1	1	1	1	1	1	1
50–64	2	3.5	<1	3	3	4	4	4	4	4
65+	2	1.5	<1	1	1	1	2	2	2	2
2. MULTIPLE DX										
0–19 Years	2	1.4	<1	1	1	1	1	3	3	3
20–34	17	4.7	25	1	2	2	4	14	17	17
35–49	65	2.4	3	1	1	2	3	5	5	9
50–64	67	3.3	10	1	1	2	4	7	9	18
65+	52	4.2	12	1	2	3	5	9	13	17
TOTAL SINGLE DX	8	2.0	1	1	1	1	3	3	4	4
TOTAL MULTIPLE DX	203	3.3	10	1	1	2	4	7	9	17
TOTAL										
0–19 Years	4	1.8	1	1	1	1	3	3	3	3
20–34	18	4.5	24	1	1	2	4	14	17	17
35–49	66	2.4	3	1	1	2	3	5	5	9
50–64	69	3.3	10	1	1	3	4	7	9	18
65+	54	4.1	12	1	2	3	5	9	13	17
GRAND TOTAL	211	3.3	9	1	1	2	4	7	9	17

65.6: BILAT SALPINGO-OOPHORECT

Type of Patients	Observed Patients	Avg. Stay	Vari-ance	10th	25th	50th	75th	90th	95th	99th
1. SINGLE DX										
0–19 Years	4	1.7	2	1	1	1	1	4	4	4
20–34	11	2.6	2	1	1	2	4	4	5	5
35–49	32	2.1	<1	1	1	2	2	3	4	4
50–64	40	1.9	<1	1	1	2	2	3	5	5
65+	17	1.8	<1	1	1	2	2	3	4	4
2. MULTIPLE DX										
0–19 Years	3	1.5	<1	1	1	1	2	3	3	3
20–34	169	2.8	8	1	2	2	3	5	6	23
35–49	1,229	2.8	5	1	2	2	3	5	6	13
50–64	1,398	3.3	15	1	2	2	3	6	9	16
65+	1,121	4.4	19	1	2	3	5	9	12	20
TOTAL SINGLE DX	104	2.0	1	1	1	2	3	3	4	5
TOTAL MULTIPLE DX	3,920	3.4	13	1	2	3	4	6	9	18
TOTAL										
0–19 Years	7	1.6	1	1	1	1	2	3	4	4
20–34	180	2.8	8	1	2	2	3	5	6	23
35–49	1,261	2.8	5	1	2	2	3	5	6	13
50–64	1,438	3.2	14	1	2	2	3	6	8	16
65+	1,138	4.4	18	1	2	3	5	8	12	20
GRAND TOTAL	4,024	3.4	13	1	2	3	4	6	9	18

LOS by Diagnosis and Operation, Western Region, 45th Edition

Western Region, October 2007–September 2008 Data, by Operation

65.61: RMVL BOTH OV & FALL NEC

Type of Patients	Observed Patients	Avg. Stay	Variance	Percentiles						
				10th	25th	50th	75th	90th	95th	99th
1. SINGLE DX										
0–19 Years	1	4.0	0	4	4	4	4	4	4	4
20–34	8	2.9	2	1	2	2	4	5	5	5
35–49	17	2.6	<1	2	2	3	3	4	4	4
50–64	16	2.8	1	1	2	2	3	5	5	5
65+	8	2.2	<1	1	2	2	2	4	4	4
2. MULTIPLE DX										
0–19 Years	1	3.0	0	3	3	3	3	3	3	3
20–34	90	3.6	13	2	2	3	4	5	8	27
35–49	754	3.2	5	2	2	3	3	5	7	14
50–64	953	3.9	19	2	2	3	4	7	11	21
65+	816	5.1	21	2	3	4	6	9	13	23
TOTAL SINGLE DX	50	2.7	1	2	2	2	3	4	5	5
TOTAL MULTIPLE DX	2,614	4.1	16	2	2	3	4	8	11	20
TOTAL										
0–19 Years	2	3.5	<1	3	3	3	4	4	4	4
20–34	98	3.6	12	2	2	3	4	5	8	23
35–49	771	3.2	5	2	2	3	3	5	7	14
50–64	969	3.9	19	2	2	3	4	7	11	21
65+	824	5.1	21	2	3	4	6	9	13	23
GRAND TOTAL	2,664	4.1	16	2	2	3	4	7	11	20

65.62: RMVL REM OV & FALL NEC

Type of Patients	Observed Patients	Avg. Stay	Variance	Percentiles						
				10th	25th	50th	75th	90th	95th	99th
1. SINGLE DX										
0–19 Years	0									
20–34	1	3.0	0	3	3	3	3	3	3	3
35–49	6	2.2	<1	2	2	2	3	3	3	3
50–64	1	2.0	0	2	2	2	2	2	2	2
65+	0									
2. MULTIPLE DX										
0–19 Years	0									
20–34	25	2.1	<1	1	2	2	3	3	3	4
35–49	113	3.3	8	2	2	3	3	5	6	20
50–64	57	3.1	6	2	2	3	3	4	6	15
65+	49	4.7	12	2	3	4	5	10	13	18
TOTAL SINGLE DX	8	2.3	<1	1	2	2	3	3	3	3
TOTAL MULTIPLE DX	244	3.4	8	2	2	3	3	6	8	18
TOTAL										
0–19 Years	0									
20–34	26	2.2	<1	1	2	2	3	3	3	4
35–49	119	3.3	8	2	2	3	3	5	6	20
50–64	58	3.0	6	2	2	3	3	4	6	15
65+	49	4.7	12	2	3	4	5	10	13	18
GRAND TOTAL	252	3.4	8	2	2	3	3	6	8	18

65.63: LAPSCP RMVL BOTH OV/FALL

Type of Patients	Observed Patients	Avg. Stay	Variance	Percentiles						
				10th	25th	50th	75th	90th	95th	99th
1. SINGLE DX										
0–19 Years	3	1.0	0	1	1	1	1	1	1	1
20–34	1	2.0	0	2	2	2	2	2	2	2
35–49	9	1.0	0	1	1	1	1	1	1	1
50–64	23	1.3	<1	1	1	1	1	2	2	2
65+	9	1.5	<1	1	1	1	1	3	3	3
2. MULTIPLE DX										
0–19 Years	1	2.0	0	2	2	2	2	2	2	2
20–34	39	1.9	2	1	1	1	2	4	5	6
35–49	306	1.8	2	1	1	1	2	3	4	6
50–64	370	1.7	2	1	1	1	2	3	4	7
65+	244	2.0	5	1	1	1	2	4	5	11
TOTAL SINGLE DX	45	1.2	<1	1	1	1	1	2	2	3
TOTAL MULTIPLE DX	960	1.8	3	1	1	1	2	3	4	7
TOTAL										
0–19 Years	4	1.3	<1	1	1	1	2	2	2	2
20–34	40	1.9	2	1	1	1	2	3	5	6
35–49	315	1.8	2	1	1	1	2	3	4	6
50–64	393	1.7	1	1	1	1	2	3	4	7
65+	253	2.0	4	1	1	1	2	4	5	11
GRAND TOTAL	1,005	1.8	3	1	1	1	2	3	4	7

65.7: REPAIR OF OVARY

Type of Patients	Observed Patients	Avg. Stay	Variance	Percentiles						
				10th	25th	50th	75th	90th	95th	99th
1. SINGLE DX										
0–19 Years	4	1.1	<1	1	1	1	1	2	2	2
20–34	3	1.7	1	1	1	1	3	3	3	3
35–49	2	1.0	0	1	1	1	1	1	1	1
50–64	0									
65+	0									
2. MULTIPLE DX										
0–19 Years	10	2.7	2	1	1	3	4	5	5	5
20–34	34	2.6	3	1	2	2	3	4	7	9
35–49	12	2.7	1	1	1	3	3	4	5	5
50–64	2	1.0	0	2	2	1	1	1	1	1
65+	1	2.0	0	2	2	2	2	2	2	2
TOTAL SINGLE DX	9	1.3	<1	1	1	1	1	2	3	3
TOTAL MULTIPLE DX	59	2.6	2	1	1	2	3	4	5	9
TOTAL										
0–19 Years	14	2.2	2	1	1	2	3	4	5	5
20–34	37	2.6	3	1	1	3	3	4	7	9
35–49	14	2.4	2	1	1	1	3	4	5	5
50–64	2	1.0	0	2	2	1	1	1	1	1
65+	1	2.0	0	2	2	2	2	2	2	2
GRAND TOTAL	68	2.4	2	1	1	2	3	4	5	9

LOS by Diagnosis and Operation, Western Region, 45th Edition

Western Region, October 2007–September 2008 Data, by Operation

65.8: TUBO-OVARIAN ADHESIO

Type of Patients	Observed Patients	Avg. Stay	Variance	10th	25th	50th	75th	90th	95th	99th
1. SINGLE DX										
0–19 Years	1	1.0	0							
20–34	3	1.7	<1	1	1	2	2	2	2	2
35–49	1	2.0	0	2	2	2	2	2	2	2
50–64	1	4.0	0	4	4	4	4	4	4	4
65+	0									
2. MULTIPLE DX										
0–19 Years	10	2.3	3	1	1	2	3	5	6	6
20–34	92	2.7	3	1	1	2	3	5	6	8
35–49	123	3.0	4	1	2	3	4	5	6	11
50–64	39	3.4	10	1	2	4	4	7	14	14
65+	8	2.3	2	1	1	2	3	5	5	5
TOTAL SINGLE DX	6	2.0	1	1	1	2	2	4	4	4
TOTAL MULTIPLE DX	272	2.9	4	1	2	2	3	5	7	11
TOTAL										
0–19 Years	11	2.2	3	1	1	1	3	5	6	6
20–34	95	2.6	3	1	1	2	3	5	6	8
35–49	124	3.0	4	1	2	3	4	5	6	11
50–64	40	3.4	9	1	2	4	4	7	10	14
65+	8	2.3	2	1	1	2	3	5	5	5
GRAND TOTAL	278	2.9	4	1	2	2	3	5	7	11

65.89: ADHESIO OV/FALL TUBE NEC

Type of Patients	Observed Patients	Avg. Stay	Variance	10th	25th	50th	75th	90th	95th	99th
1. SINGLE DX										
0–19 Years	0									
20–34	1	2.0	0	2	2	2	2	2	2	2
35–49	1	2.0	0	2	2	2	2	2	2	2
50–64	1	4.0	0	4	4	4	4	4	4	4
65+	0									
2. MULTIPLE DX										
0–19 Years	2	4.0	8	2	2	4	6	6	6	6
20–34	42	2.9	3	1	2	3	3	6	7	8
35–49	70	3.3	4	2	2	3	4	5	9	11
50–64	23	4.2	14	2	2	3	5	10	14	14
65+	4	3.3	2	2	2	3	5	5	5	5
TOTAL SINGLE DX	3	2.7	1	2	2	2	4	4	4	4
TOTAL MULTIPLE DX	141	3.3	5	1	2	3	3	6	8	14
TOTAL										
0–19 Years	2	4.0	8	2	2	4	6	6	6	6
20–34	43	2.9	3	1	2	3	3	6	7	8
35–49	71	3.3	4	2	2	3	4	5	9	11
50–64	24	4.2	13	2	2	3	4	10	14	14
65+	4	3.3	2	2	2	3	5	5	5	5
GRAND TOTAL	144	3.3	5	1	2	3	3	6	8	14

65.81: LAPSCP ADHESIO OV/FALL

Type of Patients	Observed Patients	Avg. Stay	Variance	10th	25th	50th	75th	90th	95th	99th
1. SINGLE DX										
0–19 Years	1	1.0	0	1	1	1	1	1	1	1
20–34	2	1.5	<1	1	1	2	2	2	2	2
35–49	0									
50–64	0									
65+	0									
2. MULTIPLE DX										
0–19 Years	8	2.0	2	1	1	1	3	4	5	5
20–34	50	2.5	3	1	1	2	3	5	6	7
35–49	53	2.6	4	1	1	2	3	5	5	11
50–64	16	2.1	2	1	1	2	3	4	5	5
65+	4	1.3	<1	1	1	1	2	2	2	2
TOTAL SINGLE DX	3	1.3	<1	1	1	1	2	2	2	2
TOTAL MULTIPLE DX	131	2.4	3	1	1	2	3	5	5	9
TOTAL										
0–19 Years	9	1.9	2	1	1	1	3	4	5	5
20–34	52	2.4	3	1	1	2	3	5	6	7
35–49	53	2.6	4	1	1	2	3	5	5	11
50–64	16	2.1	2	1	1	2	3	4	5	5
65+	4	1.3	<1	1	1	1	2	2	2	2
GRAND TOTAL	134	2.4	3	1	1	2	3	5	5	9

65.9: OTHER OVARIAN OPERATIONS

Type of Patients	Observed Patients	Avg. Stay	Variance	10th	25th	50th	75th	90th	95th	99th
1. SINGLE DX										
0–19 Years	20	1.3	<1	1	1	1	1	2	3	4
20–34	25	1.7	<1	1	1	1	2	3	3	5
35–49	5	3.0	4	1	1	3	4	6	6	6
50–64	0									
65+	0									
2. MULTIPLE DX										
0–19 Years	63	2.4	2	1	1	2	3	5	6	7
20–34	188	2.4	4	1	1	2	3	5	6	10
35–49	93	3.1	8	1	1	2	4	6	8	19
50–64	18	2.4	1	1	2	2	3	4	4	4
65+	12	4.0	11	1	2	3	6	10	11	11
TOTAL SINGLE DX	50	1.6	1	1	1	1	2	3	4	6
TOTAL MULTIPLE DX	374	2.6	5	1	1	2	3	5	7	10
TOTAL										
0–19 Years	83	2.1	2	1	1	2	2	4	6	7
20–34	213	2.3	4	1	1	2	3	4	6	10
35–49	98	3.1	7	1	1	2	4	6	8	19
50–64	18	2.4	1	1	2	2	3	4	4	4
65+	12	4.0	11	1	2	3	6	10	11	11
GRAND TOTAL	424	2.5	4	1	1	2	3	5	6	10

LOS by Diagnosis and Operation, Western Region, 45th Edition

Western Region, October 2007–September 2008 Data, by Operation

65.91: ASPIRATION OF OVARY

Type of Patients	Observed Patients	Avg. Stay	Vari-ance	Percentiles						
				10th	25th	50th	75th	90th	95th	99th
1. SINGLE DX										
0–19 Years	18	1.4	<1	1	1	1	2	2	3	4
20–34	20	1.6	<1	1	1	1	2	3	3	5
35–49	3	2.7	8	1	1	1	6	6	6	6
50–64	0									
65+	0									
2. MULTIPLE DX										
0–19 Years	41	2.3	1	1	2	2	3	4	5	7
20–34	149	2.6	5	1	1	2	3	5	6	10
35–49	88	3.2	8	1	2	2	4	7	8	19
50–64	18	2.4	1	1	2	2	3	4	4	4
65+	10	4.1	14	1	1	3	6	11	11	11
TOTAL SINGLE DX	41	1.5	1	1	1	1	2	3	4	6
TOTAL MULTIPLE DX	306	2.7	5	1	1	2	3	5	7	10
TOTAL										
0–19 Years	59	1.9	1	1	1	2	2	3	4	7
20–34	169	2.5	4	1	1	2	3	5	6	10
35–49	91	3.2	8	1	1	2	4	6	8	19
50–64	18	2.4	1	1	2	2	3	4	4	4
65+	10	4.1	14	1	1	3	6	11	11	11
GRAND TOTAL	347	2.6	5	1	1	2	3	5	7	10

66.02: SALPINGOSTOMY

Type of Patients	Observed Patients	Avg. Stay	Vari-ance	Percentiles						
				10th	25th	50th	75th	90th	95th	99th
1. SINGLE DX										
0–19 Years	11	1.6	<1	1	1	2	2	2	2	2
20–34	131	1.6	<1	1	1	1	2	3	4	5
35–49	21	1.7	<1	1	1	1	2	3	3	4
50–64	1	1.0	0	1	1	1	1	1	1	1
65+	0									
2. MULTIPLE DX										
0–19 Years	25	1.6	<1	1	1	1	2	3	3	4
20–34	272	1.7	<1	1	1	1	2	3	3	5
35–49	38	1.8	1	1	1	1	3	3	4	4
50–64	4	1.8	2	1	1	1	4	4	4	4
65+	0									
TOTAL SINGLE DX	164	1.6	<1	1	1	1	2	3	4	5
TOTAL MULTIPLE DX	339	1.7	<1	1	1	1	2	3	4	5
TOTAL										
0–19 Years	36	1.6	<1	1	1	2	2	2	3	4
20–34	403	1.7	<1	1	1	1	3	3	4	5
35–49	59	1.8	<1	1	1	1	2	3	4	4
50–64	5	1.6	2	1	1	1	1	4	4	4
65+	0									
GRAND TOTAL	503	1.7	<1	1	1	1	2	3	4	5

66.0: SALPINGOSTOMY/SALPINGOT

Type of Patients	Observed Patients	Avg. Stay	Vari-ance	Percentiles						
				10th	25th	50th	75th	90th	95th	99th
1. SINGLE DX										
0–19 Years	13	1.9	<1	1	1	2	3	3	3	3
20–34	155	1.6	<1	1	1	1	2	3	3	5
35–49	26	1.6	<1	1	1	1	2	3	3	4
50–64	1	1.0	0	1	1	1	1	1	1	1
65+	0									
2. MULTIPLE DX										
0–19 Years	31	1.7	<1	1	1	2	2	3	4	4
20–34	350	1.8	1	1	1	2	2	3	4	5
35–49	45	1.8	<1	1	1	1	2	3	4	4
50–64	4	1.8	2	1	1	1	4	4	4	4
65+	0									
TOTAL SINGLE DX	195	1.6	<1	1	1	1	2	3	3	4
TOTAL MULTIPLE DX	430	1.8	1	1	1	1	2	3	4	5
TOTAL										
0–19 Years	44	1.8	<1	1	1	2	2	3	3	4
20–34	505	1.7	1	1	1	1	2	3	4	5
35–49	71	1.7	<1	1	1	1	2	3	4	4
50–64	5	1.6	2	1	1	1	1	4	4	4
65+	0									
GRAND TOTAL	625	1.7	1	1	1	2	2	3	4	5

66.1: FALLOPIAN TUBE DXTIC PX

Type of Patients	Observed Patients	Avg. Stay	Vari-ance	Percentiles						
				10th	25th	50th	75th	90th	95th	99th
1. SINGLE DX										
0–19 Years	0									
20–34	0									
35–49	0									
50–64	0									
65+	0									
2. MULTIPLE DX										
0–19 Years	0									
20–34	2	3.0	8	1	1	1	5	5	5	5
35–49	1	2.0	0	2	2	2	2	2	2	2
50–64	3	2.3	5	1	1	1	5	5	5	5
65+	0									
TOTAL SINGLE DX	0									
TOTAL MULTIPLE DX	6	2.5	4	1	1	1	5	5	5	5
TOTAL										
0–19 Years	0									
20–34	2	3.0	8	1	1	1	5	5	5	5
35–49	1	2.0	0	2	2	2	2	2	2	2
50–64	3	2.3	5	1	1	1	5	5	5	5
65+	0									
GRAND TOTAL	6	2.5	4	1	1	1	5	5	5	5

Western Region, October 2007–September 2008 Data, by Operation

66.2: BILAT ENDO OCCL FALL

Type of Patients	Observed Patients	Avg. Stay	Vari-ance	Percentiles						
				10th	25th	50th	75th	90th	95th	99th
1. SINGLE DX										
0–19 Years	0									
20–34	4	1.5	<1	1	1	2	2	2	2	2
35–49	6	1.0	0	1	1	1	1	1	1	1
50–64	0									
65+	0									
2. MULTIPLE DX										
0–19 Years	1	2.0	0	2	2	2	2	2	2	2
20–34	284	2.0	<1	2	2	2	2	3	3	5
35–49	135	1.9	<1	1	1	2	2	3	3	5
50–64	19	1.9	1	1	1	2	2	3	6	6
65+	0									
TOTAL SINGLE DX	10	1.2	<1	1	1	1	1	2	2	2
TOTAL MULTIPLE DX	439	2.0	<1	1	1	2	2	3	3	5
TOTAL										
0–19 Years	1	2.0	0	2	2	2	2	2	2	2
20–34	288	2.0	<1	2	2	2	2	3	3	5
35–49	141	1.8	<1	1	1	2	2	3	3	5
50–64	19	1.9	1	1	1	2	2	3	6	6
65+	0									
GRAND TOTAL	449	2.0	<1	1	1	2	2	3	3	5

66.22: BILAT ENDO LIG/DIV FALL

Type of Patients	Observed Patients	Avg. Stay	Vari-ance	Percentiles						
				10th	25th	50th	75th	90th	95th	99th
1. SINGLE DX										
0–19 Years	0									
20–34	0									
35–49	0									
50–64	0									
65+	0									
2. MULTIPLE DX										
0–19 Years	0									
20–34	148	2.1	<1	1	2	2	2	3	3	5
35–49	53	2.3	<1	1	2	2	3	3	4	5
50–64	4	2.3	<1	2	2	2	3	3	3	3
65+	0									
TOTAL SINGLE DX	0									
TOTAL MULTIPLE DX	205	2.1	<1	1	2	2	2	3	3	5
TOTAL										
0–19 Years	0									
20–34	148	2.1	<1	1	2	2	2	3	3	5
35–49	53	2.3	<1	1	2	2	3	3	4	5
50–64	4	2.3	<1	2	2	2	3	3	3	3
65+	0									
GRAND TOTAL	205	2.1	<1	1	2	2	2	3	3	5

66.29: BILAT ENDO OCCL FALL NEC

Type of Patients	Observed Patients	Avg. Stay	Vari-ance	Percentiles						
				10th	25th	50th	75th	90th	95th	99th
1. SINGLE DX										
0–19 Years	0									
20–34	4	1.5	<1	1	1	2	2	2	2	2
35–49	6	1.0	0	1	1	1	1	1	1	1
50–64	0									
65+	0									
2. MULTIPLE DX										
0–19 Years	1	2.0	0	2	2	2	2	2	2	2
20–34	133	2.0	1	1	1	2	2	3	4	6
35–49	81	1.6	<1	1	1	2	2	3	3	6
50–64	15	1.8	2	1	1	2	2	2	6	6
65+	0									
TOTAL SINGLE DX	10	1.2	<1	1	1	1	1	2	2	2
TOTAL MULTIPLE DX	230	1.9	<1	1	1	2	2	3	3	6
TOTAL										
0–19 Years	1	2.0	0	2	2	2	2	2	2	2
20–34	137	2.0	1	1	1	2	2	3	4	6
35–49	87	1.6	<1	1	1	2	2	3	3	6
50–64	15	1.8	2	1	1	2	2	2	6	6
65+	0									
GRAND TOTAL	240	1.8	<1	1	1	2	2	3	3	6

66.3: OTH BILAT FALL DESTR/EXC

Type of Patients	Observed Patients	Avg. Stay	Vari-ance	Percentiles						
				10th	25th	50th	75th	90th	95th	99th
1. SINGLE DX										
0–19 Years	0									
20–34	21	1.6	<1	1	1	2	2	3	3	3
35–49	6	2.0	<1	2	2	2	2	3	3	3
50–64	1	2.0	0	2	2	2	2	2	2	2
65+	0									
2. MULTIPLE DX										
0–19 Years	6	2.0	<1	1	1	2	2	3	3	3
20–34	6,764	2.2	2	1	2	2	3	3	3	5
35–49	2,405	2.4	5	1	2	2	3	3	3	6
50–64	114	2.2	<1	1	2	2	2	3	3	6
65+	0									
TOTAL SINGLE DX	28	1.7	<1	1	1	2	2	3	3	3
TOTAL MULTIPLE DX	9,289	2.2	2	1	2	2	3	3	3	5
TOTAL										
0–19 Years	6	2.0	<1	1	1	2	2	3	3	3
20–34	6,785	2.2	2	1	2	2	3	3	3	5
35–49	2,411	2.4	5	1	2	2	3	3	3	6
50–64	115	2.2	<1	1	2	2	2	3	3	6
65+	0									
GRAND TOTAL	9,317	2.2	2	1	2	2	3	3	3	5

LOS by Diagnosis and Operation, Western Region, 45th Edition

Western Region, October 2007–September 2008 Data, by Operation

66.32: BILAT FALL LIG & DIV NEC

Type of Patients	Observed Patients	Avg. Stay	Vari-ance	Percentiles						
				10th	25th	50th	75th	90th	95th	99th
1. SINGLE DX										
0–19 Years	0									
20–34	13	1.8	<1	1	1	2	2	3	3	3
35–49	2	1.5	<1	1	1	1	2	2	2	2
50–64	1	2.0	0	2	2	2	2	2	2	2
65+	0									
2. MULTIPLE DX										
0–19 Years	6	2.0	<1	1	1	2	3	3	3	3
20–34	4,941	2.2	2	1	2	2	2	3	3	5
35–49	1,704	2.4	7	1	2	2	3	3	3	6
50–64	80	2.2	<1	1	2	2	3	3	4	6
65+	0									
TOTAL SINGLE DX	16	1.8	<1	1	1	2	2	2	3	3
TOTAL MULTIPLE DX	6,731	2.3	3	1	2	2	3	3	3	5
TOTAL										
0–19 Years	6	2.0	<1	1	1	2	2	3	3	3
20–34	4,954	2.2	2	1	2	2	2	3	3	5
35–49	1,706	2.4	7	1	2	2	3	3	3	6
50–64	81	2.2	<1	1	2	2	3	3	4	6
65+	0									
GRAND TOTAL	6,747	2.3	3	1	2	2	3	3	3	5

66.39: BILAT FALL DESTR NEC

Type of Patients	Observed Patients	Avg. Stay	Vari-ance	Percentiles						
				10th	25th	50th	75th	90th	95th	99th
1. SINGLE DX										
0–19 Years	0									
20–34	8	1.5	<1	1	1	2	2	2	2	2
35–49	4	2.3	<1	2	2	2	3	3	3	3
50–64	0									
65+	0									
2. MULTIPLE DX										
0–19 Years	0									
20–34	1,779	2.2	2	1	2	2	2	3	3	4
35–49	678	2.3	2	1	2	2	3	3	4	6
50–64	34	2.0	<1	1	2	2	3	3	3	3
65+	0									
TOTAL SINGLE DX	12	1.7	<1	1	1	2	2	2	3	3
TOTAL MULTIPLE DX	2,491	2.2	2	1	2	2	3	3	3	5
TOTAL										
0–19 Years	0									
20–34	1,787	2.2	2	1	2	2	2	3	3	4
35–49	682	2.3	2	1	2	2	3	3	4	6
50–64	34	2.0	<1	1	2	2	3	3	3	3
65+	0									
GRAND TOTAL	2,503	2.2	2	1	2	2	3	3	3	5

66.4: TOT UNILAT SALPINGECTOMY

Type of Patients	Observed Patients	Avg. Stay	Vari-ance	Percentiles						
				10th	25th	50th	75th	90th	95th	99th
1. SINGLE DX										
0–19 Years	11	2.1	1	1	1	2	3	3	4	4
20–34	49	1.8	<1	1	1	2	2	3	3	4
35–49	26	1.7	<1	1	1	1	2	3	4	4
50–64	2	1.5	<1	1	1	2	2	2	2	2
65+	0									
2. MULTIPLE DX										
0–19 Years	40	3.1	9	1	1	2	3	9	11	11
20–34	189	2.5	12	1	1	2	3	4	5	7
35–49	138	2.8	6	1	2	2	3	6	9	12
50–64	25	2.4	1	1	2	2	3	4	4	5
65+	8	4.5	9	1	2	4	6	9	9	9
TOTAL SINGLE DX	88	1.8	<1	1	1	2	2	3	3	4
TOTAL MULTIPLE DX	400	2.7	9	1	1	2	3	4	6	11
TOTAL										
0–19 Years	51	2.9	7	1	1	2	3	4	11	11
20–34	238	2.3	10	1	1	2	3	5	4	7
35–49	164	2.7	5	1	1	2	3	5	9	12
50–64	27	2.3	1	1	2	2	3	4	4	5
65+	8	4.5	9	1	2	4	6	9	9	9
GRAND TOTAL	488	2.5	7	1	1	2	3	4	6	11

66.5: TOT BILAT SALPINGECTOMY

Type of Patients	Observed Patients	Avg. Stay	Vari-ance	Percentiles						
				10th	25th	50th	75th	90th	95th	99th
1. SINGLE DX										
0–19 Years	0									
20–34	2	1.5	<1	1	1	2	2	2	2	2
35–49	4	2.2	3	1	2	2	2	5	5	5
50–64	1	2.0	0	2	2	2	2	2	2	2
65+	0									
2. MULTIPLE DX										
0–19 Years	3	3.0	4	1	1	3	5	5	5	5
20–34	44	2.4	7	1	1	2	3	3	5	16
35–49	65	2.5	3	1	1	2	3	5	6	8
50–64	19	2.5	3	1	1	2	4	5	6	6
65+	5	3.8	18	1	1	2	4	11	11	11
TOTAL SINGLE DX	7	2.0	2	1	1	2	2	5	5	5
TOTAL MULTIPLE DX	136	2.5	4	1	1	2	3	5	6	11
TOTAL										
0–19 Years	3	3.0	4	1	1	3	5	5	5	5
20–34	46	2.4	7	1	1	2	3	3	5	16
35–49	69	2.5	3	1	1	2	3	5	6	8
50–64	20	2.5	2	1	1	2	4	4	6	6
65+	5	3.8	18	1	1	2	4	11	11	11
GRAND TOTAL	143	2.5	4	1	1	2	3	5	6	11

Western Region, October 2007–September 2008 Data, by Operation

66.51: RMVL BOTH FALL TUBES

Type of Patients	Observed Patients	Avg. Stay	Vari- ance	Percentiles						
				10th	25th	50th	75th	90th	95th	99th
1. SINGLE DX										
0–19 Years	0									
20–34	2	1.5	<1	1	1	2	2	2	2	2
35–49	4	2.2	3	1	1	2	2	5	5	5
50–64	1	2.0	0	2	2	2	2	2	2	2
65+	0									
2. MULTIPLE DX										
0–19 Years	2	4.0	2	3	3	4	5	5	5	5
20–34	30	2.8	9	1	1	2	3	5	10	16
35–49	59	2.6	3	1	1	2	3	5	7	8
50–64	19	2.5	2	1	1	2	4	4	6	6
65+	5	3.8	18	1	1	2	4	11	11	11
TOTAL SINGLE DX	7	2.0	2	1	1	2	2	5	5	5
TOTAL MULTIPLE DX	115	2.7	5	1	1	2	3	5	7	11
TOTAL										
0–19 Years	2	4.0	2	3	3	4	5	5	5	5
20–34	32	2.8	9	1	1	2	3	5	10	16
35–49	63	2.5	3	1	1	2	3	5	6	8
50–64	20	2.5	2	1	1	2	4	4	6	6
65+	5	3.8	18	1	1	2	4	11	11	11
GRAND TOTAL	122	2.7	5	1	1	2	3	5	6	11

66.6: OTHER SALPINGECTOMY

Type of Patients	Observed Patients	Avg. Stay	Vari- ance	Percentiles						
				10th	25th	50th	75th	90th	95th	99th
1. SINGLE DX										
0–19 Years	57	1.7	<1	1	1	2	2	3	3	4
20–34	749	1.7	<1	1	1	1	2	3	3	4
35–49	224	1.7	<1	1	1	1	2	3	3	5
50–64	14	1.4	<1	1	1	1	1	3	3	3
65+	0									
2. MULTIPLE DX										
0–19 Years	155	2.0	1	1	1	2	2	3	4	5
20–34	1,985	2.0	2	1	1	2	3	3	4	6
35–49	777	2.1	4	1	1	2	3	3	4	9
50–64	53	2.1	<1	1	1	2	3	3	4	5
65+	6	2.8	2	2	2	3	4	5	5	5
TOTAL SINGLE DX	1,044	1.7	<1	1	1	1	2	3	3	4
TOTAL MULTIPLE DX	2,976	2.0	2	1	1	2	3	3	4	6
TOTAL										
0–19 Years	212	1.9	<1	1	1	2	2	3	4	5
20–34	2,734	1.9	1	1	1	2	2	3	4	6
35–49	1,001	2.0	3	1	1	2	3	3	4	8
50–64	67	1.9	<1	1	1	2	3	3	3	5
65+	6	2.8	2	2	2	3	4	5	5	5
GRAND TOTAL	4,020	1.9	2	1	1	2	2	3	4	6

66.61: EXC/DESTR FALL LES

Type of Patients	Observed Patients	Avg. Stay	Vari- ance	Percentiles						
				10th	25th	50th	75th	90th	95th	99th
1. SINGLE DX										
0–19 Years	10	1.6	<1	1	1	2	2	2	2	2
20–34	11	1.6	<1	1	1	2	2	2	3	3
35–49	7	1.6	<1	1	1	1	2	3	3	3
50–64	0									
65+	0									
2. MULTIPLE DX										
0–19 Years	40	2.1	2	1	1	2	2	4	4	8
20–34	71	2.5	3	1	1	2	3	5	6	9
35–49	49	2.4	4	1	1	2	3	4	8	11
50–64	9	2.1	1	1	1	2	3	4	4	4
65+	4	3.5	2	2	2	4	5	5	5	5
TOTAL SINGLE DX	28	1.6	<1	1	1	2	2	2	3	3
TOTAL MULTIPLE DX	173	2.4	3	1	1	2	3	4	6	10
TOTAL										
0–19 Years	50	2.1	2	1	1	2	2	4	4	8
20–34	82	2.4	3	1	1	2	3	4	6	9
35–49	56	2.3	4	1	1	2	3	3	8	11
50–64	9	2.1	1	1	1	2	3	4	4	4
65+	4	3.5	2	2	2	4	5	5	5	5
GRAND TOTAL	201	2.3	3	1	1	2	3	4	5	9

66.62: RMVL FALL & TUBAL PREG

Type of Patients	Observed Patients	Avg. Stay	Vari- ance	Percentiles						
				10th	25th	50th	75th	90th	95th	99th
1. SINGLE DX										
0–19 Years	42	1.7	<1	1	1	2	2	3	3	4
20–34	680	1.6	<1	1	1	1	2	3	3	4
35–49	205	1.7	<1	1	1	1	2	3	3	5
50–64	13	1.4	<1	1	1	1	1	3	3	3
65+	0									
2. MULTIPLE DX										
0–19 Years	101	1.9	<1	1	1	2	2	3	3	4
20–34	1,731	1.9	1	1	1	2	3	3	4	6
35–49	637	2.0	2	1	1	2	3	3	4	6
50–64	32	1.9	<1	1	1	2	3	3	3	4
65+	0									
TOTAL SINGLE DX	940	1.6	<1	1	1	1	2	3	3	4
TOTAL MULTIPLE DX	2,501	2.0	1	1	1	2	3	3	4	6
TOTAL										
0–19 Years	143	1.9	<1	1	1	2	2	3	3	4
20–34	2,411	1.9	1	1	1	2	2	3	4	5
35–49	842	1.9	1	1	1	2	2	3	4	6
50–64	45	1.8	<1	1	1	2	2	3	3	4
65+	0									
GRAND TOTAL	3,441	1.9	1	1	1	2	2	3	4	5

LOS by Diagnosis and Operation, Western Region, 45th Edition

66.69: PARTIAL FALL RMVL NEC

Type of Patients	Observed Patients	Avg. Stay	Vari-ance	Percentiles						
				10th	25th	50th	75th	90th	95th	99th
1. SINGLE DX										
0–19 Years	5	1.5	<1	1	1	2	2	2	2	2
20–34	58	1.9	<1	1	1	2	2	3	3	5
35–49	12	1.9	1	1	1	1	3	3	4	4
50–64	1	1.0	0	1	1	1	1	1	1	1
65+	0									
2. MULTIPLE DX										
0–19 Years	14	1.9	1	1	1	1	3	3	4	4
20–34	167	2.4	3	1	1	2	3	4	4	13
35–49	79	3.0	21	1	1	2	3	4	8	40
50–64	12	2.1	1	1	1	2	2	3	5	5
65+	2	1.5	<1	1	1	1	2	2	2	2
TOTAL SINGLE DX	76	1.9	<1	1	1	2	2	3	3	5
TOTAL MULTIPLE DX	274	2.5	8	1	1	2	3	4	4	13
TOTAL										
0–19 Years	19	1.8	<1	1	1	2	2	3	4	4
20–34	225	2.2	2	1	1	2	3	4	4	7
35–49	91	2.9	18	1	1	2	3	4	6	40
50–64	13	2.0	1	1	1	2	2	3	5	5
65+	2	1.5	<1	1	1	2	2	2	2	2
GRAND TOTAL	350	2.3	6	1	1	2	3	4	4	11

66.79: FALL TUBE REPAIR NEC

Type of Patients	Observed Patients	Avg. Stay	Vari-ance	Percentiles						
				10th	25th	50th	75th	90th	95th	99th
1. SINGLE DX										
0–19 Years	0									
20–34	7	1.3	<1	1	1	1	2	2	2	2
35–49	9	1.5	<1	1	1	1	2	2	3	3
50–64	1	2.0	0	2	2	2	2	2	2	2
65+	0									
2. MULTIPLE DX										
0–19 Years	2	3.0	2	2	2	3	4	4	4	4
20–34	14	1.7	<1	1	1	2	2	2	3	3
35–49	21	1.7	<1	1	1	2	2	2	3	3
50–64	0									
65+	0									
TOTAL SINGLE DX	17	1.5	<1	1	1	1	2	2	3	3
TOTAL MULTIPLE DX	37	1.8	<1	1	1	2	2	3	3	4
TOTAL										
0–19 Years	2	3.0	2	2	2	3	4	4	4	4
20–34	21	1.6	<1	1	1	2	2	2	2	3
35–49	30	1.6	<1	1	1	2	2	2	3	3
50–64	1	2.0	0	2	2	2	2	2	2	2
65+	0									
GRAND TOTAL	54	1.7	<1	1	1	2	2	2	3	4

66.7: REPAIR OF FALLOPIAN TUBE

Type of Patients	Observed Patients	Avg. Stay	Vari-ance	Percentiles						
				10th	25th	50th	75th	90th	95th	99th
1. SINGLE DX										
0–19 Years	0									
20–34	8	1.3	<1	1	1	1	1	2	2	2
35–49	9	1.5	<1	1	1	2	2	2	3	3
50–64	1	2.0	0	2	2	2	2	2	2	2
65+	0									
2. MULTIPLE DX										
0–19 Years	2	3.0	2	2	2	3	3	4	4	4
20–34	18	1.8	<1	1	1	2	2	3	3	3
35–49	23	1.9	2	1	1	2	2	3	3	7
50–64	0									
65+	1	1.0	0	1	1	1	1	1	1	1
TOTAL SINGLE DX	18	1.4	<1	1	1	1	2	2	3	3
TOTAL MULTIPLE DX	44	1.9	1	1	1	2	2	3	3	7
TOTAL										
0–19 Years	2	3.0	2	2	2	3	4	4	4	4
20–34	26	1.6	<1	1	1	2	2	3	3	3
35–49	32	1.8	2	1	1	2	2	3	3	7
50–64	1	2.0	0	2	2	2	2	2	2	2
65+	1	1.0	0	1	1	1	1	1	1	1
GRAND TOTAL	62	1.7	<1	1	1	2	2	3	3	7

66.8: FALL TUBE INSUFFLATION

Type of Patients	Observed Patients	Avg. Stay	Vari-ance	Percentiles						
				10th	25th	50th	75th	90th	95th	99th
1. SINGLE DX										
0–19 Years	0									
20–34	1	1.0	0	1	1	1	1	1	1	1
35–49	0									
50–64	0									
65+	0									
2. MULTIPLE DX										
0–19 Years	0									
20–34	2	2.0	2	1	1	1	3	3	3	3
35–49	1	2.0	0	2	2	2	2	2	2	2
50–64	0									
65+	0									
TOTAL SINGLE DX	1	1.0	0	1	1	1	1	1	1	1
TOTAL MULTIPLE DX	3	2.0	1	1	1	2	3	3	3	3
TOTAL										
0–19 Years	0									
20–34	3	1.7	1	1	1	1	3	3	3	3
35–49	1	2.0	0	2	2	2	2	2	2	2
50–64	0									
65+	0									
GRAND TOTAL	4	1.8	<1	1	1	1	3	3	3	3

LOS by Diagnosis and Operation, Western Region, 45th Edition

Western Region, October 2007–September 2008 Data, by Operation

66.9: OTHER FALLOPIAN TUBE OPS

Type of Patients	Observed Patients	Avg. Stay	Variance	10th	25th	50th	75th	90th	95th	99th
1. SINGLE DX										
0–19 Years	1	1.0	0	1	1	1	1	1	1	1
20–34	8	1.3	<1	1	1	1	1	2	2	2
35–49	2	3.5	12	1	1	1	6	6	6	6
50–64	1	2.0	0	2	2	2	2	2	2	2
65+	0									
2. MULTIPLE DX										
0–19 Years	2	2.5	4	1	1	1	4	4	4	4
20–34	57	2.0	<1	1	1	2	2	3	3	4
35–49	26	2.4	1	1	2	2	3	4	4	5
50–64	1	3.0	0	3	3	3	3	3	3	3
65+	0									
TOTAL SINGLE DX	12	1.7	2	1	1	1	2	2	6	6
TOTAL MULTIPLE DX	86	2.1	<1	1	2	2	3	3	4	5
TOTAL										
0–19 Years	3	2.0	3	1	1	1	4	4	4	4
20–34	65	1.9	<1	1	1	2	2	3	3	4
35–49	28	2.5	2	1	2	3	3	4	4	6
50–64	2	2.5	<1	2	3	3	3	3	3	3
65+	0									
GRAND TOTAL	98	2.1	<1	1	1	2	2	3	4	6

67.1: CERVICAL DIAGNOSTIC PX

Type of Patients	Observed Patients	Avg. Stay	Variance	10th	25th	50th	75th	90th	95th	99th
1. SINGLE DX										
0–19 Years	0									
20–34	5	1.8	<1			2	2	3	3	3
35–49	0									
50–64	2	1.0	0	1	1	1	1	1	1	1
65+	0									
2. MULTIPLE DX										
0–19 Years	2	5.0	2	4	4	4	6	6	6	6
20–34	35	3.0	4	1	1	3	3	6	7	9
35–49	121	4.5	33	1	1	3	5	9	14	31
50–64	87	6.1	64	1	2	4	8	13	18	65
65+	71	6.8	87	2	2	4	8	12	20	71
TOTAL SINGLE DX	7	1.6	<1	1	1	1	2	3	3	3
TOTAL MULTIPLE DX	316	5.3	52	1	2	3	6	12	16	31
TOTAL										
0–19 Years	2	5.0	2	4	4	4	6	6	6	6
20–34	40	2.9	4	1	1	2	3	6	6	9
35–49	121	4.5	33	1	1	3	5	9	14	31
50–64	89	6.0	63	1	2	4	8	13	18	65
65+	71	6.8	87	2	2	4	8	12	20	71
GRAND TOTAL	323	5.2	51	1	2	3	6	11	16	31

67.0: CERVICAL CANAL DILATION

Type of Patients	Observed Patients	Avg. Stay	Variance	10th	25th	50th	75th	90th	95th	99th
1. SINGLE DX										
0–19 Years	1	2.0	0	2	2	2	2	2	2	2
20–34	0									
35–49	1	1.0	0	1	1	1	1	1	1	1
50–64	0									
65+	0									
2. MULTIPLE DX										
0–19 Years	1	5.0	0	5	5	5	5	5	5	5
20–34	4	1.5	<1	1	1	1	1	3	3	3
35–49	3	1.0	0	1	1	1	1	1	1	1
50–64	2	1.0	0	1	1	1	1	1	1	1
65+	3	5.0	13	1	1	6	8	8	8	8
TOTAL SINGLE DX	2	1.5	<1	1	1	1	2	2	2	2
TOTAL MULTIPLE DX	13	2.4	6	1	1	1	3	6	8	8
TOTAL										
0–19 Years	2	3.5	4	2	2	5	5	5	5	5
20–34	4	1.5	<1	1	1	1	1	3	3	3
35–49	4	1.0	0	1	1	1	1	1	1	1
50–64	2	1.0	0	1	1	1	1	1	1	1
65+	3	5.0	13	1	1	6	8	8	8	8
GRAND TOTAL	15	2.3	5	1	1	1	3	6	8	8

67.12: CERVICAL BIOPSY NEC

Type of Patients	Observed Patients	Avg. Stay	Variance	10th	25th	50th	75th	90th	95th	99th
1. SINGLE DX										
0–19 Years	0									
20–34	1	1.0	0	1	1	1	1	1	1	1
35–49	0									
50–64	1	1.0	0	1	1	1	1	1	1	1
65+	0									
2. MULTIPLE DX										
0–19 Years	2	5.0	2	4	4	4	6	6	6	6
20–34	27	3.1	5	1	1	2	5	6	7	9
35–49	86	5.3	41	1	2	3	4	10	18	40
50–64	57	6.1	29	1	2	4	9	13	19	24
65+	49	7.0	113	1	2	4	8	15	20	71
TOTAL SINGLE DX	2	1.0	0	1	1	1	1	1	1	1
TOTAL MULTIPLE DX	221	5.6	50	1	2	3	7	11	18	31
TOTAL										
0–19 Years	2	5.0	2	4	4	4	6	6	6	6
20–34	28	3.0	5	1	1	2	5	6	7	9
35–49	86	5.3	41	1	2	3	4	10	18	40
50–64	58	6.0	29	1	2	4	9	13	19	24
65+	49	7.0	113	1	2	4	8	15	20	71
GRAND TOTAL	223	5.6	50	1	2	3	7	11	18	31

LOS by Diagnosis and Operation, Western Region, 45th Edition

Western Region, October 2007–September 2008 Data, by Operation

67.2: CONIZATION OF CERVIX

Type of Patients	Observed Patients	Avg. Stay	Vari-ance	Percentiles						
				10th	25th	50th	75th	90th	95th	99th
1. SINGLE DX										
0–19 Years	0									
20–34	1	1.0	0	1	1	1	1	1	1	1
35–49	2	1.0	0	1	1	1	1	1	1	1
50–64	1	1.0	0	1	1	1	1	1	1	1
65+	0									
2. MULTIPLE DX										
0–19 Years	0									
20–34	8	1.0	0	1	1	1	1	1	1	1
35–49	7	1.1	<1	1	1	1	1	2	2	2
50–64	9	2.5	13	1	1	1	2	12	12	12
65+	4	2.5	4	1	1	2	5	5	5	5
TOTAL SINGLE DX	4	1.0	0	1	1	1	1	1	1	1
TOTAL MULTIPLE DX	28	1.7	5	1	1	1	1	3	5	12
TOTAL										
0–19 Years	0									
20–34	9	1.0	0	1	1	1	1	1	1	1
35–49	9	1.1	<1	1	1	1	1	2	2	2
50–64	10	2.4	12	1	1	1	2	3	12	12
65+	4	2.5	4	1	1	2	5	5	5	5
GRAND TOTAL	32	1.7	4	1	1	1	1	3	5	12

67.3: EXC/DESTR CERV LES NEC

Type of Patients	Observed Patients	Avg. Stay	Vari-ance	Percentiles						
				10th	25th	50th	75th	90th	95th	99th
1. SINGLE DX										
0–19 Years	0									
20–34	3	1.7	1	1	1	1	3	3	3	3
35–49	7	1.4	<1	1	1	1	2	3	3	3
50–64	0									
65+	0									
2. MULTIPLE DX										
0–19 Years	6	2.2	<1	2	2	2	2	3	3	3
20–34	44	2.0	4	1	2	2	2	3	4	14
35–49	50	2.4	6	1	1	1	2	5	6	13
50–64	33	2.2	5	1	1	2	2	6	7	10
65+	12	5.3	31	1	1	2	8	12	17	17
TOTAL SINGLE DX	10	1.5	<1	1	1	1	2	3	3	3
TOTAL MULTIPLE DX	145	2.5	8	1	1	2	2	5	8	14
TOTAL										
0–19 Years	6	2.2	<1	2	2	2	2	3	3	3
20–34	47	2.0	4	1	1	1	2	3	4	14
35–49	57	2.3	6	1	1	1	2	5	6	13
50–64	33	2.2	5	1	1	1	2	6	7	10
65+	12	5.3	31	1	1	2	8	12	17	17
GRAND TOTAL	155	2.4	7	1	1	1	2	5	8	14

67.4: AMPUTATION OF CERVIX

Type of Patients	Observed Patients	Avg. Stay	Vari-ance	Percentiles						
				10th	25th	50th	75th	90th	95th	99th
1. SINGLE DX										
0–19 Years	0									
20–34	3	1.3	<1	1	1	1	2	2	2	2
35–49	2	1.5	<1	1	1	1	2	2	2	2
50–64	2	1.5	<1	1	2	2	2	2	2	2
65+	1	2.0	0	2	2	2	2	2	2	2
2. MULTIPLE DX										
0–19 Years	0									
20–34	23	1.7	<1	1	1	2	2	3	3	3
35–49	73	1.7	<1	1	1	1	2	3	4	5
50–64	51	2.7	6	1	2	2	3	5	8	12
65+	18	2.5	2	2	2	2	3	5	6	6
TOTAL SINGLE DX	8	1.5	<1	1	1	1	2	2	2	2
TOTAL MULTIPLE DX	165	2.1	3	1	1	2	3	4	5	11
TOTAL										
0–19 Years	0									
20–34	26	1.7	<1	1	1	1	2	3	3	3
35–49	75	1.7	<1	1	1	1	2	3	4	5
50–64	53	2.7	6	1	2	2	3	5	8	12
65+	19	2.5	2	2	2	2	3	5	6	6
GRAND TOTAL	173	2.1	3	1	1	2	3	4	5	11

67.5: INT CERVICAL OS REPAIR

Type of Patients	Observed Patients	Avg. Stay	Vari-ance	Percentiles						
				10th	25th	50th	75th	90th	95th	99th
1. SINGLE DX										
0–19 Years	17	4.0	54	1	1	2	3	7	32	32
20–34	232	2.0	3	1	1	1	2	4	5	8
35–49	37	1.6	1	1	1	1	2	3	5	6
50–64	2	3.0	2	2	2	3	4	4	4	4
65+	0									
2. MULTIPLE DX										
0–19 Years	29	5.0	79	1	1	2	4	7	30	42
20–34	477	4.9	92	1	1	2	4	8	15	63
35–49	250	5.5	146	1	1	1	5	8	21	67
50–64	16	10.0	360	1	1	1	6	56	58	58
65+	0									
TOTAL SINGLE DX	288	2.0	6	1	1	1	2	4	5	9
TOTAL MULTIPLE DX	772	5.2	114	1	1	2	4	8	17	63
TOTAL										
0–19 Years	46	4.7	69	1	1	2	4	7	30	42
20–34	709	3.9	65	1	1	2	4	7	10	48
35–49	287	5.0	129	1	1	2	4	8	15	67
50–64	18	9.3	323	1	2	2	4	56	58	58
65+	0									
GRAND TOTAL	1,060	4.3	87	1	1	2	4	7	13	59

LOS by Diagnosis and Operation, Western Region, 45th Edition

Western Region, October 2007–September 2008 Data, by Operation

67.59: INT CERVICAL OS REP NEC

Type of Patients	Observed Patients	Avg. Stay	Vari-ance	Percentiles						
				10th	25th	50th	75th	90th	95th	99th
1. SINGLE DX										
0–19 Years	17	4.0	54	1	1	2	3	7	32	32
20–34	228	1.9	3	1	1	1	2	4	5	8
35–49	37	1.6	1	1	1	1	2	3	5	6
50–64	2	3.0	2	2	2	3	4	4	4	4
65+	0									
2. MULTIPLE DX										
0–19 Years	29	5.0	79	1	1	2	4	7	30	42
20–34	466	4.9	94	1	1	2	4	8	15	63
35–49	245	5.6	149	1	1	2	5	9	21	67
50–64	16	10.0	360	1	1	2	6	56	58	58
65+	0									
TOTAL SINGLE DX	284	2.0	6	1	1	1	2	4	5	9
TOTAL MULTIPLE DX	756	5.2	116	1	1	2	4	8	19	63
TOTAL										
0–19 Years	46	4.7	69	1	1	2	4	7	30	42
20–34	694	3.9	66	1	1	2	4	7	10	48
35–49	282	5.1	131	1	1	2	4	8	15	67
50–64	18	9.3	323	1	1	2	4	56	58	58
65+	0									
GRAND TOTAL	1,040	4.4	88	1	1	2	4	7	14	59

67.6: OTHER REPAIR OF CERVIX

Type of Patients	Observed Patients	Avg. Stay	Vari-ance	Percentiles						
				10th	25th	50th	75th	90th	95th	99th
1. SINGLE DX										
0–19 Years	0									
20–34	2	1.5	<1	1	1	1	2	2	2	2
35–49	1	1.0	0	1	1	1	1	1	1	1
50–64	0									
65+	0									
2. MULTIPLE DX										
0–19 Years	1	2.0	0	2	2	2	2	2	2	2
20–34	15	1.5	<1	1	1	1	2	3	3	3
35–49	11	2.6	26	1	1	1	1	2	18	18
50–64	2	1.0	0	1	1	1	1	1	1	1
65+	0									
TOTAL SINGLE DX	3	1.3	<1	1	1	1	2	2	2	2
TOTAL MULTIPLE DX	29	1.9	10	1	1	1	2	3	3	18
TOTAL										
0–19 Years	1	2.0	0	2	2	2	2	2	2	2
20–34	17	1.5	<1	1	1	1	2	3	3	3
35–49	12	2.5	24	1	1	1	1	2	18	18
50–64	2	1.0	0	1	1	1	1	1	1	1
65+	0									
GRAND TOTAL	32	1.9	9	1	1	1	2	2	3	18

68.0: HYSTEROTOMY

Type of Patients	Observed Patients	Avg. Stay	Vari-ance	Percentiles						
				10th	25th	50th	75th	90th	95th	99th
1. SINGLE DX										
0–19 Years	1	1.0	0	1	1	1	1	1	1	1
20–34	0									
35–49	0									
50–64	0									
65+	0									
2. MULTIPLE DX										
0–19 Years	1	5.0	0	5	5	5	5	5	5	5
20–34	13	3.2	3	2	2	3	3	6	8	8
35–49	4	3.3	7	1	1	2	7	7	7	7
50–64	2	1.0	0	1	1	1	1	1	1	1
65+	0									
TOTAL SINGLE DX	1	1.0	0	1	1	1	1	1	1	1
TOTAL MULTIPLE DX	20	3.1	4	1	2	3	3	6	7	8
TOTAL										
0–19 Years	2	3.0	8	1	1	1	5	5	5	5
20–34	13	3.2	3	2	2	3	3	6	8	8
35–49	4	3.3	7	1	1	2	7	7	7	7
50–64	2	1.0	0	1	1	1	1	1	1	1
65+	0									
GRAND TOTAL	21	3.0	4	1	2	3	3	6	7	8

68.1: UTER/ADNEXA DXTIC PX

Type of Patients	Observed Patients	Avg. Stay	Vari-ance	Percentiles						
				10th	25th	50th	75th	90th	95th	99th
1. SINGLE DX										
0–19 Years	0									
20–34	5	1.4	<1	1	1	1	1	3	3	3
35–49	2	1.0	0	1	1	1	3	3	3	1
50–64	1	3.0	0	3	3	3	3	3	3	3
65+	1	1.0	0	1	1	1	1	1	1	1
2. MULTIPLE DX										
0–19 Years	3	1.0	0	1	1	1	1	1	1	1
20–34	44	2.9	6	1	1	2	4	6	8	11
35–49	174	2.7	7	1	1	3	5	6	9	14
50–64	102	5.2	49	1	1	3	5	13	20	33
65+	57	6.2	43	1	2	5	7	13	20	37
TOTAL SINGLE DX	9	1.4	<1	1	1	1	1	3	3	3
TOTAL MULTIPLE DX	380	3.9	26	1	1	2	5	8	12	31
TOTAL										
0–19 Years	3	1.0	0	1	1	1	1	1	1	1
20–34	49	2.8	6	1	1	2	4	6	8	11
35–49	176	2.7	7	1	1	3	5	6	9	14
50–64	103	5.1	49	1	1	3	5	13	20	33
65+	58	6.1	42	2	2	4	7	13	20	37
GRAND TOTAL	389	3.8	25	1	1	2	4	8	12	31

LOS by Diagnosis and Operation, Western Region, 45th Edition

Western Region, October 2007–September 2008 Data, by Operation

68.16: CLOSED UTERINE BIOPSY

Type of Patients	Observed Patients	Avg. Stay	Variance	10th	25th	50th	75th	90th	95th	99th
1. SINGLE DX										
0–19 Years	0									
20–34	4	1.5	<1	1	1	1	3	3	3	3
35–49	2	1.0	0	1	1	1	1	1	1	1
50–64	1	3.0	0	3	3	3	3	3	3	3
65+	0									
2. MULTIPLE DX										
0–19 Years	1	1.0	0	1	1	1	1	1	1	1
20–34	30	2.5	5	1	1	2	3	6	7	11
35–49	158	2.7	8	1	1	1	3	6	9	14
50–64	94	5.4	52	1	1	3	5	14	23	41
65+	54	6.0	35	1	2	5	7	12	17	37
TOTAL SINGLE DX	7	1.6	<1	1	1	1	3	3	3	3
TOTAL MULTIPLE DX	337	4.0	26	1	1	2	5	9	13	31
TOTAL										
0–19 Years	1	1.0	0	1	1	1	1	1	1	1
20–34	34	2.4	5	1	1	1	3	5	7	11
35–49	160	2.7	8	1	1	1	3	6	9	14
50–64	95	5.3	52	1	1	3	5	14	23	41
65+	54	6.0	35	1	2	5	7	12	17	37
GRAND TOTAL	344	3.9	26	1	1	2	5	8	13	31

68.2: UTERINE LES EXC/DESTR

Type of Patients	Observed Patients	Avg. Stay	Variance	10th	25th	50th	75th	90th	95th	99th
1. SINGLE DX										
0–19 Years	3	3.3	10	1	1	2	7	7	7	7
20–34	223	2.1	<1	1	2	2	3	3	3	4
35–49	339	2.1	<1	1	2	2	3	3	3	4
50–64	48	2.0	<1	1	1	2	3	3	3	4
65+	0									
2. MULTIPLE DX										
0–19 Years	8	3.1	4	1	1	2	5	6	6	6
20–34	1,223	2.4	2	1	2	2	3	4	4	8
35–49	2,507	2.4	2	1	2	2	3	4	5	8
50–64	560	2.5	4	1	1	2	3	4	5	11
65+	47	3.8	12	1	1	2	4	10	11	15
TOTAL SINGLE DX	613	2.1	<1	1	2	2	3	3	3	4
TOTAL MULTIPLE DX	4,345	2.4	3	1	2	2	3	4	4	9
TOTAL										
0–19 Years	11	3.2	5	1	1	2	5	6	7	7
20–34	1,446	2.4	2	1	2	2	3	3	4	7
35–49	2,846	2.3	2	1	2	2	3	3	4	8
50–64	608	2.4	4	1	1	2	3	4	5	10
65+	47	3.8	12	1	1	2	4	10	11	15
GRAND TOTAL	4,958	2.4	2	1	2	2	3	3	4	9

68.23: ENDOMETRIAL ABLATION

Type of Patients	Observed Patients	Avg. Stay	Variance	10th	25th	50th	75th	90th	95th	99th
1. SINGLE DX										
0–19 Years	0									
20–34	7	1.4	<1	1	1	1	2	3	3	3
35–49	3	1.3	<1	1	1	1	2	2	2	2
50–64	2	1.0	0	1	1	1	1	1	1	1
65+	0									
2. MULTIPLE DX										
0–19 Years	1	2.0	0	2	2	2	2	2	2	2
20–34	77	2.1	3	1	1	2	2	4	6	10
35–49	305	2.2	10	1	1	1	2	4	6	15
50–64	83	2.5	10	1	1	1	3	5	10	17
65+	6	3.7	13	1	1	2	6	10	10	10
TOTAL SINGLE DX	12	1.3	<1	1	1	1	2	2	3	3
TOTAL MULTIPLE DX	472	2.3	9	1	1	1	2	4	7	16
TOTAL										
0–19 Years	1	2.0	0	2	2	2	2	2	2	2
20–34	84	2.1	3	1	1	1	2	4	6	10
35–49	308	2.2	10	1	1	1	2	4	6	15
50–64	85	2.5	10	1	1	1	3	5	10	17
65+	6	3.7	13	1	1	2	6	10	10	10
GRAND TOTAL	484	2.3	9	1	1	1	2	4	7	16

68.29: UTER LES EXC/DESTR NEC

Type of Patients	Observed Patients	Avg. Stay	Variance	10th	25th	50th	75th	90th	95th	99th
1. SINGLE DX										
0–19 Years	3	3.3	10	1	1	2	7	7	7	7
20–34	215	2.2	<1	1	2	2	3	3	3	4
35–49	333	2.1	<1	1	2	2	3	3	3	4
50–64	46	2.0	<1	1	1	2	3	3	3	4
65+	0									
2. MULTIPLE DX										
0–19 Years	7	3.3	5	1	1	4	5	6	6	6
20–34	1,143	2.4	2	1	2	2	3	4	4	7
35–49	2,202	2.4	1	1	2	2	3	3	4	7
50–64	477	2.5	3	1	2	2	3	4	5	9
65+	40	3.7	12	1	1	2	4	10	11	15
TOTAL SINGLE DX	597	2.1	<1	1	2	2	3	3	3	4
TOTAL MULTIPLE DX	3,869	2.4	2	1	2	2	3	4	4	8
TOTAL										
0–19 Years	10	3.3	6	1	1	4	5	6	7	7
20–34	1,358	2.4	1	1	2	2	3	3	4	7
35–49	2,535	2.4	1	1	2	2	3	3	4	7
50–64	523	2.4	3	1	2	2	3	4	4	9
65+	40	3.7	12	1	1	2	4	10	11	15
GRAND TOTAL	4,466	2.4	2	1	2	2	3	3	4	7

LOS by Diagnosis and Operation, Western Region, 45th Edition

Western Region, October 2007–September 2008 Data, by Operation

68.3: SUBTOT ABD HYSTERECTOMY

Type of Patients	Observed Patients	Avg. Stay	Vari-ance	Percentiles						
				10th	25th	50th	75th	90th	95th	99th
1. SINGLE DX										
0–19 Years	0									
20–34	30	1.7	<1	1	1	2	2	3	4	4
35–49	270	1.8	<1	1	1	2	2	3	3	4
50–64	98	1.9	<1	1	1	2	3	3	3	5
65+	5	3.0	0	3	3	3	3	3	3	3
2. MULTIPLE DX										
0–19 Years	4	2.5	2	1	1	3	4	4	4	4
20–34	650	2.3	3	1	1	2	3	4	5	10
35–49	6,183	2.1	2	1	1	2	3	3	4	7
50–64	2,537	2.4	6	1	1	2	3	4	5	11
65+	259	4.9	36	1	2	3	5	9	13	40
TOTAL SINGLE DX	403	1.8	<1	1	1	2	2	3	3	4
TOTAL MULTIPLE DX	9,633	2.3	4	1	1	2	3	4	5	9
TOTAL										
0–19 Years	4	2.5	2	1	1	3	4	4	4	4
20–34	680	2.3	3	1	1	2	3	4	5	10
35–49	6,453	2.1	2	1	1	2	3	3	4	7
50–64	2,635	2.4	6	1	1	2	3	4	5	11
65+	264	4.8	35	1	2	3	5	9	13	40
GRAND TOTAL	10,036	2.3	4	1	1	2	3	4	5	9

68.31: LSH

Type of Patients	Observed Patients	Avg. Stay	Vari-ance	Percentiles						
				10th	25th	50th	75th	90th	95th	99th
1. SINGLE DX										
0–19 Years	0									
20–34	21	1.4	<1	1	1	1	2	2	2	2
35–49	141	1.3	<1	1	1	1	1	2	2	3
50–64	47	1.2	<1	1	1	1	1	2	2	3
65+	0									
2. MULTIPLE DX										
0–19 Years	1	1.0	0	1	1	1	1	1	1	1
20–34	333	1.4	<1	1	1	1	2	2	3	4
35–49	2,807	1.4	1	1	1	1	2	2	3	5
50–64	990	1.4	<1	1	1	1	2	2	3	4
65+	75	1.7	<1	1	1	2	3	3	3	4
TOTAL SINGLE DX	209	1.3	<1	1	1	1	1	2	2	3
TOTAL MULTIPLE DX	4,206	1.4	<1	1	1	1	2	2	3	4
TOTAL										
0–19 Years	1	1.0	0	1	1	1	1	1	1	1
20–34	354	1.4	<1	1	1	1	2	2	3	4
35–49	2,948	1.4	<1	1	1	1	2	2	3	5
50–64	1,037	1.4	<1	1	1	1	2	2	3	4
65+	75	1.7	<1	1	1	2	2	3	3	4
GRAND TOTAL	4,415	1.4	<1	1	1	1	2	2	3	4

68.39: SUBTOT ABD HYST NEC&NOS

Type of Patients	Observed Patients	Avg. Stay	Vari-ance	Percentiles						
				10th	25th	50th	75th	90th	95th	99th
1. SINGLE DX										
0–19 Years	0									
20–34	9	2.6	1	1	2	2	3	4	4	4
35–49	129	2.4	<1	2	2	2	3	3	3	4
50–64	51	2.5	<1	2	3	2	3	3	4	5
65+	5	3.0	0	3	3	3	3	3	3	3
2. MULTIPLE DX										
0–19 Years	3	3.0	<1	2	2	3	4	4	4	4
20–34	317	3.2	4	2	2	3	4	5	7	13
35–49	3,376	2.8	2	2	2	3	3	4	5	8
50–64	1,547	3.1	8	2	3	3	3	4	6	13
65+	184	6.1	45	2	3	4	7	11	18	43
TOTAL SINGLE DX	194	2.4	<1	2	2	2	3	3	4	4
TOTAL MULTIPLE DX	5,427	3.0	6	2	2	3	3	4	6	12
TOTAL										
0–19 Years	3	3.0	<1	2	2	3	4	4	4	4
20–34	326	3.2	4	2	2	3	4	5	7	13
35–49	3,505	2.7	2	2	2	3	3	4	5	8
50–64	1,598	3.0	8	2	3	3	3	4	6	13
65+	189	6.0	44	2	3	4	7	11	18	43
GRAND TOTAL	5,621	3.0	6	2	2	3	3	4	6	12

68.4: TOTAL ABD HYSTERECTOMY

Type of Patients	Observed Patients	Avg. Stay	Vari-ance	Percentiles						
				10th	25th	50th	75th	90th	95th	99th
1. SINGLE DX										
0–19 Years	0									
20–34	124	2.4	<1	1	2	2	3	3	4	5
35–49	799	2.5	<1	2	2	2	3	3	4	5
50–64	475	2.5	<1	2	2	2	3	3	4	5
65+	95	2.9	2	2	2	3	3	4	5	9
2. MULTIPLE DX										
0–19 Years	12	6.1	9	2	2	6	9	9	11	11
20–34	2,679	2.9	4	2	2	3	3	4	5	11
35–49	21,828	2.8	6	2	2	3	3	5	5	8
50–64	11,596	3.1	6	2	2	3	3	5	6	12
65+	3,613	4.4	19	2	3	4	5	8	11	21
TOTAL SINGLE DX	1,493	2.5	<1	2	2	2	3	3	4	5
TOTAL MULTIPLE DX	39,728	3.0	6	2	2	3	3	4	6	12
TOTAL										
0–19 Years	12	6.1	9	2	2	6	9	9	11	11
20–34	2,803	2.8	4	2	2	3	3	4	5	10
35–49	22,627	2.7	2	2	2	3	3	4	5	8
50–64	12,071	3.1	6	2	2	3	5	5	6	12
65+	3,708	4.4	19	2	2	3	5	8	11	20
GRAND TOTAL	41,221	3.0	5	2	2	3	3	4	6	12

LOS by Diagnosis and Operation, Western Region, 45th Edition

Western Region, October 2007–September 2008 Data, by Operation

68.41: TLH

Type of Patients	Observed Patients	Avg. Stay	Variance	Percentiles						
				10th	25th	50th	75th	90th	95th	99th
1. SINGLE DX										
0–19 Years	0									
20–34	10	1.5	<1	1	1	1	2	3	3	3
35–49	44	1.7	5	1	1	1	2	3	3	15
50–64	53	1.4	<1	1	1	1	2	2	3	4
65+	12	1.4	<1	1	1	1	2	3	3	2
2. MULTIPLE DX										
0–19 Years	1	11.0	0	11	11	11	11	11	11	11
20–34	183	1.5	<1	1	1	1	2	2	3	6
35–49	1,259	1.6	1	1	1	1	2	2	3	5
50–64	862	1.6	1	1	1	2	2	3	3	7
65+	353	2.0	3	1	1	2	2	4	5	10
TOTAL SINGLE DX	119	1.5	2	1	1	1	2	2	3	4
TOTAL MULTIPLE DX	2,658	1.6	1	1	1	1	2	3	4	7
TOTAL										
0–19 Years	1	11.0	0	11	11	11	11	11	11	11
20–34	193	1.5	<1	1	1	1	2	2	3	6
35–49	1,303	1.6	1	1	1	1	2	3	3	5
50–64	915	1.6	1	1	1	2	2	3	3	7
65+	365	2.0	3	1	1	2	2	3	5	10
GRAND TOTAL	2,777	1.6	2	1	1	1	2	3	4	6

68.49: TAH NEC & NOS

Type of Patients	Observed Patients	Avg. Stay	Variance	Percentiles						
				10th	25th	50th	75th	90th	95th	99th
1. SINGLE DX										
0–19 Years	0									
20–34	114	2.5	<1	2	2	3	3	3	4	5
35–49	755	2.6	<1	2	2	3	3	3	4	5
50–64	422	2.6	<1	2	2	3	3	3	4	5
65+	83	3.1	1	2	2	3	3	4	5	9
2. MULTIPLE DX										
0–19 Years	11	5.9	8	2	2	6	9	9	9	11
20–34	2,496	3.0	5	2	2	3	3	4	5	11
35–49	20,569	2.8	2	2	2	3	3	4	5	8
50–64	10,734	3.3	7	2	2	3	3	5	7	13
65+	3,260	4.7	20	2	3	3	5	8	12	21
TOTAL SINGLE DX	1,374	2.6	<1	2	2	3	3	3	4	5
TOTAL MULTIPLE DX	37,070	3.1	6	2	2	3	3	4	6	12
TOTAL										
0–19 Years	11	5.9	8	2	2	6	9	9	9	11
20–34	2,610	2.9	4	2	2	3	3	4	5	11
35–49	21,324	2.8	2	2	2	3	3	4	5	8
50–64	11,156	3.2	6	2	2	3	3	5	6	13
65+	3,343	4.6	20	2	3	3	5	8	11	21
GRAND TOTAL	38,444	3.1	6	2	2	3	3	4	6	12

68.5: VAGINAL HYSTERECTOMY

Type of Patients	Observed Patients	Avg. Stay	Variance	Percentiles						
				10th	25th	50th	75th	90th	95th	99th
1. SINGLE DX										
0–19 Years	0									
20–34	160	1.5	<1	1	1	1	2	2	2	3
35–49	585	1.5	<1	1	1	1	2	2	2	3
50–64	438	1.6	<1	1	1	1	2	2	3	3
65+	152	1.9	<1	1	1	2	2	3	3	4
2. MULTIPLE DX										
0–19 Years	3	2.3	1	1	1	3	3	3	3	3
20–34	2,775	1.6	<1	1	1	1	2	2	3	5
35–49	14,493	1.6	<1	1	1	1	2	3	3	4
50–64	7,832	1.8	1	1	1	2	2	3	3	5
65+	3,525	2.1	2	1	1	2	2	3	4	7
TOTAL SINGLE DX	1,335	1.6	<1	1	1	1	2	2	3	3
TOTAL MULTIPLE DX	28,628	1.7	1	1	1	2	2	3	3	5
TOTAL										
0–19 Years	3	2.3	1	1	1	3	3	3	3	3
20–34	2,935	1.6	<1	1	1	1	2	2	3	5
35–49	15,078	1.6	<1	1	1	1	2	3	3	4
50–64	8,270	1.8	<1	1	1	2	2	3	3	5
65+	3,677	2.1	2	1	1	2	2	3	4	7
GRAND TOTAL	29,963	1.7	<1	1	1	2	2	3	3	5

68.51: LAVH

Type of Patients	Observed Patients	Avg. Stay	Variance	Percentiles						
				10th	25th	50th	75th	90th	95th	99th
1. SINGLE DX										
0–19 Years	0									
20–34	51	1.5	<1	1	1	1	2	2	2	3
35–49	177	1.4	<1	1	1	1	2	2	2	4
50–64	131	1.5	<1	1	1	1	2	2	3	4
65+	33	1.9	<1	1	1	2	2	3	4	4
2. MULTIPLE DX										
0–19 Years	3	2.3	1	1	1	3	3	3	3	3
20–34	1,172	1.6	<1	1	1	1	2	2	3	5
35–49	5,938	1.6	<1	1	1	1	2	2	3	4
50–64	2,837	1.6	<1	1	1	1	2	3	3	4
65+	764	2.1	3	1	1	2	2	3	4	10
TOTAL SINGLE DX	392	1.5	<1	1	1	1	2	2	2	4
TOTAL MULTIPLE DX	10,714	1.6	<1	1	1	1	2	3	3	5
TOTAL										
0–19 Years	3	2.3	1	1	1	3	3	3	3	3
20–34	1,223	1.6	<1	1	1	1	2	2	3	5
35–49	6,115	1.6	<1	1	1	1	2	2	3	4
50–64	2,968	1.6	<1	1	1	1	2	3	3	4
65+	797	2.1	3	1	1	2	2	3	4	9
GRAND TOTAL	11,106	1.6	<1	1	1	1	2	3	3	5

Western Region, October 2007–September 2008 Data, by Operation

68.59: VAG HYST NEC & NOS

Type of Patients	Observed Patients	Avg. Stay	Vari-ance	Percentiles						
				10th	25th	50th	75th	90th	95th	99th
1. SINGLE DX										
0–19 Years	0									
20–34	109	1.5	<1	1	1	1	2	2	2	3
35–49	408	1.5	<1	1	1	1	2	2	3	3
50–64	307	1.6	<1	1	1	2	2	2	3	3
65+	119	1.9	<1	1	1	2	2	3	3	3
2. MULTIPLE DX										
0–19 Years	0									
20–34	1,603	1.7	1	1	1	1	2	2	3	5
35–49	8,555	1.7	<1	1	1	2	2	3	3	5
50–64	4,995	1.8	1	1	1	2	2	3	3	5
65+	2,761	2.2	2	1	2	2	3	3	4	6
TOTAL SINGLE DX	943	1.6	<1	1	1	2	2	2	3	3
TOTAL MULTIPLE DX	17,914	1.8	1	1	1	2	2	3	3	5
TOTAL										
0–19 Years	0									
20–34	1,712	1.6	<1	1	1	1	2	2	3	5
35–49	8,963	1.7	<1	1	1	2	2	3	3	4
50–64	5,302	1.8	1	1	1	2	2	3	3	5
65+	2,880	2.1	2	1	2	2	3	3	4	6
GRAND TOTAL	18,857	1.8	1	1	1	2	2	3	3	5

68.61: TLRH

Type of Patients	Observed Patients	Avg. Stay	Vari-ance	Percentiles						
				10th	25th	50th	75th	90th	95th	99th
1. SINGLE DX										
0–19 Years	1	1.0	0							1
20–34	5	2.0	<1	1	2	2	2	3	3	3
35–49	18	1.9	<1	1	1	2	2	3	3	3
50–64	15	1.7	1	1	1	1	2	4	5	5
65+	6	2.2	4	1	1	1	2	6	6	6
2. MULTIPLE DX										
0–19 Years	0									
20–34	23	1.8	<1	1	1	2	2	3	4	4
35–49	141	2.1	4	1	1	2	2	3	4	12
50–64	154	2.1	2	1	1	2	3	4	5	8
65+	64	2.7	4	1	1	2	3	6	7	8
TOTAL SINGLE DX	45	1.9	1	1	1	2	2	3	4	6
TOTAL MULTIPLE DX	382	2.2	3	1	1	2	3	4	5	9
TOTAL										
0–19 Years	1	1.0	0							1
20–34	28	1.9	<1	1	1	2	2	3	4	4
35–49	159	2.0	4	1	1	2	2	3	4	12
50–64	169	2.0	2	1	1	2	3	4	5	8
65+	70	2.6	4	1	1	2	3	6	7	8
GRAND TOTAL	427	2.1	3	1	1	2	2	4	5	8

68.6: RADICAL ABD HYSTERECTOMY

Type of Patients	Observed Patients	Avg. Stay	Vari-ance	Percentiles						
				10th	25th	50th	75th	90th	95th	99th
1. SINGLE DX										
0–19 Years	1	1.0	0	1	1	1	1	1	1	1
20–34	21	3.1	1	2	2	3	4	4	5	6
35–49	58	2.9	1	1	2	3	3	4	5	6
50–64	42	2.9	2	1	2	3	4	5	5	6
65+	11	2.7	3	1	1	3	3	5	6	6
2. MULTIPLE DX										
0–19 Years	1	5.0	0	5	5	5	5	5	5	5
20–34	108	3.7	5	1	3	3	4	6	7	13
35–49	431	3.7	7	1	2	3	4	6	8	17
50–64	533	4.4	26	1	2	4	5	7	10	18
65+	306	5.3	13	2	3	4	6	10	14	18
TOTAL SINGLE DX	133	2.9	2	1	2	3	4	5	5	6
TOTAL MULTIPLE DX	1,379	4.3	16	1	2	4	5	8	10	18
TOTAL										
0–19 Years	2	3.0	8	1	1	3	5	5	5	5
20–34	129	3.6	4	1	2	3	4	6	7	13
35–49	489	3.6	7	1	2	3	4	6	8	17
50–64	575	4.3	25	1	2	3	5	7	10	18
65+	317	5.2	13	2	3	4	6	9	14	18
GRAND TOTAL	1,512	4.2	15	1	2	3	5	7	10	17

68.69: RAD ABD HYST NEC & NOS

Type of Patients	Observed Patients	Avg. Stay	Vari-ance	Percentiles						
				10th	25th	50th	75th	90th	95th	99th
1. SINGLE DX										
0–19 Years	0									
20–34	16	3.4	1	2	3	3	4	5	6	6
35–49	40	3.4	1	2	3	3	4	5	6	6
50–64	27	3.5	<1	2	3	3	4	5	6	6
65+	5	3.4		3	3	3	3	5	5	5
2. MULTIPLE DX										
0–19 Years	1	5.0	0	5	5	5	5	5	5	5
20–34	85	4.2	4	2	3	4	5	6	8	14
35–49	290	4.5	7	3	3	4	6	7	9	17
50–64	379	5.4	33	3	3	4	6	9	12	25
65+	242	6.0	13	3	4	5	7	12	14	18
TOTAL SINGLE DX	88	3.4	1	2	3	3	4	5	6	6
TOTAL MULTIPLE DX	997	5.2	19	3	3	4	6	8	12	18
TOTAL										
0–19 Years	1	5.0	0	5	5	5	5	5	5	5
20–34	101	4.1	4	2	3	4	5	6	7	13
35–49	330	4.4	6	3	3	4	5	7	8	17
50–64	406	5.2	31	3	3	4	5	9	12	20
65+	247	5.9	13	3	4	5	7	12	14	18
GRAND TOTAL	1,085	5.0	17	3	3	4	5	8	12	18

LOS by Diagnosis and Operation, Western Region, 45th Edition

Western Region, October 2007–September 2008 Data, by Operation

68.7: RADICAL VAG HYSTERECTOMY

Type of Patients	Observed Patients	Avg. Stay	Variance	Percentiles						
				10th	25th	50th	75th	90th	95th	99th
1. SINGLE DX										
0–19 Years	0									
20–34	1	3.0	0	3	3	3	3	3	3	3
35–49	9	2.0	1	1	1	2	2	3	4	4
50–64	11	1.6	<1	1	1	1	2	2	3	3
65+	2	3.0	0	3	3	3	3	3	3	3
2. MULTIPLE DX										
0–19 Years	0									
20–34	15	3.9	49	1	2	2	2	5	29	29
35–49	98	2.2	1	1	1	2	3	3	4	7
50–64	84	2.3	2	1	2	2	3	4	4	8
65+	45	2.9	8	1	2	2	3	4	5	18
TOTAL SINGLE DX	23	1.9	<1	1	1	2	3	3	3	4
TOTAL MULTIPLE DX	242	2.5	6	1	1	2	3	4	5	10
TOTAL										
0–19 Years	0									
20–34	16	3.8	46	1	2	2	2	5	29	29
35–49	107	2.1	1	1	2	2	3	3	4	7
50–64	95	2.3	2	1	1	2	3	4	4	8
65+	47	2.9	7	1	2	2	3	4	5	18
GRAND TOTAL	265	2.4	5	1	2	2	3	4	4	10

68.79: RAD VAG HYST NEC & NOS

Type of Patients	Observed Patients	Avg. Stay	Variance	Percentiles						
				10th	25th	50th	75th	90th	95th	99th
1. SINGLE DX										
0–19 Years	0									
20–34	0									
35–49	4	2.8	<1	2	2	3	4	4	4	4
50–64	6	1.7	<1	1	1	2	2	3	3	3
65+	1	3.0	0	3	3	3	3	3	3	3
2. MULTIPLE DX										
0–19 Years	0									
20–34	10	5.0	72	2	2	2	3	29	29	29
35–49	49	2.3	2	1	1	2	3	4	5	7
50–64	45	2.8	2	1	2	2	4	4	5	8
65+	26	2.8	3	1	2	2	3	5	5	10
TOTAL SINGLE DX	11	2.2	<1	1	1	2	3	3	4	4
TOTAL MULTIPLE DX	130	2.8	7	1	2	2	3	4	5	10
TOTAL										
0–19 Years	0									
20–34	10	5.0	72	2	2	2	3	29	29	29
35–49	53	2.4	2	2	2	2	3	4	5	7
50–64	51	2.7	2	1	2	2	4	4	5	8
65+	27	2.8	3	2	2	3	3	5	5	10
GRAND TOTAL	141	2.7	7	1	2	2	3	4	5	10

68.8: PELVIC EVISCERATION

Type of Patients	Observed Patients	Avg. Stay	Variance	Percentiles						
				10th	25th	50th	75th	90th	95th	99th
1. SINGLE DX										
0–19 Years	0									
20–34	0									
35–49	0									
50–64	1	9.0	0	9	9	9	9	9	9	9
65+	0									
2. MULTIPLE DX										
0–19 Years	1	18.0	0	18	18	18	18	18	18	18
20–34	2	13.0	31	9	9	17	17	17	17	17
35–49	48	13.4	79	4	8	11	18	23	28	46
50–64	73	13.5	73	7	8	11	17	24	30	48
65+	62	14.9	87	7	9	13	17	24	34	50
TOTAL SINGLE DX	1	9.0	0	9	9	9	9	9	9	9
TOTAL MULTIPLE DX	186	14.0	77	6	8	11	18	24	30	50
TOTAL										
0–19 Years	1	18.0	0	18	18	18	18	18	18	18
20–34	2	13.0	31	9	9	17	17	17	17	17
35–49	48	13.4	79	4	8	11	18	23	28	46
50–64	74	13.4	72	7	8	11	17	24	30	48
65+	62	14.9	87	7	9	13	17	24	34	50
GRAND TOTAL	187	14.0	76	6	8	11	18	24	30	50

68.9: HYSTERECTOMY NEC & NOS

Type of Patients	Observed Patients	Avg. Stay	Variance	Percentiles						
				10th	25th	50th	75th	90th	95th	99th
1. SINGLE DX										
0–19 Years	0									
20–34	0									
35–49	1	1.0	0	1	1	1	1	1	1	1
50–64	0									
65+	1	1.0	0	1	1	1	1	1	1	1
2. MULTIPLE DX										
0–19 Years	1	5.0	0	5	5	5	5	5	5	5
20–34	11	2.7	2	1	2	2	4	4	5	5
35–49	45	2.7	2	1	2	2	3	4	5	6
50–64	28	2.9	2	1	2	2	4	5	5	6
65+	10	8.0	60	2	3	4	16	19	22	22
TOTAL SINGLE DX	2	1.0	0	1	1	1	1	1	1	1
TOTAL MULTIPLE DX	95	3.4	10	1	2	3	4	5	6	19
TOTAL										
0–19 Years	1	5.0	0	5	5	5	5	5	5	5
20–34	11	2.7	2	1	2	2	4	4	5	5
35–49	46	2.6	2	1	2	2	3	4	5	6
50–64	28	2.9	2	1	2	2	4	5	5	6
65+	11	7.4	58	2	2	4	16	19	22	22
GRAND TOTAL	97	3.3	10	1	2	3	4	5	6	19

LOS by Diagnosis and Operation, Western Region, 45th Edition

Western Region, October 2007–September 2008 Data, by Operation

69.0: UTERINE D&C

Type of Patients	Observed Patients	Avg. Stay	Variance	Percentiles						
				10th	25th	50th	75th	90th	95th	99th
1. SINGLE DX										
0–19 Years	121	1.3	<1	1	1	1	1	2	3	4
20–34	841	1.3	<1	1	1	1	1	2	3	4
35–49	271	1.2	<1	1	1	1	1	2	2	4
50–64	19	1.1	<1	1	1	1	1	1	2	2
65+	2	1.0	0	1	1	1	1	1	1	1
2. MULTIPLE DX										
0–19 Years	333	2.6	8	1	1	2	3	4	5	15
20–34	2,665	2.5	8	1	1	2	3	4	5	14
35–49	1,461	2.4	9	1	1	2	3	4	6	12
50–64	388	3.0	14	1	1	2	3	7	10	29
65+	194	4.6	15	1	2	4	7	9	13	19
TOTAL SINGLE DX	1,254	1.3	<1	1	1	1	1	2	2	4
TOTAL MULTIPLE DX	5,041	2.6	10	1	1	2	3	4	7	15
TOTAL										
0–19 Years	454	2.2	6	1	1	2	3	4	5	15
20–34	3,506	2.2	7	1	1	2	3	4	5	11
35–49	1,732	2.2	8	1	1	2	3	4	5	11
50–64	407	2.9	14	1	1	2	3	7	9	22
65+	196	4.6	15	2	2	4	7	9	13	19
GRAND TOTAL	6,295	2.3	8	1	1	2	3	4	6	13

69.01: D&C FOR TERM OF PREG

Type of Patients	Observed Patients	Avg. Stay	Variance	Percentiles						
				10th	25th	50th	75th	90th	95th	99th
1. SINGLE DX										
0–19 Years	0									
20–34	10	1.3	<1	1	1	1	2	2	2	2
35–49	3	1.7	<1	1	1	2	2	2	2	2
50–64	0									
65+	0									
2. MULTIPLE DX										
0–19 Years	6	5.2	30	1	1	3	10	14	14	14
20–34	61	3.8	22	1	1	2	4	8	13	28
35–49	24	4.6	106	1	1	2	3	7	7	52
50–64	5	2.4	10	1	1	1	1	8	8	8
65+	0									
TOTAL SINGLE DX	13	1.4	<1	1	1	1	2	2	2	2
TOTAL MULTIPLE DX	96	4.0	42	1	1	2	4	8	14	52
TOTAL										
0–19 Years	6	5.2	30	1	1	3	10	14	14	14
20–34	71	3.4	20	1	1	2	4	6	13	28
35–49	27	4.2	94	1	1	2	3	7	7	52
50–64	5	2.4	10	1	1	1	1	8	8	8
65+	0									
GRAND TOTAL	109	3.7	38	1	1	2	4	8	13	28

69.02: D&C POST DEL OR AB

Type of Patients	Observed Patients	Avg. Stay	Variance	Percentiles						
				10th	25th	50th	75th	90th	95th	99th
1. SINGLE DX										
0–19 Years	109	1.3	<1	1	1	1	1	2	3	4
20–34	771	1.3	<1	1	1	1	1	2	2	4
35–49	241	1.2	<1	1	1	1	1	2	2	4
50–64	12	1.1	<1	1	1	1	1	1	2	2
65+	0									
2. MULTIPLE DX										
0–19 Years	288	2.6	8	1	1	2	3	4	5	16
20–34	2,264	2.6	9	1	1	2	3	4	5	15
35–49	808	2.4	6	1	1	2	3	4	5	10
50–64	36	2.5	4	1	1	2	3	5	8	9
65+	0									
TOTAL SINGLE DX	1,133	1.3	<1	1	1	1	1	2	2	4
TOTAL MULTIPLE DX	3,396	2.5	8	1	1	2	3	4	5	14
TOTAL										
0–19 Years	397	2.3	6	1	1	2	3	4	5	15
20–34	3,035	2.2	7	1	1	2	3	4	5	10
35–49	1,049	2.1	5	1	1	2	2	4	5	9
50–64	48	2.1	4	1	1	1	2	5	7	9
65+	0									
GRAND TOTAL	4,529	2.2	6	1	1	2	3	4	5	10

69.09: D&C NEC

Type of Patients	Observed Patients	Avg. Stay	Variance	Percentiles						
				10th	25th	50th	75th	90th	95th	99th
1. SINGLE DX										
0–19 Years	12	1.3	<1	1	1	1	1	2	3	3
20–34	60	1.5	<1	1	1	1	2	3	3	4
35–49	27	1.3	<1	1	1	1	1	2	2	3
50–64	7	1.0	0	1	1	1	1	1	1	1
65+	2	1.0	0	1	1	1	1	1	1	1
2. MULTIPLE DX										
0–19 Years	39	2.0	2	1	1	2	2	4	6	6
20–34	340	2.1	3	1	1	2	3	4	5	8
35–49	629	2.4	10	1	1	2	3	7	7	12
50–64	347	3.1	15	2	2	2	3	7	11	29
65+	194	4.6	15	1	2	4	7	9	13	19
TOTAL SINGLE DX	108	1.4	<1	1	1	1	2	3	3	3
TOTAL MULTIPLE DX	1,549	2.7	11	1	1	2	3	6	8	16
TOTAL										
0–19 Years	51	1.8	1	1	1	1	2	3	4	6
20–34	400	2.0	3	1	1	1	3	4	4	7
35–49	656	2.3	9	1	1	1	3	4	7	12
50–64	354	3.0	15	1	2	2	3	7	11	29
65+	196	4.6	15	1	2	4	7	9	13	19
GRAND TOTAL	1,657	2.6	10	1	1	2	3	5	8	16

LOS by Diagnosis and Operation, Western Region, 45th Edition

Western Region, October 2007–September 2008 Data, by Operation

69.1: EXC/DESTR UTER/SUPP LES

Type of Patients	Observed Patients	Avg. Stay	Vari-ance	Percentiles						
				10th	25th	50th	75th	90th	95th	99th
1. SINGLE DX										
0–19 Years	10	2.2	1	1	1	2	3	3	4	4
20–34	16	2.5	<1	1	2	3	3	3	4	4
35–49	8	2.3	<1	1	2	2	3	3	3	3
50–64	2	2.0	2	1	1	3	3	3	3	3
65+	0									
2. MULTIPLE DX										
0–19 Years	38	2.8	5	1	2	2	3	5	7	13
20–34	105	2.4	3	1	1	2	3	4	5	9
35–49	75	2.3	4	1	1	2	3	4	5	14
50–64	28	3.3	10	1	1	2	4	7	9	16
65+	9	6.3	30	3	3	4	5	19	19	19
TOTAL SINGLE DX	36	2.4	<1	1	2	2	3	3	4	4
TOTAL MULTIPLE DX	255	2.7	6	1	1	2	3	5	7	14
TOTAL										
0–19 Years	48	2.7	4	1	2	2	3	5	5	13
20–34	121	2.4	3	1	1	2	3	4	5	9
35–49	83	2.3	3	1	1	2	3	4	5	14
50–64	30	3.2	9	1	1	2	4	7	9	16
65+	9	6.3	30	3	3	4	5	19	19	19
GRAND TOTAL	291	2.6	5	1	1	2	3	4	6	13

69.19: EXC UTER/SUPP STRUCT NEC

Type of Patients	Observed Patients	Avg. Stay	Vari-ance	Percentiles						
				10th	25th	50th	75th	90th	95th	99th
1. SINGLE DX										
0–19 Years	10	2.2	1	1	1	2	3	3	4	4
20–34	16	2.5	<1	1	2	3	3	3	4	4
35–49	8	2.3	<1	1	2	2	3	3	3	3
50–64	2	2.0	2	1	1	3	3	3	3	3
65+	0									
2. MULTIPLE DX										
0–19 Years	38	2.8	5	1	2	2	3	5	7	13
20–34	105	2.4	3	1	1	2	3	4	5	9
35–49	75	2.3	4	1	1	2	3	4	5	14
50–64	28	3.3	10	1	1	2	4	7	9	16
65+	9	6.3	30	3	3	4	5	19	19	19
TOTAL SINGLE DX	36	2.4	<1	1	2	2	3	3	4	4
TOTAL MULTIPLE DX	255	2.7	6	1	1	2	3	5	7	14
TOTAL										
0–19 Years	48	2.7	4	1	2	2	3	5	5	13
20–34	121	2.4	3	1	1	2	3	4	5	9
35–49	83	2.3	3	1	1	2	3	4	5	14
50–64	30	3.2	9	1	1	2	4	7	9	16
65+	9	6.3	30	3	3	4	5	19	19	19
GRAND TOTAL	291	2.6	5	1	1	2	3	4	6	13

69.2: UTERINE SUPP STRUCT REP

Type of Patients	Observed Patients	Avg. Stay	Vari-ance	Percentiles						
				10th	25th	50th	75th	90th	95th	99th
1. SINGLE DX										
0–19 Years	0									
20–34	0									
35–49	1	1.0	0	1	1	1	1	1	1	1
50–64	2	1.5	<1	1	1	2	2	2	2	2
65+	0									
2. MULTIPLE DX										
0–19 Years	2	1.5	<1	1	1	2	2	2	2	2
20–34	4	1.5	<1	1	1	1	2	2	2	2
35–49	8	2.1	2	1	1	2	2	5	5	5
50–64	16	1.4	<1	1	1	1	2	2	3	3
65+	11	2.1	2	1	1	2	3	3	5	5
TOTAL SINGLE DX	3	1.3	<1	1	1	1	2	2	2	2
TOTAL MULTIPLE DX	41	1.8	1	1	1	1	2	3	4	5
TOTAL										
0–19 Years	2	1.5	<1	1	1	2	2	2	2	2
20–34	4	1.5	<1	1	1	1	2	2	2	2
35–49	9	2.0	2	1	1	1	2	5	5	5
50–64	18	1.4	<1	1	1	1	2	2	3	3
65+	11	2.1	2	1	1	2	3	3	5	5
GRAND TOTAL	44	1.7	1	1	1	1	2	3	4	5

69.3: PARACERV UTERINE DENERV

Type of Patients	Observed Patients	Avg. Stay	Vari-ance	Percentiles						
				10th	25th	50th	75th	90th	95th	99th
1. SINGLE DX										
0–19 Years	0									
20–34	0									
35–49	0									
50–64	0									
65+	0									
2. MULTIPLE DX										
0–19 Years	0									
20–34	0									
35–49	1	5.0	0	5	5	5	5	5	5	5
50–64	0									
65+	0									
TOTAL SINGLE DX	0									
TOTAL MULTIPLE DX	1	5.0	0	5	5	5	5	5	5	5
TOTAL										
0–19 Years	0									
20–34	0									
35–49	1	5.0	0	5	5	5	5	5	5	5
50–64	0									
65+	0									
GRAND TOTAL	1	5.0	0	5	5	5	5	5	5	5

LOS by Diagnosis and Operation, Western Region, 45th Edition

Western Region, October 2007–September 2008 Data, by Operation

69.4: UTERINE REPAIR

Type of Patients	Observed Patients	Avg. Stay	Vari-ance	Percentiles						
				10th	25th	50th	75th	90th	95th	99th
1. SINGLE DX										
0–19 Years	0									
20–34	4	3.0	2	2	2	2	3	5	5	5
35–49	0									
50–64	0									
65+	0									
2. MULTIPLE DX										
0–19 Years	1	5.0	0	5	5	5	5	5	5	5
20–34	27	5.1	100	1	2	3	4	6	11	54
35–49	11	2.9	1	1	2	2	4	4	4	4
50–64	3	3.7	14	1	1	2	8	8	8	8
65+	1	11.0	0	11	11	11	11	11	11	11
TOTAL SINGLE DX	4	3.0	2	2	2	2	3	5	5	5
TOTAL MULTIPLE DX	43	4.6	65	1	2	3	4	6	11	54
TOTAL										
0–19 Years	1	5.0	0	5	5	5	5	5	5	5
20–34	31	4.8	87	2	2	3	4	6	11	54
35–49	11	2.9	1	1	2	2	4	4	4	4
50–64	3	3.7	14	1	1	2	8	8	8	8
65+	1	11.0	0	11	11	11	11	11	11	11
GRAND TOTAL	47	4.4	60	1	2	3	4	6	11	54

69.51: ASP CURETTAGE-PREG TERM

Type of Patients	Observed Patients	Avg. Stay	Vari-ance	Percentiles						
				10th	25th	50th	75th	90th	95th	99th
1. SINGLE DX										
0–19 Years	3	2.0	<1	1	1	2	3	3	3	3
20–34	19	1.2	<1	1	1	1	1	2	2	2
35–49	7	1.0	0	1	1	1	1	1	1	1
50–64	0									
65+	0									
2. MULTIPLE DX										
0–19 Years	13	2.5	4	1	1	2	3	3	8	8
20–34	104	3.7	17	1	1	2	4	7	9	19
35–49	41	2.5	5	1	1	2	3	6	7	9
50–64	9	1.7	1	1	1	1	2	4	4	4
65+	0									
TOTAL SINGLE DX	29	1.2	<1	1	1	1	1	2	2	3
TOTAL MULTIPLE DX	167	3.2	13	1	1	2	4	7	9	19
TOTAL										
0–19 Years	16	2.4	3	1	1	2	3	3	8	8
20–34	123	3.3	15	1	1	2	4	7	9	19
35–49	48	2.3	4	1	1	2	3	6	7	9
50–64	9	1.7	1	1	1	1	2	4	4	4
65+	0									
GRAND TOTAL	196	2.9	11	1	1	2	3	7	9	19

69.5: ASP CURETTAGE UTERUS

Type of Patients	Observed Patients	Avg. Stay	Vari-ance	Percentiles						
				10th	25th	50th	75th	90th	95th	99th
1. SINGLE DX										
0–19 Years	147	1.3	<1	1	1	1	1	2	3	4
20–34	851	1.2	<1	1	1	1	1	2	2	3
35–49	275	1.2	<1	1	1	1	1	2	2	4
50–64	18	1.4	<1	1	1	1	1	3	4	4
2. MULTIPLE DX										
0–19 Years	183	2.3	7	1	1	2	3	4	5	9
20–34	1,449	2.2	9	1	1	1	2	4	5	14
35–49	626	2.0	4	1	1	1	2	4	5	10
50–64	59	2.2	6	1	1	1	3	4	7	15
65+	17	4.6	13	2	2	3	6	10	13	13
TOTAL SINGLE DX	1,291	1.2	<1	1	1	1	1	2	2	4
TOTAL MULTIPLE DX	2,334	2.2	7	1	1	1	2	4	5	12
TOTAL										
0–19 Years	330	1.8	5	1	1	1	2	3	5	8
20–34	2,300	1.8	6	1	1	1	2	3	4	9
35–49	901	1.7	3	1	1	1	2	3	4	8
50–64	77	2.0	5	1	1	1	3	4	5	15
65+	17	4.6	13	1	2	3	6	10	13	13
GRAND TOTAL	3,625	1.8	5	1	1	1	2	3	4	9

69.52: ASP CURETTE POST DEL/AB

Type of Patients	Observed Patients	Avg. Stay	Vari-ance	Percentiles						
				10th	25th	50th	75th	90th	95th	99th
1. SINGLE DX										
0–19 Years	120	1.3	<1	1	1	1	2	2	3	4
20–34	747	1.2	<1	1	1	1	1	2	2	3
35–49	243	1.2	<1	1	1	1	1	2	2	3
50–64	15	1.4	<1	1	1	1	1	3	4	4
2. MULTIPLE DX										
0–19 Years	140	2.3	9	1	1	2	3	5	5	9
20–34	1,208	2.0	8	1	1	1	2	3	4	10
35–49	467	1.9	4	1	1	1	2	3	5	11
50–64	22	1.7	<1	1	1	1	3	3	3	3
65+	0									
TOTAL SINGLE DX	1,125	1.2	<1	1	1	1	1	2	2	4
TOTAL MULTIPLE DX	1,837	2.0	7	1	1	1	2	3	4	10
TOTAL										
0–19 Years	260	1.8	5	1	1	1	2	3	5	8
20–34	1,955	1.7	5	1	1	1	2	3	4	7
35–49	710	1.7	3	1	1	1	2	3	4	8
50–64	37	1.6	<1	1	1	1	2	3	3	4
65+	0									
GRAND TOTAL	2,962	1.7	5	1	1	1	2	3	4	8

LOS by Diagnosis and Operation, Western Region, 45th Edition

Western Region, October 2007–September 2008 Data, by Operation

69.59: ASP CURETTAGE UTERUS NEC

Type of Patients	Observed Patients	Avg. Stay	Vari-ance	Percentiles						
				10th	25th	50th	75th	90th	95th	99th
1. SINGLE DX										
0–19 Years	24	1.3	<1	1	1	1	1	2	3	3
20–34	85	1.2	<1	1	1	1	1	2	2	2
35–49	25	1.5	2	1	1	1	1	2	2	8
50–64	3	1.0	0	1	1	1	1	1	1	1
65+	0									
2. MULTIPLE DX										
0–19 Years	30	2.2	1	1	1	2	3	4	4	6
20–34	137	2.2	8	1	1	1	3	4	5	20
35–49	118	1.9	3	1	1	1	2	3	5	8
50–64	28	2.8	11	1	1	1	3	7	11	15
65+	17	4.6	13	1	2	3	6	10	13	13
TOTAL SINGLE DX	137	1.3	<1	1	1	1	1	2	2	3
TOTAL MULTIPLE DX	330	2.3	6	1	1	1	3	4	6	13
TOTAL										
0–19 Years	54	1.8	1	1	1	1	2	3	4	6
20–34	222	1.8	5	1	1	1	2	3	4	8
35–49	143	1.8	3	1	1	1	2	3	5	8
50–64	31	2.6	10	1	1	1	3	5	11	15
65+	17	4.6	13	1	2	3	6	10	13	13
GRAND TOTAL	467	2.0	5	1	1	1	2	3	5	12

69.6: MENSTRUAL EXTRACTION

Type of Patients	Observed Patients	Avg. Stay	Vari-ance	Percentiles						
				10th	25th	50th	75th	90th	95th	99th
1. SINGLE DX										
0–19 Years	0									
20–34	0									
35–49	0									
50–64	0									
65+	0									
2. MULTIPLE DX										
0–19 Years	0									
20–34	0									
35–49	1	1.0	0	1	1	1	1	1	1	1
50–64	0									
65+	0									
TOTAL SINGLE DX	0									
TOTAL MULTIPLE DX	1	1.0	0	1	1	1	1	1	1	1
TOTAL										
0–19 Years	0									
20–34	0									
35–49	1	1.0	0	1	1	1	1	1	1	1
50–64	0									
65+	0									
GRAND TOTAL	1	1.0	0	1	1	1	1	1	1	1

69.7: INSERTION OF IUD

Type of Patients	Observed Patients	Avg. Stay	Vari-ance	Percentiles						
				10th	25th	50th	75th	90th	95th	99th
1. SINGLE DX										
0–19 Years	0									
20–34	0									
35–49	0									
50–64	0									
65+	0									
2. MULTIPLE DX										
0–19 Years	1	4.0	0	4	4	4	4	4	4	4
20–34	2	6.0	18	3	3	9	9	9	9	9
35–49	4	15.9	429	1	4	12	46	46	46	46
50–64	0									
65+	0									
TOTAL SINGLE DX	0									
TOTAL MULTIPLE DX	7	11.3	249	1	3	4	12	46	46	46
TOTAL										
0–19 Years	1	4.0	0	4	4	4	4	4	4	4
20–34	2	6.0	18	3	3	9	9	9	9	9
35–49	4	15.9	429	1	4	12	46	46	46	46
50–64	0									
65+	0									
GRAND TOTAL	7	11.3	249	1	3	4	12	46	46	46

69.9: OTHER OPS UTERUS/ADNEXA

Type of Patients	Observed Patients	Avg. Stay	Vari-ance	Percentiles						
				10th	25th	50th	75th	90th	95th	99th
1. SINGLE DX										
0–19 Years	2	1.0	0	1	1	1	1	1	1	1
20–34	37	1.3	<1	1	1	1	1	2	3	3
35–49	5	1.0	0	1	1	1	1	1	1	1
50–64	0									
65+	0									
2. MULTIPLE DX										
0–19 Years	6	9.4	284	1	2	2	5	44	44	44
20–34	126	3.9	54	1	1	2	3	9	13	38
35–49	46	3.1	12	1	1	2	3	9	12	16
50–64	6	4.0	21	1	1	3	4	13	13	13
65+	1	1.0	0	1	1	1	1	1	1	1
TOTAL SINGLE DX	44	1.3	<1	1	1	1	1	2	3	3
TOTAL MULTIPLE DX	185	3.8	49	1	1	2	3	9	13	44
TOTAL										
0–19 Years	8	7.3	217	1	1	2	3	44	44	44
20–34	163	3.3	43	1	1	1	2	6	12	38
35–49	51	2.9	11	1	1	1	3	6	12	16
50–64	6	4.0	21	1	1	3	4	13	13	13
65+	1	1.0	0	1	1	1	1	1	1	1
GRAND TOTAL	229	3.3	40	1	1	1	3	6	12	38

Western Region, October 2007–September 2008 Data, by Operation

69.96: RMVL CERVICAL CERCLAGE

Type of Patients	Observed Patients	Avg. Stay	Variance	Percentiles						
				10th	25th	50th	75th	90th	95th	99th
1. SINGLE DX										
0–19 Years	0									
20–34	27	1.3	<1	1	1	1	1	3	3	3
35–49	1	1.0	0	1	1	1	1	1	1	1
50–64	0									
65+	0									
2. MULTIPLE DX										
0–19 Years	4	12.6	429	2	2	3	3	44	44	44
20–34	74	5.2	86	1	1	2	4	13	27	57
35–49	26	2.9	10	1	1	1	3	9	11	12
50–64	1	1.0	0	1	1	1	1	1	1	1
65+	0									
TOTAL SINGLE DX	28	1.3	<1	1	1	1	1	2	3	3
TOTAL MULTIPLE DX	105	4.9	78	1	1	2	3	12	21	44
TOTAL										
0–19 Years	4	12.6	429	2	2	3	3	44	44	44
20–34	101	4.1	65	1	1	1	3	10	21	38
35–49	27	2.8	10	1	1	1	3	9	11	12
50–64	1	1.0	0	1	1	1	1	1	1	1
65+	0									
GRAND TOTAL	133	4.1	64	1	1	1	3	10	21	44

70.0: CULDOCENTESIS

Type of Patients	Observed Patients	Avg. Stay	Variance	Percentiles						
				10th	25th	50th	75th	90th	95th	99th
1. SINGLE DX										
0–19 Years	0									
20–34	3	1.0	0	1	1	1	1	1	1	1
35–49	0									
50–64	0									
65+	0									
2. MULTIPLE DX										
0–19 Years	3	4.0	9	1	2	4	7	7	7	7
20–34	9	5.9	20	1	2	7	9	12	12	12
35–49	9	4.8	4	2	3	5	6	9	9	9
50–64	2	3.0	8	1	1	5	5	5	5	5
65+	1	3.0	0	3	3	3	3	3	3	3
TOTAL SINGLE DX	3	1.0	0	1	1	1	1	1	1	1
TOTAL MULTIPLE DX	24	4.9	10	1	2	5	7	9	11	12
TOTAL										
0–19 Years	3	4.0	9	1	1	4	7	7	7	7
20–34	12	4.7	19	1	1	2	8	11	12	12
35–49	9	4.8	4	2	3	5	6	9	9	9
50–64	2	3.0	8	1	1	5	5	5	5	5
65+	1	3.0	0	3	3	3	3	3	3	3
GRAND TOTAL	27	4.5	11	1	1	4	7	9	11	12

70.1: INC VAGINA & CUL-DE-SAC

Type of Patients	Observed Patients	Avg. Stay	Variance	Percentiles						
				10th	25th	50th	75th	90th	95th	99th
1. SINGLE DX										
0–19 Years	3	4.3	33	1	1	1	11	11	11	11
20–34	5	1.8	<1	1	1	2	2	3	3	3
35–49	9	2.0	2	1	1	2	2	5	5	5
50–64	2	2.5	<1	2	2	3	3	3	3	3
65+	3	1.7	1	1	1	1	3	3	3	3
2. MULTIPLE DX										
0–19 Years	26	4.2	26	1	1	2	5	8	15	26
20–34	76	3.4	8	1	1	2	4	8	10	15
35–49	105	4.7	11	1	3	4	6	8	11	18
50–64	56	3.6	18	1	1	2	4	7	15	25
65+	41	4.6	32	1	1	2	6	10	13	26
TOTAL SINGLE DX	22	2.3	5	1	1	2	2	3	5	11
TOTAL MULTIPLE DX	304	4.1	16	1	1	3	5	9	11	23
TOTAL										
0–19 Years	29	4.2	26	1	1	2	5	8	15	26
20–34	81	3.3	8	1	1	2	4	8	9	15
35–49	114	4.5	11	1	2	4	6	8	11	18
50–64	58	3.6	17	1	1	2	4	7	15	25
65+	44	4.4	30	1	1	2	5	10	13	26
GRAND TOTAL	326	4.0	16	1	1	3	5	8	11	23

70.12: CULDOTOMY

Type of Patients	Observed Patients	Avg. Stay	Variance	Percentiles						
				10th	25th	50th	75th	90th	95th	99th
1. SINGLE DX										
0–19 Years	1	11.0	0	11	11	11	11	11	11	11
20–34	2	2.0	0	2	2	2	2	2	2	2
35–49	2	3.5	4	2	2	5	5	5	5	5
50–64	0									
65+	0									
2. MULTIPLE DX										
0–19 Years	3	8.7	49	2	2	4	15	15	15	15
20–34	34	5.1	12	1	3	5	8	10	10	15
35–49	46	5.8	15	3	4	4	8	11	14	19
50–64	16	5.3	29	1	3	4	5	5	25	25
65+	10	10.3	71	1	3	9	13	26	26	26
TOTAL SINGLE DX	5	4.4	15	2	2	2	5	11	11	11
TOTAL MULTIPLE DX	109	6.0	23	2	3	5	8	11	15	25
TOTAL										
0–19 Years	4	9.2	38	2	4	11	15	15	15	15
20–34	36	4.9	11	2	3	4	7	10	10	15
35–49	48	5.7	14	3	4	4	7	11	14	19
50–64	16	5.3	29	2	4	4	5	5	25	25
65+	10	10.3	71	1	3	9	13	26	26	26
GRAND TOTAL	114	6.0	22	2	3	5	8	11	15	25

LOS by Diagnosis and Operation, Western Region, 45th Edition

Western Region, October 2007–September 2008 Data, by Operation

70.14: VAGINOTOMY NEC

Type of Patients	Observed Patients	Avg. Stay	Vari-ance	10th	25th	50th	75th	90th	95th	99th
1. SINGLE DX										
0–19 Years	0									
20–34	2	2.0	2	1	1	3	3	3	3	3
35–49	7	1.6	<1	1	1	2	2	2	2	2
50–64	2	2.5	<1	2	2	3	3	3	3	3
65+	3	1.7	1	1	1	1	3	3	3	3
2. MULTIPLE DX										
0–19 Years	12	5.7	32	1	2	5	8	8	26	26
20–34	37	2.0	1	1	1	2	2	3	4	7
35–49	58	3.8	7	1	2	3	5	8	10	13
50–64	32	3.3	15	1	1	2	3	9	15	15
65+	29	2.4	5	1	1	1	3	6	7	10
TOTAL SINGLE DX	14	1.8	<1	1	1	2	2	3	3	3
TOTAL MULTIPLE DX	168	3.3	10	1	1	2	4	7	9	15
TOTAL										
0–19 Years	12	5.7	32	1	2	5	8	8	26	26
20–34	39	2.0	1	1	1	2	2	3	4	7
35–49	65	3.5	6	1	2	3	4	6	9	13
50–64	34	3.3	14	1	2	2	3	9	15	15
65+	32	2.3	4	1	1	1	3	5	7	10
GRAND TOTAL	182	3.2	10	1	1	2	4	7	9	15

70.24: VAGINAL BIOPSY

Type of Patients	Observed Patients	Avg. Stay	Vari-ance	10th	25th	50th	75th	90th	95th	99th
1. SINGLE DX										
0–19 Years	2	2.0	0	2	2	2	2	2	2	2
20–34	0									
35–49	0									
50–64	0									
65+	0									
2. MULTIPLE DX										
0–19 Years	0									
20–34	7	4.3	12	2	2	3	6	12	12	12
35–49	12	5.9	48	1	1	3	6	15	24	24
50–64	25	8.5	49	2	4	7	13	14	18	33
65+	40	6.0	36	1	3	5	7	12	13	31
TOTAL SINGLE DX	2	2.0	0	2	2	2	2	2	2	2
TOTAL MULTIPLE DX	84	6.6	40	1	3	5	8	14	18	33
TOTAL										
0–19 Years	2	2.0	0	2	2	2	2	2	2	2
20–34	7	4.3	12	2	2	3	6	12	12	12
35–49	12	5.9	48	1	1	3	6	15	24	24
50–64	25	8.5	49	2	4	7	13	14	18	33
65+	40	6.0	36	1	3	5	7	12	13	31
GRAND TOTAL	86	6.4	39	1	2	4	8	14	18	33

70.2: VAG/CUL-DE-SAC DXTIC PX

Type of Patients	Observed Patients	Avg. Stay	Vari-ance	10th	25th	50th	75th	90th	95th	99th
1. SINGLE DX										
0–19 Years	3	1.7	<1	1	1	1	2	2	2	2
20–34	1	1.0	0	1	1	1	1	1	1	1
35–49	0									
50–64	0									
65+	0									
2. MULTIPLE DX										
0–19 Years	9	3.4	2	2	2	3	5	5	6	7
20–34	15	2.9	8	1	1	2	4	6	12	12
35–49	16	4.8	40	1	2	3	5	15	24	24
50–64	28	7.8	48	1	4	5	11	14	18	33
65+	44	5.8	34	1	3	5	7	12	13	31
TOTAL SINGLE DX	4	1.6	<1	1	1	1	2	2	2	2
TOTAL MULTIPLE DX	112	5.3	31	1	2	3	6	13	14	31
TOTAL										
0–19 Years	12	3.1	2	2	2	3	3	5	6	7
20–34	16	2.8	7	1	1	2	4	6	12	12
35–49	16	4.8	40	1	1	3	4	15	24	24
50–64	28	7.8	48	1	4	5	11	14	18	33
65+	44	5.8	34	1	3	5	7	12	13	31
GRAND TOTAL	116	5.2	30	1	2	3	6	12	14	31

70.3: LOC EXC/DESTR VAG/CUL

Type of Patients	Observed Patients	Avg. Stay	Vari-ance	10th	25th	50th	75th	90th	95th	99th
1. SINGLE DX										
0–19 Years	3	2.0	3	1	1	1	4	4	4	4
20–34	10	1.3	<1	1	1	1	1	3	3	3
35–49	3	1.7	<1	1	1	2	2	2	2	2
50–64	3	1.8	2	1	1	1	4	4	4	4
65+	0									
2. MULTIPLE DX										
0–19 Years	44	2.4	2	1	2	2	3	4	6	7
20–34	247	1.9	1	1	1	2	2	3	3	7
35–49	72	2.0	5	1	1	2	2	3	4	19
50–64	58	2.0	3	1	1	1	2	3	6	10
65+	58	2.0	3	1	1	1	2	5	7	8
TOTAL SINGLE DX	19	1.6	1	1	1	1	2	4	4	4
TOTAL MULTIPLE DX	479	2.0	2	1	1	2	2	3	4	7
TOTAL										
0–19 Years	47	2.3	2	1	1	2	3	4	6	7
20–34	257	1.9	1	1	1	2	2	3	3	7
35–49	75	2.0	5	1	1	2	2	3	4	19
50–64	61	2.0	3	1	1	2	2	4	6	10
65+	58	2.0	3	1	1	2	2	5	7	8
GRAND TOTAL	498	2.0	2	1	1	2	2	3	4	7

LOS by Diagnosis and Operation, Western Region, 45th Edition

Western Region, October 2007–September 2008 Data, by Operation

70.33: EXC/DESTR VAGINAL LESION

Type of Patients	Observed Patients	Avg. Stay	Vari-ance	Percentiles						
				10th	25th	50th	75th	90th	95th	99th
1. SINGLE DX										
0–19 Years	2	2.5	4	1	1	1	4	4	4	4
20–34	6	1.0	0	1	1	1	1	1	1	1
35–49	2	1.5	<1	1	1	2	2	2	2	2
50–64	3	1.8	2	1	1	1	2	4	4	4
65+	0									
2. MULTIPLE DX										
0–19 Years	32	2.4	2	1	2	2	3	4	6	7
20–34	182	1.9	<1	1	1	2	2	3	3	7
35–49	57	1.8	<1	1	1	2	2	3	4	6
50–64	51	2.0	3	1	1	1	2	4	6	10
65+	53	2.0	3	1	1	1	2	4	7	8
TOTAL SINGLE DX	13	1.5	1	1	1	1	1	4	4	4
TOTAL MULTIPLE DX	375	1.9	2	1	1	2	2	3	4	7
TOTAL										
0–19 Years	34	2.4	2	1	2	2	3	4	4	7
20–34	188	1.8	<1	1	1	2	2	3	3	7
35–49	59	1.7	<1	1	1	1	2	3	4	6
50–64	54	2.0	3	1	1	1	2	4	6	10
65+	53	2.0	3	1	1	1	2	4	7	8
GRAND TOTAL	388	1.9	2	1	1	2	2	3	4	7

70.4: VAGINAL OBLITERATION

Type of Patients	Observed Patients	Avg. Stay	Vari-ance	Percentiles						
				10th	25th	50th	75th	90th	95th	99th
1. SINGLE DX										
0–19 Years	0									
20–34	0									
35–49	0									
50–64	2	5.5	4	4	4	7	7	7	7	7
65+	0									
2. MULTIPLE DX										
0–19 Years	0									
20–34	0									
35–49	3	2.3	<1	2	2	2	3	3	3	3
50–64	14	2.7	3	1	1	3	4	5	6	6
65+	41	3.6	15	1	1	2	4	7	14	16
TOTAL SINGLE DX	2	5.5	4	4	4	7	7	7	7	7
TOTAL MULTIPLE DX	58	3.3	12	1	1	2	4	6	14	16
TOTAL										
0–19 Years	0									
20–34	0									
35–49	3	2.3	<1	2	2	2	3	3	3	3
50–64	16	3.0	4	1	1	3	4	6	7	7
65+	41	3.6	15	1	1	2	4	7	14	16
GRAND TOTAL	60	3.4	11	1	1	2	4	6	12	16

70.5: CYSTOCELE/RECTOCELE REP

Type of Patients	Observed Patients	Avg. Stay	Vari-ance	Percentiles						
				10th	25th	50th	75th	90th	95th	99th
1. SINGLE DX										
0–19 Years	1	4.0	0	4	4	4	4	4	4	4
20–34	8	1.1	<1	1	1	1	1	1	2	2
35–49	47	1.2	<1	1	1	1	1	2	2	3
50–64	144	1.3	<1	1	1	1	1	2	3	3
65+	94	1.4	<1	1	1	1	2	2	2	3
2. MULTIPLE DX										
0–19 Years	0									
20–34	135	1.5	<1	1	1	1	2	2	3	4
35–49	960	1.5	<1	1	1	1	2	2	3	4
50–64	2,290	1.5	<1	1	1	1	2	3	3	4
65+	2,683	1.7	3	1	1	1	2	3	3	7
TOTAL SINGLE DX	294	1.3	<1	1	1	1	2	2	2	3
TOTAL MULTIPLE DX	6,068	1.6	2	1	1	1	2	2	3	5
TOTAL										
0–19 Years	1	4.0	0	4	4	4	4	4	4	4
20–34	143	1.5	<1	1	1	1	2	2	3	4
35–49	1,007	1.5	<1	1	1	1	2	2	3	4
50–64	2,434	1.5	<1	1	1	1	2	3	3	4
65+	2,777	1.7	3	1	1	1	2	3	3	7
GRAND TOTAL	6,362	1.6	2	1	1	1	2	2	3	5

70.50: REP CYSTOCELE/RECTOCELE

Type of Patients	Observed Patients	Avg. Stay	Vari-ance	Percentiles						
				10th	25th	50th	75th	90th	95th	99th
1. SINGLE DX										
0–19 Years	0									
20–34	2	1.0	0	1	1	1	1	1	1	1
35–49	11	1.5	<1	1	1	1	2	2	3	3
50–64	27	1.5	<1	1	1	1	2	3	3	4
65+	22	1.6	<1	1	1	1	2	2	2	3
2. MULTIPLE DX										
0–19 Years	0									
20–34	59	1.5	<1	1	1	1	2	2	3	3
35–49	358	1.6	<1	1	1	1	2	2	3	4
50–64	802	1.6	<1	1	1	1	2	2	3	4
65+	873	1.8	3	1	1	2	2	3	3	7
TOTAL SINGLE DX	62	1.5	<1	1	1	1	2	2	3	4
TOTAL MULTIPLE DX	2,092	1.7	2	1	1	1	2	3	3	5
TOTAL										
0–19 Years	0									
20–34	61	1.5	<1	1	1	1	2	2	3	3
35–49	369	1.6	<1	1	1	1	2	2	3	4
50–64	829	1.6	<1	1	1	1	2	3	3	4
65+	895	1.8	3	1	1	2	2	3	3	7
GRAND TOTAL	2,154	1.7	2	1	1	1	2	3	3	5

LOS by Diagnosis and Operation, Western Region, 45th Edition

70.51: CYSTOCELE REPAIR

Type of Patients	Observed Patients	Avg. Stay	Variance	Percentiles						
				10th	25th	50th	75th	90th	95th	99th
1. SINGLE DX										
0–19 Years	1	4.0	0	4	4	4	4	4	4	4
20–34	3	1.3	<1	1	1	1	2	2	2	2
35–49	11	1.2	<1	1	1	1	1	2	2	2
50–64	32	1.2	<1	1	1	1	1	2	2	2
65+	26	1.4	<1	1	1	1	2	2	2	3
2. MULTIPLE DX										
0–19 Years	0									
20–34	27	1.3	<1	1	1	1	2	2	2	2
35–49	213	1.3	<1	1	1	1	1	2	2	4
50–64	516	1.3	1	1	1	1	2	2	2	3
65+	683	1.5	1	1	1	1	2	2	3	6
TOTAL SINGLE DX	73	1.3	<1	1	1	1	1	2	2	4
TOTAL MULTIPLE DX	1,439	1.4	<1	1	1	1	2	2	3	5
TOTAL										
0–19 Years	1	4.0	0	4	4	4	4	4	4	4
20–34	30	1.3	<1	1	1	1	2	2	2	2
35–49	224	1.3	<1	1	1	1	1	2	2	4
50–64	548	1.3	<1	1	1	1	2	2	2	3
65+	709	1.5	1	1	1	1	2	2	3	5
GRAND TOTAL	1,512	1.4	<1	1	1	1	2	2	3	4

70.53: CYST&RECT REP-GFT/PROSTH

Type of Patients	Observed Patients	Avg. Stay	Variance	Percentiles						
				10th	25th	50th	75th	90th	95th	99th
1. SINGLE DX										
0–19 Years	0									
20–34	1	1.0	0	1	1	1	1	1	1	1
35–49	3	1.3	<1	1	1	1	2	2	2	2
50–64	6	1.3	<1	1	1	1	2	2	2	2
65+	13	1.6	<1	1	1	1	2	3	3	3
2. MULTIPLE DX										
0–19 Years	0									
20–34	14	1.6	<1	1	1	1	2	2	4	4
35–49	92	1.8	<1	1	1	2	2	3	3	6
50–64	259	1.6	<1	1	1	1	2	3	3	4
65+	355	2.1	5	1	1	2	2	3	4	10
TOTAL SINGLE DX	23	1.5	<1	1	1	1	2	2	3	3
TOTAL MULTIPLE DX	720	1.9	3	1	1	2	2	3	3	6
TOTAL										
0–19 Years	0									
20–34	15	1.6	<1	1	1	1	2	2	4	4
35–49	95	1.8	<1	1	1	2	2	3	3	6
50–64	265	1.6	<1	1	1	1	2	3	3	4
65+	368	2.1	5	1	1	2	2	3	4	10
GRAND TOTAL	743	1.9	3	1	1	2	2	3	3	6

70.52: RECTOCELE REPAIR

Type of Patients	Observed Patients	Avg. Stay	Variance	Percentiles						
				10th	25th	50th	75th	90th	95th	99th
1. SINGLE DX										
0–19 Years	0									
20–34	2	1.0	0	1	1	1	1	1	1	1
35–49	18	1.2	<1	1	1	1	1	2	2	2
50–64	48	1.3	<1	1	1	1	1	2	2	2
65+	15	1.2	<1	1	1	1	2	2	2	2
2. MULTIPLE DX										
0–19 Years	0									
20–34	23	1.6	<1	1	1	1	2	2	2	2
35–49	185	1.5	<1	1	1	1	2	3	3	4
50–64	385	1.5	1	1	1	1	2	2	3	3
65+	344	1.6	2	1	1	1	2	2	3	6
TOTAL SINGLE DX	83	1.2	<1	1	1	1	1	2	2	3
TOTAL MULTIPLE DX	937	1.5	1	1	1	1	2	2	3	5
TOTAL										
0–19 Years	0									
20–34	25	1.6	<1	1	1	1	2	3	3	4
35–49	203	1.5	<1	1	1	1	2	2	3	4
50–64	433	1.4	<1	1	1	1	2	2	3	7
65+	359	1.6	2	1	1	1	2	2	3	6
GRAND TOTAL	1,020	1.5	1	1	1	1	2	2	3	5

70.54: CYSTOCELE REP-GFT/PROSTH

Type of Patients	Observed Patients	Avg. Stay	Variance	Percentiles						
				10th	25th	50th	75th	90th	95th	99th
1. SINGLE DX										
0–19 Years	0									
20–34	0									
35–49	2	1.0	0	1	1	1	1	1	1	1
50–64	23	1.3	<1	1	1	1	2	2	2	2
65+	15	1.1	<1	1	1	1	1	2	2	2
2. MULTIPLE DX										
0–19 Years	0									
20–34	9	1.8	<1	1	1	1	2	3	3	3
35–49	76	1.5	<1	1	1	1	2	3	3	4
50–64	224	1.4	1	1	1	1	2	2	3	5
65+	321	1.7	3	1	1	1	2	3	3	10
TOTAL SINGLE DX	40	1.2	<1	1	1	1	1	2	2	2
TOTAL MULTIPLE DX	630	1.6	2	1	1	1	2	2	3	8
TOTAL										
0–19 Years	0									
20–34	9	1.8	<1	1	1	1	2	3	3	3
35–49	78	1.5	<1	1	1	1	2	2	3	4
50–64	247	1.4	1	1	1	1	2	2	3	5
65+	336	1.7	3	1	1	1	2	3	3	10
GRAND TOTAL	670	1.5	2	1	1	1	2	2	3	8

LOS by Diagnosis and Operation, Western Region, 45th Edition

Western Region, October 2007–September 2008 Data, by Operation

70.55: RECTOCELE REP-GFT/PROSTH

Type of Patients	Observed Patients	Avg. Stay	Variance	10th	25th	50th	75th	90th	95th	99th
1. SINGLE DX										
0–19 Years	0									
20–34	0									
35–49	2	1.0	0	1	1	1	1	1	1	1
50–64	8	1.3	<1	1	1	1	2	2	2	2
65+	3	1.3	<1	1	1	1	2	2	2	2
2. MULTIPLE DX										
0–19 Years	0									
20–34	3	1.0	0	1	1	1	1	1	1	1
35–49	36	1.6	1	1	1	1	2	2	4	7
50–64	104	1.4	<1	1	1	1	2	2	3	4
65+	107	1.7	1	1	1	1	2	2	3	5
TOTAL SINGLE DX	13	1.2	<1	1	1	1	1	2	2	2
TOTAL MULTIPLE DX	250	1.6	1	1	1	1	2	2	3	5
TOTAL										
0–19 Years	0									
20–34	3	1.0	0	1	1	1	1	1	1	1
35–49	38	1.5	<1	1	1	1	2	2	3	7
50–64	112	1.4	<1	1	1	1	2	2	3	4
65+	110	1.7	1	1	1	1	2	2	3	5
GRAND TOTAL	263	1.5	1	1	1	1	2	2	3	5

70.6: VAGINAL CONSTR/RECONST

Type of Patients	Observed Patients	Avg. Stay	Variance	10th	25th	50th	75th	90th	95th	99th
1. SINGLE DX										
0–19 Years	0									
20–34	0									
35–49	0									
50–64	0									
65+	0									
2. MULTIPLE DX										
0–19 Years	10	4.4	11	1	2	2	8	8	11	11
20–34	3	5.7	1	5	5	5	7	7	7	7
35–49	3	1.7	1	1	1	1	2	3	3	3
50–64	13	4.2	59	1	1	2	2	8	29	29
65+	6	1.3	<1	1	1	1	2	2	2	2
TOTAL SINGLE DX	0									
TOTAL MULTIPLE DX	35	3.8	23	1	1	2	5	8	8	29
TOTAL										
0–19 Years	10	4.4	11	1	2	2	8	8	11	11
20–34	3	5.7	1	5	5	5	7	7	7	7
35–49	3	1.7	1	1	1	1	2	3	3	3
50–64	13	4.2	59	1	1	2	2	8	29	29
65+	6	1.3	<1	1	1	1	2	2	2	2
GRAND TOTAL	35	3.8	23	1	1	2	5	8	8	29

70.7: OTHER VAGINAL REPAIR

Type of Patients	Observed Patients	Avg. Stay	Variance	10th	25th	50th	75th	90th	95th	99th
1. SINGLE DX										
0–19 Years	14	1.8	<1	1	1	1	3	3	3	3
20–34	23	2.0	1	1	1	2	2	4	4	4
35–49	26	1.6	<1	1	1	1	2	3	3	5
50–64	39	1.6	<1	1	1	1	2	3	3	4
65+	19	1.6	<1	1	1	1	2	3	4	4
2. MULTIPLE DX										
0–19 Years	71	3.2	11	1	1	2	3	9	9	17
20–34	122	2.2	4	1	1	2	3	4	5	8
35–49	297	2.8	10	1	1	2	3	5	7	16
50–64	670	2.4	7	1	1	2	3	4	5	17
65+	805	2.7	8	1	1	2	3	5	8	16
TOTAL SINGLE DX	121	1.7	<1	1	1	1	2	3	3	4
TOTAL MULTIPLE DX	1,965	2.6	8	1	1	2	3	5	7	17
TOTAL										
0–19 Years	85	3.0	10	1	1	2	3	7	9	17
20–34	145	2.1	4	1	1	2	3	4	5	8
35–49	323	2.7	10	1	1	2	3	5	7	16
50–64	709	2.4	7	1	1	2	3	4	5	16
65+	824	2.7	8	1	1	2	3	5	8	16
GRAND TOTAL	2,086	2.6	8	1	1	2	3	5	7	17

70.71: SUTURE VAGINA LACERATION

Type of Patients	Observed Patients	Avg. Stay	Variance	10th	25th	50th	75th	90th	95th	99th
1. SINGLE DX										
0–19 Years	6	1.0	0	1	1	1	1	1	1	1
20–34	7	1.1	<1	1	1	1	1	2	2	2
35–49	8	1.2	<1	1	1	1	1	2	2	2
50–64	3	1.0	0	1	1	1	1	1	1	1
65+	1	2.0	0	2	2	2	2	2	2	2
2. MULTIPLE DX										
0–19 Years	27	1.5	1	1	1	1	1	3	3	7
20–34	37	2.4	10	1	1	1	3	4	8	19
35–49	38	1.8	1	1	1	1	2	3	5	5
50–64	26	1.7	1	1	1	1	2	3	3	6
65+	18	2.1	2	2	2	2	2	5	7	7
TOTAL SINGLE DX	25	1.1	<1	1	1	1	1	2	2	2
TOTAL MULTIPLE DX	146	1.9	3	1	1	1	2	3	4	8
TOTAL										
0–19 Years	33	1.4	1	1	1	1	1	3	3	7
20–34	44	2.2	9	1	1	1	3	4	4	19
35–49	46	1.7	1	1	1	1	2	3	4	5
50–64	29	1.6	1	1	1	1	2	3	3	6
65+	19	2.1	2	2	2	2	2	5	7	7
GRAND TOTAL	171	1.8	3	1	1	1	2	3	4	8

LOS by Diagnosis and Operation, Western Region, 45th Edition

Western Region, October 2007–September 2008 Data, by Operation

70.73: REP RECTOVAGINAL FISTULA

Type of Patients	Observed Patients	Avg. Stay	Variance	Percentiles						
				10th	25th	50th	75th	90th	95th	99th
1. SINGLE DX										
0–19 Years	2	3.0	0	3	3	3	3	3	3	3
20–34	12	2.2	<1	1	1	2	3	3	3	3
35–49	8	2.0	2	1	1	1	3	5	5	5
50–64	9	1.5	<1	1	1	1	2	2	2	2
65+	1	1.0	0	1	1	1	1	1	1	1
2. MULTIPLE DX										
0–19 Years	8	3.7	11	1	2	3	4	7	14	14
20–34	40	2.2	3	1	1	2	3	5	5	6
35–49	48	4.1	31	1	1	2	5	8	10	34
50–64	51	3.8	11	1	1	3	5	7	13	16
65+	28	5.9	20	1	2	6	9	12	14	18
TOTAL SINGLE DX	32	2.1	1	1	1	2	3	3	4	5
TOTAL MULTIPLE DX	175	3.9	17	1	1	3	5	8	11	22
TOTAL										
0–19 Years	10	3.5	7	2	2	3	4	4	7	14
20–34	52	2.2	2	1	1	2	3	4	5	6
35–49	56	3.8	28	1	1	3	5	7	10	34
50–64	60	3.4	10	1	1	3	4	7	13	16
65+	29	5.8	20	1	2	5	8	12	14	18
GRAND TOTAL	207	3.6	14	1	1	3	4	7	10	18

70.77: VAGINAL SUSP & FIXATION

Type of Patients	Observed Patients	Avg. Stay	Variance	Percentiles						
				10th	25th	50th	75th	90th	95th	99th
1. SINGLE DX										
0–19 Years	0									
20–34	0									
35–49	1	2.0	0	2	2	2	2	2	2	2
50–64	4	2.3	2	1	2	2	4	4	4	4
65+	3	1.7	1	1	1	1	3	3	3	3
2. MULTIPLE DX										
0–19 Years	0									
20–34	2	1.5	<1	1	1	1	2	2	2	2
35–49	43	2.0	2	1	1	2	3	3	3	7
50–64	166	2.1	2	1	1	2	3	3	4	6
65+	197	2.0	2	1	1	2	2	4	5	6
TOTAL SINGLE DX	8	2.0	1	1	1	2	3	4	4	4
TOTAL MULTIPLE DX	408	2.0	2	1	1	2	2	3	5	6
TOTAL										
0–19 Years	0									
20–34	2	1.5	<1	1	1	1	2	2	2	2
35–49	44	2.0	1	1	1	2	2	3	3	7
50–64	170	2.1	2	1	1	2	3	3	4	6
65+	200	2.0	2	1	1	2	2	4	5	6
GRAND TOTAL	416	2.0	2	1	1	2	2	3	4	6

70.78: VAG SUSP/FIX-GRFT/PROSTH

Type of Patients	Observed Patients	Avg. Stay	Variance	Percentiles						
				10th	25th	50th	75th	90th	95th	99th
1. SINGLE DX										
0–19 Years	0									
20–34	0									
35–49	1	2.0	0	2	2	2	2	2	2	2
50–64	14	1.9	<1	1	1	2	3	3	3	3
65+	12	1.7	<1	1	1	1	2	3	4	4
2. MULTIPLE DX										
0–19 Years	0									
20–34	3	1.3	<1	1	1	1	2	2	2	2
35–49	52	2.1	1	1	1	2	3	3	4	6
50–64	262	2.0	1	1	1	2	3	3	4	5
65+	356	2.3	3	1	1	2	3	4	5	8
TOTAL SINGLE DX	27	1.8	<1	1	1	2	2	3	3	4
TOTAL MULTIPLE DX	673	2.1	2	1	1	2	3	3	4	7
TOTAL										
0–19 Years	0									
20–34	3	1.3	<1	1	1	1	2	2	2	2
35–49	53	2.1	1	1	1	2	3	3	4	6
50–64	276	2.0	1	1	1	2	3	3	4	5
65+	368	2.3	3	1	1	2	3	4	5	8
GRAND TOTAL	700	2.1	2	1	1	2	3	3	4	7

70.79: VAGINAL REPAIR NEC

Type of Patients	Observed Patients	Avg. Stay	Variance	Percentiles						
				10th	25th	50th	75th	90th	95th	99th
1. SINGLE DX										
0–19 Years	5	1.5	<1	1	1	1	2	2	2	2
20–34	4	3.0	1	2	2	2	4	4	4	4
35–49	7	1.4	<1	1	1	1	2	2	2	2
50–64	8	1.3	<1	1	1	1	1	1	1	2
65+	2	1.0	0	1	1	1	1	1	1	1
2. MULTIPLE DX										
0–19 Years	33	4.1	16	1	2	2	5	9	9	17
20–34	36	2.0	2	1	1	2	3	4	5	7
35–49	96	2.3	4	1	1	2	3	4	5	8
50–64	137	1.9	4	1	1	2	2	3	3	9
65+	145	2.1	8	1	1	1	2	4	4	23
TOTAL SINGLE DX	26	1.6	<1	1	1	1	2	2	4	4
TOTAL MULTIPLE DX	447	2.4	7	1	1	2	3	4	7	17
TOTAL										
0–19 Years	38	3.8	15	1	2	2	4	9	9	17
20–34	40	2.1	2	1	1	2	3	4	5	7
35–49	103	2.2	2	1	1	1	2	3	3	7
50–64	145	1.9	4	1	1	1	2	3	4	9
65+	147	2.1	8	1	1	2	2	3	4	23
GRAND TOTAL	473	2.3	7	1	1	2	2	4	6	17

Western Region, October 2007–September 2008 Data, by Operation

70.8: VAGINAL VAULT OBLIT

Type of Patients	Observed Patients	Avg. Stay	Variance	10th	25th	50th	75th	90th	95th	99th
1. SINGLE DX										
0–19 Years	0									
20–34	0									
35–49	0									
50–64	0									
65+	4	1.0	0	1	1		1	1	1	1
2. MULTIPLE DX										
0–19 Years	0									
20–34	0									
35–49	0									
50–64	6	2.7	6	1	2	2	2	8	8	8
65+	194	2.0	5	1	1	1	2	3	4	13
TOTAL SINGLE DX	4	1.0	0	1	1	1	1	1	1	1
TOTAL MULTIPLE DX	200	2.0	5	1	1	1	2	3	4	9
TOTAL										
0–19 Years	0									
20–34	0									
35–49	0									
50–64	6	2.7	6	1	2	2	2	8	8	8
65+	198	1.9	5	1	1	1	2	3	4	13
GRAND TOTAL	204	2.0	5	1	1	1	2	3	4	9

70.92: CUL-DE-SAC OPERATION NEC

Type of Patients	Observed Patients	Avg. Stay	Variance	10th	25th	50th	75th	90th	95th	99th
1. SINGLE DX										
0–19 Years	0									
20–34	1	1.0	0	1	1	1	1	1	1	1
35–49	1	1.0	0	1	1	1	1	1	1	1
50–64	7	1.0	0	1	1	1	1	1	1	1
65+	6	1.7	<1	1	1	2	2	2	2	2
2. MULTIPLE DX										
0–19 Years	1	3.0	0	3	3	3	3	3	3	3
20–34	10	1.5	<1	1	1	1	2	3	3	3
35–49	112	1.8	1	1	1	2	2	3	3	4
50–64	496	1.7	<1	1	1	2	2	3	3	5
65+	896	1.8	1	1	1	2	2	3	3	6
TOTAL SINGLE DX	15	1.3	<1	1	1	1	1	2	2	2
TOTAL MULTIPLE DX	1,515	1.8	1	1	1	2	2	3	3	5
TOTAL										
0–19 Years	1	3.0	0	3	3	3	3	3	3	3
20–34	11	1.5	<1	1	1	1	2	3	3	3
35–49	113	1.8	1	1	1	2	2	3	3	4
50–64	503	1.7	<1	1	1	2	2	3	3	5
65+	902	1.8	1	1	1	2	2	3	3	6
GRAND TOTAL	1,530	1.8	1	1	1	2	2	3	3	5

70.9: OTH VAG & CUL-DE-SAC OPS

Type of Patients	Observed Patients	Avg. Stay	Variance	10th	25th	50th	75th	90th	95th	99th
1. SINGLE DX										
0–19 Years	0									
20–34	1	1.0	0	1	1	1	1	1	1	1
35–49	2	1.0	0	1	1	1	1	1	1	1
50–64	10	1.1	<1	1	1	1	1	1	2	2
65+	9	1.6	<1	1	1	2	2	2	2	2
2. MULTIPLE DX										
0–19 Years	1	3.0	0	3	3	3	3	3	3	3
20–34	15	1.7	<1	1	1	1	3	3	3	3
35–49	152	1.8	1	1	1	2	2	3	3	4
50–64	631	1.7	2	1	1	2	2	3	3	5
65+	1,147	1.8	1	1	1	2	2	3	3	6
TOTAL SINGLE DX	22	1.3	<1	1	1	1	2	2	2	2
TOTAL MULTIPLE DX	1,946	1.8	1	1	1	2	2	3	3	5
TOTAL										
0–19 Years	1	3.0	0	3	3	3	3	3	3	3
20–34	16	1.7	<1	1	1	1	3	3	3	3
35–49	154	1.8	1	1	1	2	2	3	3	4
50–64	641	1.7	2	1	1	1	2	3	3	5
65+	1,156	1.8	1	1	1	2	2	3	3	6
GRAND TOTAL	1,968	1.8	1	1	1	2	2	3	3	5

70.93: CUL OP NEC-GRAFT/PROSTH

Type of Patients	Observed Patients	Avg. Stay	Variance	10th	25th	50th	75th	90th	95th	99th
1. SINGLE DX										
0–19 Years	0									
20–34	0									
35–49	0									
50–64	2	1.5	<1	1	1	1	2	2	2	2
65+	3	1.3	<1	1	1	1	2	2	2	2
2. MULTIPLE DX										
0–19 Years	0									
20–34	4	2.3	<1	1	2	3	3	3	3	3
35–49	38	1.7	<1	1	1	1	2	3	4	4
50–64	129	1.7	<1	1	1	1	2	3	3	4
65+	248	1.7	1	1	1	1	2	3	3	6
TOTAL SINGLE DX	5	1.4	<1	1	1	1	2	2	2	2
TOTAL MULTIPLE DX	419	1.7	1	1	1	1	2	3	3	6
TOTAL										
0–19 Years	0									
20–34	4	2.3	<1	1	2	3	3	3	4	4
35–49	38	1.7	<1	1	1	1	2	3	3	4
50–64	131	1.6	<1	1	1	1	2	3	3	4
65+	251	1.7	1	1	1	1	2	3	3	6
GRAND TOTAL	424	1.7	1	1	1	1	2	3	3	6

LOS by Diagnosis and Operation, Western Region, 45th Edition

Western Region, October 2007–September 2008 Data, by Operation

71.0: INC VULVA & PERINEUM

Type of Patients	Observed Patients	Avg. Stay	Vari-ance	Percentiles						
				10th	25th	50th	75th	90th	95th	99th
1. SINGLE DX										
0–19 Years	34	2.4	3	1	1	2	3	4	4	14
20–34	10	1.6	1	1	1	1	2	4	4	4
35–49	8	2.3	2	1	1	2	3	4	4	4
50–64	4	1.8	<1	1	1	2	3	3	3	3
65+	0									
2. MULTIPLE DX										
0–19 Years	210	3.3	4	1	2	3	4	6	6	11
20–34	154	3.8	18	1	2	3	4	7	9	25
35–49	150	4.5	17	1	2	4	5	9	11	22
50–64	157	5.9	34	2	3	4	7	12	19	42
65+	111	6.4	59	2	3	5	7	13	16	27
TOTAL SINGLE DX	56	2.3	2	1	1	2	3	4	4	5
TOTAL MULTIPLE DX	782	4.4	21	1	2	3	5	8	11	25
TOTAL										
0–19 Years	244	3.2	4	1	2	3	4	6	6	11
20–34	164	3.7	17	1	2	3	4	7	8	25
35–49	158	4.4	17	1	2	4	5	9	11	22
50–64	161	5.8	34	1	3	4	7	12	16	42
65+	111	6.4	59	2	3	5	7	13	16	27
GRAND TOTAL	838	4.2	19	1	2	3	5	7	11	23

71.1: VULVAR DIAGNOSTIC PX

Type of Patients	Observed Patients	Avg. Stay	Vari-ance	Percentiles						
				10th	25th	50th	75th	90th	95th	99th
1. SINGLE DX										
0–19 Years	0									
20–34	1	1.0	0	1	1	1	1	1	1	1
35–49	1	1.0	0	1	1	1	1	1	1	1
50–64	0									
65+	0									
2. MULTIPLE DX										
0–19 Years	5	5.1	3	2	4	6	6	7	7	7
20–34	15	2.1	<1	1	2	2	2	3	5	5
35–49	14	4.2	18	1	1	2	9	11	13	13
50–64	22	2.6	9	1	1	1	3	7	10	12
65+	34	6.0	29	1	2	5	8	13	18	23
TOTAL SINGLE DX	2	1.0	0	1	1	1	1	1	1	1
TOTAL MULTIPLE DX	90	4.2	18	1	1	2	6	10	13	23
TOTAL										
0–19 Years	5	5.1	3	2	4	6	6	7	7	7
20–34	16	2.1	<1	1	1	2	2	3	5	5
35–49	15	4.0	18	1	1	2	4	11	13	13
50–64	22	2.6	9	1	1	1	3	7	10	12
65+	34	6.0	29	1	2	5	8	13	18	23
GRAND TOTAL	92	4.2	18	1	1	2	6	10	13	23

71.09: INC VULVA/PERINEUM NEC

Type of Patients	Observed Patients	Avg. Stay	Vari-ance	Percentiles						
				10th	25th	50th	75th	90th	95th	99th
1. SINGLE DX										
0–19 Years	34	2.4	3	1	1	2	3	4	4	14
20–34	10	1.6	1	1	1	1	2	4	4	4
35–49	8	2.3	2	1	1	2	3	4	4	4
50–64	4	1.8	<1	1	1	2	3	3	3	3
65+	0									
2. MULTIPLE DX										
0–19 Years	206	3.4	4	1	2	3	4	6	6	11
20–34	151	3.9	18	1	2	3	4	7	9	25
35–49	150	4.5	17	1	2	4	5	9	11	22
50–64	157	5.9	34	2	3	4	7	12	19	42
65+	109	6.5	60	2	3	5	7	13	16	27
TOTAL SINGLE DX	56	2.3	2	1	1	2	3	4	4	5
TOTAL MULTIPLE DX	773	4.4	21	1	2	3	5	8	11	25
TOTAL										
0–19 Years	240	3.2	4	1	2	3	4	6	6	11
20–34	161	3.8	18	1	2	3	4	7	8	25
35–49	158	4.4	17	1	2	3	5	9	11	22
50–64	161	5.8	34	1	3	4	7	12	16	42
65+	109	6.5	60	2	3	5	7	13	16	27
GRAND TOTAL	829	4.2	19	1	2	3	5	7	11	23

71.11: VULVAR BIOPSY

Type of Patients	Observed Patients	Avg. Stay	Vari-ance	Percentiles						
				10th	25th	50th	75th	90th	95th	99th
1. SINGLE DX										
0–19 Years	0									
20–34	1	1.0	0	1	1	1	1	1	1	1
35–49	1	1.0	0	1	1	1	1	1	1	1
50–64	0									
65+	0									
2. MULTIPLE DX										
0–19 Years	4	5.3	3	2	4	6	6	7	7	7
20–34	14	2.1	<1	1	2	2	2	3	5	5
35–49	14	4.2	18	1	1	2	9	11	13	13
50–64	22	2.6	9	1	1	1	3	7	10	12
65+	34	6.0	29	1	2	5	8	13	18	23
TOTAL SINGLE DX	2	1.0	0	1	1	1	1	1	1	1
TOTAL MULTIPLE DX	88	4.2	18	1	1	2	6	10	13	23
TOTAL										
0–19 Years	4	5.3	3	2	4	6	6	7	7	7
20–34	15	2.0	1	1	1	2	2	3	5	5
35–49	15	4.0	18	1	1	2	4	11	13	13
50–64	22	2.6	9	1	1	1	3	7	10	12
65+	34	6.0	29	1	2	5	8	13	18	23
GRAND TOTAL	90	4.2	18	1	1	2	6	10	13	23

LOS by Diagnosis and Operation, Western Region, 45th Edition

Western Region, October 2007–September 2008 Data, by Operation

71.2: BARTHOLIN'S GLAND OPS

Type of Patients	Observed Patients	Avg. Stay	Variance	10th	25th	50th	75th	90th	95th	99th
1. SINGLE DX										
0–19 Years	4	2.1	2	1	1	2	2	5	5	5
20–34	7	1.0	0	1	1	1	1	1	1	1
35–49	8	1.8	1	1	1	1	2	4	4	4
50–64	2	1.0	0	1	1	1	1	1	1	1
65+	0									
2. MULTIPLE DX										
0–19 Years	13	2.8	18	1	1	2	2	4	17	17
20–34	78	2.1	2	1	1	2	3	3	5	8
35–49	42	3.9	39	1	1	2	4	7	9	34
50–64	19	4.1	40	1	1	2	5	9	28	28
65+	7	2.2	2	1	1	2	3	5	5	5
TOTAL SINGLE DX	21	1.6	1	1	1	1	2	3	4	5
TOTAL MULTIPLE DX	159	2.9	18	1	1	2	3	5	8	28
TOTAL										
0–19 Years	17	2.6	12	1	1	2	2	4	5	17
20–34	85	2.0	2	1	1	2	3	3	4	8
35–49	50	3.5	33	1	1	2	3	7	9	34
50–64	21	3.8	37	1	1	1	3	8	9	28
65+	7	2.2	2	1	1	2	3	5	5	5
GRAND TOTAL	180	2.7	16	1	1	2	3	5	7	28

71.22: INC BARTHOLIN'S GLAND

Type of Patients	Observed Patients	Avg. Stay	Variance	10th	25th	50th	75th	90th	95th	99th
1. SINGLE DX										
0–19 Years	2	2.6	2	2	2	2	2	5	5	5
20–34	3	1.0	0	1	1	1	1	1	1	1
35–49	4	2.5	2	1	1	2	3	4	4	4
50–64	0									
65+	0									
2. MULTIPLE DX										
0–19 Years	10	3.1	22	1	1	1	3	4	17	17
20–34	47	2.2	2	1	1	2	3	4	5	8
35–49	18	4.7	32	1	1	3	5	9	25	25
50–64	9	6.3	74	1	1	3	7	28	28	28
65+	2	4.0	2	3	3	4	5	5	5	5
TOTAL SINGLE DX	9	2.2	2	1	1	2	2	4	5	5
TOTAL MULTIPLE DX	86	3.3	19	1	1	2	3	6	8	28
TOTAL										
0–19 Years	12	2.9	15	1	1	2	3	5	17	17
20–34	50	2.2	2	1	1	2	3	3	5	8
35–49	22	4.3	27	1	1	3	5	8	9	25
50–64	9	6.3	74	1	1	3	7	28	28	28
65+	2	4.0	2	3	3	4	5	5	5	5
GRAND TOTAL	95	3.2	17	1	1	2	3	5	8	28

71.3: LOC VULVAR/PERI EXC NEC

Type of Patients	Observed Patients	Avg. Stay	Variance	10th	25th	50th	75th	90th	95th	99th
1. SINGLE DX										
0–19 Years	4	1.5	<1	1	1	1	1	3	3	3
20–34	6	1.8	3	1	1	1	2	5	5	5
35–49	5	1.2	<1	1	1	1	1	2	2	2
50–64	2	1.0	0	1	1	1	1	1	1	1
65+	4	1.0	0	1	1	1	1	1	1	1
2. MULTIPLE DX										
0–19 Years	43	3.9	125	1	1	2	3	4	6	80
20–34	356	2.1	1	1	2	2	2	3	3	6
35–49	118	3.1	25	1	1	2	3	5	8	26
50–64	77	5.6	97	1	1	2	4	18	22	66
65+	69	3.9	15	1	1	2	5	10	13	16
TOTAL SINGLE DX	21	1.4	<1	1	1	1	1	2	3	5
TOTAL MULTIPLE DX	663	3.0	28	1	1	2	3	4	8	22
TOTAL										
0–19 Years	47	3.7	116	1	1	2	3	4	6	80
20–34	362	2.1	1	1	2	2	2	3	3	6
35–49	123	3.0	24	1	1	2	3	5	8	26
50–64	79	5.5	95	1	1	2	4	18	22	66
65+	73	3.7	15	1	1	2	4	9	13	16
GRAND TOTAL	684	2.9	27	1	1	2	3	4	8	22

71.4: OPERATIONS ON CLITORIS

Type of Patients	Observed Patients	Avg. Stay	Variance	10th	25th	50th	75th	90th	95th	99th
1. SINGLE DX										
0–19 Years	1	2.0	0	2	2	2	2	2	2	2
20–34	0									
35–49	0									
50–64	0									
65+	0									
2. MULTIPLE DX										
0–19 Years	6	1.4	<1	1	1	1	1	2	4	4
20–34	6	1.7	<1	1	1	2	2	3	3	3
35–49	2	1.5	<1	1	1	1	2	2	2	2
50–64	0									
65+	0									
TOTAL SINGLE DX	1	2.0	0	2	2	2	2	2	2	2
TOTAL MULTIPLE DX	14	1.5	<1	1	1	1	2	2	3	4
TOTAL										
0–19 Years	7	1.6	<1	1	1	1	2	2	4	4
20–34	6	1.7	<1	1	1	2	2	3	3	3
35–49	2	1.5	<1	1	1	1	2	2	2	2
50–64	0									
65+	0									
GRAND TOTAL	15	1.6	<1	1	1	1	2	2	3	4

311

LOS by Diagnosis and Operation, Western Region, 45th Edition

Western Region, October 2007–September 2008 Data, by Operation

71.5: RADICAL VULVECTOMY

Type of Patients	Observed Patients	Avg. Stay	Variance	10th	25th	50th	75th	90th	95th	99th
1. SINGLE DX										
0–19 Years	0									
20–34	0									
35–49	0									
50–64	4	2.0	2	1	1	2	4	4	4	4
65+	2	4.5	<1	4	4	5	5	5	5	5
2. MULTIPLE DX										
0–19 Years	0									
20–34	1	4.0	0	4	4	4	4	4	4	4
35–49	30	4.8	22	2	2	3	4	10	18	19
50–64	55	3.8	9	1	2	3	5	9	10	14
65+	111	5.0	26	1	3	3	6	8	12	32
TOTAL SINGLE DX	6	2.8	3	1	1	4	4	5	5	5
TOTAL MULTIPLE DX	197	4.6	21	1	2	3	6	9	12	21
TOTAL										
0–19 Years	0									
20–34	1	4.0	0	4	4	4	4	4	4	4
35–49	30	4.8	22	2	2	3	4	10	18	19
50–64	59	3.7	9	1	2	3	5	9	10	14
65+	113	5.0	26	1	3	3	6	8	12	32
GRAND TOTAL	203	4.6	20	1	2	3	6	9	11	21

71.6: OTHER VULVECTOMY

Type of Patients	Observed Patients	Avg. Stay	Variance	10th	25th	50th	75th	90th	95th	99th
1. SINGLE DX										
0–19 Years	0									
20–34	4	2.7	6	1	1	1	3	6	6	6
35–49	4	1.5	<1	1	1	2	2	2	2	2
50–64	13	1.5	<1	1	1	1	2	3	3	3
65+	7	1.6	2	1	1	1	1	5	5	5
2. MULTIPLE DX										
0–19 Years	0									
20–34	5	1.8	<1	1	1	2	2	3	3	3
35–49	49	2.0	2	1	1	2	2	3	4	9
50–64	85	3.5	17	1	1	2	4	8	15	19
65+	148	3.0	23	1	1	2	3	5	8	13
TOTAL SINGLE DX	28	1.7	2	1	1	1	2	3	5	6
TOTAL MULTIPLE DX	287	2.9	17	1	1	2	3	5	9	17
TOTAL										
0–19 Years	0									
20–34	9	2.2	3	1	1	2	3	6	6	6
35–49	53	2.0	2	1	1	2	3	3	4	9
50–64	98	3.2	15	1	1	2	3	7	15	19
65+	155	2.9	22	1	1	2	3	5	8	13
GRAND TOTAL	315	2.8	16	1	1	2	3	5	8	16

71.61: UNILATERAL VULVECTOMY

Type of Patients	Observed Patients	Avg. Stay	Variance	10th	25th	50th	75th	90th	95th	99th
1. SINGLE DX										
0–19 Years	0									
20–34	4	2.7	6	1	1	1	3	6	6	6
35–49	3	1.7	<1	1	1	2	2	2	2	2
50–64	12	1.4	<1	1	1	1	2	2	3	3
65+	5	1.8	3	1	1	1	1	5	5	5
2. MULTIPLE DX										
0–19 Years	0									
20–34	3	1.7	1	1	1	1	3	3	3	3
35–49	35	2.1	2	1	1	2	3	3	4	9
50–64	63	3.4	16	1	1	2	4	7	14	19
65+	123	3.0	27	1	1	2	3	5	9	13
TOTAL SINGLE DX	24	1.8	2	1	1	1	2	3	5	6
TOTAL MULTIPLE DX	224	3.0	20	1	1	2	3	5	9	16
TOTAL										
0–19 Years	0									
20–34	7	2.3	4	1	1	1	3	6	6	6
35–49	38	2.1	2	1	1	2	3	3	4	9
50–64	75	3.1	14	1	1	2	3	6	14	19
65+	128	3.0	26	1	1	2	3	5	9	13
GRAND TOTAL	248	2.8	18	1	1	2	3	5	9	16

71.7: VULVAR & PERINEAL REPAIR

Type of Patients	Observed Patients	Avg. Stay	Variance	10th	25th	50th	75th	90th	95th	99th
1. SINGLE DX										
0–19 Years	22	1.6	<1	1	1	1	2	2	4	4
20–34	15	1.6	<1	1	1	2	2	2	3	3
35–49	6	1.5	<1	1	1	1	2	2	2	2
50–64	3	2.0	1	1	1	2	3	3	3	3
65+	3	1.0	0	1	1	1	1	1	1	1
2. MULTIPLE DX										
0–19 Years	23	2.3	2	1	1	2	3	4	5	5
20–34	57	2.0	2	1	1	2	2	3	4	9
35–49	142	1.8	2	1	1	1	2	3	3	8
50–64	176	1.8	2	1	1	1	2	3	3	7
65+	229	2.0	5	1	1	2	2	3	4	16
TOTAL SINGLE DX	49	1.6	<1	1	1	1	2	2	4	4
TOTAL MULTIPLE DX	627	1.9	3	1	1	2	2	3	4	9
TOTAL										
0–19 Years	45	2.0	1	1	1	1	3	4	4	5
20–34	72	1.9	2	1	1	2	2	3	3	9
35–49	148	1.8	1	1	1	1	2	3	3	8
50–64	179	1.8	2	1	1	2	2	3	3	7
65+	232	2.0	4	1	1	2	2	3	4	16
GRAND TOTAL	676	1.9	2	1	1	1	2	3	4	9

LOS by Diagnosis and Operation, Western Region, 45th Edition

Western Region, October 2007–September 2008 Data, by Operation

71.71: SUTURE VULVAR/PERI LAC

Type of Patients	Observed Patients	Avg. Stay	Vari-ance	10th	25th	50th	75th	90th	95th	99th
1. SINGLE DX										
0–19 Years	17	1.3	<1	1	1	1	2	2	2	2
20–34	5	1.7	<1	1	1	2	2	3	3	3
35–49	1	1.0	0	1	1	1	1	1	1	1
50–64	0									
65+	1	1.0	0	1	1	1	1	1	1	1
2. MULTIPLE DX										
0–19 Years	18	1.9	1	1	1	1	3	4	4	4
20–34	15	1.9	1	1	1	2	3	4	4	4
35–49	35	1.8	2	1	1	1	2	3	5	9
50–64	50	1.9	3	1	1	1	2	3	3	12
65+	81	1.9	4	1	1	1	2	3	3	16
TOTAL SINGLE DX	24	1.4	<1	1	1	1	2	2	2	3
TOTAL MULTIPLE DX	199	1.9	3	1	1	1	2	3	4	11
TOTAL										
0–19 Years	35	1.6	<1	1	1	1	2	3	4	4
20–34	20	1.9	1	1	1	2	2	3	4	4
35–49	36	1.8	2	1	1	1	2	3	5	9
50–64	50	1.9	3	1	1	1	2	3	3	12
65+	82	1.9	4	1	1	1	2	3	3	16
GRAND TOTAL	223	1.8	2	1	1	1	2	3	4	11

71.79: VULVAR/PERINEUM REP NEC

Type of Patients	Observed Patients	Avg. Stay	Vari-ance	10th	25th	50th	75th	90th	95th	99th
1. SINGLE DX										
0–19 Years	4	2.9	2	1	1	4	4	4	4	4
20–34	9	1.6	<1	1	1	2	2	2	2	2
35–49	5	1.6	<1	1	1	2	2	2	3	3
50–64	3	2.0	1	1	1	2	3	3	3	3
65+	2	1.0	0	1	1	1	1	1	1	1
2. MULTIPLE DX										
0–19 Years	4	2.9	<1	2	2	3	3	4	4	4
20–34	41	2.0	2	1	1	2	2	3	3	9
35–49	103	1.7	2	1	1	1	2	3	3	6
50–64	123	1.7	1	1	1	1	2	3	3	7
65+	148	2.0	5	1	1	2	2	3	4	17
TOTAL SINGLE DX	23	1.9	1	1	1	2	2	4	4	4
TOTAL MULTIPLE DX	419	1.9	3	1	1	2	2	3	3	8
TOTAL										
0–19 Years	8	2.9	1	1	2	2	4	4	4	4
20–34	50	1.9	2	1	1	2	2	3	3	9
35–49	108	1.7	1	1	1	1	2	3	3	6
50–64	126	1.7	1	1	1	1	2	3	3	7
65+	150	2.0	5	1	1	2	2	3	4	17
GRAND TOTAL	442	1.9	2	1	1	2	2	3	4	8

71.8: VULVAR OPERATIONS NEC

Type of Patients	Observed Patients	Avg. Stay	Vari-ance	10th	25th	50th	75th	90th	95th	99th
1. SINGLE DX										
0–19 Years	0									
20–34	1	1.0	0	1	1	1	1	1	1	1
35–49	0									
50–64	0									
65+	0									
2. MULTIPLE DX										
0–19 Years	1	2.0	0	2	2	2	2	2	2	2
20–34	2	2.5	4	1	1	1	4	4	4	4
35–49	0									
50–64	1	1.0	0	1	1	1	1	1	1	1
65+	2	3.0	8	1	1	3	5	5	5	5
TOTAL SINGLE DX	1	1.0	0	1	1	1	1	1	1	1
TOTAL MULTIPLE DX	6	2.3	3	1	1	1	4	5	5	5
TOTAL										
0–19 Years	1	2.0	0	2	2	2	2	2	2	2
20–34	3	2.0	3	1	1	1	4	4	4	4
35–49	0									
50–64	1	1.0	0	1	1	1	1	1	1	1
65+	2	3.0	8	1	1	3	5	5	5	5
GRAND TOTAL	7	2.1	3	1	1	1	4	5	5	5

71.9: FEMALE GENITAL OPS NEC

Type of Patients	Observed Patients	Avg. Stay	Vari-ance	10th	25th	50th	75th	90th	95th	99th
1. SINGLE DX										
0–19 Years	0									
20–34	0									
35–49	0									
50–64	0									
65+	0									
2. MULTIPLE DX										
0–19 Years	1	3.0	0	3	3	3	3	3	3	3
20–34	3	3.0	0	3	3	3	3	3	3	3
35–49	1	1.0	0	1	1	1	1	1	1	1
50–64	1	9.0	0	9	9	9	9	9	9	9
65+	0									
TOTAL SINGLE DX	0									
TOTAL MULTIPLE DX	6	3.7	8	1	3	3	3	9	9	9
TOTAL										
0–19 Years	1	3.0	0	3	3	3	3	3	3	3
20–34	3	3.0	0	3	3	3	3	3	3	3
35–49	1	1.0	0	1	1	1	1	1	1	1
50–64	1	9.0	0	9	9	9	9	9	9	9
65+	0									
GRAND TOTAL	6	3.7	8	1	3	3	3	9	9	9

LOS by Diagnosis and Operation, Western Region, 45th Edition

Western Region, October 2007–September 2008 Data, by Operation

72.0: LOW FORCEPS OPERATION

Type of Patients	Observed Patients	Avg. Stay	Variance	Percentiles						
				10th	25th	50th	75th	90th	95th	99th
1. SINGLE DX										
0–19 Years	3	2.3	<1	2	2	2	3	3	3	3
20–34	50	1.8	<1	1	1	2	2	3	3	3
35–49	3	2.0	0	2	2	2	2	2	2	2
50–64	0									
65+	0									
2. MULTIPLE DX										
0–19 Years	160	2.4	<1	2	2	2	3	3	4	6
20–34	1,181	2.4	2	1	2	2	3	3	4	5
35–49	299	2.6	3	1	2	2	3	3	4	10
50–64	13	2.5	2	2	2	2	3	4	6	6
65+	0									
TOTAL SINGLE DX	56	1.9	<1	1	1	2	2	3	3	3
TOTAL MULTIPLE DX	1,653	2.5	2	1	2	2	3	3	4	6
TOTAL										
0–19 Years	163	2.4	<1	2	2	2	3	3	4	6
20–34	1,231	2.4	2	1	2	2	3	3	4	5
35–49	302	2.6	3	1	2	2	3	3	4	10
50–64	13	2.5	2	2	2	2	3	4	6	6
65+	0									
GRAND TOTAL	1,709	2.4	2	1	2	2	3	3	4	6

72.1: LOW FORCEPS W EPISIOTOMY

Type of Patients	Observed Patients	Avg. Stay	Variance	Percentiles						
				10th	25th	50th	75th	90th	95th	99th
1. SINGLE DX										
0–19 Years	21	2.2	<1	2	2	2	2	3	3	3
20–34	161	2.0	<1	1	1	2	2	3	3	3
35–49	11	2.0	<1	1	2	2	2	2	2	2
50–64	0									
65+	0									
2. MULTIPLE DX										
0–19 Years	173	2.4	<1	2	2	2	3	3	4	5
20–34	892	2.4	3	1	2	2	3	3	4	5
35–49	171	2.4	<1	2	2	2	3	3	4	5
50–64	5	2.6	<1	2	2	3	3	3	3	3
65+	0									
TOTAL SINGLE DX	193	2.0	<1	1	2	2	2	3	3	4
TOTAL MULTIPLE DX	1,241	2.4	2	1	2	2	3	3	4	5
TOTAL										
0–19 Years	194	2.4	<1	2	2	2	3	3	4	5
20–34	1,053	2.3	3	1	2	2	3	3	4	5
35–49	182	2.4	<1	2	2	2	3	3	4	5
50–64	5	2.6	<1	2	2	3	3	3	3	3
65+	0									
GRAND TOTAL	1,434	2.3	2	1	2	2	3	3	4	5

72.2: MID FORCEPS OPERATION

Type of Patients	Observed Patients	Avg. Stay	Variance	Percentiles						
				10th	25th	50th	75th	90th	95th	99th
1. SINGLE DX										
0–19 Years	4	2.0	<1	1	2	2	3	3	3	3
20–34	21	1.8	<1	1	1	2	2	3	3	3
35–49	3	2.0	0	2	2	2	2	2	2	2
50–64	0									
65+	0									
2. MULTIPLE DX										
0–19 Years	19	2.6	1	2	2	2	3	4	6	6
20–34	150	2.6	13	1	2	2	3	4	4	12
35–49	34	2.6	<1	1	2	3	3	3	4	5
50–64	2	3.0	0	3	3	3	3	3	3	3
65+	0									
TOTAL SINGLE DX	28	1.8	<1	1	1	2	2	3	3	3
TOTAL MULTIPLE DX	205	2.6	10	1	2	2	3	4	4	12
TOTAL										
0–19 Years	23	2.5	1	2	2	2	3	3	4	6
20–34	171	2.5	12	1	2	2	3	3	4	12
35–49	37	2.5	<1	1	2	3	3	3	4	5
50–64	2	3.0	0	3	3	3	3	3	3	3
65+	0									
GRAND TOTAL	233	2.5	9	1	2	2	3	3	4	12

72.21: MID FORCEPS W EPISIOTOMY

Type of Patients	Observed Patients	Avg. Stay	Variance	Percentiles						
				10th	25th	50th	75th	90th	95th	99th
1. SINGLE DX										
0–19 Years	4	2.0	<1	1	2	2	3	3	3	3
20–34	18	1.8	<1	1	1	2	2	3	3	3
35–49	3	2.0	0	2	2	2	2	2	2	2
50–64	0									
65+	0									
2. MULTIPLE DX										
0–19 Years	15	2.4	<1	2	2	2	3	4	4	4
20–34	82	2.6	21	1	2	2	3	3	4	43
35–49	13	2.8	<1	3	3	3	3	4	5	5
50–64	1	3.0	0	3	3	3	3	3	3	3
65+	0									
TOTAL SINGLE DX	25	1.8	<1	1	1	2	2	3	3	3
TOTAL MULTIPLE DX	111	2.6	16	1	2	2	3	3	4	5
TOTAL										
0–19 Years	19	2.3	<1	1	2	2	3	4	4	4
20–34	100	2.5	18	1	2	2	3	3	4	43
35–49	16	2.6	<1	2	3	3	3	4	5	5
50–64	1	3.0	0	3	3	3	3	3	3	3
65+	0									
GRAND TOTAL	136	2.5	13	1	2	2	3	3	4	5

314

LOS by Diagnosis and Operation, Western Region, 45th Edition

Western Region, October 2007–September 2008 Data, by Operation

72.3: HIGH FORCEPS OPERATION

Type of Patients	Observed Patients	Avg. Stay	Vari- ance	Percentiles						
				10th	25th	50th	75th	90th	95th	99th
1. SINGLE DX										
0–19 Years	0									
20–34	0									
35–49	0									
50–64	0									
65+	0									
2. MULTIPLE DX										
0–19 Years	2	2.5	<1	2	2	2	3	3	3	3
20–34	9	2.2	<1	1	2	2	3	3	3	3
35–49	0									
50–64	0									
65+	0									
TOTAL SINGLE DX	**0**									
TOTAL MULTIPLE DX	**11**	**2.3**	**<1**	**1**	**2**	**2**	**3**	**3**	**3**	**3**
TOTAL										
0–19 Years	2	2.5	<1	2	2	2	3	3	3	3
20–34	9	2.2	<1	1	2	2	3	3	3	3
35–49	0									
50–64	0									
65+	0									
GRAND TOTAL	**11**	**2.3**	**<1**	**1**	**2**	**2**	**3**	**3**	**3**	**3**

72.4: FORCEPS ROT FETAL HEAD

Type of Patients	Observed Patients	Avg. Stay	Vari- ance	Percentiles						
				10th	25th	50th	75th	90th	95th	99th
1. SINGLE DX										
0–19 Years	0									
20–34	4	1.3	<1	1	1	1	1	2	2	2
35–49	1	1.0	0	1	1	1	1	1	1	1
50–64	0									
65+	0									
2. MULTIPLE DX										
0–19 Years	4	6.9	74	2	2	3	3	20	20	20
20–34	17	2.1	<1	1	2	2	3	3	4	4
35–49	2	1.5	<1	1	1	1	2	2	2	2
50–64	0									
65+	0									
TOTAL SINGLE DX	**5**	**1.2**	**<1**	**1**	**1**	**1**	**1**	**2**	**2**	**2**
TOTAL MULTIPLE DX	**23**	**2.9**	**14**	**1**	**2**	**2**	**3**	**3**	**4**	**20**
TOTAL										
0–19 Years	4	6.9	74	2	2	3	3	20	20	20
20–34	21	2.0	<1	1	1	2	2	3	3	4
35–49	3	1.3	<1	1	1	1	2	2	2	2
50–64	0									
65+	0									
GRAND TOTAL	**28**	**2.6**	**12**	**1**	**1**	**2**	**3**	**3**	**4**	**20**

72.5: BREECH EXTRACTION

Type of Patients	Observed Patients	Avg. Stay	Vari- ance	Percentiles						
				10th	25th	50th	75th	90th	95th	99th
1. SINGLE DX										
0–19 Years	2	1.5	<1	1	1	2	2	2	2	2
20–34	10	2.0	<1	1	2	2	2	3	3	3
35–49	2	2.0	2	1	1	3	3	3	3	3
50–64	0									
65+	0									
2. MULTIPLE DX										
0–19 Years	23	2.6	9	1	1	2	3	4	4	16
20–34	217	2.8	7	1	2	2	3	5	7	15
35–49	70	2.4	2	1	2	2	3	4	5	8
50–64	2	2.5	<1	2	2	3	3	3	3	3
65+	0									
TOTAL SINGLE DX	**14**	**1.9**	**<1**	**1**	**2**	**2**	**2**	**3**	**3**	**3**
TOTAL MULTIPLE DX	**312**	**2.7**	**6**	**1**	**2**	**2**	**3**	**5**	**6**	**15**
TOTAL										
0–19 Years	25	2.5	9	1	1	2	3	4	4	16
20–34	227	2.7	7	1	2	2	3	5	7	15
35–49	72	2.4	2	1	2	2	3	4	5	8
50–64	2	2.5	<1	2	2	2	3	3	3	3
65+	0									
GRAND TOTAL	**326**	**2.6**	**6**	**1**	**2**	**2**	**3**	**4**	**6**	**15**

72.54: TOT BREECH EXTRACT NEC

Type of Patients	Observed Patients	Avg. Stay	Vari- ance	Percentiles						
				10th	25th	50th	75th	90th	95th	99th
1. SINGLE DX										
0–19 Years	2	1.5	<1	1	1	2	2	2	2	2
20–34	9	2.0	<1	1	2	2	2	3	3	3
35–49	1	3.0	0	3	3	3	3	3	3	3
50–64	0									
65+	0									
2. MULTIPLE DX										
0–19 Years	14	3.2	15	1	2	2	3	4	16	16
20–34	165	2.8	8	1	1	2	3	5	8	17
35–49	41	2.2	2	1	3	3	3	3	4	8
50–64	1	3.0	0	3	3	3	3	3	3	3
65+	0									
TOTAL SINGLE DX	**12**	**2.0**	**<1**	**1**	**2**	**2**	**2**	**3**	**3**	**3**
TOTAL MULTIPLE DX	**221**	**2.7**	**7**	**1**	**2**	**2**	**3**	**5**	**7**	**16**
TOTAL										
0–19 Years	16	3.0	13	1	2	2	3	4	16	16
20–34	174	2.8	7	1	2	2	3	5	8	17
35–49	42	2.3	2	1	1	2	3	3	4	8
50–64	1	3.0	0	3	3	3	3	3	3	3
65+	0									
GRAND TOTAL	**233**	**2.7**	**7**	**1**	**2**	**2**	**3**	**5**	**7**	**16**

LOS by Diagnosis and Operation, Western Region, 45th Edition

315

Western Region, October 2007–September 2008 Data, by Operation

72.6: FORCEPS-AFTERCOMING HEAD

Type of Patients	Observed Patients	Avg. Stay	Variance	10th	25th	50th	75th	90th	95th	99th
1. SINGLE DX										
0–19 Years	0									
20–34	0									
35–49	0									
50–64	0									
65+	0									
2. MULTIPLE DX										
0–19 Years	5	4.6	17	2	2	3	4	12	12	12
20–34	11	2.4	<1	2	2	2	2	4	4	4
35–49	4	2.5	1	2	2	2	4	4	4	4
50–64	0									
65+	0									
TOTAL SINGLE DX	0									
TOTAL MULTIPLE DX	20	2.9	5	2	2	2	3	4	4	12
TOTAL										
0–19 Years	5	4.6	17	2	2	3	4	12	12	12
20–34	11	2.4	<1	2	2	2	2	4	4	4
35–49	4	2.5	1	2	2	2	4	4	4	4
50–64	0									
65+	0									
GRAND TOTAL	20	2.9	5	2	2	2	3	4	4	12

72.71: VED W EPISIOTOMY

Type of Patients	Observed Patients	Avg. Stay	Variance	10th	25th	50th	75th	90th	95th	99th
1. SINGLE DX										
0–19 Years	531	2.1	<1	1	2	2	2	3	3	4
20–34	2,328	2.0	<1	1	2	2	2	3	3	4
35–49	102	2.0	<1	1	2	2	2	3	3	3
50–64	5	2.0	<1	1	2	2	2	3	3	3
65+	0									
2. MULTIPLE DX										
0–19 Years	1,822	2.3	<1	1	2	2	3	3	4	5
20–34	8,668	2.3	1	1	2	2	3	3	3	5
35–49	1,623	2.3	<1	1	2	2	3	3	3	4
50–64	82	2.3	<1	2	2	2	3	3	3	4
65+	0									
TOTAL SINGLE DX	2,966	2.0	<1	1	2	2	2	3	3	4
TOTAL MULTIPLE DX	12,195	2.3	1	1	2	3	3	3	3	5
TOTAL										
0–19 Years	2,353	2.2	<1	1	2	2	3	3	3	4
20–34	10,996	2.2	1	1	2	2	3	3	3	4
35–49	1,725	2.3	<1	1	2	2	3	3	3	4
50–64	87	2.3	<1	1	2	2	3	3	3	4
65+	0									
GRAND TOTAL	15,161	2.2	<1	1	2	2	3	3	3	4

72.7: VACUUM EXTRACTION DEL

Type of Patients	Observed Patients	Avg. Stay	Variance	10th	25th	50th	75th	90th	95th	99th
1. SINGLE DX										
0–19 Years	713	2.0	<1	1	2	2	2	3	3	4
20–34	3,678	2.0	<1	1	1	2	2	3	3	4
35–49	177	1.9	<1	1	1	2	2	3	3	4
50–64	9	1.8	<1	1	1	2	2	2	3	3
65+	0									
2. MULTIPLE DX										
0–19 Years	3,900	2.3	<1	1	2	2	3	3	4	5
20–34	22,253	2.2	1	1	2	2	3	3	3	5
35–49	4,573	2.2	1	1	2	2	3	3	3	5
50–64	211	2.3	<1	2	2	2	3	3	3	4
65+	0									
TOTAL SINGLE DX	4,577	2.0	<1	1	2	2	2	3	3	4
TOTAL MULTIPLE DX	30,937	2.2	1	1	2	2	3	3	3	5
TOTAL										
0–19 Years	4,613	2.2	<1	1	2	2	3	3	4	5
20–34	25,931	2.2	1	1	2	2	3	3	3	4
35–49	4,750	2.2	<1	1	2	2	3	3	3	5
50–64	220	2.3	<1	2	2	2	3	3	3	4
65+	0									
GRAND TOTAL	35,514	2.2	1	1	2	2	3	3	3	5

72.79: VACUUM EXTRACT DEL NEC

Type of Patients	Observed Patients	Avg. Stay	Variance	10th	25th	50th	75th	90th	95th	99th
1. SINGLE DX										
0–19 Years	182	2.0	<1	1	1	2	2	3	3	6
20–34	1,350	1.8	<1	1	1	2	2	3	3	3
35–49	75	1.9	<1	1	1	2	2	3	3	4
50–64	4	1.6	<1	1	1	2	2	2	2	2
65+	0									
2. MULTIPLE DX										
0–19 Years	2,078	2.3	1	1	2	2	3	3	4	5
20–34	13,585	2.2	1	1	2	2	3	3	3	5
35–49	2,950	2.2	1	1	2	2	3	3	4	5
50–64	129	2.3	<1	2	2	2	3	3	3	5
65+	0									
TOTAL SINGLE DX	1,611	1.9	<1	1	1	2	2	3	3	4
TOTAL MULTIPLE DX	18,742	2.2	1	1	2	2	3	3	3	5
TOTAL										
0–19 Years	2,260	2.3	1	1	2	2	3	3	4	5
20–34	14,935	2.2	1	1	2	2	3	3	3	5
35–49	3,025	2.2	1	1	2	2	3	3	3	5
50–64	133	2.3	<1	2	2	2	3	4	4	5
65+	0									
GRAND TOTAL	20,353	2.2	1	1	2	2	3	3	3	5

LOS by Diagnosis and Operation, Western Region, 45th Edition

Western Region, October 2007–September 2008 Data, by Operation

72.8: INSTRUMENTAL DEL NEC

Type of Patients	Observed Patients	Avg. Stay	Variance	Percentiles						
				10th	25th	50th	75th	90th	95th	99th
1. SINGLE DX										
0–19 Years	0									
20–34	2	1.5	<1	1	1	1	2	2	2	2
35–49	1	1.0	0	1	1	1	1	1	1	1
50–64	0									
65+	0									
2. MULTIPLE DX										
0–19 Years	1	3.0	0	3	3	3	3	3	3	3
20–34	12	2.4	<1	1	2	3	3	3	4	4
35–49	2	2.0	0	2	2	2	2	2	2	2
50–64	0									
65+	0									
TOTAL SINGLE DX	**3**	**1.3**	**<1**	**1**	**1**	**1**	**2**	**2**	**2**	**2**
TOTAL MULTIPLE DX	**15**	**2.4**	**<1**	**1**	**2**	**2**	**3**	**3**	**4**	**4**
TOTAL										
0–19 Years	1	3.0	0	3	3	3	3	3	3	3
20–34	14	2.3	<1	1	2	2	3	3	4	4
35–49	3	1.7	<1	1	1	2	2	2	2	2
50–64	0									
65+	0									
GRAND TOTAL	**18**	**2.2**	**<1**	**1**	**2**	**2**	**3**	**3**	**4**	**4**

72.9: INSTRUMENTAL DEL NOS

Type of Patients	Observed Patients	Avg. Stay	Variance	Percentiles						
				10th	25th	50th	75th	90th	95th	99th
1. SINGLE DX										
0–19 Years	3	1.7	<1	1	1	2	2	2	2	2
20–34	10	2.2	<1	1	1	2	3	3	4	4
35–49	0									
50–64	0									
65+	0									
2. MULTIPLE DX										
0–19 Years	18	2.3	<1	2	2	2	3	3	3	3
20–34	104	2.4	2	1	2	3	3	3	4	6
35–49	14	2.6	<1	2	2	3	3	4	4	4
50–64	1	3.0	0	3	3	3	3	3	3	3
65+	0									
TOTAL SINGLE DX	**13**	**2.1**	**<1**	**1**	**1**	**2**	**3**	**3**	**4**	**4**
TOTAL MULTIPLE DX	**137**	**2.4**	**1**	**2**	**2**	**2**	**3**	**3**	**3**	**6**
TOTAL										
0–19 Years	21	2.2	<1	2	2	2	3	3	3	3
20–34	114	2.4	1	1	2	2	3	3	4	6
35–49	14	2.6	<1	2	2	3	3	3	4	4
50–64	1	3.0	0	3	3	3	3	3	3	3
65+	0									
GRAND TOTAL	**150**	**2.4**	**1**	**1**	**2**	**2**	**3**	**3**	**3**	**6**

73.0: ARTIFICIAL RUPT MEMBRANE

Type of Patients	Observed Patients	Avg. Stay	Variance	Percentiles						
				10th	25th	50th	75th	90th	95th	99th
1. SINGLE DX										
0–19 Years	596	1.9	<1	1	1	2	2	3	3	3
20–34	4,053	1.7	<1	1	1	2	2	2	3	3
35–49	233	1.7	<1	1	1	2	2	2	2	3
50–64	14	2.0	<1	1	2	2	2	3	3	3
65+	0									
2. MULTIPLE DX										
0–19 Years	1,090	2.1	<1	1	2	2	3	3	3	5
20–34	7,183	2.0	3	1	1	2	2	3	3	4
35–49	1,130	2.0	<1	1	1	2	2	3	3	5
50–64	34	2.0	<1	1	2	2	3	3	3	4
65+	0									
TOTAL SINGLE DX	**4,896**	**1.7**	**<1**	**1**	**1**	**2**	**2**	**2**	**3**	**3**
TOTAL MULTIPLE DX	**9,437**	**2.0**	**2**	**1**	**1**	**2**	**2**	**3**	**3**	**5**
TOTAL										
0–19 Years	1,686	2.0	<1	1	2	2	3	3	3	5
20–34	11,236	1.9	2	1	1	2	2	3	3	4
35–49	1,363	1.9	<1	1	1	2	2	3	3	5
50–64	48	2.0	<1	1	2	2	3	3	3	4
65+	0									
GRAND TOTAL	**14,333**	**1.9**	**2**	**1**	**1**	**2**	**2**	**3**	**3**	**4**

73.01: INDUCTION LABOR BY AROM

Type of Patients	Observed Patients	Avg. Stay	Variance	Percentiles						
				10th	25th	50th	75th	90th	95th	99th
1. SINGLE DX										
0–19 Years	47	1.9	<1	1	1	2	2	3	3	3
20–34	373	1.6	<1	1	1	2	2	3	3	3
35–49	26	1.5	<1	1	1	2	2	2	2	2
50–64	2	2.0	0	2	2	2	2	2	2	2
65+	0									
2. MULTIPLE DX										
0–19 Years	87	2.3	<1	1	2	2	3	4	4	5
20–34	849	2.0	1	1	1	2	2	3	3	4
35–49	171	2.0	<1	1	1	2	3	4	4	5
50–64	9	2.2	<1	1	2	2	3	4	4	4
65+	0									
TOTAL SINGLE DX	**448**	**1.6**	**<1**	**1**	**1**	**2**	**2**	**2**	**3**	**3**
TOTAL MULTIPLE DX	**1,116**	**2.0**	**1**	**1**	**1**	**2**	**3**	**3**	**3**	**5**
TOTAL										
0–19 Years	134	2.1	<1	1	1	2	3	3	4	4
20–34	1,222	1.9	<1	1	1	2	2	3	3	4
35–49	197	2.0	<1	1	1	2	3	4	4	5
50–64	11	2.2	<1	2	2	2	3	4	4	4
65+	0									
GRAND TOTAL	**1,564**	**1.9**	**<1**	**1**	**1**	**2**	**2**	**3**	**3**	**4**

LOS by Diagnosis and Operation, Western Region, 45th Edition

Western Region, October 2007–September 2008 Data, by Operation

73.09: ARTIF RUPT MEMBRANES NEC

Type of Patients	Observed Patients	Avg. Stay	Vari-ance	Percentiles						
				10th	25th	50th	75th	90th	95th	99th
1. SINGLE DX										
0–19 Years	549	1.9	<1	1	1	2	2	3	3	3
20–34	3,680	1.7	<1	1	1	2	2	2	3	3
35–49	207	1.7	<1	1	1	2	2	2	2	3
50–64	12	2.0	<1	1	2	2	2	3	3	3
65+	0									
2. MULTIPLE DX										
0–19 Years	1,003	2.1	<1	1	2	2	2	3	3	5
20–34	6,334	2.0	3	1	1	2	2	3	3	4
35–49	959	1.9	<1	1	1	2	2	3	3	5
50–64	25	1.9	<1	1	1	2	2	3	3	3
65+	0									
TOTAL SINGLE DX	4,448	1.7	<1	1	1	2	2	2	3	3
TOTAL MULTIPLE DX	8,321	2.0	2	1	1	2	2	3	3	5
TOTAL										
0–19 Years	1,552	2.0	<1	1	2	2	2	3	3	5
20–34	10,014	1.9	2	1	1	2	2	3	3	4
35–49	1,166	1.9	<1	1	1	2	2	3	3	4
50–64	37	1.9	<1	1	2	2	2	3	3	3
65+	0									
GRAND TOTAL	12,769	1.9	2	1	1	2	2	3	3	4

73.1: SURG INDUCTION LABOR NEC

Type of Patients	Observed Patients	Avg. Stay	Vari-ance	Percentiles						
				10th	25th	50th	75th	90th	95th	99th
1. SINGLE DX										
0–19 Years	19	2.3	<1	1	2	2	3	3	3	3
20–34	74	1.9	<1	1	1	2	2	3	3	4
35–49	4	1.8	<1	1	1	2	3	3	3	3
50–64	0									
65+	0									
2. MULTIPLE DX										
0–19 Years	64	2.9	3	2	2	3	3	4	5	13
20–34	324	2.5	1	1	2	2	3	4	5	6
35–49	57	2.4	1	1	2	2	3	3	5	6
50–64	4	2.0	<1	1	2	2	3	3	3	3
65+	0									
TOTAL SINGLE DX	97	2.0	<1	1	1	2	3	3	3	4
TOTAL MULTIPLE DX	449	2.5	2	1	2	2	3	4	5	6
TOTAL										
0–19 Years	83	2.7	2	2	2	3	3	4	5	13
20–34	398	2.4	1	1	2	2	3	4	4	6
35–49	61	2.4	1	1	2	2	3	3	5	6
50–64	4	2.0	<1	1	2	2	3	3	3	3
65+	0									
GRAND TOTAL	546	2.4	2	1	2	2	3	4	4	6

73.2: INT/COMB VERSION/EXTRACT

Type of Patients	Observed Patients	Avg. Stay	Vari-ance	Percentiles						
				10th	25th	50th	75th	90th	95th	99th
1. SINGLE DX										
0–19 Years	0									
20–34	7	1.0	0	1	1	1	1	1	1	1
35–49	0									
50–64	0									
65+	0									
2. MULTIPLE DX										
0–19 Years	2	3.5	4	2	2	5	5	5	5	5
20–34	32	1.8	<1	1	1	2	2	3	3	3
35–49	7	2.1	<1	1	2	2	3	3	3	3
50–64	0									
65+	0									
TOTAL SINGLE DX	7	1.0	0	1	1	1	1	1	1	1
TOTAL MULTIPLE DX	41	1.9	<1	1	1	2	2	3	3	5
TOTAL										
0–19 Years	2	3.5	4	2	2	5	5	5	5	5
20–34	39	1.6	<1	1	1	1	2	3	3	3
35–49	7	2.1	<1	1	2	2	3	3	3	3
50–64	0									
65+	0									
GRAND TOTAL	48	1.8	<1	1	1	2	2	3	3	5

73.3: FAILED FORCEPS

Type of Patients	Observed Patients	Avg. Stay	Vari-ance	Percentiles						
				10th	25th	50th	75th	90th	95th	99th
1. SINGLE DX										
0–19 Years	0									
20–34	2	2.5	<1	2	2	2	3	3	3	3
35–49	0									
50–64	0									
65+	0									
2. MULTIPLE DX										
0–19 Years	0									
20–34	1	1.0	0	1	1	1	1	1	1	1
35–49	0									
50–64	0									
65+	0									
TOTAL SINGLE DX	2	2.5	<1	2	2	2	3	3	3	3
TOTAL MULTIPLE DX	1	1.0	0	1	1	1	1	1	1	1
TOTAL										
0–19 Years	0									
20–34	3	2.0	<1	1	1	2	3	3	3	3
35–49	0									
50–64	0									
65+	0									
GRAND TOTAL	3	2.0	<1	1	1	2	3	3	3	3

Western Region, October 2007–September 2008 Data, by Operation

73.4: MEDICAL INDUCTION LABOR

Type of Patients	Observed Patients	Avg. Stay	Vari-ance	Percentiles						
				10th	25th	50th	75th	90th	95th	99th
1. SINGLE DX										
0–19 Years	243	2.0	2	1	1	2	2	3	3	4
20–34	2,009	1.7	<1	1	1	2	2	3	3	3
35–49	141	1.6	<1	1	1	1	2	2	3	3
50–64	4	2.7	<1	2	2	2	3	4	4	4
65+	0									
2. MULTIPLE DX										
0–19 Years	1,030	2.5	4	1	2	2	3	4	4	11
20–34	7,869	2.2	2	1	2	2	3	3	4	6
35–49	1,571	2.1	1	1	1	2	3	3	4	6
50–64	48	2.3	1	1	2	2	3	3	5	5
65+	0									
TOTAL SINGLE DX	2,397	1.7	<1	1	1	2	2	3	3	4
TOTAL MULTIPLE DX	10,518	2.2	2	1	2	2	3	3	4	6
TOTAL										
0–19 Years	1,273	2.4	4	1	2	2	3	3	4	10
20–34	9,878	2.1	2	1	1	2	2	3	4	5
35–49	1,712	2.1	1	1	1	2	3	3	4	5
50–64	52	2.3	1	1	2	2	3	4	5	5
65+	0									
GRAND TOTAL	12,915	2.1	2	1	1	2	3	3	4	6

73.5: MANUALLY ASSISTED DEL

Type of Patients	Observed Patients	Avg. Stay	Vari-ance	Percentiles						
				10th	25th	50th	75th	90th	95th	99th
1. SINGLE DX										
0–19 Years	13,361	1.9	<1	1	1	2	2	3	3	4
20–34	98,284	1.8	<1	1	1	2	2	3	3	3
35–49	6,260	1.8	<1	1	1	2	2	2	3	3
50–64	392	1.9	<1	1	1	2	2	3	3	3
65+	0									
2. MULTIPLE DX										
0–19 Years	23,676	2.3	3	1	2	2	3	3	4	6
20–34	175,681	2.1	2	1	1	2	2	3	3	5
35–49	38,477	2.1	3	1	2	2	2	3	3	6
50–64	2,205	2.1	3	1	2	2	2	3	3	5
65+	0									
TOTAL SINGLE DX	118,297	1.8	<1	1	1	2	2	3	3	3
TOTAL MULTIPLE DX	240,039	2.1	3	1	2	2	2	3	3	5
TOTAL										
0–19 Years	37,037	2.2	2	1	2	2	3	3	3	5
20–34	273,965	2.0	2	1	1	2	2	3	3	4
35–49	44,737	2.1	3	1	1	2	2	3	3	5
50–64	2,597	2.1	2	1	2	2	2	3	3	5
65+	0									
GRAND TOTAL	358,336	2.0	2	1	1	2	2	3	3	5

73.51: MANUAL ROT FETAL HEAD

Type of Patients	Observed Patients	Avg. Stay	Vari-ance	Percentiles						
				10th	25th	50th	75th	90th	95th	99th
1. SINGLE DX										
0–19 Years	5	1.8	<1	1	2		2	2	2	2
20–34	29	1.8	<1	1	1		2	2	2	3
35–49	3	2.0	<1	1	1		3	3	3	3
50–64	0									
65+	0									
2. MULTIPLE DX										
0–19 Years	17	2.2	1	1	1	2	3	4	5	5
20–34	204	2.1	<1	1	2	2	3	3	3	4
35–49	73	2.2	<1	1	2	2	3	3	3	5
50–64	3	1.8	<1	1	1	2	3	3	3	3
65+	0									
TOTAL SINGLE DX	37	1.8	<1	1	1	2	2	3	3	3
TOTAL MULTIPLE DX	297	2.2	<1	1	2	2	3	3	3	5
TOTAL										
0–19 Years	22	2.1	1	1	1	2	2	3	4	5
20–34	233	2.1	<1	1	2	2	3	3	3	4
35–49	76	2.2	<1	1	2	2	3	3	3	5
50–64	3	1.8	<1	1	1	2	3	3	3	3
65+	0									
GRAND TOTAL	334	2.1	<1	1	2	2	3	3	3	5

73.59: MANUAL ASSISTED DEL NEC

Type of Patients	Observed Patients	Avg. Stay	Vari-ance	Percentiles						
				10th	25th	50th	75th	90th	95th	99th
1. SINGLE DX										
0–19 Years	13,356	1.9	<1	1	1	2	2	3	3	4
20–34	98,255	1.8	<1	1	1	2	2	3	3	3
35–49	6,257	1.8	<1	1	1	2	2	3	3	3
50–64	392	1.9	<1	1	1	2	2	3	3	3
65+	0									
2. MULTIPLE DX										
0–19 Years	23,659	2.3	3	1	2	2	3	3	4	6
20–34	175,477	2.1	2	1	1	2	2	3	3	5
35–49	38,404	2.1	3	1	2	2	2	3	3	6
50–64	2,202	2.1	3	1	2	2	2	3	3	5
65+	0									
TOTAL SINGLE DX	118,260	1.8	<1	1	1	2	2	3	3	3
TOTAL MULTIPLE DX	239,742	2.1	3	1	2	2	3	3	3	5
TOTAL										
0–19 Years	37,015	2.2	2	1	2	2	3	3	3	5
20–34	273,732	2.0	2	1	1	2	2	3	3	4
35–49	44,661	2.1	3	1	1	2	2	3	3	5
50–64	2,594	2.1	2	1	2	2	2	3	3	5
65+	0									
GRAND TOTAL	358,002	2.0	2	1	1	2	2	3	3	5

LOS by Diagnosis and Operation, Western Region, 45th Edition

Western Region, October 2007–September 2008 Data, by Operation

73.6: EPISIOTOMY

Type of Patients	Observed Patients	Avg. Stay	Variance	Percentiles						
				10th	25th	50th	75th	90th	95th	99th
1. SINGLE DX										
0–19 Years	2,490	2.0	<1	1	2	2	2	3	3	4
20–34	10,732	1.9	<1	1	1	2	2	3	3	3
35–49	863	1.9	<1	1	1	2	2	3	3	3
50–64	56	1.9	<1	1	2	2	2	3	3	3
65+	0									
2. MULTIPLE DX										
0–19 Years	2,662	2.3	3	1	2	2	3	3	3	5
20–34	13,026	2.2	2	1	2	2	2	3	3	5
35–49	2,766	2.1	2	1	2	2	2	3	3	4
50–64	107	2.1	<1	1	2	2	2	3	4	4
65+	0									
TOTAL SINGLE DX	14,141	1.9	<1	1	1	2	2	3	3	3
TOTAL MULTIPLE DX	18,561	2.2	2	1	2	2	3	3	3	5
TOTAL										
0–19 Years	5,152	2.1	2	1	2	2	2	3	3	4
20–34	23,758	2.0	1	1	2	2	2	3	3	4
35–49	3,629	2.0	1	1	2	2	2	3	3	4
50–64	163	2.1	<1	1	2	2	2	3	3	4
65+	0									
GRAND TOTAL	32,702	2.0	2	1	2	2	2	3	3	4

73.9: OTH OPS ASSISTING DEL

Type of Patients	Observed Patients	Avg. Stay	Variance	Percentiles						
				10th	25th	50th	75th	90th	95th	99th
1. SINGLE DX										
0–19 Years	4	1.5	<1	1	1	2	2	2	2	2
20–34	49	1.4	<1	1	1	1	2	2	2	3
35–49	4	1.8	<1	1	1	2	3	3	3	3
50–64	1	2.0	0	2	2	2	2	2	2	2
65+	0									
2. MULTIPLE DX										
0–19 Years	13	1.9	<1	1	2	2	2	3	3	3
20–34	102	2.0	2	1	1	2	2	3	4	9
35–49	31	2.0	1	1	1	2	3	4	4	5
50–64	1	3.0	0	3	3	3	3	3	3	3
65+	0									
TOTAL SINGLE DX	58	1.4	<1	1	1	1	2	2	2	3
TOTAL MULTIPLE DX	147	2.0	2	1	1	2	2	3	4	9
TOTAL										
0–19 Years	17	1.8	<1	1	1	2	2	3	3	3
20–34	151	1.8	<1	1	1	1	2	3	4	9
35–49	35	2.0	1	1	1	2	3	4	4	5
50–64	2	2.5	<1	2	2	3	3	3	3	3
65+	0									
GRAND TOTAL	205	1.8	2	1	1	2	2	3	4	7

73.8: FETAL OPS-FACILITATE DEL

Type of Patients	Observed Patients	Avg. Stay	Variance	Percentiles						
				10th	25th	50th	75th	90th	95th	99th
1. SINGLE DX										
0–19 Years	0									
20–34	2	1.5	<1	1	1	1	2	2	2	2
35–49	0									
50–64	0									
65+	0									
2. MULTIPLE DX										
0–19 Years	0									
20–34	3	1.3	<1	1	1	1	2	2	2	2
35–49	1	2.0	0	2	2	2	2	2	2	2
50–64	0									
65+	0									
TOTAL SINGLE DX	2	1.5	<1	1	1	1	2	2	2	2
TOTAL MULTIPLE DX	4	1.5	<1	1	1	2	2	2	2	2
TOTAL										
0–19 Years	0									
20–34	5	1.4	<1	1	1	1	2	2	2	2
35–49	1	2.0	0	2	2	2	2	2	2	2
50–64	0									
65+	0									
GRAND TOTAL	6	1.5	<1	1	1	1	2	2	2	2

74.0: CLASSICAL CD

Type of Patients	Observed Patients	Avg. Stay	Variance	Percentiles						
				10th	25th	50th	75th	90th	95th	99th
1. SINGLE DX										
0–19 Years	6	2.7	<1	2	2	3	3	3	3	3
20–34	55	2.9	<1	2	3	3	3	4	4	5
35–49	3	2.7	1	2	2	2	4	4	4	4
50–64	0									
65+	0									
2. MULTIPLE DX										
0–19 Years	101	5.6	27	2	3	4	6	11	16	22
20–34	1,011	6.7	61	2	3	4	7	14	21	43
35–49	438	7.2	79	3	3	4	7	16	22	50
50–64	34	6.4	27	3	3	4	7	13	14	25
65+	0									
TOTAL SINGLE DX	64	2.9	<1	2	2	3	3	4	4	5
TOTAL MULTIPLE DX	1,584	6.8	63	2	3	4	7	14	21	43
TOTAL										
0–19 Years	107	5.5	26	2	3	4	6	11	16	22
20–34	1,066	6.6	58	2	3	4	7	13	21	41
35–49	441	7.2	79	2	3	4	7	16	22	50
50–64	34	6.4	27	3	3	4	7	13	14	25
65+	0									
GRAND TOTAL	1,648	6.6	61	2	3	4	7	14	21	43

LOS by Diagnosis and Operation, Western Region, 45th Edition

Western Region, October 2007–September 2008 Data, by Operation

74.1: LOW CERVICAL CD

Type of Patients	Observed Patients	Avg. Stay	Variance	10th	25th	50th	75th	90th	95th	99th
1. SINGLE DX										
0–19 Years	2,229	3.0	1	2	2	3	3	4	4	5
20–34	30,506	2.9	<1	2	2	3	3	4	4	5
35–49	1,627	3.0	<1	2	2	3	3	4	4	5
50–64	88	3.1	<1	2	3	3	4	4	4	4
65+	0									
2. MULTIPLE DX										
0–19 Years	14,323	3.7	6	2	3	3	4	5	6	11
20–34	157,495	3.5	8	2	3	3	4	5	5	12
35–49	51,816	3.7	11	2	3	3	4	5	5	15
50–64	3,070	4.1	20	2	3	3	4	5	6	23
65+	0									
TOTAL SINGLE DX	34,450	2.9	<1	2	2	3	3	4	4	5
TOTAL MULTIPLE DX	226,704	3.6	9	2	3	3	4	5	5	13
TOTAL										
0–19 Years	16,552	3.6	5	2	3	3	4	5	5	10
20–34	188,001	3.4	7	2	3	3	4	5	5	11
35–49	53,443	3.7	11	2	3	3	4	5	5	14
50–64	3,158	4.0	19	2	3	3	4	5	6	23
65+	0									
GRAND TOTAL	261,154	3.5	8	2	3	3	4	5	5	11

74.2: EXTRAPERITONEAL CD

Type of Patients	Observed Patients	Avg. Stay	Variance	10th	25th	50th	75th	90th	95th	99th
1. SINGLE DX										
0–19 Years	1	4.0	0	4	4	4	4	4	4	4
20–34	6	2.3	<1	1	2	3	3	3	3	3
35–49	0									
50–64	0									
65+	0									
2. MULTIPLE DX										
0–19 Years	3	6.3	10	4	4	5	10	10	10	10
20–34	62	3.4	2	2	3	3	4	5	6	12
35–49	12	3.7	1	3	3	3	4	4	7	7
50–64	3	4.3	<1	4	4	4	5	5	5	5
65+	0									
TOTAL SINGLE DX	7	2.6	<1	1	2	3	3	4	4	4
TOTAL MULTIPLE DX	80	3.6	3	2	3	3	4	5	7	12
TOTAL										
0–19 Years	4	5.7	8	4	4	4	5	10	10	10
20–34	68	3.3	2	2	3	3	4	5	6	12
35–49	12	3.7	1	3	3	3	4	4	7	7
50–64	3	4.3	<1	4	4	4	5	5	5	5
65+	0									
GRAND TOTAL	87	3.5	3	2	3	3	4	5	7	12

74.3: RMVL EXTRATUBAL PREG

Type of Patients	Observed Patients	Avg. Stay	Variance	10th	25th	50th	75th	90th	95th	99th
1. SINGLE DX										
0–19 Years	4	1.5	<1	1	1	2	2	2	2	2
20–34	38	2.4	<1	1	1	2	3	4	4	7
35–49	10	2.3	<1	1	2	3	3	3	3	3
50–64	0									
65+	0									
2. MULTIPLE DX										
0–19 Years	8	2.1	<1	1	1	2	3	4	4	4
20–34	104	2.3	3	1	1	2	3	4	5	8
35–49	45	2.3	3	1	1	2	3	3	5	10
50–64	0									
65+	0									
TOTAL SINGLE DX	52	2.3	1	1	1	2	3	3	4	7
TOTAL MULTIPLE DX	157	2.3	3	1	1	2	3	4	5	10
TOTAL										
0–19 Years	12	1.9	<1	1	1	2	2	3	4	4
20–34	142	2.3	3	1	1	2	3	4	5	8
35–49	55	2.3	2	1	1	2	3	3	5	10
50–64	0									
65+	0									
GRAND TOTAL	209	2.3	2	1	1	2	3	4	5	8

74.4: CESAREAN SECTION NEC

Type of Patients	Observed Patients	Avg. Stay	Variance	10th	25th	50th	75th	90th	95th	99th
1. SINGLE DX										
0–19 Years	2	3.0	0	3	3	3	3	3	3	3
20–34	29	2.5	<1	2	2	2	3	3	3	4
35–49	2	3.5	<1	3	3	4	4	4	4	4
50–64	0									
65+	0									
2. MULTIPLE DX										
0–19 Years	25	3.6	5	2	2	3	4	5	9	12
20–34	313	4.2	20	2	3	3	4	6	10	25
35–49	118	5.4	51	2	3	3	4	9	19	41
50–64	7	3.6	<1	3	3	3	4	5	5	5
65+	0									
TOTAL SINGLE DX	33	2.6	<1	2	2	3	3	3	4	4
TOTAL MULTIPLE DX	463	4.5	27	2	3	3	4	6	10	33
TOTAL										
0–19 Years	27	3.6	5	2	2	3	4	5	9	12
20–34	342	4.1	18	2	3	3	4	6	10	25
35–49	120	5.3	51	2	3	4	4	7	13	41
50–64	7	3.6	<1	3	3	3	4	5	5	5
65+	0									
GRAND TOTAL	496	4.4	25	2	3	3	4	6	10	33

LOS by Diagnosis and Operation, Western Region, 45th Edition

Western Region, October 2007–September 2008 Data, by Operation

74.9: CESAREAN SECTION NOS

Type of Patients	Observed Patients	Avg. Stay	Variance	10th	25th	50th	75th	90th	95th	99th
1. SINGLE DX										
0–19 Years	4	2.5	<1	2	2	2	3	3	3	3
20–34	51	2.7	<1	2	2	3	3	3	4	5
35–49	5	3.0	2	2	2	2	4	5	5	5
50–64	0									
65+	0									
2. MULTIPLE DX										
0–19 Years	27	4.4	26	2	3	3	4	4	19	25
20–34	256	3.1	2	2	2	3	4	4	5	12
35–49	77	3.5	4	2	2	3	4	5	7	12
50–64	7	3.3	<1	2	3	3	5	5	5	5
65+	0									
TOTAL SINGLE DX	60	2.7	<1	2	2	3	3	4	5	5
TOTAL MULTIPLE DX	367	3.3	4	2	2	3	4	4	5	13
TOTAL										
0–19 Years	31	4.2	23	2	3	3	4	4	19	25
20–34	307	3.1	2	2	2	3	4	4	5	6
35–49	82	3.4	3	2	2	3	4	5	7	12
50–64	7	3.3	<1	2	3	3	4	5	5	5
65+	0									
GRAND TOTAL	427	3.2	4	2	2	3	4	4	5	12

74.99: OTHER CD TYPE NOS

Type of Patients	Observed Patients	Avg. Stay	Variance	10th	25th	50th	75th	90th	95th	99th
1. SINGLE DX										
0–19 Years	4	2.5	<1	2	2	2	3	3	3	3
20–34	50	2.7	<1	2	2	3	3	4	4	5
35–49	4	2.5	<1	2	2	2	2	4	4	4
50–64	0									
65+	0									
2. MULTIPLE DX										
0–19 Years	27	4.4	26	2	3	3	4	4	19	25
20–34	249	3.1	2	2	2	3	4	4	5	12
35–49	70	3.4	3	2	2	3	4	5	7	12
50–64	5	3.4	1	2	3	3	4	5	5	5
65+	0									
TOTAL SINGLE DX	58	2.7	<1	2	2	3	3	4	4	5
TOTAL MULTIPLE DX	351	3.3	4	2	2	3	4	4	5	13
TOTAL										
0–19 Years	31	4.2	23	2	2	3	4	4	19	25
20–34	299	3.1	2	2	2	3	3	4	5	6
35–49	74	3.3	3	2	2	3	4	4	7	12
50–64	5	3.4	1	2	3	3	4	5	5	5
65+	0									
GRAND TOTAL	409	3.2	4	2	2	3	4	4	5	12

75.0: INTRA-AMNIO INJECT-AB

Type of Patients	Observed Patients	Avg. Stay	Variance	10th	25th	50th	75th	90th	95th	99th
1. SINGLE DX										
0–19 Years	0									
20–34	2	1.0	0	1	1	1	1	1	1	1
35–49	0									
50–64	0									
65+	0									
2. MULTIPLE DX										
0–19 Years	2	2.0	0	2	2	2	2	2	2	2
20–34	39	1.8	2	1	1	1	2	3	4	7
35–49	12	1.3	<1	1	1	1	2	2	2	2
50–64	2	1.5	<1	1	1	1	2	2	2	2
65+	0									
TOTAL SINGLE DX	2	1.0	0	1	1	1	1	1	1	1
TOTAL MULTIPLE DX	55	1.7	1	1	1	1	2	3	4	7
TOTAL										
0–19 Years	2	2.0	0	2	2	2	2	2	2	2
20–34	41	1.7	2	1	1	1	2	3	4	7
35–49	12	1.3	<1	1	1	1	2	2	2	2
50–64	2	1.5	<1	1	1	1	2	2	2	2
65+	0									
GRAND TOTAL	57	1.6	1	1	1	1	2	3	4	7

75.1: DIAGNOSTIC AMNIOCENTESIS

Type of Patients	Observed Patients	Avg. Stay	Variance	10th	25th	50th	75th	90th	95th	99th
1. SINGLE DX										
0–19 Years	11	4.8	70	1	1	2	4	9	29	29
20–34	56	3.7	26	1	1	2	3	10	18	24
35–49	7	1.1	<1	1	1	1	1	2	2	2
50–64	0									
65+	0									
2. MULTIPLE DX										
0–19 Years	61	4.7	33	1	1	3	5	15	18	29
20–34	370	5.4	66	1	2	3	5	12	19	49
35–49	96	5.3	79	1	1	3	5	10	14	65
50–64	3	3.4	8	1	1	1	6	6	6	6
65+	0									
TOTAL SINGLE DX	74	3.7	30	1	1	2	3	10	18	29
TOTAL MULTIPLE DX	530	5.3	64	1	1	3	5	11	18	49
TOTAL										
0–19 Years	72	4.7	37	1	1	2	5	15	20	29
20–34	426	5.2	61	1	1	3	5	12	19	36
35–49	103	5.0	74	1	1	3	5	10	12	54
50–64	3	3.4	8	1	1	1	6	6	6	6
65+	0									
GRAND TOTAL	604	5.1	60	1	1	3	5	11	18	36

LOS by Diagnosis and Operation, Western Region, 45th Edition

75.2: INTRAUTERINE TRANSFUSION

Type of Patients	Observed Patients	Avg. Stay	Vari-ance	Percentiles						
				10th	25th	50th	75th	90th	95th	99th
1. SINGLE DX										
0–19 Years	0									
20–34	5	1.2	<1	1	1	1	1	2	2	2
35–49	2	1.0	0	1	1	1	1	1	1	1
50–64	0									
65+	0									
2. MULTIPLE DX										
0–19 Years	2	2.5	4	1	1	1	4	4	4	4
20–34	18	2.7	8	1	1	2	2	7	12	12
35–49	16	2.1	9	1	1	1	2	4	13	13
50–64	0									
65+	0									
TOTAL SINGLE DX	7	1.1	<1	1	1	1	1	2	2	2
TOTAL MULTIPLE DX	36	2.4	8	1	1	1	2	6	12	13
TOTAL										
0–19 Years	2	2.5	4	1	1	1	4	4	4	4
20–34	23	2.4	7	1	1	1	2	6	7	12
35–49	18	2.0	8	1	1	1	1	4	13	13
50–64	0									
65+	0									
GRAND TOTAL	43	2.2	7	1	1	1	2	4	7	13

75.32: FETAL EKG

Type of Patients	Observed Patients	Avg. Stay	Vari-ance	Percentiles						
				10th	25th	50th	75th	90th	95th	99th
1. SINGLE DX										
0–19 Years	7	2.1	<1	2	2	2	2	3	3	3
20–34	72	1.8	<1	1	1	2	2	3	3	3
35–49	1	1.0	0	1	1	1	1	1	1	1
50–64	0									
65+	0									
2. MULTIPLE DX										
0–19 Years	30	2.7	2	1	2	2	3	4	6	6
20–34	188	2.2	2	1	2	2	2	3	4	6
35–49	41	2.0	<1	1	1	2	2	3	4	5
50–64	2	2.5	<1	2	2	2	3	3	3	3
65+	0									
TOTAL SINGLE DX	80	1.8	<1	1	1	2	2	3	3	3
TOTAL MULTIPLE DX	261	2.2	1	1	2	2	3	3	4	6
TOTAL										
0–19 Years	37	2.6	2	1	2	2	3	4	6	6
20–34	260	2.1	1	1	1	2	2	3	3	6
35–49	42	2.0	<1	1	1	2	2	3	4	5
50–64	2	2.5	<1	2	2	2	3	3	3	3
65+	0									
GRAND TOTAL	341	2.1	1	1	2	2	2	3	4	6

75.3: IU OPS FETUS & AMNIO NEC

Type of Patients	Observed Patients	Avg. Stay	Vari-ance	Percentiles						
				10th	25th	50th	75th	90th	95th	99th
1. SINGLE DX										
0–19 Years	276	1.9	3	1	1	1	2	3	5	11
20–34	1,457	1.8	6	1	1	1	2	3	4	9
35–49	119	1.5	2	1	1	1	2	2	3	5
50–64	5	1.3	<1	1	1	1	2	2	2	2
65+	0									
2. MULTIPLE DX										
0–19 Years	671	3.0	22	1	1	2	3	5	9	23
20–34	4,131	3.0	25	1	1	2	3	5	8	28
35–49	1,105	3.5	54	1	1	2	3	6	11	52
50–64	46	4.5	49	1	1	2	4	10	22	37
65+	0									
TOTAL SINGLE DX	1,857	1.8	5	1	1	1	2	3	4	9
TOTAL MULTIPLE DX	5,953	3.1	30	1	1	2	3	5	8	30
TOTAL										
0–19 Years	947	2.7	17	1	1	2	3	5	7	18
20–34	5,588	2.7	21	1	1	2	3	4	7	22
35–49	1,224	3.3	49	1	1	2	3	5	10	42
50–64	51	4.1	44	1	1	2	4	7	22	37
65+	0									
GRAND TOTAL	7,810	2.8	25	1	1	2	3	5	7	24

75.34: FETAL MONITORING NEC

Type of Patients	Observed Patients	Avg. Stay	Vari-ance	Percentiles						
				10th	25th	50th	75th	90th	95th	99th
1. SINGLE DX										
0–19 Years	259	1.9	4	1	1	1	2	4	5	11
20–34	1,313	1.8	7	1	1	1	2	3	4	9
35–49	114	1.5	2	1	1	1	2	2	3	5
50–64	4	1.3	<1	1	1	1	2	2	2	2
65+	0									
2. MULTIPLE DX										
0–19 Years	580	3.1	24	1	1	2	3	5	9	27
20–34	3,564	3.1	26	1	1	2	3	5	8	29
35–49	975	3.7	60	1	1	2	3	6	12	56
50–64	42	4.8	53	1	1	2	4	10	22	37
65+	0									
TOTAL SINGLE DX	1,690	1.8	6	1	1	1	2	3	5	9
TOTAL MULTIPLE DX	5,161	3.2	33	1	1	2	3	6	9	31
TOTAL										
0–19 Years	839	2.7	18	1	1	2	3	5	7	21
20–34	4,877	2.7	21	1	1	2	3	5	7	23
35–49	1,089	3.5	54	1	1	2	3	6	12	52
50–64	46	4.4	48	1	1	2	4	10	22	37
65+	0									
GRAND TOTAL	6,851	2.9	27	1	1	2	3	5	8	27

LOS by Diagnosis and Operation, Western Region, 45th Edition

Western Region, October 2007–September 2008 Data, by Operation

75.4: MAN RMVL OF RET PLACENTA

Type of Patients	Observed Patients	Avg. Stay	Vari-ance	Percentiles						
				10th	25th	50th	75th	90th	95th	99th
1. SINGLE DX										
0–19 Years	14	1.5	<1	1	1	2	2	2	2	2
20–34	165	1.4	<1	1	1	1	2	2	2	3
35–49	20	1.6	<1	1	1	2	2	2	2	2
50–64	2	1.5	<1	1	1	1	2	2	2	2
65+	0									
2. MULTIPLE DX										
0–19 Years	46	2.0	<1	1	1	2	2	3	3	5
20–34	412	2.2	21	1	1	2	2	3	3	8
35–49	98	2.9	61	1	1	2	2	3	5	77
50–64	2	3.5	<1	3	3	4	4	4	4	4
65+	0									
TOTAL SINGLE DX	201	1.4	<1	1	1	1	2	2	2	2
TOTAL MULTIPLE DX	558	2.3	26	1	1	2	2	3	3	13
TOTAL										
0–19 Years	60	1.9	<1	1	1	2	2	3	3	5
20–34	577	2.0	15	1	1	2	2	3	3	7
35–49	118	2.7	51	1	1	2	2	3	4	20
50–64	4	2.5	2	3	3	2	4	4	4	4
65+	0									
GRAND TOTAL	759	2.1	19	1	1	2	2	3	3	7

75.5: REP CURRENT OB LAC UTER

Type of Patients	Observed Patients	Avg. Stay	Vari-ance	Percentiles						
				10th	25th	50th	75th	90th	95th	99th
1. SINGLE DX										
0–19 Years	7	2.0	0	2	2	2	2	2	2	2
20–34	23	1.8	<1	1	1	2	2	3	3	4
35–49	1	1.0	0	1	1	1	1	1	1	1
50–64	0									
65+	0									
2. MULTIPLE DX										
0–19 Years	73	2.8	3	2	2	2	3	4	6	13
20–34	347	2.5	14	1	2	2	3	3	4	7
35–49	79	2.5	1	1	2	3	3	4	5	6
50–64	3	2.7	<1	2	2	3	3	3	3	3
65+	0									
TOTAL SINGLE DX	31	1.8	<1	1	1	2	2	3	3	4
TOTAL MULTIPLE DX	502	2.5	10	1	2	2	3	3	4	7
TOTAL										
0–19 Years	80	2.7	3	2	2	2	3	4	5	13
20–34	370	2.4	13	1	2	2	3	3	4	7
35–49	80	2.5	1	1	2	3	3	4	4	6
50–64	3	2.7	<1	2	2	3	3	3	3	3
65+	0									
GRAND TOTAL	533	2.5	9	1	2	2	3	3	4	7

75.35: DXTIC PX FETUS/AMNIO NEC

Type of Patients	Observed Patients	Avg. Stay	Vari-ance	Percentiles						
				10th	25th	50th	75th	90th	95th	99th
1. SINGLE DX										
0–19 Years	10	1.6	<1	1	1	2	2	3	3	3
20–34	41	1.8	4	1	1	1	2	2	3	14
35–49	2	1.0	0	1	1	1	1	1	1	1
50–64	0									
65+	0									
2. MULTIPLE DX										
0–19 Years	43	2.8	9	1	1	2	3	5	11	14
20–34	237	3.0	40	1	1	2	3	4	5	42
35–49	54	2.6	8	1	1	2	3	3	8	20
50–64	0									
65+	0									
TOTAL SINGLE DX	53	1.7	4	1	1	1	2	2	3	14
TOTAL MULTIPLE DX	334	2.9	31	1	1	2	3	4	7	24
TOTAL										
0–19 Years	53	2.6	8	1	1	2	3	4	11	14
20–34	278	2.9	35	1	1	2	3	3	5	42
35–49	56	2.5	8	1	1	2	3	3	8	20
50–64	0									
65+	0									
GRAND TOTAL	387	2.8	27	1	1	2	3	3	5	24

75.37: AMNIOINFUSION

Type of Patients	Observed Patients	Avg. Stay	Vari-ance	Percentiles						
				10th	25th	50th	75th	90th	95th	99th
1. SINGLE DX										
0–19 Years	0									
20–34	21	1.7	<1	1	2	2	2	3	3	3
35–49	1	2.0	0	2	2	2	2	2	2	2
50–64	0									
65+	0									
2. MULTIPLE DX										
0–19 Years	15	2.8	3	1	2	3	3	4	8	8
20–34	98	2.1	<1	1	2	2	3	3	3	5
35–49	19	2.4	<1	1	2	2	3	3	4	4
50–64	0									
65+	0									
TOTAL SINGLE DX	22	1.7	<1	1	1	2	2	3	3	3
TOTAL MULTIPLE DX	132	2.2	<1	1	2	2	3	3	3	5
TOTAL										
0–19 Years	15	2.8	3	1	2	3	3	4	8	8
20–34	119	2.0	<1	1	1	2	3	3	3	4
35–49	20	2.4	<1	2	2	2	3	3	4	4
50–64	0									
65+	0									
GRAND TOTAL	154	2.1	<1	1	2	2	3	3	3	5

Western Region, October 2007–September 2008 Data, by Operation

75.51: REP CURRENT OB LAC CERV

Type of Patients	Observed Patients	Avg. Stay	Variance	10th	25th	50th	75th	90th	95th	99th
1. SINGLE DX										
0–19 Years	7	2.0	0	2	2	2	2	2	2	2
20–34	23	1.8	<1	1	1	2	2	3	3	4
35–49	1	1.0	0	1	1	1	1	1	1	1
50–64	0									
65+	0									
2. MULTIPLE DX										
0–19 Years	72	2.8	3	2	2	2	3	4	6	13
20–34	338	2.5	14	1	2	2	3	3	4	7
35–49	77	2.5	1	2	2	2	3	4	5	6
50–64	2	2.5	<1	2	2	3	3	3	3	3
65+	0									
TOTAL SINGLE DX	31	1.8	<1	1	1	2	2	3	3	4
TOTAL MULTIPLE DX	489	2.5	10	1	2	2	3	3	4	10
TOTAL										
0–19 Years	79	2.7	3	2	2	2	3	4	6	13
20–34	361	2.4	13	1	2	2	3	3	4	7
35–49	78	2.4	1	1	2	2	3	4	5	6
50–64	2	2.5	<1	2	2	3	3	3	3	3
65+	0									
GRAND TOTAL	520	2.5	10	1	2	2	3	3	4	7

75.6: REP OTH CURRENT OB LAC

Type of Patients	Observed Patients	Avg. Stay	Variance	10th	25th	50th	75th	90th	95th	99th
1. SINGLE DX										
0–19 Years	2,850	1.9	<1	1	1	2	2	3	3	3
20–34	18,911	1.8	<1	1	1	2	2	3	3	3
35–49	834	1.7	<1	1	1	2	2	2	3	3
50–64	39	1.9	<1	1	2	2	2	3	3	3
65+	0									
2. MULTIPLE DX										
0–19 Years	11,082	2.2	2	1	2	2	3	3	3	5
20–34	68,880	2.1	2	1	2	2	2	3	3	4
35–49	13,332	2.0	1	1	1	2	2	3	4	4
50–64	466	2.0	<1	2	2	3	3	3	3	4
65+	0									
TOTAL SINGLE DX	22,634	1.8	<1	1	1	2	2	3	3	3
TOTAL MULTIPLE DX	93,760	2.1	2	1	2	2	2	3	3	4
TOTAL										
0–19 Years	13,932	2.1	2	1	2	2	2	3	3	5
20–34	87,791	2.0	1	1	1	2	2	3	3	4
35–49	14,166	2.0	1	1	1	2	2	3	3	4
50–64	505	2.0	<1	1	1	2	2	3	3	4
65+	0									
GRAND TOTAL	116,394	2.0	1	1	2	2	3	3	4	4

75.61: REP OB LAC BLAD/URETHRA

Type of Patients	Observed Patients	Avg. Stay	Variance	10th	25th	50th	75th	90th	95th	99th
1. SINGLE DX										
0–19 Years	38	2.0	<1	1	2	2	2	3	3	3
20–34	156	1.8	<1	1	1	2	2	3	3	3
35–49	6	2.0	0	2	2	2	2	2	2	2
50–64	0									
65+	0									
2. MULTIPLE DX										
0–19 Years	230	2.3	2	1	2	2	3	3	4	5
20–34	972	2.0	2	1	2	2	3	3	4	4
35–49	134	2.0	<1	1	2	2	3	3	4	5
50–64	3	2.0	0	2	2	3	3	4	4	4
65+	0									
TOTAL SINGLE DX	200	1.9	<1	1	1	2	2	3	3	4
TOTAL MULTIPLE DX	1,339	2.1	2	1	2	2	3	3	3	5
TOTAL										
0–19 Years	268	2.2	2	1	2	2	3	3	4	5
20–34	1,128	2.0	1	1	2	2	3	3	3	4
35–49	140	2.0	<1	1	2	2	3	3	4	5
50–64	3	2.0	0	2	2	3	3	4	4	4
65+	0									
GRAND TOTAL	1,539	2.0	1	1	2	2	3	3	3	4

75.62: REP OB LAC RECTUM/ANUS

Type of Patients	Observed Patients	Avg. Stay	Variance	10th	25th	50th	75th	90th	95th	99th
1. SINGLE DX										
0–19 Years	141	2.0	<1	1	2	2	2	3	3	4
20–34	742	2.0	<1	1	2	2	2	3	3	4
35–49	27	2.1	<1	1	2	2	3	3	3	3
50–64	2	2.5	<1	2	2	3	3	3	3	3
65+	0									
2. MULTIPLE DX										
0–19 Years	592	2.3	<1	1	2	2	3	3	4	5
20–34	3,870	2.3	1	1	2	2	3	3	4	4
35–49	547	2.3	<1	1	2	2	3	3	4	5
50–64	17	2.7	<1	2	2	3	3	4	4	4
65+	0									
TOTAL SINGLE DX	912	2.0	<1	1	2	2	2	3	3	4
TOTAL MULTIPLE DX	5,026	2.3	<1	1	2	2	3	3	4	5
TOTAL										
0–19 Years	733	2.2	<1	1	2	2	3	3	4	5
20–34	4,612	2.2	<1	1	2	2	3	3	4	4
35–49	574	2.3	<1	1	2	2	3	3	4	5
50–64	19	2.7	<1	2	2	3	3	4	4	4
65+	0									
GRAND TOTAL	5,938	2.2	<1	1	2	2	3	3	3	4

LOS by Diagnosis and Operation, Western Region, 45th Edition

Western Region, October 2007–September 2008 Data, by Operation

75.69: REP CURRENT OB LAC NEC

Type of Patients	Observed Patients	Avg. Stay	Vari-ance	10th	25th	50th	75th	90th	95th	99th
1. SINGLE DX										
0–19 Years	2,671	1.9	<1	1	1	1	2	2	3	3
20–34	18,013	1.7	<1	1	1	2	2	2	3	3
35–49	801	1.7	<1	1	1	2	2	2	3	3
50–64	37	1.9	<1	1	2	2	2	3	3	3
65+	0									
2. MULTIPLE DX										
0–19 Years	10,260	2.2	2	1	2	2	3	3	3	5
20–34	64,038	2.0	2	1	2	2	2	3	3	4
35–49	12,651	2.0	2	1	1	2	2	3	3	4
50–64	446	2.0	<1	1	1	2	2	3	3	4
65+	0									
TOTAL SINGLE DX	21,522	1.8	<1	1	1	2	2	3	3	3
TOTAL MULTIPLE DX	87,395	2.1	2	1	2	2	2	3	3	4
TOTAL										
0–19 Years	12,931	2.1	2	1	2	2	2	3	3	5
20–34	82,051	2.0	1	1	1	2	2	3	3	4
35–49	13,452	2.0	1	1	1	2	2	3	3	4
50–64	483	1.9	<1	1	1	2	2	3	3	4
65+	0									
GRAND TOTAL	108,917	2.0	1	1	1	2	2	3	3	4

75.8: OB TAMPONADE UTERUS/VAG

Type of Patients	Observed Patients	Avg. Stay	Vari-ance	10th	25th	50th	75th	90th	95th	99th
1. SINGLE DX										
0–19 Years	0									
20–34	0									
35–49	0									
50–64	0									
65+	0									
2. MULTIPLE DX										
0–19 Years	0									
20–34	3	3.3	5	2	2	2	6	6	6	6
35–49	0									
50–64	0									
65+	0									
TOTAL SINGLE DX	0									
TOTAL MULTIPLE DX	3	3.3	5	2	2	2	6	6	6	6
TOTAL										
0–19 Years	0									
20–34	3	3.3	5	2	2	2	6	6	6	6
35–49	0									
50–64	0									
65+	0									
GRAND TOTAL	3	3.3	5	2	2	2	6	6	6	6

75.7: PP MANUAL EXPL UTERUS

Type of Patients	Observed Patients	Avg. Stay	Vari-ance	10th	25th	50th	75th	90th	95th	99th
1. SINGLE DX										
0–19 Years	1	1.0	0	1	1	1	1	1	1	1
20–34	10	1.4	<1	1	1	1	2	2	2	2
35–49	0									
50–64	0									
65+	0									
2. MULTIPLE DX										
0–19 Years	9	2.3	<1	1	2	3	3	3	3	3
20–34	37	2.0	<1	1	1	2	3	3	4	4
35–49	13	1.8	<1	1	1	2	2	2	3	3
50–64	1	1.0	0	1	1	1	1	1	1	1
65+	0									
TOTAL SINGLE DX	11	1.4	<1	1	1	1	2	2	2	2
TOTAL MULTIPLE DX	60	2.0	<1	1	1	2	3	3	3	4
TOTAL										
0–19 Years	10	2.2	<1	1	1	3	3	3	3	3
20–34	47	1.9	<1	1	1	2	2	3	3	4
35–49	13	1.8	<1	1	1	2	2	2	3	3
50–64	1	1.0	0	1	1	1	1	1	1	1
65+	0									
GRAND TOTAL	71	1.9	<1	1	1	2	2	3	3	4

75.9: OTHER OBSTETRICAL OPS

Type of Patients	Observed Patients	Avg. Stay	Vari-ance	10th	25th	50th	75th	90th	95th	99th
1. SINGLE DX										
0–19 Years	1	4.0	0	4	4	4	4	4	4	4
20–34	17	1.7	<1	1	1	2	2	2	2	2
35–49	2	2.0	0	2	2	2	2	2	2	2
50–64	0									
65+	0									
2. MULTIPLE DX										
0–19 Years	15	3.1	2	1	2	3	4	5	5	5
20–34	94	2.6	2	1	2	2	3	4	5	9
35–49	26	2.7	6	1	1	1	3	5	7	12
50–64	1	1.0	0	1	1	1	1	1	1	1
65+	0									
TOTAL SINGLE DX	20	1.9	<1	1	2	2	2	2	2	4
TOTAL MULTIPLE DX	136	2.7	3	1	2	2	3	4	5	9
TOTAL										
0–19 Years	16	3.2	2	1	2	3	4	5	5	5
20–34	111	2.5	2	1	2	2	3	4	5	7
35–49	28	2.6	5	1	1	1	3	5	7	12
50–64	1	1.0	0	1	1	1	1	1	1	1
65+	0									
GRAND TOTAL	156	2.6	2	1	2	2	3	4	5	9

LOS by Diagnosis and Operation, Western Region, 45th Edition

Western Region, October 2007–September 2008 Data, by Operation

76.0: FACIAL BONE INCISION

Type of Patients	Observed Patients	Avg. Stay	Vari-ance	10th	25th	50th	75th	90th	95th	99th
1. SINGLE DX										
0–19 Years	0									
20–34	0									
35–49	0									
50–64	1	1.0	0	1	1	1	1	1	1	1
65+	0									
2. MULTIPLE DX										
0–19 Years	2	4.5	12	2	2	7	7	7	7	7
20–34	6	5.5	54	1	2	2	6	20	20	20
35–49	9	4.1	13	1	2	2	7	11	11	11
50–64	10	3.7	4	2	2	4	5	6	7	7
65+	3	6.0	21	1	1	7	10	10	10	10
TOTAL SINGLE DX	1	1.0	0	1	1	1	1	1	1	1
TOTAL MULTIPLE DX	30	4.5	17	1	2	3	7	8	11	20
TOTAL										
0–19 Years	2	4.5	12	2	2	7	7	7	7	7
20–34	6	5.5	54	1	2	2	6	20	20	20
35–49	9	4.1	13	1	2	2	7	11	11	11
50–64	11	3.5	4	1	2	3	5	6	7	7
65+	3	6.0	21	1	1	7	10	10	10	10
GRAND TOTAL	31	4.4	17	1	2	2	7	8	11	20

76.1: DXTIC PX FACIAL BONE/JT

Type of Patients	Observed Patients	Avg. Stay	Vari-ance	10th	25th	50th	75th	90th	95th	99th
1. SINGLE DX										
0–19 Years	3	1.9	1	1	1	1	3	3	3	3
20–34	0									
35–49	0									
50–64	0									
65+	0									
2. MULTIPLE DX										
0–19 Years	3	5.3	12	4	4	4	4	13	13	13
20–34	7	7.0	43	1	1	5	12	18	18	18
35–49	6	6.0	12	2	3	6	10	10	10	10
50–64	10	7.1	66	1	1	2	11	15	26	26
65+	7	3.3	5	1	2	2	5	7	7	7
TOTAL SINGLE DX	3	1.9	1	1	1	1	3	3	3	3
TOTAL MULTIPLE DX	33	5.9	30	1	2	4	8	13	18	26
TOTAL										
0–19 Years	6	3.3	8	1	1	3	4	4	13	13
20–34	7	7.0	43	1	1	5	12	18	18	18
35–49	6	6.0	12	2	3	6	10	10	10	10
50–64	10	7.1	66	1	1	2	11	15	26	26
65+	7	3.3	5	1	2	2	5	7	7	7
GRAND TOTAL	36	5.1	27	2	2	3	7	12	15	26

76.2: EXC/DESTR FAC BONE LES

Type of Patients	Observed Patients	Avg. Stay	Vari-ance	10th	25th	50th	75th	90th	95th	99th
1. SINGLE DX										
0–19 Years	12	1.9	<1	1	1	2	3	3	3	4
20–34	4	1.8	<1	1	1	2	3	3	3	3
35–49	13	1.6	1	1	1	1	2	3	5	5
50–64	6	1.7	<1	1	1	1	2	3	3	3
65+	2	1.0	0	1	1	1	1	1	1	1
2. MULTIPLE DX										
0–19 Years	18	2.6	5	1	1	1	3	7	7	7
20–34	40	4.4	11	1	2	4	6	9	14	15
35–49	30	4.9	46	1	1	2	6	12	15	33
50–64	52	4.1	27	1	1	2	4	11	18	25
65+	56	4.1	17	1	1	2	5	11	14	18
TOTAL SINGLE DX	37	1.8	<1	1	1	1	2	3	3	5
TOTAL MULTIPLE DX	196	4.0	21	1	1	2	5	9	14	19
TOTAL										
0–19 Years	30	2.3	3	1	1	1	3	6	7	7
20–34	44	4.1	11	1	2	3	6	9	14	15
35–49	43	3.9	35	1	1	2	5	12	15	33
50–64	58	3.8	24	1	1	2	3	11	18	25
65+	58	4.0	17	1	1	2	5	11	14	18
GRAND TOTAL	233	3.6	18	1	1	2	4	8	13	19

76.3: PARTIAL FACIAL OSTECTOMY

Type of Patients	Observed Patients	Avg. Stay	Vari-ance	10th	25th	50th	75th	90th	95th	99th
1. SINGLE DX										
0–19 Years	4	1.0	0	1	1	1	1	1	1	1
20–34	5	1.4	<1	1	1	1	2	2	2	2
35–49	6	1.3	<1	1	1	1	3	3	3	3
50–64	4	2.7	3	1	1	2	5	5	5	5
65+	3	2.4	2	1	1	2	4	4	4	4
2. MULTIPLE DX										
0–19 Years	23	3.4	4	1	2	3	4	7	8	8
20–34	23	3.9	20	1	1	2	4	8	15	18
35–49	39	6.5	91	1	2	5	7	14	22	55
50–64	83	7.5	73	1	2	5	9	16	25	48
65+	135	7.0	48	1	2	5	9	16	22	29
TOTAL SINGLE DX	22	1.5	<1	1	1	1	2	3	4	5
TOTAL MULTIPLE DX	303	6.3	53	1	2	4	8	14	22	38
TOTAL										
0–19 Years	27	2.9	4	1	1	2	4	5	8	8
20–34	28	3.4	17	1	1	3	6	8	15	18
35–49	45	5.8	82	1	2	3	9	14	19	55
50–64	87	7.3	71	1	2	5	9	16	25	48
65+	138	6.9	47	1	2	5	9	16	22	29
GRAND TOTAL	325	5.9	50	1	1	4	7	14	22	38

LOS by Diagnosis and Operation, Western Region, 45th Edition

76.31: PARTIAL MANDIBULECTOMY

Type of Patients	Observed Patients	Avg. Stay	Vari-ance	Percentiles						
				10th	25th	50th	75th	90th	95th	99th
1. SINGLE DX										
0–19 Years	3	1.0	0	1	1	1	1	1	1	1
20–34	1	1.0	0	1	1	1	1	1	1	1
35–49	4	1.5	<1	1	1	1	1	3	3	3
50–64	3	3.3	2	2	2	3	5	5	5	5
65+	1	2.0	0	2	2	2	2	2	2	2
2. MULTIPLE DX										
0–19 Years	11	3.5	3	2	2	4	5	5	5	7
20–34	19	3.9	24	1	1	2	4	15	18	18
35–49	26	7.1	121	1	3	4	7	14	19	55
50–64	65	8.6	84	2	3	6	10	24	26	48
65+	97	8.3	57	1	3	7	11	20	24	42
TOTAL SINGLE DX	12	1.6	1	1	1	1	2	3	5	5
TOTAL MULTIPLE DX	218	7.5	67	1	2	5	9	17	24	42
TOTAL										
0–19 Years	14	2.7	3	1	1	2	4	5	5	7
20–34	20	3.7	23	1	1	2	3	8	18	18
35–49	30	6.4	108	1	1	3	7	14	19	55
50–64	68	8.4	82	1	3	6	10	24	26	48
65+	98	8.2	57	1	3	7	11	20	24	42
GRAND TOTAL	230	7.0	64	1	2	5	8	16	24	42

76.4: FACIAL BONE EXC/RECONST

Type of Patients	Observed Patients	Avg. Stay	Vari-ance	Percentiles						
				10th	25th	50th	75th	90th	95th	99th
1. SINGLE DX										
0–19 Years	14	3.5	3	1	3	3	5	6	6	6
20–34	8	2.3	6	1	1	1	3	8	8	8
35–49	1	2.0	0	2	2	2	2	2	2	2
50–64	6	5.0	25	2	2	3	5	15	15	15
65+	1	1.0	0	1	1	1	1	1	1	1
2. MULTIPLE DX										
0–19 Years	55	3.2	6	1	1	3	4	5	6	11
20–34	30	1.7	1	1	1	1	2	3	5	5
35–49	20	6.0	38	1	2	2	13	15	18	18
50–64	29	4.8	33	1	2	4	6	17	17	19
65+	20	5.5	42	1	2	4	6	10	18	27
TOTAL SINGLE DX	30	3.4	7	1	1	3	5	6	8	15
TOTAL MULTIPLE DX	154	3.7	17	1	1	2	4	8	14	19
TOTAL										
0–19 Years	69	3.3	6	1	1	3	4	5	6	11
20–34	38	1.8	2	1	1	1	2	3	5	8
35–49	21	5.8	36	1	2	2	13	15	15	18
50–64	35	4.9	31	1	1	2	6	15	17	19
65+	21	5.3	41	1	2	3	6	10	18	27
GRAND TOTAL	184	3.7	15	1	1	2	4	7	13	19

76.39: PART FACIAL OSTECT NEC

Type of Patients	Observed Patients	Avg. Stay	Vari-ance	Percentiles						
				10th	25th	50th	75th	90th	95th	99th
1. SINGLE DX										
0–19 Years	1	1.0	0	1	1	1	1	1	1	1
20–34	4	1.5	<1	1	1	1	1	2	2	2
35–49	2	1.0	0	1	1	1	1	1	1	1
50–64	1	1.0	0	1	1	1	1	1	1	1
65+	2	2.5	4	1	1	4	4	4	4	4
2. MULTIPLE DX										
0–19 Years	12	3.3	6	1	2	2	4	8	8	8
20–34	4	3.8	3	2	2	3	6	6	6	6
35–49	13	5.3	37	1	1	4	6	13	22	22
50–64	18	8.4	13	1	1	2	5	10	14	14
65+	38	3.9	11	1	1	3	6	8	13	13
TOTAL SINGLE DX	10	1.4	<1	1	1	1	1	2	4	4
TOTAL MULTIPLE DX	85	3.8	13	1	1	3	5	8	11	14
TOTAL										
0–19 Years	13	3.0	5	1	1	2	4	8	8	8
20–34	8	2.6	3	1	1	2	3	6	6	6
35–49	15	4.7	34	1	1	2	6	13	22	22
50–64	19	3.4	13	1	1	2	5	10	14	14
65+	40	3.8	11	1	1	3	6	8	13	13
GRAND TOTAL	95	3.6	12	1	1	2	4	8	11	14

76.5: TMJ ARTHROPLASTY

Type of Patients	Observed Patients	Avg. Stay	Vari-ance	Percentiles						
				10th	25th	50th	75th	90th	95th	99th
1. SINGLE DX										
0–19 Years	2	1.0	0	1	1	1	1	1	1	1
20–34	5	1.2	<1	1	1	1	1	2	2	2
35–49	1	1.0	0	1	1	1	1	1	1	1
50–64	7	1.7	2	1	1	1	3	4	4	4
65+	0									
2. MULTIPLE DX										
0–19 Years	6	4.9	38	2	2	3	5	5	24	24
20–34	9	1.6	<1	1	1	1	2	3	3	3
35–49	14	2.2	<1	1	1	1	3	3	5	5
50–64	26	1.7	<1	1	1	1	2	3	3	5
65+	3	1.3	<1	1	1	1	2	2	2	2
TOTAL SINGLE DX	15	1.4	<1	1	1	1	1	3	4	4
TOTAL MULTIPLE DX	58	2.4	9	1	1	2	2	5	5	24
TOTAL										
0–19 Years	8	4.4	34	1	2	2	5	5	24	24
20–34	14	1.4	<1	1	1	1	2	3	3	3
35–49	15	2.1	1	1	1	2	2	3	5	5
50–64	33	1.7	1	1	1	1	2	3	4	5
65+	3	1.3	<1	1	1	1	2	2	2	2
GRAND TOTAL	73	2.2	8	1	1	2	2	4	5	24

Western Region, October 2007–September 2008 Data, by Operation

76.6: OTHER FACIAL BONE REPAIR

Type of Patients	Observed Patients	Avg. Stay	Variance	10th	25th	50th	75th	90th	95th	99th
1. SINGLE DX										
0–19 Years	115	1.5	<1	1	1	1	2	2	4	5
20–34	145	1.3	<1	1	1	1	1	2	2	4
35–49	51	1.3	<1	1	1	1	1	2	2	3
50–64	31	1.4	<1	1	1	1	2	2	2	4
65+	0									
2. MULTIPLE DX										
0–19 Years	585	2.6	27	1	1	1	2	4	6	29
20–34	525	1.6	1	1	1	1	2	3	3	6
35–49	217	1.9	1	1	1	1	2	3	4	7
50–64	184	1.8	2	1	1	2	2	3	4	10
65+	5	1.0	0	1	1	1	1	1	1	1
TOTAL SINGLE DX	342	1.4	<1	1	1	1	2	2	3	5
TOTAL MULTIPLE DX	1,516	2.1	14	1	1	1	2	3	4	25
TOTAL										
0–19 Years	700	2.4	24	1	1	1	2	3	6	29
20–34	670	1.6	1	1	1	1	2	2	3	5
35–49	268	1.7	1	1	1	1	2	3	4	7
50–64	215	1.7	2	1	1	1	2	3	4	6
65+	5	1.0	0	1	1	1	1	1	1	1
GRAND TOTAL	1,858	2.0	12	1	1	1	2	3	4	11

76.62: OPEN OSTY MAND RAMUS

Type of Patients	Observed Patients	Avg. Stay	Variance	10th	25th	50th	75th	90th	95th	99th
1. SINGLE DX										
0–19 Years	27	1.2	<1	1	1	1	1	2	2	2
20–34	47	1.1	<1	1	1	1	1	2	2	2
35–49	12	1.1	<1	1	1	1	1	1	2	2
50–64	13	1.2	<1	1	1	1	1	2	2	2
65+	0									
2. MULTIPLE DX										
0–19 Years	117	1.8	2	1	1	1	2	3	4	9
20–34	80	1.4	<1	1	1	1	2	2	3	5
35–49	32	1.3	<1	1	1	1	2	2	3	3
50–64	42	1.6	1	1	1	1	2	3	3	6
65+	0									
TOTAL SINGLE DX	99	1.2	<1	1	1	1	1	2	2	2
TOTAL MULTIPLE DX	271	1.6	1	1	1	1	2	3	4	8
TOTAL										
0–19 Years	144	1.7	2	1	1	1	2	3	4	9
20–34	127	1.3	<1	1	1	1	1	2	2	4
35–49	44	1.3	<1	1	1	1	2	2	2	3
50–64	55	1.5	<1	1	1	1	2	2	3	6
65+	0									
GRAND TOTAL	370	1.5	1	1	1	1	2	3	3	6

76.64: MAND ORTHOGNATHIC OP NEC

Type of Patients	Observed Patients	Avg. Stay	Variance	10th	25th	50th	75th	90th	95th	99th
1. SINGLE DX										
0–19 Years	30	1.3	<1	1	1	1	2	2	2	2
20–34	14	1.1	<1	1	1	1	1	1	2	2
35–49	14	1.5	<1	1	1	1	2	2	2	2
50–64	4	1.3	<1	1	1	1	1	2	2	2
65+	0									
2. MULTIPLE DX										
0–19 Years	87	5.9	119	1	1	2	4	25	34	48
20–34	46	1.8	<1	1	1	2	2	3	3	9
35–49	35	2.3	2	1	1	2	3	4	5	8
50–64	44	1.6	2	1	1	1	1	3	3	4
65+	2	1.0	0	1	1	1	1	1	1	1
TOTAL SINGLE DX	62	1.3	<1	1	1	1	2	2	2	2
TOTAL MULTIPLE DX	214	3.8	60	1	1	2	3	7	13	48
TOTAL										
0–19 Years	117	4.7	92	1	1	1	3	8	29	48
20–34	60	1.6	1	1	1	1	2	2	3	9
35–49	49	2.1	2	1	1	1	2	3	4	8
50–64	48	1.6	<1	1	1	1	2	3	3	4
65+	2	1.0	0	1	1	1	1	1	1	1
GRAND TOTAL	276	3.2	48	1	1	1	2	4	8	48

76.65: SEG OSTEOPLASTY MAXILLA

Type of Patients	Observed Patients	Avg. Stay	Variance	10th	25th	50th	75th	90th	95th	99th
1. SINGLE DX										
0–19 Years	38	1.4	<1	1	1	1	2	2	2	4
20–34	53	1.2	<1	1	1	1	1	2	3	3
35–49	19	1.3	<1	1	1	1	1	3	3	3
50–64	6	1.8	1	1	1	2	2	4	4	4
65+	0									
2. MULTIPLE DX										
0–19 Years	238	1.8	2	1	1	2	2	3	3	11
20–34	293	1.7	1	1	1	1	2	3	3	5
35–49	95	1.8	1	1	1	2	2	3	4	7
50–64	64	2.1	2	1	1	2	2	3	5	10
65+	1	1.0	0	1	1	1	1	1	1	1
TOTAL SINGLE DX	116	1.3	<1	1	1	1	2	2	3	4
TOTAL MULTIPLE DX	691	1.8	2	1	1	1	2	3	3	7
TOTAL										
0–19 Years	276	1.7	2	1	1	1	2	3	3	11
20–34	346	1.6	1	1	1	1	2	3	3	5
35–49	114	1.7	1	1	1	2	2	3	4	5
50–64	70	2.1	2	1	1	1	2	3	5	10
65+	1	1.0	0	1	1	1	1	1	1	1
GRAND TOTAL	807	1.7	1	1	1	1	2	3	3	6

LOS by Diagnosis and Operation, Western Region, 45th Edition

Western Region, October 2007–September 2008 Data, by Operation

76.66: TOT OSTEOPLASTY MAXILLA

Type of Patients	Observed Patients	Avg. Stay	Vari-ance	10th	25th	50th	75th	90th	95th	99th
1. SINGLE DX										
0–19 Years	9	1.8	<1	1	1	2	3	3	3	3
20–34	14	2.3	4	1	1	2	2	3	3	9
35–49	3	3.0	0	1	1	1	1	1	1	1
50–64	1	1.0	0	1	1	1	1	1	1	1
65+	0									
2. MULTIPLE DX										
0–19 Years	99	1.7	1	1	1	1	2	3	4	6
20–34	70	1.7	1	1	1	1	2	3	4	7
35–49	23	2.3	1	1	1	2	3	4	5	5
50–64	12	1.7	<1	1	1	1	2	3	4	4
65+	0									
TOTAL SINGLE DX	27	1.9	2	1	1	2	2	3	3	9
TOTAL MULTIPLE DX	204	1.8	1	1	1	1	2	3	4	6
TOTAL										
0–19 Years	108	1.7	1	1	1	1	2	3	4	6
20–34	84	1.8	2	1	1	2	2	3	4	9
35–49	26	2.1	3	1	1	2	2	4	5	5
50–64	13	1.6	<1	1	1	1	2	3	4	4
65+	0									
GRAND TOTAL	231	1.8	1	1	1	1	2	3	4	6

76.72: OPEN RED MALAR/ZMC FX

Type of Patients	Observed Patients	Avg. Stay	Vari-ance	10th	25th	50th	75th	90th	95th	99th
1. SINGLE DX										
0–19 Years	4	2.3	4	1	1	1	5	5	5	5
20–34	26	1.4	<1	1	1	1	1	2	3	5
35–49	6	1.3	<1	1	1	1	2	2	2	2
50–64	6	1.8	2	1	1	1	3	4	4	4
65+	1	1.0	0	1	1	1	1	1	1	1
2. MULTIPLE DX										
0–19 Years	52	3.2	11	1	1	2	4	7	10	18
20–34	157	4.0	18	1	1	2	5	9	14	19
35–49	143	4.7	34	1	2	3	6	9	15	36
50–64	91	5.9	80	1	2	3	6	10	26	51
65+	29	7.1	38	1	2	5	10	15	18	28
TOTAL SINGLE DX	43	1.5	1	1	1	1	2	3	4	5
TOTAL MULTIPLE DX	472	4.6	35	1	1	3	6	10	15	34
TOTAL										
0–19 Years	56	3.1	11	1	1	2	4	7	10	18
20–34	183	3.6	16	1	1	2	4	8	13	19
35–49	149	4.6	33	1	1	3	6	9	15	36
50–64	97	5.7	76	1	2	3	5	10	26	51
65+	30	6.9	38	1	2	5	10	15	18	28
GRAND TOTAL	515	4.4	33	1	1	2	5	9	14	32

76.7: REDUCTION OF FACIAL FX

Type of Patients	Observed Patients	Avg. Stay	Vari-ance	10th	25th	50th	75th	90th	95th	99th
1. SINGLE DX										
0–19 Years	90	1.7	<1	1	1	2	2	3	3	3
20–34	188	1.9	2	1	1	2	2	3	9	9
35–49	48	2.1	3	1	1	1	2	5	6	7
50–64	24	1.4	<1	1	1	1	2	3	3	4
65+	3	1.3	<1	1	1	1	2	2	2	2
2. MULTIPLE DX										
0–19 Years	619	3.2	26	1	1	2	3	6	8	23
20–34	1,534	3.5	25	1	1	2	4	7	10	27
35–49	854	4.4	31	1	2	3	5	8	13	32
50–64	459	5.4	60	1	2	3	6	11	17	51
65+	184	5.8	52	1	2	4	7	11	18	48
TOTAL SINGLE DX	353	1.8	2	1	1	1	2	3	4	8
TOTAL MULTIPLE DX	3,650	4.0	33	1	1	2	4	8	12	31
TOTAL										
0–19 Years	709	3.0	23	1	1	2	3	6	8	19
20–34	1,722	3.4	23	1	1	2	4	6	10	26
35–49	902	4.3	30	1	2	3	5	8	12	32
50–64	483	5.2	58	1	2	3	6	11	16	51
65+	187	5.7	51	1	2	4	7	11	18	48
GRAND TOTAL	4,003	3.8	30	1	1	2	4	7	11	30

76.74: OPEN RED MAXILLARY FX

Type of Patients	Observed Patients	Avg. Stay	Vari-ance	10th	25th	50th	75th	90th	95th	99th
1. SINGLE DX										
0–19 Years	2	1.5	<1	1	1	2	2	2	2	2
20–34	4	1.3	<1	1	1	1	2	2	2	2
35–49	2	1.5	<1	1	1	1	2	2	2	2
50–64	0									
65+	0									
2. MULTIPLE DX										
0–19 Years	36	4.6	34	1	2	3	6	8	12	37
20–34	107	4.5	33	1	2	4	4	11	15	30
35–49	67	7.3	91	2	3	5	7	22	26	46
50–64	41	8.2	132	2	3	7	9	13	22	59
65+	16	7.4	24	1	5	7	9	15	19	19
TOTAL SINGLE DX	8	1.4	<1	1	1	1	2	2	2	2
TOTAL MULTIPLE DX	267	5.9	63	1	2	3	7	13	22	46
TOTAL										
0–19 Years	38	4.5	33	1	1	2	6	8	12	37
20–34	111	4.4	32	1	2	3	4	9	15	30
35–49	69	7.1	90	1	2	3	6	22	26	46
50–64	41	8.2	132	2	3	5	9	13	22	59
65+	16	7.4	24	1	5	7	9	15	19	19
GRAND TOTAL	275	5.8	62	1	2	3	7	12	20	46

LOS by Diagnosis and Operation, Western Region, 45th Edition

Western Region, October 2007–September 2008 Data, by Operation

76.75: CLSD RED MANDIBULAR FX

Type of Patients	Observed Patients	Avg. Stay	Vari-ance	10th	25th	50th	75th	90th	95th	99th
1. SINGLE DX										
0–19 Years	20	1.9	1	1	1	2	2	4	4	4
20–34	34	1.7	2	1	1	1	2	2	4	9
35–49	3	1.3	<1	1	1	1	2	2	2	2
50–64	4	1.0	0	1	1	1	1	1	1	1
65+	0									
2. MULTIPLE DX										
0–19 Years	87	2.3	3	1	1	2	2	4	6	9
20–34	167	2.6	6	1	1	2	3	6	7	12
35–49	80	2.6	3	1	2	2	3	5	6	9
50–64	40	2.7	6	1	2	2	4	5	5	14
65+	11	3.3	8	1	2	3	4	4	11	11
TOTAL SINGLE DX	61	1.7	2	1	1	1	2	3	4	9
TOTAL MULTIPLE DX	385	2.5	4	1	1	2	3	5	6	11
TOTAL										
0–19 Years	107	2.2	3	1	1	2	2	4	5	9
20–34	201	2.5	5	1	1	2	3	5	7	11
35–49	83	2.6	3	1	1	2	3	5	6	9
50–64	44	2.5	5	1	1	2	3	5	5	14
65+	11	3.3	8	1	2	3	4	4	11	11
GRAND TOTAL	446	2.4	4	1	1	2	3	5	6	11

76.76: OPEN RED MANDIBULAR FX

Type of Patients	Observed Patients	Avg. Stay	Vari-ance	10th	25th	50th	75th	90th	95th	99th
1. SINGLE DX										
0–19 Years	48	1.7	<1	1	1	1	2	3	4	5
20–34	94	2.1	3	1	1	2	2	4	6	11
35–49	30	2.2	3	1	1	2	2	5	6	7
50–64	10	1.8	<1	1	1	2	2	3	3	3
65+	1	1.0	0	1	1	1	1	1	1	1
2. MULTIPLE DX										
0–19 Years	321	3.6	40	1	1	2	3	6	8	49
20–34	830	3.5	31	1	1	3	4	6	9	30
35–49	383	4.3	29	1	2	3	5	8	12	32
50–64	173	5.6	58	1	2	3	7	12	19	50
65+	62	6.4	96	1	2	4	6	10	18	61
TOTAL SINGLE DX	183	2.0	2	1	1	2	2	3	5	9
TOTAL MULTIPLE DX	1,769	4.0	38	1	1	2	4	7	11	39
TOTAL										
0–19 Years	369	3.4	36	1	1	2	3	6	8	49
20–34	924	3.4	28	1	1	2	3	6	9	30
35–49	413	4.2	27	1	2	3	5	8	12	27
50–64	183	5.4	56	1	2	3	6	11	18	50
65+	63	6.3	94	1	2	4	6	10	18	61
GRAND TOTAL	1,952	3.8	35	1	1	2	4	7	11	31

76.79: OPEN RED FACIAL FX NEC

Type of Patients	Observed Patients	Avg. Stay	Vari-ance	10th	25th	50th	75th	90th	95th	99th
1. SINGLE DX										
0–19 Years	15	1.2	<1	1	1	1	1	2	3	3
20–34	26	2.2	2	1	1	2	3	4	5	6
35–49	7	3.0	6	1	1	2	6	7	7	7
50–64	3	2.0	<1	1	2	2	3	3	3	3
65+	1	2.0	0	2	2	2	2	2	2	2
2. MULTIPLE DX										
0–19 Years	85	3.0	14	1	1	2	3	7	8	14
20–34	255	3.4	19	1	1	2	4	7	10	18
35–49	172	4.2	22	1	2	3	5	7	11	32
50–64	102	4.7	37	1	2	3	6	9	13	17
65+	55	4.8	31	1	2	3	6	11	21	29
TOTAL SINGLE DX	52	1.8	2	1	1	1	2	4	5	7
TOTAL MULTIPLE DX	669	3.8	22	1	1	2	4	8	11	21
TOTAL										
0–19 Years	100	2.7	12	1	1	2	3	6	8	14
20–34	281	3.3	17	1	1	2	4	7	9	18
35–49	179	4.1	21	1	2	3	5	9	11	32
50–64	105	4.6	36	1	2	3	6	9	13	17
65+	56	4.7	31	2	2	3	6	11	21	29
GRAND TOTAL	721	3.6	21	1	1	2	4	8	11	21

76.9: OTH OPS FACIAL BONE/JT

Type of Patients	Observed Patients	Avg. Stay	Vari-ance	10th	25th	50th	75th	90th	95th	99th
1. SINGLE DX										
0–19 Years	23	1.4	<1	1	1	1	2	2	3	3
20–34	9	1.7	2	1	1	1	4	4	4	4
35–49	10	1.2	<1	1	1	1	2	2	2	2
50–64	8	1.5	<1	1	1	1	2	3	3	3
65+	0									
2. MULTIPLE DX										
0–19 Years	142	2.1	10	1	1	1	2	3	6	19
20–34	76	3.1	32	1	1	2	3	6	8	43
35–49	84	3.7	42	1	1	1	4	7	9	50
50–64	73	3.4	37	1	1	3	5	7	13	47
65+	33	3.0	3	1	1	3	5	5	6	7
TOTAL SINGLE DX	50	1.4	<1	1	1	1	2	2	3	4
TOTAL MULTIPLE DX	408	2.8	22	1	1	2	2	5	7	28
TOTAL										
0–19 Years	165	2.0	9	1	1	1	2	3	4	19
20–34	85	3.0	29	1	1	2	3	6	8	43
35–49	94	3.4	38	1	1	2	3	7	9	50
50–64	81	3.3	34	1	1	3	5	7	10	47
65+	33	3.0	3	1	1	3	5	5	6	7
GRAND TOTAL	458	2.6	20	1	1	1	2	5	7	28

LOS by Diagnosis and Operation, Western Region, 45th Edition

Western Region, October 2007–September 2008 Data, by Operation

76.91: BONE GRAFT TO FACE BONE

Type of Patients	Observed Patients	Avg. Stay	Variance	10th	25th	50th	75th	90th	95th	99th
1. SINGLE DX										
0–19 Years	18	1.2	<1	1	1	1	1	2	2	2
20–34	2	1.0	0	1	1	1	1	1	1	1
35–49	3	1.0	0	1	1	1	1	1	1	1
50–64	4	1.3	<1	1	1	1	2	2	2	2
65+	0									
2. MULTIPLE DX										
0–19 Years	76	1.4	<1	1	1	1	2	2	2	3
20–34	11	1.9	2	1	1	1	3	3	6	6
35–49	14	2.0	2	1	1	2	2	4	5	5
50–64	16	2.1	16	1	1	1	1	2	17	17
65+	2	1.0	0	1	1	1	2	1	1	1
TOTAL SINGLE DX	27	1.2	<1	1	1	1	1	2	2	2
TOTAL MULTIPLE DX	119	1.6	2	1	1	1	2	2	3	6
TOTAL										
0–19 Years	94	1.4	<1	1	1	1	2	2	2	3
20–34	13	1.8	2	1	1	1	3	3	6	6
35–49	17	1.8	2	1	1	1	2	4	5	5
50–64	20	1.9	13	1	1	1	1	2	2	17
65+	2	1.0	0	1	1	1	2	1	1	1
GRAND TOTAL	146	1.5	2	1	1	1	2	2	2	5

76.97: RMVL INT FIX FACE BONE

Type of Patients	Observed Patients	Avg. Stay	Variance	10th	25th	50th	75th	90th	95th	99th
1. SINGLE DX										
0–19 Years	2	1.8	<1	1	2	2	2	2	2	2
20–34	2	1.0	0	1	1	1	1	1	1	1
35–49	3	1.0	0	1	1	1	1	1	1	1
50–64	0									
65+	0									
2. MULTIPLE DX										
0–19 Years	42	3.5	31	1	1	2	3	6	19	36
20–34	31	4.1	64	1	1	2	3	7	28	43
35–49	43	4.8	74	1	1	2	5	8	9	50
50–64	29	4.2	76	1	1	2	3	7	13	47
65+	11	2.4	3	1	1	1	4	5	5	5
TOTAL SINGLE DX	7	1.4	<1	1	1	1	2	2	2	2
TOTAL MULTIPLE DX	156	3.9	52	1	1	2	4	7	13	47
TOTAL										
0–19 Years	44	3.4	29	1	1	2	3	6	19	36
20–34	33	3.9	61	1	1	2	3	7	28	43
35–49	46	4.5	70	1	1	2	4	8	9	50
50–64	29	4.2	76	1	1	2	3	7	13	47
65+	11	2.4	3	1	1	1	4	5	5	5
GRAND TOTAL	163	3.8	49	1	1	2	3	7	12	47

77.0: SEQUESTRECTOMY

Type of Patients	Observed Patients	Avg. Stay	Variance	10th	25th	50th	75th	90th	95th	99th
1. SINGLE DX										
0–19 Years	2	1.5	<1	1	1		2	2	2	2
20–34	1	15.0	0	15	15	15	15	15	15	15
35–49	1	3.0	0	3	3	3	3	3	3	3
50–64	2	2.5	<1	2	2	2	3	3	3	3
65+	0									
2. MULTIPLE DX										
0–19 Years	7	8.5	25	2	4	8	14	14	14	14
20–34	14	3.7	7	1	1	4	5	7	10	10
35–49	26	8.1	176	1	3	6	9	11	13	71
50–64	29	5.9	26	2	4	4	7	9	17	27
65+	25	5.6	18	1	2	4	7	13	15	15
TOTAL SINGLE DX	6	4.3	28	1	2	2	3	15	15	15
TOTAL MULTIPLE DX	101	6.3	60	1	3	5	7	13	14	27
TOTAL										
0–19 Years	9	7.3	28	2	2	5	14	14	14	14
20–34	15	4.5	15	1	1	4	6	10	15	15
35–49	27	7.9	170	1	3	6	9	11	13	71
50–64	31	5.7	25	2	3	4	7	8	17	27
65+	25	5.6	18	1	2	4	7	13	15	15
GRAND TOTAL	107	6.2	58	1	3	4	7	13	15	27

77.1: BONE INC NEC W/O DIV

Type of Patients	Observed Patients	Avg. Stay	Variance	10th	25th	50th	75th	90th	95th	99th
1. SINGLE DX										
0–19 Years	17	3.1	12	1	1	2	3	13	13	13
20–34	8	2.9	6	1	1	2	3	8	8	8
35–49	3	4.3	4	2	2	5	6	6	6	6
50–64	3	2.0	<1	1	1	2	3	3	3	3
65+	0									
2. MULTIPLE DX										
0–19 Years	93	6.7	59	1	2	4	7	16	21	33
20–34	23	5.1	27	1	1	4	7	9	13	24
35–49	41	5.2	82	1	2	4	6	10	12	56
50–64	37	6.8	58	1	2	5	7	21	23	36
65+	30	6.8	59	1	2	4	8	13	27	35
TOTAL SINGLE DX	31	3.1	10	1	1	2	3	6	13	13
TOTAL MULTIPLE DX	224	6.5	59	1	2	4	7	15	21	36
TOTAL										
0–19 Years	110	6.2	54	1	2	4	7	15	20	33
20–34	31	4.5	22	1	1	3	6	8	13	24
35–49	44	5.2	76	1	1	3	6	10	12	56
50–64	40	6.5	56	1	2	5	7	17	21	36
65+	30	6.8	59	1	2	4	8	13	27	35
GRAND TOTAL	255	6.0	54	1	2	4	7	14	20	35

Western Region, October 2007–September 2008 Data, by Operation

77.2: WEDGE OSTEOTOMY

Type of Patients	Observed Patients	Avg. Stay	Vari-ance	Percentiles						
				10th	25th	50th	75th	90th	95th	99th
1. SINGLE DX										
0–19 Years	32	1.9	<1	1	1	2	2	3	4	4
20–34	4	2.5	<1	2	2	3	3	3	3	3
35–49	2	2.5	<1	2	2	3	3	3	3	3
50–64	6	2.5	5	1	1	1	3	7	7	7
65+	0									
2. MULTIPLE DX										
0–19 Years	201	2.9	6	1	1	2	3	5	6	15
20–34	43	3.2	4	1	2	3	5	6	8	8
35–49	49	3.0	26	1	1	2	3	4	5	37
50–64	68	2.4	2	1	1	2	3	4	5	7
65+	12	3.3	3	2	2	3	3	7	7	7
TOTAL SINGLE DX	44	2.0	<1	1	1	2	2	3	4	4
TOTAL MULTIPLE DX	373	2.9	7	1	1	2	3	5	6	15
TOTAL										
0–19 Years	233	2.8	5	1	1	2	3	4	6	15
20–34	47	3.0	4	1	2	3	5	5	8	8
35–49	51	3.0	25	1	1	2	3	4	5	37
50–64	74	2.4	<1	1	1	2	3	4	5	7
65+	12	3.3	3	2	2	3	3	7	7	7
GRAND TOTAL	417	2.8	6	1	1	2	3	5	6	15

77.25: FEMORAL WEDGE OSTEOTOMY

Type of Patients	Observed Patients	Avg. Stay	Vari-ance	Percentiles						
				10th	25th	50th	75th	90th	95th	99th
1. SINGLE DX										
0–19 Years	10	2.1	<1	2	2	2	2	3	3	3
20–34	2	2.5	<1	2	2	3	3	3	3	3
35–49	1	2.0	0	2	2	2	2	2	2	2
50–64	0									
65+	0									
2. MULTIPLE DX										
0–19 Years	120	3.4	6	2	2	3	4	5	7	20
20–34	16	4.2	6	1	2	3	6	8	8	8
35–49	7	2.7	2	1	1	2	4	4	4	4
50–64	7	2.7	<1	2	2	3	3	4	4	4
65+	3	5.3	8	2	2	7	7	7	7	7
TOTAL SINGLE DX	13	2.1	<1	2	2	2	2	3	3	3
TOTAL MULTIPLE DX	153	3.4	6	1	2	3	4	6	7	20
TOTAL										
0–19 Years	130	3.3	6	1	2	3	4	5	6	20
20–34	18	4.0	6	2	2	3	5	8	8	8
35–49	8	2.4	1	1	1	2	3	4	4	4
50–64	7	2.7	<1	2	2	3	3	4	5	4
65+	3	5.3	8	2	2	7	7	7	7	7
GRAND TOTAL	166	3.3	6	2	2	3	4	5	7	17

77.27: TIB & FIB WEDGE OSTY

Type of Patients	Observed Patients	Avg. Stay	Vari-ance	Percentiles						
				10th	25th	50th	75th	90th	95th	99th
1. SINGLE DX										
0–19 Years	9	1.9	1	1	1	2	2	4	4	4
20–34	2	2.5	<1	2	2	3	3	3	3	3
35–49	1	3.0	0	3	3	3	3	3	3	3
50–64	6	2.5	5	1	1	1	3	7	7	7
65+	0									
2. MULTIPLE DX										
0–19 Years	40	2.5	6	1	1	2	3	4	6	15
20–34	18	2.6	3	1	1	2	4	5	5	5
35–49	34	3.4	37	1	2	2	3	5	6	37
50–64	45	2.4	2	1	1	2	3	4	5	7
65+	5	2.6	<1	2	2	3	3	3	3	3
TOTAL SINGLE DX	18	2.0	2	1	1	2	2	4	4	7
TOTAL MULTIPLE DX	142	2.6	9	1	1	2	3	4	6	15
TOTAL										
0–19 Years	49	2.4	6	1	1	2	3	4	6	15
20–34	20	2.6	2	1	2	2	4	5	5	5
35–49	35	3.4	36	1	2	2	3	5	6	37
50–64	51	2.4	2	1	1	2	3	4	6	7
65+	5	2.6	<1	2	2	3	3	3	3	3
GRAND TOTAL	160	2.6	8	1	2	2	3	4	5	15

77.3: OTHER DIVISION OF BONE

Type of Patients	Observed Patients	Avg. Stay	Vari-ance	Percentiles						
				10th	25th	50th	75th	90th	95th	99th
1. SINGLE DX										
0–19 Years	125	1.7	<1	1	1	1	2	3	3	6
20–34	10	3.5	5	1	1	4	5	6	7	7
35–49	11	2.2	<1	1	1	2	3	3	4	4
50–64	8	1.8	<1	1	1	2	2	3	3	3
65+	0									
2. MULTIPLE DX										
0–19 Years	406	2.6	4	1	1	2	3	4	5	11
20–34	85	3.8	14	1	2	3	5	6	7	28
35–49	107	4.7	56	1	2	3	5	8	13	31
50–64	115	3.2	11	1	2	3	3	5	8	17
65+	58	3.2	4	1	2	3	4	6	8	9
TOTAL SINGLE DX	154	1.8	1	1	1	1	2	3	3	6
TOTAL MULTIPLE DX	771	2.9	9	1	1	2	3	5	7	13
TOTAL										
0–19 Years	531	2.4	4	1	2	2	3	4	5	10
20–34	95	3.7	13	1	2	3	5	6	7	22
35–49	118	4.4	51	1	2	3	4	8	12	31
50–64	123	3.1	11	1	2	2	3	5	7	17
65+	58	3.2	4	1	2	3	4	6	8	9
GRAND TOTAL	925	2.7	8	1	1	2	3	5	6	12

LOS by Diagnosis and Operation, Western Region, 45th Edition

Western Region, October 2007–September 2008 Data, by Operation

77.35: FEMORAL DIVISION NEC

Type of Patients	Observed Patients	Avg. Stay	Variance	Percentiles						
				10th	25th	50th	75th	90th	95th	99th
1. SINGLE DX										
0–19 Years	49	2.0	<1	1	1	2	2	3	3	4
20–34	1	4.0	0	4	4	4	4	4	4	4
35–49	3	3.0	<1	2	2	3	3	4	4	4
50–64	2	2.5	<1	2	2	2	2	3	3	3
65+	0									
2. MULTIPLE DX										
0–19 Years	212	3.0	5	1	2	3	3	5	7	13
20–34	16	5.6	32	2	3	4	6	9	28	28
35–49	34	4.8	17	2	2	4	6	8	12	23
50–64	19	3.2	5	1	2	2	4	8	9	9
65+	12	4.6	3	3	3	4	6	7	8	8
TOTAL SINGLE DX	55	2.1	<1	1	2	2	3	3	3	4
TOTAL MULTIPLE DX	293	3.2	7	1	2	3	4	5	7	13
TOTAL										
0–19 Years	261	2.8	5	1	2	2	3	4	6	11
20–34	17	5.5	30	3	3	4	6	6	9	28
35–49	37	4.7	16	2	2	4	6	8	12	23
50–64	21	3.1	4	2	2	2	3	5	8	9
65+	12	4.6	3	3	3	4	6	7	8	8
GRAND TOTAL	348	3.0	6	1	2	3	3	5	7	13

77.4: BIOPSY OF BONE

Type of Patients	Observed Patients	Avg. Stay	Variance	Percentiles						
				10th	25th	50th	75th	90th	95th	99th
1. SINGLE DX										
0–19 Years	65	3.8	21	1	1	2	5	7	9	29
20–34	23	2.1	3	1	1	2	2	5	6	7
35–49	9	2.0	2	1	1	2	2	5	5	5
50–64	15	1.6	1	1	1	1	2	2	5	5
65+	24	1.4	2	1	1	1	1	2	3	7
2. MULTIPLE DX										
0–19 Years	234	8.2	72	2	3	5	11	17	21	36
20–34	157	7.9	61	1	3	6	10	17	23	49
35–49	328	9.5	107	2	4	7	11	18	29	61
50–64	1,114	8.0	74	1	3	6	10	16	23	48
65+	3,171	6.1	35	1	2	5	8	13	17	26
TOTAL SINGLE DX	136	3.2	16	1	1	2	5	6	7	29
TOTAL MULTIPLE DX	5,004	7.0	54	1	2	5	9	15	19	36
TOTAL										
0–19 Years	299	7.3	65	1	3	5	9	15	21	36
20–34	180	7.2	58	1	2	5	9	16	23	49
35–49	337	9.3	106	1	3	7	11	18	29	61
50–64	1,129	7.9	73	1	3	6	10	16	23	48
65+	3,195	6.1	35	1	2	5	8	13	16	26
GRAND TOTAL	5,140	6.9	53	1	2	5	9	14	19	36

77.37: TIBIA/FIBULA DIV NEC

Type of Patients	Observed Patients	Avg. Stay	Variance	Percentiles						
				10th	25th	50th	75th	90th	95th	99th
1. SINGLE DX										
0–19 Years	45	1.6	1	1	1	1	2	3	3	6
20–34	4	3.5	7	1	1	2	4	7	7	7
35–49	7	2.0	<1	1	1	2	3	3	3	3
50–64	5	1.6	<1	1	1	2	2	2	2	2
65+	0									
2. MULTIPLE DX										
0–19 Years	119	2.1	2	1	1	2	2	4	5	10
20–34	27	2.6	4	1	1	2	3	6	6	10
35–49	41	3.3	13	1	2	3	3	5	13	16
50–64	65	3.2	14	1	2	3	3	5	7	30
65+	14	3.2	3	2	2	3	4	5	8	8
TOTAL SINGLE DX	61	1.7	1	1	1	1	2	3	3	6
TOTAL MULTIPLE DX	266	2.4	5	1	1	2	3	4	5	10
TOTAL										
0–19 Years	164	2.0	2	1	1	2	2	3	4	9
20–34	31	2.7	4	1	1	2	3	6	7	10
35–49	48	3.1	11	1	2	2	3	6	13	16
50–64	70	3.1	13	1	2	3	3	5	7	30
65+	14	3.2	3	2	3	3	4	5	8	8
GRAND TOTAL	327	2.2	4	1	1	2	3	4	5	10

77.41: CHEST CAGE BONE BIOPSY

Type of Patients	Observed Patients	Avg. Stay	Variance	Percentiles						
				10th	25th	50th	75th	90th	95th	99th
1. SINGLE DX										
0–19 Years	1	1.0	0	1	1	1	1	1	1	1
20–34	1	7.0	0	7	7	7	7	7	7	7
35–49	1	1.0	0	1	1	1	1	1	1	1
50–64	1	2.0	0	2	2	2	2	2	2	2
65+	1	7.0	0	7	7	7	7	7	7	7
2. MULTIPLE DX										
0–19 Years	9	5.4	15	1	1	5	8	12	12	12
20–34	8	6.6	17	1	5	7	9	14	14	14
35–49	10	18.1	265	2	4	17	28	55	55	55
50–64	84	7.7	40	2	3	6	10	15	16	35
65+	105	8.0	21	3	4	7	11	15	17	19
TOTAL SINGLE DX	5	2.6	7	1	1	1	2	7	7	7
TOTAL MULTIPLE DX	216	8.0	42	2	4	7	11	15	17	30
TOTAL										
0–19 Years	10	4.8	15	1	1	4	8	12	12	12
20–34	9	6.7	15	1	3	7	9	14	14	14
35–49	11	16.6	265	1	3	15	28	30	55	55
50–64	85	7.6	40	2	3	6	10	15	16	35
65+	106	8.0	21	3	4	7	11	15	17	19
GRAND TOTAL	221	7.8	42	1	4	6	11	15	17	30

Western Region, October 2007–September 2008 Data, by Operation

77.42: HUMERUS BIOPSY

Type of Patients	Observed Patients	Avg. Stay	Variance	10th	25th	50th	75th	90th	95th	99th
1. SINGLE DX										
0–19 Years	8	3.3	4	1	2	4	5	5	5	7
20–34	5	3.0	5	1	1	2	5	6	6	6
35–49	0									
50–64	3	1.3	<1	1	1	1	2	2	2	2
65+	0									
2. MULTIPLE DX										
0–19 Years	24	8.9	34	2	5	6	13	17	21	25
20–34	9	5.3	53	1	2	2	6	24	24	24
35–49	7	4.3	4	1	3	4	6	7	7	7
50–64	36	5.3	43	1	1	3	6	16	22	29
65+	62	5.0	19	1	2	3	7	11	13	22
TOTAL SINGLE DX	16	3.0	4	1	1	2	5	5	6	7
TOTAL MULTIPLE DX	138	6.6	34	1	2	5	10	16	18	25
TOTAL										
0–19 Years	32	7.8	33	1	4	6	12	16	21	25
20–34	14	4.5	36	1	1	2	6	6	24	24
35–49	7	4.3	4	1	3	4	6	7	7	7
50–64	39	5.0	41	1	1	3	6	16	22	29
65+	62	5.0	19	1	2	3	7	11	13	22
GRAND TOTAL	154	6.2	31	1	2	5	9	13	17	24

77.45: FEMORAL BIOPSY

Type of Patients	Observed Patients	Avg. Stay	Variance	10th	25th	50th	75th	90th	95th	99th
1. SINGLE DX										
0–19 Years	26	4.6	40	1	2	2	5	7	29	29
20–34	6	1.7	<1	1	1	2	2	2	2	2
35–49	2	3.5	4	2	2	4	5	5	5	5
50–64	2	1.5	<1	2	2	1	2	2	2	2
65+	1	2.0	0	2	2	2	2	2	2	2
2. MULTIPLE DX										
0–19 Years	70	7.7	44	1	3	6	12	17	18	36
20–34	31	7.9	32	1	3	7	13	14	18	20
35–49	45	6.4	15	2	4	6	9	12	14	17
50–64	115	7.3	36	2	4	6	9	15	19	32
65+	174	7.2	32	3	4	6	8	13	16	37
TOTAL SINGLE DX	37	4.3	36	1	2	2	5	7	10	29
TOTAL MULTIPLE DX	435	7.4	35	2	4	6	10	14	18	36
TOTAL										
0–19 Years	96	6.8	45	1	2	5	9	15	18	36
20–34	37	7.0	33	1	3	6	12	14	18	20
35–49	47	6.3	15	2	4	6	9	12	14	17
50–64	117	7.2	36	2	3	6	9	15	19	32
65+	175	7.2	32	3	4	6	8	13	16	37
GRAND TOTAL	472	7.0	37	2	3	5	9	14	18	33

77.47: TIBIA & FIBULA BIOPSY

Type of Patients	Observed Patients	Avg. Stay	Variance	10th	25th	50th	75th	90th	95th	99th
1. SINGLE DX										
0–19 Years	20	3.4	7	1	1	3	5	9	9	9
20–34	8	1.6	<1	1	1	2	2	3	3	3
35–49	0									
50–64	2	2.0	0	2	2	2	2	2	2	2
65+	0									
2. MULTIPLE DX										
0–19 Years	57	7.6	141	1	3	5	7	12	18	74
20–34	29	4.8	19	1	2	3	7	10	11	22
35–49	25	7.8	36	2	3	6	10	16	21	22
50–64	56	7.4	51	2	3	5	10	19	24	33
65+	50	8.2	35	2	4	7	11	17	20	27
TOTAL SINGLE DX	30	3.1	6	1	1	2	5	8	9	9
TOTAL MULTIPLE DX	217	7.4	89	1	3	5	8	15	21	74
TOTAL										
0–19 Years	77	6.7	114	1	2	5	7	10	15	74
20–34	37	4.1	17	1	2	2	5	9	11	22
35–49	25	7.8	36	2	3	6	10	16	21	22
50–64	58	7.2	50	2	4	7	10	19	24	33
65+	50	8.2	35	2	4	7	11	17	20	27
GRAND TOTAL	247	6.8	79	1	2	5	8	13	18	74

77.48: METATARSAL/TARSAL BIOPSY

Type of Patients	Observed Patients	Avg. Stay	Variance	10th	25th	50th	75th	90th	95th	99th
1. SINGLE DX										
0–19 Years	1	3.0	0	3	3	3	3	3	3	3
20–34	0									
35–49	0									
50–64	0									
65+	0									
2. MULTIPLE DX										
0–19 Years	6	15.4	136	4	4	9	26	26	36	36
20–34	10	8.4	99	2	4	5	8	36	36	36
35–49	33	7.8	63	3	4	6	8	11	32	41
50–64	57	7.6	49	2	3	6	11	15	17	45
65+	48	7.8	26	2	3	7	10	14	19	22
TOTAL SINGLE DX	1	3.0	0	3	3	3	3	3	3	3
TOTAL MULTIPLE DX	154	8.3	57	2	4	6	10	16	26	41
TOTAL										
0–19 Years	7	14.5	136	4	4	9	26	26	36	36
20–34	10	8.4	99	2	4	6	8	36	36	36
35–49	33	7.8	63	3	4	6	8	11	32	41
50–64	57	7.6	49	2	3	6	11	15	17	45
65+	48	7.8	26	2	3	7	10	14	19	22
GRAND TOTAL	155	8.3	57	2	4	6	10	16	26	41

LOS by Diagnosis and Operation, Western Region, 45th Edition

Western Region, October 2007–September 2008 Data, by Operation

77.49: BONE BIOPSY NEC

Type of Patients	Observed Patients	Avg. Stay	Variance	10th	25th	50th	75th	90th	95th	99th
1. SINGLE DX										
0–19 Years	3	4.0	5	1	1	5	6	6	6	6
20–34	3	1.3	<1	1	1	1	2	2	2	2
35–49	6	1.7	<1	1	1	2	2	3	3	3
50–64	7	1.6	2	1	1	1	1	5	5	5
65+	22	1.1	<1	1	1	1	1	1	1	3
2. MULTIPLE DX										
0–19 Years	59	9.1	63	2	4	6	12	19	25	36
20–34	66	10.0	92	2	5	7	11	23	40	>99
35–49	207	10.4	133	1	4	7	13	20	36	68
50–64	751	8.3	85	1	3	6	11	17	25	55
65+	2,723	6.0	36	1	1	5	8	13	16	26
TOTAL SINGLE DX	41	2.0	3	1	1	1	2	5	6	6
TOTAL MULTIPLE DX	3,806	6.8	55	1	2	5	9	14	19	39
TOTAL										
0–19 Years	62	8.7	60	2	3	6	12	18	25	36
20–34	69	9.6	91	1	4	6	11	23	40	>99
35–49	213	10.1	132	1	4	7	12	19	36	68
50–64	758	8.3	85	1	3	6	10	17	24	55
65+	2,745	5.9	36	1	1	5	8	13	16	26
GRAND TOTAL	3,847	6.8	54	1	2	5	9	14	19	38

77.5: TOE DEFORMITY EXC/REP

Type of Patients	Observed Patients	Avg. Stay	Variance	10th	25th	50th	75th	90th	95th	99th
1. SINGLE DX										
0–19 Years	12	1.3	<1	1	1	1	2	2	2	2
20–34	0									
35–49	2	1.0	0	1	1	3	3	3	3	3
50–64	2	2.0	0	1	1	1	1	1	1	1
65+	1	1.0		1	1	1	1	1	1	1
2. MULTIPLE DX										
0–19 Years	32	1.8	1	1	1	1	2	3	4	4
20–34	16	1.6	<1	1	1	1	2	3	3	3
35–49	44	2.6	3	1	1	2	4	5	5	8
50–64	122	2.4	5	1	1	2	3	5	6	11
65+	98	2.6	9	1	1	2	3	4	6	28
TOTAL SINGLE DX	17	1.3	<1	1	1	1	2	2	2	3
TOTAL MULTIPLE DX	312	2.3	4	1	1	2	3	4	5	10
TOTAL										
0–19 Years	44	1.7	<1	1	1	1	2	3	4	4
20–34	16	1.6	<1	1	1	1	2	3	3	3
35–49	46	2.5	3	1	1	2	4	5	5	8
50–64	124	2.4	5	1	1	2	3	5	6	11
65+	99	2.6	8	1	1	2	3	4	6	28
GRAND TOTAL	329	2.2	4	1	1	2	3	4	5	9

77.6: LOC EXC BONE LESION

Type of Patients	Observed Patients	Avg. Stay	Variance	10th	25th	50th	75th	90th	95th	99th
1. SINGLE DX										
0–19 Years	129	1.7	1	1	1	1	2	3	4	6
20–34	60	1.6	<1	1	1	1	2	3	3	5
35–49	37	2.2	2	1	1	2	3	4	5	6
50–64	10	3.0	13	1	1	2	3	13	13	13
65+	4	1.8	<1	1	1	2	3	3	3	3
2. MULTIPLE DX										
0–19 Years	277	6.6	102	1	1	4	8	16	22	50
20–34	357	6.9	89	1	2	4	7	18	26	67
35–49	675	7.6	81	1	3	5	9	16	24	46
50–64	1,134	7.9	70	1	3	6	10	17	24	42
65+	932	8.2	62	2	4	6	10	16	22	42
TOTAL SINGLE DX	240	1.7	2	1	1	1	2	3	4	6
TOTAL MULTIPLE DX	3,375	7.6	77	1	3	5	9	16	23	46
TOTAL										
0–19 Years	406	4.8	71	1	1	2	5	11	19	39
20–34	417	6.2	80	1	2	3	6	15	24	46
35–49	712	7.4	78	1	3	5	8	15	23	45
50–64	1,144	7.9	70	1	3	6	10	17	24	42
65+	936	8.2	62	2	4	6	10	16	22	42
GRAND TOTAL	3,615	7.0	72	1	2	4	8	15	22	43

77.61: EXC CHEST CAGE BONE LES

Type of Patients	Observed Patients	Avg. Stay	Variance	10th	25th	50th	75th	90th	95th	99th
1. SINGLE DX										
0–19 Years	7	1.6	<1	1	1	1	3	3	3	3
20–34	4	2.0	<1	1	1	2	3	3	3	3
35–49	1	1.0	0	1	1	1	1	1	1	1
50–64	2	2.5	<1	2	2	2	3	3	3	3
65+	0									
2. MULTIPLE DX										
0–19 Years	13	3.6	14	1	1	3	6	8	10	18
20–34	10	5.9	45	1	2	4	6	20	20	20
35–49	26	9.7	119	1	2	3	19	29	30	34
50–64	94	9.2	81	2	2	6	14	23	27	42
65+	105	10.7	116	2	4	7	12	25	35	42
TOTAL SINGLE DX	14	1.8	<1	1	1	1	3	3	3	3
TOTAL MULTIPLE DX	248	9.1	94	1	2	6	12	23	29	42
TOTAL										
0–19 Years	20	2.9	11	1	1	2	3	6	8	18
20–34	14	4.8	34	1	2	3	5	16	20	20
35–49	27	9.4	117	1	2	3	19	29	30	34
50–64	96	9.0	80	1	2	5	13	23	27	42
65+	105	10.7	116	2	4	7	12	25	35	42
GRAND TOTAL	262	8.6	91	1	2	5	11	23	29	42

Western Region, October 2007–September 2008 Data, by Operation

77.62: LOC EXC HUMERUS LESION

Type of Patients	Observed Patients	Avg. Stay	Vari-ance	10th	25th	50th	75th	90th	95th	99th
1. SINGLE DX										
0–19 Years	12	1.1	<1	1	1	1	1	2	2	2
20–34	2	1.5	<1	1	1	2	2	2	2	2
35–49	4	1.5	<1	1	1	1	1	3	3	3
50–64	0									
65+	0									
2. MULTIPLE DX										
0–19 Years	17	4.8	12	1	1	4	7	10	10	10
20–34	17	3.6	6	1	2	3	4	8	9	9
35–49	28	4.6	10	1	2	4	6	10	10	13
50–64	43	4.5	23	1	2	5	6	10	11	27
65+	27	5.9	23	2	3	5	8	13	14	23
TOTAL SINGLE DX	18	1.2	<1	1	1	1	1	2	2	3
TOTAL MULTIPLE DX	132	4.7	16	1	2	4	6	10	10	23
TOTAL										
0–19 Years	29	2.9	9	1	1	1	4	10	10	10
20–34	19	3.3	5	1	2	3	4	8	9	9
35–49	32	4.2	10	1	2	4	5	8	10	13
50–64	43	4.5	23	1	2	3	6	10	11	27
65+	27	5.9	23	2	3	5	8	13	14	23
GRAND TOTAL	150	3.9	15	1	1	3	5	10	10	23

77.63: LOC EXC RADIUS/ULNA LES

Type of Patients	Observed Patients	Avg. Stay	Vari-ance	10th	25th	50th	75th	90th	95th	99th
1. SINGLE DX										
0–19 Years	11	1.5	<1	1	1	1	2	2	2	6
20–34	5	1.2	<1	1	1	1	1	2	2	2
35–49	4	2.0	0	2	2	2	2	2	2	2
50–64	3	1.0	0	1	1	1	1	1	1	1
65+	0									
2. MULTIPLE DX										
0–19 Years	19	7.4	139	1	2	3	4	39	39	39
20–34	29	4.8	66	1	1	3	5	6	21	42
35–49	38	4.5	13	1	2	4	7	11	14	14
50–64	30	5.8	59	1	2	4	8	11	15	42
65+	22	8.8	144	2	4	5	8	13	43	46
TOTAL SINGLE DX	23	1.5	<1	1	1	1	2	2	2	6
TOTAL MULTIPLE DX	138	6.1	79	1	2	4	6	11	39	43
TOTAL										
0–19 Years	30	4.7	83	1	1	2	3	6	39	39
20–34	34	4.3	58	1	2	3	4	6	21	42
35–49	42	4.3	13	1	2	3	6	10	13	14
50–64	33	5.4	55	1	2	4	6	11	15	42
65+	22	8.8	144	2	4	5	8	13	43	46
GRAND TOTAL	161	5.1	66	1	1	3	5	10	15	43

77.65: LOCAL EXC FEMUR LESION

Type of Patients	Observed Patients	Avg. Stay	Vari-ance	10th	25th	50th	75th	90th	95th	99th
1. SINGLE DX										
0–19 Years	46	1.4	<1	1	1	1	2	3	3	4
20–34	11	1.5	<1	1	1	1	2	2	3	3
35–49	9	2.0	1	1	1	2	3	4	4	4
50–64	3	2.3	2	1	1	2	4	4	4	4
65+	0									
2. MULTIPLE DX										
0–19 Years	48	4.3	28	1	1	2	6	10	20	21
20–34	35	3.6	16	1	1	2	6	9	21	>99
35–49	72	6.5	113	1	2	3	7	15	21	81
50–64	88	6.4	57	1	2	3	8	18	23	>99
65+	80	8.3	72	2	4	6	9	16	22	51
TOTAL SINGLE DX	69	1.5	<1	1	1	1	2	3	3	4
TOTAL MULTIPLE DX	323	5.9	59	1	1	3	8	13	21	50
TOTAL										
0–19 Years	94	2.8	16	1	1	1	2	8	10	21
20–34	46	3.1	13	1	1	2	4	8	12	>99
35–49	81	6.0	103	1	2	3	8	14	20	81
50–64	91	6.3	56	1	2	3	8	17	23	>99
65+	80	8.3	72	2	4	6	9	16	22	51
GRAND TOTAL	392	4.6	46	1	1	2	6	10	20	41

77.67: LOC EXC TIBIA/FIBULA LES

Type of Patients	Observed Patients	Avg. Stay	Vari-ance	10th	25th	50th	75th	90th	95th	99th
1. SINGLE DX										
0–19 Years	30	1.8	2	1	1	1	2	4	5	11
20–34	17	1.8	<1	1	1	2	2	3	3	3
35–49	5	2.0	<1	2	2	2	2	3	3	3
50–64	2	7.5	59	3	3	8	13	13	13	13
65+	1	3.0	0	3	3	3	3	3	3	3
2. MULTIPLE DX										
0–19 Years	66	5.5	32	1	1	4	7	14	19	22
20–34	90	8.7	104	1	3	5	9	25	42	>99
35–49	107	7.6	75	1	3	5	9	18	23	50
50–64	153	7.2	63	1	3	5	9	16	23	41
65+	75	7.0	36	2	3	5	9	14	18	39
TOTAL SINGLE DX	55	1.9	3	1	1	1	2	3	5	11
TOTAL MULTIPLE DX	491	7.0	60	1	2	4	9	17	22	45
TOTAL										
0–19 Years	96	4.2	25	1	1	2	5	11	17	22
20–34	107	7.5	93	1	2	4	8	22	28	46
35–49	112	7.4	73	1	2	4	7	17	23	50
50–64	155	7.2	63	1	3	5	9	16	23	41
65+	76	7.0	36	2	3	5	9	14	18	39
GRAND TOTAL	546	6.2	55	1	2	4	8	15	21	45

LOS by Diagnosis and Operation, Western Region, 45th Edition

Western Region, October 2007–September 2008 Data, by Operation

77.68: LOCAL EXC MT/TARSAL LES

Type of Patients	Observed Patients	Avg. Stay	Vari-ance	10th	25th	50th	75th	90th	95th	99th
1. SINGLE DX										
0–19 Years	5	1.4	<1	1	1	1	1	3	3	3
20–34	0									
35–49	3	3.0	7	1	1	2	6	6	6	6
50–64	0									
65+	0									
2. MULTIPLE DX										
0–19 Years	19	2.9	3	1	1	3	4	5	7	7
20–34	32	7.4	51	1	3	5	9	18	24	31
35–49	126	8.2	52	2	4	6	10	15	21	40
50–64	247	8.4	37	2	4	7	11	16	21	31
65+	211	7.9	30	3	4	7	10	15	18	30
TOTAL SINGLE DX	8	1.8	2	1	1	1	2	3	6	6
TOTAL MULTIPLE DX	635	7.8	38	2	4	6	10	15	20	34
TOTAL										
0–19 Years	24	2.6	3	1	1	3	3	5	7	7
20–34	32	7.4	51	1	3	5	9	18	24	31
35–49	129	8.1	52	1	4	6	10	15	21	40
50–64	247	8.4	37	2	4	7	11	16	21	31
65+	211	7.9	30	3	4	7	10	15	18	30
GRAND TOTAL	643	7.7	38	2	4	6	10	15	20	34

77.69: LOC EXC BONE LESION NEC

Type of Patients	Observed Patients	Avg. Stay	Vari-ance	10th	25th	50th	75th	90th	95th	99th
1. SINGLE DX										
0–19 Years	17	2.8	1	1	2	3	4	4	5	6
20–34	17	1.7	2	1	1	1	2	4	5	5
35–49	10	2.7	3	1	1	1	4	5	5	5
50–64	0									
65+	3	1.3	<1	1	1	2	2	2	2	2
2. MULTIPLE DX										
0–19 Years	89	11.1	241	1	2	6	13	25	50	85
20–34	124	8.2	135	1	2	5	8	19	31	67
35–49	249	8.6	105	1	3	6	10	17	30	56
50–64	436	8.6	99	1	3	6	10	18	31	50
65+	375	8.4	68	2	4	6	10	18	24	42
TOTAL SINGLE DX	47	2.4	2	1	1	2	4	4	5	6
TOTAL MULTIPLE DX	1,273	8.8	114	1	3	6	10	19	29	56
TOTAL										
0–19 Years	106	9.7	210	1	2	4	10	22	28	85
20–34	141	7.4	123	1	2	4	8	16	27	67
35–49	259	8.4	103	1	3	5	10	17	30	56
50–64	436	8.6	99	1	3	6	10	18	31	50
65+	378	8.4	68	2	4	6	10	18	24	42
GRAND TOTAL	1,320	8.6	110	1	3	5	10	18	28	50

77.7: EXC BONE FOR GRAFT

Type of Patients	Observed Patients	Avg. Stay	Vari-ance	10th	25th	50th	75th	90th	95th	99th
1. SINGLE DX										
0–19 Years	25	2.5	14	1	1	1	2	3	16	16
20–34	17	1.4	<1	1	1	1	2	2	3	4
35–49	19	2.2	<1	1	1	2	3	4	4	4
50–64	17	1.7	<1	1	1	2	2	2	3	3
65+	7	2.4	3	1	1	2	4	5	5	5
2. MULTIPLE DX										
0–19 Years	57	2.0	1	1	1	2	3	3	4	6
20–34	96	2.7	9	1	1	2	3	5	10	21
35–49	147	2.1	4	1	1	2	3	3	5	10
50–64	222	2.7	42	1	1	2	3	4	6	10
65+	134	2.7	6	1	2	2	3	4	6	14
TOTAL SINGLE DX	85	2.2	8	1	1	2	2	3	4	16
TOTAL MULTIPLE DX	656	2.5	18	1	1	2	3	4	6	12
TOTAL										
0–19 Years	82	2.2	7	1	1	1	3	3	4	16
20–34	113	2.5	8	1	1	2	3	5	9	13
35–49	166	2.1	4	1	1	2	2	3	4	10
50–64	239	2.7	40	1	1	2	3	4	6	10
65+	141	2.7	6	1	2	2	3	4	6	14
GRAND TOTAL	741	2.5	16	1	1	2	3	4	6	16

77.77: EXC TIB/FIB FOR GRAFT

Type of Patients	Observed Patients	Avg. Stay	Vari-ance	10th	25th	50th	75th	90th	95th	99th
1. SINGLE DX										
0–19 Years	0									
20–34	2	1.5	<1	1	1	2	2	2	2	2
35–49	2	2.0	0	2	2	2	2	2	2	2
50–64	4	1.3	<1	1	1	1	2	2	2	2
65+	2	1.5	<1	1	1	1	2	2	2	2
2. MULTIPLE DX										
0–19 Years	4	4.0	5	2	2	6	6	6	6	6
20–34	21	2.1	3	1	1	2	2	3	5	9
35–49	38	2.3	3	1	1	2	2	4	7	10
50–64	75	2.3	4	1	1	2	3	4	8	10
65+	53	2.3	1	2	2	2	3	3	4	7
TOTAL SINGLE DX	10	1.5	<1	1	1	2	2	2	2	2
TOTAL MULTIPLE DX	191	2.3	3	1	1	2	3	4	6	10
TOTAL										
0–19 Years	4	4.0	5	2	2	6	6	6	6	6
20–34	23	2.0	3	1	1	2	2	3	5	9
35–49	40	2.0	3	1	1	2	2	3	4	10
50–64	79	2.3	4	1	1	2	3	4	8	10
65+	55	2.3	1	2	2	2	3	3	4	7
GRAND TOTAL	201	2.2	3	1	1	2	3	3	6	10

LOS by Diagnosis and Operation, Western Region, 45th Edition

Western Region, October 2007–September 2008 Data, by Operation

77.79: EXC BONE FOR GRAFT NEC

Type of Patients	Observed Patients	Avg. Stay	Vari-ance	Percentiles						
				10th	25th	50th	75th	90th	95th	99th
1. SINGLE DX										
0–19 Years	21	2.7	18	1	1	1	2	4	16	16
20–34	12	1.5	<1	1	1	1	2	2	3	3
35–49	14	2.4	1	1	2	2	3	4	4	4
50–64	12	1.8	<1	1	1	2	2	2	3	3
65+	5	2.8	3	1	1	3	4	5	5	5
2. MULTIPLE DX										
0–19 Years	46	1.8	1	1	1	1	3	3	4	4
20–34	70	2.6	6	1	1	2	3	5	9	13
35–49	101	2.0	1	1	1	2	3	3	4	6
50–64	131	2.3	2	1	1	2	3	5	5	6
65+	75	2.8	7	1	2	2	3	5	6	20
TOTAL SINGLE DX	**64**	**2.4**	**10**	**1**	**1**	**2**	**2**	**4**	**5**	**16**
TOTAL MULTIPLE DX	**423**	**2.3**	**3**	**1**	**1**	**2**	**3**	**4**	**5**	**11**
TOTAL										
0–19 Years	67	2.2	8	1	1	1	2	3	4	16
20–34	82	2.4	5	1	1	2	3	4	6	13
35–49	115	2.0	1	1	1	2	3	3	4	6
50–64	143	2.3	2	1	1	2	3	4	5	6
65+	80	2.8	7	1	2	2	3	5	6	20
GRAND TOTAL	**487**	**2.3**	**4**	**1**	**1**	**2**	**3**	**4**	**5**	**13**

77.8: OTHER PARTIAL OSTECTOMY

Type of Patients	Observed Patients	Avg. Stay	Vari-ance	Percentiles						
				10th	25th	50th	75th	90th	95th	99th
1. SINGLE DX										
0–19 Years	64	1.5	2	1	1	1	1	3	3	10
20–34	22	2.1	1	1	1	2	3	3	4	5
35–49	17	2.0	2	1	1	1	2	5	5	5
50–64	13	2.5	7	1	1	1	3	5	10	10
65+	2	2.0	0	2	2	2	2	2	2	2
2. MULTIPLE DX										
0–19 Years	117	3.4	17	1	1	2	3	8	15	22
20–34	162	5.6	52	1	1	3	7	12	16	40
35–49	312	6.3	49	1	2	4	7	14	21	37
50–64	589	6.6	70	1	2	5	8	13	19	47
65+	516	6.4	49	2	3	5	8	13	18	34
TOTAL SINGLE DX	**118**	**1.7**	**3**	**1**	**1**	**1**	**2**	**3**	**5**	**10**
TOTAL MULTIPLE DX	**1,696**	**5.9**	**52**	**1**	**2**	**4**	**7**	**12**	**17**	**41**
TOTAL										
0–19 Years	181	2.7	13	1	1	1	3	5	11	22
20–34	184	5.2	47	1	1	3	6	11	16	40
35–49	329	6.0	47	1	2	4	7	13	21	37
50–64	602	6.5	69	1	2	4	8	13	18	46
65+	518	6.4	48	1	3	5	8	13	18	34
GRAND TOTAL	**1,814**	**5.5**	**48**	**1**	**1**	**3**	**7**	**12**	**16**	**39**

77.81: CHEST CAGE OSTECTOMY NEC

Type of Patients	Observed Patients	Avg. Stay	Vari-ance	Percentiles						
				10th	25th	50th	75th	90th	95th	99th
1. SINGLE DX										
0–19 Years	4	1.4	<1	1	1	1	2	2	2	2
20–34	2	2.5	<1	2	2	2	3	3	3	3
35–49	2	1.5	<1	1	1	1	2	2	2	2
50–64	1	1.0	0	1	1	1	1	1	1	1
65+	0									
2. MULTIPLE DX										
0–19 Years	5	4.8	12	1	3	4	5	11	11	11
20–34	21	2.9	15	1	1	2	3	4	10	21
35–49	28	6.8	96	1	1	2	7	24	34	38
50–64	84	6.4	79	1	1	3	7	14	22	56
65+	54	6.1	72	1	1	2	8	13	23	49
TOTAL SINGLE DX	**9**	**1.5**	**<1**	**1**	**1**	**1**	**2**	**2**	**3**	**3**
TOTAL MULTIPLE DX	**192**	**5.8**	**69**	**1**	**1**	**2**	**7**	**13**	**22**	**41**
TOTAL										
0–19 Years	9	2.7	7	1	1	2	3	5	11	11
20–34	23	2.8	14	1	1	2	3	4	10	21
35–49	30	6.4	91	1	1	3	7	16	34	38
50–64	85	6.3	79	1	1	3	7	14	22	56
65+	54	6.1	72	1	1	2	8	13	23	49
GRAND TOTAL	**201**	**5.5**	**65**	**1**	**1**	**2**	**6**	**13**	**22**	**41**

77.85: PART OSTECTOMY FEMUR

Type of Patients	Observed Patients	Avg. Stay	Vari-ance	Percentiles						
				10th	25th	50th	75th	90th	95th	99th
1. SINGLE DX										
0–19 Years	6	1.9	2	1	1	1	2	5	5	5
20–34	3	2.7	<1	2	2	3	3	3	3	3
35–49	1	1.0	0	1	1	1	1	1	1	1
50–64	2	1.5	<1	1	1	2	2	2	2	2
65+	0									
2. MULTIPLE DX										
0–19 Years	44	4.1	14	1	2	3	4	11	15	15
20–34	29	6.3	44	1	3	3	8	20	22	24
35–49	39	8.9	115	1	4	6	11	18	37	56
50–64	68	11.0	192	2	4	6	12	22	37	95
65+	54	9.6	144	3	5	6	12	15	29	77
TOTAL SINGLE DX	**12**	**1.9**	**2**	**1**	**1**	**1**	**3**	**4**	**5**	**5**
TOTAL MULTIPLE DX	**234**	**7.6**	**102**	**1**	**3**	**4**	**9**	**15**	**24**	**56**
TOTAL										
0–19 Years	50	4.0	13	1	2	3	4	11	15	15
20–34	32	6.0	41	1	3	3	7	15	22	24
35–49	40	8.7	114	1	3	5	10	17	37	56
50–64	70	10.7	189	2	3	6	12	20	37	95
65+	54	9.6	144	3	5	6	9	15	29	77
GRAND TOTAL	**246**	**7.3**	**99**	**1**	**2**	**4**	**8**	**15**	**22**	**45**

LOS by Diagnosis and Operation, Western Region, 45th Edition

Western Region, October 2007–September 2008 Data, by Operation

77.86: PARTIAL PATELLECTOMY

Type of Patients	Observed Patients	Avg. Stay	Variance	10th	25th	50th	75th	90th	95th	99th
1. SINGLE DX										
0–19 Years	1	1.0	0	1	1	1	1	1	1	1
20–34	5	3.0	2	2	2	2	4	5	5	5
35–49	2	4.5	<1	4	4	5	5	5	5	5
50–64	4	2.3	<1	1	2	2	3	3	3	3
65+	1	2.0	0	2	2	2	2	2	2	2
2. MULTIPLE DX										
0–19 Years	0									
20–34	29	5.7	106	1	1	3	6	11	15	56
35–49	30	3.3	4	1	2	3	4	7	7	9
50–64	66	3.3	7	1	2	3	5	6	7	18
65+	96	4.6	16	2	3	3	5	8	10	24
TOTAL SINGLE DX	13	2.8	2	1	2	2	4	5	5	5
TOTAL MULTIPLE DX	221	4.2	24	1	2	3	5	7	9	24
TOTAL										
0–19 Years	1	1.0	0	1	1	1	1	1	1	1
20–34	34	5.3	91	1	1	3	4	10	15	56
35–49	32	3.4	4	1	2	3	4	6	7	9
50–64	70	3.3	7	1	2	3	4	6	7	18
65+	97	4.6	16	2	3	3	5	8	10	24
GRAND TOTAL	234	4.1	23	1	2	3	5	7	9	24

77.87: PART OSTECTOMY TIB/FIB

Type of Patients	Observed Patients	Avg. Stay	Variance	10th	25th	50th	75th	90th	95th	99th
1. SINGLE DX										
0–19 Years	10	2.9	12	1	1	1	3	10	10	10
20–34	2	1.5	<1	1	1	2	2	2	2	2
35–49	2	3.5	4	2	2	5	5	5	5	5
50–64	2	5.5	40	1	1	1	10	10	10	10
65+	0									
2. MULTIPLE DX										
0–19 Years	17	2.3	2	1	1	3	3	4	4	7
20–34	16	11.3	156	2	2	5	16	34	40	40
35–49	30	4.9	30	2	2	3	6	9	21	23
50–64	21	5.3	24	2	2	3	5	13	15	19
65+	18	6.6	17	3	3	6	11	15	>99	>99
TOTAL SINGLE DX	16	3.0	12	1	1	1	3	10	10	10
TOTAL MULTIPLE DX	102	5.2	40	1	2	3	5	14	19	40
TOTAL										
0–19 Years	27	2.5	5	1	1	1	3	4	10	10
20–34	18	10.2	147	1	2	5	15	34	40	40
35–49	32	4.8	28	1	2	3	6	9	21	23
50–64	23	5.3	24	2	2	3	6	13	15	19
65+	18	6.6	17	3	3	6	11	15	>99	>99
GRAND TOTAL	118	4.8	35	1	1	3	5	11	16	40

77.88: PART OSTECTOMY MT/TARSAL

Type of Patients	Observed Patients	Avg. Stay	Variance	10th	25th	50th	75th	90th	95th	99th
1. SINGLE DX										
0–19 Years	28	1.0	0	1	1	1	1		1	1
20–34	0									
35–49	0									
50–64	0									
2. MULTIPLE DX										
0–19 Years	31	2.2	19	1	1	1	1	2	11	22
20–34	22	7.1	15	2	4	7	10	11	14	15
35–49	91	7.0	33	2	3	6	8	15	19	>99
50–64	187	6.6	33	2	3	6	8	11	15	46
65+	153	7.0	39	2	4	5	8	13	17	32
TOTAL SINGLE DX	28	1.0	0	1	1	1	1	1	1	1
TOTAL MULTIPLE DX	484	6.1	34	1	2	5	8	12	16	32
TOTAL										
0–19 Years	59	1.6	10	1	1	1	1	2	2	22
20–34	22	7.1	15	2	4	7	10	11	14	15
35–49	91	7.0	33	2	3	6	8	15	19	>99
50–64	187	6.6	33	2	3	6	8	11	15	46
65+	153	7.0	39	2	4	5	8	13	17	32
GRAND TOTAL	512	5.3	33	1	1	4	7	11	15	27

77.89: PARTIAL OSTECTOMY NEC

Type of Patients	Observed Patients	Avg. Stay	Variance	10th	25th	50th	75th	90th	95th	99th
1. SINGLE DX										
0–19 Years	11	2.1	1	1	1	2	3	3	3	5
20–34	7	1.4	<1	1	1	1	2	3	3	3
35–49	6	1.3	<1	1	1	1	1	3	3	3
50–64	2	3.0	8	1	1	1	5	5	5	5
65+	0									
2. MULTIPLE DX										
0–19 Years	13	6.5	39	1	2	3	9	15	15	27
20–34	31	4.8	15	1	2	3	6	10	14	16
35–49	64	6.7	45	1	2	5	8	13	24	37
50–64	124	7.2	97	1	2	5	8	16	21	87
65+	109	6.7	40	1	2	5	9	14	20	31
TOTAL SINGLE DX	26	1.9	1	1	1	1	3	3	5	5
TOTAL MULTIPLE DX	341	6.7	59	1	2	5	8	14	20	39
TOTAL										
0–19 Years	24	4.4	26	1	1	3	5	15	15	27
20–34	38	4.2	14	1	2	4	6	10	14	16
35–49	70	6.2	43	1	2	4	8	12	24	37
50–64	126	7.1	96	1	2	5	8	16	21	87
65+	109	6.7	40	1	2	5	9	14	20	31
GRAND TOTAL	367	6.2	55	1	2	4	8	13	17	39

LOS by Diagnosis and Operation, Western Region, 45th Edition

Western Region, October 2007–September 2008 Data, by Operation

77.9: TOTAL OSTECTOMY

Type of Patients	Observed Patients	Avg. Stay	Vari-ance	10th	25th	50th	75th	90th	95th	99th
1. SINGLE DX										
0–19 Years	9	2.2	3	1	1	1	4	5	5	5
20–34	26	1.9	1	1	1	1	3	3	3	6
35–49	34	1.8	2	1	1	2	2	2	6	7
50–64	20	1.8	<1	1	1	1	2	3	3	5
65+	2	1.0	0	1	1	1	1	1	1	1
2. MULTIPLE DX										
0–19 Years	31	2.6	4	1	1	2	3	6	7	9
20–34	105	3.6	25	1	1	2	4	7	10	11
35–49	138	3.6	12	1	1	3	5	7	10	20
50–64	117	6.0	61	1	2	3	6	14	26	36
65+	103	5.7	31	1	2	4	7	13	17	25
TOTAL SINGLE DX	91	1.9	2	1	1	1	2	3	5	6
TOTAL MULTIPLE DX	494	4.5	30	1	2	3	5	9	15	31
TOTAL										
0–19 Years	40	2.5	4	1	1	2	3	5	7	9
20–34	131	3.3	21	1	1	2	3	7	9	11
35–49	172	3.3	10	1	1	3	5	6	8	20
50–64	137	5.4	55	1	2	3	5	14	23	36
65+	105	5.6	31	1	2	3	7	13	17	25
GRAND TOTAL	585	4.1	27	1	1	2	5	8	13	28

78.0: BONE GRAFT

Type of Patients	Observed Patients	Avg. Stay	Vari-ance	10th	25th	50th	75th	90th	95th	99th
1. SINGLE DX										
0–19 Years	52	1.4	<1	1	1	1	2	2	3	4
20–34	21	1.8	1	1	1	1	2	2	3	4
35–49	21	2.3	3	1	1	2	2	4	5	8
50–64	17	2.0	2	1	1	1	3	4	4	4
65+	3	1.7	1	1	1	1	3	3	3	3
2. MULTIPLE DX										
0–19 Years	69	2.1	2	1	1	2	3	4	5	7
20–34	107	2.8	6	1	1	2	3	7	8	11
35–49	147	2.9	8	1	1	2	3	6	8	14
50–64	181	3.4	13	1	1	3	4	6	10	24
65+	87	3.2	7	1	2	3	4	6	7	18
TOTAL SINGLE DX	114	1.6	1	1	1	1	2	3	4	4
TOTAL MULTIPLE DX	591	2.9	7	1	1	2	4	6	7	15
TOTAL										
0–19 Years	121	1.8	2	1	1	2	2	4	4	7
20–34	128	2.6	6	1	1	2	3	6	8	11
35–49	168	2.9	7	1	1	2	3	6	8	14
50–64	198	3.3	12	1	1	3	4	6	9	24
65+	90	3.1	7	1	2	3	4	6	7	18
GRAND TOTAL	705	2.6	6	1	1	2	3	5	7	14

77.91: TOT CHEST CAGE OSTECTOMY

Type of Patients	Observed Patients	Avg. Stay	Vari-ance	10th	25th	50th	75th	90th	95th	99th
1. SINGLE DX										
0–19 Years	7	2.7	3	1	1	3	5	5	5	5
20–34	21	1.9	2	1	1	1	3	3	3	6
35–49	31	1.7	<1	1	1	2	2	2	3	6
50–64	16	1.8	1	1	1	1	2	3	5	5
65+	1	1.0	0	1	1	1	1	1	1	1
2. MULTIPLE DX										
0–19 Years	24	3.4	5	1	2	3	4	7	8	9
20–34	93	2.8	4	1	1	2	3	6	8	10
35–49	94	3.2	7	1	1	3	5	7	8	20
50–64	73	4.7	49	1	2	3	4	11	18	44
65+	22	7.5	75	2	3	4	9	17	25	36
TOTAL SINGLE DX	76	1.9	2	1	1	1	2	3	5	6
TOTAL MULTIPLE DX	306	3.8	22	1	1	3	4	7	10	25
TOTAL										
0–19 Years	31	3.2	4	1	1	3	5	6	7	9
20–34	114	2.6	4	1	1	2	3	6	7	10
35–49	125	2.8	6	1	1	2	4	5	7	10
50–64	89	4.2	42	1	1	2	4	9	14	44
65+	23	7.2	74	1	2	4	7	17	25	36
GRAND TOTAL	382	3.4	18	1	1	2	4	6	9	25

78.05: BONE GRAFT TO FEMUR

Type of Patients	Observed Patients	Avg. Stay	Vari-ance	10th	25th	50th	75th	90th	95th	99th
1. SINGLE DX										
0–19 Years	26	1.3	<1	1	1	1	1	2	2	3
20–34	7	1.9	1	1	1	2	2	4	4	4
35–49	7	2.4	2	1	2	2	3	5	5	5
50–64	8	2.4	2	1	1	2	4	4	4	4
65+	0									
2. MULTIPLE DX										
0–19 Years	28	1.9	1	1	1	1	2	4	4	6
20–34	40	3.7	9	1	1	3	5	8	11	13
35–49	49	3.1	6	1	1	2	4	6	8	14
50–64	65	3.8	18	1	1	2	4	8	15	24
65+	45	3.8	10	1	2	3	5	7	8	18
TOTAL SINGLE DX	48	1.5	<1	1	1	1	2	3	4	5
TOTAL MULTIPLE DX	227	3.1	9	1	1	2	4	6	8	16
TOTAL										
0–19 Years	54	1.6	1	1	1	1	2	4	4	4
20–34	47	3.5	9	1	1	2	4	8	11	13
35–49	56	3.0	6	1	1	2	4	6	8	14
50–64	73	3.6	17	1	2	2	4	7	15	24
65+	45	3.8	10	1	2	3	5	7	8	18
GRAND TOTAL	275	2.7	8	1	1	2	3	5	8	16

LOS by Diagnosis and Operation, Western Region, 45th Edition

Western Region, October 2007–September 2008 Data, by Operation

78.07: BONE GRAFT TIBIA/FIBULA

Type of Patients	Observed Patients	Avg. Stay	Variance	10th	25th	50th	75th	90th	95th	99th
1. SINGLE DX										
0–19 Years	20	1.6	<1	1	1	1	2	3	4	4
20–34	10	2.1	3	1	1	2	3	3	4	4
35–49	7	2.6	7	1	2	2	4	8	8	8
50–64	6	1.7	<1	1	1	2	2	3	3	3
65+	1	1.0	0	1	1	1	1	1	1	1
2. MULTIPLE DX										
0–19 Years	30	2.7	3	1	1	2	4	5	7	7
20–34	47	2.2	3	1	1	2	3	5	6	7
35–49	73	3.1	10	1	1	2	3	7	14	15
50–64	85	2.8	4	1	1	2	3	5	6	10
65+	22	2.6	4	1	1	2	3	6	6	7
TOTAL SINGLE DX	44	1.7	1	1	1	1	2	3	4	8
TOTAL MULTIPLE DX	257	2.8	5	1	1	2	4	5	7	14
TOTAL										
0–19 Years	50	2.2	2	1	1	1	3	4	5	7
20–34	57	2.2	3	1	1	2	3	4	6	7
35–49	80	3.1	10	1	1	2	4	7	14	15
50–64	91	2.7	4	1	1	2	3	5	6	10
65+	23	2.6	4	1	1	2	3	6	6	7
GRAND TOTAL	301	2.5	4	1	1	2	3	5	7	14

78.13: APPL EXT FIX RAD/ULNA

Type of Patients	Observed Patients	Avg. Stay	Variance	10th	25th	50th	75th	90th	95th	99th
1. SINGLE DX										
0–19 Years	4	1.0	0	1	1	1	1	1	1	1
20–34	2	1.0	0	1	1	1	1	1	1	1
35–49	8	2.1	2	1	1	2	4	4	4	4
50–64	5	1.6	<1	1	1	1	2	3	3	3
65+	4	1.0	0	1	1	1	1	1	1	1
2. MULTIPLE DX										
0–19 Years	3	8.0	37	1	1	11	12	12	12	12
20–34	25	3.2	9	1	1	3	3	6	10	13
35–49	22	5.6	50	1	2	3	5	19	22	26
50–64	47	3.9	12	1	1	3	5	9	11	15
65+	77	3.4	8	1	1	3	4	7	9	19
TOTAL SINGLE DX	23	1.5	<1	1	1	1	2	3	4	4
TOTAL MULTIPLE DX	174	3.9	15	1	1	3	5	8	11	22
TOTAL										
0–19 Years	7	4.0	26	1	1	1	11	12	12	12
20–34	27	3.0	9	1	1	2	3	6	10	13
35–49	30	4.7	39	1	1	2	4	7	22	26
50–64	52	3.7	11	1	1	2	5	8	11	15
65+	81	3.2	8	1	1	3	4	7	9	19
GRAND TOTAL	197	3.6	14	1	1	2	4	7	11	22

78.1: APPL EXT FIXATOR DEVICE

Type of Patients	Observed Patients	Avg. Stay	Variance	10th	25th	50th	75th	90th	95th	99th
1. SINGLE DX										
0–19 Years	33	1.9	1	1	1	2	2	3	5	5
20–34	33	2.3	3	1	1	2	3	3	6	9
35–49	40	2.9	4	1	2	2	4	6	8	11
50–64	25	3.7	11	1	1	3	5	8	10	14
65+	6	1.3	<1	1	1	1	1	3	3	3
2. MULTIPLE DX										
0–19 Years	64	7.4	84	2	2	4	8	25	31	>99
20–34	216	8.4	97	2	2	5	11	18	30	56
35–49	305	8.2	107	2	3	5	9	18	28	62
50–64	308	7.6	94	2	2	4	8	16	28	45
65+	198	6.3	51	1	2	4	7	14	20	49
TOTAL SINGLE DX	137	2.5	4	1	1	2	3	5	6	11
TOTAL MULTIPLE DX	1,091	7.6	90	2	2	4	9	17	27	52
TOTAL										
0–19 Years	97	5.6	63	1	2	3	5	11	25	48
20–34	249	7.6	89	1	2	4	10	18	28	56
35–49	345	7.5	98	2	2	4	9	16	26	62
50–64	333	7.3	89	1	2	4	8	15	26	45
65+	204	6.1	51	1	2	4	7	13	20	43
GRAND TOTAL	1,228	7.1	83	1	2	4	8	16	25	50

78.15: APPL EXT FIX DEV FEMUR

Type of Patients	Observed Patients	Avg. Stay	Variance	10th	25th	50th	75th	90th	95th	99th
1. SINGLE DX										
0–19 Years	14	2.0	2	1	1	1	3	4	5	5
20–34	0									
35–49	0									
50–64	0									
65+	0									
2. MULTIPLE DX										
0–19 Years	23	8.6	96	2	2	4	9	25	34	>99
20–34	32	16.6	185	5	8	14	20	41	68	>99
35–49	28	18.6	292	5	9	14	20	44	52	78
50–64	23	16.6	340	3	4	10	25	26	54	81
65+	16	10.1	102	4	4	7	14	24	42	42
TOTAL SINGLE DX	14	2.0	2	1	1	1	3	4	5	5
TOTAL MULTIPLE DX	122	14.3	213	3	5	9	19	34	52	>99
TOTAL										
0–19 Years	37	6.1	70	1	2	3	5	25	31	48
20–34	32	16.6	185	5	8	14	20	41	68	56
35–49	28	18.6	292	5	9	14	25	44	52	78
50–64	23	16.6	340	3	4	10	25	26	54	81
65+	16	10.1	102	4	4	7	14	24	42	43
GRAND TOTAL	136	12.6	203	2	4	7	17	30	44	50

LOS by Diagnosis and Operation, Western Region, 45th Edition

Western Region, October 2007–September 2008 Data, by Operation

78.17: APPL EXT FIX DEV TIB/FIB

Type of Patients	Observed Patients	Avg. Stay	Variance				Percentiles			
				10th	25th	50th	75th	90th	95th	99th
1. SINGLE DX										
0–19 Years	10	2.4	<1	2	2	2	3	3	5	5
20–34	27	2.5	0	1	2	2	3	4	6	9
35–49	32	3.1	5	1	2	2	3	6	8	11
50–64	19	4.3	13	1	1	3	6	10	14	14
65+	2	2.0	2	1	1	3	3	3	3	3
2. MULTIPLE DX										
0–19 Years	31	7.0	98	2	2	4	8	10	22	48
20–34	122	6.5	48	1	2	4	8	14	18	35
35–49	228	6.7	64	2	3	4	8	14	21	62
50–64	218	7.1	72	2	3	4	8	14	28	45
65+	85	6.6	38	2	3	5	8	14	19	>99
TOTAL SINGLE DX	90	3.0	6	1	2	2	3	6	8	14
TOTAL MULTIPLE DX	684	6.8	62	2	3	4	8	14	21	48
TOTAL										
0–19 Years	41	5.8	78	2	2	3	5	8	22	48
20–34	149	5.8	42	1	2	3	7	13	18	35
35–49	260	6.2	58	2	2	4	7	13	16	62
50–64	237	6.9	68	2	2	4	8	14	21	45
65+	87	6.5	38	2	3	5	8	14	19	>99
GRAND TOTAL	774	6.3	57	2	2	4	7	13	19	48

78.2: LIMB SHORTENING PX

Type of Patients	Observed Patients	Avg. Stay	Variance				Percentiles			
				10th	25th	50th	75th	90th	95th	99th
1. SINGLE DX										
0–19 Years	48	1.4	<1	1	1	1	1	2	3	4
20–34	1	4.0	0	4	4	4	4	4	4	4
35–49	0									
50–64	1	1.0	0	1	1	1	1	1	1	1
65+	0									
2. MULTIPLE DX										
0–19 Years	162	1.8	2	1	1	1	2	3	5	7
20–34	11	2.2	3	1	1	1	3	5	6	6
35–49	6	3.2	7	1	1	3	4	8	8	8
50–64	14	2.8	5	1	1	3	4	5	8	8
65+	5	2.6	5	1	1	1	4	6	6	6
TOTAL SINGLE DX	50	1.4	<1	1	1	1	1	2	3	4
TOTAL MULTIPLE DX	198	1.8	2	1	1	1	2	3	5	7
TOTAL										
0–19 Years	210	1.7	2	1	1	1	2	3	4	7
20–34	12	2.3	3	1	1	1	3	5	6	6
35–49	6	3.2	7	1	1	3	4	8	8	8
50–64	15	2.7	4	1	1	2	4	5	8	8
65+	5	2.6	5	1	1	1	4	6	6	6
GRAND TOTAL	248	1.7	2	1	1	1	2	3	5	7

78.25: LIMB SHORT PX FEMUR

Type of Patients	Observed Patients	Avg. Stay	Variance				Percentiles			
				10th	25th	50th	75th	90th	95th	99th
1. SINGLE DX										
0–19 Years	34	1.5	<1	1	1	1	2	3	3	5
20–34	1	4.0	0	4	4	4	4	4	4	4
35–49	0									
50–64	0									
65+	0									
2. MULTIPLE DX										
0–19 Years	111	1.8	2	1	1	1	2	3	5	7
20–34	8	2.6	4	1	1	2	5	5	6	6
35–49	4	4.3	7	2	3	4	8	8	8	8
50–64	4	3.3	3	1	3	4	4	4	5	5
65+	1	4.0	0	4	4	4	4	4	4	4
TOTAL SINGLE DX	35	1.5	<1	1	1	1	2	3	3	5
TOTAL MULTIPLE DX	128	1.9	2	1	1	1	2	4	5	7
TOTAL										
0–19 Years	145	1.7	1	1	1	1	2	3	5	7
20–34	9	2.7	4	1	1	2	5	5	6	6
35–49	4	4.3	7	2	3	4	8	8	8	8
50–64	4	3.3	3	1	3	4	4	4	5	5
65+	1	4.0	0	4	4	4	4	4	4	4
GRAND TOTAL	163	1.8	2	1	1	1	2	3	5	7

78.3: LIMB LENGTHENING PX

Type of Patients	Observed Patients	Avg. Stay	Variance				Percentiles			
				10th	25th	50th	75th	90th	95th	99th
1. SINGLE DX										
0–19 Years	21	1.8	2	1	1	1	2	2	6	7
20–34	1	3.0	2	2	2	4	4	4	4	4
35–49	1	2.0	0	2	2	2	2	2	2	2
50–64	0									
65+	0									
2. MULTIPLE DX										
0–19 Years	95	2.7	2	1	2	2	4	5	6	9
20–34	11	2.9	2	1	1	3	4	5	5	5
35–49	10	2.5	1	2	2	2	3	3	5	5
50–64	14	3.7	10	1	1	3	4	5	14	14
65+	2	1.5	<1	1	1	2	2	2	2	2
TOTAL SINGLE DX	24	1.9	2	1	1	1	2	4	5	7
TOTAL MULTIPLE DX	132	2.8	3	1	2	2	4	5	6	9
TOTAL										
0–19 Years	116	2.5	2	1	1	2	3	5	6	7
20–34	13	2.9	2	1	2	3	4	5	5	5
35–49	11	2.5	1	2	2	3	4	3	5	5
50–64	14	3.7	10	2	2	3	4	5	14	14
65+	2	1.5	<1	1	1	2	2	2	2	2
GRAND TOTAL	156	2.6	3	1	1	2	3	5	6	9

LOS by Diagnosis and Operation, Western Region, 45th Edition

343

Western Region, October 2007–September 2008 Data, by Operation

78.35: LIMB LENGTH PX FEMUR

Type of Patients	Observed Patients	Avg. Stay	Variance	10th	25th	50th	75th	90th	95th	99th
1. SINGLE DX										
0–19 Years	12	2.4	3	1	1	2	3	6	7	7
20–34	0									
35–49	0									
50–64	0									
65+	0									
2. MULTIPLE DX										
0–19 Years	38	3.3	3	2	2	3	4	6	6	9
20–34	5	3.6	2	1	4	4	4	5	5	5
35–49	7	2.6	2	1	2	2	3	5	5	5
50–64	2	3.0	0	3	3	3	3	3	3	3
65+	0									
TOTAL SINGLE DX	12	2.4	3	1	1	2	3	6	7	7
TOTAL MULTIPLE DX	52	3.3	3	2	2	3	4	6	6	9
TOTAL										
0–19 Years	50	3.2	3	1	2	2	4	6	6	9
20–34	5	3.6	2	1	4	4	4	5	5	5
35–49	7	2.6	2	1	2	2	3	5	5	5
50–64	2	3.0	0	3	3	3	3	3	3	3
65+	0									
GRAND TOTAL	64	3.1	3	1	2	2	4	6	6	9

78.4: OTHER BONE REPAIR

Type of Patients	Observed Patients	Avg. Stay	Variance	10th	25th	50th	75th	90th	95th	99th
1. SINGLE DX										
0–19 Years	15	1.6	<1	1	1	1	3	3	3	3
20–34	11	1.7	2	1	1	1	3	4	4	4
35–49	7	1.6	<1	1	1	1	2	2	2	2
50–64	5	1.6	<1	1	1	1	2	3	3	3
65+	1	3.0	0	3	3	3	3	3	3	3
2. MULTIPLE DX										
0–19 Years	91	2.4	12	1	1	1	3	4	6	18
20–34	72	3.0	5	1	1	2	5	6	7	9
35–49	94	3.1	13	1	1	2	4	6	7	29
50–64	83	5.7	130	1	2	3	5	9	17	74
65+	49	4.0	25	1	2	3	5	8	9	34
TOTAL SINGLE DX	39	1.7	<1	1	1	1	3	3	3	4
TOTAL MULTIPLE DX	389	3.2	31	1	1	2	3	6	8	27
TOTAL										
0–19 Years	106	2.3	11	1	1	2	3	4	6	18
20–34	83	2.9	4	1	1	2	4	6	7	9
35–49	101	3.0	12	1	1	2	4	6	7	16
50–64	88	5.5	124	1	1	3	4	9	17	74
65+	50	3.9	24	1	2	3	5	7	9	34
GRAND TOTAL	428	3.1	28	1	1	2	3	6	7	21

78.45: FEMORAL REPAIR NEC

Type of Patients	Observed Patients	Avg. Stay	Variance	10th	25th	50th	75th	90th	95th	99th
1. SINGLE DX										
0–19 Years	8	1.9	1	1	1	1	3	3	3	3
20–34	7	1.3	<1	1	1	1	1	3	3	3
35–49	2	2.0	0	2	2	2	2	2	2	2
50–64	2	2.0	2	1	1	2	3	3	3	3
65+	0									
2. MULTIPLE DX										
0–19 Years	21	3.3	4	1	2	3	4	5	7	12
20–34	36	3.5	5	1	1	3	6	6	7	9
35–49	49	2.6	4	1	1	1	5	6	7	7
50–64	14	10.0	386	1	1	2	12	21	74	74
65+	7	4.1	7	1	2	3	7	8	8	8
TOTAL SINGLE DX	19	1.8	<1	1	1	1	3	3	3	3
TOTAL MULTIPLE DX	127	3.8	43	1	1	2	5	6	7	21
TOTAL										
0–19 Years	29	2.7	3	1	1	3	3	5	5	12
20–34	43	3.2	5	1	1	2	5	6	7	9
35–49	51	2.6	4	1	1	2	5	6	7	7
50–64	16	9.0	342	1	1	2	3	21	74	74
65+	7	4.1	7	1	2	3	7	8	8	8
GRAND TOTAL	146	3.4	36	1	1	2	4	6	7	21

78.47: TIBIA/FIBULA REPAIR NEC

Type of Patients	Observed Patients	Avg. Stay	Variance	10th	25th	50th	75th	90th	95th	99th
1. SINGLE DX										
0–19 Years	3	1.0	0	1	1	1	1	1	1	1
20–34	2	2.5	4	1	1	4	4	4	4	4
35–49	3	1.7	<1	2	2	2	2	2	2	2
50–64	0									
65+	1	3.0	0	3	3	3	3	3	3	3
2. MULTIPLE DX										
0–19 Years	15	1.9	2	1	1	2	2	3	3	8
20–34	19	2.3	2	1	1	2	2	4	5	5
35–49	26	3.2	30	1	1	2	3	6	6	29
50–64	26	3.5	10	1	2	3	4	7	8	16
65+	9	3.3	4	1	2	3	3	8	8	8
TOTAL SINGLE DX	9	1.6	<1	1	1	1	1	3	4	4
TOTAL MULTIPLE DX	95	2.8	11	1	1	2	3	5	7	16
TOTAL										
0–19 Years	18	1.8	2	1	1	2	2	3	3	8
20–34	21	2.3	2	1	1	2	3	4	4	5
35–49	29	3.1	27	1	1	2	3	6	6	29
50–64	26	3.5	10	1	2	3	4	7	8	16
65+	10	3.3	4	1	2	3	3	8	8	8
GRAND TOTAL	104	2.7	10	1	1	2	3	5	7	16

Western Region, October 2007–September 2008 Data, by Operation

78.5: INT FIX W/O FX REDUCTION

Type of Patients	Observed Patients	Avg. Stay	Vari-ance	10th	25th	50th	75th	90th	95th	99th
1. SINGLE DX										
0–19 Years	290	1.8	2	1	1	1	2	3	4	5
20–34	117	2.3	1	1	1	2	3	4	6	6
35–49	97	2.4	3	1	1	2	3	4	5	12
50–64	73	2.2	2	1	1	2	3	3	4	9
65+	37	3.3	3	2	2	3	4	5	8	10
2. MULTIPLE DX										
0–19 Years	407	2.8	9	1	1	2	3	6	8	18
20–34	422	4.6	30	1	2	3	5	9	13	25
35–49	527	4.8	40	1	2	3	5	10	17	33
50–64	1,083	5.0	27	1	2	4	6	9	14	30
65+	3,624	5.2	12	3	3	4	6	9	12	20
TOTAL SINGLE DX	614	2.0	2	1	1	2	2	3	4	6
TOTAL MULTIPLE DX	6,063	4.8	18	1	3	4	6	9	12	22
TOTAL										
0–19 Years	697	2.4	7	1	1	2	3	4	6	16
20–34	539	4.1	24	1	2	3	4	8	12	25
35–49	624	4.5	35	1	2	3	4	9	15	29
50–64	1,156	4.8	25	1	2	3	6	9	13	30
65+	3,661	5.2	12	3	3	4	6	9	11	20
GRAND TOTAL	6,677	4.5	17	1	2	4	5	8	11	21

78.52: INT FIX W/O RED HUMERUS

Type of Patients	Observed Patients	Avg. Stay	Vari-ance	10th	25th	50th	75th	90th	95th	99th
1. SINGLE DX										
0–19 Years	13	1.6	1	1	1	1	2	2	4	5
20–34	3	2.7	4	1	1	2	5	5	5	5
35–49	8	1.9	1	1	1	2	3	4	4	4
50–64	4	2.8	<1	2	2	2	4	4	4	4
65+	2	1.0	0	1	1	1	1	1	1	1
2. MULTIPLE DX										
0–19 Years	11	3.2	9	1	1	2	3	6	8	11
20–34	21	3.6	26	1	2	3	3	4	6	25
35–49	28	2.6	5	1	1	3	5	5	5	12
50–64	97	3.4	14	1	1	3	4	7	14	22
65+	140	4.2	14	3	3	4	6	9	11	20
TOTAL SINGLE DX	30	1.9	1	1	1	2	2	3	4	5
TOTAL MULTIPLE DX	297	3.7	14	1	1	3	4	7	12	17
TOTAL										
0–19 Years	24	2.5	6	1	1	2	3	5	11	11
20–34	24	3.5	23	1	2	3	3	5	6	25
35–49	36	2.4	4	1	1	2	3	5	5	12
50–64	101	3.4	13	1	1	2	4	7	11	17
65+	142	4.2	14	2	2	3	5	8	14	20
GRAND TOTAL	327	3.5	13	1	1	2	4	7	12	17

78.55: INT FIX W/O RED FEMUR

Type of Patients	Observed Patients	Avg. Stay	Vari-ance	10th	25th	50th	75th	90th	95th	99th
1. SINGLE DX										
0–19 Years	226	1.8	2	1	1	1	2	3	4	5
20–34	34	2.5	2	1	2	2	3	4	6	6
35–49	28	2.6	5	1	1	2	4	4	5	12
50–64	32	2.2	1	1	1	2	3	3	4	6
65+	29	3.6	3	2	3	3	4	6	8	10
2. MULTIPLE DX										
0–19 Years	277	2.7	9	1	1	2	3	5	7	18
20–34	187	5.6	28	2	3	4	7	10	16	24
35–49	236	6.0	62	1	2	4	6	13	19	43
50–64	685	5.5	29	2	3	4	6	10	15	33
65+	3,272	5.2	11	3	3	4	6	9	11	19
TOTAL SINGLE DX	349	2.0	2	1	1	2	2	3	4	6
TOTAL MULTIPLE DX	4,657	5.0	17	2	3	4	6	9	12	22
TOTAL										
0–19 Years	503	2.3	6	1	1	2	2	4	5	15
20–34	221	5.1	26	2	2	4	6	10	14	24
35–49	264	5.7	57	1	2	4	6	12	19	43
50–64	717	5.3	28	2	3	4	6	10	14	31
65+	3,301	5.2	11	3	3	4	6	9	11	19
GRAND TOTAL	5,006	4.7	16	1	3	4	6	8	11	21

78.57: INT FIX W/O RED TIB/FIB

Type of Patients	Observed Patients	Avg. Stay	Vari-ance	10th	25th	50th	75th	90th	95th	99th
1. SINGLE DX										
0–19 Years	36	2.3	2	1	1	2	3	4	5	7
20–34	72	2.1	1	1	1	2	3	3	4	5
35–49	52	2.4	2	1	1	2	3	4	5	6
50–64	33	2.1	<1	2	2	2	3	3	4	9
65+	4	2.8	<1	2	2	2	3	4	4	4
2. MULTIPLE DX										
0–19 Years	70	2.5	4	1	1	2	3	5	6	9
20–34	167	3.8	29	1	2	3	4	7	9	29
35–49	219	3.6	12	1	2	3	5	6	10	21
50–64	217	4.0	13	1	2	3	5	8	11	21
65+	125	4.4	14	2	3	4	5	7	9	21
TOTAL SINGLE DX	197	2.2	2	1	1	2	3	4	4	6
TOTAL MULTIPLE DX	798	3.7	15	1	2	3	4	7	10	21
TOTAL										
0–19 Years	106	2.5	3	1	1	2	3	5	6	9
20–34	239	3.3	21	1	2	3	4	5	8	19
35–49	271	3.4	10	1	2	3	4	6	8	21
50–64	250	3.7	12	1	2	3	4	7	10	21
65+	129	4.4	13	2	3	4	5	7	9	21
GRAND TOTAL	995	3.4	13	1	2	3	4	6	9	20

LOS by Diagnosis and Operation, Western Region, 45th Edition

Western Region, October 2007–September 2008 Data, by Operation

78.59: INT FIX W/O FX RED NEC

Type of Patients	Observed Patients	Avg. Stay	Variance	10th	25th	50th	75th	90th	95th	99th
1. SINGLE DX										
0–19 Years	6	1.7	1	1	1	1	2	4	4	4
20–34	2	3.5	4	2	2	5	5	5	5	5
35–49	5	2.4	2	1	1	2	4	4	4	4
50–64	1	1.0	0	1	1	1	1	1	1	1
65+	2	2.5	<1	2	2	2	3	3	3	3
2. MULTIPLE DX										
0–19 Years	39	3.3	16	1	1	3	4	7	16	16
20–34	19	5.7	38	1	2	5	8	16	25	25
35–49	28	6.2	53	1	2	5	8	17	21	34
50–64	48	6.4	54	1	2	4	7	15	29	30
65+	54	6.9	29	1	3	6	9	16	20	22
TOTAL SINGLE DX	16	2.2	2	1	1	2	4	4	5	5
TOTAL MULTIPLE DX	188	5.2	34	1	1	3	7	14	16	30
TOTAL										
0–19 Years	45	3.2	15	1	1	2	4	7	12	16
20–34	21	5.5	35	1	2	3	7	12	16	25
35–49	33	5.7	47	1	2	3	7	11	21	34
50–64	49	6.3	53	1	2	4	7	15	29	30
65+	56	6.7	29	1	3	5	9	16	20	22
GRAND TOTAL	204	5.0	33	1	1	3	6	12	16	30

78.62: RMVL IMPL DEV HUMERUS

Type of Patients	Observed Patients	Avg. Stay	Variance	10th	25th	50th	75th	90th	95th	99th
1. SINGLE DX										
0–19 Years	5	1.5	<1	1	1	1	2	3	3	3
20–34	0									
35–49	2	2.0	2			3	3	3	3	3
50–64	4	1.0	0	1	1	1	1	1	1	1
65+	1	1.0	0	1	1	1	1	1	1	1
2. MULTIPLE DX										
0–19 Years	11	6.3	18	1	2	5	9	9	15	15
20–34	15	4.5	10	2	2	3	6	10	12	12
35–49	30	2.5	5	1	1	2	3	4	7	11
50–64	66	4.0	11	1	1	3	5	7	11	20
65+	52	5.2	39	1	1	4	6	9	16	36
TOTAL SINGLE DX	12	1.4	<1	1	1	1	2	3	3	3
TOTAL MULTIPLE DX	174	4.3	19	1	2	3	5	9	12	26
TOTAL										
0–19 Years	16	4.3	16	1	2	2	9	9	15	15
20–34	15	4.5	10	2	2	3	6	10	12	12
35–49	32	2.5	4	1	1	3	3	4	7	11
50–64	70	3.8	11	1	1	3	5	7	11	20
65+	53	5.1	38	1	1	4	6	9	16	36
GRAND TOTAL	186	4.1	18	1	1	3	5	9	12	26

78.6: RMVL IMPL DEV FROM BONE

Type of Patients	Observed Patients	Avg. Stay	Variance	10th	25th	50th	75th	90th	95th	99th
1. SINGLE DX										
0–19 Years	93	1.6	4	1	1	1	2	2	4	12
20–34	104	1.9	3	1	1	1	2	4	4	10
35–49	75	2.4	11	1	1	2	3	4	5	23
50–64	71	2.5	9	1	1	2	3	4	8	19
65+	21	1.8	1	1	1	1	3	3	3	4
2. MULTIPLE DX										
0–19 Years	311	3.7	54	1	1	1	3	7	13	42
20–34	534	3.8	20	1	1	2	5	8	11	19
35–49	881	3.8	25	1	1	2	4	8	13	28
50–64	1,278	4.3	35	1	1	2	5	9	14	31
65+	1,012	4.3	22	1	1	3	5	10	14	23
TOTAL SINGLE DX	364	2.0	5	1	1	1	2	3	5	13
TOTAL MULTIPLE DX	4,016	4.0	31	1	1	2	4	9	13	30
TOTAL										
0–19 Years	404	3.3	46	1	1	1	3	6	11	42
20–34	638	3.5	18	1	1	2	4	8	10	19
35–49	956	3.7	24	1	1	2	4	8	12	23
50–64	1,349	4.2	34	1	1	2	5	9	14	30
65+	1,033	4.3	21	1	1	3	5	9	13	23
GRAND TOTAL	4,380	3.9	29	1	1	2	4	8	13	29

78.63: RMVL IMPL DEV RAD/ULNA

Type of Patients	Observed Patients	Avg. Stay	Variance	10th	25th	50th	75th	90th	95th	99th
1. SINGLE DX										
0–19 Years	9	1.2	<1	1	1	1	1	2	2	2
20–34	11	1.9	2	1	1	1	3	4	5	5
35–49	5	1.4	<1	1	1	1	2	2	2	2
50–64	11	1.5	1	1	1	1	2	3	4	4
65+	3	1.7	1	1	1	1	3	3	3	3
2. MULTIPLE DX										
0–19 Years	23	2.0	7	1	1	1	2	3	4	17
20–34	47	3.1	8	1	1	2	4	7	8	15
35–49	64	4.6	61	1	1	3	4	6	8	47
50–64	92	5.3	66	1	1	3	5	10	23	46
65+	77	3.8	16	1	1	3	5	7	10	29
TOTAL SINGLE DX	39	1.6	1	1	1	1	2	3	4	5
TOTAL MULTIPLE DX	303	4.1	38	1	1	2	4	8	10	40
TOTAL										
0–19 Years	32	1.9	6	1	1	1	2	3	3	17
20–34	58	2.9	7	1	1	2	4	6	8	15
35–49	69	4.3	57	1	1	2	4	6	8	47
50–64	103	4.9	61	1	1	2	5	9	14	40
65+	80	3.7	16	1	1	3	4	7	8	29
GRAND TOTAL	342	3.8	35	1	1	2	4	7	10	40

LOS by Diagnosis and Operation, Western Region, 45th Edition

Western Region, October 2007–September 2008 Data, by Operation

78.65: RMVL IMPL DEV FEMUR

Type of Patients	Observed Patients	Avg. Stay	Variance	10th	25th	50th	75th	90th	95th	99th
1. SINGLE DX										
0–19 Years	33	1.2	<1	1	1	1	1	2	2	3
20–34	20	2.1	4	1	1	1	2	5	10	10
35–49	5	3.2	10	1	1	2	5	8	8	8
50–64	8	2.1	1	1	1	2	3	4	4	4
65+	5	1.4	<1	1	1	1	1	3	3	3
2. MULTIPLE DX										
0–19 Years	103	2.3	18	1	1	1	2	3	6	30
20–34	58	4.2	18	1	1	3	6	11	18	>99
35–49	71	4.3	42	1	1	2	5	8	14	42
50–64	144	4.9	48	1	1	3	5	10	19	40
65+	250	4.5	23	1	1	3	6	10	14	29
TOTAL SINGLE DX	71	1.5	2	1	1	1	1	2	3	8
TOTAL MULTIPLE DX	626	3.8	28	1	1	2	4	9	13	31
TOTAL										
0–19 Years	136	2.1	14	1	1	1	2	3	5	30
20–34	78	3.7	15	1	1	2	5	10	13	>99
35–49	76	4.2	40	1	1	2	5	8	14	42
50–64	152	4.7	46	1	1	3	5	10	19	40
65+	255	4.4	23	1	1	3	6	10	14	29
GRAND TOTAL	697	3.5	25	1	1	2	4	8	13	30

78.67: RMVL IMPL DEV TIB & FIB

Type of Patients	Observed Patients	Avg. Stay	Variance	10th	25th	50th	75th	90th	95th	99th
1. SINGLE DX										
0–19 Years	21	2.2	3	1	1	1	2	5	6	6
20–34	24	2.1	6	1	1	1	2	4	5	12
35–49	29	3.1	25	1	1	2	2	5	18	23
50–64	16	2.9	19	1	1	2	3	3	9	19
65+	4	2.0	2	1	1	2	4	4	4	4
2. MULTIPLE DX										
0–19 Years	45	2.8	11	1	1	2	3	8	8	23
20–34	140	4.9	42	1	1	3	6	10	14	42
35–49	205	5.4	34	2	2	3	7	13	16	28
50–64	292	4.8	27	1	1	3	6	11	14	28
65+	209	5.9	32	2	2	4	7	12	18	24
TOTAL SINGLE DX	94	2.5	13	1	1	1	2	5	6	23
TOTAL MULTIPLE DX	891	5.0	31	1	2	3	6	11	15	28
TOTAL										
0–19 Years	66	2.6	9	1	1	1	3	6	8	23
20–34	164	4.5	37	1	1	3	6	10	13	42
35–49	234	5.1	33	1	2	3	7	13	16	28
50–64	308	4.7	27	1	2	3	6	11	14	26
65+	213	5.8	32	1	2	4	7	12	18	24
GRAND TOTAL	985	4.8	30	1	1	3	6	11	15	28

78.68: RMVL IMPL DEV MT/TARSAL

Type of Patients	Observed Patients	Avg. Stay	Variance	10th	25th	50th	75th	90th	95th	99th
1. SINGLE DX										
0–19 Years	0									
20–34	5	1.6	<1	1	1	2	2	2	2	2
35–49	3	3.0	<1	2	2	3	4	4	4	4
50–64	2	7.5	39	3	3	3	12	12	12	12
65+	1	1.0	0	1	1	1	1	1	1	1
2. MULTIPLE DX										
0–19 Years	8	3.9	15	1	2	3	4	13	14	14
20–34	44	3.7	16	1	1	2	5	8	11	18
35–49	71	3.7	13	1	2	3	5	8	11	22
50–64	96	4.6	76	1	2	3	5	8	10	63
65+	66	3.6	9	1	2	3	4	7	9	17
TOTAL SINGLE DX	11	3.0	10	1	1	2	3	4	12	12
TOTAL MULTIPLE DX	285	4.0	33	1	2	3	4	8	11	22
TOTAL										
0–19 Years	8	3.9	15	1	2	3	4	13	14	14
20–34	49	3.5	15	1	1	2	3	8	11	18
35–49	74	3.7	13	1	2	3	4	8	11	22
50–64	98	4.7	75	1	2	3	5	8	12	63
65+	67	3.6	8	1	2	3	4	7	9	17
GRAND TOTAL	296	4.0	32	1	2	3	4	8	11	18

78.69: RMVL IMPL DEV SITE NEC

Type of Patients	Observed Patients	Avg. Stay	Variance	10th	25th	50th	75th	90th	95th	99th
1. SINGLE DX										
0–19 Years	20	2.3	15	1	1	1	2	4	12	19
20–34	29	1.9	1	1	1	2	2	4	4	4
35–49	26	1.8	<1	1	1	2	2	3	4	4
50–64	27	2.6	7	1	1	2	3	5	8	13
65+	6	2.3	1	1	1	3	3	3	3	3
2. MULTIPLE DX										
0–19 Years	105	5.6	119	1	1	2	4	11	29	57
20–34	196	3.0	8	1	1	2	3	7	9	13
35–49	389	3.0	16	1	1	2	4	6	10	14
50–64	519	3.6	26	1	1	2	4	8	13	23
65+	320	3.4	14	1	1	2	4	7	12	18
TOTAL SINGLE DX	108	2.2	6	1	1	1	3	4	4	13
TOTAL MULTIPLE DX	1,529	3.6	33	1	1	2	4	8	12	26
TOTAL										
0–19 Years	125	5.2	108	1	1	2	3	11	23	57
20–34	225	2.8	7	1	1	2	3	6	9	13
35–49	415	2.9	15	1	1	2	3	6	10	14
50–64	546	3.6	25	1	1	2	4	8	13	23
65+	326	3.4	14	1	1	2	4	7	12	18
GRAND TOTAL	1,637	3.5	31	1	1	2	3	7	12	26

LOS by Diagnosis and Operation, Western Region, 45th Edition

Western Region, October 2007–September 2008 Data, by Operation

78.7: OSTEOCLASIS

Type of Patients	Observed Patients	Avg. Stay	Variance	10th	25th	50th	75th	90th	95th	99th
1. SINGLE DX										
0–19 Years	1	1.0	0	1	1	1	1	1	1	1
20–34	1	1.0	0	1	1	1	1	1	1	1
35–49	0									
50–64	1	11.0	0	11	11	11	11	11	11	11
65+	0									
2. MULTIPLE DX										
0–19 Years	7	2.4	5	1	1	1	6	6	6	6
20–34	1	4.0	0	4	4	4	4	4	4	4
35–49	3	1.7	<1	1	1	2	2	2	2	2
50–64	4	4.7	32	1	1	1	4	13	13	13
65+	1	4.0	0	4	4	4	4	4	4	4
TOTAL SINGLE DX	3	4.3	33	1	1	1	11	11	11	11
TOTAL MULTIPLE DX	16	2.8	8	1	1	1	4	6	6	13
TOTAL										
0–19 Years	8	2.3	5	1	1	1	2	6	6	6
20–34	2	2.5	4	1	1	1	4	4	4	4
35–49	3	1.7	<1	1	1	2	2	2	2	2
50–64	5	6.0	32	1	1	4	11	13	13	13
65+	1	4.0	0	4	4	4	4	4	4	4
GRAND TOTAL	19	3.0	10	1	1	1	4	6	11	13

78.8: OTHER BONE DIAGNOSTIC PX

Type of Patients	Observed Patients	Avg. Stay	Variance	10th	25th	50th	75th	90th	95th	99th
1. SINGLE DX										
0–19 Years	0									
20–34	0									
35–49	0									
50–64	0									
65+	0									
2. MULTIPLE DX										
0–19 Years	1	7.0	0	7	7	7	7	7	7	7
20–34	0									
35–49	1	1.0	0	1	1	1	1	1	1	1
50–64	1	3.0	0	3	3	3	3	3	3	3
65+	0									
TOTAL SINGLE DX	0									
TOTAL MULTIPLE DX	3	3.7	9	1	1	3	7	7	7	7
TOTAL										
0–19 Years	1	7.0	0	7	7	7	7	7	7	7
20–34	0									
35–49	1	1.0	0	1	1	1	1	1	1	1
50–64	1	3.0	0	3	3	3	3	3	3	3
65+	0									
GRAND TOTAL	3	3.7	9	1	1	3	7	7	7	7

78.9: INSERT BONE GROWTH STIM

Type of Patients	Observed Patients	Avg. Stay	Variance	10th	25th	50th	75th	90th	95th	99th
1. SINGLE DX										
0–19 Years	0									
20–34	0									
35–49	1	3.0	0	3	3	3	3	3	3	3
50–64	0									
65+	0									
2. MULTIPLE DX										
0–19 Years	1	3.0	0	3	3	3	3	3	3	3
20–34	1	2.0	0	2	2	2	2	2	2	2
35–49	3	2.7	1	2	2	2	2	4	4	4
50–64	10	1.8	<1	1	1	2	2	3	3	3
65+	3	4.0	7	1	1	5	6	6	6	6
TOTAL SINGLE DX	1	3.0	0	3	3	3	3	3	3	3
TOTAL MULTIPLE DX	18	2.4	2	1	1	2	3	5	6	6
TOTAL										
0–19 Years	1	3.0	0	3	3	3	3	3	3	3
20–34	1	2.0	0	2	2	2	2	2	2	2
35–49	4	2.8	<1	2	2	2	3	4	4	4
50–64	10	1.8	<1	1	1	2	2	3	3	3
65+	3	4.0	7	1	1	5	6	6	6	6
GRAND TOTAL	19	2.4	2	1	1	2	3	5	6	6

79.0: CLSD FX RED W/O INT FIX

Type of Patients	Observed Patients	Avg. Stay	Variance	10th	25th	50th	75th	90th	95th	99th
1. SINGLE DX										
0–19 Years	984	1.3	<1	1	1	1	1	2	2	4
20–34	109	1.5	<1	1	1	1	2	3	4	5
35–49	75	1.7	1	1	1	1	2	3	3	7
50–64	48	1.7	1	1	1	1	2	3	3	7
65+	17	1.5	<1	1	1	1	2	3	4	4
2. MULTIPLE DX										
0–19 Years	568	2.2	6	1	1	2	2	4	6	15
20–34	287	2.9	18	1	1	2	3	5	8	22
35–49	321	3.7	21	1	1	2	4	7	11	22
50–64	556	3.9	27	1	1	2	4	8	11	22
65+	1,151	4.3	15	1	2	3	5	8	11	19
TOTAL SINGLE DX	1,233	1.3	<1	1	1	1	1	2	3	5
TOTAL MULTIPLE DX	2,883	3.5	16	1	1	2	4	7	10	20
TOTAL										
0–19 Years	1,552	1.6	3	1	1	1	2	3	4	8
20–34	396	2.5	14	1	1	1	3	5	7	21
35–49	396	3.3	18	1	1	2	4	7	10	22
50–64	604	3.7	25	1	1	2	5	8	10	22
65+	1,168	4.3	15	1	2	3	5	8	11	19
GRAND TOTAL	4,116	2.7	12	1	1	2	3	5	8	16

LOS by Diagnosis and Operation, Western Region, 45th Edition

Western Region, October 2007–September 2008 Data, by Operation

79.01: CLSD FX RED HUMERUS

Type of Patients	Observed Patients	Avg. Stay	Vari-ance	10th	25th	50th	75th	90th	95th	99th
1. SINGLE DX										
0–19 Years	65	1.1	<1	1	1	1	1	2	2	2
20–34	8	1.6	<1	1	1	1	3	3	3	3
35–49	3	3.3	10	1	1	2	7	7	7	7
50–64	7	1.6	<1	1	1	2	2	2	2	2
65+	1	1.0	0	1	1	1	1	1	1	1
2. MULTIPLE DX										
0–19 Years	41	1.9	2	1	1	1	2	3	4	7
20–34	41	3.0	9	1	1	2	4	6	9	15
35–49	53	3.6	14	1	2	2	4	6	15	19
50–64	102	3.9	20	1	2	3	6	9	12	22
65+	290	4.1	13	1	2	3	5	8	11	16
TOTAL SINGLE DX	84	1.3	<1	1	1	1	1	2	2	4
TOTAL MULTIPLE DX	527	3.7	14	1	1	3	5	8	11	19
TOTAL										
0–19 Years	106	1.4	<1	1	1	1	2	2	3	7
20–34	49	2.8	8	1	1	2	3	6	9	15
35–49	56	3.6	14	1	2	2	5	6	15	19
50–64	109	3.7	19	1	2	2	5	9	12	22
65+	291	4.1	13	1	2	3	5	8	11	16
GRAND TOTAL	611	3.4	12	1	1	2	4	7	10	16

79.02: CLSD FX RED RADIUS/ULNA

Type of Patients	Observed Patients	Avg. Stay	Vari-ance	10th	25th	50th	75th	90th	95th	99th
1. SINGLE DX										
0–19 Years	335	1.1	<1	1	1	1	1	1	2	2
20–34	14	1.1	<1	1	1	1	1	1	2	3
35–49	18	1.3	<1	1	1	1	1	3	3	3
50–64	16	1.5	<1	1	1	1	2	2	3	3
65+	9	1.1	<1	1	1	1	1	2	2	2
2. MULTIPLE DX										
0–19 Years	164	1.6	2	1	1	1	2	3	4	7
20–34	65	2.0	2	1	1	1	3	4	4	7
35–49	67	3.0	6	1	1	2	4	7	7	12
50–64	137	2.8	6	1	1	2	3	5	8	13
65+	389	3.6	7	2	2	3	4	6	8	15
TOTAL SINGLE DX	392	1.1	<1	1	1	1	1	1	2	3
TOTAL MULTIPLE DX	822	2.8	6	1	1	2	4	5	7	13
TOTAL										
0–19 Years	499	1.3	<1	1	1	1	1	2	3	4
20–34	79	1.8	2	1	1	1	3	4	4	7
35–49	85	2.7	5	1	1	2	3	6	7	12
50–64	153	2.6	5	1	1	2	3	5	7	13
65+	398	3.6	7	1	2	3	4	6	8	15
GRAND TOTAL	1,214	2.2	4	1	1	1	3	5	6	12

79.05: CLSD FX RED FEMUR

Type of Patients	Observed Patients	Avg. Stay	Vari-ance	10th	25th	50th	75th	90th	95th	99th
1. SINGLE DX										
0–19 Years	333	1.5	1	1	1	1	2	2	3	4
20–34	8	2.3	2	1	1	1	4	4	4	4
35–49	2	1.0	0	1	1	1	1	1	1	1
50–64	1	2.0	0	2	2	2	2	2	2	2
65+	2	2.5	<1	2	2	2	3	3	3	3
2. MULTIPLE DX										
0–19 Years	180	2.4	7	1	1	2	2	4	6	15
20–34	13	4.1	7	2	2	3	5	9	10	10
35–49	11	5.1	48	1	1	2	7	10	24	24
50–64	17	7.2	62	1	3	4	9	11	35	35
65+	98	5.5	38	2	3	4	6	9	12	58
TOTAL SINGLE DX	341	1.5	1	1	1	1	2	2	3	4
TOTAL MULTIPLE DX	319	3.3	17	1	1	2	4	6	9	16
TOTAL										
0–19 Years	513	1.8	3	1	1	1	2	3	4	11
20–34	16	3.8	7	1	2	3	5	9	10	10
35–49	13	4.5	43	1	1	4	5	10	24	24
50–64	18	6.9	60	1	3	4	9	11	35	35
65+	100	5.5	37	2	3	4	6	9	12	58
GRAND TOTAL	660	2.2	9	1	1	1	4	4	6	15

79.06: CLSD FX RED TIBIA/FIBULA

Type of Patients	Observed Patients	Avg. Stay	Vari-ance	10th	25th	50th	75th	90th	95th	99th
1. SINGLE DX										
0–19 Years	241	1.3	<1	1	1	1	2	2	3	5
20–34	73	1.6	1	1	1	1	3	3	4	5
35–49	48	1.8	1	1	1	1	3	3	3	6
50–64	22	1.9	3	1	1	3	4	4	6	7
65+	3	2.7	2	1	1	3	4	4	4	4
2. MULTIPLE DX										
0–19 Years	151	2.5	10	1	1	2	3	4	7	22
20–34	107	2.7	24	1	1	2	3	5	5	13
35–49	125	4.0	20	1	2	3	5	8	11	22
50–64	245	4.4	41	2	2	3	5	8	12	25
65+	315	4.5	15	2	2	3	5	8	11	19
TOTAL SINGLE DX	387	1.4	<1	1	1	1	2	2	3	5
TOTAL MULTIPLE DX	943	3.8	22	1	1	3	4	7	10	22
TOTAL										
0–19 Years	392	1.7	4	1	1	1	2	3	4	8
20–34	180	2.2	15	1	1	2	4	4	5	13
35–49	173	3.4	16	1	1	2	4	6	7	22
50–64	267	4.2	39	1	2	3	5	8	10	25
65+	318	4.5	14	1	2	3	5	8	11	19
GRAND TOTAL	1,330	2.9	16	1	1	2	3	6	8	19

LOS by Diagnosis and Operation, Western Region, 45th Edition

Western Region, October 2007–September 2008 Data, by Operation

79.09: CLOSED FX REDUCTION NEC

Type of Patients	Observed Patients	Avg. Stay	Vari-ance	10th	25th	50th	75th	90th	95th	99th
1. SINGLE DX										
0–19 Years	5	1.2	<1	1	1	1	1	2	2	2
20–34	3	2.3	<1	2	2	2	3	3	3	3
35–49	0									
50–64	0									
65+	0									
2. MULTIPLE DX										
0–19 Years	7	3.6	3	1	2	4	4	6	6	6
20–34	20	7.0	60	2	3	4	8	11	21	34
35–49	18	5.0	19	1	2	3	5	13	14	14
50–64	12	5.7	20	1	1	4	7	13	15	15
65+	21	7.7	47	3	3	6	10	12	14	33
TOTAL SINGLE DX	8	1.6	<1	1	1	2	2	3	3	3
TOTAL MULTIPLE DX	78	6.2	36	1	3	4	7	13	15	34
TOTAL										
0–19 Years	12	2.6	3	1	1	2	4	4	6	6
20–34	23	6.4	54	2	2	4	7	11	21	34
35–49	18	5.0	19	1	2	3	5	13	14	14
50–64	12	5.7	20	1	1	4	7	13	15	15
65+	21	7.7	47	3	3	6	10	12	14	33
GRAND TOTAL	86	5.8	35	1	2	4	7	12	14	34

79.11: CRIF HUMERUS

Type of Patients	Observed Patients	Avg. Stay	Vari-ance	10th	25th	50th	75th	90th	95th	99th
1. SINGLE DX										
0–19 Years	1,648	1.2	<1	1	1	1	1	2	2	2
20–34	6	3.8	25	1	1	2	3	14	14	14
35–49	7	1.7	1	1	1	1	2	4	4	4
50–64	5	2.4	2	1	1	2	4	4	4	4
65+	4	1.5	<1	1	1	2	2	2	2	2
2. MULTIPLE DX										
0–19 Years	577	1.6	4	1	1	1	2	2	2	8
20–34	28	3.4	6	1	2	3	5	6	9	11
35–49	33	4.3	35	1	2	3	4	8	22	29
50–64	74	5.0	37	1	2	3	6	11	18	36
65+	196	4.9	30	1	2	3	6	10	12	42
TOTAL SINGLE DX	1,670	1.2	<1	1	1	1	1	2	2	2
TOTAL MULTIPLE DX	908	2.4	12	1	1	1	2	4	7	18
TOTAL										
0–19 Years	2,225	1.3	<1	1	1	1	1	2	2	3
20–34	34	3.5	9	1	2	3	4	6	11	14
35–49	40	3.9	30	1	2	3	4	8	22	29
50–64	79	4.9	35	1	2	3	6	11	18	36
65+	200	4.9	30	1	2	3	6	9	12	42
GRAND TOTAL	2,578	1.6	4	1	1	1	2	2	3	9

79.1: CLSD FX RED W INT FIX

Type of Patients	Observed Patients	Avg. Stay	Vari-ance	10th	25th	50th	75th	90th	95th	99th
1. SINGLE DX										
0–19 Years	2,239	1.3	<1	1	1	1	2	2	2	4
20–34	261	2.2	2	1	1	2	3	4	5	6
35–49	166	2.3	2	1	1	2	3	4	5	7
50–64	149	2.4	2	1	1	2	3	4	5	8
65+	52	2.8	4	1	1	3	4	4	7	11
2. MULTIPLE DX										
0–19 Years	1,169	2.5	9	1	1	2	2	5	7	17
20–34	842	5.1	48	1	2	3	6	9	15	32
35–49	903	5.0	37	1	2	3	5	10	17	32
50–64	1,875	5.5	42	2	3	4	6	10	14	35
65+	8,387	5.4	13	3	4	5	6	9	11	19
TOTAL SINGLE DX	2,867	1.5	<1	1	1	1	2	2	3	5
TOTAL MULTIPLE DX	13,176	5.0	21	1	3	4	6	9	12	23
TOTAL										
0–19 Years	3,408	1.7	3	1	1	1	2	3	4	9
20–34	1,103	4.5	39	1	1	3	5	8	12	27
35–49	1,069	4.6	32	1	2	3	5	10	16	32
50–64	2,024	5.3	40	2	3	4	6	10	14	34
65+	8,439	5.4	13	3	4	5	6	9	11	19
GRAND TOTAL	16,043	4.1	18	1	1	3	5	8	10	20

79.12: CRIF RADIUS/ULNA

Type of Patients	Observed Patients	Avg. Stay	Vari-ance	10th	25th	50th	75th	90th	95th	99th
1. SINGLE DX										
0–19 Years	206	1.3	<1	1	1	1	1	2	3	3
20–34	20	1.6	2	1	1	1	2	5	5	5
35–49	16	1.8	1	1	1	1	2	3	4	4
50–64	24	1.4	<1	1	1	1	2	2	2	5
65+	12	1.4	<1	1	1	1	2	2	4	4
2. MULTIPLE DX										
0–19 Years	94	1.5	<1	1	1	1	2	2	3	5
20–34	52	2.8	6	1	1	2	4	6	8	11
35–49	59	2.5	7	1	1	2	3	5	10	15
50–64	149	3.2	22	1	1	2	3	6	8	10
65+	285	3.0	5	1	2	2	4	6	7	11
TOTAL SINGLE DX	278	1.3	<1	1	1	1	1	2	3	5
TOTAL MULTIPLE DX	639	2.7	8	1	1	2	3	5	7	11
TOTAL										
0–19 Years	300	1.4	<1	1	1	1	2	2	3	5
20–34	72	2.5	5	1	1	1	3	5	8	11
35–49	75	2.3	6	1	1	2	3	4	8	15
50–64	173	2.9	20	1	1	2	3	5	7	10
65+	297	3.0	5	1	1	2	4	6	7	11
GRAND TOTAL	917	2.2	6	1	1	1	3	4	6	10

Western Region, October 2007–September 2008 Data, by Operation

79.13: CRIF MC/CARPALS

Type of Patients	Observed Patients	Avg. Stay	Vari-ance	10th	25th	50th	75th	90th	95th	99th
1. SINGLE DX										
0–19 Years	9	1.9	3	1	1	1	1	4	7	7
20–34	11	1.3	<1	1	1	1	2	2	2	2
35–49	3	3.0	3	2	2	2	5	5	5	5
50–64	0									
65+	0									
2. MULTIPLE DX										
0–19 Years	10	1.5	3	1	1	1	1	2	8	8
20–34	36	2.3	5	1	1	1	3	6	8	11
35–49	30	4.7	25	1	2	2	7	11	17	19
50–64	18	5.9	41	1	2	3	8	16	25	25
65+	7	4.5	6	1	2	6	6	7	7	7
TOTAL SINGLE DX	23	1.8	2	1	1	1	2	4	5	7
TOTAL MULTIPLE DX	101	3.7	18	1	1	2	5	9	12	19
TOTAL										
0–19 Years	19	1.7	3	1	1	1	1	4	7	8
20–34	47	2.1	4	1	1	1	2	4	7	11
35–49	33	4.6	23	1	2	2	6	11	17	19
50–64	18	5.9	41	1	2	3	8	16	25	25
65+	7	4.5	6	1	2	6	6	7	7	7
GRAND TOTAL	124	3.3	16	1	1	2	3	8	11	19

79.14: CRIF FINGER

Type of Patients	Observed Patients	Avg. Stay	Vari-ance	10th	25th	50th	75th	90th	95th	99th
1. SINGLE DX										
0–19 Years	10	1.2	<1	1	1	1	1	2	4	4
20–34	9	1.8	<1	1	1	2	2	3	3	3
35–49	5	1.4	<1	1	1	1	2	2	2	2
50–64	4	1.8	2	1	1	1	4	4	4	4
65+	0									
2. MULTIPLE DX										
0–19 Years	14	2.1	4	1	1	1	2	7	8	8
20–34	26	2.0	3	1	1	1	2	5	7	7
35–49	27	2.2	2	1	1	2	2	4	5	8
50–64	25	2.2	2	1	1	2	3	5	5	6
65+	12	5.1	57	1	1	3	4	7	28	28
TOTAL SINGLE DX	28	1.4	<1	1	1	1	2	3	4	4
TOTAL MULTIPLE DX	104	2.4	9	1	1	2	3	5	7	8
TOTAL										
0–19 Years	24	1.6	3	1	1	1	2	3	7	8
20–34	35	2.0	2	1	1	2	2	3	7	7
35–49	32	1.9	2	1	1	2	2	3	5	8
50–64	29	2.1	2	1	1	2	3	5	5	6
65+	12	5.1	57	1	1	3	4	7	28	28
GRAND TOTAL	132	2.2	7	1	1	1	2	4	7	8

79.15: CRIF FEMUR

Type of Patients	Observed Patients	Avg. Stay	Vari-ance	10th	25th	50th	75th	90th	95th	99th
1. SINGLE DX										
0–19 Years	219	2.2	3	1	1	2	2	4	4	8
20–34	82	2.6	2	1	2	2	3	4	5	6
35–49	53	2.7	2	1	2	2	3	4	5	7
50–64	65	2.9	3	1	2	3	4	5	5	11
65+	34	3.5	4	2	2	3	4	5	8	11
2. MULTIPLE DX										
0–19 Years	318	4.5	18	2	2	3	5	9	13	26
20–34	371	6.4	54	2	3	4	7	12	18	41
35–49	399	6.5	52	2	3	4	7	14	20	40
50–64	1,237	6.0	43	2	3	5	6	11	15	34
65+	7,693	5.5	12	3	4	5	6	9	11	19
TOTAL SINGLE DX	453	2.4	3	1	1	2	3	4	5	8
TOTAL MULTIPLE DX	10,018	5.6	19	3	3	5	6	9	12	23
TOTAL										
0–19 Years	537	3.5	12	1	2	2	4	6	9	21
20–34	453	5.7	47	2	2	4	6	10	17	38
35–49	452	6.1	47	2	3	4	7	12	18	35
50–64	1,302	5.8	41	2	3	4	6	10	14	34
65+	7,727	5.5	12	3	4	5	6	9	11	19
GRAND TOTAL	10,471	5.4	19	2	3	4	6	9	12	23

79.16: CRIF TIBIA & FIBULA

Type of Patients	Observed Patients	Avg. Stay	Vari-ance	10th	25th	50th	75th	90th	95th	99th
1. SINGLE DX										
0–19 Years	141	1.7	<1	1	1	1	2	3	3	4
20–34	119	2.2	1	1	1	2	3	4	4	5
35–49	76	2.3	2	1	1	2	3	4	5	8
50–64	45	2.5	1	1	1	2	3	4	5	6
65+	2	2.0	2	1	1	2	3	3	3	3
2. MULTIPLE DX										
0–19 Years	129	3.2	7	1	1	2	4	6	8	15
20–34	268	4.4	49	1	2	3	4	8	13	32
35–49	304	4.0	23	1	2	3	4	7	12	22
50–64	329	4.9	34	1	2	3	5	9	13	35
65+	166	4.8	13	2	3	4	5	8	13	18
TOTAL SINGLE DX	383	2.0	1	1	1	2	3	3	4	6
TOTAL MULTIPLE DX	1,196	4.3	28	1	2	3	5	8	12	26
TOTAL										
0–19 Years	270	2.3	4	1	1	2	3	4	6	13
20–34	387	3.8	35	1	2	2	4	6	9	26
35–49	380	3.7	19	1	2	3	4	7	10	22
50–64	374	4.6	31	1	2	3	5	8	13	35
65+	168	4.7	13	2	3	4	5	8	13	18
GRAND TOTAL	1,579	3.7	22	1	2	3	4	7	10	22

351

LOS by Diagnosis and Operation, Western Region, 45th Edition

Western Region, October 2007–September 2008 Data, by Operation

79.17: CRIF METATARSAL/TARSAL

Type of Patients	Observed Patients	Avg. Stay	Variance	Percentiles						
				10th	25th	50th	75th	90th	95th	99th
1. SINGLE DX										
0–19 Years	3	1.3	<1	1	1	1	2	2	2	2
20–34	11	1.6	<1	1	1	1	2	3	3	3
35–49	5	1.8	<1	1	2	2	2	3	2	2
50–64	4	1.5	<1	1	1	1	1	3	3	3
65+	0									
2. MULTIPLE DX										
0–19 Years	14	2.7	2	1	2	3	3	4	7	7
20–34	30	5.4	166	1	2	2	5	10	13	72
35–49	36	2.9	4	1	2	3	4	5	6	11
50–64	29	5.7	50	1	2	4	6	16	23	33
65+	7	3.0	2	1	2	3	4	5	5	5
TOTAL SINGLE DX	23	1.6	<1	1	1	1	2	3	3	3
TOTAL MULTIPLE DX	116	4.2	56	1	2	3	4	6	11	33
TOTAL										
0–19 Years	17	2.4	2	1	1	3	3	3	4	7
20–34	41	4.4	124	1	1	2	3	5	10	72
35–49	41	2.7	3	1	2	3	3	5	6	11
50–64	33	5.2	46	1	1	4	5	11	23	33
65+	7	3.0	2	1	2	3	4	5	5	5
GRAND TOTAL	139	3.8	48	1	1	2	4	6	10	33

79.22: OPEN RED RADIUS/ULNA FX

Type of Patients	Observed Patients	Avg. Stay	Variance	Percentiles						
				10th	25th	50th	75th	90th	95th	99th
1. SINGLE DX										
0–19 Years	20	1.2	<1	1	1	1	1	2	2	2
20–34	0									
35–49	2	2.5	<1	2	2	2	3	3	3	3
50–64	0									
65+	2	1.0	0	1	1	1	1	1	1	1
2. MULTIPLE DX										
0–19 Years	17	2.8	1	1	2	3	4	4	4	4
20–34	8	3.5	13	1	1	2	7	11	11	11
35–49	18	3.6	7	1	2	3	4	7	12	12
50–64	12	2.7	<1	2	2	3	3	4	4	4
65+	33	3.2	6	1	2	3	3	5	8	14
TOTAL SINGLE DX	24	1.3	<1	1	1	1	2	2	2	3
TOTAL MULTIPLE DX	88	3.1	5	1	2	3	4	5	7	14
TOTAL										
0–19 Years	37	1.9	1	1	1	2	3	4	4	4
20–34	8	3.5	13	1	1	2	7	11	11	11
35–49	20	3.5	7	1	2	3	4	6	7	12
50–64	12	2.7	<1	2	2	3	3	4	4	4
65+	35	3.1	6	1	2	3	3	5	8	14
GRAND TOTAL	112	2.6	4	1	1	2	3	4	6	12

79.2: OPEN FRACTURE REDUCTION

Type of Patients	Observed Patients	Avg. Stay	Variance	Percentiles						
				10th	25th	50th	75th	90th	95th	99th
1. SINGLE DX										
0–19 Years	61	1.9	2	1	1	1	2	2	2	2
20–34	15	2.7	6	1	1	1	2	3	3	3
35–49	10	2.4	6	1	2	2	2	3	2	2
50–64	12	2.9	6	1	1	2	3	3	3	3
65+	6	1.8	1	1	1	1	1	4	3	3
2. MULTIPLE DX										
0–19 Years	75	5.0	103	1	1	3	4	9	18	89
20–34	93	5.8	61	1	2	2	7	11	23	51
35–49	111	5.9	34	2	2	4	7	14	20	24
50–64	113	7.0	137	1	2	4	6	15	20	65
65+	143	5.2	25	1	2	4	6	10	16	26
TOTAL SINGLE DX	104	2.1	3	1	1	1	2	4	7	9
TOTAL MULTIPLE DX	535	5.8	69	1	2	3	6	12	20	38
TOTAL										
0–19 Years	136	3.5	57	1	1	2	4	6	9	32
20–34	108	5.4	55	1	2	3	6	11	21	38
35–49	121	5.6	32	1	2	3	7	13	20	24
50–64	125	6.6	126	1	2	3	6	15	20	65
65+	149	5.1	24	1	2	4	6	10	16	26
GRAND TOTAL	639	5.1	59	1	2	3	5	10	18	35

79.26: OPEN RED TIBIA/FIB FX

Type of Patients	Observed Patients	Avg. Stay	Variance	Percentiles						
				10th	25th	50th	75th	90th	95th	99th
1. SINGLE DX										
0–19 Years	20	2.6	2	1	1	2	4	5	5	6
20–34	5	3.2	5	2	2	2	3	7	7	7
35–49	8	5.0	31	1	1	5	9	9	9	9
50–64	8	2.9	7	1	1	2	3	9	9	9
65+	0									
2. MULTIPLE DX										
0–19 Years	25	5.5	37	1	1	4	7	10	24	26
20–34	36	6.9	64	1	2	4	8	14	28	38
35–49	51	6.0	32	2	3	5	9	13	19	30
50–64	49	8.0	192	2	3	5	7	15	19	90
65+	38	6.4	37	2	2	4	7	16	21	26
TOTAL SINGLE DX	35	2.9	5	1	1	2	4	6	9	9
TOTAL MULTIPLE DX	199	6.6	77	1	2	4	7	14	19	38
TOTAL										
0–19 Years	45	4.4	25	1	1	3	5	9	13	26
20–34	41	6.4	58	1	2	4	8	11	24	38
35–49	53	5.9	31	2	2	4	9	13	19	30
50–64	57	7.3	168	1	3	4	6	14	19	90
65+	38	6.4	37	2	2	4	7	16	21	26
GRAND TOTAL	234	6.1	68	1	2	4	7	13	19	38

Western Region, October 2007–September 2008 Data, by Operation

79.3: OP FX REDUCTION INT FIX

Type of Patients	Observed Patients	Avg. Stay	Vari-ance	Percentiles						
				10th	25th	50th	75th	90th	95th	99th
1. SINGLE DX										
0–19 Years	2,347	1.7	<1	1	1	1	2	3	3	5
20–34	2,206	2.2	1	1	1	2	3	4	5	8
35–49	1,615	2.2	2	1	1	2	3	4	5	8
50–64	1,219	2.2	3	1	1	2	3	4	5	9
65+	371	2.4	3	1	1	2	3	4	5	7
2. MULTIPLE DX										
0–19 Years	2,644	3.3	19	1	1	2	4	7	9	22
20–34	6,187	4.4	29	1	2	3	5	9	13	28
35–49	7,257	4.6	35	1	2	3	5	9	14	30
50–64	11,800	4.8	32	1	2	3	5	9	14	30
65+	25,093	5.3	15	2	3	4	6	9	12	21
TOTAL SINGLE DX	7,758	2.0	2	1	1	2	2	3	4	7
TOTAL MULTIPLE DX	52,981	4.9	24	1	2	4	6	9	12	24
TOTAL										
0–19 Years	4,991	2.5	10	1	1	2	3	4	7	16
20–34	8,393	3.8	23	1	1	3	4	8	11	23
35–49	8,872	4.1	30	1	2	3	5	8	13	27
50–64	13,019	4.6	29	1	2	3	5	9	13	28
65+	25,464	5.3	15	2	3	4	6	9	12	21
GRAND TOTAL	60,739	4.4	22	1	2	3	5	8	12	23

79.31: ORIF HUMERUS

Type of Patients	Observed Patients	Avg. Stay	Vari-ance	Percentiles						
				10th	25th	50th	75th	90th	95th	99th
1. SINGLE DX										
0–19 Years	561	1.4	<1	1	1	1	2	2	2	3
20–34	124	1.9	1	1	1	2	2	3	4	6
35–49	96	2.0	2	1	1	2	3	4	5	8
50–64	100	1.8	2	1	1	2	2	3	4	7
65+	56	1.8	1	1	1	2	2	3	4	8
2. MULTIPLE DX										
0–19 Years	385	2.3	5	1	1	2	2	4	6	13
20–34	506	4.2	23	1	2	3	5	9	12	25
35–49	588	3.9	17	1	2	3	4	8	10	23
50–64	1,307	3.6	14	1	2	3	4	7	11	18
65+	2,054	4.3	13	2	2	3	5	8	11	19
TOTAL SINGLE DX	937	1.5	<1	1	1	1	2	2	3	5
TOTAL MULTIPLE DX	4,840	3.8	14	1	2	3	5	8	10	19
TOTAL										
0–19 Years	946	1.7	2	1	1	1	2	3	4	8
20–34	630	3.7	19	1	1	2	4	8	10	21
35–49	684	3.6	16	1	1	2	4	7	10	22
50–64	1,407	3.5	14	1	1	2	4	7	10	18
65+	2,110	4.2	13	1	2	3	5	8	11	18
GRAND TOTAL	5,777	3.3	12	1	1	2	4	7	9	18

79.32: ORIF RADIUS/ULNA

Type of Patients	Observed Patients	Avg. Stay	Vari-ance	Percentiles						
				10th	25th	50th	75th	90th	95th	99th
1. SINGLE DX										
0–19 Years	638	1.5	<1	1	1	1	2	2	3	4
20–34	349	1.8	1	1	1	2	2	3	4	6
35–49	236	1.8	2	1	1	1	2	3	4	8
50–64	205	1.5	<1	1	1	1	2	3	3	4
65+	71	1.6	<1	1	1	1	2	3	4	4
2. MULTIPLE DX										
0–19 Years	511	2.2	6	1	1	2	2	4	6	13
20–34	906	3.9	28	1	1	2	4	8	12	28
35–49	863	3.6	29	1	1	2	4	7	10	30
50–64	1,231	3.3	20	1	1	2	4	6	9	23
65+	1,651	3.4	9	2	3	3	4	7	9	17
TOTAL SINGLE DX	1,499	1.6	<1	1	1	1	2	3	3	5
TOTAL MULTIPLE DX	5,162	3.3	18	1	1	2	4	7	9	23
TOTAL										
0–19 Years	1,149	1.8	3	1	1	1	2	3	4	10
20–34	1,255	3.3	22	1	1	2	3	7	11	23
35–49	1,099	3.2	23	1	1	2	3	6	9	28
50–64	1,436	3.0	17	1	1	2	3	6	8	21
65+	1,722	3.3	9	1	1	3	4	7	9	16
GRAND TOTAL	6,661	2.9	14	1	1	2	3	6	8	19

79.33: ORIF CARPALS/METACARPALS

Type of Patients	Observed Patients	Avg. Stay	Vari-ance	Percentiles						
				10th	25th	50th	75th	90th	95th	99th
1. SINGLE DX										
0–19 Years	22	1.5	<1	1	1	1	2	2	3	4
20–34	50	1.4	<1	1	1	1	2	3	3	5
35–49	16	1.3	<1	1	1	1	1	2	2	2
50–64	8	1.8	<1	1	1	2	3	3	3	3
65+	0									
2. MULTIPLE DX										
0–19 Years	51	3.7	22	1	1	2	4	7	16	25
20–34	184	3.2	17	1	1	2	3	6	10	24
35–49	89	3.5	36	1	1	2	4	7	9	54
50–64	79	3.3	11	1	1	2	4	8	11	20
65+	33	3.1	7	1	2	2	4	7	10	11
TOTAL SINGLE DX	96	1.5	<1	1	1	1	2	3	3	5
TOTAL MULTIPLE DX	436	3.4	19	1	1	2	4	7	10	20
TOTAL										
0–19 Years	73	3.1	17	1	1	2	3	6	16	25
20–34	234	2.8	14	1	1	2	3	6	9	20
35–49	105	3.2	31	1	1	2	3	6	9	14
50–64	87	3.2	11	1	1	2	3	7	9	20
65+	33	3.1	7	1	2	2	4	7	10	11
GRAND TOTAL	532	3.0	17	1	1	2	3	6	9	20

LOS by Diagnosis and Operation, Western Region, 45th Edition

Western Region, October 2007–September 2008 Data, by Operation

79.34: ORIF FINGER

Type of Patients	Observed Patients	Avg. Stay	Vari-ance	10th	25th	50th	75th	90th	95th	99th
1. SINGLE DX										
0–19 Years	31	1.5	2	1	1	1	1	2	6	6
20–34	37	1.4	<1	1	1	1	2	2	3	4
35–49	22	1.3	<1	1	1	1	1	2	2	3
50–64	21	1.7	<1	1	1	1	2	2	3	5
65+	1	1.0	0	1	1	1	2	1	1	1
2. MULTIPLE DX										
0–19 Years	69	1.8	2	1	1	1	2	4	5	9
20–34	199	2.2	8	1	1	1	2	4	6	12
35–49	149	2.6	8	1	1	2	3	6	8	17
50–64	157	2.2	4	1	1	1	3	4	6	9
65+	51	2.0	4	1	1	1	2	5	6	11
TOTAL SINGLE DX	112	1.5	1	1	1	1	2	2	3	6
TOTAL MULTIPLE DX	625	2.2	6	1	1	1	2	5	6	12
TOTAL										
0–19 Years	100	1.7	2	1	1	1	2	3	5	7
20–34	236	2.1	7	1	1	1	3	4	6	12
35–49	171	2.4	7	1	1	1	3	5	7	17
50–64	178	2.1	3	1	1	1	2	4	6	9
65+	52	2.0	4	1	1	1	2	5	6	11
GRAND TOTAL	737	2.1	5	1	1	1	2	4	6	12

79.35: ORIF FEMUR

Type of Patients	Observed Patients	Avg. Stay	Vari-ance	10th	25th	50th	75th	90th	95th	99th
1. SINGLE DX										
0–19 Years	285	2.4	1	1	2	2	3	4	4	6
20–34	119	3.1	3	1	2	3	4	5	8	8
35–49	88	3.2	4	1	2	3	4	6	8	10
50–64	96	3.8	4	2	2	3	5	6	8	13
65+	66	3.6	2	2	3	4	4	5	6	7
2. MULTIPLE DX										
0–19 Years	608	5.1	39	1	2	3	6	9	15	38
20–34	862	6.8	46	2	3	5	8	14	19	40
35–49	978	7.2	65	2	3	5	8	14	21	48
50–64	2,779	7.0	48	3	4	5	8	13	19	39
65+	16,269	5.9	15	3	4	5	7	9	12	21
TOTAL SINGLE DX	654	2.8	2	1	2	3	4	5	6	8
TOTAL MULTIPLE DX	21,496	6.1	24	3	4	5	7	10	14	26
TOTAL										
0–19 Years	893	4.1	28	1	2	3	4	7	10	31
20–34	981	6.4	42	2	3	5	7	13	18	39
35–49	1,066	6.9	61	2	3	5	7	13	20	47
50–64	2,875	6.9	47	3	4	5	8	12	18	38
65+	16,335	5.9	15	3	4	5	7	9	12	21
GRAND TOTAL	22,150	6.0	23	3	4	5	7	10	13	25

79.36: ORIF TIBIA & FIBULA

Type of Patients	Observed Patients	Avg. Stay	Vari-ance	10th	25th	50th	75th	90th	95th	99th
1. SINGLE DX										
0–19 Years	696	1.7	1	1	1	1	2	3	4	5
20–34	1,275	2.3	3	1	1	2	3	4	5	9
35–49	995	2.3	3	1	1	2	3	4	5	9
50–64	682	2.3	3	1	1	2	3	4	5	8
65+	165	2.4	3	1	1	2	3	4	5	9
2. MULTIPLE DX										
0–19 Years	827	2.8	11	1	2	2	3	5	8	16
20–34	2,841	3.6	18	1	2	3	4	7	10	20
35–49	3,834	4.1	28	1	2	3	5	8	12	26
50–64	5,490	4.2	25	2	2	3	5	8	12	25
65+	4,728	4.4	15	2	2	3	5	8	10	21
TOTAL SINGLE DX	3,813	2.1	2	1	1	2	3	4	5	8
TOTAL MULTIPLE DX	17,720	4.1	21	1	2	3	5	8	11	23
TOTAL										
0–19 Years	1,523	2.3	6	1	1	2	3	4	5	11
20–34	4,116	3.2	13	1	1	2	4	6	9	17
35–49	4,829	3.7	23	1	2	3	4	7	11	24
50–64	6,172	4.0	23	1	2	3	4	8	11	24
65+	4,893	4.4	14	2	2	3	5	8	10	21
GRAND TOTAL	21,533	3.7	18	1	2	3	4	7	10	21

79.37: ORIF METATARSAL/TARSAL

Type of Patients	Observed Patients	Avg. Stay	Vari-ance	10th	25th	50th	75th	90th	95th	99th
1. SINGLE DX										
0–19 Years	50	1.6	1	1	1	1	2	3	4	5
20–34	162	2.3	4	1	1	2	2	4	5	13
35–49	113	2.2	<1	1	1	2	3	3	5	5
50–64	69	2.0	<1	1	1	2	3	3	4	5
65+	7	1.6	<1	1	1	1	2	3	3	3
2. MULTIPLE DX										
0–19 Years	79	3.3	11	1	2	2	4	6	8	21
20–34	340	4.0	22	1	2	3	4	10	13	18
35–49	395	4.2	33	1	2	3	4	9	14	27
50–64	377	3.8	16	1	2	3	4	9	12	19
65+	122	3.8	10	1	2	3	5	7	9	16
TOTAL SINGLE DX	401	2.1	2	1	1	2	2	4	4	8
TOTAL MULTIPLE DX	1,313	3.9	22	1	2	2	4	8	13	21
TOTAL										
0–19 Years	129	2.6	8	1	1	2	3	4	7	20
20–34	502	3.4	17	1	2	2	3	7	12	17
35–49	508	3.8	27	1	2	2	4	7	12	22
50–64	446	3.5	14	1	2	3	4	8	12	19
65+	129	3.7	10	1	2	3	5	7	9	16
GRAND TOTAL	1,714	3.5	18	1	1	2	4	7	12	19

Western Region, October 2007–September 2008 Data, by Operation

79.38: ORIF TOE

Type of Patients	Observed Patients	Avg. Stay	Variance	10th	25th	50th	75th	90th	95th	99th
1. SINGLE DX										
0–19 Years	7	1.8	<1	1	1	2	2	2	4	4
20–34	5	1.2	<1	1	1	2	1	2	2	2
35–49	3	1.7	<1	1	1	2	2	2	2	2
50–64	1	1.0	0	1	1	1	1	1	1	1
65+	0									
2. MULTIPLE DX										
0–19 Years	14	2.3	3	1	1	2	3	5	7	7
20–34	19	3.4	20	1	1	2	3	6	21	21
35–49	20	3.3	6	1	2	2	3	8	10	10
50–64	16	2.6	3	1	1	2	4	5	6	6
65+	17	3.5	6	1	1	3	4	8	8	8
TOTAL SINGLE DX	16	1.6	<1	1	1	1	2	2	2	4
TOTAL MULTIPLE DX	86	3.0	8	1	1	2	4	6	8	21
TOTAL										
0–19 Years	21	2.1	2	1	1	2	2	4	5	7
20–34	24	2.9	17	1	1	2	3	5	6	21
35–49	23	3.0	5	1	2	2	3	6	8	10
50–64	17	2.5	3	1	1	2	3	5	6	6
65+	17	3.5	6	1	1	3	4	8	8	8
GRAND TOTAL	102	2.7	7	1	1	2	3	5	7	10

79.39: ORIF BONE NEC X FACIAL

Type of Patients	Observed Patients	Avg. Stay	Variance	10th	25th	50th	75th	90th	95th	99th
1. SINGLE DX										
0–19 Years	56	1.5	2	1	1	2	2	2	3	8
20–34	83	2.0	4	1	1	1	2	3	6	13
35–49	45	1.9	4	1	1	1	2	4	6	12
50–64	37	3.1	9	1	1	1	2	5	10	10
65+	5	2.2	3	1	1	2	2	5	5	5
2. MULTIPLE DX										
0–19 Years	100	7.7	50	1	2	6	9	17	22	34
20–34	329	7.9	83	1	3	6	10	16	21	51
35–49	341	7.4	64	1	2	5	10	17	22	36
50–64	362	8.1	76	1	2	6	11	16	24	44
65+	167	8.5	61	1	4	7	11	18	24	>99
TOTAL SINGLE DX	226	2.0	4	1	1	1	2	4	7	10
TOTAL MULTIPLE DX	1,299	7.9	71	1	2	6	10	16	23	46
TOTAL										
0–19 Years	156	5.2	40	1	1	2	7	14	20	34
20–34	412	6.7	73	1	2	4	9	15	19	44
35–49	386	6.7	60	1	2	5	9	15	21	36
50–64	399	7.6	72	1	2	6	10	15	23	44
65+	172	8.3	60	1	3	7	11	16	24	>99
GRAND TOTAL	1,525	7.0	65	1	2	5	9	15	21	41

79.4: CR SEP EPIPHYSIS

Type of Patients	Observed Patients	Avg. Stay	Variance	10th	25th	50th	75th	90th	95th	99th
1. SINGLE DX										
0–19 Years	119	1.6	<1	1	1	1	2	2	3	4
20–34	1	1.5	<1	2	2	2	2	2	2	2
35–49	2	2.0	0	2	2	2	2	2	2	2
50–64	2	1.5	<1	1	1	2	2	2	2	2
65+	0									
2. MULTIPLE DX										
0–19 Years	65	2.1	2	1	1	2	3	4	5	7
20–34	6	2.7	4	1	1	2	4	6	6	6
35–49	4	4.3	3	2	4	5	6	6	6	6
50–64	5	7.6	31	1	4	7	11	15	15	15
65+	11	4.7	5	2	3	5	7	7	8	8
TOTAL SINGLE DX	124	1.6	<1	1	1	1	2	2	3	4
TOTAL MULTIPLE DX	91	2.6	5	1	1	2	4	5	7	11
TOTAL										
0–19 Years	184	1.8	1	1	1	1	2	3	4	5
20–34	8	2.4	3	1	1	2	2	5	6	6
35–49	5	3.8	3	2	2	4	5	6	6	6
50–64	7	5.9	29	1	1	4	11	15	15	15
65+	11	4.7	5	2	3	5	7	7	8	8
GRAND TOTAL	215	2.0	3	1	1	1	2	4	5	8

79.5: OPEN RED SEP EPIPHYSIS

Type of Patients	Observed Patients	Avg. Stay	Variance	10th	25th	50th	75th	90th	95th	99th
1. SINGLE DX										
0–19 Years	92	1.8	1	1	1	1	2	3	4	6
20–34	12	2.2	2	1	1	2	3	4	6	6
35–49	12	2.9	1	2	2	3	4	4	5	5
50–64	6	3.0	<1	2	2	3	4	4	4	4
65+	3	2.3	<1	2	2	2	3	3	3	3
2. MULTIPLE DX										
0–19 Years	60	3.0	4	1	1	3	4	5	8	10
20–34	18	2.7	1	1	2	2	3	5	5	5
35–49	35	3.1	4	1	2	3	4	5	8	9
50–64	48	4.2	21	1	2	5	5	8	10	31
65+	56	5.4	27	1	3	4	6	10	20	27
TOTAL SINGLE DX	125	1.9	1	1	1	2	2	3	4	6
TOTAL MULTIPLE DX	217	3.7	12	1	2	3	4	7	8	22
TOTAL										
0–19 Years	152	2.3	3	1	1	2	3	4	5	9
20–34	30	2.5	2	1	2	3	3	4	5	6
35–49	47	3.0	3	1	2	3	4	5	6	9
50–64	54	4.1	19	1	2	3	5	7	10	31
65+	59	5.2	26	1	3	4	6	10	20	27
GRAND TOTAL	342	2.9	8	1	1	2	4	5	8	17

LOS by Diagnosis and Operation, Western Region, 45th Edition

79.56: OP RED SEP EPIPH TIB/FIB

Type of Patients	Observed Patients	Avg. Stay	Variance	Percentiles						
				10th	25th	50th	75th	90th	95th	99th
1. SINGLE DX										
0–19 Years	45	1.6	1	1	1	1	2	3	3	9
20–34	10	2.2	3	1	1	2	3	6	6	6
35–49	8	2.6	<1	1	2	3	3	4	4	4
50–64	4	2.8	<1	2	2	2	4	4	4	4
65+	3	2.3	<1	2	2	2	3	3	3	3
2. MULTIPLE DX										
0–19 Years	18	2.8	3	1	1	2	4	5	6	8
20–34	8	2.5	1	1	2	2	4	4	4	4
35–49	25	3.4	4	1	2	3	4	6	8	9
50–64	22	5.0	41	1	1	3	5	10	11	31
65+	16	4.1	16	2	2	3	4	8	17	17
TOTAL SINGLE DX	70	1.8	2	1	1	1	2	3	4	6
TOTAL MULTIPLE DX	89	3.7	14	1	2	3	4	7	9	31
TOTAL										
0–19 Years	63	1.9	2	1	1	1	2	3	5	8
20–34	18	2.3	2	1	1	2	3	4	6	6
35–49	33	3.2	11	1	1	3	4	5	8	9
50–64	26	4.7	36	1	2	3	5	10	11	31
65+	19	3.8	14	1	2	3	4	8	17	17
GRAND TOTAL	159	2.7	8	1	1	2	3	4	7	11

79.6: OPEN FX SITE DEBRIDEMENT

Type of Patients	Observed Patients	Avg. Stay	Variance	Percentiles						
				10th	25th	50th	75th	90th	95th	99th
1. SINGLE DX										
0–19 Years	103	2.2	3	1	1	1	3	4	4	7
20–34	70	2.8	4	1	2	2	3	5	6	15
35–49	37	2.9	11	1	1	3	3	5	5	15
50–64	21	2.1	2	1	1	2	3	4	5	6
65+	3	1.3	<1	1	1	1	2	2	2	2
2. MULTIPLE DX										
0–19 Years	196	4.7	49	1	1	3	6	11	20	>99
20–34	374	6.5	93	1	2	3	7	16	24	67
35–49	286	6.5	104	1	2	3	6	16	27	71
50–64	250	7.9	95	1	2	4	9	21	27	51
65+	158	6.5	81	1	2	4	8	12	18	49
TOTAL SINGLE DX	234	2.5	4	1	1	2	3	4	5	15
TOTAL MULTIPLE DX	1,264	6.5	87	1	2	3	7	15	24	67
TOTAL										
0–19 Years	299	3.8	34	1	1	2	4	9	12	>99
20–34	444	5.9	80	1	2	3	6	15	20	67
35–49	323	6.1	94	1	2	3	6	15	22	63
50–64	271	7.4	91	1	2	4	8	20	27	51
65+	161	6.4	80	1	2	4	7	12	18	49
GRAND TOTAL	1,498	5.8	76	1	2	3	6	14	21	60

79.61: DEBRIDE OPEN FX HUMERUS

Type of Patients	Observed Patients	Avg. Stay	Variance	Percentiles						
				10th	25th	50th	75th	90th	95th	99th
1. SINGLE DX										
0–19 Years	4	1.3	<1	1	1	1	1	2	2	2
20–34	4	3.3	2	2	3	3	5	5	5	5
35–49	0									
50–64	1	4.0	0	4	4	4	4	4	4	4
65+	1	1.0	0	1	1	1	1	1	1	1
2. MULTIPLE DX										
0–19 Years	14	5.7	59	2	2	3	4	16	29	29
20–34	17	10.0	261	1	2	3	9	27	67	67
35–49	19	7.9	81	2	3	5	7	19	40	40
50–64	15	10.2	119	2	3	6	17	21	42	42
65+	17	5.8	8	2	4	5	8	10	12	12
TOTAL SINGLE DX	10	2.3	2	1	1	2	3	5	5	5
TOTAL MULTIPLE DX	82	7.9	105	2	3	5	8	17	27	67
TOTAL										
0–19 Years	18	4.7	49	1	2	2	4	16	29	29
20–34	21	8.7	217	1	3	3	8	15	27	67
35–49	19	7.9	81	2	3	5	7	19	40	40
50–64	16	9.9	114	2	4	6	17	21	42	42
65+	18	5.5	9	1	4	5	8	10	12	12
GRAND TOTAL	92	7.3	97	1	2	4	8	17	27	67

79.62: DEBRIDE OPEN FX RAD/ULNA

Type of Patients	Observed Patients	Avg. Stay	Variance	Percentiles						
				10th	25th	50th	75th	90th	95th	99th
1. SINGLE DX										
0–19 Years	57	1.6	<1	1	1	1	2	3	4	4
20–34	7	2.3	1	1	1	2	3	4	4	4
35–49	2	2.0	2	1	1	1	1	3	3	3
50–64	5	1.4	<1	1	1	1	2	2	2	2
65+	0									
2. MULTIPLE DX										
0–19 Years	32	3.2	10	1	1	2	4	10	10	11
20–34	32	5.5	49	1	1	3	6	12	20	33
35–49	32	3.3	6	1	1	3	4	5	8	14
50–64	29	4.8	39	1	1	3	5	13	23	27
65+	37	4.7	17	1	2	3	5	9	18	19
TOTAL SINGLE DX	71	1.7	<1	1	1	1	2	3	4	4
TOTAL MULTIPLE DX	162	4.2	23	1	2	3	4	10	13	27
TOTAL										
0–19 Years	89	2.2	5	1	1	1	3	4	10	11
20–34	39	4.9	42	1	1	3	4	12	20	33
35–49	34	3.2	6	1	2	3	4	5	8	14
50–64	34	4.3	35	1	1	2	4	8	23	27
65+	37	4.7	17	1	2	3	5	9	18	19
GRAND TOTAL	233	3.4	17	1	1	2	3	7	11	23

LOS by Diagnosis and Operation, Western Region, 45th Edition

79.64: DEBRIDE OPEN FX FINGER

Type of Patients	Observed Patients	Avg. Stay	Variance	10th	25th	50th	75th	90th	95th	99th
1. SINGLE DX										
0–19 Years	4	1.0	0	1	1	1	1	1	1	1
20–34	6	1.3	<1	1	1	1	1	3	3	3
35–49	9	1.3	<1	1	1	1	1	3	3	3
50–64	5	1.6	<1	1	1	1	2	3	3	3
65+	0									
2. MULTIPLE DX										
0–19 Years	30	2.0	6	1	1	1	2	4	10	11
20–34	53	2.0	3	1	1	1	2	5	6	7
35–49	53	1.7	1	1	1	1	2	3	4	6
50–64	46	2.4	3	1	1	2	4	4	6	7
65+	19	1.7	1	1	1	1	2	3	5	5
TOTAL SINGLE DX	**24**	**1.3**	**<1**	**1**	**1**	**1**	**1**	**3**	**3**	**3**
TOTAL MULTIPLE DX	**201**	**2.0**	**3**	**1**	**1**	**1**	**2**	**4**	**5**	**7**
TOTAL										
0–19 Years	34	1.9	5	1	1	1	2	4	10	11
20–34	59	2.0	3	1	1	1	2	5	6	7
35–49	62	1.7	1	1	1	1	2	3	4	6
50–64	51	2.3	3	1	1	2	4	4	6	7
65+	19	1.7	1	1	1	1	2	3	5	5
GRAND TOTAL	**225**	**1.9**	**3**	**1**	**1**	**1**	**2**	**4**	**5**	**7**

79.65: DEBRIDE OPEN FEMUR FX

Type of Patients	Observed Patients	Avg. Stay	Variance	10th	25th	50th	75th	90th	95th	99th
1. SINGLE DX										
0–19 Years	2	3.4	2	1	4	4	4	4	4	4
20–34	5	1.6	<1	1	1	2	2	2	2	2
35–49	0									
50–64	0									
65+	0									
2. MULTIPLE DX										
0–19 Years	15	9.8	120	1	3	7	9	22	43	43
20–34	46	12.7	175	2	4	8	16	34	49	>99
35–49	19	17.5	451	1	3	10	19	63	76	76
50–64	25	15.0	210	3	6	11	18	36	53	55
65+	18	16.2	472	4	6	9	12	49	89	89
TOTAL SINGLE DX	**7**	**2.5**	**2**	**1**	**1**	**2**	**4**	**4**	**4**	**4**
TOTAL MULTIPLE DX	**123**	**14.1**	**258**	**2**	**4**	**9**	**17**	**36**	**53**	**89**
TOTAL										
0–19 Years	17	8.2	96	1	3	4	7	20	22	43
20–34	51	11.6	169	2	2	7	16	27	49	>99
35–49	19	17.5	451	1	3	10	19	63	76	76
50–64	25	15.0	210	3	6	11	18	36	53	55
65+	18	16.2	472	4	6	9	12	49	89	89
GRAND TOTAL	**130**	**13.2**	**248**	**2**	**4**	**8**	**16**	**34**	**53**	**89**

79.66: DEBRIDE OPN FX TIBIA/FIB

Type of Patients	Observed Patients	Avg. Stay	Variance	10th	25th	50th	75th	90th	95th	99th
1. SINGLE DX										
0–19 Years	26	3.4	4	2	2	3	4	5	6	11
20–34	24	3.0	2	2	2	3	4	5	5	6
35–49	15	4.7	20	1	2	4	5	15	15	15
50–64	7	2.6	4	1	1	2	4	6	6	6
65+	2	1.5	<1	1	1	2	2	2	2	2
2. MULTIPLE DX										
0–19 Years	60	5.1	38	1	2	3	6	15	>99	>99
20–34	136	6.9	66	2	3	4	8	17	23	60
35–49	112	8.0	107	2	3	4	9	17	34	71
50–64	93	10.1	97	3	3	5	14	24	30	51
65+	46	6.9	24	2	4	6	8	12	16	27
TOTAL SINGLE DX	**74**	**3.4**	**6**	**1**	**2**	**3**	**4**	**5**	**6**	**15**
TOTAL MULTIPLE DX	**447**	**7.5**	**75**	**2**	**3**	**4**	**9**	**18**	**28**	**>99**
TOTAL										
0–19 Years	86	4.6	28	1	2	3	6	12	20	>99
20–34	160	6.3	58	2	3	4	7	15	19	60
35–49	127	7.6	98	1	2	4	9	17	29	71
50–64	100	9.5	94	2	3	5	14	23	28	51
65+	48	6.6	24	2	3	6	8	12	16	27
GRAND TOTAL	**521**	**6.9**	**67**	**2**	**3**	**4**	**8**	**17**	**25**	**>99**

79.67: DEBRIDE OPN FX MT/TARSAL

Type of Patients	Observed Patients	Avg. Stay	Variance	10th	25th	50th	75th	90th	95th	99th
1. SINGLE DX										
0–19 Years	5	2.8	7	1	1	1	4	7	7	7
20–34	12	2.8	2	1	2	3	3	5	6	6
35–49	3	2.7	2	1	1	3	4	4	4	4
50–64	2	3.0	8	1	1	5	5	5	5	5
65+	0									
2. MULTIPLE DX										
0–19 Years	17	7.2	241	1	2	2	4	14	66	66
20–34	37	5.6	151	1	2	3	5	9	12	77
35–49	19	6.0	50	1	2	4	6	14	30	30
50–64	12	5.7	21	2	4	5	6	7	19	19
65+	3	11.7	59	3	3	14	18	18	18	18
TOTAL SINGLE DX	**22**	**2.8**	**3**	**1**	**1**	**2**	**4**	**5**	**6**	**7**
TOTAL MULTIPLE DX	**88**	**6.2**	**123**	**1**	**2**	**3**	**5**	**13**	**18**	**77**
TOTAL										
0–19 Years	22	6.2	188	1	2	2	4	9	14	66
20–34	49	4.9	115	1	2	3	5	7	12	77
35–49	22	5.6	44	1	2	3	5	13	14	30
50–64	14	5.3	19	1	3	5	6	7	19	19
65+	3	11.7	59	3	3	14	18	18	18	18
GRAND TOTAL	**110**	**5.5**	**100**	**1**	**2**	**3**	**5**	**11**	**14**	**66**

Western Region, October 2007–September 2008 Data, by Operation

79.7: CLOSED RED DISLOCATION

Type of Patients	Observed Patients	Avg. Stay	Vari-ance	Percentiles						
				10th	25th	50th	75th	90th	95th	99th
1. SINGLE DX										
0–19 Years	50	1.3	1	1	1	1	1	2	2	9
20–34	49	1.5	1	1	1	1	2	3	4	6
35–49	23	1.4	<1	1	1	1	2	2	2	2
50–64	14	1.7	<1	1	1	1	2	3	4	4
65+	7	1.1	<1	1	1	1	1	2	2	2
2. MULTIPLE DX										
0–19 Years	71	3.0	34	1	1	2	3	5	7	57
20–34	233	2.5	6	1	1	2	3	5	7	14
35–49	210	3.3	26	1	1	2	3	6	10	34
50–64	493	2.7	8	1	1	2	3	5	8	14
65+	1,378	3.2	11	1	2	2	4	6	8	17
TOTAL SINGLE DX	143	1.4	<1	1	1	1	1	2	3	6
TOTAL MULTIPLE DX	2,385	3.0	12	1	1	2	4	6	8	16
TOTAL										
0–19 Years	121	2.2	20	1	1	1	2	4	7	9
20–34	282	2.3	5	1	1	2	3	4	7	14
35–49	233	3.1	24	1	1	2	3	6	9	34
50–64	507	2.7	8	1	1	2	3	5	8	14
65+	1,385	3.2	11	1	2	2	4	6	8	17
GRAND TOTAL	2,528	2.9	12	1	1	2	3	6	8	16

79.72: CLSD RED ELBOW DISLOC

Type of Patients	Observed Patients	Avg. Stay	Vari-ance	Percentiles						
				10th	25th	50th	75th	90th	95th	99th
1. SINGLE DX										
0–19 Years	6	1.0	0	1	1	1	1	1	1	1
20–34	5	1.0	0	1	1	1	1	1	1	1
35–49	3	1.3	<1	1	1	1	2	2	2	2
50–64	0									
65+	0									
2. MULTIPLE DX										
0–19 Years	9	1.2	<1	1	1	1	1	3	3	3
20–34	22	2.1	3	1	1	1	2	4	6	6
35–49	19	1.9	2	1	1	2	2	4	4	6
50–64	16	3.2	10	1	1	2	3	9	12	12
65+	22	3.2	4	1	2	3	3	7	7	8
TOTAL SINGLE DX	14	1.1	<1	1	1	1	1	1	2	2
TOTAL MULTIPLE DX	88	2.4	4	1	1	2	3	6	7	12
TOTAL										
0–19 Years	15	1.1	<1	1	1	1	2	3	3	3
20–34	27	1.9	2	1	1	1	2	4	6	6
35–49	22	1.9	2	1	1	2	2	3	4	6
50–64	16	3.2	10	1	1	2	3	9	12	12
65+	22	3.2	4	1	2	3	3	7	7	8
GRAND TOTAL	102	2.2	4	1	1	1	3	4	6	9

79.71: CLSD RED SHOULDER DISLOC

Type of Patients	Observed Patients	Avg. Stay	Vari-ance	Percentiles						
				10th	25th	50th	75th	90th	95th	99th
1. SINGLE DX										
0–19 Years	2	1.0	0	1	1	1	1	1	1	1
20–34	16	1.5	2	1	1	1	2	2	6	6
35–49	6	1.3	<1	1	1	1	2	2	2	2
50–64	4	1.3	<1	1	1	1	2	2	2	2
65+	1	1.0	0	1	1	1	1	1	1	1
2. MULTIPLE DX										
0–19 Years	12	3.2	7	1	1	2	7	7	7	7
20–34	69	2.2	6	1	1	1	2	6	7	15
35–49	64	4.0	51	1	1	2	4	9	9	41
50–64	76	3.1	15	1	1	2	4	6	8	31
65+	294	3.7	14	1	2	3	4	7	9	17
TOTAL SINGLE DX	29	1.4	<1	1	1	1	1	2	2	6
TOTAL MULTIPLE DX	515	3.5	17	1	1	2	4	7	9	17
TOTAL										
0–19 Years	14	3.0	7	1	1	1	7	7	7	7
20–34	85	2.0	5	1	1	1	2	5	7	15
35–49	70	3.8	47	1	1	2	3	9	9	41
50–64	80	3.0	15	1	1	2	4	6	8	31
65+	295	3.7	14	1	2	3	4	7	9	17
GRAND TOTAL	544	3.3	17	1	1	2	4	7	8	17

79.74: CLSD RED HAND/FINGER DIS

Type of Patients	Observed Patients	Avg. Stay	Vari-ance	Percentiles						
				10th	25th	50th	75th	90th	95th	99th
1. SINGLE DX										
0–19 Years	7	1.0	0	1	1	1	1	1	1	1
20–34	3	1.3	<1	1	1	1	2	2	2	2
35–49	1	1.0	0	1	1	1	1	1	1	1
50–64	1	1.0	0	1	1	1	1	1	1	1
65+	0									
2. MULTIPLE DX										
0–19 Years	2	1.0	0	1	1	1	1	1	1	1
20–34	11	2.2	2	1	1	2	2	5	5	5
35–49	26	3.8	41	1	1	2	4	6	7	34
50–64	24	3.3	9	1	1	2	4	6	7	15
65+	34	4.0	11	1	3	3	6	8	11	13
TOTAL SINGLE DX	12	1.1	<1	1	1	1	1	1	2	2
TOTAL MULTIPLE DX	97	3.5	17	1	1	2	4	7	11	34
TOTAL										
0–19 Years	9	1.0	0	1	1	1	1	1	1	1
20–34	14	2.0	2	1	1	2	2	5	5	5
35–49	27	3.7	39	1	1	2	4	6	7	34
50–64	25	3.2	9	1	1	2	4	6	7	15
65+	34	4.0	11	1	3	3	6	8	11	13
GRAND TOTAL	109	3.2	15	1	1	2	4	6	8	15

LOS by Diagnosis and Operation, Western Region, 45th Edition

Western Region, October 2007–September 2008 Data, by Operation

79.75: CLSD RED HIP DISLOC

Type of Patients	Observed Patients	Avg. Stay	Variance	10th	25th	50th	75th	90th	95th	99th
1. SINGLE DX										
0–19 Years	25	1.4	2	1	1	1	1	2	3	9
20–34	10	1.7	1	1	1	1	2	4	4	4
35–49	5	1.4	<1	1	1	1	2	2	2	2
50–64	7	1.7	1	1	1	1	2	4	4	4
65+	6	1.2	<1	1	1	1	1	2	2	2
2. MULTIPLE DX										
0–19 Years	28	3.7	75	1	1	2	3	5	5	57
20–34	78	2.7	7	1	1	2	3	5	7	14
35–49	75	2.7	9	1	1	1	3	5	10	16
50–64	326	2.6	7	1	1	2	3	5	8	14
65+	988	3.0	11	1	1	2	3	6	8	17
TOTAL SINGLE DX	53	1.4	1	1	1	1	1	2	3	9
TOTAL MULTIPLE DX	1,495	2.9	11	1	1	2	3	6	8	16
TOTAL										
0–19 Years	53	2.6	41	1	1	1	2	4	5	57
20–34	88	2.6	6	1	1	2	3	5	7	14
35–49	80	2.6	9	1	1	2	3	5	8	16
50–64	333	2.6	7	1	1	2	3	5	8	14
65+	994	3.0	11	1	1	2	3	6	8	17
GRAND TOTAL	1,548	2.8	11	1	1	2	3	5	8	16

79.76: CLSD RED KNEE DISLOC

Type of Patients	Observed Patients	Avg. Stay	Variance	10th	25th	50th	75th	90th	95th	99th
1. SINGLE DX										
0–19 Years	2	1.8	<1	1	2	2	2	2	2	2
20–34	4	2.3	2	1	2	2	3	4	4	4
35–49	1	2.0	0	2	2	2	2	2	2	2
50–64	1	3.0	0	3	3	3	3	3	3	3
65+	0									
2. MULTIPLE DX										
0–19 Years	6	1.7	1	1	1	1	2	4	4	4
20–34	17	4.3	16	1	2	3	4	10	17	17
35–49	9	4.3	18	1	1	3	3	13	13	13
50–64	29	2.6	9	1	1	2	3	5	11	14
65+	21	2.8	3	1	1	2	4	5	6	7
TOTAL SINGLE DX	8	2.1	<1	1	2	2	2	3	4	4
TOTAL MULTIPLE DX	82	3.1	9	1	1	2	4	6	10	17
TOTAL										
0–19 Years	8	1.7	<1	1	1	2	2	3	4	4
20–34	21	3.9	14	1	2	3	4	7	10	17
35–49	10	4.1	16	1	2	3	3	13	13	13
50–64	30	2.6	8	1	1	2	3	4	11	14
65+	21	2.8	3	1	1	2	4	5	6	7
GRAND TOTAL	90	3.0	8	1	1	2	3	5	10	17

79.8: OPEN RED DISLOCATION

Type of Patients	Observed Patients	Avg. Stay	Variance	10th	25th	50th	75th	90th	95th	99th
1. SINGLE DX										
0–19 Years	126	1.5	<1	1	1	1	2	3	3	6
20–34	38	1.6	1	1	1	1	2	3	4	6
35–49	17	1.8	3	1	1	1	2	4	7	7
50–64	2	1.5	<1	1	1	1	2	2	2	2
65+	2	1.0	0	1	1	1	1	1	1	1
2. MULTIPLE DX										
0–19 Years	156	2.8	5	1	1	2	3	5	8	10
20–34	85	3.6	17	1	1	2	4	8	11	>99
35–49	102	4.9	28	1	2	3	7	10	15	26
50–64	125	4.8	29	1	3	3	5	9	14	29
65+	133	5.1	17	1	3	4	7	10	12	19
TOTAL SINGLE DX	185	1.5	1	1	1	1	2	3	4	6
TOTAL MULTIPLE DX	601	3.8	16	1	1	3	5	8	10	21
TOTAL										
0–19 Years	282	2.2	4	1	1	1	3	4	6	10
20–34	123	3.0	13	1	1	2	3	6	8	26
35–49	119	4.5	25	1	2	3	5	10	15	26
50–64	127	4.8	29	1	2	3	5	9	14	29
65+	135	5.1	17	1	2	4	7	10	12	19
GRAND TOTAL	786	3.1	12	1	1	2	4	7	9	19

79.85: OPEN RED HIP DISLOC

Type of Patients	Observed Patients	Avg. Stay	Variance	10th	25th	50th	75th	90th	95th	99th
1. SINGLE DX										
0–19 Years	101	1.6	1	1	1	1	2	3	4	6
20–34	3	2.0	<1	1	1	2	3	3	3	3
35–49	0									
50–64	0									
65+	0									
2. MULTIPLE DX										
0–19 Years	131	2.8	4	1	1	2	3	5	8	10
20–34	10	6.6	49	3	4	4	8	26	>99	>99
35–49	14	6.9	46	2	4	5	5	10	29	29
50–64	26	5.3	55	2	3	5	5	9	9	40
65+	75	5.7	19	2	3	5	7	10	12	32
TOTAL SINGLE DX	104	1.6	1	1	1	1	2	3	4	6
TOTAL MULTIPLE DX	256	3.6	13	1	2	3	4	7	9	26
TOTAL										
0–19 Years	232	2.3	3	1	1	2	3	4	6	10
20–34	13	5.6	41	2	3	4	5	26	>99	>99
35–49	14	6.9	46	2	4	5	5	10	29	29
50–64	26	5.3	55	2	3	4	5	9	9	40
65+	75	5.7	19	2	3	5	7	10	12	32
GRAND TOTAL	360	2.9	10	1	1	2	3	6	8	12

LOS by Diagnosis and Operation, Western Region, 45th Edition

Western Region, October 2007–September 2008 Data, by Operation

79.87: OPEN RED ANKLE DISLOC

Type of Patients	Observed Patients	Avg. Stay	Vari-ance	Percentiles						
				10th	25th	50th	75th	90th	95th	99th
1. SINGLE DX										
0–19 Years	2	1.0	0	1	1	1	1	1	1	1
20–34	6	1.7	1	1	1	1	2	4	4	4
35–49	3	3.0	12	1	1	1	7	7	7	7
50–64	0									
65+	0									
2. MULTIPLE DX										
0–19 Years	5	2.1	4	1	1	1	2	7	7	7
20–34	23	2.9	9	1	1	2	3	6	8	14
35–49	27	4.0	21	1	1	2	5	9	17	19
50–64	26	2.7	4	1	1	2	3	6	7	9
65+	8	4.6	6	1	2	6	7	8	8	8
TOTAL SINGLE DX	11	1.9	4	1	1	1	2	4	7	7
TOTAL MULTIPLE DX	89	3.3	11	1	1	2	4	7	9	19
TOTAL										
0–19 Years	7	1.9	4	1	1	1	2	7	7	7
20–34	29	2.6	8	1	1	2	3	6	8	14
35–49	30	3.9	20	1	1	2	5	7	17	19
50–64	26	2.7	4	1	1	2	3	6	7	9
65+	8	4.6	6	1	2	6	7	8	8	8
GRAND TOTAL	100	3.1	10	1	1	2	4	7	8	17

80.0: ARTHROTOMY RMVL PROSTH

Type of Patients	Observed Patients	Avg. Stay	Vari-ance	Percentiles						
				10th	25th	50th	75th	90th	95th	99th
1. SINGLE DX										
0–19 Years	0									
20–34	2	2.0	0	2	2	2	2	2	2	2
35–49	0									
50–64	6	3.2	1	2	2	3	4	5	5	5
65+	2	2.0	2	1	1	1	3	3	3	3
2. MULTIPLE DX										
0–19 Years	2	2.5	<1	2	2	3	3	3	3	3
20–34	9	5.9	15	3	3	4	8	12	12	12
35–49	95	7.3	37	3	4	5	9	15	23	>99
50–64	455	7.5	55	3	4	5	8	15	21	42
65+	738	7.6	42	3	4	6	9	14	19	34
TOTAL SINGLE DX	10	2.7	1	2	2	2	3	5	5	5
TOTAL MULTIPLE DX	1,299	7.5	46	3	4	6	9	14	20	39
TOTAL										
0–19 Years	2	2.5	<1	2	2	3	3	3	3	3
20–34	11	5.2	14	2	3	3	8	12	12	12
35–49	95	7.3	37	3	4	5	9	15	23	>99
50–64	461	7.5	54	3	4	5	8	15	21	42
65+	740	7.6	42	3	4	6	9	14	19	34
GRAND TOTAL	1,309	7.5	46	3	4	6	8	14	20	38

79.9: BONE INJURY OP NOS

Type of Patients	Observed Patients	Avg. Stay	Vari-ance	Percentiles						
				10th	25th	50th	75th	90th	95th	99th
1. SINGLE DX										
0–19 Years	0									
20–34	0									
35–49	0									
50–64	0									
65+	0									
2. MULTIPLE DX										
0–19 Years	0									
20–34	0									
35–49	0									
50–64	0									
65+	1	5.0	0	5	5	5	5	5	5	5
TOTAL SINGLE DX	0									
TOTAL MULTIPLE DX	1	5.0	0	5	5	5	5	5	5	5
TOTAL										
0–19 Years	0									
20–34	0									
35–49	0									
50–64	0									
65+	1	5.0	0	5	5	5	5	5	5	5
GRAND TOTAL	1	5.0	0	5	5	5	5	5	5	5

80.05: RMVL PROSTH HIP INC

Type of Patients	Observed Patients	Avg. Stay	Vari-ance	Percentiles						
				10th	25th	50th	75th	90th	95th	99th
1. SINGLE DX										
0–19 Years	0									
20–34	0									
35–49	0									
50–64	0									
65+	0									
2. MULTIPLE DX										
0–19 Years	0									
20–34	5	7.8	18	3	4	8	12	12	12	12
35–49	31	9.4	55	4	5	7	12	23	33	>99
50–64	147	9.0	53	4	5	7	10	20	24	40
65+	260	9.6	61	4	5	7	11	20	25	41
TOTAL SINGLE DX	0									
TOTAL MULTIPLE DX	443	9.4	57	4	5	7	11	20	25	41
TOTAL										
0–19 Years	0									
20–34	5	7.8	18	3	4	8	12	12	12	12
35–49	31	9.4	55	4	5	7	12	23	33	>99
50–64	147	9.0	53	4	5	7	10	20	24	40
65+	260	9.6	61	4	5	7	11	20	25	41
GRAND TOTAL	443	9.4	57	4	5	7	11	20	25	41

LOS by Diagnosis and Operation, Western Region, 45th Edition

Western Region, October 2007–September 2008 Data, by Operation

80.06: RMVL PROSTH KNEE INC

Type of Patients	Observed Patients	Avg. Stay	Vari-ance	Percentiles 10th	25th	50th	75th	90th	95th	99th
1. SINGLE DX										
0–19 Years	0									
20–34	0									
35–49	0									
50–64	3	4.0	<1	3	3	4	5	5	5	5
65+	1	3.0	0	3	3					3
2. MULTIPLE DX										
0–19 Years	0									
20–34	2	4.0	2	3	3	5	5	5	5	5
35–49	40	6.5	17	3	4	5	8	10	16	22
50–64	248	7.6	63	3	4	5	8	15	20	44
65+	389	6.9	29	3	4	6	8	11	15	28
TOTAL SINGLE DX	4	3.8	<1	3	3	4	5	5	5	5
TOTAL MULTIPLE DX	679	7.1	41	3	4	6	8	13	16	38
TOTAL										
0–19 Years	0									
20–34	2	4.0	2	3	3	5	5	5	5	5
35–49	40	6.5	17	3	4	5	8	10	16	22
50–64	251	7.6	62	3	4	5	8	14	20	44
65+	390	6.8	29	3	4	6	8	11	15	28
GRAND TOTAL	683	7.1	40	3	4	6	8	12	16	38

80.1: OTHER ARTHROTOMY

Type of Patients	Observed Patients	Avg. Stay	Vari-ance	Percentiles 10th	25th	50th	75th	90th	95th	99th
1. SINGLE DX										
0–19 Years	83	4.1	10	1	2	3	5	8	11	13
20–34	39	3.2	20	1	1	2	4	5	11	28
35–49	28	3.1	3	1	2	3	4	7	7	8
50–64	23	2.7	6	1	1	2	3	4	9	11
65+	8	2.3	2	1	1	2	3	5	5	5
2. MULTIPLE DX										
0–19 Years	376	8.1	67	2	3	5	9	17	27	43
20–34	446	4.9	27	1	3	3	6	10	14	29
35–49	684	6.5	58	1	3	4	7	13	18	43
50–64	1,000	6.8	60	2	3	5	7	13	20	46
65+	1,031	7.0	33	2	3	5	8	14	18	29
TOTAL SINGLE DX	181	3.6	10	1	2	3	4	7	11	13
TOTAL MULTIPLE DX	3,537	6.8	51	2	3	5	8	14	20	39
TOTAL										
0–19 Years	459	7.4	59	2	3	5	8	15	27	40
20–34	485	4.8	27	1	2	3	5	10	14	29
35–49	712	6.3	57	1	3	4	7	12	18	40
50–64	1,023	6.7	59	2	3	5	7	13	20	46
65+	1,039	6.9	33	2	3	5	8	14	18	29
GRAND TOTAL	3,718	6.6	49	2	3	5	8	13	19	39

80.11: ARTHROTOMY NEC SHOULDER

Type of Patients	Observed Patients	Avg. Stay	Vari-ance	Percentiles 10th	25th	50th	75th	90th	95th	99th
1. SINGLE DX										
0–19 Years	3	5.0	13	1	1	6	8	8	8	8
20–34	0									
35–49	0									
50–64	1	2.0	0	2	2	2	2	2	2	2
65+	1	3.0	0	3	3	3	3	3	3	3
2. MULTIPLE DX										
0–19 Years	4	5.7	7	2	2	6	8	8	8	8
20–34	20	8.4	195	1	2	4	6	30	60	60
35–49	30	6.7	26	1	3	6	8	15	16	21
50–64	86	8.5	82	2	4	6	9	18	23	48
65+	109	7.3	44	1	3	5	10	17	23	28
TOTAL SINGLE DX	5	4.0	8	1	2	3	6	8	8	8
TOTAL MULTIPLE DX	249	7.7	66	2	3	5	9	17	23	46
TOTAL										
0–19 Years	7	5.4	8	1	2	6	8	8	8	8
20–34	20	8.4	195	1	3	4	6	30	60	60
35–49	30	6.7	26	2	4	6	8	15	16	21
50–64	87	8.5	81	2	4	6	9	18	23	48
65+	110	7.3	44	1	3	5	10	17	23	28
GRAND TOTAL	254	7.7	65	2	3	5	9	17	23	46

80.12: ARTHROTOMY NEC ELBOW

Type of Patients	Observed Patients	Avg. Stay	Vari-ance	Percentiles 10th	25th	50th	75th	90th	95th	99th
1. SINGLE DX										
0–19 Years	4	4.8	8	1	1	4	7	7	7	7
20–34	2	2.5	<1	2	2	3	3	3	3	3
35–49	1	3.0	0	3	3	3	3	3	3	3
50–64	4	4.3	21	1	2	3	11	11	11	11
65+	0									
2. MULTIPLE DX										
0–19 Years	18	4.9	7	2	3	5	6	7	9	14
20–34	34	4.1	9	1	2	3	6	7	9	16
35–49	53	5.8	20	2	3	4	7	11	18	24
50–64	64	6.2	67	1	2	4	6	12	15	47
65+	51	5.6	29	2	2	4	6	9	17	28
TOTAL SINGLE DX	11	4.0	10	1	2	3	7	7	11	11
TOTAL MULTIPLE DX	220	5.5	30	2	3	4	6	10	14	28
TOTAL										
0–19 Years	22	4.9	7	1	3	5	7	7	9	14
20–34	36	4.1	8	2	2	3	6	7	9	16
35–49	54	5.8	20	2	3	4	7	11	18	24
50–64	68	6.1	64	1	2	4	6	12	15	47
65+	51	5.6	29	2	2	4	6	9	17	28
GRAND TOTAL	231	5.4	29	2	3	4	6	10	14	28

LOS by Diagnosis and Operation, Western Region, 45th Edition

Western Region, October 2007–September 2008 Data, by Operation

80.15: ARTHROTOMY NEC HIP

Type of Patients	Observed Patients	Avg. Stay	Vari-ance	Percentiles						
				10th	25th	50th	75th	90th	95th	99th
1. SINGLE DX										
0–19 Years	23	4.6	9	2	3	4	5	8	13	13
20–34	2	3.0	2	2	2	3	4	4	4	4
35–49	6	2.7	7	1	1	2	3	8	8	8
50–64	1	1.0	0	1	1	1	1	1	1	1
65+	1	5.0	0	5	5	5	5	5	5	5
2. MULTIPLE DX										
0–19 Years	125	10.0	84	3	4	7	12	22	28	43
20–34	51	6.7	37	1	3	4	9	14	19	29
35–49	73	9.3	63	2	4	7	12	18	23	46
50–64	137	8.0	75	2	3	6	9	17	23	52
65+	186	7.9	33	3	4	6	9	14	21	33
TOTAL SINGLE DX	33	4.3	9	2	2	4	5	8	13	13
TOTAL MULTIPLE DX	572	8.7	64	2	4	6	11	17	26	43
TOTAL										
0–19 Years	148	9.0	75	2	4	6	11	21	28	43
20–34	53	6.6	37	1	3	4	8	14	19	29
35–49	79	8.8	61	1	4	7	11	18	23	46
50–64	138	8.0	75	2	3	6	9	17	23	52
65+	187	7.9	32	3	4	6	9	14	21	33
GRAND TOTAL	605	8.4	61	2	4	6	10	17	25	43

80.16: ARTHROTOMY NEC KNEE

Type of Patients	Observed Patients	Avg. Stay	Vari-ance	Percentiles						
				10th	25th	50th	75th	90th	95th	99th
1. SINGLE DX										
0–19 Years	39	3.9	12	1	2	3	4	7	11	23
20–34	21	2.4	2	1	1	2	4	4	5	6
35–49	14	3.1	2	1	2	3	3	4	7	7
50–64	13	2.8	5	1	2	2	3	4	9	9
65+	4	1.8	<1	1	1	2	2	3	3	3
2. MULTIPLE DX										
0–19 Years	144	7.5	65	2	4	5	8	15	27	39
20–34	155	5.1	17	2	2	4	6	9	14	21
35–49	290	6.7	78	2	3	5	7	11	21	64
50–64	473	6.9	63	2	3	5	7	13	22	45
65+	472	7.0	32	2	4	5	8	14	18	29
TOTAL SINGLE DX	91	3.4	9	1	2	3	4	6	9	11
TOTAL MULTIPLE DX	1,534	6.8	53	2	3	5	8	13	19	40
TOTAL										
0–19 Years	183	6.8	57	1	3	5	7	14	21	39
20–34	176	4.7	16	1	3	4	6	9	14	21
35–49	304	6.5	75	2	3	4	7	11	18	46
50–64	486	6.8	62	2	3	5	7	12	21	45
65+	476	7.0	32	2	3	5	8	14	18	29
GRAND TOTAL	1,625	6.6	51	2	3	5	7	13	18	39

80.13: ARTHROTOMY NEC WRIST

Type of Patients	Observed Patients	Avg. Stay	Vari-ance	Percentiles						
				10th	25th	50th	75th	90th	95th	99th
1. SINGLE DX										
0–19 Years	3	2.3	1	1	1	3	3	3	3	3
20–34	0									
35–49	2	5.0	8	3	3	7	7	7	7	7
50–64	1	1.0	0	1	1	1	1	1	1	1
65+	0									
2. MULTIPLE DX										
0–19 Years	5	5.5	64	1	3	3	5	>99	>99	>99
20–34	11	5.1	22	1	2	4	8	12	15	15
35–49	27	7.2	67	2	3	5	7	15	28	38
50–64	49	7.1	74	1	2	4	8	18	31	43
65+	70	6.5	43	2	3	5	8	11	21	34
TOTAL SINGLE DX	6	3.0	5	1	1	3	3	7	7	7
TOTAL MULTIPLE DX	162	6.7	55	2	2	4	8	15	27	43
TOTAL										
0–19 Years	8	4.7	48	1	1	3	5	25	>99	>99
20–34	11	5.1	22	1	2	4	8	12	15	15
35–49	29	7.0	63	2	3	5	7	15	28	38
50–64	50	6.9	74	1	2	4	8	18	31	43
65+	70	6.5	43	2	3	5	8	11	21	34
GRAND TOTAL	168	6.5	54	1	2	4	7	14	27	43

80.14: ARTHROTOMY NEC HAND/FING

Type of Patients	Observed Patients	Avg. Stay	Vari-ance	Percentiles						
				10th	25th	50th	75th	90th	95th	99th
1. SINGLE DX										
0–19 Years	5	1.3	<1	1	1	1	2	2	2	2
20–34	12	4.9	60	1	1	2	3	11	28	28
35–49	1	3.0	0	3	3	3	3	3	3	3
50–64	1	2.0	0	2	2	2	2	2	2	2
65+	2	1.5	<1	1	1	2	2	2	2	2
2. MULTIPLE DX										
0–19 Years	38	2.8	3	1	1	2	4	6	6	6
20–34	129	3.2	9	1	2	3	5	5	7	11
35–49	129	3.7	10	1	2	3	5	7	9	13
50–64	88	3.8	7	1	2	3	5	7	8	19
65+	66	4.1	12	1	2	3	5	8	11	18
TOTAL SINGLE DX	23	3.2	30	1	1	2	3	4	11	28
TOTAL MULTIPLE DX	450	3.6	9	1	2	3	4	6	8	15
TOTAL										
0–19 Years	43	2.6	3	1	1	2	4	5	6	6
20–34	141	3.4	13	1	2	3	5	5	7	28
35–49	132	3.7	10	1	2	3	5	7	9	13
50–64	89	3.8	7	1	2	3	5	7	8	19
65+	68	4.1	12	1	2	3	5	8	11	18
GRAND TOTAL	473	3.6	10	1	2	3	4	6	8	18

LOS by Diagnosis and Operation, Western Region, 45th Edition

Western Region, October 2007–September 2008 Data, by Operation

80.17: ARTHROTOMY NEC ANKLE

Type of Patients	Observed Patients	Avg. Stay	Vari-ance	Percentiles						
				10th	25th	50th	75th	90th	95th	99th
1. SINGLE DX										
0–19 Years	5	4.6	6	2	2	4	4	9	9	9
20–34	2	2.0	0	2	2	2	2	2	2	2
35–49	2	2.5	5	1	1	3	4	4	4	4
50–64	2	1.0	0	1	1	1	1	1	1	1
65+	0									
2. MULTIPLE DX										
0–19 Years	33	9.4	66	4	5	7	10	19	35	35
20–34	36	5.6	19	3	3	4	9	12	14	18
35–49	59	7.3	65	1	3	5	9	19	26	43
50–64	67	6.6	41	2	3	5	7	12	14	47
65+	49	7.4	25	1	4	7	9	14	18	22
TOTAL SINGLE DX	11	3.4	6	1	2	4	4	8	9	9
TOTAL MULTIPLE DX	244	7.4	47	2	3	5	9	14	20	35
TOTAL										
0–19 Years	38	8.8	61	3	5	7	8	19	35	35
20–34	38	5.4	19	1	2	4	9	12	14	18
35–49	61	7.2	63	1	3	4	8	17	25	43
50–64	69	6.4	41	2	3	5	7	12	14	47
65+	49	7.4	25	1	4	7	9	14	18	22
GRAND TOTAL	255	7.2	45	2	3	5	9	14	19	35

80.2: ARTHROSCOPY

Type of Patients	Observed Patients	Avg. Stay	Vari-ance	Percentiles						
				10th	25th	50th	75th	90th	95th	99th
1. SINGLE DX										
0–19 Years	4	1.5	<1	1	1	1	1	3	3	3
20–34	9	2.8	9	1	1	1	2	9	9	9
35–49	5	1.8	1	1	1	1	3	3	3	3
50–64	3	1.0	0	1	1	1	1	1	1	1
65+	5	1.0	0	1	1	1	1	1	1	1
2. MULTIPLE DX										
0–19 Years	17	2.5	8	1	1	1	3	8	8	14
20–34	22	5.6	74	1	1	3	4	16	23	36
35–49	49	4.5	38	1	1	2	5	7	15	33
50–64	85	4.6	37	1	1	2	6	11	16	40
65+	89	3.8	32	1	1	2	3	9	17	36
TOTAL SINGLE DX	26	1.8	3	1	1	1	2	3	7	9
TOTAL MULTIPLE DX	262	4.1	34	1	1	2	4	8	16	36
TOTAL										
0–19 Years	21	2.3	7	1	1	1	3	6	8	14
20–34	31	4.8	56	1	1	2	4	9	23	36
35–49	54	4.3	35	1	1	2	5	7	15	33
50–64	88	4.5	36	1	1	2	6	11	16	40
65+	94	3.7	31	1	1	2	3	8	17	36
GRAND TOTAL	288	3.9	32	1	1	2	4	8	16	33

80.21: SHOULDER ARTHROSCOPY

Type of Patients	Observed Patients	Avg. Stay	Vari-ance	Percentiles						
				10th	25th	50th	75th	90th	95th	99th
1. SINGLE DX										
0–19 Years	1	1.0	0	1	1	1	1	1	1	1
20–34	3	1.0	0	1	1	1	1	1	1	1
35–49	3	1.7	1	1	1	1	3	3	3	3
50–64	1	1.0	0	1	1	1	1	1	1	1
65+	3	1.0	0	1	1	1	1	1	1	1
2. MULTIPLE DX										
0–19 Years	7	1.4	1	1	1	1	1	2	2	6
20–34	8	8.7	179	1	1	2	23	36	36	36
35–49	24	3.6	35	1	1	2	2	5	15	28
50–64	55	3.1	32	1	1	1	2	6	10	40
65+	61	2.1	6	1	1	1	2	3	6	17
TOTAL SINGLE DX	11	1.1	<1	1	1	1	1	1	3	3
TOTAL MULTIPLE DX	155	2.8	27	1	1	1	2	5	9	36
TOTAL										
0–19 Years	8	1.3	<1	1	1	1	1	2	2	6
20–34	11	6.6	138	1	1	1	4	23	36	36
35–49	27	3.4	31	1	1	2	3	5	15	28
50–64	56	3.0	32	1	1	1	2	6	10	40
65+	64	2.1	6	1	1	1	2	3	6	17
GRAND TOTAL	166	2.7	25	1	1	1	2	5	8	36

80.26: KNEE ARTHROSCOPY

Type of Patients	Observed Patients	Avg. Stay	Vari-ance	Percentiles						
				10th	25th	50th	75th	90th	95th	99th
1. SINGLE DX										
0–19 Years	2	1.0	0	1	1	1	1	1	1	1
20–34	6	3.7	12	1	1	2	7	9	9	9
35–49	1	1.0	0	1	1	1	1	1	1	1
50–64	2	1.0	0	1	1	1	1	1	1	1
65+	2	1.0	0	1	1	1	1	1	1	1
2. MULTIPLE DX										
0–19 Years	9	4.1	14	1	1	3	8	8	14	14
20–34	10	3.2	1	2	3	3	3	6	6	6
35–49	20	5.8	51	1	2	4	7	14	33	33
50–64	25	6.8	32	2	3	5	8	19	19	20
65+	25	7.9	77	1	3	5	9	23	26	36
TOTAL SINGLE DX	13	2.2	7	1	1	1	2	7	9	9
TOTAL MULTIPLE DX	89	6.0	42	1	2	4	7	14	20	33
TOTAL										
0–19 Years	11	3.8	13	1	1	3	8	8	8	14
20–34	16	3.4	5	1	2	3	4	7	9	9
35–49	21	5.5	49	1	2	4	7	7	14	33
50–64	27	6.4	32	2	2	5	8	19	19	20
65+	27	7.4	74	1	2	4	9	23	26	36
GRAND TOTAL	102	5.6	39	1	2	3	7	12	19	33

LOS by Diagnosis and Operation, Western Region, 45th Edition

Western Region, October 2007–September 2008 Data, by Operation

80.3: BIOPSY JOINT STRUCTURE

Type of Patients	Observed Patients	Avg. Stay	Variance	10th	25th	50th	75th	90th	95th	99th
1. SINGLE DX										
0–19 Years	14	3.0	4	1	2	2	3	8	8	8
20–34	0									
35–49	1	1.0	0	1	1	1	1	1	1	1
50–64	2	2.5	4	1	1	1	4	4	4	4
65+	1	12.0	0	12	12	12	12	12	12	12
2. MULTIPLE DX										
0–19 Years	20	4.3	10	2	2	3	6	7	8	18
20–34	17	5.4	19	2	3	5	6	11	19	19
35–49	65	7.8	61	2	3	6	10	16	19	47
50–64	135	8.0	56	2	4	6	9	17	21	44
65+	234	7.8	41	2	4	6	10	15	20	27
TOTAL SINGLE DX	18	3.2	6	1	2	2	3	8	8	12
TOTAL MULTIPLE DX	471	7.4	45	2	3	6	9	15	19	37
TOTAL										
0–19 Years	34	3.8	8	1	2	3	5	7	8	18
20–34	17	5.4	19	2	3	5	6	11	19	19
35–49	66	7.7	61	2	3	6	10	16	19	47
50–64	137	7.9	56	2	4	6	9	17	21	44
65+	235	7.8	41	2	4	6	10	15	20	27
GRAND TOTAL	489	7.1	43	2	3	5	9	14	19	32

80.36: KNEE JOINT BIOPSY

Type of Patients	Observed Patients	Avg. Stay	Variance	10th	25th	50th	75th	90th	95th	99th
1. SINGLE DX										
0–19 Years	4	2.4	<1	2	2	3	3	3	3	3
20–34	0									
35–49	1	1.0	0	1	1	1	1	1	1	1
50–64	0									
65+	0									
2. MULTIPLE DX										
0–19 Years	6	3.7	6	2	2	3	3	7	10	10
20–34	6	4.2	5	2	2	3	6	7	7	7
35–49	11	4.0	9	1	1	3	6	6	11	11
50–64	20	5.1	11	2	3	5	7	8	16	16
65+	63	6.0	24	2	3	5	7	10	15	32
TOTAL SINGLE DX	5	2.3	<1	1	2	2	3	3	3	3
TOTAL MULTIPLE DX	106	5.3	18	2	3	5	6	9	12	19
TOTAL										
0–19 Years	10	3.1	4	2	2	3	3	6	7	10
20–34	6	4.2	5	2	2	3	6	7	7	7
35–49	12	3.8	9	1	1	3	6	6	11	11
50–64	20	5.1	11	2	3	5	7	8	16	16
65+	63	6.0	24	2	3	5	7	10	15	32
GRAND TOTAL	111	5.0	17	2	2	4	6	8	11	19

80.39: JOINT BIOPSY NEC

Type of Patients	Observed Patients	Avg. Stay	Variance	10th	25th	50th	75th	90th	95th	99th
1. SINGLE DX										
0–19 Years	2	3.0	0	3	3	3	3	3	3	3
20–34	0									
35–49	0									
50–64	1	4.0	0	4	4	4	4	4	4	4
65+	0									
2. MULTIPLE DX										
0–19 Years	3	5.3	1	3	5	6	6	6	6	6
20–34	2	11.1	126	3	3	19	19	19	19	19
35–49	34	9.9	91	4	5	7	10	19	37	47
50–64	75	9.3	81	3	4	8	12	18	21	56
65+	109	9.8	53	3	5	8	13	18	22	27
TOTAL SINGLE DX	3	3.3	<1	3	3	3	4	4	4	4
TOTAL MULTIPLE DX	223	9.6	66	3	5	7	12	18	21	47
TOTAL										
0–19 Years	5	4.8	2	3	3	6	5	6	6	6
20–34	2	11.1	126	3	3	19	19	19	19	19
35–49	34	9.9	91	4	5	7	10	19	37	47
50–64	76	9.2	80	3	4	8	11	18	21	56
65+	109	9.8	53	3	5	8	13	18	22	27
GRAND TOTAL	226	9.5	66	3	5	7	12	18	21	47

80.4: JT CAPSULE/LIG/CART DIV

Type of Patients	Observed Patients	Avg. Stay	Variance	10th	25th	50th	75th	90th	95th	99th
1. SINGLE DX										
0–19 Years	57	1.3	<1	1	1	1	1	2	2	4
20–34	12	1.7	<1	1	1	1	2	3	3	3
35–49	6	2.3	3	1	1	2	2	6	6	6
50–64	10	1.8	2	1	1	1	2	5	5	5
65+	2	2.5	<1	2	2	2	3	3	3	3
2. MULTIPLE DX										
0–19 Years	118	2.2	8	1	1	1	2	4	7	22
20–34	74	4.0	124	1	1	2	4	7	8	98
35–49	104	2.6	3	1	1	2	3	4	5	10
50–64	170	2.9	7	1	1	2	3	6	7	15
65+	123	2.9	6	1	1	2	4	5	6	10
TOTAL SINGLE DX	87	1.4	<1	1	1	1	2	2	3	5
TOTAL MULTIPLE DX	589	2.7	18	1	1	2	3	5	7	14
TOTAL										
0–19 Years	175	2.0	6	1	1	1	2	4	5	14
20–34	86	3.7	108	1	1	2	3	7	8	98
35–49	110	2.6	3	1	1	2	3	5	5	10
50–64	180	2.8	7	1	1	2	3	6	7	15
65+	125	2.9	6	1	2	2	3	5	6	10
GRAND TOTAL	676	2.4	15	1	1	2	3	4	7	14

LOS by Diagnosis and Operation, Western Region, 45th Edition

Western Region, October 2007–September 2008 Data, by Operation

80.50: IV DISC EXC/DESTR NOS

Type of Patients	Observed Patients	Avg. Stay	Variance	10th	25th	50th	75th	90th	95th	99th
1. SINGLE DX										
0–19 Years	0									
20–34	5	1.0	0	1	1	1	1	1	1	1
35–49	6	1.3	<1	1	1	1	2	2	2	2
50–64	4	1.0	0	1	1	1	1	1	1	1
65+	4	1.5	<1	1	1	1	2	2	2	2
2. MULTIPLE DX										
0–19 Years	0									
20–34	9	3.1	13	1	1	1	3	11	11	11
35–49	17	1.9	6	1	1	1	2	4	11	11
50–64	43	2.1	4	1	1	1	2	5	7	9
65+	32	2.5	9	1	1	1	3	4	10	14
TOTAL SINGLE DX	19	1.2	<1	1	1	1	1	2	2	2
TOTAL MULTIPLE DX	101	2.3	6	1	1	1	2	5	9	11
TOTAL										
0–19 Years	0									
20–34	14	2.4	9	1	1	1	2	7	11	11
35–49	23	1.8	5	1	1	1	2	2	4	11
50–64	47	2.0	4	1	1	1	2	5	7	9
65+	36	2.4	8	1	1	1	2	4	10	14
GRAND TOTAL	120	2.1	6	1	1	1	2	5	9	11

80.51: IV DISC EXCISION

Type of Patients	Observed Patients	Avg. Stay	Variance	10th	25th	50th	75th	90th	95th	99th
1. SINGLE DX										
0–19 Years	66	1.5	<1	1	1	1	2	3	3	4
20–34	940	1.4	1	1	1	1	1	2	3	6
35–49	1,488	1.4	<1	1	1	1	1	2	3	5
50–64	877	1.4	<1	1	1	1	1	2	3	5
65+	204	1.5	1	1	1	1	2	3	3	5
2. MULTIPLE DX										
0–19 Years	74	4.5	30	1	1	3	5	8	11	28
20–34	1,998	2.0	5	1	1	1	2	4	6	11
35–49	4,521	2.0	6	1	1	1	2	4	5	11
50–64	5,575	2.2	11	1	1	1	2	4	6	13
65+	3,921	2.7	13	1	1	2	3	6	8	16
TOTAL SINGLE DX	3,575	1.4	<1	1	1	1	1	2	3	5
TOTAL MULTIPLE DX	16,089	2.3	10	1	1	1	2	4	6	14
TOTAL										
0–19 Years	140	3.3	21	1	1	2	4	7	8	28
20–34	2,938	1.8	4	1	1	1	2	4	5	9
35–49	6,009	1.9	5	1	1	1	2	4	5	10
50–64	6,452	2.1	10	1	1	1	2	4	6	12
65+	4,125	2.7	12	1	1	2	3	5	7	16
GRAND TOTAL	19,664	2.1	8	1	1	1	2	4	6	12

80.46: KNEE STRUCTURE DIVISION

Type of Patients	Observed Patients	Avg. Stay	Variance	10th	25th	50th	75th	90th	95th	99th
1. SINGLE DX										
0–19 Years	10	2.2	<1	1	1	2	4	4	4	4
20–34	10	1.7	<1	1	1	1	2	3	3	3
35–49	6	2.3	3	1	1	2	2	6	6	6
50–64	5	1.4	<1	1	1	1	1	3	3	3
65+	2	2.5	<1	2	2	2	3	3	3	3
2. MULTIPLE DX										
0–19 Years	26	3.4	12	1	1	2	5	7	14	14
20–34	46	3.0	5	1	1	2	4	7	8	8
35–49	63	2.4	2	1	1	2	3	4	4	11
50–64	107	2.7	4	1	1	2	3	5	6	8
65+	83	2.8	7	1	1	2	3	5	5	23
TOTAL SINGLE DX	33	2.0	1	1	1	2	2	4	4	6
TOTAL MULTIPLE DX	325	2.8	6	1	1	2	3	5	7	14
TOTAL										
0–19 Years	36	3.1	10	1	1	2	4	7	14	14
20–34	56	2.8	4	1	1	2	3	7	8	8
35–49	69	2.4	3	1	1	2	3	4	5	11
50–64	112	2.7	4	1	1	2	3	5	6	8
65+	85	2.8	7	1	1	2	3	5	5	23
GRAND TOTAL	358	2.7	6	1	1	2	3	5	7	14

80.5: IV DISC EXC/DESTRUCTION

Type of Patients	Observed Patients	Avg. Stay	Variance	10th	25th	50th	75th	90th	95th	99th
1. SINGLE DX										
0–19 Years	67	1.5	<1	1	1	1	2	3	3	4
20–34	945	1.4	1	1	1	1	1	2	3	6
35–49	1,500	1.4	<1	1	1	1	1	2	3	5
50–64	885	1.4	<1	1	1	1	1	2	3	5
65+	209	1.5	1	2	2	2	2	3	3	5
2. MULTIPLE DX										
0–19 Years	75	4.5	30	1	1	3	5	8	11	28
20–34	2,014	2.0	5	1	1	1	2	4	6	11
35–49	4,549	2.0	6	1	1	1	2	4	5	11
50–64	5,635	2.2	11	1	1	1	2	4	6	13
65+	3,981	2.7	13	1	1	2	3	6	8	16
TOTAL SINGLE DX	3,606	1.4	<1	1	1	1	1	2	3	5
TOTAL MULTIPLE DX	16,254	2.3	10	1	1	1	2	4	6	14
TOTAL										
0–19 Years	142	3.3	20	1	1	2	4	7	8	28
20–34	2,959	1.8	4	1	1	1	2	4	5	10
35–49	6,049	1.9	5	1	1	1	2	4	5	10
50–64	6,520	2.1	10	1	1	1	2	4	6	12
65+	4,190	2.7	12	1	1	2	3	5	7	16
GRAND TOTAL	19,860	2.1	8	1	1	1	2	4	6	12

LOS by Diagnosis and Operation, Western Region, 45th Edition

Western Region, October 2007–September 2008 Data, by Operation

80.76: KNEE SYNOVECTOMY

Type of Patients	Observed Patients	Avg. Stay	Variance	Percentiles						
				10th	25th	50th	75th	90th	95th	99th
1. SINGLE DX										
0–19 Years	4	2.1	5	1	1	1	3	7	7	7
20–34	11	2.6	1	2	2	2	4	4	5	5
35–49	8	2.5	<1	1	2	2	3	4	4	4
50–64	7	2.6	2	1	1	3	3	5	5	5
65+	0									
2. MULTIPLE DX										
0–19 Years	30	4.5	35	1	1	2	5	17	>99	>99
20–34	88	4.5	18	1	2	3	6	8	13	30
35–49	149	6.0	36	1	2	4	8	14	18	30
50–64	269	6.6	36	2	3	5	8	14	17	36
65+	290	7.0	46	2	3	5	8	13	18	42
TOTAL SINGLE DX	30	2.5	2	1	1	2	3	4	5	7
TOTAL MULTIPLE DX	826	6.3	38	2	3	4	8	13	18	42
TOTAL										
0–19 Years	34	4.2	32	1	1	2	5	17	>99	>99
20–34	99	4.3	17	1	2	3	6	8	13	30
35–49	157	5.8	34	1	2	4	7	12	18	30
50–64	276	6.5	36	2	3	5	8	13	17	36
65+	290	7.0	46	2	3	5	8	13	18	42
GRAND TOTAL	856	6.1	37	1	2	4	8	13	18	42

80.8: OTH EXC/DESTR JOINT LES

Type of Patients	Observed Patients	Avg. Stay	Variance	Percentiles						
				10th	25th	50th	75th	90th	95th	99th
1. SINGLE DX										
0–19 Years	32	2.5	3	1	1	2	3	5	6	9
20–34	38	2.2	2	1	1	2	3	4	6	6
35–49	30	2.1	2	1	1	2	3	4	5	5
50–64	14	1.9	2	1	1	1	2	4	5	5
65+	6	1.8	3	1	1	1	2	5	5	5
2. MULTIPLE DX										
0–19 Years	125	6.9	74	1	2	4	7	17	27	38
20–34	267	4.7	36	1	2	3	5	8	11	41
35–49	503	5.6	44	1	2	3	7	12	18	31
50–64	930	5.6	63	1	2	3	6	12	16	43
65+	1,020	5.5	33	1	2	4	7	11	15	28
TOTAL SINGLE DX	120	2.3	3	1	1	2	3	5	6	9
TOTAL MULTIPLE DX	2,845	5.6	48	1	2	4	7	12	17	38
TOTAL										
0–19 Years	157	6.0	62	1	1	3	6	17	27	38
20–34	305	4.4	32	1	1	3	5	8	11	36
35–49	533	5.4	42	1	1	3	7	11	18	31
50–64	944	5.6	62	1	2	3	6	12	16	43
65+	1,026	5.5	33	1	2	4	7	11	15	28
GRAND TOTAL	2,965	5.4	46	1	2	3	6	11	17	38

80.6: EXC KNEE SEMILUNAR CART

Type of Patients	Observed Patients	Avg. Stay	Variance	Percentiles						
				10th	25th	50th	75th	90th	95th	99th
1. SINGLE DX										
0–19 Years	8	1.5	<1	1	1	1	2	3	3	3
20–34	9	1.3	<1	1	1	1	1	3	3	3
35–49	5	1.4	<1	1	1	1	1	3	3	3
50–64	4	1.5	<1	1	1	1	1	3	3	3
65+	3	1.3	<1	1	1	1	2	2	2	2
2. MULTIPLE DX										
0–19 Years	29	1.5	<1	1	1	1	2	2	3	5
20–34	81	2.6	9	1	1	2	3	4	7	22
35–49	184	3.4	33	1	1	2	3	7	12	40
50–64	292	3.4	19	1	1	2	4	8	12	25
65+	218	4.6	19	1	1	3	6	10	13	19
TOTAL SINGLE DX	29	1.4	<1	1	1	1	2	3	3	3
TOTAL MULTIPLE DX	804	3.5	21	1	1	2	4	8	12	24
TOTAL										
0–19 Years	37	1.5	<1	1	1	1	2	2	3	5
20–34	90	2.5	8	1	1	2	3	4	7	22
35–49	189	3.3	32	1	1	2	3	7	12	40
50–64	296	3.4	19	1	1	2	4	8	12	25
65+	221	4.6	19	1	1	3	6	10	13	19
GRAND TOTAL	833	3.5	20	1	1	2	4	8	11	24

80.7: SYNOVECTOMY

Type of Patients	Observed Patients	Avg. Stay	Variance	Percentiles						
				10th	25th	50th	75th	90th	95th	99th
1. SINGLE DX										
0–19 Years	7	2.0	3	1	1	2	2	3	7	7
20–34	12	2.5	2	1	2	2	4	4	5	5
35–49	11	2.2	<1	1	1	2	3	3	4	4
50–64	8	2.4	2	1	1	2	3	5	5	5
65+	1	2.0	0	2	2	2	2	2	2	2
2. MULTIPLE DX										
0–19 Years	36	4.3	32	1	1	2	5	17	>99	>99
20–34	122	4.5	19	1	2	3	5	8	13	27
35–49	209	5.7	44	1	2	3	7	11	18	30
50–64	331	6.2	34	1	3	4	8	12	16	31
65+	352	6.6	41	2	3	5	8	13	18	38
TOTAL SINGLE DX	39	2.2	2	1	1	2	3	4	5	7
TOTAL MULTIPLE DX	1,050	5.9	37	1	2	4	7	12	17	38
TOTAL										
0–19 Years	43	3.9	28	1	1	2	4	17	>99	>99
20–34	134	4.3	18	1	2	3	5	8	13	27
35–49	220	5.5	42	1	2	3	7	11	18	30
50–64	339	6.1	34	1	3	4	8	12	16	31
65+	353	6.6	41	2	3	5	8	13	18	38
GRAND TOTAL	1,089	5.8	36	1	2	4	7	12	17	36

LOS by Diagnosis and Operation, Western Region, 45th Edition

Western Region, October 2007–September 2008 Data, by Operation

80.81: EXC/DESTR SHOULD LES NEC

Type of Patients	Observed Patients	Avg. Stay	Variance	10th	25th	50th	75th	90th	95th	99th
1. SINGLE DX										
0–19 Years	2	1.0	0	1	1	1	1	1	1	1
20–34	2	2.5	4	1	1	1	4	4	4	4
35–49	5	1.2	<1	1	1	1	1	2	2	2
50–64	5	2.0	3	1	1	1	2	5	5	5
65+	2	1.0	0	1	1	1	1	1	1	1
2. MULTIPLE DX										
0–19 Years	9	11.5	98	1	1	6	17	27	27	27
20–34	26	4.8	66	1	1	2	5	10	10	42
35–49	108	3.1	17	1	1	2	3	7	12	18
50–64	330	4.6	71	1	1	2	4	9	14	50
65+	417	4.1	26	1	1	2	5	9	13	22
TOTAL SINGLE DX	16	1.5	1	1	1	1	1	4	5	5
TOTAL MULTIPLE DX	890	4.3	45	1	1	2	5	9	14	40
TOTAL										
0–19 Years	11	9.5	96	1	1	6	17	27	27	27
20–34	28	4.7	62	1	1	2	4	10	10	42
35–49	113	3.0	17	1	1	2	3	6	12	18
50–64	335	4.5	70	1	1	2	4	9	14	50
65+	419	4.1	26	1	1	2	5	9	13	22
GRAND TOTAL	906	4.3	45	1	1	2	5	9	14	40

80.82: EXC/DESTR ELBOW LES NEC

Type of Patients	Observed Patients	Avg. Stay	Variance	10th	25th	50th	75th	90th	95th	99th
1. SINGLE DX										
0–19 Years	4	1.1	<1	1	1	1	1	1	2	2
20–34	2	1.5	<1	1	1	2	2	2	2	2
35–49	1	9.0	0	9	9	9	9	9	9	9
50–64	0									
65+	2	3.0	8	1	1	1	5	5	5	5
2. MULTIPLE DX										
0–19 Years	18	2.9	9	1	1	2	4	5	10	18
20–34	21	6.7	112	1	1	3	6	12	17	49
35–49	49	4.7	21	1	2	4	6	12	15	22
50–64	52	5.7	138	1	1	4	5	10	21	78
65+	42	5.5	17	2	3	4	7	11	15	17
TOTAL SINGLE DX	9	1.8	4	1	1	1	1	5	9	9
TOTAL MULTIPLE DX	182	5.0	57	1	2	3	5	10	15	37
TOTAL										
0–19 Years	22	2.5	8	1	1	1	3	4	6	18
20–34	23	6.2	104	1	1	4	6	12	17	49
35–49	50	4.8	21	1	2	4	6	12	15	22
50–64	52	5.7	138	1	1	3	5	10	21	78
65+	44	5.4	16	2	3	4	7	11	15	17
GRAND TOTAL	191	4.7	54	1	1	3	5	9	15	37

80.84: EXC/DESTR HAND LES NEC

Type of Patients	Observed Patients	Avg. Stay	Variance	10th	25th	50th	75th	90th	95th	99th
1. SINGLE DX										
0–19 Years	4	2.2	4	1	1	1	2	5	5	5
20–34	3	2.3	1	1	1	3	3	3	3	3
35–49	2	2.0	2	1	1	1	3	3	3	3
50–64	2	1.5	<1	1	1	2	2	2	2	2
65+	0									
2. MULTIPLE DX										
0–19 Years	5	3.4	<1	3	3	3	3	5	5	5
20–34	40	3.6	5	3	3	3	4	7	8	10
35–49	36	3.8	4	2	2	3	6	7	7	8
50–64	33	4.0	6	1	2	4	6	7	8	12
65+	31	5.1	26	1	2	4	6	8	22	23
TOTAL SINGLE DX	11	2.1	2	1	1	2	3	3	5	5
TOTAL MULTIPLE DX	145	4.1	10	2	2	3	5	7	8	22
TOTAL										
0–19 Years	9	2.9	2	1	2	3	3	5	5	5
20–34	43	3.5	5	1	2	3	4	7	8	10
35–49	38	3.7	4	2	2	3	6	7	7	8
50–64	35	3.9	6	1	2	3	6	7	8	12
65+	31	5.1	26	1	2	4	6	8	22	23
GRAND TOTAL	156	3.9	9	1	2	3	5	7	8	22

80.85: EXC/DESTR HIP LESION NEC

Type of Patients	Observed Patients	Avg. Stay	Variance	10th	25th	50th	75th	90th	95th	99th
1. SINGLE DX										
0–19 Years	3	5.0	16	1	1	5	9	9	9	9
20–34	4	2.5	6	1	1	2	2	6	6	6
35–49	8	1.9	2	1	1	1	4	4	4	4
50–64	2	1.5	<1	1	1	2	2	2	2	2
65+	0									
2. MULTIPLE DX										
0–19 Years	26	9.9	77	2	5	6	15	29	29	29
20–34	28	5.5	90	1	1	2	5	11	35	41
35–49	50	5.9	43	1	2	4	8	15	22	28
50–64	109	5.8	35	1	3	4	8	14	15	23
65+	122	6.8	53	2	3	5	8	12	16	46
TOTAL SINGLE DX	17	2.5	5	1	1	1	4	6	9	9
TOTAL MULTIPLE DX	335	6.7	53	1	2	5	8	15	21	40
TOTAL										
0–19 Years	29	9.6	74	2	5	6	12	29	29	29
20–34	32	5.1	80	1	1	3	5	8	35	41
35–49	58	5.4	39	1	1	4	6	15	22	28
50–64	111	5.7	35	1	2	4	8	13	15	23
65+	122	6.8	53	2	3	5	8	12	16	46
GRAND TOTAL	352	6.5	52	1	2	5	8	14	21	40

LOS by Diagnosis and Operation, Western Region, 45th Edition

Western Region, October 2007–September 2008 Data, by Operation

80.86: EXC/DESTR KNEE LES NEC

Type of Patients	Observed Patients	Avg. Stay	Variance	10th	25th	50th	75th	90th	95th	99th
1. SINGLE DX										
0–19 Years	14	3.3	2	1	2	3	4	6	6	6
20–34	23	2.3	2	1	1	2	3	4	4	6
35–49	10	2.2	2	1	1	2	3	4	5	5
50–64	3	1.3	<1	1	1	2	2	2	2	2
65+	2	1.5	<1	1	1	2	2	2	2	2
2. MULTIPLE DX										
0–19 Years	45	6.6	78	1	2	3	6	17	38	38
20–34	94	4.3	9	2	2	4	6	8	11	17
35–49	152	7.5	66	1	3	5	10	15	25	42
50–64	257	6.9	62	1	3	4	8	14	19	45
65+	276	6.7	30	2	3	5	8	14	17	31
TOTAL SINGLE DX	52	2.6	2	1	1	3	3	4	6	6
TOTAL MULTIPLE DX	824	6.7	48	2	3	5	8	14	17	38
TOTAL										
0–19 Years	59	5.7	60	1	2	3	6	12	20	38
20–34	117	3.9	8	1	2	3	5	7	11	14
35–49	162	7.2	63	1	2	5	10	14	23	42
50–64	260	6.9	62	2	3	4	8	14	17	45
65+	278	6.7	30	2	3	5	8	14	17	31
GRAND TOTAL	876	6.4	46	1	3	4	8	13	17	38

80.87: EXC/DESTR ANKLE LES NEC

Type of Patients	Observed Patients	Avg. Stay	Variance	10th	25th	50th	75th	90th	95th	99th
1. SINGLE DX										
0–19 Years	4	3.3	4	1	2	5	5	5	5	5
20–34	3	2.0	<1	1	1	2	3	3	3	3
35–49	3	2.3	<1	1	2	2	3	3	3	3
50–64	1	3.0	0	3	3	3	3	3	3	3
65+	0									
2. MULTIPLE DX										
0–19 Years	15	7.4	112	2	3	3	9	12	12	60
20–34	39	4.6	39	1	2	3	5	8	19	36
35–49	71	5.6	57	1	2	3	7	12	20	49
50–64	85	5.1	33	1	2	3	6	12	16	32
65+	62	5.9	22	1	3	4	8	11	12	29
TOTAL SINGLE DX	11	2.7	2	1	2	2	3	5	5	5
TOTAL MULTIPLE DX	272	5.6	45	1	2	3	7	12	16	36
TOTAL										
0–19 Years	19	6.9	101	2	2	3	7	12	12	60
20–34	42	4.4	36	1	2	3	4	7	13	36
35–49	74	5.4	55	1	1	3	6	12	20	49
50–64	86	5.1	33	1	2	3	6	12	16	32
65+	62	5.9	22	1	3	4	8	11	12	29
GRAND TOTAL	283	5.5	44	1	2	3	7	12	16	36

80.88: EXC/DESTR FT JT LES NEC

Type of Patients	Observed Patients	Avg. Stay	Variance	10th	25th	50th	75th	90th	95th	99th
1. SINGLE DX										
0–19 Years	0									
20–34	1	1.0	0	1	1	1	1	1	1	1
35–49	0									
50–64	0									
65+	0									
2. MULTIPLE DX										
0–19 Years	3	1.8	3	1	1	1	2	5	5	5
20–34	9	4.4	5	1	3	4	6	8	8	8
35–49	23	8.8	47	2	3	7	11	20	25	26
50–64	43	7.5	92	2	3	5	9	14	16	61
65+	36	7.2	48	1	3	6	10	13	20	36
TOTAL SINGLE DX	1	1.0	0	1	1	1	1	1	1	1
TOTAL MULTIPLE DX	114	7.1	60	1	3	5	9	14	20	36
TOTAL										
0–19 Years	3	1.8	3	1	1	1	2	5	5	5
20–34	10	4.1	6	1	2	4	6	7	8	8
35–49	23	8.8	47	2	3	7	11	20	25	26
50–64	43	7.5	92	2	3	5	9	14	16	61
65+	36	7.2	48	1	3	6	10	13	20	36
GRAND TOTAL	115	7.1	60	1	3	5	9	14	20	36

80.9: OTHER JOINT EXCISION

Type of Patients	Observed Patients	Avg. Stay	Variance	10th	25th	50th	75th	90th	95th	99th
1. SINGLE DX										
0–19 Years	1	9.0	0	9	9	9	9	9	9	9
20–34	2	1.5	<1	1	1	2	2	2	2	2
35–49	3	3.3	2	2	2	3	5	5	5	5
50–64	5	2.8	6	1	2	3	2	7	7	7
65+	0									
2. MULTIPLE DX										
0–19 Years	18	14.4	226	2	4	12	17	47	47	60
20–34	27	11.6	434	1	2	4	9	71	80	>99
35–49	64	7.3	89	1	2	4	8	20	29	47
50–64	119	7.7	85	1	2	5	10	16	28	68
65+	82	8.9	116	1	3	6	12	19	28	78
TOTAL SINGLE DX	11	4.5	11	1	2	3	9	9	9	9
TOTAL MULTIPLE DX	310	9.1	142	1	2	5	11	21	34	78
TOTAL										
0–19 Years	19	13.9	208	2	5	12	17	47	47	60
20–34	29	10.9	409	1	2	4	8	71	80	>99
35–49	67	7.1	86	1	2	4	8	20	29	47
50–64	124	7.5	83	1	2	5	10	16	28	68
65+	82	8.9	116	1	3	6	12	19	28	78
GRAND TOTAL	321	8.9	138	1	2	5	11	21	33	78

Western Region, October 2007–September 2008 Data, by Operation

80.99: EXCISION OF JOINT NEC

Type of Patients	Observed Patients	Avg. Stay	Vari-ance	10th	25th	50th	75th	90th	95th	99th
1. SINGLE DX										
0–19 Years	0									
20–34	0									
35–49	3	3.3	2	2	2	3	5	5	5	5
50–64	2	4.5	12	2	2	7	7	7	7	7
65+	0									
2. MULTIPLE DX										
0–19 Years	9	14.1	175	2	5	12	17	24	60	60
20–34	14	19.3	730	1	2	5	44	80	>99	>99
35–49	37	8.4	127	1	2	3	8	29	34	47
50–64	64	9.3	134	1	2	5	11	27	29	68
65+	44	9.9	174	1	2	6	13	21	28	78
TOTAL SINGLE DX	5	3.8	5	2	2	3	5	7	7	7
TOTAL MULTIPLE DX	168	10.5	196	1	2	6	13	28	36	80
TOTAL										
0–19 Years	9	14.1	175	2	5	12	17	24	60	60
20–34	14	19.3	730	1	2	5	44	80	>99	>99
35–49	40	8.0	119	1	2	3	8	26	34	47
50–64	66	9.2	131	1	2	5	11	27	29	68
65+	44	9.9	174	1	2	6	13	21	28	78
GRAND TOTAL	173	10.4	192	1	2	5	13	28	34	80

81.00: SPINAL FUSION NOS

Type of Patients	Observed Patients	Avg. Stay	Vari-ance	10th	25th	50th	75th	90th	95th	99th
1. SINGLE DX										
0–19 Years	2	4.2	<1	4	4	4	4	5	5	5
20–34	0									
35–49	5	1.2	<1	1	1	1	1	2	2	2
50–64	5	3.0	12	1	1	1	3	9	9	9
65+	1	1.0	0	1	1	1	1	1	1	1
2. MULTIPLE DX										
0–19 Years	7	5.9	23	3	3	5	6	7	22	22
20–34	8	4.5	5	1	1	4	7	7	7	7
35–49	21	6.4	49	1	3	5	8	11	23	28
50–64	68	4.6	23	1	2	3	5	11	15	24
65+	44	5.1	19	1	2	3	7	10	15	21
TOTAL SINGLE DX	13	2.7	5	1	1	2	4	5	9	9
TOTAL MULTIPLE DX	148	5.1	24	1	2	3	6	10	15	24
TOTAL										
0–19 Years	9	5.4	17	3	4	5	5	7	22	22
20–34	8	4.5	5	1	3	4	7	7	7	7
35–49	26	5.4	43	1	1	3	6	11	23	28
50–64	73	4.5	22	1	2	3	5	10	15	24
65+	45	5.0	19	1	2	3	7	10	15	21
GRAND TOTAL	161	4.9	23	1	2	3	6	10	15	24

81.0: SPINAL FUSION

Type of Patients	Observed Patients	Avg. Stay	Vari-ance	10th	25th	50th	75th	90th	95th	99th
1. SINGLE DX										
0–19 Years	356	5.0	4	3	4	5	5	6	8	10
20–34	340	2.8	3	1	1	2	4	5	6	10
35–49	1,338	1.9	2	1	1	2	3	4	5	7
50–64	1,136	2.2	2	1	1	2	3	4	5	7
65+	266	2.3	2	1	1	2	3	4	5	7
2. MULTIPLE DX										
0–19 Years	1,256	7.1	34	4	5	6	7	11	15	37
20–34	2,576	4.9	35	1	2	3	5	9	13	32
35–49	11,335	3.3	16	1	2	3	4	6	8	19
50–64	19,825	3.8	19	1	2	3	4	7	10	21
65+	14,931	4.8	22	1	2	4	6	9	12	23
TOTAL SINGLE DX	3,436	2.8	4	1	1	2	4	5	6	8
TOTAL MULTIPLE DX	49,923	4.3	22	1	2	3	5	8	11	23
TOTAL										
0–19 Years	1,612	6.6	28	4	4	5	7	10	13	35
20–34	2,916	4.7	32	1	2	3	5	9	13	31
35–49	12,673	3.2	15	1	1	2	4	6	8	18
50–64	20,961	3.8	18	1	1	3	4	7	9	21
65+	15,197	4.8	21	1	2	4	6	9	12	23
GRAND TOTAL	53,359	4.2	21	1	2	3	5	8	11	22

81.01: ATLAS-AXIS SPINAL FUSION

Type of Patients	Observed Patients	Avg. Stay	Vari-ance	10th	25th	50th	75th	90th	95th	99th
1. SINGLE DX										
0–19 Years	2	7.0	0	7	7	7	7	7	7	7
20–34	1	10.0	0	10	10	10	10	10	10	10
35–49	5	2.0	1	1	1	2	3	3	3	3
50–64	3	1.7	1	2	2	2	3	3	3	3
65+	4	3.0	2	2	2	2	3	5	5	5
2. MULTIPLE DX										
0–19 Years	21	11.5	207	3	4	6	12	15	55	67
20–34	24	6.7	35	2	3	5	9	14	16	27
35–49	64	5.8	30	1	2	4	8	15	17	21
50–64	120	7.6	130	2	3	4	8	14	22	80
65+	235	8.5	76	2	3	6	10	16	23	39
TOTAL SINGLE DX	15	3.6	8	1	1	3	5	7	10	10
TOTAL MULTIPLE DX	464	8.0	92	2	3	6	9	15	22	55
TOTAL										
0–19 Years	23	11.1	192	3	5	6	12	15	55	67
20–34	25	6.8	34	2	3	5	9	14	16	27
35–49	69	5.5	29	1	2	5	8	15	17	21
50–64	123	7.5	128	2	3	4	8	14	22	80
65+	239	8.4	76	2	3	6	10	16	23	39
GRAND TOTAL	479	7.9	90	2	3	5	9	15	22	55

LOS by Diagnosis and Operation, Western Region, 45th Edition

Western Region, October 2007–September 2008 Data, by Operation

81.02: ANT CERVICAL FUSION NEC

Type of Patients	Observed Patients	Avg. Stay	Vari-ance	Percentiles						
				10th	25th	50th	75th	90th	95th	99th
1. SINGLE DX										
0–19 Years	4	1.9	2	1	1	1	2	5	5	5
20–34	135	1.5	1	1	1	1	2	2	3	7
35–49	884	1.4	<1	1	1	1	2	2	3	5
50–64	703	1.5	1	1	1	1	2	3	3	7
65+	128	1.5	<1	1	1	1	2	3	3	5
2. MULTIPLE DX										
0–19 Years	46	9.3	161	1	3	5	10	20	42	64
20–34	689	3.4	42	1	1	1	3	6	11	38
35–49	5,386	2.0	7	1	1	1	2	3	5	12
50–64	7,918	2.4	12	1	1	1	2	4	7	17
65+	3,408	3.3	24	1	1	2	3	7	12	25
TOTAL SINGLE DX	1,854	1.5	<1	1	1	1	2	2	3	6
TOTAL MULTIPLE DX	17,447	2.5	15	1	1	1	2	5	7	19
TOTAL										
0–19 Years	50	8.5	149	1	2	4	10	17	32	64
20–34	824	3.1	36	1	1	1	3	6	9	34
35–49	6,270	2.0	6	1	1	1	2	3	5	12
50–64	8,621	2.3	12	1	1	1	2	4	6	16
65+	3,536	3.3	24	1	1	2	3	7	12	25
GRAND TOTAL	19,301	2.4	14	1	1	1	2	4	7	18

81.03: POST CERVICAL FUSION NEC

Type of Patients	Observed Patients	Avg. Stay	Vari-ance	Percentiles						
				10th	25th	50th	75th	90th	95th	99th
1. SINGLE DX										
0–19 Years	4	4.0	2	1	3	5	5	5	5	5
20–34	6	2.8	3	1	1	3	4	5	5	5
35–49	27	3.1	5	1	2	3	4	5	8	11
50–64	30	3.6	3	1	2	4	5	6	6	8
65+	14	2.9	4	1	1	3	4	6	7	7
2. MULTIPLE DX										
0–19 Years	26	6.4	87	2	2	4	7	14	19	>99
20–34	75	10.0	134	2	3	5	12	23	38	68
35–49	357	5.2	32	2	2	4	6	11	15	32
50–64	848	5.0	28	2	2	4	6	9	13	25
65+	838	6.5	46	2	3	5	8	12	16	36
TOTAL SINGLE DX	81	3.3	4	1	2	3	4	5	6	11
TOTAL MULTIPLE DX	2,144	5.8	42	2	3	4	6	11	16	36
TOTAL										
0–19 Years	30	6.1	75	2	2	5	7	10	19	>99
20–34	81	9.5	128	2	3	5	10	23	33	68
35–49	384	5.0	31	1	2	3	5	11	15	32
50–64	878	4.9	27	2	2	4	6	9	13	25
65+	852	6.4	46	2	3	5	7	12	16	36
GRAND TOTAL	2,225	5.7	40	2	3	4	6	11	15	34

81.04: ANTERIOR DORSAL FUSION

Type of Patients	Observed Patients	Avg. Stay	Vari-ance	Percentiles						
				10th	25th	50th	75th	90th	95th	99th
1. SINGLE DX										
0–19 Years	19	6.3	36	3	4	5	7	9	9	42
20–34	4	4.8	2	3	5	5	5	6	6	6
35–49	0									
50–64	4	2.8	2	1	1	4	4	4	4	4
65+	0									
2. MULTIPLE DX										
0–19 Years	93	9.4	66	4	5	7	9	14	22	42
20–34	58	10.3	94	4	5	8	12	19	31	60
35–49	82	9.9	164	2	3	7	11	20	27	99
50–64	191	10.3	66	2	4	8	14	21	28	34
65+	103	10.4	47	4	6	9	13	20	25	30
TOTAL SINGLE DX	27	5.9	31	3	4	5	6	9	9	42
TOTAL MULTIPLE DX	527	9.9	77	3	5	7	12	20	28	42
TOTAL										
0–19 Years	112	8.9	63	4	5	7	9	13	22	42
20–34	62	9.9	90	3	5	7	10	19	31	60
35–49	82	9.9	164	2	3	7	11	20	27	99
50–64	195	10.1	66	2	4	8	14	21	28	34
65+	103	10.4	47	4	6	9	13	20	25	30
GRAND TOTAL	554	9.6	75	3	5	7	11	19	27	42

81.05: POSTERIOR DORSAL FUSION

Type of Patients	Observed Patients	Avg. Stay	Vari-ance	Percentiles						
				10th	25th	50th	75th	90th	95th	99th
1. SINGLE DX										
0–19 Years	293	5.0	2	4	4	5	6	6	8	9
20–34	24	5.0	4	3	3	4	6	9	10	10
35–49	9	5.3	5	2	3	5	7	9	9	9
50–64	8	5.3	14	2	3	4	7	14	14	14
65+	4	4.7	5	2	2	4	7	7	7	7
2. MULTIPLE DX										
0–19 Years	887	7.0	25	4	5	6	7	10	15	33
20–34	274	8.7	61	3	5	7	10	15	21	45
35–49	294	9.4	88	3	5	7	11	20	29	>99
50–64	637	9.0	75	3	4	6	11	18	24	46
65+	741	8.8	47	3	5	7	11	16	22	38
TOTAL SINGLE DX	338	5.0	2	4	4	5	6	6	8	10
TOTAL MULTIPLE DX	2,833	7.9	44	4	5	6	8	14	20	39
TOTAL										
0–19 Years	1,180	6.5	20	4	5	5	7	9	12	29
20–34	298	8.4	58	3	4	6	10	15	21	45
35–49	303	9.0	86	3	4	6	11	20	29	76
50–64	645	9.0	74	3	4	6	10	18	24	46
65+	745	8.8	47	3	5	7	11	16	22	38
GRAND TOTAL	3,171	7.4	38	4	5	6	8	12	18	37

LOS by Diagnosis and Operation, Western Region, 45th Edition

Western Region, October 2007–September 2008 Data, by Operation

81.06: ANTERIOR LUMBAR FUSION

Type of Patients	Observed Patients	Avg. Stay	Variance	Percentiles						
				10th	25th	50th	75th	90th	95th	99th
1. SINGLE DX										
0–19 Years	3	9.5	15	4	5	12	12	12	12	12
20–34	53	3.6	3	2	3	3	4	5	7	11
35–49	130	3.0	2	1	2	3	4	5	5	7
50–64	100	3.1	2	1	2	3	4	5	6	9
65+	11	2.4	2	1	1	2	4	4	4	4
2. MULTIPLE DX										
0–19 Years	37	6.7	54	3	3	6	8	9	13	60
20–34	474	4.4	17	2	3	4	5	7	8	22
35–49	1,581	4.3	13	2	3	4	5	7	9	18
50–64	2,241	4.9	17	2	3	4	6	8	11	18
65+	973	5.7	27	2	3	4	7	11	15	27
TOTAL SINGLE DX	297	3.3	3	1	2	3	4	5	6	12
TOTAL MULTIPLE DX	5,306	4.8	18	2	3	4	6	8	11	22
TOTAL										
0–19 Years	40	6.9	51	3	3	6	8	12	13	60
20–34	527	4.3	16	2	3	4	5	6	8	20
35–49	1,711	4.2	12	2	3	4	5	7	8	17
50–64	2,341	4.8	16	2	3	4	6	8	11	17
65+	984	5.7	27	2	3	4	7	11	15	27
GRAND TOTAL	5,603	4.8	17	2	3	4	5	8	11	22

81.07: LAT TRANS LUMBAR FUSION

Type of Patients	Observed Patients	Avg. Stay	Variance	Percentiles						
				10th	25th	50th	75th	90th	95th	99th
1. SINGLE DX										
0–19 Years	1	4.0	0	4	4	4	4	4	4	4
20–34	10	2.7	<1	1	2	3	3	3	4	4
35–49	22	2.6	2	1	1	2	3	4	4	6
50–64	23	2.9	3	1	2	2	4	6	6	7
65+	13	2.3	<1	1	2	2	4	3	4	4
2. MULTIPLE DX										
0–19 Years	6	9.1	27	2	5	12	14	14	14	14
20–34	78	5.0	22	1	2	3	6	12	13	27
35–49	253	4.4	43	2	3	4	5	6	8	20
50–64	661	4.3	10	2	3	4	5	7	9	20
65+	743	4.7	17	2	3	4	6	7	9	16
TOTAL SINGLE DX	69	2.7	2	1	2	3	3	4	6	7
TOTAL MULTIPLE DX	1,741	4.5	19	2	3	4	5	7	10	20
TOTAL										
0–19 Years	7	8.6	26	2	4	6	14	14	14	14
20–34	88	4.7	20	1	2	3	6	10	13	27
35–49	275	4.2	40	2	2	3	4	6	8	20
50–64	684	4.3	10	2	3	4	5	7	9	20
65+	756	4.6	17	2	3	4	5	7	9	16
GRAND TOTAL	1,810	4.5	18	2	3	4	5	7	9	19

81.08: POSTERIOR LUMBAR FUSION

Type of Patients	Observed Patients	Avg. Stay	Variance	Percentiles						
				10th	25th	50th	75th	90th	95th	99th
1. SINGLE DX										
0–19 Years	28	3.8	1	2	3	4	5	5	5	8
20–34	107	3.3	2	2	3	3	4	5	5	9
35–49	256	3.1	2	1	2	3	4	5	5	7
50–64	260	3.4	2	2	2	3	4	5	6	7
65+	91	3.2	2	1	2	3	4	5	6	8
2. MULTIPLE DX										
0–19 Years	133	5.3	12	3	3	5	6	8	9	21
20–34	896	4.2	8	3	3	4	5	7	9	16
35–49	3,297	4.0	11	2	3	3	4	6	8	14
50–64	7,141	4.3	12	2	3	4	5	7	8	17
65+	7,846	4.6	10	2	3	4	5	7	10	17
TOTAL SINGLE DX	742	3.3	2	2	2	3	4	5	6	8
TOTAL MULTIPLE DX	19,313	4.4	11	2	3	4	5	7	9	17
TOTAL										
0–19 Years	161	5.0	10	3	3	4	6	8	9	21
20–34	1,003	4.1	7	2	3	4	5	7	9	14
35–49	3,553	3.9	11	2	3	4	4	6	8	14
50–64	7,401	4.2	12	2	3	4	5	7	8	17
65+	7,937	4.6	10	2	3	4	5	7	10	17
GRAND TOTAL	20,055	4.3	11	2	3	4	5	7	9	17

81.1: FOOT & ANKLE ARTHRODESIS

Type of Patients	Observed Patients	Avg. Stay	Variance	Percentiles						
				10th	25th	50th	75th	90th	95th	99th
1. SINGLE DX										
0–19 Years	10	2.0	<1	1	1	2	3	3	3	3
20–34	19	2.1	<1	1	1	2	3	3	4	4
35–49	31	2.0	1	1	1	2	2	3	5	6
50–64	55	1.6	<1	1	1	2	3	3	3	4
65+	15	2.0	1	1	1	2	3	3	4	4
2. MULTIPLE DX										
0–19 Years	78	4.0	126	1	1	2	3	4	6	74
20–34	134	2.7	23	1	1	2	3	4	5	7
35–49	403	2.4	2	1	1	2	3	4	6	10
50–64	925	2.7	7	1	1	2	3	4	6	9
65+	744	2.7	4	1	2	2	3	4	5	9
TOTAL SINGLE DX	130	1.9	<1	1	1	2	2	3	3	5
TOTAL MULTIPLE DX	2,284	2.7	15	1	1	2	3	4	5	10
TOTAL										
0–19 Years	88	3.8	115	1	1	2	3	4	6	74
20–34	153	2.6	20	1	1	2	3	4	5	7
35–49	434	2.4	2	1	1	2	3	4	5	10
50–64	980	2.6	7	1	1	2	3	4	6	9
65+	759	2.6	4	1	2	2	3	4	5	9
GRAND TOTAL	2,414	2.7	14	1	1	2	3	4	5	10

LOS by Diagnosis and Operation, Western Region, 45th Edition

Western Region, October 2007–September 2008 Data, by Operation

81.11: ANKLE FUSION

Type of Patients	Observed Patients	Avg. Stay	Vari-ance	10th	25th	50th	75th	90th	95th	99th
1. SINGLE DX										
0–19 Years	1	1.0	0	1	1	1	1	1	1	1
20–34	9	2.1	1	1	1	2	3	4	4	4
35–49	21	2.2	2	1	1	2	2	4	5	6
50–64	37	1.7	<1	1	1	2	2	3	3	4
65+	12	2.1	<1	1	1	2	3	3	4	4
2. MULTIPLE DX										
0–19 Years	10	1.5	<1	1	1	1	2	2	3	3
20–34	66	2.4	1	1	2	2	3	4	4	5
35–49	204	2.5	3	1	2	2	3	4	6	10
50–64	460	2.8	11	1	2	2	3	5	7	11
65+	383	2.7	6	1	2	2	3	4	5	16
TOTAL SINGLE DX	80	1.9	1	1	1	2	2	3	4	6
TOTAL MULTIPLE DX	1,123	2.7	7	1	2	2	3	4	6	11
TOTAL										
0–19 Years	11	1.4	<1	1	1	1	2	2	3	3
20–34	75	2.4	1	1	2	2	3	4	4	5
35–49	225	2.5	3	1	2	2	3	4	6	10
50–64	497	2.7	11	1	2	2	3	4	6	11
65+	395	2.7	6	1	2	2	3	4	5	16
GRAND TOTAL	1,203	2.6	7	1	1	2	3	4	6	11

81.12: TRIPLE ARTHRODESIS

Type of Patients	Observed Patients	Avg. Stay	Vari-ance	10th	25th	50th	75th	90th	95th	99th
1. SINGLE DX										
0–19 Years	4	2.4	<1	2	2	3	3	3	3	3
20–34	4	2.3	<1	1	2	3	3	3	3	3
35–49	3	1.7	<1	1	1	2	2	2	2	2
50–64	10	1.8	<1	1	1	2	2	3	3	3
65+	0									
2. MULTIPLE DX										
0–19 Years	47	5.0	176	1	2	2	3	6	7	74
20–34	32	2.5	2	1	2	2	3	4	6	7
35–49	91	2.4	3	1	1	2	3	4	5	12
50–64	246	2.7	2	1	2	2	3	4	5	8
65+	199	2.8	2	1	2	3	3	4	5	7
TOTAL SINGLE DX	21	2.1	<1	1	1	2	3	3	3	3
TOTAL MULTIPLE DX	615	3.1	32	1	2	2	3	4	6	10
TOTAL										
0–19 Years	51	4.8	162	1	2	2	3	5	7	74
20–34	36	2.4	3	1	2	2	3	4	5	7
35–49	94	2.4	3	1	1	2	3	4	5	12
50–64	256	2.6	2	1	2	2	3	4	5	8
65+	199	2.8	2	1	2	3	3	4	5	7
GRAND TOTAL	636	3.0	31	1	2	2	3	4	5	8

81.13: SUBTALAR FUSION

Type of Patients	Observed Patients	Avg. Stay	Vari-ance	10th	25th	50th	75th	90th	95th	99th
1. SINGLE DX										
0–19 Years	3	1.3	<1	1	1	1	2	2	2	2
20–34	4	1.8	<1	1	2	1	2	2	2	2
35–49	6	1.3	<1	1	1	1	2	2	2	2
50–64	5	1.2	<1	1	1	1	1	1	1	1
65+	1	1.0	0	1	1	1	1	1	1	1
2. MULTIPLE DX										
0–19 Years	11	1.3	<1	1	1	1	2	2	2	2
20–34	19	1.8	<1	1	1	2	2	3	4	4
35–49	58	2.1	1	1	1	2	3	4	5	5
50–64	97	2.4	4	1	1	2	3	4	6	17
65+	64	2.4	2	1	1	2	3	5	6	7
TOTAL SINGLE DX	19	1.4	<1	1	1	1	2	2	2	2
TOTAL MULTIPLE DX	249	2.2	3	1	1	2	3	4	5	7
TOTAL										
0–19 Years	14	1.3	<1	1	1	1	2	2	2	2
20–34	23	1.8	<1	1	1	2	2	3	3	4
35–49	64	2.1	1	1	1	2	3	4	5	5
50–64	102	2.4	4	1	1	2	3	4	6	8
65+	65	2.4	2	1	1	2	3	5	6	7
GRAND TOTAL	268	2.2	3	1	1	2	3	4	5	7

81.2: ARTHRODESIS OF OTH JOINT

Type of Patients	Observed Patients	Avg. Stay	Vari-ance	10th	25th	50th	75th	90th	95th	99th
1. SINGLE DX										
0–19 Years	2	2.0	0	2	2	2	2	2	2	2
20–34	4	1.8	<1	1	1	1	3	3	3	3
35–49	7	1.6	<1	2	2	1	3	3	3	3
50–64	2	2.5	<1	1	1	2	3	3	3	3
65+	2	1.5	<1	1	1	2	2	2	2	2
2. MULTIPLE DX										
0–19 Years	19	2.1	2	1	1	2	3	4	4	6
20–34	24	3.6	10	1	1	2	5	9	11	11
35–49	59	3.0	8	1	1	3	4	6	10	14
50–64	95	4.2	21	1	1	3	5	9	13	26
65+	80	4.2	9	1	2	3	6	9	11	12
TOTAL SINGLE DX	17	1.8	<1	1	1	2	2	3	3	3
TOTAL MULTIPLE DX	277	3.6	12	1	1	3	5	8	11	17
TOTAL										
0–19 Years	21	2.1	1	1	1	2	2	4	4	6
20–34	28	3.3	9	1	1	2	5	9	11	11
35–49	66	2.9	7	1	1	2	4	6	9	14
50–64	97	4.1	20	1	2	3	5	9	13	26
65+	82	4.1	9	1	2	3	6	9	11	12
GRAND TOTAL	294	3.5	11	1	1	3	4	7	10	17

LOS by Diagnosis and Operation, Western Region, 45th Edition

Western Region, October 2007–September 2008 Data, by Operation

81.22: ARTHRODESIS OF KNEE

Type of Patients	Observed Patients	Avg. Stay	Variance	Percentiles						
				10th	25th	50th	75th	90th	95th	99th
1. SINGLE DX										
0–19 Years	1	2.0	0	2	2	2	2	2	2	2
20–34	1	2.0	0	2	2	2	2	2	2	2
35–49	0									
50–64	1	2.0	0	2	2	2	2	2	2	2
65+	0									
2. MULTIPLE DX										
0–19 Years	4	3.0	1	2	2	4	4	4	4	4
20–34	4	8.8	11	4	4	11	11	11	11	11
35–49	13	6.2	13	3	4	5	6	13	14	14
50–64	42	6.1	27	2	3	5	7	11	17	26
65+	47	5.6	8	3	3	5	8	11	11	12
TOTAL SINGLE DX	3	2.0	0	2	2	2	2	2	2	2
TOTAL MULTIPLE DX	110	5.7	16	2	3	4	7	11	13	22
TOTAL										
0–19 Years	5	2.7	<1	2	2	2	4	4	4	4
20–34	5	7.4	17	2	4	9	11	11	11	11
35–49	13	6.2	13	3	4	5	6	13	14	14
50–64	43	6.0	27	2	3	5	7	11	17	26
65+	47	5.6	8	3	3	5	8	11	11	12
GRAND TOTAL	113	5.5	16	2	3	4	7	11	12	22

81.3: SPINAL REFUSION

Type of Patients	Observed Patients	Avg. Stay	Variance	Percentiles						
				10th	25th	50th	75th	90th	95th	99th
1. SINGLE DX										
0–19 Years	4	2.2	<1	1	2	2	2	2	4	4
20–34	10	2.8	2	1	2	2	3	6	6	6
35–49	31	2.4	2	1	1	2	3	4	4	7
50–64	37	2.7	3	1	2	2	4	5	7	7
65+	7	1.9	<1	1	1	2	2	3	3	3
2. MULTIPLE DX										
0–19 Years	75	8.6	118	2	3	5	7	24	42	51
20–34	124	4.5	14	2	2	4	5	8	11	22
35–49	693	3.5	11	1	2	3	4	6	9	18
50–64	1,242	4.4	15	1	2	3	5	8	11	22
65+	761	5.3	24	2	3	4	6	9	12	21
TOTAL SINGLE DX	89	2.5	2	1	2	2	3	4	5	7
TOTAL MULTIPLE DX	2,895	4.7	25	1	2	4	5	8	12	26
TOTAL										
0–19 Years	79	8.4	116	2	3	5	7	24	42	51
20–34	134	4.4	14	2	2	4	5	7	11	22
35–49	724	3.5	10	1	2	3	4	6	9	17
50–64	1,279	4.3	15	1	2	3	5	8	11	22
65+	768	5.2	24	2	3	4	6	9	12	21
GRAND TOTAL	2,984	4.7	25	1	2	4	5	8	12	25

81.32: ANT CERV REFUSION NEC

Type of Patients	Observed Patients	Avg. Stay	Variance	Percentiles						
				10th	25th	50th	75th	90th	95th	99th
1. SINGLE DX										
0–19 Years	0									
20–34	1	2.0	0	2	2	2	2	2	2	2
35–49	8	1.5	<1	1	1	1	2	3	3	3
50–64	9	1.6	<1	1	1	1	2	3	3	3
65+	1	2.0	0	2	2	2	2	2	2	2
2. MULTIPLE DX										
0–19 Years	0									
20–34	13	2.1	1	1	1	2	2	4	4	4
35–49	201	2.4	4	1	2	2	3	4	5	14
50–64	256	2.7	6	1	2	2	3	5	8	13
65+	69	3.9	17	1	2	2	5	10	12	19
TOTAL SINGLE DX	19	1.6	<1	1	1	1	2	3	3	3
TOTAL MULTIPLE DX	539	2.7	7	1	1	2	3	5	7	14
TOTAL										
0–19 Years	0									
20–34	14	2.1	1	1	1	2	2	4	4	4
35–49	209	2.4	4	1	1	2	3	4	5	10
50–64	265	2.6	6	1	2	2	3	5	8	13
65+	70	3.9	16	1	2	2	5	10	12	19
GRAND TOTAL	558	2.7	6	1	1	2	3	5	7	14

81.33: POST CERV REFUSION NEC

Type of Patients	Observed Patients	Avg. Stay	Variance	Percentiles						
				10th	25th	50th	75th	90th	95th	99th
1. SINGLE DX										
0–19 Years	0									
20–34	2	2.5	<1	2	2	2	3	3	3	3
35–49	2	2.5	<1	2	2	3	3	3	3	3
50–64	6	2.8	3	1	1	2	5	5	5	5
65+	1	2.0	0	2	2	2	2	2	2	2
2. MULTIPLE DX										
0–19 Years	0									
20–34	5	2.2	3	1	1	2	2	5	5	5
35–49	88	2.9	6	1	2	3	4	5	5	21
50–64	118	4.0	18	1	2	3	4	8	14	22
65+	45	3.9	3	2	3	4	5	7	8	8
TOTAL SINGLE DX	11	2.6	2	1	2	2	3	5	5	5
TOTAL MULTIPLE DX	256	3.6	11	1	2	3	4	6	8	21
TOTAL										
0–19 Years	0									
20–34	7	2.3	2	1	1	2	3	5	5	5
35–49	90	2.9	5	1	2	3	3	5	5	21
50–64	124	3.9	18	1	2	3	4	7	13	22
65+	46	3.9	3	2	3	4	5	7	8	8
GRAND TOTAL	267	3.5	11	1	2	3	4	6	8	21

LOS by Diagnosis and Operation, Western Region, 45th Edition

Western Region, October 2007–September 2008 Data, by Operation

81.35: POST DORSAL REFUSION

Type of Patients	Observed Patients	Avg. Stay	Vari-ance	10th	25th	50th	75th	90th	95th	99th
1. SINGLE DX										
0–19 Years	2	2.0	0	2	2	2	2	2	2	2
20–34	3	4.0	3	3	3	3	6	6	6	6
35–49	0									
50–64	0									
65+	1	1.0	0	1	1	1	1	1	1	1
2. MULTIPLE DX										
0–19 Years	52	9.8	143	2	4	5	8	24	44	51
20–34	19	5.2	8	2	4	4	6	7	9	16
35–49	31	6.4	12	3	4	6	9	10	13	15
50–64	99	7.1	27	3	4	6	9	13	21	26
65+	87	8.1	98	3	4	5	9	14	19	61
TOTAL SINGLE DX	6	2.6	2	1	2	2	3	6	6	6
TOTAL MULTIPLE DX	288	8.2	88	2	4	5	8	14	25	51
TOTAL										
0–19 Years	54	9.6	140	2	4	5	8	24	42	51
20–34	22	5.1	7	2	4	4	6	7	9	16
35–49	31	6.4	12	3	4	6	9	10	13	15
50–64	99	7.1	27	3	4	6	9	13	21	26
65+	88	8.0	97	3	4	5	9	14	19	61
GRAND TOTAL	294	8.1	87	2	4	5	8	14	25	51

81.36: ANT LUMBAR REFUSION

Type of Patients	Observed Patients	Avg. Stay	Vari-ance	10th	25th	50th	75th	90th	95th	99th
1. SINGLE DX										
0–19 Years	0									
20–34	1	4.0	0	4	4	4	4	4	4	4
35–49	4	3.3	<1	2	3	3	4	4	4	4
50–64	5	4.0	7	2	2	2	7	7	7	7
65+	0									
2. MULTIPLE DX										
0–19 Years	2	5.5	3	4	4	7	7	7	7	7
20–34	18	4.1	19	2	2	3	4	6	21	21
35–49	70	5.2	20	2	3	4	6	11	17	23
50–64	119	5.2	22	2	3	4	5	9	14	23
65+	69	5.4	16	2	3	4	7	9	11	29
TOTAL SINGLE DX	10	3.7	4	2	2	3	4	7	7	7
TOTAL MULTIPLE DX	278	5.2	19	2	3	4	6	9	13	23
TOTAL										
0–19 Years	2	5.5	3	4	4	7	7	7	7	7
20–34	19	4.1	18	2	2	3	4	6	21	21
35–49	74	5.1	19	2	3	4	6	11	17	23
50–64	124	5.2	21	2	3	4	5	9	12	23
65+	69	5.4	16	2	3	4	7	9	11	29
GRAND TOTAL	288	5.1	19	2	3	4	6	9	13	23

81.37: LAT TRANS LUMB REFUSION

Type of Patients	Observed Patients	Avg. Stay	Vari-ance	10th	25th	50th	75th	90th	95th	99th
1. SINGLE DX										
0–19 Years	0									
20–34	0									
35–49	1	7.0	0	7	7	7	7	7	7	7
50–64	1	4.0	0	4	4	4	4	4	4	4
65+	1	1.0	0	1	1	1	1	1	1	1
2. MULTIPLE DX										
0–19 Years	1	2.0	0	2	2	2	2	2	2	2
20–34	4	4.7	3	3	3	4	6	7	7	7
35–49	8	3.9	1	2	3	4	5	5	5	5
50–64	39	4.5	13	2	3	3	5	9	13	19
65+	28	4.4	5	2	3	4	6	7	9	10
TOTAL SINGLE DX	3	4.0	9	1	1	4	7	7	7	7
TOTAL MULTIPLE DX	80	4.4	8	2	3	4	5	7	10	19
TOTAL										
0–19 Years	1	2.0	0	2	2	2	2	2	2	2
20–34	4	4.7	3	3	3	4	6	7	7	7
35–49	9	4.2	13	2	2	3	5	7	7	7
50–64	40	4.5	13	2	3	3	5	9	13	19
65+	29	4.3	5	2	3	4	6	7	9	10
GRAND TOTAL	83	4.4	8	2	3	4	5	7	9	19

81.38: POST LUMBAR REFUSION

Type of Patients	Observed Patients	Avg. Stay	Vari-ance	10th	25th	50th	75th	90th	95th	99th
1. SINGLE DX										
0–19 Years	2	2.5	4	1	1	4	4	4	4	4
20–34	3	1.7	<1	1	1	2	2	2	2	2
35–49	15	2.3	<1	1	2	2	3	3	4	4
50–64	16	2.8	1	2	2	2	4	4	5	5
65+	3	2.3	<1	2	2	2	3	3	3	3
2. MULTIPLE DX										
0–19 Years	10	5.1	53	2	2	3	3	12	27	27
20–34	54	4.4	13	2	2	4	5	7	10	23
35–49	286	3.8	13	1	2	3	4	7	9	19
50–64	581	4.5	10	2	3	4	5	8	10	20
65+	442	5.1	11	2	3	4	6	8	12	19
TOTAL SINGLE DX	39	2.5	1	1	2	2	3	4	4	5
TOTAL MULTIPLE DX	1,373	4.5	12	2	3	4	5	8	11	19
TOTAL										
0–19 Years	12	4.9	49	2	2	3	3	12	27	27
20–34	57	4.2	13	2	2	3	5	7	10	23
35–49	301	3.8	12	1	2	3	4	6	8	17
50–64	597	4.4	10	2	3	4	5	7	10	19
65+	445	5.1	11	2	3	4	6	8	12	19
GRAND TOTAL	1,412	4.5	12	2	3	4	5	7	11	19

LOS by Diagnosis and Operation, Western Region, 45th Edition

Western Region, October 2007–September 2008 Data, by Operation

81.4: OTHER LOW LIMB JOINT REP

Type of Patients	Observed Patients	Avg. Stay	Vari-ance	10th	25th	50th	75th	90th	95th	99th
1. SINGLE DX										
0–19 Years	138	1.4	<1	1	1	1	2	2	3	5
20–34	77	1.4	<1	1	1	1	1	3	3	4
35–49	50	1.7	1	1	1	1	2	3	3	6
50–64	35	2.5	2	1	1	2	3	4	7	7
65+	14	2.4	1	1	1	2	4	4	4	4
2. MULTIPLE DX										
0–19 Years	372	2.0	2	1	1	2	2	4	4	7
20–34	493	2.6	8	1	1	2	3	5	7	16
35–49	535	2.8	10	1	1	2	3	5	8	15
50–64	531	3.4	13	1	2	3	4	6	9	18
65+	330	4.0	13	2	2	3	4	7	12	20
TOTAL SINGLE DX	314	1.5	<1	1	1	1	2	3	3	5
TOTAL MULTIPLE DX	2,261	2.7	8	1	1	2	3	5	7	15
TOTAL										
0–19 Years	510	1.8	2	1	1	1	2	3	4	6
20–34	570	2.4	7	1	1	2	3	5	7	16
35–49	585	2.7	9	1	1	2	3	5	7	15
50–64	566	3.3	12	1	2	3	4	6	8	18
65+	344	3.9	13	2	2	3	4	6	11	20
GRAND TOTAL	2,575	2.5	7	1	1	2	3	5	6	14

81.40: HIP REPAIR NEC

Type of Patients	Observed Patients	Avg. Stay	Vari-ance	10th	25th	50th	75th	90th	95th	99th
1. SINGLE DX										
0–19 Years	28	2.3	<1	1	2	2	3	3	5	5
20–34	4	2.3	2	1	2	2	3	4	4	4
35–49	6	2.3	4	1	2	2	3	6	6	6
50–64	1	2.0	0	2	2	2	2	2	2	2
65+	0									
2. MULTIPLE DX										
0–19 Years	72	2.9	2	2	2	3	4	4	6	7
20–34	25	3.2	3	1	1	3	4	5	6	10
35–49	23	3.0	20	1	1	1	5	5	15	18
50–64	20	4.5	36	1	1	3	5	8	23	23
65+	27	4.8	12	1	3	4	5	12	13	15
TOTAL SINGLE DX	39	2.3	1	1	2	2	3	3	5	6
TOTAL MULTIPLE DX	167	3.2	6	1	2	3	4	5	6	15
TOTAL										
0–19 Years	100	2.8	2	2	2	3	3	4	6	7
20–34	29	3.1	3	1	1	3	4	5	6	10
35–49	29	2.9	16	1	1	1	4	6	15	18
50–64	21	4.3	34	1	1	2	4	8	19	23
65+	27	4.8	12	1	3	4	5	12	13	15
GRAND TOTAL	206	3.0	5	1	2	3	3	5	6	15

81.44: PATELLAR STABILIZATION

Type of Patients	Observed Patients	Avg. Stay	Vari-ance	10th	25th	50th	75th	90th	95th	99th
1. SINGLE DX										
0–19 Years	28	1.5	<1	1	1	1	2	2	2	4
20–34	7	1.7	<1	1	1	1	3	3	3	3
35–49	2	1.5	<1	1	1	2	2	2	2	2
50–64	2	3.0	8	1	1	5	5	5	5	5
65+	1	1.0	0	1	1	1	1	1	1	1
2. MULTIPLE DX										
0–19 Years	66	1.8	1	1	1	1	2	3	3	7
20–34	38	2.3	13	1	1	1	2	5	6	23
35–49	17	2.2	3	1	1	2	2	4	8	8
50–64	26	3.4	5	1	2	3	4	6	7	11
65+	39	3.5	6	2	2	3	4	5	10	14
TOTAL SINGLE DX	40	1.5	<1	1	1	1	2	2	3	5
TOTAL MULTIPLE DX	186	2.3	4	1	1	2	3	4	5	11
TOTAL										
0–19 Years	94	1.7	1	1	1	1	2	3	3	7
20–34	45	2.2	11	1	1	1	2	3	5	23
35–49	19	2.2	3	1	1	2	2	4	8	8
50–64	28	3.3	5	1	2	3	5	6	7	11
65+	40	3.4	6	1	2	3	4	5	8	14
GRAND TOTAL	226	2.1	4	1	1	2	2	4	5	10

81.45: CRUCIATE LIG REPAIR NEC

Type of Patients	Observed Patients	Avg. Stay	Vari-ance	10th	25th	50th	75th	90th	95th	99th
1. SINGLE DX										
0–19 Years	63	1.1	<1	1	1	1	1	1	2	2
20–34	39	1.2	<1	1	1	1	1	2	3	3
35–49	16	1.1	<1	1	1	1	1	2	2	2
50–64	5	1.0	0	1	1	1	1	1	1	1
65+	0									
2. MULTIPLE DX										
0–19 Years	145	1.4	2	1	1	1	1	2	2	6
20–34	215	2.2	7	1	1	1	2	4	6	17
35–49	176	2.1	5	1	1	1	2	4	6	14
50–64	71	2.0	3	1	1	1	2	4	5	9
65+	9	2.8	2	1	2	3	4	5	5	5
TOTAL SINGLE DX	123	1.1	<1	1	1	1	1	1	2	3
TOTAL MULTIPLE DX	616	1.8	4	1	1	1	2	3	4	11
TOTAL										
0–19 Years	208	1.3	2	1	1	1	1	2	2	5
20–34	254	2.0	6	1	1	1	2	4	6	17
35–49	192	2.0	4	1	1	1	2	4	5	14
50–64	76	2.0	3	1	1	1	2	4	5	9
65+	9	2.8	2	1	2	3	4	5	5	5
GRAND TOTAL	739	1.7	3	1	1	1	2	3	4	9

375

LOS by Diagnosis and Operation, Western Region, 45th Edition

Western Region, October 2007–September 2008 Data, by Operation

81.47: REPAIR OF KNEE NEC

Type of Patients	Observed Patients	Avg. Stay	Variance	10th	25th	50th	75th	90th	95th	99th
1. SINGLE DX										
0–19 Years	15	1.4	<1	1	1	1	2	2	3	3
20–34	20	1.3	<1	1	1	1	2	2	3	3
35–49	23	1.9	<1	1	1	2	3	3	3	4
50–64	24	2.8	2	1	2	3	4	4	7	7
65+	10	2.8	2	1	2	3	4	4	4	4
2. MULTIPLE DX										
0–19 Years	61	2.0	2	1	1	1	3	4	4	6
20–34	147	3.0	7	1	1	2	4	6	9	13
35–49	243	3.2	13	1	1	2	4	6	8	15
50–64	340	3.8	15	1	2	3	4	7	10	18
65+	229	4.1	16	2	2	3	4	7	12	24
TOTAL SINGLE DX	92	2.0	1	1	1	2	3	3	4	7
TOTAL MULTIPLE DX	1,020	3.4	13	1	2	3	4	6	9	16
TOTAL										
0–19 Years	76	1.9	2	1	1	1	3	4	4	6
20–34	167	2.8	7	1	1	2	3	6	8	13
35–49	266	3.1	12	1	1	2	4	5	8	15
50–64	364	3.7	14	1	2	3	4	7	9	18
65+	239	4.0	16	2	2	3	4	7	12	24
GRAND TOTAL	1,112	3.3	12	1	1	3	4	6	9	16

81.5: JOINT REPL LOWER EXT

Type of Patients	Observed Patients	Avg. Stay	Variance	10th	25th	50th	75th	90th	95th	99th
1. SINGLE DX										
0–19 Years	7	5.7	4	3	5	5	8	8	8	8
20–34	52	2.9	1	2	2	3	3	4	5	6
35–49	639	2.8	<1	2	2	3	3	4	4	6
50–64	2,743	2.9	1	2	3	3	3	4	4	6
65+	1,960	3.1	1	2	3	3	4	4	5	6
2. MULTIPLE DX										
0–19 Years	95	5.8	15	2	3	5	7	9	11	21
20–34	607	3.8	8	2	3	3	4	6	7	14
35–49	6,584	3.4	4	2	3	3	4	5	6	11
50–64	44,647	3.4	3	2	3	3	4	5	6	10
65+	87,928	4.0	6	2	3	3	4	6	8	14
TOTAL SINGLE DX	5,401	3.0	1	2	2	3	3	4	5	6
TOTAL MULTIPLE DX	139,861	3.8	5	2	3	3	4	6	7	13
TOTAL										
0–19 Years	102	5.8	14	2	3	5	8	9	11	21
20–34	659	3.7	7	2	3	3	4	6	7	14
35–49	7,223	3.3	4	2	3	3	4	5	6	10
50–64	47,390	3.4	4	2	3	3	4	5	6	10
65+	89,888	4.0	6	2	3	3	4	6	8	13
GRAND TOTAL	145,262	3.8	5	2	3	3	4	6	7	12

81.49: REPAIR OF ANKLE NEC

Type of Patients	Observed Patients	Avg. Stay	Variance	10th	25th	50th	75th	90th	95th	99th
1. SINGLE DX										
0–19 Years	4	1.3	<1	1	1	1	1	2	2	2
20–34	4	1.5	1	1	1	1	3	3	3	3
35–49	3	1.3	<1	1	1	1	2	2	2	2
50–64	3	2.0	0	2	2	2	2	3	3	3
65+	2	1.5	<1	1	1	1	2	2	2	2
2. MULTIPLE DX										
0–19 Years	13	1.4	<1	1	1	1	2	2	3	4
20–34	35	2.1	2	1	1	2	4	4	5	7
35–49	40	2.7	3	1	1	2	4	6	6	9
50–64	46	2.2	3	1	1	2	4	5	5	10
65+	18	3.1	2	2	2	3	4	6	6	6
TOTAL SINGLE DX	16	1.5	<1	1	1	1	2	2	3	3
TOTAL MULTIPLE DX	152	2.3	2	1	1	2	3	5	6	7
TOTAL										
0–19 Years	17	1.4	<1	1	1	1	2	2	3	4
20–34	39	2.0	2	1	1	2	4	4	5	7
35–49	43	2.6	2	1	1	2	4	5	6	6
50–64	49	2.2	3	1	1	2	4	5	5	10
65+	20	3.0	2	1	2	3	4	6	6	6
GRAND TOTAL	168	2.2	2	1	1	2	3	4	5	7

81.51: TOTAL HIP REPLACEMENT

Type of Patients	Observed Patients	Avg. Stay	Variance	10th	25th	50th	75th	90th	95th	99th
1. SINGLE DX										
0–19 Years	2	3.0	0	3	3	3	3	3	3	3
20–34	39	2.9	1	2	2	3	3	4	6	6
35–49	297	2.8	<1	2	2	3	3	4	4	5
50–64	956	2.9	<1	2	2	3	3	4	4	6
65+	594	3.1	<1	2	3	3	4	4	4	6
2. MULTIPLE DX										
0–19 Years	45	5.2	11	2	3	4	8	9	10	20
20–34	447	3.7	7	2	3	3	4	5	7	13
35–49	3,104	3.3	3	2	3	3	4	5	6	10
50–64	14,156	3.4	3	2	3	3	4	5	6	9
65+	23,276	3.7	4	2	3	3	4	5	7	11
TOTAL SINGLE DX	1,888	2.9	<1	2	2	3	3	4	4	6
TOTAL MULTIPLE DX	41,028	3.6	4	2	3	3	4	5	6	11
TOTAL										
0–19 Years	47	5.2	11	2	3	3	8	9	10	20
20–34	486	3.6	7	2	3	3	4	5	7	13
35–49	3,401	3.3	3	2	3	3	4	5	6	10
50–64	15,112	3.3	3	2	3	3	4	5	6	9
65+	23,870	3.7	4	2	3	3	4	5	7	11
GRAND TOTAL	42,916	3.5	4	2	3	3	4	5	6	11

LOS by Diagnosis and Operation, Western Region, 45th Edition

Western Region, October 2007–September 2008 Data, by Operation

81.52: PARTIAL HIP REPLACEMENT

Type of Patients	Observed Patients	Avg. Stay	Variance	10th	25th	50th	75th	90th	95th	99th
1. SINGLE DX										
0–19 Years	2	5.0	8	3	3	7	7	7	7	7
20–34	2	2.5	<1	2	2	3	3	3	3	3
35–49	8	3.0	<1	2	2	3	4	4	4	4
50–64	27	4.5	16	2	2	4	4	6	8	23
65+	61	4.4	5	3	3	4	5	6	8	17
2. MULTIPLE DX										
0–19 Years	19	5.0	15	1	2	4	6	9	17	17
20–34	23	7.0	37	3	4	5	7	13	22	27
35–49	174	6.9	37	3	4	5	8	14	21	32
50–64	1,171	6.8	27	3	4	5	8	12	16	27
65+	14,608	6.0	14	3	4	5	7	10	13	21
TOTAL SINGLE DX	100	4.3	8	2	3	4	5	6	8	23
TOTAL MULTIPLE DX	15,995	6.1	16	3	4	5	7	10	13	22
TOTAL										
0–19 Years	21	5.0	15	1	2	4	6	9	17	17
20–34	25	6.6	36	2	3	5	7	13	22	27
35–49	182	6.8	36	2	4	5	8	14	20	32
50–64	1,198	6.7	27	3	4	5	8	12	16	27
65+	14,669	6.0	14	3	4	5	7	10	13	21
GRAND TOTAL	16,095	6.1	16	3	4	5	7	10	13	22

81.53: HIP REPL REVISION NOS

Type of Patients	Observed Patients	Avg. Stay	Variance	10th	25th	50th	75th	90th	95th	99th
1. SINGLE DX										
0–19 Years	0									
20–34	0									
35–49	1	3.0	0	3	3	3	3	3	3	3
50–64	0									
65+	1	3.0	0	3	3	3	3	3	3	3
2. MULTIPLE DX										
0–19 Years	1	4.0	0	4	4	4	4	4	4	4
20–34	4	3.5	<1	3	3	4	4	4	4	4
35–49	24	4.0	3	2	3	4	5	7	8	8
50–64	86	4.5	16	2	3	4	5	7	9	35
65+	209	5.9	19	3	3	4	7	10	16	22
TOTAL SINGLE DX	2	3.0	0	3	3	3	3	3	3	3
TOTAL MULTIPLE DX	324	5.4	17	2	3	4	6	9	14	22
TOTAL										
0–19 Years	1	4.0	0	4	4	4	4	4	4	4
20–34	4	3.5	<1	3	3	4	4	4	4	4
35–49	25	4.0	3	2	3	4	5	7	8	8
50–64	86	4.5	16	2	3	4	5	7	9	35
65+	210	5.9	19	3	3	4	7	10	16	22
GRAND TOTAL	326	5.4	17	2	3	4	6	9	14	22

81.54: TOTAL KNEE REPLACEMENT

Type of Patients	Observed Patients	Avg. Stay	Variance	10th	25th	50th	75th	90th	95th	99th
1. SINGLE DX										
0–19 Years	3	6.4	2	5	5	6	8	8	8	8
20–34	11	2.6	1	1	1	3	4	4	4	4
35–49	331	2.9	1	2	2	3	3	4	4	6
50–64	1,750	2.9	<1	2	2	3	3	4	4	6
65+	1,294	3.1	<1	2	3	3	4	4	5	5
2. MULTIPLE DX										
0–19 Years	28	7.2	17	3	5	6	8	11	21	21
20–34	120	3.6	3	2	3	3	4	6	7	13
35–49	3,235	3.2	2	2	3	3	4	4	5	8
50–64	28,938	3.3	2	2	3	3	4	5	5	8
65+	49,417	3.5	2	2	3	3	4	5	6	9
TOTAL SINGLE DX	3,389	3.0	<1	2	2	3	3	4	5	6
TOTAL MULTIPLE DX	81,738	3.4	2	2	3	3	4	5	6	8
TOTAL										
0–19 Years	31	7.1	15	4	5	6	8	11	21	21
20–34	131	3.5	3	2	3	3	4	5	7	13
35–49	3,566	3.2	2	2	3	3	4	4	5	8
50–64	30,688	3.3	2	2	3	3	4	4	5	8
65+	50,711	3.5	2	2	3	3	4	5	6	9
GRAND TOTAL	85,127	3.4	2	2	3	3	4	5	6	8

81.55: KNEE REPL REVISION NOS

Type of Patients	Observed Patients	Avg. Stay	Variance	10th	25th	50th	75th	90th	95th	99th
1. SINGLE DX										
0–19 Years	0									
20–34	0									
35–49	1	1.0	0	1	1	1	1	1	1	1
50–64	1	2.0	0	2	2	2	2	2	2	2
65+	4	2.8	<1	2	2	3	4	4	4	4
2. MULTIPLE DX										
0–19 Years	2	4.5	12	2	2	2	7	7	7	7
20–34	6	5.0	15	1	3	5	6	12	12	12
35–49	26	5.5	24	2	3	4	5	16	19	19
50–64	178	5.4	11	2	3	3	5	7	12	28
65+	280	4.8	13	2	3	4	6	8	11	21
TOTAL SINGLE DX	6	2.3	1	1	2	2	3	4	4	4
TOTAL MULTIPLE DX	492	4.7	13	2	3	4	5	8	12	24
TOTAL										
0–19 Years	2	4.5	12	2	2	2	7	7	7	7
20–34	6	5.0	15	1	3	5	6	12	12	12
35–49	27	5.4	24	2	3	4	5	16	19	19
50–64	179	5.4	11	2	3	3	5	7	12	28
65+	284	4.8	13	2	3	4	5	8	11	21
GRAND TOTAL	498	4.7	13	2	3	4	5	8	12	24

LOS by Diagnosis and Operation, Western Region, 45th Edition

Western Region, October 2007–September 2008 Data, by Operation

81.56: TOTAL ANKLE REPLACEMENT

Type of Patients	Observed Patients	Avg. Stay	Variance	10th	25th	50th	75th	90th	95th	99th
1. SINGLE DX										
0–19 Years	0									
20–34	0									
35–49	0									
50–64	9	2.3	<1	2	2	2	3	3	3	3
65+	5	1.8	<1	1	2	2	2	2	2	2
2. MULTIPLE DX										
0–19 Years	0									
20–34	5	2.2	<1	1	2	2	3	3	3	3
35–49	17	2.7	<1	2	2	3	3	4	4	4
50–64	99	2.6	1	2	2	2	3	4	5	7
65+	121	2.8	4	2	2	3	3	4	4	6
TOTAL SINGLE DX	14	2.1	<1	2	2	2	2	3	3	3
TOTAL MULTIPLE DX	242	2.7	2	2	2	2	3	4	4	7
TOTAL										
0–19 Years	0									
20–34	5	2.2	<1	1	2	2	3	3	3	3
35–49	17	2.7	<1	2	2	3	3	4	4	4
50–64	108	2.5	1	2	2	2	3	4	5	7
65+	126	2.7	4	2	2	3	3	4	4	6
GRAND TOTAL	256	2.6	2	2	2	2	3	4	4	7

81.6: OTH SPINAL PROCEDURES

Type of Patients	Observed Patients	Avg. Stay	Variance	10th	25th	50th	75th	90th	95th	99th
1. SINGLE DX										
0–19 Years	0									
20–34	3	2.7	2	1	1	3	4	4	4	4
35–49	3	2.4	5	1	1	1	5	5	5	5
50–64	15	1.8	2	1	1	1	2	5	5	5
65+	34	1.2	<1	1	1	1	1	2	2	3
2. MULTIPLE DX										
0–19 Years	4	5.2	16	1	1	3	7	10	10	10
20–34	16	3.5	5	1	2	3	5	7	8	8
35–49	106	6.9	130	1	1	3	8	14	19	75
50–64	470	5.4	34	1	1	4	7	13	17	30
65+	4,375	4.8	18	1	1	4	7	10	13	19
TOTAL SINGLE DX	55	1.5	1	1	1	1	2	3	5	5
TOTAL MULTIPLE DX	4,971	4.9	22	1	1	4	7	10	13	21
TOTAL										
0–19 Years	4	5.2	16	1	1	3	7	10	10	10
20–34	19	3.4	4	1	2	3	5	7	8	8
35–49	109	6.8	127	1	1	3	8	14	19	75
50–64	485	5.3	34	1	1	4	7	12	17	30
65+	4,409	4.8	18	1	1	4	7	10	13	19
GRAND TOTAL	5,026	4.9	22	1	1	4	7	10	13	20

81.65: VERTEBROPLASTY

Type of Patients	Observed Patients	Avg. Stay	Variance	10th	25th	50th	75th	90th	95th	99th
1. SINGLE DX										
0–19 Years	0									
20–34	0									
35–49	1	1.0	0	1	1	1	1	1	1	1
50–64	2	3.5	4	2	2	2	5	5	5	5
65+	10	1.5	<1	1	1	1	2	3	3	3
2. MULTIPLE DX										
0–19 Years	0									
20–34	2	6.5	4	5	5	8	8	8	8	8
35–49	34	8.9	164	2	4	7	9	11	30	76
50–64	154	6.6	31	1	3	5	8	14	18	28
65+	1,671	5.6	15	1	3	5	7	11	14	18
TOTAL SINGLE DX	13	1.8	1	1	1	1	2	3	5	5
TOTAL MULTIPLE DX	1,861	5.7	20	1	3	5	7	11	14	20
TOTAL										
0–19 Years	0									
20–34	2	6.5	4	5	5	8	8	8	8	8
35–49	35	8.7	161	2	3	5	8	11	30	76
50–64	156	6.6	31	1	3	5	8	14	18	28
65+	1,681	5.6	15	1	3	5	7	11	13	18
GRAND TOTAL	1,874	5.7	20	1	3	5	7	11	14	20

81.66: KYPHOPLASTY

Type of Patients	Observed Patients	Avg. Stay	Variance	10th	25th	50th	75th	90th	95th	99th
1. SINGLE DX										
0–19 Years	0									
20–34	1	1.0	0	1	1	1	1	1	1	1
35–49	2	3.0	8	1	1	5	5	5	5	5
50–64	12	1.6	1	1	1	1	2	5	5	5
65+	24	1.0	<1	1	1	1	1	2	2	2
2. MULTIPLE DX										
0–19 Years	2	4.0	18	1	1	3	7	7	7	7
20–34	12	3.2	4	1	1	2	5	6	7	7
35–49	68	5.9	117	1	1	3	6	14	19	75
50–64	310	4.8	35	1	1	3	7	11	17	30
65+	2,696	4.4	19	1	1	3	6	9	12	20
TOTAL SINGLE DX	39	1.3	<1	1	1	1	1	2	5	5
TOTAL MULTIPLE DX	3,088	4.5	22	1	1	3	6	10	13	21
TOTAL										
0–19 Years	2	4.0	18	1	1	3	7	7	7	7
20–34	13	3.0	4	1	1	2	4	6	7	7
35–49	70	5.9	114	1	1	3	6	13	19	75
50–64	322	4.7	34	1	1	3	6	11	17	30
65+	2,720	4.3	19	1	1	3	6	9	12	19
GRAND TOTAL	3,127	4.4	22	1	1	3	6	10	13	21

LOS by Diagnosis and Operation, Western Region, 45th Edition

Western Region, October 2007–September 2008 Data, by Operation

81.7: HAND/FINGER ARTHROPLASTY

Type of Patients	Observed Patients	Avg. Stay	Variance	Percentiles						
				10th	25th	50th	75th	90th	95th	99th
1. SINGLE DX										
0–19 Years	5	1.5	<1	1	1	1	2	2	2	2
20–34	4	1.8	<1	1	1	1	2	2	2	2
35–49	4	1.8	<1	1	1	1	3	2	3	2
50–64	10	1.6	<1	1	1	1	2	3	3	3
65+	2	1.5	<1	1	1	1	2	2	2	2
2. MULTIPLE DX										
0–19 Years	17	1.6	<1	1	1	1	2	3	3	4
20–34	55	2.7	9	1	1	2	3	7	8	19
35–49	38	1.8	1	1	1	1	2	4	4	5
50–64	81	2.2	5	1	1	1	2	5	5	15
65+	70	2.2	4	1	1	1	2	5	7	12
TOTAL SINGLE DX	25	1.6	<1	1	1	1	2	2	3	3
TOTAL MULTIPLE DX	261	2.2	5	1	1	1	2	4	7	12
TOTAL										
0–19 Years	22	1.5	<1	1	1	1	2	3	3	4
20–34	59	2.7	9	1	1	2	3	7	8	19
35–49	42	1.8	1	1	1	1	2	4	4	5
50–64	91	2.1	5	1	1	1	2	4	5	15
65+	72	2.2	4	1	1	1	2	5	7	12
GRAND TOTAL	286	2.1	4	1	1	1	2	4	6	10

81.8: SHOULD/ELB ARTHROPLASTY

Type of Patients	Observed Patients	Avg. Stay	Variance	Percentiles						
				10th	25th	50th	75th	90th	95th	99th
1. SINGLE DX										
0–19 Years	19	1.5	1	1	1	1	1	5	5	5
20–34	51	1.6	1	1	1	1	2	3	5	7
35–49	82	1.7	<1	1	1	1	2	3	3	6
50–64	197	1.9	2	1	1	2	2	3	4	9
65+	147	1.9	1	1	1	2	2	3	4	5
2. MULTIPLE DX										
0–19 Years	57	2.5	10	1	1	1	2	6	10	16
20–34	188	2.9	10	1	1	2	3	7	9	15
35–49	580	2.5	7	1	1	2	3	4	7	16
50–64	2,484	2.3	7	1	1	2	3	4	5	10
65+	5,567	2.7	6	1	2	2	3	4	6	11
TOTAL SINGLE DX	496	1.8	1	1	1	1	2	3	4	5
TOTAL MULTIPLE DX	8,876	2.6	6	1	1	2	3	4	6	11
TOTAL										
0–19 Years	76	2.3	8	1	1	1	2	5	7	16
20–34	239	2.6	8	1	1	2	3	6	9	13
35–49	662	2.4	8	1	1	2	3	4	6	15
50–64	2,681	2.3	7	1	1	2	3	4	5	10
65+	5,714	2.7	5	1	2	2	3	4	6	11
GRAND TOTAL	9,372	2.5	6	1	1	2	3	4	6	11

81.80: TOTAL SHOULDER REPL

Type of Patients	Observed Patients	Avg. Stay	Variance	Percentiles						
				10th	25th	50th	75th	90th	95th	99th
1. SINGLE DX										
0–19 Years	1	5.0	0	5	5	5	5	5	5	5
20–34	1	2.0	0	2	2	2	2	2	2	2
35–49	21	1.6	<1	1	1	2	2	2	2	2
50–64	83	1.7	<1	1	1	2	2	3	3	3
65+	82	2.0	1	1	1	2	2	3	4	4
2. MULTIPLE DX										
0–19 Years	3	5.2	2	4	4	4	6	7	7	7
20–34	10	2.6	3	1	2	2	3	3	7	7
35–49	108	2.6	7	1	1	2	3	4	5	18
50–64	1,007	2.1	2	1	1	2	2	3	4	5
65+	3,001	2.3	2	1	1	2	3	4	4	7
TOTAL SINGLE DX	188	1.9	1	1	1	2	2	3	4	5
TOTAL MULTIPLE DX	4,129	2.2	2	1	1	2	3	4	4	7
TOTAL										
0–19 Years	4	5.1	1	4	4	5	6	7	7	7
20–34	11	2.6	3	1	2	2	3	3	7	7
35–49	129	2.4	6	1	1	2	3	4	5	18
50–64	1,090	2.0	2	1	1	2	2	3	4	5
65+	3,083	2.3	2	1	1	2	3	4	4	7
GRAND TOTAL	4,317	2.2	2	1	1	2	3	3	4	7

81.81: PARTIAL SHOULDER REPL

Type of Patients	Observed Patients	Avg. Stay	Variance	Percentiles						
				10th	25th	50th	75th	90th	95th	99th
1. SINGLE DX										
0–19 Years	0									
20–34	4	2.3	4	1	1	2	2	5	5	5
35–49	24	2.0	1	1	1	2	2	3	4	6
50–64	70	2.1	2	1	1	2	3	3	4	9
65+	42	2.0	<1	1	1	2	3	3	3	4
2. MULTIPLE DX										
0–19 Years	10	7.7	26	2	3	5	10	16	16	16
20–34	34	2.8	3	1	1	2	4	6	6	7
35–49	202	2.7	14	1	1	2	3	4	7	15
50–64	895	2.6	8	1	1	2	3	4	7	15
65+	1,951	3.3	10	1	2	2	4	6	8	14
TOTAL SINGLE DX	140	2.0	1	1	1	2	3	3	4	6
TOTAL MULTIPLE DX	3,092	3.1	10	1	2	2	3	6	8	15
TOTAL										
0–19 Years	10	7.7	26	2	3	5	10	16	16	16
20–34	38	2.8	3	1	1	2	4	5	6	7
35–49	226	2.6	13	1	1	2	3	4	7	15
50–64	965	2.6	8	1	1	2	3	4	6	10
65+	1,993	3.2	10	1	2	2	4	6	8	14
GRAND TOTAL	3,232	3.0	10	1	2	2	3	5	8	15

LOS by Diagnosis and Operation, Western Region, 45th Edition

Western Region, October 2007–September 2008 Data, by Operation

81.82: RECUR SHOULD DISLOC REP

Type of Patients	Observed Patients	Avg. Stay	Vari-ance	Percentiles						
				10th	25th	50th	75th	90th	95th	99th
1. SINGLE DX										
0–19 Years	11	1.1	<1	1	1	1	1	2	2	2
20–34	25	1.4	<1	1	1	1	1	3	3	5
35–49	10	1.3	<1	1	1	1	1	2	3	3
50–64	1	1.0	0	1	1	1	1	1	1	1
65+	1	1.0	0	1	1	1	1	1	1	1
2. MULTIPLE DX										
0–19 Years	17	1.2	<1	1	1	1	1	2	2	3
20–34	33	1.7	3	1	1	1	1	3	7	9
35–49	23	1.7	6	1	1	1	1	2	4	12
50–64	29	3.0	9	1	1	2	3	9	10	14
65+	20	3.7	12	1	1	3	5	10	14	14
TOTAL SINGLE DX	**48**	**1.3**	**<1**	**1**	**1**	**1**	**1**	**2**	**3**	**5**
TOTAL MULTIPLE DX	**122**	**2.1**	**6**	**1**	**1**	**1**	**2**	**4**	**7**	**14**
TOTAL										
0–19 Years	28	1.2	<1	1	1	1	1	2	2	3
20–34	58	1.6	2	1	1	1	1	3	5	9
35–49	33	1.6	4	1	1	1	1	2	4	12
50–64	30	2.9	9	1	1	2	3	5	10	14
65+	21	3.5	12	1	1	3	5	7	10	14
GRAND TOTAL	**170**	**1.8**	**4**	**1**	**1**	**1**	**2**	**3**	**5**	**12**

81.83: SHOULD ARTHROPLASTY NEC

Type of Patients	Observed Patients	Avg. Stay	Vari-ance	Percentiles						
				10th	25th	50th	75th	90th	95th	99th
1. SINGLE DX										
0–19 Years	4	1.0	0	1	1	1	1	1	1	1
20–34	9	1.1	<1	1	1	1	1	2	2	2
35–49	13	1.4	<1	1	1	1	1	2	4	4
50–64	28	1.5	<1	1	1	1	2	3	4	4
65+	18	1.6	<1	1	1	1	2	3	4	4
2. MULTIPLE DX										
0–19 Years	12	1.6	2	1	1	1	2	2	6	6
20–34	36	2.2	6	1	1	1	2	4	10	10
35–49	144	1.7	3	1	1	1	2	3	3	9
50–64	343	2.0	19	1	1	1	2	3	4	10
65+	393	2.1	2	1	1	2	3	4	5	9
TOTAL SINGLE DX	**72**	**1.4**	**<1**	**1**	**1**	**1**	**1**	**2**	**3**	**4**
TOTAL MULTIPLE DX	**928**	**2.0**	**9**	**1**	**1**	**1**	**2**	**3**	**4**	**10**
TOTAL										
0–19 Years	16	1.4	1	1	1	1	1	2	2	6
20–34	45	2.0	5	1	1	1	2	3	9	10
35–49	157	1.7	3	1	1	1	2	3	4	9
50–64	371	2.0	18	1	1	1	2	3	4	10
65+	411	2.1	2	1	1	2	3	4	5	8
GRAND TOTAL	**1,000**	**2.0**	**8**	**1**	**1**	**1**	**2**	**3**	**4**	**9**

81.84: TOTAL ELBOW REPLACEMENT

Type of Patients	Observed Patients	Avg. Stay	Vari-ance	Percentiles						
				10th	25th	50th	75th	90th	95th	99th
1. SINGLE DX										
0–19 Years	0									
20–34	7	2.6	4	1	1	2	3	7	7	7
35–49	9	2.0	1	1	1	2	3	4	4	4
50–64	9	3.3	17	2	2	2	3	14	14	14
65+	2	2.0	0	2	2	2	2	2	2	2
2. MULTIPLE DX										
0–19 Years	1	7.0	0	7	7	7	7	7	7	7
20–34	36	3.7	8	1	2	3	4	9	10	10
35–49	56	3.3	14	1	1	2	4	6	10	24
50–64	135	3.0	5	1	2	3	4	5	8	12
65+	149	3.7	14	1	2	3	4	7	11	19
TOTAL SINGLE DX	**27**	**2.6**	**7**	**1**	**1**	**2**	**3**	**4**	**7**	**14**
TOTAL MULTIPLE DX	**377**	**3.4**	**10**	**1**	**2**	**3**	**4**	**6**	**10**	**17**
TOTAL										
0–19 Years	1	7.0	0	7	7	7	7	7	7	7
20–34	43	3.5	7	1	2	3	4	7	10	10
35–49	65	3.1	12	1	2	2	3	6	9	24
50–64	144	3.0	6	1	2	2	3	5	8	14
65+	151	3.6	14	1	2	3	4	6	11	19
GRAND TOTAL	**404**	**3.3**	**10**	**1**	**2**	**2**	**4**	**6**	**10**	**15**

81.85: ELBOW ARTHROPLASTY NEC

Type of Patients	Observed Patients	Avg. Stay	Vari-ance	Percentiles						
				10th	25th	50th	75th	90th	95th	99th
1. SINGLE DX										
0–19 Years	3	1.3	<1	1	1	1	2	2	2	2
20–34	5	1.4	<1	1	1	1	2	2	2	2
35–49	5	1.6	<1	1	1	1	2	3	3	3
50–64	6	2.0	2	1	1	2	2	5	5	5
65+	2	1.5	<1	1	1	2	2	2	2	2
2. MULTIPLE DX										
0–19 Years	14	1.3	<1	1	1	1	1	2	2	5
20–34	39	4.0	25	1	1	2	4	12	15	26
35–49	47	2.6	4	1	1	2	4	5	5	8
50–64	75	2.4	4	1	1	2	3	5	6	8
65+	53	3.4	31	1	1	2	3	5	7	41
TOTAL SINGLE DX	**21**	**1.6**	**<1**	**1**	**1**	**1**	**2**	**2**	**3**	**5**
TOTAL MULTIPLE DX	**228**	**2.8**	**13**	**1**	**1**	**2**	**3**	**5**	**7**	**15**
TOTAL										
0–19 Years	17	1.3	<1	1	1	1	1	2	2	5
20–34	44	3.7	23	1	1	2	4	9	13	26
35–49	52	2.5	2	1	1	2	4	5	5	8
50–64	81	2.4	4	1	1	2	3	5	6	8
65+	55	3.3	30	1	1	2	3	5	7	41
GRAND TOTAL	**249**	**2.7**	**12**	**1**	**1**	**2**	**3**	**5**	**7**	**15**

Western Region, October 2007–September 2008 Data, by Operation

81.9: OTHER JOINT STRUCTURE OP

Type of Patients	Observed Patients	Avg. Stay	Variance	10th	25th	50th	75th	90th	95th	99th
1. SINGLE DX										
0–19 Years	78	2.8	4	1	2	3	3	4	6	7
20–34	39	2.3	1	1	2	2	3	3	5	6
35–49	34	2.3	2	1	1	2	3	5	5	6
50–64	14	1.9	<1	1	1	2	2	3	4	4
65+	13	2.7	3	1	1	2	5	5	5	5
2. MULTIPLE DX										
0–19 Years	210	5.5	31	1	2	4	7	13	18	33
20–34	356	4.8	20	1	2	4	6	9	11	27
35–49	861	5.2	29	1	2	4	6	10	15	30
50–64	1,584	5.1	25	1	2	4	6	10	14	26
65+	3,856	5.4	19	2	3	4	7	10	13	22
TOTAL SINGLE DX	178	2.6	3	1	1	2	3	4	5	7
TOTAL MULTIPLE DX	6,867	5.3	23	2	2	4	6	10	14	25
TOTAL										
0–19 Years	288	4.8	25	1	2	3	5	10	16	23
20–34	395	4.6	19	1	2	3	6	9	11	27
35–49	895	5.1	29	1	2	4	6	10	15	30
50–64	1,598	5.1	25	1	2	4	6	10	14	26
65+	3,869	5.4	19	2	3	4	7	10	13	22
GRAND TOTAL	7,045	5.2	22	1	2	4	6	10	14	24

81.92: INJECTION INTO JOINT

Type of Patients	Observed Patients	Avg. Stay	Variance	10th	25th	50th	75th	90th	95th	99th
1. SINGLE DX										
0–19 Years	1	2.0	0	2	2		2	2	2	2
20–34	4	2.8	<1	2	2	3	3	3	3	3
35–49	2	2.0	2	1	1	2	3	3	3	3
50–64	0									
65+	2	1.5	<1	1	1	2	2	2	2	2
2. MULTIPLE DX										
0–19 Years	9	4.5	16	1	2	4	7	7	18	18
20–34	27	4.7	6	2	3	4	7	8	8	11
35–49	94	6.7	65	2	2	5	7	13	24	51
50–64	170	6.1	28	2	3	5	7	11	15	29
65+	851	6.0	25	2	3	5	7	11	14	27
TOTAL SINGLE DX	9	2.2	<1	1	2	2	3	3	3	3
TOTAL MULTIPLE DX	1,151	6.0	28	2	3	5	7	11	15	29
TOTAL										
0–19 Years	10	4.1	14	1	2	3	4	7	7	18
20–34	31	4.5	5	2	3	4	6	8	8	11
35–49	96	6.6	64	2	3	5	7	13	24	51
50–64	170	6.1	28	2	3	5	7	11	15	29
65+	853	6.0	25	2	3	5	7	11	14	27
GRAND TOTAL	1,160	6.0	28	2	3	5	7	11	15	29

81.91: ARTHROCENTESIS

Type of Patients	Observed Patients	Avg. Stay	Variance	10th	25th	50th	75th	90th	95th	99th
1. SINGLE DX										
0–19 Years	71	2.9	4	1	2	3	4	5	6	7
20–34	26	2.3	<1	1	2	2	3	3	4	5
35–49	24	2.4	2	1	1	2	3	5	5	6
50–64	11	1.6	<1	1	1	1	2	3	3	3
65+	6	3.3	4	1	1	5	5	5	5	5
2. MULTIPLE DX										
0–19 Years	189	5.7	33	1	2	4	7	14	21	33
20–34	295	5.0	21	1	2	4	6	9	13	27
35–49	708	5.1	22	1	2	4	6	10	14	24
50–64	1,155	5.5	28	1	3	4	7	11	15	28
65+	2,670	5.5	18	2	3	4	7	10	14	21
TOTAL SINGLE DX	138	2.7	3	1	2	2	3	5	6	7
TOTAL MULTIPLE DX	5,017	5.5	22	2	3	4	7	10	14	24
TOTAL										
0–19 Years	260	5.0	27	1	2	3	6	11	16	27
20–34	321	4.8	20	1	2	3	6	9	11	26
35–49	732	5.0	22	1	2	4	6	10	14	24
50–64	1,166	5.5	28	1	3	4	7	11	15	28
65+	2,676	5.5	18	2	3	4	7	10	14	21
GRAND TOTAL	5,155	5.4	22	2	3	4	7	10	14	24

81.97: REV JOINT REPL UE

Type of Patients	Observed Patients	Avg. Stay	Variance	10th	25th	50th	75th	90th	95th	99th
1. SINGLE DX										
0–19 Years	0									
20–34	3	3.7	4	2	2	3	6	6	6	6
35–49	7	2.3	3	1	1	2	4	5	5	5
50–64	3	2.7	1	1	2	2	4	4	4	4
65+	4	2.5	<1	2	2	2	3	3	3	3
2. MULTIPLE DX										
0–19 Years	1	3.0	0	3	3	3	3	3	3	3
20–34	8	2.4	3	1	2	2	3	6	6	6
35–49	33	2.6	6	1	2	2	3	4	10	12
50–64	229	2.5	3	1	2	2	3	4	6	9
65+	326	2.7	3	1	2	2	3	5	6	9
TOTAL SINGLE DX	17	2.7	2	1	2	2	3	5	6	6
TOTAL MULTIPLE DX	597	2.6	3	1	2	2	3	4	6	10
TOTAL										
0–19 Years	1	3.0	0	3	3	3	3	3	3	3
20–34	11	2.7	3	1	2	2	3	6	6	6
35–49	40	2.6	5	1	1	2	3	5	10	12
50–64	232	2.5	3	1	2	2	3	4	6	9
65+	330	2.7	3	1	2	2	3	5	6	9
GRAND TOTAL	614	2.6	3	1	2	2	3	4	6	10

LOS by Diagnosis and Operation, Western Region, 45th Edition

Western Region, October 2007–September 2008 Data, by Operation

82.0: INC HAND SOFT TISSUE

Type of Patients	Observed Patients	Avg. Stay	Vari-ance	Percentiles						
				10th	25th	50th	75th	90th	95th	99th
1. SINGLE DX										
0–19 Years	9	2.3	4	1	1	1	3	7	7	7
20–34	23	2.1	2	1	1	2	3	5	5	5
35–49	18	2.8	3	1	2	2	4	6	8	8
50–64	12	2.6	2	1	2	2	3	5	6	6
65+	3	2.7	4	1	1	2	5	5	5	5
2. MULTIPLE DX										
0–19 Years	56	3.7	9	1	2	3	4	9	11	18
20–34	201	3.5	6	1	2	3	4	6	7	14
35–49	266	4.4	18	1	2	3	5	9	12	20
50–64	219	4.2	16	1	2	3	5	8	11	21
65+	129	4.4	9	2	3	4	5	9	12	14
TOTAL SINGLE DX	65	2.5	3	1	1	2	3	5	6	8
TOTAL MULTIPLE DX	871	4.1	13	1	2	3	5	8	11	20
TOTAL										
0–19 Years	65	3.6	9	1	2	3	4	9	11	18
20–34	224	3.3	6	1	2	3	4	6	7	10
35–49	284	4.3	18	1	2	3	5	8	12	20
50–64	231	4.1	15	1	2	3	5	8	11	21
65+	132	4.4	9	2	3	4	5	9	12	14
GRAND TOTAL	936	4.0	13	1	2	3	5	7	10	18

82.01: EXPL TENDON SHEATH HAND

Type of Patients	Observed Patients	Avg. Stay	Vari-ance	Percentiles						
				10th	25th	50th	75th	90th	95th	99th
1. SINGLE DX										
0–19 Years	3	1.7	1	1	1	1	3	3	3	3
20–34	12	2.5	3	1	1	2	3	5	5	5
35–49	16	2.9	4	1	2	2	4	6	8	8
50–64	6	2.5	3	1	2	2	2	6	6	6
65+	3	2.7	4	1	1	2	5	5	5	5
2. MULTIPLE DX										
0–19 Years	26	2.7	1	1	2	3	3	4	5	5
20–34	132	3.4	3	2	2	3	4	6	7	10
35–49	172	3.9	10	1	2	3	5	7	12	18
50–64	133	4.1	20	1	2	3	5	7	10	30
65+	81	3.9	6	2	2	3	5	7	9	14
TOTAL SINGLE DX	40	2.6	3	1	1	2	3	5	6	8
TOTAL MULTIPLE DX	544	3.7	10	1	2	3	4	7	9	18
TOTAL										
0–19 Years	29	2.6	1	1	2	3	3	4	5	5
20–34	144	3.3	3	1	2	3	4	6	7	10
35–49	188	3.8	9	1	2	3	4	7	11	18
50–64	139	4.1	19	1	2	3	5	7	9	30
65+	84	3.8	6	2	2	3	5	7	9	14
GRAND TOTAL	584	3.7	9	1	2	3	4	7	8	18

82.09: INC SOFT TISSUE HAND NEC

Type of Patients	Observed Patients	Avg. Stay	Vari-ance	Percentiles						
				10th	25th	50th	75th	90th	95th	99th
1. SINGLE DX										
0–19 Years	5	2.6	7	1	1	1	3	7	7	7
20–34	7	1.9	1	1	1	1	3	3	3	3
35–49	2	2.5	4	1	2	3	4	4	4	4
50–64	6	2.7	2	1	2	3	3	5	5	5
65+	0									
2. MULTIPLE DX										
0–19 Years	25	4.5	15	2	2	3	6	11	11	18
20–34	50	3.7	15	1	2	3	5	7	8	25
35–49	76	5.5	37	1	2	4	6	10	16	43
50–64	66	4.3	11	1	2	3	6	9	11	18
65+	38	5.0	13	2	3	5	6	12	13	18
TOTAL SINGLE DX	20	2.4	3	1	1	2	3	5	5	7
TOTAL MULTIPLE DX	255	4.7	20	1	2	3	6	10	12	24
TOTAL										
0–19 Years	30	4.3	14	1	2	3	6	11	11	18
20–34	57	3.5	14	1	1	3	4	7	8	25
35–49	78	5.4	36	1	2	3	6	10	16	43
50–64	72	4.2	10	1	2	3	5	8	11	18
65+	38	5.0	13	2	3	5	6	12	13	18
GRAND TOTAL	275	4.5	19	1	2	3	6	9	12	24

82.1: DIV HAND MUSC/TEND/FASC

Type of Patients	Observed Patients	Avg. Stay	Vari-ance	Percentiles						
				10th	25th	50th	75th	90th	95th	99th
1. SINGLE DX										
0–19 Years	2	2.0	2	1	1	3	3	3	3	3
20–34	3	3.5	<1	3	3	4	4	4	4	4
35–49	3	2.0	3	1	1	1	4	4	4	4
50–64	3	2.7	2	1	1	3	4	4	4	4
65+	0									
2. MULTIPLE DX										
0–19 Years	7	3.1	17	1	2	2	2	4	17	17
20–34	21	5.0	21	1	2	4	5	9	15	19
35–49	31	6.8	66	1	3	5	7	14	15	45
50–64	30	6.8	99	2	3	4	8	10	24	54
65+	13	4.5	13	1	2	3	5	11	12	12
TOTAL SINGLE DX	10	2.5	2	1	1	3	4	4	4	4
TOTAL MULTIPLE DX	102	5.7	54	1	2	4	6	12	15	45
TOTAL										
0–19 Years	9	3.0	15	1	2	2	2	4	17	17
20–34	23	4.8	19	1	2	5	5	9	15	19
35–49	34	6.4	62	1	2	5	7	14	15	45
50–64	33	6.5	91	2	3	4	6	10	24	54
65+	13	4.5	13	1	2	3	5	11	12	12
GRAND TOTAL	112	5.4	50	1	2	4	5	11	15	45

LOS by Diagnosis and Operation, Western Region, 45th Edition

Western Region, October 2007–September 2008 Data, by Operation

82.2: EXC LES HAND SOFT TISSUE

Type of Patients	Observed Patients	Avg. Stay	Variance	Percentiles						
				10th	25th	50th	75th	90th	95th	99th
1. SINGLE DX										
0–19 Years	3	1.3	<1	1	1	1	1	3	3	3
20–34	5	1.8	3	1	1	1	1	5	5	5
35–49	3	3.3	5	2	2	2	6	6	6	6
50–64	3	3.0	3	1	1	2	4	4	4	4
65+	0									
2. MULTIPLE DX										
0–19 Years	16	5.0	39	1	2	3	5	6	24	24
20–34	44	3.2	11	1	2	3	3	5	9	18
35–49	51	4.1	9	2	2	3	5	8	9	18
50–64	57	4.9	18	1	2	4	7	11	16	>99
65+	38	5.3	11	2	3	4	8	11	12	12
TOTAL SINGLE DX	14	2.1	3	1	1	1	3	5	6	6
TOTAL MULTIPLE DX	206	4.4	15	1	2	3	5	9	12	24
TOTAL										
0–19 Years	19	4.2	33	1	1	3	4	6	24	24
20–34	49	3.1	10	1	2	2	3	5	9	18
35–49	54	4.0	9	2	2	3	5	8	9	18
50–64	60	4.8	18	2	2	4	7	11	16	>99
65+	38	5.3	11	2	3	4	8	11	12	12
GRAND TOTAL	220	4.3	15	1	2	3	5	9	12	24

82.3: OTH EXC HAND SOFT TISSUE

Type of Patients	Observed Patients	Avg. Stay	Variance	Percentiles						
				10th	25th	50th	75th	90th	95th	99th
1. SINGLE DX										
0–19 Years	2	1.5	<1	1	1	2	2	2	2	2
20–34	5	2.8	6	1	1	2	3	7	7	7
35–49	4	2.3	4	1	1	2	2	5	5	5
50–64	4	1.3	<1	1	1	1	2	2	2	2
65+	1	7.0	0	7	7	7	7	7	7	7
2. MULTIPLE DX										
0–19 Years	12	3.7	3	1	2	4	5	6	6	6
20–34	27	3.4	5	1	2	3	6	7	8	8
35–49	47	6.7	46	2	3	4	7	19	22	34
50–64	55	5.3	29	1	3	4	6	9	18	34
65+	53	4.8	11	1	2	4	7	9	12	13
TOTAL SINGLE DX	16	2.4	4	1	1	2	3	7	7	7
TOTAL MULTIPLE DX	194	5.1	24	1	2	4	6	9	12	34
TOTAL										
0–19 Years	14	3.5	3	1	2	4	5	6	6	6
20–34	32	3.3	5	1	2	2	6	7	8	8
35–49	51	6.4	44	1	3	4	7	12	22	34
50–64	59	5.0	28	1	2	4	6	9	18	34
65+	54	4.8	11	1	2	4	7	9	12	13
GRAND TOTAL	210	4.9	23	1	2	4	6	9	12	25

82.29: EXC LES SFT TISS HND NEC

Type of Patients	Observed Patients	Avg. Stay	Variance	Percentiles						
				10th	25th	50th	75th	90th	95th	99th
1. SINGLE DX										
0–19 Years	1	1.0	0	1	1	1	1	1	1	1
20–34	3	2.4	5	1	1	1	5	5	5	5
35–49	3	6.0	0	6	6	6	6	6	6	6
50–64	2	2.5	4	1	1	3	4	4	4	4
65+	0									
2. MULTIPLE DX										
0–19 Years	8	2.7	1	2	2	3	3	3	5	5
20–34	34	3.4	13	1	2	3	3	7	14	18
35–49	33	3.9	11	1	2	3	5	8	10	18
50–64	34	3.6	10	1	2	3	5	10	14	>99
65+	27	5.7	11	2	3	5	9	11	12	12
TOTAL SINGLE DX	7	2.2	4	1	1	1	4	5	6	6
TOTAL MULTIPLE DX	136	4.0	11	1	2	3	5	9	12	18
TOTAL										
0–19 Years	9	2.3	1	1	1	2	3	3	5	5
20–34	37	3.3	12	1	1	2	3	7	14	18
35–49	34	4.0	11	2	2	3	5	8	10	18
50–64	36	3.6	9	1	2	3	5	10	14	>99
65+	27	5.7	11	2	3	5	9	11	12	12
GRAND TOTAL	143	3.9	11	1	2	3	5	9	11	18

82.33: HAND TENONECTOMY NEC

Type of Patients	Observed Patients	Avg. Stay	Variance	Percentiles						
				10th	25th	50th	75th	90th	95th	99th
1. SINGLE DX										
0–19 Years	0									
20–34	2	2.5	<1	2	2	3	3	3	3	3
35–49	2	1.5	<1	1	1	2	2	2	2	2
50–64	0									
65+	0									
2. MULTIPLE DX										
0–19 Years	1	4.0	0	4	4	4	4	4	4	4
20–34	12	3.3	5	1	2	3	6	6	7	7
35–49	23	6.0	24	3	3	4	6	12	19	20
50–64	27	5.3	20	2	2	4	6	11	18	18
65+	30	5.3	12	2	2	4	7	10	13	13
TOTAL SINGLE DX	4	2.0	<1	1	2	2	3	3	3	3
TOTAL MULTIPLE DX	93	5.2	16	2	3	4	6	10	13	20
TOTAL										
0–19 Years	1	4.0	0	4	4	4	4	4	4	4
20–34	14	3.2	4	1	3	3	6	6	7	7
35–49	25	5.6	24	3	3	4	6	12	19	20
50–64	27	5.3	20	2	3	4	6	11	18	18
65+	30	5.3	12	2	2	4	7	10	13	13
GRAND TOTAL	97	5.0	16	2	3	4	6	10	13	19

LOS by Diagnosis and Operation, Western Region, 45th Edition

Western Region, October 2007–September 2008 Data, by Operation

82.4: SUTURE HAND SOFT TISSUE

Type of Patients	Observed Patients	Avg. Stay	Variance	10th	25th	50th	75th	90th	95th	99th
1. SINGLE DX										
0–19 Years	14	1.3	<1	1	1	1	1	2	2	2
20–34	45	1.8	2	1	1	1	2	4	4	6
35–49	21	1.6	2	1	1	1	1	3	5	6
50–64	8	1.1	<1	1	1	1	1	2	2	2
65+	1	1.0	0	1	1	1	1	1	1	1
2. MULTIPLE DX										
0–19 Years	56	2.1	6	1	1	1	2	4	7	14
20–34	170	2.0	2	1	1	1	2	4	5	9
35–49	115	2.4	4	1	1	2	3	6	6	10
50–64	71	2.7	7	1	1	2	3	6	9	14
65+	41	3.5	12	1	1	2	4	8	9	19
TOTAL SINGLE DX	89	1.6	1	1	1	1	2	3	4	6
TOTAL MULTIPLE DX	453	2.4	5	1	1	1	3	5	7	12
TOTAL										
0–19 Years	70	1.9	4	1	1	1	2	3	6	14
20–34	215	2.0	2	1	1	1	2	4	5	7
35–49	136	2.3	4	1	1	1	3	5	6	10
50–64	79	2.5	7	1	1	1	3	6	9	14
65+	42	3.4	12	1	1	2	4	8	9	19
GRAND TOTAL	542	2.2	5	1	1	1	3	5	6	12

82.44: SUT FLEXOR TEND HAND NEC

Type of Patients	Observed Patients	Avg. Stay	Variance	10th	25th	50th	75th	90th	95th	99th
1. SINGLE DX										
0–19 Years	4	1.4	<1	1	1	1	2	2	2	2
20–34	21	2.2	2	1	1	2	3	4	5	6
35–49	8	2.4	4	1	1	1	3	6	6	6
50–64	3	1.3	<1	1	1	1	2	2	2	2
65+	1	1.0	0	1	1	1	1	1	1	1
2. MULTIPLE DX										
0–19 Years	28	1.9	5	1	1	1	2	3	7	11
20–34	70	2.0	3	1	1	1	2	5	5	9
35–49	51	2.4	6	1	1	1	3	6	6	12
50–64	18	2.7	5	1	1	2	3	6	9	9
65+	16	2.6	4	1	1	2	3	5	8	8
TOTAL SINGLE DX	37	2.0	2	1	1	1	2	4	5	6
TOTAL MULTIPLE DX	183	2.2	4	1	1	1	3	5	6	11
TOTAL										
0–19 Years	32	1.8	3	1	1	1	2	2	5	11
20–34	91	2.1	2	1	1	1	2	4	5	9
35–49	59	2.4	5	1	1	1	3	6	6	12
50–64	21	2.5	4	1	1	2	3	5	6	9
65+	17	2.5	4	1	1	2	3	5	8	8
GRAND TOTAL	220	2.2	4	1	1	1	3	5	6	10

82.45: SUTURE HAND TENDON NEC

Type of Patients	Observed Patients	Avg. Stay	Variance	10th	25th	50th	75th	90th	95th	99th
1. SINGLE DX										
0–19 Years	7	1.1	<1	1	1	1	1	2	2	2
20–34	22	1.4	<1	1	1	1	1	2	3	4
35–49	8	1.3	<1	1	1	1	1	3	3	3
50–64	5	1.0	0	1	1	1	1	1	1	1
65+	0									
2. MULTIPLE DX										
0–19 Years	21	2.4	9	1	1	1	2	4	6	14
20–34	63	1.8	2	1	1	1	2	4	5	6
35–49	42	2.4	3	1	1	2	3	5	6	7
50–64	34	2.3	6	1	1	2	2	5	6	14
65+	22	3.0	6	1	1	2	4	7	7	10
TOTAL SINGLE DX	42	1.3	<1	1	1	1	1	2	3	4
TOTAL MULTIPLE DX	182	2.2	4	1	1	1	3	5	6	14
TOTAL										
0–19 Years	28	2.1	7	1	1	1	2	4	6	14
20–34	85	1.7	1	1	1	1	2	3	4	6
35–49	50	2.2	3	1	1	1	3	5	6	7
50–64	39	2.1	6	1	1	1	2	5	6	14
65+	22	3.0	6	1	1	2	4	7	7	10
GRAND TOTAL	224	2.1	4	1	1	1	2	4	6	10

82.5: HAND MUSC/TEND TRANSPL

Type of Patients	Observed Patients	Avg. Stay	Variance	10th	25th	50th	75th	90th	95th	99th
1. SINGLE DX										
0–19 Years	3	1.1	<1	1	1	1	1	2	2	2
20–34	0									
35–49	0									
50–64	1	1.0	0	1	1	1	1	1	1	1
65+	0									
2. MULTIPLE DX										
0–19 Years	2	1.0	0	1	1	1	1	1	1	1
20–34	5	5.4	36	1	3	3	4	16	16	16
35–49	6	1.8	<1	1	1	2	2	3	3	3
50–64	6	1.7	<1	1	1	2	2	2	2	2
65+	2	2.5	4	1	1	1	4	4	4	4
TOTAL SINGLE DX	4	1.1	<1	1	1	1	1	1	2	2
TOTAL MULTIPLE DX	21	2.6	10	1	1	2	3	4	4	16
TOTAL										
0–19 Years	5	1.1	<1	1	1	1	1	1	2	2
20–34	5	5.4	36	1	3	3	4	16	16	16
35–49	6	1.8	<1	1	1	2	2	3	3	3
50–64	7	1.6	<1	1	1	1	2	2	2	2
65+	2	2.5	4	1	1	1	4	4	4	4
GRAND TOTAL	25	2.1	7	1	1	1	2	3	4	16

Western Region, October 2007–September 2008 Data, by Operation

82.6: RECONSTRUCTION OF THUMB

Type of Patients	Observed Patients	Avg. Stay	Variance	10th	25th	50th	75th	90th	95th	99th
1. SINGLE DX										
0–19 Years	2	1.5	<1	1	1	1	2	2	2	2
20–34	0									
35–49	0									
50–64	0									
65+	0									
2. MULTIPLE DX										
0–19 Years	11	1.0	0	1	1	1	1	1	1	1
20–34	2	9.0	18	6	6	12	12	12	12	12
35–49	1	9.0	0	9	9	9	9	9	9	9
50–64	3	4.7	12	1	1	5	8	8	8	8
65+	0									
TOTAL SINGLE DX	2	1.5	<1	1	1	1	2	2	2	2
TOTAL MULTIPLE DX	17	1.9	6	1	1	1	1	6	9	12
TOTAL										
0–19 Years	13	1.0	<1	1	1	1	1	1	2	2
20–34	2	9.0	18	6	6	12	12	12	12	12
35–49	1	9.0	0	9	9	9	9	9	9	9
50–64	3	4.7	12	1	1	5	8	8	8	8
65+	0									
GRAND TOTAL	19	1.9	6	1	1	1	1	5	8	12

82.7: PLASTIC OP HND GRFT/IMPL

Type of Patients	Observed Patients	Avg. Stay	Variance	10th	25th	50th	75th	90th	95th	99th
1. SINGLE DX										
0–19 Years	3	2.0	<1	1	1	2	3	3	3	3
20–34	1	1.0	0	1	1	1	1	1	1	1
35–49	3	3.4	10	1	1	2	7	7	7	7
50–64	1	5.0	0	5	5	5	5	5	5	5
65+	0									
2. MULTIPLE DX										
0–19 Years	2	1.0	0	1	1	1	1	1	1	1
20–34	11	2.0	1	1	1	2	3	3	4	4
35–49	5	7.3	20	3	3	7	12	12	12	12
50–64	5	1.8	3	1	1	1	1	5	5	5
65+	1	1.0	0	1	1	1	1	1	1	1
TOTAL SINGLE DX	8	2.8	5	1	1	2	5	7	7	7
TOTAL MULTIPLE DX	22	2.4	6	1	1	1	3	5	7	12
TOTAL										
0–19 Years	5	1.4	<1	1	1	1	3	3	3	3
20–34	12	1.9	1	1	1	1	3	3	4	4
35–49	6	5.4	17	2	2	7	7	12	12	12
50–64	6	2.3	4	1	1	1	5	5	5	5
65+	1	1.0	0	1	1	1	1	1	1	1
GRAND TOTAL	30	2.5	6	1	1	1	3	5	7	12

82.8: OTHER PLASTIC OPS HAND

Type of Patients	Observed Patients	Avg. Stay	Variance	10th	25th	50th	75th	90th	95th	99th
1. SINGLE DX										
0–19 Years	2	1.0	0	1	1	1	1	1	1	1
20–34	4	1.3	<1	1	1	1	1	2	2	2
35–49	0									
50–64	0									
65+	0									
2. MULTIPLE DX										
0–19 Years	3	1.7	<1	2	2	2	2	2	2	2
20–34	9	1.6	2	1	1	1	1	5	5	5
35–49	6	1.8	<1	1	1	1	3	3	3	3
50–64	9	1.5	<1	1	1	1	2	2	2	2
65+	4	2.5	4	5	5	5	5	5	5	5
TOTAL SINGLE DX	6	1.1	<1	1	1	1	1	2	2	2
TOTAL MULTIPLE DX	31	1.7	1	1	1	1	2	3	5	5
TOTAL										
0–19 Years	5	1.3	<1	1	1	1	1	2	2	2
20–34	13	1.5	1	1	1	1	1	2	5	5
35–49	6	1.8	<1	1	1	1	3	3	3	3
50–64	9	1.5	<1	1	1	1	2	2	2	2
65+	4	2.5	4	5	5	5	5	5	5	5
GRAND TOTAL	37	1.6	1	1	1	1	2	3	3	5

82.9: OTH HAND SOFT TISSUE OPS

Type of Patients	Observed Patients	Avg. Stay	Variance	10th	25th	50th	75th	90th	95th	99th
1. SINGLE DX										
0–19 Years	0									
20–34	1	2.0	0	2	2	2	2	2	2	2
35–49	2	3.0	8	1	1	3	5	5	5	5
50–64	1	1.0	0	1	1	1	1	1	1	1
65+	0									
2. MULTIPLE DX										
0–19 Years	0									
20–34	2	3.0	8	1	1	4	5	5	5	5
35–49	1	4.0	0	4	4	4	4	4	4	4
50–64	4	1.8	<1	1	2	2	2	3	3	3
65+	5	4.4	7	1	1	4	6	8	8	8
TOTAL SINGLE DX	4	2.2	4	1	1	2	2	5	5	5
TOTAL MULTIPLE DX	12	3.2	5	1	1	3	4	6	8	8
TOTAL										
0–19 Years	0									
20–34	3	2.7	4	1	1	2	5	5	5	5
35–49	3	3.3	4	1	1	4	5	5	5	5
50–64	5	1.6	<1	1	1	1	2	3	3	3
65+	5	4.4	7	1	1	4	6	8	8	8
GRAND TOTAL	16	3.0	5	1	1	2	4	6	8	8

LOS by Diagnosis and Operation, Western Region, 45th Edition

Western Region, October 2007–September 2008 Data, by Operation

83.0: INC MUSC/TEND/FASC/BURSA

Type of Patients	Observed Patients	Avg. Stay	Vari-ance	Percentiles						
				10th	25th	50th	75th	90th	95th	99th
1. SINGLE DX										
0–19 Years	40	2.3	<1	1	1	2	3	3	5	5
20–34	42	3.1	5	1	1	3	4	6	8	11
35–49	34	2.3	3	1	1	3	3	5	6	7
50–64	32	2.6	6	1	1	2	3	4	8	12
65+	4	1.5	1	1	1	1	3	3	3	3
2. MULTIPLE DX										
0–19 Years	290	6.3	53	2	3	4	7	10	15	47
20–34	543	5.9	39	1	2	4	7	12	17	32
35–49	852	6.6	48	2	3	5	8	14	18	31
50–64	942	6.9	44	2	3	5	9	13	19	39
65+	674	6.8	37	2	3	5	8	13	18	27
TOTAL SINGLE DX	152	2.5	3	1	1	2	3	5	6	11
TOTAL MULTIPLE DX	3,301	6.6	44	2	3	5	8	13	18	37
TOTAL										
0–19 Years	330	5.9	49	1	3	4	7	10	15	47
20–34	585	5.7	38	1	2	4	7	11	16	32
35–49	886	6.5	47	2	3	5	8	13	18	31
50–64	974	6.7	44	2	3	5	9	13	19	39
65+	678	6.8	37	2	3	5	8	13	18	27
GRAND TOTAL	3,453	6.4	43	2	3	5	8	12	17	37

83.02: MYOTOMY

Type of Patients	Observed Patients	Avg. Stay	Vari-ance	Percentiles						
				10th	25th	50th	75th	90th	95th	99th
1. SINGLE DX										
0–19 Years	8	1.4	<1	1	1	1	2	2	2	2
20–34	5	2.2	1	1	1	3	3	3	3	3
35–49	7	2.4	3	1	1	2	4	5	5	5
50–64	3	1.7	1	1	1	2	3	3	3	5
65+	1	1.0	0	1	1	1	1	1	1	1
2. MULTIPLE DX										
0–19 Years	51	9.1	113	2	4	6	9	16	37	47
20–34	91	7.5	89	1	2	5	9	15	28	>99
35–49	141	7.3	45	2	3	5	9	16	21	29
50–64	146	7.9	50	2	3	6	10	16	23	43
65+	99	7.8	57	1	3	7	9	16	21	59
TOTAL SINGLE DX	24	1.9	1	1	1	1	3	3	4	5
TOTAL MULTIPLE DX	528	7.9	67	1	3	6	9	16	23	47
TOTAL										
0–19 Years	59	8.5	108	1	3	6	9	14	37	47
20–34	96	7.2	86	1	2	5	9	15	28	>99
35–49	148	7.1	44	1	3	5	9	16	21	29
50–64	149	7.8	50	1	3	6	10	16	23	43
65+	100	7.7	57	1	3	6	9	15	21	59
GRAND TOTAL	552	7.6	65	1	3	6	9	16	23	47

83.03: BURSOTOMY

Type of Patients	Observed Patients	Avg. Stay	Vari-ance	Percentiles						
				10th	25th	50th	75th	90th	95th	99th
1. SINGLE DX										
0–19 Years	3	2.7	<1	2	2	3	3	3	3	3
20–34	3	3.7	1	2	2	3	5	5	5	5
35–49	6	2.8	2	1	2	4	4	4	4	4
50–64	3	1.0	0	1	1	1	1	1	1	1
65+	2	2.0	2	1	1	3	3	3	3	3
2. MULTIPLE DX										
0–19 Years	27	4.5	5	2	3	4	6	7	8	11
20–34	64	4.3	10	2	2	4	5	8	8	19
35–49	100	5.3	29	2	3	4	6	9	13	47
50–64	128	5.5	20	2	3	5	7	11	12	23
65+	111	5.2	12	2	3	5	7	9	11	20
TOTAL SINGLE DX	17	2.5	2	1	1	3	3	4	5	5
TOTAL MULTIPLE DX	430	5.1	17	2	3	4	6	9	11	22
TOTAL										
0–19 Years	30	4.4	4	2	3	4	6	6	7	11
20–34	67	4.2	9	2	2	4	5	8	8	19
35–49	106	5.1	28	2	3	4	6	9	13	20
50–64	131	5.3	20	2	3	4	7	10	12	23
65+	113	5.2	12	2	3	5	7	9	11	20
GRAND TOTAL	447	5.0	17	2	3	4	6	9	11	22

83.09: SOFT TISSUE INCISION NEC

Type of Patients	Observed Patients	Avg. Stay	Vari-ance	Percentiles						
				10th	25th	50th	75th	90th	95th	99th
1. SINGLE DX										
0–19 Years	28	2.5	2	1	1	3	3	5	5	5
20–34	34	3.2	6	1	1	2	4	6	8	11
35–49	19	2.3	3	1	1	2	3	6	7	7
50–64	24	3.0	7	1	1	2	4	7	8	12
65+	1	1.0	0	1	1	1	1	1	1	1
2. MULTIPLE DX										
0–19 Years	210	5.8	42	2	3	4	7	10	15	39
20–34	379	5.8	33	1	2	4	7	12	17	29
35–49	587	6.8	52	2	3	5	8	14	18	32
50–64	646	7.0	48	2	3	5	9	13	19	40
65+	447	7.0	38	2	3	5	8	13	18	27
TOTAL SINGLE DX	106	2.7	4	1	1	2	3	5	7	11
TOTAL MULTIPLE DX	2,269	6.6	44	2	3	5	8	13	18	35
TOTAL										
0–19 Years	238	5.4	38	1	3	4	7	9	12	39
20–34	413	5.6	31	1	3	5	7	11	16	28
35–49	606	6.6	51	2	3	5	8	13	18	31
50–64	670	6.9	47	2	3	5	9	13	18	40
65+	448	7.0	38	2	3	5	8	13	18	27
GRAND TOTAL	2,375	6.4	43	2	3	5	8	12	17	35

LOS by Diagnosis and Operation, Western Region, 45th Edition

Western Region, October 2007–September 2008 Data, by Operation

83.1: MUSC/TEND/FASC DIVISION

Type of Patients	Observed Patients	Avg. Stay	Vari-ance	10th	25th	50th	75th	90th	95th	99th
1. SINGLE DX										
0–19 Years	91	1.6	2	1	1	1	2	3	4	9
20–34	16	2.1	2	1	1	1	3	4	6	6
35–49	16	2.1	6	1	1	1	2	5	10	10
50–64	7	1.9	2	1	1	1	3	5	5	5
65+	1	5.0	0	5	5	5	5	5	5	5
2. MULTIPLE DX										
0–19 Years	394	2.6	13	1	1	1	3	5	8	21
20–34	182	6.9	43	1	2	5	9	17	21	29
35–49	212	8.8	136	1	3	5	10	20	29	66
50–64	248	6.9	58	1	2	4	9	16	24	31
65+	220	6.8	59	1	2	4	9	13	22	42
TOTAL SINGLE DX	**131**	**1.7**	**2**	**1**	**1**	**1**	**2**	**3**	**4**	**9**
TOTAL MULTIPLE DX	**1,256**	**4.8**	**48**	**1**	**1**	**2**	**6**	**11**	**19**	**31**
TOTAL										
0–19 Years	485	2.4	11	1	1	1	2	4	7	21
20–34	198	6.5	42	1	2	4	8	17	20	29
35–49	228	8.3	130	1	2	4	10	19	28	66
50–64	255	6.8	57	1	2	4	9	15	24	31
65+	221	6.8	58	1	2	4	9	13	22	42
GRAND TOTAL	**1,387**	**4.4**	**43**	**1**	**1**	**2**	**5**	**10**	**17**	**29**

83.12: ADDUCTOR TENOTOMY OF HIP

Type of Patients	Observed Patients	Avg. Stay	Vari-ance	10th	25th	50th	75th	90th	95th	99th
1. SINGLE DX										
0–19 Years	19	1.6	2	1	1	1	2	2	3	10
20–34	0									
35–49	0									
50–64	0									
2. MULTIPLE DX										
0–19 Years	121	2.5	7	1	1	2	3	4	6	20
20–34	6	4.0	5	1	1	5	6	6	7	7
35–49	2	1.0	0	1	1	1	1	1	1	1
50–64	2	2.5	4	1	1	4	4	4	4	4
65+	6	5.4	11	2	3	6	7	11	11	11
TOTAL SINGLE DX	**19**	**1.6**	**2**	**1**	**1**	**1**	**2**	**2**	**3**	**10**
TOTAL MULTIPLE DX	**136**	**2.6**	**7**	**1**	**1**	**2**	**3**	**5**	**6**	**20**
TOTAL										
0–19 Years	140	2.3	6	1	1	2	3	4	6	20
20–34	6	4.0	5	1	1	5	6	6	7	7
35–49	1	1.0	0	1	1	1	1	1	1	1
50–64	2	2.5	4	1	1	4	4	4	4	4
65+	6	5.4	11	2	3	6	7	11	11	11
GRAND TOTAL	**155**	**2.4**	**6**	**1**	**1**	**2**	**3**	**4**	**6**	**20**

83.13: TENOTOMY NEC

Type of Patients	Observed Patients	Avg. Stay	Vari-ance	10th	25th	50th	75th	90th	95th	99th
1. SINGLE DX										
0–19 Years	22	1.2	<1	1	1	1	1	2	2	4
20–34	3	1.7	<1	1	1	1	2	2	2	2
35–49	8	1.4	<1	1	1	1	2	2	2	2
50–64	1	1.0	0	1	1	1	1	1	1	1
65+	0									
2. MULTIPLE DX										
0–19 Years	126	1.7	2	1	1	1	2	3	4	8
20–34	29	2.9	5	1	1	2	4	7	8	9
35–49	45	3.5	13	1	2	3	4	8	8	21
50–64	74	4.0	25	1	1	3	4	9	13	27
65+	86	3.7	9	1	1	3	5	9	10	13
TOTAL SINGLE DX	**34**	**1.2**	**<1**	**1**	**1**	**1**	**1**	**2**	**2**	**4**
TOTAL MULTIPLE DX	**360**	**2.5**	**8**	**1**	**1**	**1**	**3**	**6**	**8**	**13**
TOTAL										
0–19 Years	148	1.7	2	1	1	1	2	3	4	8
20–34	32	2.8	5	1	1	2	4	6	8	9
35–49	53	3.2	11	1	1	2	4	8	8	21
50–64	75	4.0	25	1	1	3	4	9	13	27
65+	86	3.7	9	1	1	3	5	9	10	13
GRAND TOTAL	**394**	**2.4**	**7**	**1**	**1**	**1**	**3**	**5**	**8**	**11**

83.14: FASCIOTOMY

Type of Patients	Observed Patients	Avg. Stay	Vari-ance	10th	25th	50th	75th	90th	95th	99th
1. SINGLE DX										
0–19 Years	30	2.3	5	1	1	1	3	4	9	9
20–34	12	2.1	3	1	1	1	3	4	6	6
35–49	7	3.2	11	1	1	2	5	10	10	10
50–64	3	2.3	5	1	1	1	5	5	5	5
65+	1	5.0	0	5	5	5	5	5	5	5
2. MULTIPLE DX										
0–19 Years	93	5.2	44	1	1	3	5	15	23	29
20–34	131	8.0	47	2	4	6	10	18	23	29
35–49	149	10.6	174	2	3	6	12	21	34	67
50–64	148	8.7	74	2	3	6	11	19	27	36
65+	112	9.1	82	2	3	6	11	22	29	48
TOTAL SINGLE DX	**53**	**2.4**	**5**	**1**	**1**	**1**	**3**	**5**	**9**	**10**
TOTAL MULTIPLE DX	**633**	**8.3**	**89**	**1**	**3**	**5**	**10**	**19**	**26**	**50**
TOTAL										
0–19 Years	123	4.3	34	1	1	2	4	10	17	29
20–34	143	7.5	46	1	3	6	10	18	22	29
35–49	156	10.2	169	1	3	6	12	21	34	67
50–64	151	8.6	73	2	4	6	11	17	27	36
65+	113	9.1	82	2	3	6	11	22	29	48
GRAND TOTAL	**686**	**7.7**	**83**	**1**	**2**	**5**	**9**	**18**	**25**	**48**

LOS by Diagnosis and Operation, Western Region, 45th Edition

Western Region, October 2007–September 2008 Data, by Operation

83.2: SOFT TISSUE DXTIC PX

Type of Patients	Observed Patients	Avg. Stay	Variance	10th	25th	50th	75th	90th	95th	99th
1. SINGLE DX										
0–19 Years	25	3.9	4	2	2	3	5	7	8	8
20–34	31	2.0	6	1	1	1	2	3	5	14
35–49	8	2.6	2	1	2	2	4	5	5	5
50–64	8	1.4	<1	1	1	1	2	3	3	3
65+	4	2.0	4	1	1	1	5	5	5	5
2. MULTIPLE DX										
0–19 Years	147	13.1	232	1	3	9	18	29	36	85
20–34	121	9.8	141	2	4	6	11	20	30	60
35–49	253	9.7	86	2	4	7	12	21	29	52
50–64	535	9.9	89	2	4	7	12	20	28	49
65+	672	8.9	46	2	4	7	12	17	21	36
TOTAL SINGLE DX	**76**	**3.0**	**5**	**1**	**1**	**2**	**4**	**6**	**7**	**8**
TOTAL MULTIPLE DX	**1,728**	**10.1**	**104**	**2**	**4**	**7**	**12**	**21**	**28**	**51**
TOTAL										
0–19 Years	172	11.8	211	1	3	7	15	28	36	85
20–34	152	8.3	123	1	3	5	10	17	25	60
35–49	261	9.5	85	2	4	7	12	21	29	52
50–64	543	9.7	89	2	4	7	12	20	28	49
65+	676	8.8	46	2	4	7	12	17	21	36
GRAND TOTAL	**1,804**	**9.7**	**101**	**2**	**4**	**7**	**12**	**21**	**28**	**50**

83.3: EXC LESION SOFT TISSUE

Type of Patients	Observed Patients	Avg. Stay	Variance	10th	25th	50th	75th	90th	95th	99th
1. SINGLE DX										
0–19 Years	92	1.5	<1	1	1	1	2	3	4	4
20–34	66	2.3	4	1	1	2	3	4	5	13
35–49	72	1.5	<1	1	1	1	2	2	3	5
50–64	63	2.1	7	1	1	1	2	4	5	19
65+	18	1.7	<1	1	1	1	2	4	4	4
2. MULTIPLE DX										
0–19 Years	133	5.4	38	1	1	3	7	14	17	24
20–34	297	6.2	49	1	2	4	8	13	18	43
35–49	569	6.1	40	1	2	4	7	14	19	34
50–64	954	6.3	60	1	2	4	7	13	19	43
65+	895	6.4	49	1	2	4	8	14	18	36
TOTAL SINGLE DX	**311**	**1.7**	**2**	**1**	**1**	**1**	**2**	**3**	**4**	**6**
TOTAL MULTIPLE DX	**2,848**	**6.2**	**50**	**1**	**2**	**4**	**8**	**14**	**19**	**36**
TOTAL										
0–19 Years	225	3.6	24	1	1	2	4	8	14	24
20–34	363	5.5	43	1	2	3	7	13	16	38
35–49	641	5.6	38	1	2	4	7	13	18	34
50–64	1,017	6.0	57	1	2	4	7	12	19	43
65+	913	6.3	48	1	2	4	8	14	18	35
GRAND TOTAL	**3,159**	**5.6**	**46**	**1**	**2**	**4**	**7**	**13**	**18**	**34**

83.21: SOFT TISSUE BIOPSY

Type of Patients	Observed Patients	Avg. Stay	Variance	10th	25th	50th	75th	90th	95th	99th
1. SINGLE DX										
0–19 Years	25	3.9	4	2	2	3	5	7	8	8
20–34	31	2.0	6	1	1	1	2	3	5	14
35–49	8	2.6	2	1	2	2	4	5	5	5
50–64	8	1.4	<1	1	1	1	2	3	3	3
65+	4	2.0	4	1	1	1	5	5	5	5
2. MULTIPLE DX										
0–19 Years	147	13.1	232	1	3	9	18	29	36	85
20–34	121	9.8	141	2	4	6	11	20	30	60
35–49	252	9.8	86	2	4	7	12	21	29	52
50–64	533	9.9	90	2	4	7	12	20	28	49
65+	672	8.9	46	2	4	7	12	17	21	36
TOTAL SINGLE DX	**76**	**3.0**	**5**	**1**	**1**	**2**	**4**	**6**	**7**	**8**
TOTAL MULTIPLE DX	**1,725**	**10.1**	**104**	**2**	**4**	**7**	**12**	**21**	**28**	**51**
TOTAL										
0–19 Years	172	11.8	211	1	3	7	15	28	36	85
20–34	152	8.3	123	1	3	5	10	17	25	60
35–49	260	9.5	85	2	4	7	12	21	29	52
50–64	541	9.7	89	2	4	7	12	20	28	49
65+	676	8.8	46	2	4	7	12	17	21	36
GRAND TOTAL	**1,801**	**9.7**	**101**	**2**	**4**	**7**	**12**	**21**	**28**	**50**

83.32: EXC MUSCLE LESION

Type of Patients	Observed Patients	Avg. Stay	Variance	10th	25th	50th	75th	90th	95th	99th
1. SINGLE DX										
0–19 Years	18	1.1	<1	1	1	1	1	1	2	2
20–34	22	2.5	6	1	1	2	3	5	5	13
35–49	24	1.7	1	1	1	1	2	3	3	5
50–64	20	1.6	1	1	1	1	2	3	5	5
65+	3	2.3	2	1	1	2	4	4	4	4
2. MULTIPLE DX										
0–19 Years	12	5.2	19	2	2	4	5	13	13	16
20–34	41	4.9	37	1	2	3	5	12	13	32
35–49	91	4.1	19	1	1	3	5	8	12	23
50–64	153	4.2	25	1	1	3	5	10	12	27
65+	139	5.4	35	1	2	3	7	14	21	26
TOTAL SINGLE DX	**87**	**1.6**	**2**	**1**	**1**	**1**	**2**	**3**	**3**	**5**
TOTAL MULTIPLE DX	**436**	**4.7**	**28**	**1**	**1**	**3**	**5**	**11**	**16**	**26**
TOTAL										
0–19 Years	30	2.4	10	1	1	1	2	5	13	16
20–34	63	4.0	26	1	2	2	4	9	13	32
35–49	115	3.6	16	1	1	2	4	7	10	22
50–64	173	3.9	23	1	1	2	4	8	12	27
65+	142	5.3	34	1	2	3	7	12	21	26
GRAND TOTAL	**523**	**4.0**	**23**	**1**	**1**	**2**	**5**	**9**	**13**	**25**

LOS by Diagnosis and Operation, Western Region, 45th Edition

83.39: EXC LES SOFT TISSUE NEC

Type of Patients	Observed Patients	Avg. Stay	Variance	10th	25th	50th	75th	90th	95th	99th
1. SINGLE DX										
0–19 Years	74	1.6	<1	1	1	1	2	3	4	4
20–34	42	2.2	2	1	1	1	3	4	4	9
35–49	46	1.3	<1	1	1	1	2	2	2	3
50–64	43	2.3	9	1	1	1	2	5	6	19
65+	15	1.5	<1	1	1	1	2	2	4	4
2. MULTIPLE DX										
0–19 Years	120	5.4	40	1	1	3	7	14	20	24
20–34	250	6.4	51	1	2	4	8	13	18	43
35–49	468	6.6	44	1	2	5	8	14	20	36
50–64	783	6.8	66	1	2	5	8	14	20	45
65+	738	6.6	52	1	2	5	8	14	18	36
TOTAL SINGLE DX	220	1.8	2	1	1	1	2	3	4	6
TOTAL MULTIPLE DX	2,359	6.5	54	1	2	4	8	14	19	39
TOTAL										
0–19 Years	194	3.8	27	1	1	2	4	10	15	24
20–34	292	5.8	46	1	2	4	7	13	16	43
35–49	514	6.1	43	1	2	4	8	14	19	34
50–64	826	6.5	64	1	2	4	8	14	20	43
65+	753	6.5	52	1	2	4	8	14	18	36
GRAND TOTAL	2,579	6.0	50	1	2	4	7	13	18	38

83.42: TENONECTOMY NEC

Type of Patients	Observed Patients	Avg. Stay	Variance	10th	25th	50th	75th	90th	95th	99th
1. SINGLE DX										
0–19 Years	0									
20–34	0									
35–49	2	7.4	83	1	1	1	14	14	14	14
50–64	1	3.0	0	3	3	3	3	3	3	3
65+	0									
2. MULTIPLE DX										
0–19 Years	0									
20–34	7	8.4	35	1	5	7	15	18	18	18
35–49	28	4.1	15	1	1	2	6	9	13	16
50–64	38	5.5	30	1	2	3	8	13	16	29
65+	40	6.9	38	1	2	5	12	15	23	24
TOTAL SINGLE DX	3	5.9	48	1	1	3	14	14	14	14
TOTAL MULTIPLE DX	113	5.8	30	1	2	4	8	13	16	24
TOTAL										
0–19 Years	0									
20–34	7	8.4	35	1	5	7	15	18	18	18
35–49	30	4.4	17	1	1	2	6	9	14	16
50–64	39	5.4	29	1	2	3	8	13	16	29
65+	40	6.9	38	1	2	5	12	15	23	24
GRAND TOTAL	116	5.8	30	1	2	4	8	14	16	24

83.4: OTHER EXC MUSC/TEND/FASC

Type of Patients	Observed Patients	Avg. Stay	Variance	10th	25th	50th	75th	90th	95th	99th
1. SINGLE DX										
0–19 Years	14	3.2	5	1	1	2	2	3	4	4
20–34	21	2.5	2	1	1	2	3	4	4	9
35–49	24	2.6	10	1	1	1	2	2	2	3
50–64	16	2.2	1	1	1	1	2	5	6	19
65+	5	2.0	<1	1	2	2	2	2	4	4
2. MULTIPLE DX										
0–19 Years	87	6.3	83	1	2	3	7	14	24	30
20–34	260	9.0	124	2	3	6	9	21	35	65
35–49	504	8.1	76	1	3	6	10	17	26	44
50–64	662	9.9	120	2	3	7	12	21	29	64
65+	749	8.9	72	2	4	7	11	17	25	39
TOTAL SINGLE DX	80	2.6	5	1	1	2	3	5	7	14
TOTAL MULTIPLE DX	2,262	8.9	94	2	3	6	11	19	27	55
TOTAL										
0–19 Years	101	5.9	73	1	1	3	7	10	24	30
20–34	281	8.5	118	2	3	6	8	19	35	65
35–49	528	7.9	74	1	3	6	10	16	25	44
50–64	678	9.7	119	2	3	6	12	21	29	64
65+	754	8.9	72	2	4	6	11	17	25	39
GRAND TOTAL	2,342	8.6	92	1	3	6	10	18	26	55

83.44: FASCIECTOMY NEC

Type of Patients	Observed Patients	Avg. Stay	Variance	10th	25th	50th	75th	90th	95th	99th
1. SINGLE DX										
0–19 Years	0									
20–34	0									
35–49	0									
50–64	1	2.0	0	2	2	2	2	2	2	2
65+	1	2.0	0	2	2	2	2	2	2	2
2. MULTIPLE DX										
0–19 Years	5	6.4	33	2	2	5	7	16	16	16
20–34	13	8.7	56	3	6	7	8	16	31	31
35–49	40	8.9	96	2	4	6	11	17	18	60
50–64	39	9.7	105	1	2	6	14	21	42	45
65+	31	10.3	100	3	4	6	12	23	40	42
TOTAL SINGLE DX	2	2.0	0	2	2	2	2	2	2	2
TOTAL MULTIPLE DX	127	9.4	92	2	4	6	12	20	24	45
TOTAL										
0–19 Years	5	6.4	33	2	2	5	7	16	16	16
20–34	13	8.7	56	3	6	7	8	16	31	31
35–49	40	8.9	96	2	4	6	11	17	18	60
50–64	39	9.5	103	1	2	6	14	21	42	45
65+	32	10.0	99	3	4	6	12	23	40	42
GRAND TOTAL	129	9.2	91	2	4	6	11	20	24	45

LOS by Diagnosis and Operation, Western Region, 45th Edition

Western Region, October 2007–September 2008 Data, by Operation

83.45: MYECTOMY NEC

Type of Patients	Observed Patients	Avg. Stay	Vari-ance	Percentiles						
				10th	25th	50th	75th	90th	95th	99th
1. SINGLE DX										
0–19 Years	11	3.5	5	1	1	4	5	7	7	7
20–34	17	2.5	3	1	1	2	4	6	6	6
35–49	19	2.3	5	1	1	1	3	7	9	9
50–64	9	2.3	2	1	1	2	4	4	4	4
65+	3	2.0	1	1	1	2	3	3	3	3
2. MULTIPLE DX										
0–19 Years	71	5.8	93	1	2	3	6	10	30	78
20–34	223	9.2	131	2	3	5	10	22	36	65
35–49	399	8.5	78	2	4	6	10	17	27	44
50–64	544	10.4	127	2	4	7	12	22	29	65
65+	610	9.3	76	2	4	7	11	18	25	39
TOTAL SINGLE DX	59	2.7	4	1	1	2	4	5	7	9
TOTAL MULTIPLE DX	1,847	9.3	99	2	4	6	11	19	27	60
TOTAL										
0–19 Years	82	5.5	81	1	2	3	6	9	23	30
20–34	240	8.8	125	2	3	5	9	21	35	65
35–49	418	8.2	76	2	3	6	10	17	27	44
50–64	553	10.2	126	2	4	7	12	22	29	65
65+	613	9.3	76	2	4	7	11	18	25	39
GRAND TOTAL	1,906	9.0	98	2	3	6	11	19	27	60

83.49: SOFT TISSUE EXC NEC

Type of Patients	Observed Patients	Avg. Stay	Vari-ance	Percentiles						
				10th	25th	50th	75th	90th	95th	99th
1. SINGLE DX										
0–19 Years	3	1.3	<1	1	1	1	2	2	2	2
20–34	4	2.3	<1	2	2	2	3	3	3	3
35–49	3	1.7	1	1	1	1	3	3	3	3
50–64	5	1.8	<1	1	1	2	2	3	3	3
65+	1	2.0	0	2	2	2	2	2	2	2
2. MULTIPLE DX										
0–19 Years	10	8.3	56	1	2	7	9	24	24	24
20–34	15	7.0	149	1	2	4	6	10	50	50
35–49	33	6.4	71	1	1	3	8	15	20	42
50–64	42	7.7	108	1	2	4	7	20	30	54
65+	64	5.9	33	1	2	4	7	12	17	33
TOTAL SINGLE DX	16	1.8	<1	1	1	2	2	3	3	3
TOTAL MULTIPLE DX	164	6.9	69	1	2	4	8	16	24	50
TOTAL										
0–19 Years	13	7.6	55	1	2	6	9	24	24	24
20–34	19	6.0	120	1	2	3	6	10	50	50
35–49	36	6.1	66	1	1	3	8	15	20	42
50–64	47	7.1	100	1	2	3	7	20	30	54
65+	65	5.8	33	1	2	4	7	12	17	33
GRAND TOTAL	180	6.4	66	1	2	4	7	15	24	50

83.5: BURSECTOMY

Type of Patients	Observed Patients	Avg. Stay	Vari-ance	Percentiles						
				10th	25th	50th	75th	90th	95th	99th
1. SINGLE DX										
0–19 Years	3	2.3	5	1	1	1	5	5	5	5
20–34	9	3.0	3	1	2	2	3	7	7	7
35–49	6	5.0	17	1	1	3	10	10	10	10
50–64	8	1.6	<1	1	1	1	2	3	3	3
65+	3	2.0	3	1	1	1	4	4	4	4
2. MULTIPLE DX										
0–19 Years	24	8.1	135	1	2	4	6	40	40	40
20–34	91	4.7	10	2	3	5	6	7	8	25
35–49	192	4.8	19	1	2	4	6	9	11	20
50–64	227	4.4	16	1	2	4	5	9	13	17
65+	232	4.6	13	1	2	4	6	9	12	17
TOTAL SINGLE DX	29	2.9	6	1	1	2	3	7	10	10
TOTAL MULTIPLE DX	766	4.8	21	1	2	4	6	9	12	25
TOTAL										
0–19 Years	27	7.7	127	1	2	4	6	40	40	40
20–34	100	4.6	9	2	2	4	6	7	8	12
35–49	198	4.8	19	1	2	4	6	9	11	20
50–64	235	4.3	15	1	2	3	5	9	13	17
65+	235	4.6	13	1	2	4	6	9	12	17
GRAND TOTAL	795	4.7	20	1	2	4	6	9	12	20

83.6: SUTURE MUSC/TENDON/FASC

Type of Patients	Observed Patients	Avg. Stay	Vari-ance	Percentiles						
				10th	25th	50th	75th	90th	95th	99th
1. SINGLE DX										
0–19 Years	54	1.4	<1	1	1	1	2	2	3	5
20–34	107	1.8	2	1	1	1	2	4	5	6
35–49	104	1.7	1	1	1	1	2	3	4	5
50–64	80	1.7	1	1	1	1	2	3	3	14
65+	28	1.5	<1	1	1	1	2	3	3	4
2. MULTIPLE DX										
0–19 Years	183	2.7	10	1	1	1	3	6	8	19
20–34	496	2.5	6	1	1	2	3	5	7	15
35–49	548	2.6	13	1	1	1	3	5	7	14
50–64	869	2.3	7	1	1	1	2	4	6	12
65+	1,015	2.2	4	1	1	2	3	4	6	11
TOTAL SINGLE DX	373	1.7	1	1	1	1	2	3	4	5
TOTAL MULTIPLE DX	3,111	2.4	7	1	1	2	3	5	7	13
TOTAL										
0–19 Years	237	2.3	8	1	1	1	2	5	7	19
20–34	603	2.4	6	1	1	1	3	5	7	15
35–49	652	2.5	11	1	1	1	3	5	7	13
50–64	949	2.2	6	1	1	1	2	4	6	12
65+	1,043	2.2	4	1	1	2	3	4	6	11
GRAND TOTAL	3,484	2.3	7	1	1	1	3	4	6	13

LOS by Diagnosis and Operation, Western Region, 45th Edition

Western Region, October 2007–September 2008 Data, by Operation

83.61: TENDON SHEATH SUTURE

Type of Patients	Observed Patients	Avg. Stay	Vari-ance	Percentiles						
				10th	25th	50th	75th	90th	95th	99th
1. SINGLE DX										
0–19 Years	1	2.0	0	2	2	2	2	2	2	2
20–34	8	1.1	<1	1	1	1	1	2	2	2
35–49	6	1.7	1	1	1	1	2	4	4	4
50–64	6	1.5	<1	1	1	1	2	3	3	4
65+	1	1.0	0	1	1	1	1	1	1	1
2. MULTIPLE DX										
0–19 Years	9	2.1	3	1	1	2	2	6	6	6
20–34	39	2.8	3	1	1	2	4	5	7	8
35–49	35	2.6	4	1	1	2	3	6	8	8
50–64	37	2.8	8	1	1	2	4	6	7	16
65+	38	3.0	5	1	1	3	4	4	9	13
TOTAL SINGLE DX	22	1.5	<1	1	1	1	2	2	3	4
TOTAL MULTIPLE DX	158	2.8	5	1	1	2	3	6	7	13
TOTAL										
0–19 Years	10	2.1	2	1	1	2	2	3	6	6
20–34	47	2.5	3	1	1	2	3	5	6	8
35–49	41	2.5	4	1	1	2	3	6	6	8
50–64	43	2.6	7	1	1	2	3	5	6	16
65+	39	3.0	5	1	1	3	4	4	9	13
GRAND TOTAL	180	2.6	5	1	1	2	3	5	6	13

83.63: ROTATOR CUFF REPAIR

Type of Patients	Observed Patients	Avg. Stay	Vari-ance	Percentiles						
				10th	25th	50th	75th	90th	95th	99th
1. SINGLE DX										
0–19 Years	0									
20–34	0									
35–49	16	1.6	<1	1	1	1	2	3	4	4
50–64	31	1.4	<1	1	1	1	2	2	3	4
65+	17	1.4	<1	1	1	1	1	3	3	3
2. MULTIPLE DX										
0–19 Years	0									
20–34	6	3.3	32	1	1	1	1	15	15	15
35–49	111	1.6	1	1	1	1	2	3	3	7
50–64	503	1.7	1	1	1	1	2	3	4	7
65+	733	1.8	3	1	1	1	2	3	4	8
TOTAL SINGLE DX	64	1.4	<1	1	1	1	2	3	3	4
TOTAL MULTIPLE DX	1,353	1.8	2	1	1	1	2	3	4	7
TOTAL										
0–19 Years	0									
20–34	6	3.3	32	1	1	1	1	15	15	15
35–49	127	1.6	1	1	1	1	2	3	3	7
50–64	534	1.7	1	1	1	1	2	3	4	6
65+	750	1.8	2	1	1	1	2	3	4	8
GRAND TOTAL	1,417	1.7	2	1	1	1	2	3	4	7

83.64: SUTURE OF TENDON NEC

Type of Patients	Observed Patients	Avg. Stay	Vari-ance	Percentiles						
				10th	25th	50th	75th	90th	95th	99th
1. SINGLE DX										
0–19 Years	28	1.2	<1	1	1	1	1	2	2	2
20–34	67	1.9	2	1	1	1	2	4	5	6
35–49	67	1.8	1	1	1	1	2	3	4	5
50–64	32	1.7	1	1	1	1	2	3	4	5
65+	8	1.9	1	1	1	2	3	4	4	4
2. MULTIPLE DX										
0–19 Years	83	1.7	2	1	1	2	2	3	4	11
20–34	243	2.4	7	1	1	2	3	4	7	16
35–49	245	2.7	19	1	1	2	3	5	7	14
50–64	195	2.6	10	1	2	2	3	6	8	20
65+	158	3.2	8	1	2	2	4	6	8	14
TOTAL SINGLE DX	202	1.7	1	1	1	1	2	3	4	5
TOTAL MULTIPLE DX	924	2.6	11	1	1	2	3	5	7	15
TOTAL										
0–19 Years	111	1.6	2	1	1	2	2	3	4	8
20–34	310	2.3	6	1	1	2	3	4	6	15
35–49	312	2.5	15	1	1	2	3	5	6	13
50–64	227	2.5	9	1	1	2	3	5	8	18
65+	166	3.1	8	1	2	2	4	6	8	14
GRAND TOTAL	1,126	2.4	9	1	1	2	3	5	7	14

83.65: MUSCLE/FASC SUTURE NEC

Type of Patients	Observed Patients	Avg. Stay	Vari-ance	Percentiles						
				10th	25th	50th	75th	90th	95th	99th
1. SINGLE DX										
0–19 Years	24	1.4	<1	1	1	1	2	3	3	4
20–34	29	1.8	2	1	1	1	2	4	5	6
35–49	12	1.8	2	1	1	1	3	3	5	5
50–64	10	2.6	16	1	1	2	2	2	14	14
65+	2	1.5	<1	1	1	2	2	2	2	2
2. MULTIPLE DX										
0–19 Years	89	3.5	16	1	1	2	5	7	12	19
20–34	205	2.6	6	1	1	2	3	6	7	10
35–49	151	3.1	12	1	1	2	4	6	9	18
50–64	118	3.7	19	1	2	2	4	7	12	17
65+	79	3.7	8	1	2	3	5	7	10	16
TOTAL SINGLE DX	77	1.7	3	1	1	1	2	3	4	14
TOTAL MULTIPLE DX	642	3.2	12	1	1	2	4	7	9	19
TOTAL										
0–19 Years	113	3.0	13	1	1	1	3	6	12	19
20–34	234	2.5	6	1	1	2	3	5	7	10
35–49	163	3.0	11	1	1	2	3	6	8	18
50–64	128	3.6	19	1	1	2	4	7	12	17
65+	81	3.6	8	1	2	3	5	7	9	16
GRAND TOTAL	719	3.0	11	1	1	2	4	6	8	18

LOS by Diagnosis and Operation, Western Region, 45th Edition

Western Region, October 2007–September 2008 Data, by Operation

83.7: MUSCLE/TENDON RECONST

Type of Patients	Observed Patients	Avg. Stay	Variance	10th	25th	50th	75th	90th	95th	99th
1. SINGLE DX										
0–19 Years	41	1.3	2	1	1	1	1	1	3	11
20–34	6	2.8	7	1	1	1	5	7	7	7
35–49	8	1.3	<1	1	1	1	2	2	2	2
50–64	7	1.3	<1	1	1	1	2	2	2	2
65+	1	3.0	0	3	3	3	3	3	3	3
2. MULTIPLE DX										
0–19 Years	156	1.6	2	1	1	1	2	3	3	9
20–34	56	2.0	2	1	1	2	2	3	4	8
35–49	103	2.4	5	1	1	2	3	4	6	12
50–64	187	2.8	8	1	1	2	3	5	6	18
65+	147	2.6	4	1	1	2	3	4	5	12
TOTAL SINGLE DX	63	1.4	2	1	1	1	1	2	3	11
TOTAL MULTIPLE DX	649	2.1	4	1	1	2	2	4	5	10
TOTAL										
0–19 Years	197	1.6	2	1	1	1	2	3	3	9
20–34	62	2.1	2	1	1	2	2	4	5	8
35–49	111	2.4	5	1	1	2	3	4	6	12
50–64	194	2.7	8	1	1	2	3	5	6	18
65+	148	2.6	4	1	1	2	3	4	5	12
GRAND TOTAL	712	2.0	4	1	1	2	2	4	5	10

83.72: TENDON RECESSION

Type of Patients	Observed Patients	Avg. Stay	Variance	10th	25th	50th	75th	90th	95th	99th
1. SINGLE DX										
0–19 Years	4	5.5	21	1	1	5	11	11	11	11
20–34	2	1.0	0	1	1	1	1	1	1	1
35–49	0									
50–64	3	1.3	<1	1	1	1	2	2	2	2
65+	0									
2. MULTIPLE DX										
0–19 Years	31	1.5	<1	1	1	1	2	2	3	3
20–34	21	1.8	<1	1	1	1	2	3	3	4
35–49	42	2.7	6	1	1	2	3	4	7	12
50–64	75	2.8	6	1	1	2	3	5	7	18
65+	44	2.5	1	1	2	2	3	4	4	5
TOTAL SINGLE DX	9	3.5	15	1	1	1	5	11	11	11
TOTAL MULTIPLE DX	213	2.3	3	1	1	2	3	4	4	11
TOTAL										
0–19 Years	35	1.8	3	1	1	1	2	3	3	11
20–34	23	1.7	<1	1	1	1	2	3	3	4
35–49	42	2.7	6	1	1	2	3	4	7	12
50–64	78	2.7	6	1	1	2	3	4	7	18
65+	44	2.5	1	1	2	3	3	4	4	5
GRAND TOTAL	222	2.3	4	1	1	2	3	4	5	11

83.75: TENDON TRANSF/TRANSPL

Type of Patients	Observed Patients	Avg. Stay	Variance	10th	25th	50th	75th	90th	95th	99th
1. SINGLE DX										
0–19 Years	24	1.1	<1	1	1	1	1	1	3	3
20–34	6	5.0	0	5	5	5	5	5	5	5
35–49	4	1.3	<1	1	1	2	2	2	2	2
50–64	2	1.5	<1	1	1	2	2	2	2	2
65+	1	3.0	0	3	3	3	3	3	3	3
2. MULTIPLE DX										
0–19 Years	91	1.6	2	1	1	1	2	3	3	9
20–34	20	2.0	3	1	1	2	2	3	6	8
35–49	40	1.7	<1	1	1	1	2	3	3	4
50–64	74	2.3	2	1	1	2	3	4	5	7
65+	73	2.5	4	1	1	2	3	4	6	12
TOTAL SINGLE DX	32	1.2	<1	1	1	1	1	2	3	5
TOTAL MULTIPLE DX	298	1.9	2	1	1	1	2	3	5	9
TOTAL										
0–19 Years	115	1.5	2	1	1	1	2	3	3	9
20–34	21	2.2	3	1	1	2	2	5	6	8
35–49	44	1.7	<1	1	1	1	2	3	3	4
50–64	76	2.3	2	1	1	2	3	4	5	7
65+	74	2.5	4	1	1	2	3	4	6	12
GRAND TOTAL	330	1.8	2	1	1	1	2	3	4	9

83.8: MUSC/TEND/FASC OP NEC

Type of Patients	Observed Patients	Avg. Stay	Variance	10th	25th	50th	75th	90th	95th	99th
1. SINGLE DX										
0–19 Years	90	1.4	<1	1	1	1	1	2	3	5
20–34	40	2.5	4	1	1	2	3	5	8	9
35–49	32	2.1	3	1	1	1	3	4	6	4
50–64	33	1.6	<1	1	1	2	2	3	4	4
65+	8	2.1	<1	1	2	2	2	4	4	4
2. MULTIPLE DX										
0–19 Years	363	1.8	6	1	1	2	2	3	4	8
20–34	105	4.7	70	1	1	4	4	10	21	53
35–49	211	3.6	24	1	1	2	4	6	12	27
50–64	503	3.3	19	1	1	2	3	7	11	25
65+	442	3.7	24	1	1	2	4	7	11	28
TOTAL SINGLE DX	203	1.6	1	1	1	1	2	3	4	6
TOTAL MULTIPLE DX	1,624	2.8	18	1	1	2	3	5	8	25
TOTAL										
0–19 Years	453	1.7	5	1	1	1	2	3	4	8
20–34	145	4.1	54	1	1	3	4	8	15	53
35–49	243	3.4	22	1	1	2	4	6	11	27
50–64	536	3.2	18	1	1	2	3	6	11	25
65+	450	3.6	23	1	1	2	4	7	11	28
GRAND TOTAL	1,827	2.7	16	1	1	1	3	5	8	22

LOS by Diagnosis and Operation, Western Region, 45th Edition

83.81: TENDON GRAFT

Type of Patients	Observed Patients	Avg. Stay	Variance	10th	25th	50th	75th	90th	95th	99th
1. SINGLE DX										
0–19 Years	1	1.0	0	1	1	1	1	1		1
20–34	6	1.5	<1	1	1	1	2	3	3	3
35–49	4	1.3	<1	1	1	1	1	2	2	2
50–64	3	1.3	<1	1	1	1	2	2	2	2
65+	0									
2. MULTIPLE DX										
0–19 Years	0									
20–34	4	2.3	4	1	1	2	5	5	5	5
35–49	13	1.7	1	1	1	1	3	3	4	4
50–64	35	2.5	3	1	1	2	3	6	6	7
65+	29	2.9	4	1	1	3	3	5	6	11
TOTAL SINGLE DX	14	1.4	<1	1	1	1	2	2	3	3
TOTAL MULTIPLE DX	81	2.5	3	1	1	2	3	5	6	11
TOTAL										
0–19 Years	1	1.0	0	1	1	1	1	1	1	1
20–34	10	1.8	2	1	1	1	2	5	5	5
35–49	17	1.6	1	1	1	1	2	3	4	4
50–64	38	2.4	3	1	1	2	3	6	6	7
65+	29	2.9	4	1	1	3	3	5	6	11
GRAND TOTAL	95	2.3	3	1	1	2	3	5	6	11

83.82: MUSCLE OR FASCIA GRAFT

Type of Patients	Observed Patients	Avg. Stay	Variance	10th	25th	50th	75th	90th	95th	99th
1. SINGLE DX										
0–19 Years	4	3.5	2	2	3	3	5	5	5	5
20–34	5	4.0	8	1	2	3	6	8	8	8
35–49	0									
50–64	1	1.0	0	1	1	1	1	1	1	1
65+	0									
2. MULTIPLE DX										
0–19 Years	11	4.6	5	1	4	4	6	8	8	8
20–34	22	13.9	203	3	6	7	21	28	53	57
35–49	29	8.4	89	1	2	5	11	22	27	42
50–64	62	8.6	89	1	2	5	12	20	27	44
65+	54	8.9	114	1	3	5	10	26	38	45
TOTAL SINGLE DX	10	3.5	4	1	2	3	5	6	8	8
TOTAL MULTIPLE DX	178	8.8	102	1	3	5	11	21	34	53
TOTAL										
0–19 Years	15	4.3	4	1	3	4	6	8	8	8
20–34	27	12.3	183	3	5	7	15	21	53	57
35–49	29	8.4	89	1	2	5	11	22	27	42
50–64	63	8.5	88	1	2	5	12	20	27	44
65+	54	8.9	114	1	3	5	10	26	38	45
GRAND TOTAL	188	8.4	96	1	3	5	10	21	28	45

83.85: CHANGE IN M/T LENGTH NEC

Type of Patients	Observed Patients	Avg. Stay	Variance	10th	25th	50th	75th	90th	95th	99th
1. SINGLE DX										
0–19 Years	56	1.3	<1	1	1	2	1	2	2	3
20–34	4	2.3	<1	1	1	3	3	3	3	3
35–49	1	3.0	0	3	3	3	3	3	3	3
50–64	1	1.0	0	1	1	1	1	1	1	1
65+	1	2.0	0	2	2	2	2	2	2	2
2. MULTIPLE DX										
0–19 Years	313	1.7	6	1	1	1	2	3	4	8
20–34	37	2.2	6	1	1	1	3	4	5	15
35–49	64	3.2	10	1	1	2	4	7	12	14
50–64	123	2.9	3	1	1	2	4	5	7	8
65+	84	3.4	11	1	2	3	3	6	11	22
TOTAL SINGLE DX	63	1.3	<1	1	1	1	1	2	2	3
TOTAL MULTIPLE DX	621	2.1	7	1	1	1	2	4	5	12
TOTAL										
0–19 Years	369	1.7	5	1	1	1	2	3	4	8
20–34	41	2.2	6	1	1	1	3	4	5	15
35–49	65	3.2	9	1	1	2	3	7	12	14
50–64	124	2.9	3	1	1	2	4	5	7	8
65+	85	3.4	11	1	2	3	3	6	11	22
GRAND TOTAL	684	2.0	6	1	1	1	2	3	5	12

83.86: QUADRICEPSPLASTY

Type of Patients	Observed Patients	Avg. Stay	Variance	10th	25th	50th	75th	90th	95th	99th
1. SINGLE DX										
0–19 Years	2	2.5	4	1	1	1	4	4	4	4
20–34	1	5.0	0	5	5	5	5	5	5	5
35–49	6	2.2	2	1	1	2	2	5	5	5
50–64	11	2.0	<1	1	1	2	2	3	4	4
65+	2	1.5	<1	1	1	1	2	2	2	2
2. MULTIPLE DX										
0–19 Years	2	1.0	0	1	1	1	1	1	1	1
20–34	2	1.5	<1	1	1	2	2	2	2	2
35–49	9	3.8	5	1	2	3	4	8	8	8
50–64	46	3.1	7	1	1	3	3	8	9	12
65+	39	3.0	4	1	2	3	4	5	8	11
TOTAL SINGLE DX	22	2.2	2	1	1	2	3	4	5	5
TOTAL MULTIPLE DX	98	3.0	6	1	1	2	3	6	8	11
TOTAL										
0–19 Years	4	1.4	1	1	1	1	1	4	4	4
20–34	3	2.7	4	1	1	2	5	5	5	5
35–49	15	3.1	5	1	2	2	4	7	9	8
50–64	57	2.9	4	1	1	2	3	6	9	12
65+	41	3.0	4	1	2	3	4	5	7	11
GRAND TOTAL	120	2.8	5	1	1	2	3	5	8	11

LOS by Diagnosis and Operation, Western Region, 45th Edition

Western Region, October 2007–September 2008 Data, by Operation

83.88: PLASTIC OPS TENDON NEC

Type of Patients	Observed Patients	Avg. Stay	Variance	10th	25th	50th	75th	90th	95th	99th
1. SINGLE DX										
0–19 Years	4	1.0	0	1	1	1	1	1	1	1
20–34	22	2.4	4	1	1	2	3	4	5	9
35–49	19	2.3	4	1	1	2	3	6	9	9
50–64	16	1.6	<1	1	1	1	2	3	4	4
65+	4	2.5	1	2	2	2	4	4	4	4
2. MULTIPLE DX										
0–19 Years	11	1.8	<1	1	1	1	2	2	3	3
20–34	33	1.9	1	1	1	1	3	4	4	5
35–49	87	2.5	13	1	1	1	3	5	5	33
50–64	215	2.2	6	1	1	1	3	4	6	12
65+	217	2.8	6	1	1	2	3	5	8	13
TOTAL SINGLE DX	65	2.1	3	1	1	1	2	4	5	9
TOTAL MULTIPLE DX	563	2.5	7	1	1	2	3	4	6	13
TOTAL										
0–19 Years	15	1.6	<1	1	1	1	2	2	3	3
20–34	55	2.1	2	1	1	1	3	4	5	9
35–49	106	2.5	12	1	1	1	3	5	6	33
50–64	231	2.2	6	1	1	1	2	4	6	12
65+	221	2.7	6	1	1	2	3	5	8	13
GRAND TOTAL	628	2.4	6	1	1	2	3	4	6	12

83.9: OTHER CONN TISSUE OPS

Type of Patients	Observed Patients	Avg. Stay	Variance	10th	25th	50th	75th	90th	95th	99th
1. SINGLE DX										
0–19 Years	4	3.6	<1	3	3	3	4	5	5	5
20–34	9	2.9	2	2	2	2	4	5	5	5
35–49	10	2.0	3	1	2	2	3	6	6	9
50–64	2	6.5	<1	6	6	7	7	7	7	7
65+	2	2.0	0	2	2	2	2	2	2	2
2. MULTIPLE DX										
0–19 Years	39	6.9	25	2	5	5	9	12	14	36
20–34	107	5.0	23	1	2	3	6	11	16	21
35–49	168	6.2	51	1	2	4	7	14	20	37
50–64	280	7.1	79	2	3	4	8	16	22	46
65+	364	7.5	60	2	3	5	9	15	21	44
TOTAL SINGLE DX	27	3.0	3	1	2	3	4	5	6	9
TOTAL MULTIPLE DX	958	6.9	58	2	3	5	8	14	20	37
TOTAL										
0–19 Years	43	6.6	24	2	3	4	8	12	14	36
20–34	116	4.8	21	2	2	3	6	11	16	21
35–49	178	6.0	49	1	2	4	7	14	20	37
50–64	282	7.1	78	2	3	4	8	16	22	46
65+	366	7.5	60	2	3	5	9	15	21	44
GRAND TOTAL	985	6.8	57	2	3	4	8	14	20	36

83.94: ASPIRATION OF BURSA

Type of Patients	Observed Patients	Avg. Stay	Variance	10th	25th	50th	75th	90th	95th	99th
1. SINGLE DX										
0–19 Years	0									
20–34	2	3.5	4	2	2	4	5	5	5	5
35–49	2	2.5	<1	2	2	2	3	3	3	3
50–64	0									
65+	0									
2. MULTIPLE DX										
0–19 Years	1	2.0	0	2	2	2	2	2	2	2
20–34	21	3.1	2	1	2	3	4	5	5	6
35–49	38	3.0	2	1	2	3	4	5	6	7
50–64	65	4.1	9	1	3	4	6	8	11	14
65+	73	5.2	47	1	3	4	6	8	11	56
TOTAL SINGLE DX	4	3.0	2	2	2	2	3	5	5	5
TOTAL MULTIPLE DX	198	4.1	21	2	2	3	5	7	9	21
TOTAL										
0–19 Years	1	2.0	0	2	2	2	2	2	2	2
20–34	23	3.1	2	1	2	3	4	5	5	6
35–49	40	3.0	2	1	2	3	4	5	6	7
50–64	65	4.1	9	1	3	4	6	8	11	14
65+	73	5.2	47	1	3	4	6	8	11	56
GRAND TOTAL	202	4.1	21	2	2	3	5	7	9	16

83.95: SOFT TISSUE ASP NEC

Type of Patients	Observed Patients	Avg. Stay	Variance	10th	25th	50th	75th	90th	95th	99th
1. SINGLE DX										
0–19 Years	4	3.6	<1	3	3	3	4	5	5	5
20–34	7	2.7	2	1	2	2	4	5	5	5
35–49	7	2.0	4	1	1	1	3	6	6	6
50–64	2	6.5	<1	6	6	7	7	7	7	7
65+	1	2.0	0	2	2	2	2	2	2	2
2. MULTIPLE DX										
0–19 Years	35	7.5	27	3	5	6	10	14	14	36
20–34	70	5.9	30	1	2	4	8	11	17	30
35–49	109	7.6	61	2	3	5	9	16	22	35
50–64	164	8.0	68	2	3	5	10	19	22	46
65+	194	9.2	76	3	4	7	11	18	23	57
TOTAL SINGLE DX	21	3.1	3	1	2	3	4	6	6	7
TOTAL MULTIPLE DX	572	8.0	61	2	3	6	10	16	22	44
TOTAL										
0–19 Years	39	7.0	25	3	4	5	9	12	14	36
20–34	77	5.6	29	1	2	3	7	11	17	30
35–49	116	7.3	59	2	3	4	9	16	22	35
50–64	166	8.0	67	2	3	5	10	19	22	46
65+	195	9.2	75	2	4	7	11	18	23	57
GRAND TOTAL	593	7.8	60	2	3	5	10	16	21	37

LOS by Diagnosis and Operation, Western Region, 45th Edition

Western Region, October 2007–September 2008 Data, by Operation

83.96: INJECTION INTO BURSA

Type of Patients	Observed Patients	Avg. Stay	Vari-ance	Percentiles						
				10th	25th	50th	75th	90th	95th	99th
1. SINGLE DX										
0–19 Years	0									
20–34	0									
35–49	0									
50–64	0									
65+	0									
2. MULTIPLE DX										
0–19 Years	1	5.0	0	5	5	5	5	5	5	5
20–34	3	4.7	8	3	3	3	8	8	8	8
35–49	6	8.7	195	2	2	3	4	37	37	37
50–64	19	9.0	67	1	4	6	10	25	31	31
65+	71	6.0	24	2	3	5	8	12	16	23
TOTAL SINGLE DX	0									
TOTAL MULTIPLE DX	100	6.6	40	2	3	5	8	13	22	31
TOTAL										
0–19 Years	1	5.0	0	5	5	5	5	5	5	5
20–34	3	4.7	8	3	3	3	8	8	8	8
35–49	6	8.7	195	2	2	3	4	37	37	37
50–64	19	9.0	67	1	4	6	10	25	31	31
65+	71	6.0	24	2	3	5	8	12	16	23
GRAND TOTAL	100	6.6	40	2	3	5	8	13	22	31

84.01: FINGER AMPUTATION

Type of Patients	Observed Patients	Avg. Stay	Vari-ance	Percentiles						
				10th	25th	50th	75th	90th	95th	99th
1. SINGLE DX										
0–19 Years	13	1.2	<1	1	1	1	1	2	2	2
20–34	25	1.9	7	1	1	1	2	3	4	14
35–49	19	1.7	7	1	1	1	2	3	5	5
50–64	15	1.3	<1	1	1	1	1	2	3	3
65+	3	1.0	0	1	1	1	1	1	1	1
2. MULTIPLE DX										
0–19 Years	43	6.4	218	1	1	1	2	8	57	57
20–34	102	3.2	19	1	1	1	4	8	11	18
35–49	151	5.1	61	1	1	2	6	12	18	33
50–64	226	5.3	37	1	1	3	7	11	16	29
65+	143	5.5	33	1	1	4	7	13	18	33
TOTAL SINGLE DX	75	1.5	2	1	1	1	2	2	3	14
TOTAL MULTIPLE DX	665	5.1	56	1	1	2	6	11	17	42
TOTAL										
0–19 Years	56	5.0	165	1	1	1	2	6	42	57
20–34	127	3.0	17	1	1	1	3	7	11	18
35–49	170	4.7	56	1	1	2	5	12	17	33
50–64	241	5.1	36	1	1	3	6	11	15	29
65+	146	5.4	33	1	1	4	7	13	18	33
GRAND TOTAL	740	4.7	51	1	1	2	5	11	16	42

84.0: AMPUTATION OF UPPER LIMB

Type of Patients	Observed Patients	Avg. Stay	Vari-ance	Percentiles						
				10th	25th	50th	75th	90th	95th	99th
1. SINGLE DX										
0–19 Years	17	2.5	12	1	1	1	2	11	11	11
20–34	39	2.2	6	1	1	1	3	4	9	14
35–49	24	1.8	1	1	1	1	2	3	4	5
50–64	22	1.2	<1	1	1	1	1	2	2	3
65+	4	1.0	0	1	1	1	1	1	1	1
2. MULTIPLE DX										
0–19 Years	52	6.0	176	1	1	2	4	16	57	>99
20–34	127	3.9	24	1	1	2	5	11	14	32
35–49	195	5.9	77	1	1	3	7	14	22	>99
50–64	289	5.7	46	1	1	3	8	13	16	39
65+	192	5.6	36	1	1	4	7	14	19	33
TOTAL SINGLE DX	106	2.0	6	1	1	1	2	3	9	11
TOTAL MULTIPLE DX	855	5.5	59	1	1	3	7	13	20	57
TOTAL										
0–19 Years	69	5.0	133	1	1	2	4	11	57	>99
20–34	166	3.5	20	1	1	2	6	10	14	32
35–49	219	5.4	71	1	1	2	6	13	21	75
50–64	311	5.4	44	1	1	3	7	13	16	29
65+	196	5.5	36	1	1	3	7	14	19	33
GRAND TOTAL	961	5.1	54	1	1	2	6	12	18	57

84.02: THUMB AMPUTATION

Type of Patients	Observed Patients	Avg. Stay	Vari-ance	Percentiles						
				10th	25th	50th	75th	90th	95th	99th
1. SINGLE DX										
0–19 Years	3	1.0	0	1	1	1	1	1	1	1
20–34	9	2.0	3	1	1	1	3	6	6	6
35–49	5	2.2	2	1	1	2	3	4	4	4
50–64	4	1.0	0	1	1	1	1	1	1	1
65+	0									
2. MULTIPLE DX										
0–19 Years	6	3.0	3	1	1	3	5	5	5	5
20–34	14	5.8	39	1	2	3	10	11	24	24
35–49	20	4.0	26	1	1	2	6	8	23	23
50–64	22	3.1	9	1	1	2	4	7	8	12
65+	21	3.1	10	1	1	1	4	6	8	13
TOTAL SINGLE DX	21	1.7	2	1	1	1	2	3	4	6
TOTAL MULTIPLE DX	83	3.8	17	1	1	2	5	8	11	24
TOTAL										
0–19 Years	9	2.6	3	1	1	2	5	5	5	5
20–34	23	4.3	27	1	1	3	5	10	11	24
35–49	25	3.7	21	1	1	2	4	7	8	23
50–64	26	2.8	8	1	1	2	3	6	8	12
65+	21	3.1	10	1	1	1	4	6	8	13
GRAND TOTAL	104	3.4	15	1	1	2	4	7	10	23

LOS by Diagnosis and Operation, Western Region, 45th Edition

Western Region, October 2007–September 2008 Data, by Operation

84.1: AMPUTATION OF LOWER LIMB

Type of Patients	Observed Patients	Avg. Stay	Variance	10th	25th	50th	75th	90th	95th	99th
1. SINGLE DX										
0–19 Years	19	1.8	3	1	1	1	1	5	6	6
20–34	12	3.6	8	1	2	3	5	7	11	11
35–49	13	4.5	13	1	2	4	6	8	13	13
50–64	7	4.0	8	1	1	3	7	7	7	7
65+	6	2.3	<1	1	2	2	3	3	3	3
2. MULTIPLE DX										
0–19 Years	70	6.3	92	1	1	3	7	15	22	53
20–34	334	10.5	113	2	4	7	13	21	34	48
35–49	2,028	9.8	80	3	4	7	12	19	26	48
50–64	5,025	10.4	92	3	5	8	13	21	28	56
65+	6,392	9.6	62	3	5	7	12	19	24	39
TOTAL SINGLE DX	57	2.7	7	1	1	1	4	6	7	13
TOTAL MULTIPLE DX	13,849	9.9	77	3	5	7	12	20	26	46
TOTAL										
0–19 Years	89	5.4	77	1	1	2	6	15	21	53
20–34	346	10.3	111	2	4	7	13	21	33	48
35–49	2,041	9.7	80	3	4	7	12	19	26	48
50–64	5,032	10.4	92	3	5	8	13	21	28	56
65+	6,398	9.6	62	3	5	7	12	19	24	39
GRAND TOTAL	13,906	9.9	77	3	5	7	12	20	26	46

84.11: TOE AMPUTATION

Type of Patients	Observed Patients	Avg. Stay	Variance	10th	25th	50th	75th	90th	95th	99th
1. SINGLE DX										
0–19 Years	10	1.2	<1	1	1	1	1	1	1	5
20–34	6	2.2	1	1	1	2	3	4	4	4
35–49	7	2.4	1	1	1	2	2	8	8	8
50–64	1	1.0	0	1	1	1	1	1	1	1
65+	3	2.0	<1	1	1	2	3	3	3	3
2. MULTIPLE DX										
0–19 Years	16	9.3	253	1	1	3	15	38	53	53
20–34	154	8.3	66	3	4	6	9	19	27	44
35–49	1,062	7.7	37	2	4	6	9	14	19	32
50–64	2,326	8.1	53	2	4	6	10	15	20	34
65+	2,093	7.4	33	2	4	6	9	14	18	28
TOTAL SINGLE DX	27	1.6	2	1	1	1	2	3	4	8
TOTAL MULTIPLE DX	5,651	7.8	44	2	4	6	9	15	20	33
TOTAL										
0–19 Years	26	6.3	174	1	1	2	9	19	53	53
20–34	160	8.1	65	1	4	6	9	19	27	44
35–49	1,069	7.6	37	2	4	6	9	14	19	32
50–64	2,327	8.1	53	2	4	6	10	15	20	34
65+	2,096	7.4	33	2	4	6	9	14	18	28
GRAND TOTAL	5,678	7.7	44	2	4	6	9	15	19	33

84.12: AMPUTATION THROUGH FOOT

Type of Patients	Observed Patients	Avg. Stay	Variance	10th	25th	50th	75th	90th	95th	99th
1. SINGLE DX										
0–19 Years	1	1.0	0	1	1	1	1	1	1	1
20–34	1	11.0	0	11	11	11	11	11	11	11
35–49	1	8.0	0	8	8	8	8	8	8	8
50–64	2	7.0	0	7	7	7	7	7	7	7
65+	0									
2. MULTIPLE DX										
0–19 Years	6	8.3	91	1	3	3	7	21	21	36
20–34	52	11.7	107	3	7	9	13	21	27	68
35–49	320	11.1	101	3	5	8	14	22	32	55
50–64	750	11.2	94	3	5	8	14	22	30	50
65+	847	10.6	75	3	5	8	14	21	28	43
TOTAL SINGLE DX	5	6.8	13	1	7	7	8	11	11	11
TOTAL MULTIPLE DX	1,975	10.9	87	3	5	8	14	22	29	50
TOTAL										
0–19 Years	7	8.0	89	1	3	3	7	21	21	36
20–34	53	11.7	105	3	7	9	13	21	27	68
35–49	321	11.1	100	3	5	8	14	22	32	55
50–64	752	11.2	94	3	5	8	14	22	30	50
65+	847	10.6	75	3	5	8	14	21	28	43
GRAND TOTAL	1,980	10.9	87	3	5	8	14	22	29	50

84.15: BK AMPUTATION NEC

Type of Patients	Observed Patients	Avg. Stay	Variance	10th	25th	50th	75th	90th	95th	99th
1. SINGLE DX										
0–19 Years	1	1.0	0	1	1	1	1	1	1	1
20–34	1	2.0	0	2	2	2	2	2	2	2
35–49	4	5.0	<1	4	4	5	5	6	6	6
50–64	3	3.3	10	1	1	2	7	7	7	7
65+	0									
2. MULTIPLE DX										
0–19 Years	12	4.1	26	1	1	3	6	11	22	22
20–34	81	11.4	174	2	3	9	15	23	36	95
35–49	497	12.2	116	3	5	9	15	24	31	50
50–64	1,378	12.6	113	4	6	10	16	25	35	67
65+	1,948	10.8	72	3	5	8	14	21	26	43
TOTAL SINGLE DX	9	3.0	5	1	1	2	5	6	7	7
TOTAL MULTIPLE DX	3,916	11.6	95	3	5	9	15	22	30	48
TOTAL										
0–19 Years	13	3.6	23	1	1	1	4	7	11	22
20–34	82	11.3	173	2	3	9	14	23	36	95
35–49	501	12.2	115	3	5	9	15	24	31	50
50–64	1,381	12.6	113	4	6	10	16	25	35	67
65+	1,948	10.8	72	3	5	8	14	21	26	43
GRAND TOTAL	3,925	11.6	95	3	5	9	15	22	30	48

Western Region, October 2007–September 2008 Data, by Operation

84.17: ABOVE KNEE AMPUTATION

Type of Patients	Observed Patients	Avg. Stay	Vari-ance	Percentiles						
				10th	25th	50th	75th	90th	95th	99th
1. SINGLE DX										
0–19 Years	3	4.3	1	3	3	5	5	5	5	5
20–34	4	4.2	5	2	2	5	5	7	7	7
35–49	0									
50–64	1	3.0	0	3	3	3	3	3	3	3
65+	3	2.7	<1	2	2	3	3	3	3	3
2. MULTIPLE DX										
0–19 Years	11	8.1	35	2	7	7	7	19	26	26
20–34	25	15.9	179	5	7	11	18	43	44	48
35–49	94	14.6	201	3	6	9	21	34	51	>99
50–64	466	13.1	144	4	6	8	16	28	36	77
65+	1,382	10.5	68	3	5	8	13	20	26	44
TOTAL SINGLE DX	11	3.7	2	2	3	3	5	5	7	7
TOTAL MULTIPLE DX	1,978	11.4	95	3	5	8	14	23	30	57
TOTAL										
0–19 Years	14	7.5	31	3	5	7	7	9	26	26
20–34	29	14.3	170	2	6	10	16	43	44	48
35–49	94	14.6	201	3	6	9	21	34	51	>99
50–64	467	13.1	144	4	6	8	16	28	36	77
65+	1,385	10.5	68	3	5	8	13	20	26	44
GRAND TOTAL	1,989	11.3	95	3	5	8	14	23	30	57

84.3: AMPUTATION STUMP REV

Type of Patients	Observed Patients	Avg. Stay	Vari-ance	Percentiles						
				10th	25th	50th	75th	90th	95th	99th
1. SINGLE DX										
0–19 Years	6	1.5	<1	1	1	2	2	2	2	2
20–34	6	1.5	<1	1	1	2	2	3	3	3
35–49	6	2.2	2	1	1	3	3	4	4	4
50–64	3	3.4	2	2	2	3	5	5	5	5
65+	1	6.0	0	6	6	6	6	6	6	6
2. MULTIPLE DX										
0–19 Years	15	2.5	4	1	2	3	3	3	4	13
20–34	54	5.6	41	1	2	3	7	13	20	30
35–49	193	6.4	35	1	3	5	8	13	18	36
50–64	364	7.6	57	2	3	5	10	15	25	43
65+	369	7.4	31	2	3	6	10	15	19	26
TOTAL SINGLE DX	22	2.1	2	1	1	2	3	4	5	6
TOTAL MULTIPLE DX	995	7.0	41	1	3	5	9	14	19	33
TOTAL										
0–19 Years	21	2.4	3	1	2	2	3	3	3	13
20–34	60	5.2	38	1	2	3	7	13	18	30
35–49	199	6.3	34	1	3	5	8	13	18	36
50–64	367	7.5	56	2	3	5	10	15	25	43
65+	370	7.4	31	2	3	6	10	15	19	26
GRAND TOTAL	1,017	6.9	41	1	3	5	9	14	19	33

84.2: EXTREMITY REATTACHMENT

Type of Patients	Observed Patients	Avg. Stay	Vari-ance	Percentiles						
				10th	25th	50th	75th	90th	95th	99th
1. SINGLE DX										
0–19 Years	4	1.4	1	1	1	1	1	1	5	5
20–34	7	3.3	2	2	2	3	5	5	5	5
35–49	4	6.0	3	4	5	7	8	8	8	8
50–64	6	3.0	6	1	1	1	6	6	6	6
65+	0									
2. MULTIPLE DX										
0–19 Years	16	6.7	14	2	4	7	9	13	13	13
20–34	25	5.3	12	2	3	5	7	8	11	18
35–49	21	6.1	14	2	4	5	8	11	12	15
50–64	28	5.9	10	2	2	6	9	10	11	11
65+	8	3.6	5	1	2	5	6	6	6	6
TOTAL SINGLE DX	21	2.9	5	1	1	2	5	6	7	8
TOTAL MULTIPLE DX	98	5.7	12	2	3	5	8	11	12	18
TOTAL										
0–19 Years	20	4.6	16	1	1	3	8	11	13	13
20–34	32	4.8	11	2	2	5	5	7	11	18
35–49	25	6.1	12	2	4	5	8	11	12	15
50–64	34	5.4	11	1	2	6	8	10	11	11
65+	8	3.6	5	1	2	5	6	6	6	6
GRAND TOTAL	119	5.1	12	1	2	5	7	10	11	15

84.4: IMPL OR FIT PROSTH LIMB

Type of Patients	Observed Patients	Avg. Stay	Vari-ance	Percentiles						
				10th	25th	50th	75th	90th	95th	99th
1. SINGLE DX										
0–19 Years	0									
20–34	0									
35–49	0									
50–64	0									
65+	0									
2. MULTIPLE DX										
0–19 Years	0									
20–34	0									
35–49	0									
50–64	0									
65+	0									
TOTAL SINGLE DX	0									
TOTAL MULTIPLE DX	0									
TOTAL										
0–19 Years	0									
20–34	0									
35–49	0									
50–64	0									
65+	0									
GRAND TOTAL	0									

LOS by Diagnosis and Operation, Western Region, 45th Edition

Western Region, October 2007–September 2008 Data, by Operation

84.5: IMPL OTH MS DEV & SUBST

Type of Patients	Observed Patients	Avg. Stay	Vari-ance	Percentiles						
				10th	25th	50th	75th	90th	95th	99th
1. SINGLE DX										
0–19 Years	3	2.7	1	2	2		4	4	4	4
20–34	1	1.0	0	1	1		1	1	1	1
35–49	0									
50–64	6	1.3	<1	1	1		1	3	3	3
65+	2	2.0	0	2	2		2	2	2	2
2. MULTIPLE DX										
0–19 Years	13	5.8	22	1	1	6	7	16	16	16
20–34	3	2.0	<1	1	1	2	3	3	3	3
35–49	21	4.7	17	2	3	3	5	9	12	18
50–64	50	4.5	13	1	2	3	5	9	12	18
65+	71	3.3	6	1	1	2	4	7	8	11
TOTAL SINGLE DX	12	1.8	<1	1	1	1	2	3	4	4
TOTAL MULTIPLE DX	158	4.2	13	1	2	3	6	9	12	18
TOTAL										
0–19 Years	16	5.5	21	1	2	4	7	16	16	16
20–34	4	1.8	<1	1	1	1	2	3	3	3
35–49	21	4.7	17	2	3	3	5	9	12	18
50–64	56	4.2	12	1	2	3	5	9	12	18
65+	73	3.2	6	1	1	2	4	7	8	11
GRAND TOTAL	170	4.1	13	1	2	3	5	9	11	18

84.6: SPINAL DISC REPLACEMENT

Type of Patients	Observed Patients	Avg. Stay	Vari-ance	Percentiles						
				10th	25th	50th	75th	90th	95th	99th
1. SINGLE DX										
0–19 Years	1	2.0	0	2	2	2	2	2	2	2
20–34	31	2.1	1	1	1	2	2	4	5	5
35–49	55	1.9	1	1	1	2	3	3	4	6
50–64	31	1.9	1	1	1	2	3	4	4	4
65+	2	2.0	2	1	1	1	3	3	3	3
2. MULTIPLE DX										
0–19 Years	2	1.0	0	1	1	1	1	1	1	1
20–34	99	3.0	21	1	1	2	3	5	6	7
35–49	327	2.1	4	1	1	2	3	4	5	8
50–64	226	2.3	4	1	1	2	3	4	5	11
65+	37	2.1	2	1	1	2	3	4	5	6
TOTAL SINGLE DX	120	1.9	1	1	1	2	2	4	4	6
TOTAL MULTIPLE DX	691	2.3	5	1	1	2	3	4	5	10
TOTAL										
0–19 Years	3	1.2	<1	1	1	1	1	2	2	2
20–34	130	2.8	16	1	1	2	3	5	5	7
35–49	382	2.0	4	1	1	2	3	4	4	8
50–64	257	2.2	4	1	1	2	3	4	5	11
65+	39	2.1	2	1	1	2	3	4	5	6
GRAND TOTAL	811	2.2	5	1	1	2	3	4	5	8

84.62: INSERT TOT C IVD PROSTH

Type of Patients	Observed Patients	Avg. Stay	Vari-ance	Percentiles						
				10th	25th	50th	75th	90th	95th	99th
1. SINGLE DX										
0–19 Years	0									
20–34	7	1.1	<1	1	1	1	1	2	2	2
35–49	23	1.1	<1	1	1	1	1	2	2	2
50–64	13	1.5	<1	1	1	1	2	3	4	4
65+	1	3.0	0	3	3	3	3	3	3	3
2. MULTIPLE DX										
0–19 Years	1	1.0	0	1	1	1	1	1	1	1
20–34	25	3.2	79	1	1	1	2	3	6	46
35–49	154	1.5	<1	1	1	1	2	3	3	5
50–64	134	1.8	4	1	1	1	2	3	5	11
65+	18	1.8	2	1	1	1	2	5	6	6
TOTAL SINGLE DX	44	1.3	<1	1	1	1	1	2	3	4
TOTAL MULTIPLE DX	332	1.8	8	1	1	1	2	3	4	10
TOTAL										
0–19 Years	1	1.0	0	1	1	1	1	1	1	1
20–34	32	2.7	62	1	1	1	2	3	6	46
35–49	177	1.5	<1	1	1	1	2	3	3	5
50–64	147	1.8	4	1	1	1	2	3	5	11
65+	19	1.9	2	1	1	1	2	5	6	6
GRAND TOTAL	376	1.7	7	1	1	1	2	3	4	10

84.65: INSERT TOT LS IVD PROSTH

Type of Patients	Observed Patients	Avg. Stay	Vari-ance	Percentiles						
				10th	25th	50th	75th	90th	95th	99th
1. SINGLE DX										
0–19 Years	0									
20–34	18	2.5	2	1	1	2	3	5	5	5
35–49	25	2.6	2	1	2	2	4	6	6	6
50–64	15	2.4	1	1	1	2	4	4	4	4
65+	0									
2. MULTIPLE DX										
0–19 Years	0									
20–34	67	3.0	2	1	2	3	4	5	6	7
35–49	131	2.8	2	1	2	3	4	6	6	9
50–64	67	2.8	2	1	2	3	4	5	5	7
65+	2	3.5	<1	3	3	3	4	4	4	4
TOTAL SINGLE DX	58	2.5	2	1	2	2	3	4	5	6
TOTAL MULTIPLE DX	267	2.9	2	1	2	3	4	4	6	8
TOTAL										
0–19 Years	0									
20–34	85	2.9	2	1	2	3	4	5	5	7
35–49	156	2.8	2	1	2	3	4	4	6	9
50–64	82	2.8	2	1	2	3	4	4	5	7
65+	2	3.5	<1	3	3	3	4	4	4	4
GRAND TOTAL	325	2.8	2	1	2	3	3	4	5	7

LOS by Diagnosis and Operation, Western Region, 45th Edition

Western Region, October 2007–September 2008 Data, by Operation

84.7: ADJUNCT CODE EXT FIX DEV

Type of Patients	Observed Patients	Avg. Stay	Vari-ance	Percentiles						
				10th	25th	50th	75th	90th	95th	99th
1. SINGLE DX										
0–19 Years	0									
20–34	1	2.0	0	2	2	2	2	2	2	2
35–49	0									
50–64	0									
65+	0									
2. MULTIPLE DX										
0–19 Years	0									
20–34	0									
35–49	1	3.0	0	3	3	3	3	3	3	3
50–64	1	1.0	0	1	1	1	1	1	1	1
65+	0									
TOTAL SINGLE DX	1	2.0	0	2	2	2	2	2	2	2
TOTAL MULTIPLE DX	2	2.0	2	1	1	3	3	3	3	3
TOTAL										
0–19 Years	0									
20–34	1	2.0	0	2	2	2	2	2	2	2
35–49	1	3.0	0	3	3	3	3	3	3	3
50–64	1	1.0	0	1	1	1	1	1	1	1
65+	0									
GRAND TOTAL	3	2.0	<1	1	1	2	3	3	3	3

84.8: INSERT/REPL/REV SPIN DEV

Type of Patients	Observed Patients	Avg. Stay	Vari-ance	Percentiles						
				10th	25th	50th	75th	90th	95th	99th
1. SINGLE DX										
0–19 Years	0									
20–34	3	2.7	4	1	1	2	5	5	5	5
35–49	4	1.3	<1	1	1	1	1	2	2	2
50–64	14	1.4	<1	1	1	1	1	3	3	3
65+	23	1.1	<1	1	1	1	1	1	2	2
2. MULTIPLE DX										
0–19 Years	2	1.8	<1	1	2	2	2	2	2	2
20–34	11	2.1	2	1	1	1	3	4	4	4
35–49	38	2.5	2	1	1	2	3	5	6	7
50–64	186	2.2	3	1	1	2	3	4	5	8
65+	852	2.0	3	1	1	1	2	4	5	8
TOTAL SINGLE DX	44	1.3	<1	1	1	1	1	2	3	5
TOTAL MULTIPLE DX	1,089	2.0	3	1	1	1	3	4	5	8
TOTAL										
0–19 Years	2	1.8	<1	1	2	2	2	2	2	2
20–34	14	2.2	2	1	1	2	3	4	5	5
35–49	42	2.4	2	1	1	2	3	4	5	7
50–64	200	2.2	3	1	1	2	3	4	5	7
65+	875	2.0	3	1	1	1	2	4	5	8
GRAND TOTAL	1,133	2.0	3	1	1	1	3	4	5	8

84.80: INS/REPL INTSP PROC DEV

Type of Patients	Observed Patients	Avg. Stay	Vari-ance	Percentiles						
				10th	25th	50th	75th	90th	95th	99th
1. SINGLE DX										
0–19 Years	0									
20–34	2	1.5	<1	1	1	2	2	2	2	2
35–49	2	1.5	<1	1	1	1	2	2	2	2
50–64	14	1.4	<1	1	1	1	1	3	3	3
65+	23	1.1	<1	1	1	1	1	1	2	2
2. MULTIPLE DX										
0–19 Years	1	1.0	0	1	1	1	1	1	1	1
20–34	7	1.4	<1	1	1	1	1	4	4	4
35–49	19	1.7	<1	1	1	1	2	3	4	4
50–64	141	1.7	<1	1	1	1	2	3	4	4
65+	807	1.9	2	1	1	1	2	3	5	8
TOTAL SINGLE DX	41	1.2	<1	1	1	1	1	2	2	3
TOTAL MULTIPLE DX	975	1.8	2	1	1	1	2	3	4	8
TOTAL										
0–19 Years	1	1.0	0	1	1	1	1	1	1	1
20–34	9	1.5	1	1	1	1	1	4	4	4
35–49	21	1.7	<1	1	1	1	2	3	3	4
50–64	155	1.6	<1	1	1	1	2	3	4	4
65+	830	1.8	2	1	1	1	2	3	5	8
GRAND TOTAL	1,016	1.8	2	1	1	1	2	3	4	7

84.9: OTHER MUSCULOSKELETAL OP

Type of Patients	Observed Patients	Avg. Stay	Vari-ance	Percentiles						
				10th	25th	50th	75th	90th	95th	99th
1. SINGLE DX										
0–19 Years	0									
20–34	1	1.0	0	1	1	1	1	1	1	1
35–49	0									
50–64	0									
65+	0									
2. MULTIPLE DX										
0–19 Years	2	29.0	0	29	29	29	29	29	29	29
20–34	1	2.0	0	2	2	2	2	2	2	2
35–49	0									
50–64	0									
65+	0									
TOTAL SINGLE DX	1	1.0	0	1	1	1	1	1	1	1
TOTAL MULTIPLE DX	3	23.2	157	2	29	29	29	29	29	29
TOTAL										
0–19 Years	2	29.0	0	29	29	29	29	29	29	29
20–34	2	1.5	<1	1	1	2	2	2	2	2
35–49	0									
50–64	0									
65+	0									
GRAND TOTAL	4	19.2	211	1	2	29	29	29	29	29

LOS by Diagnosis and Operation, Western Region, 45th Edition

Western Region, October 2007–September 2008 Data, by Operation

85.0: MASTOTOMY

Type of Patients	Observed Patients	Avg. Stay	Variance	Percentiles						
				10th	25th	50th	75th	90th	95th	99th
1. SINGLE DX										
0–19 Years	39	2.6	3	1	1	2	4	5	6	7
20–34	106	2.5	5	1	1	2	3	5	6	11
35–49	43	2.0	3	1	1	1	2	3	4	11
50–64	16	2.0	<1	1	1	2	2	4	4	10
65+	1	1.0	0	1	1	1	1	1	1	1
2. MULTIPLE DX										
0–19 Years	87	3.3	4	1	2	3	4	6	7	10
20–34	202	3.5	6	1	2	3	4	6	8	12
35–49	224	3.7	17	1	1	3	4	7	10	15
50–64	223	3.7	11	1	2	3	4	7	10	16
65+	131	4.2	9	1	2	3	6	8	10	16
TOTAL SINGLE DX	205	2.4	4	1	1	2	3	4	5	11
TOTAL MULTIPLE DX	867	3.6	10	1	2	3	4	7	9	15
TOTAL										
0–19 Years	126	3.2	4	1	2	3	4	6	6	9
20–34	308	3.1	6	1	1	2	4	6	7	12
35–49	267	3.4	15	1	1	3	4	7	9	15
50–64	239	3.6	10	1	2	3	4	7	10	16
65+	132	4.2	9	2	2	3	6	8	10	16
GRAND TOTAL	1,072	3.4	9	1	2	3	4	6	9	14

85.11: PERC BREAST BIOPSY

Type of Patients	Observed Patients	Avg. Stay	Variance	Percentiles						
				10th	25th	50th	75th	90th	95th	99th
1. SINGLE DX										
0–19 Years	2	2.6	<1	1	3	3	3	3	3	3
20–34	2	1.0	0	1	1	1	1	3	3	1
35–49	2	2.0	2	1	1	3	3	3	3	3
50–64	3	1.7	1	1	1	1	3	3	3	3
65+	0									
2. MULTIPLE DX										
0–19 Years	3	4.4	1	3	4	4	6	6	6	6
20–34	16	4.2	5	2	3	4	6	7	9	9
35–49	46	6.9	65	1	2	4	9	21	21	40
50–64	120	6.4	26	2	3	5	8	13	16	24
65+	144	7.8	71	2	4	6	9	15	17	41
TOTAL SINGLE DX	9	2.0	1	1	1	1	3	3	3	3
TOTAL MULTIPLE DX	329	6.9	50	2	3	5	8	13	17	36
TOTAL										
0–19 Years	5	3.6	2	3	3	3	4	6	6	6
20–34	18	3.8	5	1	2	4	6	7	9	9
35–49	48	6.7	63	2	3	5	9	21	21	40
50–64	123	6.2	26	2	3	5	8	12	16	24
65+	144	7.8	71	2	4	6	9	15	17	41
GRAND TOTAL	338	6.7	49	2	3	5	8	13	17	36

85.1: BREAST DIAGNOSTIC PX

Type of Patients	Observed Patients	Avg. Stay	Variance	Percentiles						
				10th	25th	50th	75th	90th	95th	99th
1. SINGLE DX										
0–19 Years	4	2.3	<1	1	1	3	3	3	3	3
20–34	8	1.5	<1	1	1	2	2	2	2	2
35–49	4	2.0	1	1	1	3	3	3	3	3
50–64	8	1.4	<1	1	1	1	1	2	3	3
65+	2	1.5	<1	1	1	2	2	2	2	2
2. MULTIPLE DX										
0–19 Years	5	3.7	3	1	3	4	4	6	6	6
20–34	53	4.4	10	1	2	4	6	7	9	16
35–49	98	5.9	39	1	2	4	8	12	21	40
50–64	184	6.1	30	1	3	5	7	13	17	28
65+	199	7.7	60	2	3	6	9	15	17	28
TOTAL SINGLE DX	26	1.7	<1	1	1	1	2	3	3	3
TOTAL MULTIPLE DX	539	6.5	41	1	3	5	8	13	17	28
TOTAL										
0–19 Years	9	3.1	2	1	2	3	3	6	6	9
20–34	61	4.0	10	1	2	4	5	7	9	16
35–49	102	5.8	38	1	2	4	8	12	15	29
50–64	192	5.9	30	1	3	5	7	12	17	28
65+	201	7.6	60	2	3	6	9	15	17	28
GRAND TOTAL	565	6.2	40	1	2	5	8	13	16	28

85.12: OPEN BIOPSY OF BREAST

Type of Patients	Observed Patients	Avg. Stay	Variance	Percentiles						
				10th	25th	50th	75th	90th	95th	99th
1. SINGLE DX										
0–19 Years	2	1.5	<1	1	1	1	2	2	2	2
20–34	6	1.7	<1	1	1	2	2	2	2	2
35–49	5	2.0	2	1	1	3	3	3	3	3
50–64	5	1.2	<1	1	1	1	1	2	2	2
65+	2	1.5	<1	1	1	2	2	2	2	2
2. MULTIPLE DX										
0–19 Years	2	1.5	<1	1	1	2	2	2	2	2
20–34	37	4.5	12	1	2	4	6	9	16	16
35–49	52	5.0	15	1	2	4	7	11	12	15
50–64	62	5.8	39	1	2	4	7	13	22	28
65+	53	7.7	34	1	4	6	11	15	20	28
TOTAL SINGLE DX	17	1.5	<1	1	1	1	2	2	3	3
TOTAL MULTIPLE DX	206	5.8	28	1	2	4	7	13	16	26
TOTAL										
0–19 Years	4	1.5	<1	1	1	1	2	2	2	2
20–34	43	4.1	12	1	2	3	5	7	9	16
35–49	54	4.9	14	1	1	4	7	11	12	15
50–64	67	5.4	38	1	2	4	7	13	22	28
65+	55	7.5	34	1	3	6	11	15	20	28
GRAND TOTAL	223	5.5	27	1	2	4	7	12	16	26

LOS by Diagnosis and Operation, Western Region, 45th Edition

85.2: EXC/DESTR BREAST TISSUE

Type of Patients	Observed Patients	Avg. Stay	Variance	10th	25th	50th	75th	90th	95th	99th
1. SINGLE DX										
0–19 Years	2	2.0	2	1	1	1	3	3	3	3
20–34	19	3.2	10	1	1	2	4	6	14	14
35–49	29	1.3	<1	1	1	1	1	3	3	4
50–64	22	1.1	<1	1	1	1	1	1	2	2
65+	15	1.1	<1	1	1	1	1	2	2	2
2. MULTIPLE DX										
0–19 Years	20	5.0	21	1	1	3	8	13	13	13
20–34	75	3.7	8	1	1	3	5	8	9	15
35–49	190	3.3	21	1	1	2	3	7	14	32
50–64	364	3.5	26	1	1	1	4	9	13	30
65+	345	2.8	15	1	1	1	2	6	10	21
TOTAL SINGLE DX	87	1.7	3	1	1	1	2	3	4	14
TOTAL MULTIPLE DX	994	3.2	20	1	1	1	3	8	13	21
TOTAL										
0–19 Years	22	4.8	20	1	1	3	7	13	13	13
20–34	94	3.6	8	1	1	3	5	8	9	15
35–49	219	3.0	19	1	1	1	3	7	11	20
50–64	386	3.4	25	1	1	1	3	9	13	30
65+	360	2.7	15	1	1	1	2	6	10	21
GRAND TOTAL	1,081	3.1	19	1	1	1	3	7	12	21

85.21: LOCAL EXC BREAST LESION

Type of Patients	Observed Patients	Avg. Stay	Variance	10th	25th	50th	75th	90th	95th	99th
1. SINGLE DX										
0–19 Years	2	2.0	2	1	1	1	3	3	3	3
20–34	17	2.7	3	1	1	2	4	6	6	6
35–49	17	1.5	<1	1	1	1	1	3	4	4
50–64	14	1.1	<1	1	1	1	1	1	2	2
65+	7	1.1	<1	1	1	1	1	2	2	2
2. MULTIPLE DX										
0–19 Years	20	5.0	21	1	1	3	8	13	13	13
20–34	69	3.8	8	1	2	3	5	8	9	15
35–49	135	3.6	24	1	1	2	4	7	14	32
50–64	253	4.2	34	1	1	2	5	11	15	33
65+	211	3.3	21	1	1	1	4	8	13	21
TOTAL SINGLE DX	57	1.7	2	1	1	1	2	4	5	6
TOTAL MULTIPLE DX	688	3.8	25	1	1	2	5	9	13	30
TOTAL										
0–19 Years	22	4.8	20	1	1	3	7	13	13	13
20–34	86	3.6	7	1	1	3	5	8	9	15
35–49	152	3.4	22	1	1	2	4	7	11	32
50–64	267	4.1	33	1	1	2	5	10	15	33
65+	218	3.2	21	1	1	1	4	8	13	21
GRAND TOTAL	745	3.7	24	1	1	2	4	8	13	26

85.23: SUBTOTAL MASTECTOMY

Type of Patients	Observed Patients	Avg. Stay	Variance	10th	25th	50th	75th	90th	95th	99th
1. SINGLE DX										
0–19 Years	0									
20–34	2	7.5	85	1	1	8	14	14	14	14
35–49	11	1.1	<1	1	1	1	1	1	2	2
50–64	7	1.1	<1	1	1	1	1	2	2	2
65+	6	1.0	0	1	1	1	1	1	1	1
2. MULTIPLE DX										
0–19 Years	0									
20–34	2	1.5	<1	1	1	2	2	2	2	2
35–49	44	2.1	12	1	1	1	1	3	4	18
50–64	94	1.6	4	1	1	1	1	2	3	15
65+	113	1.8	4	1	1	1	2	3	5	10
TOTAL SINGLE DX	26	1.6	6	1	1	1	1	2	2	14
TOTAL MULTIPLE DX	253	1.8	5	1	1	1	2	3	5	15
TOTAL										
0–19 Years	0									
20–34	4	4.5	40	1	1	2	2	14	14	14
35–49	55	1.9	10	1	1	1	1	2	4	18
50–64	101	1.6	4	1	1	1	1	2	3	14
65+	119	1.8	4	1	1	1	2	3	5	10
GRAND TOTAL	279	1.8	6	1	1	1	2	3	5	15

85.3: RED MAMMOPLASTY/ECTOMY

Type of Patients	Observed Patients	Avg. Stay	Variance	10th	25th	50th	75th	90th	95th	99th
1. SINGLE DX										
0–19 Years	14	1.2	<1	1	1	1	1	2	2	2
20–34	58	1.2	<1	1	1	1	1	2	3	4
35–49	76	1.4	<1	1	1	1	1	2	3	5
50–64	62	1.5	<1	1	1	1	1	2	3	8
65+	2	3.0	2	2	2	2	4	4	4	4
2. MULTIPLE DX										
0–19 Years	32	1.3	<1	1	1	1	2	2	2	2
20–34	150	1.6	2	1	1	1	2	3	4	9
35–49	323	1.9	4	1	1	1	2	3	5	8
50–64	434	1.7	2	1	1	1	2	3	5	7
65+	116	1.7	1	1	1	1	2	3	4	5
TOTAL SINGLE DX	212	1.3	<1	1	1	1	1	2	3	5
TOTAL MULTIPLE DX	1,055	1.7	2	1	1	1	2	3	4	7
TOTAL										
0–19 Years	46	1.2	<1	1	1	1	1	2	2	2
20–34	208	1.5	<1	1	1	1	1	2	3	6
35–49	399	1.8	3	1	1	1	2	3	5	8
50–64	496	1.7	2	1	1	1	2	3	5	7
65+	118	1.7	1	1	1	1	2	3	4	5
GRAND TOTAL	1,267	1.7	2	1	1	1	2	3	4	7

LOS by Diagnosis and Operation, Western Region, 45th Edition

401

Western Region, October 2007–September 2008 Data, by Operation

85.32: BILAT RED MAMMOPLASTY

Type of Patients	Observed Patients	Avg. Stay	Vari-ance	Percentiles						
				10th	25th	50th	75th	90th	95th	99th
1. SINGLE DX										
0–19 Years	8	1.2	<1	1	1	1	1	2	2	2
20–34	54	1.1	<1	1	1	1	1	1	2	2
35–49	54	1.1	<1	1	1	1	1	2	2	2
50–64	34	1.0	<1	1	1	1	1	1	1	2
65+	1	2.0	0	2	2	2	2	2	2	2
2. MULTIPLE DX										
0–19 Years	22	1.3	<1	1	1	1	2	2	2	2
20–34	118	1.3	<1	1	1	1	1	2	3	4
35–49	195	1.4	<1	1	1	1	2	2	3	4
50–64	261	1.4	<1	1	1	1	1	2	3	5
65+	64	1.4	<1	1	1	1	2	2	3	5
TOTAL SINGLE DX	151	1.1	<1	1	1	1	1	2	2	2
TOTAL MULTIPLE DX	660	1.4	<1	1	1	1	1	2	3	5
TOTAL										
0–19 Years	30	1.2	<1	1	1	1	1	2	2	2
20–34	172	1.2	<1	1	1	1	1	2	3	4
35–49	249	1.3	<1	1	1	1	1	2	3	4
50–64	295	1.3	<1	1	1	1	1	2	3	5
65+	65	1.4	<1	1	1	1	2	2	3	5
GRAND TOTAL	811	1.3	<1	1	1	1	1	2	3	4

85.34: UNI SUBCU MAMMECTOMY NEC

Type of Patients	Observed Patients	Avg. Stay	Vari-ance	Percentiles						
				10th	25th	50th	75th	90th	95th	99th
1. SINGLE DX										
0–19 Years	3	1.2	<1	1	1	1	1	2	2	2
20–34	3	3.3	<1	3	3	3	4	4	4	4
35–49	9	1.9	2	1	1	1	2	5	5	5
50–64	11	2.3	5	1	1	1	2	5	8	8
65+	0									
2. MULTIPLE DX										
0–19 Years	4	1.5	<1	1	1	1	2	2	2	2
20–34	12	3.1	13	1	1	2	3	9	12	12
35–49	36	2.8	4	1	1	2	4	6	7	8
50–64	54	2.3	2	1	1	2	3	4	6	7
65+	18	2.0	1	1	1	2	3	4	5	5
TOTAL SINGLE DX	26	2.0	3	1	1	1	2	5	5	8
TOTAL MULTIPLE DX	124	2.4	4	1	1	2	3	5	6	9
TOTAL										
0–19 Years	7	1.3	<1	1	1	1	1	2	2	2
20–34	15	3.1	10	1	1	2	3	9	12	12
35–49	45	2.6	3	1	1	2	4	5	7	8
50–64	65	2.3	3	1	1	2	3	5	6	8
65+	18	2.0	1	1	1	2	3	4	5	5
GRAND TOTAL	150	2.4	3	1	1	2	3	5	6	9

85.36: BILAT SUBCU MAMMECT NEC

Type of Patients	Observed Patients	Avg. Stay	Vari-ance	Percentiles						
				10th	25th	50th	75th	90th	95th	99th
1. SINGLE DX										
0–19 Years	2	1.0	0	1	1	1	1	1	1	1
20–34	0									
35–49	8	2.1	2	1	1	2	3	5	5	5
50–64	8	2.0	2	1	1	2	2	5	5	5
65+	1	4.0	0	4	4	4	4	4	4	4
2. MULTIPLE DX										
0–19 Years	2	1.5	<1	1	1	2	2	2	2	2
20–34	8	2.6	5	1	1	1	6	6	6	6
35–49	51	3.1	12	1	1	2	3	6	7	25
50–64	42	3.2	5	1	2	2	5	6	7	8
65+	12	2.5	4	1	1	1	5	5	6	6
TOTAL SINGLE DX	19	2.1	2	1	1	2	3	5	5	5
TOTAL MULTIPLE DX	115	3.0	8	1	1	2	4	6	7	8
TOTAL										
0–19 Years	4	1.3	<1	1	1	1	2	2	2	2
20–34	8	2.6	5	1	1	1	6	6	6	6
35–49	59	3.0	11	1	1	2	3	6	7	25
50–64	50	3.0	4	1	2	2	5	6	7	8
65+	13	2.6	4	1	1	2	4	5	6	6
GRAND TOTAL	134	2.9	7	1	1	2	4	6	7	8

85.4: MASTECTOMY

Type of Patients	Observed Patients	Avg. Stay	Vari-ance	Percentiles						
				10th	25th	50th	75th	90th	95th	99th
1. SINGLE DX										
0–19 Years	2	1.0	0	1	1	1	1	1	1	1
20–34	40	1.7	<1	1	1	1	2	3	4	4
35–49	285	1.5	<1	1	1	1	2	2	3	6
50–64	384	1.6	<1	1	1	1	2	3	4	5
65+	162	1.5	<1	1	1	1	2	2	3	4
2. MULTIPLE DX										
0–19 Years	3	2.7	2	1	1	3	4	4	4	4
20–34	186	2.1	4	1	1	2	2	3	5	9
35–49	1,608	2.0	3	1	1	2	2	3	5	8
50–64	2,967	2.0	4	1	1	2	2	4	5	8
65+	3,209	1.9	3	1	1	1	2	3	4	8
TOTAL SINGLE DX	873	1.6	<1	1	1	1	2	3	3	5
TOTAL MULTIPLE DX	7,973	1.9	3	1	1	1	2	3	5	8
TOTAL										
0–19 Years	5	2.0	2	1	1	2	3	4	4	4
20–34	226	2.0	3	1	1	1	2	3	5	8
35–49	1,893	1.9	2	1	1	1	2	3	4	8
50–64	3,351	1.9	3	1	1	1	2	4	5	8
65+	3,371	1.8	3	1	1	1	2	3	4	8
GRAND TOTAL	8,846	1.9	3	1	1	1	2	3	5	8

LOS by Diagnosis and Operation, Western Region, 45th Edition

Western Region, October 2007–September 2008 Data, by Operation

85.41: UNILAT SIMPLE MASTECTOMY

Type of Patients	Observed Patients	Avg. Stay	Vari-ance	Percentiles						
				10th	25th	50th	75th	90th	95th	99th
1. SINGLE DX										
0–19 Years	2	1.0	0	1	1	1	1	1	1	1
20–34	10	1.6	<1	1	1	1	2	4	4	4
35–49	72	1.5	1	1	1	1	2	2	4	6
50–64	103	1.6	1	1	1	1	2	3	4	6
65+	40	1.2	<1	1	1	1	1	2	2	3
2. MULTIPLE DX										
0–19 Years	2	2.0	2	1	1	1	3	3	3	3
20–34	21	2.2	3	1	1	1	3	5	5	6
35–49	302	1.8	2	1	1	1	2	3	5	6
50–64	664	1.9	2	1	1	1	2	4	5	7
65+	800	1.6	2	1	1	1	2	3	4	8
TOTAL SINGLE DX	227	1.5	1	1	1	1	2	2	4	6
TOTAL MULTIPLE DX	1,789	1.8	2	1	1	1	2	3	5	8
TOTAL										
0–19 Years	4	1.5	<1	1	1	1	1	3	3	3
20–34	31	2.0	2	1	1	1	3	4	5	6
35–49	374	1.8	2	1	1	1	2	3	5	6
50–64	767	1.9	3	1	1	1	2	4	5	7
65+	840	1.6	2	1	1	1	2	3	3	8
GRAND TOTAL	2,016	1.8	2	1	1	1	2	3	4	8

85.42: BILAT SIMPLE MASTECTOMY

Type of Patients	Observed Patients	Avg. Stay	Vari-ance	Percentiles						
				10th	25th	50th	75th	90th	95th	99th
1. SINGLE DX										
0–19 Years	0									
20–34	5	2.4	1	1	2	2	3	4	4	4
35–49	38	1.6	<1	1	1	1	2	3	3	4
50–64	34	2.2	<1	1	2	2	3	3	4	5
65+	5	1.6	<1	1	1	1	2	2	3	3
2. MULTIPLE DX										
0–19 Years	0									
20–34	34	2.1	2	1	1	2	2	3	5	7
35–49	304	2.1	2	1	1	2	3	4	5	8
50–64	389	2.3	2	1	1	2	3	5	5	7
65+	176	2.0	2	1	1	2	2	3	4	8
TOTAL SINGLE DX	82	1.9	<1	1	1	2	2	3	3	5
TOTAL MULTIPLE DX	903	2.1	2	1	1	2	2	4	5	8
TOTAL										
0–19 Years	0									
20–34	39	2.1	2	1	1	2	2	4	5	7
35–49	342	2.1	2	1	1	2	3	3	5	8
50–64	423	2.3	2	1	1	2	3	4	5	7
65+	181	1.9	2	1	1	2	2	3	4	8
GRAND TOTAL	985	2.1	2	1	1	2	2	4	5	8

85.43: UNILAT EXTEN SIMPLE MAST

Type of Patients	Observed Patients	Avg. Stay	Vari-ance	Percentiles						
				10th	25th	50th	75th	90th	95th	99th
1. SINGLE DX										
0–19 Years	0									
20–34	25	1.6	<1	1	1	1	2	3	3	4
35–49	154	1.5	<1	1	1	1	2	3	3	7
50–64	211	1.4	<1	1	1	1	2	2	3	5
65+	106	1.5	<1	1	1	1	2	2	3	4
2. MULTIPLE DX										
0–19 Years	0									
20–34	112	1.9	2	1	1	2	2	3	5	8
35–49	823	1.8	2	1	1	1	2	3	4	7
50–64	1,632	1.9	4	1	1	1	2	3	4	8
65+	2,043	1.9	3	1	1	1	2	3	4	8
TOTAL SINGLE DX	496	1.5	<1	1	1	1	2	2	3	5
TOTAL MULTIPLE DX	4,610	1.9	3	1	1	1	2	3	4	8
TOTAL										
0–19 Years	0									
20–34	137	1.8	2	1	1	1	2	3	4	8
35–49	977	1.8	2	1	1	1	2	3	4	7
50–64	1,843	1.8	4	1	1	1	2	3	4	8
65+	2,149	1.9	3	1	1	1	2	3	4	8
GRAND TOTAL	5,106	1.8	3	1	1	1	2	3	4	8

85.44: BILAT EXTEN SIMPLE MAST

Type of Patients	Observed Patients	Avg. Stay	Vari-ance	Percentiles						
				10th	25th	50th	75th	90th	95th	99th
1. SINGLE DX										
0–19 Years	0									
20–34	0									
35–49	14	1.8	<1	1	1	2	2	3	4	4
50–64	23	2.2	1	1	1	2	3	4	4	5
65+	7	2.0	1	1	1	2	2	4	4	4
2. MULTIPLE DX										
0–19 Years	0									
20–34	17	2.2	1	1	1	2	3	4	4	4
35–49	147	2.6	7	1	1	2	3	5	5	19
50–64	211	2.3	4	1	1	2	3	4	5	7
65+	123	2.1	2	1	1	2	2	3	5	10
TOTAL SINGLE DX	44	2.0	<1	1	1	2	2	4	4	5
TOTAL MULTIPLE DX	498	2.3	4	1	1	2	3	4	5	12
TOTAL										
0–19 Years	0									
20–34	17	2.2	1	1	1	2	3	4	4	4
35–49	161	2.6	7	1	1	2	3	4	5	19
50–64	234	2.2	2	1	1	2	3	4	5	7
65+	130	2.0	2	1	1	2	2	3	5	10
GRAND TOTAL	542	2.3	4	1	1	2	3	4	5	10

LOS by Diagnosis and Operation, Western Region, 45th Edition

85.45: UNILAT RAD MASTECTOMY

Type of Patients	Observed Patients	Avg. Stay	Vari-ance	Percentiles						
				10th	25th	50th	75th	90th	95th	99th
1. SINGLE DX										
0–19 Years	0									
20–34	0									
35–49	6	1.0	0	1	1	1	1	1	1	1
50–64	10	1.7	<1	1	1	1	1	1	1	1
65+	3	2.0	0	2	2	2	2	2	2	2
2. MULTIPLE DX										
0–19 Years	1	4.0	0	4	4	4	4	4	4	4
20–34	1	22.0	0	22	22	22	22	22	22	22
35–49	18	2.2	2	1	1	2	2	4	7	7
50–64	49	2.9	8	1	1	2	3	8	9	14
65+	57	2.6	9	1	1	1	3	6	10	18
TOTAL SINGLE DX	19	1.5	<1	1	1	1	1	2	4	4
TOTAL MULTIPLE DX	126	2.8	11	1	1	2	3	7	9	18
TOTAL										
0–19 Years	1	4.0	0	4	4	4	4	4	4	4
20–34	1	22.0	0	22	22	22	22	22	22	22
35–49	24	1.9	2	1	1	2	2	4	4	7
50–64	59	2.7	7	1	1	2	3	7	9	14
65+	60	2.6	9	1	1	2	3	6	10	18
GRAND TOTAL	145	2.7	10	1	1	2	3	6	9	18

85.6: MASTOPEXY

Type of Patients	Observed Patients	Avg. Stay	Vari-ance	Percentiles						
				10th	25th	50th	75th	90th	95th	99th
1. SINGLE DX										
0–19 Years	0									
20–34	0									
35–49	0									
50–64	1	1.0	0	1	1	1	1	1	1	1
65+	0									
2. MULTIPLE DX										
0–19 Years	2	1.0	0	1	1	1	1	1	1	1
20–34	2	1.0	0	1	1	1	1	1	1	1
35–49	26	1.1	<1	1	1	1	1	2	2	2
50–64	22	2.0	2	1	1	2	2	4	5	5
65+	8	3.4	20	1	1	2	3	14	14	14
TOTAL SINGLE DX	1	1.0	0	1	1	1	1	1	1	1
TOTAL MULTIPLE DX	60	1.7	3	1	1	1	2	3	4	14
TOTAL										
0–19 Years	2	1.0	0	1	1	1	1	1	1	1
20–34	2	1.0	0	1	1	1	1	1	1	1
35–49	26	1.1	<1	1	1	1	1	2	2	2
50–64	23	1.9	2	1	1	2	2	4	5	5
65+	8	3.4	20	1	1	2	3	14	14	14
GRAND TOTAL	61	1.7	3	1	1	1	2	3	4	14

85.5: AUGMENTATION MAMMOPLASTY

Type of Patients	Observed Patients	Avg. Stay	Vari-ance	Percentiles						
				10th	25th	50th	75th	90th	95th	99th
1. SINGLE DX										
0–19 Years	1	1.0	0	1	1	1	1	1	1	1
20–34	3	1.0	0	1	1	1	1	1	1	1
35–49	3	2.7	8	1	1	6	6	6	6	6
50–64	2	1.0	0	1	1	1	1	1	1	1
65+	0									
2. MULTIPLE DX										
0–19 Years	6	1.5	<1	1	1	2	2	2	2	2
20–34	10	1.5	<1	1	1	1	2	2	4	4
35–49	49	1.5	<1	1	1	1	2	3	3	5
50–64	59	1.5	<1	1	1	1	2	3	3	5
65+	18	1.9	1	1	1	1	3	4	4	4
TOTAL SINGLE DX	9	1.6	3	1	1	1	1	6	6	6
TOTAL MULTIPLE DX	142	1.6	<1	1	1	1	2	3	3	5
TOTAL										
0–19 Years	7	1.4	<1	1	1	1	1	2	2	2
20–34	13	1.4	<1	1	1	1	2	2	4	4
35–49	52	1.6	1	1	1	1	2	3	4	6
50–64	61	1.5	<1	1	1	1	2	2	3	5
65+	18	1.9	1	1	1	1	3	4	4	4
GRAND TOTAL	151	1.6	<1	1	1	2	2	3	3	5

85.7: TOTAL BREAST RECONST

Type of Patients	Observed Patients	Avg. Stay	Vari-ance	Percentiles						
				10th	25th	50th	75th	90th	95th	99th
1. SINGLE DX										
0–19 Years	0									
20–34	0									
35–49	7	2.6	2	1	1	2	4	4	4	4
50–64	7	3.6	2	2	2	4	5	5	5	5
65+	0									
2. MULTIPLE DX										
0–19 Years	1	4.0	0	4	4	4	4	4	4	4
20–34	23	3.8	4	1	3	4	5	6	7	9
35–49	242	4.1	5	2	3	4	5	6	7	16
50–64	354	4.2	6	1	3	4	5	6	7	16
65+	48	4.9	14	1	2	4	6	9	12	22
TOTAL SINGLE DX	14	3.1	2	2	2	4	4	5	5	5
TOTAL MULTIPLE DX	668	4.2	6	2	3	4	5	6	7	16
TOTAL										
0–19 Years	1	4.0	0	4	4	4	4	4	4	4
20–34	23	3.8	4	1	3	4	5	6	7	9
35–49	249	4.0	5	2	3	4	5	6	7	16
50–64	361	4.2	6	1	3	4	5	6	7	16
65+	48	4.9	14	1	2	4	6	9	12	22
GRAND TOTAL	682	4.1	6	2	3	4	5	6	7	16

LOS by Diagnosis and Operation, Western Region, 45th Edition

Western Region, October 2007–September 2008 Data, by Operation

85.8: OTHER BREAST REPAIR

Type of Patients	Observed Patients	Avg. Stay	Vari-ance	10th	25th	50th	75th	90th	95th	99th
1. SINGLE DX										
0–19 Years	2	1.0	0	1	1	1	1	1	1	1
20–34	2	2.0	2	1	1	3	3	3	3	3
35–49	26	2.1	2	1	1	3	3	4	4	5
50–64	21	2.3	2	1	1	2	3	4	4	5
65+	1	1.0	0	1	1	1	1	1	1	1
2. MULTIPLE DX										
0–19 Years	7	4.3	9	2	2	2	8	8	8	8
20–34	29	4.2	15	1	1	3	5	8	12	19
35–49	296	2.8	3	1	2	2	3	5	6	11
50–64	511	2.9	7	1	1	2	3	5	6	15
65+	153	2.5	4	1	1	2	3	5	7	11
TOTAL SINGLE DX	**52**	**2.1**	**1**	**1**	**1**	**2**	**3**	**4**	**4**	**5**
TOTAL MULTIPLE DX	**996**	**2.9**	**6**	**1**	**1**	**2**	**3**	**5**	**7**	**12**
TOTAL										
0–19 Years	9	3.9	9	1	2	2	8	8	8	8
20–34	31	4.1	15	1	1	3	5	8	12	19
35–49	322	2.8	3	1	2	2	3	5	6	10
50–64	532	2.8	7	1	1	2	3	5	6	15
65+	154	2.5	4	1	1	2	3	5	7	11
GRAND TOTAL	**1,048**	**2.8**	**6**	**1**	**1**	**2**	**3**	**5**	**6**	**12**

85.84: BREAST PEDICLE GRAFT

Type of Patients	Observed Patients	Avg. Stay	Vari-ance	10th	25th	50th	75th	90th	95th	99th
1. SINGLE DX										
0–19 Years	0									
20–34	0									
35–49	6	1.8	2	1	1	1	3	4	4	4
50–64	5	2.0	2	1	1	2	2	4	4	4
65+	0									
2. MULTIPLE DX										
0–19 Years	1	4.0	0	4	4	4	4	4	4	4
20–34	3	3.7	14	1	1	2	4	8	8	8
35–49	52	3.0	6	1	1	2	4	6	8	12
50–64	91	2.9	6	1	1	2	4	5	6	20
65+	42	2.4	5	1	1	2	3	5	5	13
TOTAL SINGLE DX	**11**	**1.9**	**2**	**1**	**1**	**1**	**3**	**4**	**4**	**4**
TOTAL MULTIPLE DX	**189**	**2.9**	**6**	**1**	**1**	**2**	**4**	**5**	**7**	**13**
TOTAL										
0–19 Years	1	4.0	0	4	4	4	4	4	4	4
20–34	3	3.7	14	1	1	2	4	8	8	8
35–49	58	2.9	6	1	1	2	4	6	8	12
50–64	96	2.9	6	1	1	2	4	5	6	20
65+	42	2.4	5	1	1	2	3	5	5	13
GRAND TOTAL	**200**	**2.8**	**6**	**1**	**1**	**2**	**4**	**5**	**7**	**12**

85.85: BREAST MUSCLE FLAP GRAFT

Type of Patients	Observed Patients	Avg. Stay	Vari-ance	10th	25th	50th	75th	90th	95th	99th
1. SINGLE DX										
0–19 Years	1	1.0	0	1	1	1	1	1	1	1
20–34	0									
35–49	12	2.8	1	2	2	3	4	4	5	5
50–64	10	2.8	1	1	1	3	3	4	5	5
65+	1	1.0	0	1	1	1	1	1	1	1
2. MULTIPLE DX										
0–19 Years	1	2.0	0	2	2	2	2	2	2	2
20–34	9	4.2	3	1	3	4	5	7	7	7
35–49	170	2.9	2	1	2	2	3	5	6	7
50–64	275	2.8	5	1	2	2	3	5	6	9
65+	75	2.6	3	1	1	2	3	5	6	10
TOTAL SINGLE DX	**24**	**2.7**	**1**	**1**	**2**	**2**	**3**	**4**	**5**	**5**
TOTAL MULTIPLE DX	**530**	**2.8**	**4**	**1**	**2**	**2**	**3**	**5**	**6**	**9**
TOTAL										
0–19 Years	2	1.8	<1	1	2	2	2	2	2	2
20–34	9	4.2	3	1	3	4	5	7	7	7
35–49	182	2.9	2	1	2	2	3	5	6	7
50–64	285	2.8	5	1	2	2	3	5	6	9
65+	76	2.5	3	1	1	2	3	5	6	10
GRAND TOTAL	**554**	**2.8**	**4**	**1**	**2**	**2**	**3**	**5**	**6**	**9**

85.89: MAMMOPLASTY NEC

Type of Patients	Observed Patients	Avg. Stay	Vari-ance	10th	25th	50th	75th	90th	95th	99th
1. SINGLE DX										
0–19 Years	0									
20–34	1	1.0	0	1	1	1	1	1	1	1
35–49	5	1.4	<1	1	1	1	2	2	2	2
50–64	4	1.8	2	1	1	1	4	4	4	4
65+	0									
2. MULTIPLE DX										
0–19 Years	0									
20–34	7	4.5	42	1	1	2	5	19	19	19
35–49	52	2.5	4	1	1	2	3	5	5	12
50–64	81	2.3	3	1	1	2	3	4	5	10
65+	21	1.3	<1	1	1	1	1	2	2	5
TOTAL SINGLE DX	**10**	**1.5**	**<1**	**1**	**1**	**1**	**2**	**4**	**4**	**4**
TOTAL MULTIPLE DX	**161**	**2.3**	**5**	**1**	**1**	**2**	**3**	**5**	**5**	**12**
TOTAL										
0–19 Years	0									
20–34	8	4.1	38	1	1	1	5	19	19	19
35–49	57	2.4	4	1	1	2	3	5	5	12
50–64	85	2.2	3	1	1	1	3	4	5	10
65+	21	1.3	<1	1	1	1	1	2	2	5
GRAND TOTAL	**171**	**2.3**	**5**	**1**	**1**	**2**	**3**	**4**	**5**	**12**

LOS by Diagnosis and Operation, Western Region, 45th Edition

Western Region, October 2007–September 2008 Data, by Operation

85.94: BREAST IMPLANT REMOVAL

Type of Patients	Observed Patients	Avg. Stay	Vari-ance	Percentiles						
				10th	25th	50th	75th	90th	95th	99th
1. SINGLE DX										
0–19 Years	0									
20–34	2	1.5	<1	1	1	1	2	2	2	2
35–49	2	1.0	0	1	1	1	1	1	1	1
50–64	6	1.5	<1	1	1	1	2	3	3	3
65+	6	1.7	1	1	1	1	2	4	4	4
2. MULTIPLE DX										
0–19 Years	3	2.5	13	1	1	1	1	10	10	10
20–34	17	5.2	39	1	1	2	7	15	22	22
35–49	106	3.2	5	1	1	3	4	6	8	9
50–64	167	2.8	8	1	1	1	4	6	8	13
65+	98	2.9	16	1	1	2	3	5	7	25
TOTAL SINGLE DX	16	1.5	<1	1	1	1	2	3	4	4
TOTAL MULTIPLE DX	391	3.0	10	1	1	2	4	6	8	19
TOTAL										
0–19 Years	3	2.5	13	1	1	1	1	10	10	10
20–34	19	4.9	36	1	1	3	7	15	22	22
35–49	108	3.2	5	1	1	3	4	6	8	9
50–64	173	2.7	7	1	1	1	4	6	8	13
65+	104	2.8	15	1	1	2	3	5	7	23
GRAND TOTAL	407	3.0	10	1	1	2	4	6	8	17

85.96: RMVL BRST TISS EXPANDER

Type of Patients	Observed Patients	Avg. Stay	Vari-ance	Percentiles						
				10th	25th	50th	75th	90th	95th	99th
1. SINGLE DX										
0–19 Years	0									
20–34	2	1.0	0	1	1	1	1	1	1	1
35–49	3	1.0	0	1	1	1	1	1	1	1
50–64	2	2.0	2	1	1	3	3	3	3	3
65+	0									
2. MULTIPLE DX										
0–19 Years	1	5.0	0	5	5	5	5	5	5	5
20–34	13	3.2	5	1	1	2	5	7	7	7
35–49	103	2.8	6	1	1	2	4	6	8	12
50–64	161	2.5	4	1	1	2	3	5	6	10
65+	61	2.7	10	1	1	2	3	5	7	22
TOTAL SINGLE DX	7	1.3	<1	1	1	1	1	3	3	3
TOTAL MULTIPLE DX	339	2.7	6	1	1	2	4	5	7	12
TOTAL										
0–19 Years	1	5.0	0	5	5	5	5	5	5	5
20–34	15	2.9	5	1	1	2	5	7	7	7
35–49	106	2.7	6	1	1	2	4	6	8	12
50–64	163	2.4	4	1	1	2	3	5	6	10
65+	61	2.7	10	1	1	2	3	5	7	22
GRAND TOTAL	346	2.6	6	1	1	2	4	5	7	12

85.9: OTHER BREAST OPERATIONS

Type of Patients	Observed Patients	Avg. Stay	Vari-ance	Percentiles						
				10th	25th	50th	75th	90th	95th	99th
1. SINGLE DX										
0–19 Years	3	2.8	2	2	2	2	4	5	5	5
20–34	11	1.6	1	1	1	1	2	3	4	4
35–49	12	1.5	1	1	1	1	2	2	5	5
50–64	11	1.6	<1	1	1	1	2	3	3	3
65+	7	1.6	1	1	1	1	2	4	4	4
2. MULTIPLE DX										
0–19 Years	18	3.0	8	1	1	2	5	5	10	14
20–34	71	3.8	15	1	1	3	4	7	13	22
35–49	301	3.1	6	1	1	2	4	6	8	10
50–64	451	2.8	10	1	1	2	4	6	8	12
65+	219	3.0	12	1	1	2	3	6	10	22
TOTAL SINGLE DX	44	1.7	1	1	1	1	2	4	4	5
TOTAL MULTIPLE DX	1,060	3.0	10	1	1	2	4	6	8	15
TOTAL										
0–19 Years	21	2.9	7	1	1	2	5	5	6	14
20–34	82	3.5	14	1	1	3	4	7	10	22
35–49	313	3.0	6	1	1	2	4	6	8	10
50–64	462	2.8	10	1	1	2	4	6	8	12
65+	226	3.0	12	1	1	2	3	6	9	22
GRAND TOTAL	1,104	2.9	9	1	1	2	4	6	8	15

85.91: ASPIRATION OF BREAST

Type of Patients	Observed Patients	Avg. Stay	Vari-ance	Percentiles						
				10th	25th	50th	75th	90th	95th	99th
1. SINGLE DX										
0–19 Years	3	2.8	2	2	2	2	4	5	5	5
20–34	5	2.2	2	1	1	1	3	4	4	4
35–49	6	2.0	<1	1	1	2	2	5	5	5
50–64	3	1.3		1	1	1	2	2	2	2
65+	0									
2. MULTIPLE DX										
0–19 Years	10	3.8	10	1	2	3	5	6	14	14
20–34	35	3.7	8	1	2	3	4	6	9	17
35–49	52	3.8	5	1	2	3	5	7	8	9
50–64	55	5.4	39	1	3	4	7	10	11	45
65+	35	4.7	9	2	3	3	7	9	10	13
TOTAL SINGLE DX	17	2.2	2	1	1	2	2	4	5	5
TOTAL MULTIPLE DX	187	4.4	17	1	2	3	6	8	10	17
TOTAL										
0–19 Years	13	3.6	8	2	2	3	5	5	6	14
20–34	40	3.5	7	1	2	3	4	6	8	17
35–49	58	3.6	5	1	2	3	5	7	8	9
50–64	58	5.2	38	1	2	4	6	10	11	45
65+	35	4.7	9	2	3	3	7	9	10	13
GRAND TOTAL	204	4.2	16	1	2	3	5	8	10	15

Western Region, October 2007–September 2008 Data, by Operation

86.0: INCISION SKIN & SUBCU

Type of Patients	Observed Patients	Avg. Stay	Variance	10th	25th	50th	75th	90th	95th	99th
1. SINGLE DX										
0–19 Years	813	2.8	5	1	1	2	3	5	6	12
20–34	394	2.4	4	1	1	2	3	4	5	7
35–49	294	2.5	3	1	1	2	3	5	6	8
50–64	180	2.3	3	1	1	2	3	4	5	10
65+	45	2.2	3	1	1	2	3	4	5	8
2. MULTIPLE DX										
0–19 Years	4,718	5.3	41	1	2	3	6	11	16	34
20–34	4,672	4.8	28	1	2	3	6	9	13	25
35–49	7,921	5.0	22	1	2	4	6	10	13	25
50–64	8,694	5.8	35	2	3	4	7	12	15	30
65+	6,703	6.5	36	2	3	5	8	13	17	30
TOTAL SINGLE DX	1,726	2.6	5	1	1	2	3	5	6	10
TOTAL MULTIPLE DX	32,708	5.5	33	1	2	4	6	11	15	29
TOTAL										
0–19 Years	5,531	5.0	37	1	2	3	5	10	15	32
20–34	5,066	4.6	27	1	2	3	5	9	12	24
35–49	8,215	5.0	22	1	2	4	6	9	13	25
50–64	8,874	5.7	34	1	3	4	7	11	15	29
65+	6,748	6.5	36	2	3	5	8	13	17	30
GRAND TOTAL	34,434	5.4	32	1	2	4	6	11	15	29

86.01: ASPIRATION SKIN & SUBCU

Type of Patients	Observed Patients	Avg. Stay	Variance	10th	25th	50th	75th	90th	95th	99th
1. SINGLE DX										
0–19 Years	29	3.0	2	1	2	3	4	5	5	7
20–34	18	2.0	1	1	1	2	2	4	4	4
35–49	11	2.5	2	1	1	2	3	4	6	6
50–64	3	3.3	4	1	2	4	5	5	5	5
65+	4	1.0	0	1	1	1	1	1	1	1
2. MULTIPLE DX										
0–19 Years	162	4.6	34	2	2	3	5	8	14	24
20–34	184	4.4	27	1	2	3	5	8	10	17
35–49	289	5.0	16	2	2	4	6	10	12	20
50–64	363	5.6	33	2	3	4	7	10	16	24
65+	407	5.9	22	2	3	5	8	11	14	22
TOTAL SINGLE DX	65	2.6	2	1	1	2	3	4	5	7
TOTAL MULTIPLE DX	1,405	5.2	26	2	2	4	6	10	14	23
TOTAL										
0–19 Years	191	4.4	30	1	2	3	5	8	10	23
20–34	202	4.2	25	1	2	3	5	7	10	15
35–49	300	4.9	16	1	2	4	6	10	12	20
50–64	366	5.6	33	2	3	4	6	10	16	24
65+	411	5.9	22	2	3	5	8	11	14	22
GRAND TOTAL	1,470	5.1	26	2	2	4	6	10	13	22

86.03: INCISION PILONIDAL SINUS

Type of Patients	Observed Patients	Avg. Stay	Variance	10th	25th	50th	75th	90th	95th	99th
1. SINGLE DX										
0–19 Years	46	2.0	<1	1	1	2	2	3	3	4
20–34	27	2.0	<1	1	1	2	2	3	4	5
35–49	3	1.3	<1	1	1	1	2	2	2	2
50–64	2	2.0	2	1	1	3	3	3	3	3
65+	0									
2. MULTIPLE DX										
0–19 Years	43	3.0	2	1	2	3	4	5	5	8
20–34	51	2.9	6	1	1	3	4	6	7	14
35–49	23	3.7	8	1	1	3	5	7	8	12
50–64	13	2.9	2	1	2	3	3	5	6	6
65+	8	4.1	5	2	3	3	4	9	9	9
TOTAL SINGLE DX	78	2.0	<1	1	1	2	2	3	3	4
TOTAL MULTIPLE DX	138	3.1	4	1	2	3	4	5	7	12
TOTAL										
0–19 Years	89	2.4	2	1	2	2	3	4	5	7
20–34	78	2.6	4	1	1	2	3	5	6	14
35–49	26	3.5	8	1	1	2	5	7	8	12
50–64	15	2.7	2	1	2	2	3	5	6	6
65+	8	4.1	5	2	3	3	4	9	9	9
GRAND TOTAL	216	2.6	3	1	1	2	3	5	6	9

86.04: SKIN & SUBCU I&D NEC

Type of Patients	Observed Patients	Avg. Stay	Variance	10th	25th	50th	75th	90th	95th	99th
1. SINGLE DX										
0–19 Years	599	2.7	2	1	2	2	3	5	5	7
20–34	304	2.5	2	1	1	2	3	4	6	7
35–49	245	2.6	3	1	1	2	3	5	6	8
50–64	130	2.5	4	1	1	2	3	5	6	10
65+	25	2.8	3	1	1	3	3	5	7	8
2. MULTIPLE DX										
0–19 Years	3,284	3.8	12	1	2	3	4	6	8	16
20–34	3,595	4.2	12	1	2	3	5	8	10	18
35–49	5,907	4.6	16	2	2	4	6	10	11	21
50–64	5,560	5.2	24	2	3	4	6	10	13	24
65+	3,546	5.8	25	2	3	4	7	11	14	24
TOTAL SINGLE DX	1,303	2.6	2	1	2	2	3	5	5	8
TOTAL MULTIPLE DX	21,892	4.7	18	2	2	4	6	8	12	21
TOTAL										
0–19 Years	3,883	3.6	11	1	2	3	4	6	8	15
20–34	3,899	4.1	12	1	2	3	5	7	10	18
35–49	6,152	4.5	15	1	2	4	6	8	11	20
50–64	5,690	5.1	24	2	3	4	6	10	13	24
65+	3,571	5.7	25	2	3	4	7	11	14	24
GRAND TOTAL	23,195	4.5	17	1	2	3	5	8	11	21

407

LOS by Diagnosis and Operation, Western Region, 45th Edition

Western Region, October 2007–September 2008 Data, by Operation

86.05: INC W RMVL FB/DEV SKIN

Type of Patients	Observed Patients	Avg. Stay	Vari-ance	Percentiles						
				10th	25th	50th	75th	90th	95th	99th
1. SINGLE DX										
0–19 Years	36	1.4	<1	1	1	1	1	2	3	5
20–34	26	1.2	<1	1	1	1	1	2	3	4
35–49	10	1.4	<1	1	1	1	1	3	3	3
50–64	11	1.5	<1	1	1	1	2	2	3	3
65+	1	1.0	0	1	1	1	1	1	1	1
2. MULTIPLE DX										
0–19 Years	527	9.3	94	1	3	7	12	20	28	40
20–34	344	7.9	116	1	3	5	9	17	21	83
35–49	687	6.6	41	2	3	5	8	14	18	31
50–64	1,056	6.9	39	2	3	5	8	14	17	33
65+	928	7.5	38	2	4	6	9	14	20	29
TOTAL SINGLE DX	84	1.4	<1	1	1	1	1	2	3	4
TOTAL MULTIPLE DX	3,542	7.7	62	2	3	6	9	16	21	38
TOTAL										
0–19 Years	563	8.9	92	1	3	6	11	19	28	40
20–34	370	7.4	111	1	2	5	9	16	21	83
35–49	697	6.5	41	2	3	5	8	14	18	31
50–64	1,067	6.8	39	2	3	5	8	14	17	33
65+	929	7.5	38	2	4	6	9	14	20	29
GRAND TOTAL	3,626	7.6	62	1	3	5	9	15	21	38

86.06: INSERTION INFUSION PUMP

Type of Patients	Observed Patients	Avg. Stay	Vari-ance	Percentiles						
				10th	25th	50th	75th	90th	95th	99th
1. SINGLE DX										
0–19 Years	5	2.1	<1	2	2	2	2	2	4	4
20–34	5	2.2	3	1	1	2	2	5	5	5
35–49	7	3.7	3	1	3	4	5	6	6	6
50–64	12	1.4	<1	1	1	1	1	2	4	4
65+	6	1.5	<1	1	1	1	2	3	3	3
2. MULTIPLE DX										
0–19 Years	131	4.0	28	1	2	3	4	6	10	36
20–34	112	6.0	74	1	2	3	7	13	21	33
35–49	227	4.4	36	1	1	3	5	10	16	39
50–64	372	5.0	41	1	1	3	6	12	18	36
65+	313	5.3	54	1	1	2	6	12	18	33
TOTAL SINGLE DX	35	2.1	2	1	1	2	2	4	5	6
TOTAL MULTIPLE DX	1,155	4.8	43	1	1	3	5	11	17	36
TOTAL										
0–19 Years	136	4.0	27	1	2	3	4	6	10	36
20–34	117	5.8	71	1	1	3	7	13	21	33
35–49	234	4.4	35	1	1	2	5	10	16	39
50–64	384	4.9	40	1	1	2	5	12	18	36
65+	319	5.3	53	1	1	2	6	12	18	33
GRAND TOTAL	1,190	4.7	42	1	1	3	5	11	17	36

86.07: VAD INSERTION

Type of Patients	Observed Patients	Avg. Stay	Vari-ance	Percentiles						
				10th	25th	50th	75th	90th	95th	99th
1. SINGLE DX										
0–19 Years	70	5.2	30	1	2	3	7	12	14	38
20–34	3	9.7	199	1	1	2	26	26	26	26
35–49	12	1.6	<1	1	1	1	2	2	4	4
50–64	16	1.7	<1	1	1	1	2	3	4	4
65+	7	2.0	2	1	1	1	3	5	5	5
2. MULTIPLE DX										
0–19 Years	496	9.5	85	1	3	7	13	22	28	42
20–34	275	8.5	67	2	4	6	11	19	22	42
35–49	616	7.7	51	2	3	6	10	16	24	37
50–64	1,137	8.2	74	2	3	6	10	17	23	44
65+	1,319	8.5	62	2	3	6	10	17	24	37
TOTAL SINGLE DX	108	4.6	28	1	1	3	6	10	13	38
TOTAL MULTIPLE DX	3,843	8.6	70	2	3	6	11	19	25	41
TOTAL										
0–19 Years	566	9.1	81	1	3	6	12	21	28	41
20–34	278	8.5	68	2	4	6	11	19	25	42
35–49	628	7.6	51	1	3	6	10	16	23	37
50–64	1,153	8.1	74	2	3	6	10	17	23	44
65+	1,326	8.4	62	2	3	6	10	17	24	37
GRAND TOTAL	3,951	8.4	69	2	3	6	11	18	25	40

86.09: SKIN/SUBCU INCISION NEC

Type of Patients	Observed Patients	Avg. Stay	Vari-ance	Percentiles						
				10th	25th	50th	75th	90th	95th	99th
1. SINGLE DX										
0–19 Years	27	2.2	2	1	1	2	3	4	4	7
20–34	10	1.8	<1	1	1	2	2	3	3	3
35–49	6	2.0	<1	1	2	2	2	3	3	3
50–64	5	1.4	<1	1	1	1	2	4	4	4
65+	2	1.5	<1	1	1	1	2	2	2	2
2. MULTIPLE DX										
0–19 Years	71	5.2	32	1	2	3	6	11	22	26
20–34	110	4.7	39	1	2	4	6	8	13	19
35–49	172	4.7	31	1	2	4	5	9	12	22
50–64	193	5.1	30	1	2	4	6	10	13	35
65+	181	5.3	20	1	2	4	6	11	13	24
TOTAL SINGLE DX	50	2.1	1	1	1	2	3	4	4	7
TOTAL MULTIPLE DX	727	5.0	29	1	2	4	6	10	13	24
TOTAL										
0–19 Years	98	4.5	26	1	2	3	5	11	14	26
20–34	120	4.4	36	1	2	3	5	8	12	19
35–49	178	4.6	30	1	2	3	5	9	12	22
50–64	198	5.0	30	1	2	4	6	10	13	35
65+	183	5.2	20	1	2	4	6	11	13	24
GRAND TOTAL	777	4.8	28	1	2	3	6	10	13	23

Western Region, October 2007–September 2008 Data, by Operation

86.1: SKIN & SUBCU DXTIC PX

Type of Patients	Observed Patients	Avg. Stay	Vari-ance	10th	25th	50th	75th	90th	95th	99th
1. SINGLE DX										
0–19 Years	16	2.9	4	1	1	2	4	7	7	7
20–34	6	3.0	10	1	1	1	6	8	8	8
35–49	10	1.7	<1	1	1	1	3	3	3	3
50–64	2	1.5	<1	1	1	2	2	2	2	2
65+	1	6.0	0	6	6	6	6	6	6	6
2. MULTIPLE DX										
0–19 Years	111	7.0	47	2	3	5	8	16	31	>99
20–34	171	6.5	42	2	3	4	7	13	18	45
35–49	307	7.2	52	2	3	5	9	15	19	42
50–64	453	7.3	50	2	3	5	9	15	18	40
65+	565	7.6	46	2	4	6	9	14	19	36
TOTAL SINGLE DX	35	2.8	4	1	1	2	3	6	7	8
TOTAL MULTIPLE DX	1,607	7.2	48	2	3	5	9	15	20	40
TOTAL										
0–19 Years	127	6.4	42	2	3	4	7	15	21	>99
20–34	177	6.3	42	2	3	4	7	13	18	45
35–49	317	7.0	52	2	3	5	9	15	19	42
50–64	455	7.2	50	2	3	5	9	15	18	40
65+	566	7.6	46	2	4	6	9	14	19	36
GRAND TOTAL	1,642	7.1	47	2	3	5	9	14	19	40

86.11: SKIN & SUBCU BIOPSY

Type of Patients	Observed Patients	Avg. Stay	Vari-ance	10th	25th	50th	75th	90th	95th	99th
1. SINGLE DX										
0–19 Years	15	3.1	4	1	2	2	5	7	7	7
20–34	6	3.0	10	1	1	1	6	8	8	8
35–49	10	1.7	<1	1	1	1	3	3	3	3
50–64	2	1.5	<1	1	1	2	2	2	2	2
65+	1	6.0	0	6	6	6	6	6	6	6
2. MULTIPLE DX										
0–19 Years	111	7.0	47	2	3	5	8	16	31	>99
20–34	171	6.5	42	2	3	4	7	13	18	45
35–49	307	7.2	52	2	3	5	9	15	19	42
50–64	452	7.3	50	2	3	5	9	15	18	40
65+	564	7.6	46	2	4	6	9	14	19	36
TOTAL SINGLE DX	34	2.9	4	1	1	2	4	7	7	8
TOTAL MULTIPLE DX	1,605	7.2	48	2	3	5	9	15	20	40
TOTAL										
0–19 Years	126	6.5	43	2	3	4	7	15	21	>99
20–34	177	6.3	42	2	3	4	7	13	18	45
35–49	317	7.0	52	2	3	5	9	15	19	42
50–64	454	7.2	50	2	3	5	9	15	18	40
65+	565	7.6	46	2	4	6	9	14	19	36
GRAND TOTAL	1,639	7.1	47	2	3	5	9	14	19	40

86.2: EXC/DESTR SKIN LESION

Type of Patients	Observed Patients	Avg. Stay	Vari-ance	10th	25th	50th	75th	90th	95th	99th
1. SINGLE DX										
0–19 Years	207	2.6	7	1	1	2	3	5	7	13
20–34	215	2.5	4	1	1	2	3	5	7	9
35–49	129	2.9	7	1	1	2	4	6	7	15
50–64	74	3.1	6	1	1	2	4	7	8	12
65+	13	2.6	3	1	1	2	3	5	6	6
2. MULTIPLE DX										
0–19 Years	1,713	6.1	81	1	2	3	6	13	21	55
20–34	2,672	7.1	74	1	2	4	8	16	23	47
35–49	4,952	8.2	85	2	3	5	10	17	25	56
50–64	7,342	9.1	100	2	4	6	11	19	28	59
65+	8,652	8.8	72	2	4	6	11	17	24	44
TOTAL SINGLE DX	638	2.7	6	1	1	2	3	5	7	13
TOTAL MULTIPLE DX	25,331	8.3	84	2	3	6	10	17	25	52
TOTAL										
0–19 Years	1,920	5.7	74	1	2	3	6	12	18	54
20–34	2,887	6.8	70	1	3	4	8	15	23	46
35–49	5,081	8.0	83	2	3	6	9	17	25	56
50–64	7,416	9.1	99	2	3	6	11	19	28	59
65+	8,665	8.8	71	2	4	6	11	17	24	44
GRAND TOTAL	25,969	8.2	83	2	3	6	10	17	25	52

86.21: EXCISION PILONIDAL CYST

Type of Patients	Observed Patients	Avg. Stay	Vari-ance	10th	25th	50th	75th	90th	95th	99th
1. SINGLE DX										
0–19 Years	61	1.9	3	1	1	2	2	4	4	10
20–34	30	1.4	<1	1	1	1	2	2	3	4
35–49	5	2.8	9	1	1	2	2	8	8	8
50–64	0									
65+	0									
2. MULTIPLE DX										
0–19 Years	56	3.7	11	1	1	2	4	8	8	18
20–34	45	3.4	22	1	1	2	4	5	7	24
35–49	24	2.6	3	1	3	4	7	6	6	7
50–64	17	6.3	38	1	3	4	7	17	23	23
65+	6	5.5	35	1	2	2	11	15	15	15
TOTAL SINGLE DX	96	1.9	2	1	1	1	2	3	4	10
TOTAL MULTIPLE DX	148	3.8	16	1	1	2	4	8	13	23
TOTAL										
0–19 Years	117	2.8	7	1	1	1	3	6	8	14
20–34	75	2.6	14	1	1	1	3	5	6	24
35–49	29	2.7	4	1	1	2	3	6	7	8
50–64	17	6.3	38	1	3	4	7	17	23	23
65+	6	5.5	35	1	2	2	11	15	15	15
GRAND TOTAL	244	2.9	11	1	1	2	3	6	8	18

LOS by Diagnosis and Operation, Western Region, 45th Edition

Western Region, October 2007–September 2008 Data, by Operation

86.26: LIG DERMAL APPENDAGE

Type of Patients	Observed Patients	Avg. Stay	Variance	Percentiles						
				10th	25th	50th	75th	90th	95th	99th
1. SINGLE DX										
0–19 Years	1	1.0	0	1	1	1	1	1	1	1
20–34	0									
35–49	0									
50–64	0									
65+	0									
2. MULTIPLE DX										
0–19 Years	371	2.8	13	1	1	2	3	4	6	26
20–34	0									
35–49	0									
50–64	0									
65+	0									
TOTAL SINGLE DX	1	1.0	0	1	1	1	1	1	1	1
TOTAL MULTIPLE DX	371	2.8	13	1	1	2	3	4	6	26
TOTAL										
0–19 Years	372	2.8	13	1	1	2	3	4	6	26
20–34	0									
35–49	0									
50–64	0									
65+	0									
GRAND TOTAL	372	2.8	13	1	1	2	3	4	6	26

86.27: DEBRIDEMENT OF NAIL

Type of Patients	Observed Patients	Avg. Stay	Variance	Percentiles						
				10th	25th	50th	75th	90th	95th	99th
1. SINGLE DX										
0–19 Years	1	1.0	0	1	1	1	1	1	1	1
20–34	0									
35–49	0									
50–64	1	12.0	0	12	12	12	12	12	12	12
65+	0									
2. MULTIPLE DX										
0–19 Years	4	3.7	2	1	4	4	4	5	5	5
20–34	16	14.8	407	2	3	6	18	40	80	80
35–49	42	12.4	150	2	4	9	19	36	63	>99
50–64	137	13.3	130	4	6	10	17	36	44	>99
65+	527	10.6	123	3	4	7	14	21	27	69
TOTAL SINGLE DX	2	6.4	60	1	1	1	12	12	12	12
TOTAL MULTIPLE DX	726	11.2	132	3	4	8	14	23	36	>99
TOTAL										
0–19 Years	5	3.4	2	1	4	4	4	5	5	5
20–34	16	14.8	407	2	3	6	18	40	80	80
35–49	42	12.4	150	2	4	9	19	36	63	>99
50–64	138	13.3	129	4	6	10	17	36	44	>99
65+	527	10.6	123	3	4	7	14	21	27	69
GRAND TOTAL	728	11.2	132	3	4	8	14	23	36	>99

86.22: EXC DEBRIDE WND/INFECT

Type of Patients	Observed Patients	Avg. Stay	Variance	Percentiles						
				10th	25th	50th	75th	90th	95th	99th
1. SINGLE DX										
0–19 Years	107	3.4	11	1	1	2	4	6	11	14
20–34	151	2.8	5	1	1	2	4	6	7	10
35–49	99	3.1	8	1	1	2	4	6	10	17
50–64	62	3.1	5	1	1	2	4	6	7	12
65+	13	2.6	3	1	1	2	3	5	6	6
2. MULTIPLE DX										
0–19 Years	876	8.1	124	1	3	4	9	18	29	66
20–34	2,074	7.7	82	1	3	5	9	18	26	52
35–49	3,912	8.7	95	2	3	6	10	19	28	60
50–64	5,722	9.6	108	2	4	7	11	21	30	60
65+	6,075	9.3	77	3	4	7	11	18	25	46
TOTAL SINGLE DX	432	3.1	7	1	1	2	4	6	8	13
TOTAL MULTIPLE DX	18,659	9.0	94	2	3	6	11	19	27	55
TOTAL										
0–19 Years	983	7.6	114	1	2	4	8	17	26	59
20–34	2,225	7.4	78	1	3	5	8	17	25	50
35–49	4,011	8.6	94	2	3	6	10	18	27	59
50–64	5,784	9.6	107	2	4	7	11	21	29	60
65+	6,088	9.3	77	3	4	7	11	18	25	46
GRAND TOTAL	19,091	8.9	93	2	3	6	11	19	27	55

86.23: NAIL REMOVAL

Type of Patients	Observed Patients	Avg. Stay	Variance	Percentiles						
				10th	25th	50th	75th	90th	95th	99th
1. SINGLE DX										
0–19 Years	3	1.3	<1	1	1	1	1	3	3	3
20–34	2	1.0	0	1	1	1	1	1	1	1
35–49	1	1.0	0	1	1	1	1	1	1	1
50–64	0									
65+	0									
2. MULTIPLE DX										
0–19 Years	25	8.2	96	1	2	4	8	32	32	32
20–34	27	7.0	86	1	2	3	12	12	30	44
35–49	42	5.3	36	1	2	3	6	9	29	>99
50–64	70	7.4	92	2	3	4	8	20	29	59
65+	139	8.4	57	2	4	6	10	18	26	41
TOTAL SINGLE DX	6	1.2	<1	1	1	1	1	3	3	3
TOTAL MULTIPLE DX	303	7.6	69	2	3	5	8	17	29	42
TOTAL										
0–19 Years	28	7.1	87	1	2	3	8	32	32	32
20–34	29	6.6	83	1	2	3	8	12	30	44
35–49	43	5.2	36	1	2	4	6	9	29	>99
50–64	70	7.4	92	2	3	4	8	20	29	59
65+	139	8.4	57	2	4	6	10	18	26	41
GRAND TOTAL	309	7.4	68	1	3	5	8	17	29	42

Western Region, October 2007–September 2008 Data, by Operation

86.28: NONEXC DEBRIDEMENT WOUND

Type of Patients	Observed Patients	Avg. Stay	Variance	Percentiles						
				10th	25th	50th	75th	90th	95th	99th
1. SINGLE DX										
0–19 Years	34	2.0	2	1	1	2	2	3	6	7
20–34	31	2.1	2	1	1	2	3	4	5	6
35–49	24	2.2	2	1	1	2	3	4	5	7
50–64	11	2.5	4	1	1	2	3	4	8	8
65+	0									
2. MULTIPLE DX										
0–19 Years	377	3.8	15	1	1	3	4	8	10	27
20–34	509	4.6	25	1	2	3	6	10	11	27
35–49	931	5.8	34	1	3	4	7	12	15	28
50–64	1,394	6.8	56	2	3	5	8	13	18	40
65+	1,903	6.7	36	2	3	5	8	13	17	30
TOTAL SINGLE DX	100	2.1	2	1	1	2	3	4	6	7
TOTAL MULTIPLE DX	5,114	6.1	39	1	3	4	7	12	16	32
TOTAL										
0–19 Years	411	3.6	15	1	1	2	4	7	10	21
20–34	540	4.5	24	1	2	3	6	9	11	27
35–49	955	5.7	33	1	3	4	7	11	15	28
50–64	1,405	6.8	56	2	3	5	8	13	18	40
65+	1,903	6.7	36	2	3	5	8	13	17	30
GRAND TOTAL	5,214	6.0	39	1	3	4	7	12	16	32

86.3: LOC EXC/DESTR SKIN NEC

Type of Patients	Observed Patients	Avg. Stay	Variance	Percentiles						
				10th	25th	50th	75th	90th	95th	99th
1. SINGLE DX										
0–19 Years	40	1.7	1	1	1	1	2	3	5	6
20–34	26	3.6	29	1	1	1	5	8	9	27
35–49	20	2.0	5	1	1	1	2	4	11	11
50–64	18	1.4	<1	1	1	1	2	3	3	3
65+	11	1.5	1	1	1	1	1	3	4	4
2. MULTIPLE DX										
0–19 Years	123	2.3	3	1	1	2	3	5	8	>99
20–34	143	4.0	24	1	1	2	5	9	11	19
35–49	265	4.7	28	1	1	3	6	10	16	30
50–64	389	4.6	29	1	1	3	6	10	14	23
65+	406	4.8	20	2	2	4	6	10	13	20
TOTAL SINGLE DX	115	2.0	7	1	1	1	2	4	5	11
TOTAL MULTIPLE DX	1,326	4.2	22	1	1	3	5	10	14	32
TOTAL										
0–19 Years	163	2.1	2	1	1	2	3	4	7	>99
20–34	169	3.9	25	1	1	3	6	9	11	27
35–49	285	4.5	27	1	1	3	6	10	16	30
50–64	407	4.4	28	1	1	3	6	10	14	21
65+	417	4.7	20	2	2	3	6	10	13	20
GRAND TOTAL	1,441	4.0	21	1	1	3	5	9	13	30

86.4: RAD EXCISION SKIN LESION

Type of Patients	Observed Patients	Avg. Stay	Variance	Percentiles						
				10th	25th	50th	75th	90th	95th	99th
1. SINGLE DX										
0–19 Years	22	1.8	2	1	1	1	2	4	5	5
20–34	8	3.8	18	1	1	1	4	14	14	14
35–49	25	3.5	14	1	1	2	5	10	10	16
50–64	22	1.7	2	1	1	1	2	3	4	7
65+	24	2.0	2	1	1	1	3	4	4	6
2. MULTIPLE DX										
0–19 Years	31	3.8	41	1	1	3	4	7	14	41
20–34	57	5.2	35	1	1	3	7	11	22	29
35–49	131	7.2	98	1	2	4	9	15	21	43
50–64	280	6.3	98	1	1	3	7	14	24	71
65+	515	4.6	36	1	1	3	6	10	15	29
TOTAL SINGLE DX	101	2.3	5	1	1	1	3	5	6	14
TOTAL MULTIPLE DX	1,014	5.4	61	1	1	3	6	12	19	43
TOTAL										
0–19 Years	53	2.9	25	1	1	2	3	5	7	28
20–34	65	5.1	33	1	1	3	7	11	14	29
35–49	156	6.6	85	1	2	4	8	14	19	43
50–64	302	5.9	93	1	1	3	7	11	22	60
65+	539	4.5	34	1	1	3	6	10	14	29
GRAND TOTAL	1,115	5.0	55	1	1	3	6	11	16	41

86.5: SKIN/SUBCU SUTURE/CLOSE

Type of Patients	Observed Patients	Avg. Stay	Variance	Percentiles						
				10th	25th	50th	75th	90th	95th	99th
1. SINGLE DX										
0–19 Years	98	1.3	<1	1	1	1	1	2	2	3
20–34	71	1.5	2	1	1	1	1	2	3	10
35–49	49	1.5	2	1	1	1	1	2	4	11
50–64	13	1.5	<1	1	1	1	2	2	4	4
65+	5	2.6	13	1	1	1	1	9	9	9
2. MULTIPLE DX										
0–19 Years	1,077	2.4	11	1	1	1	3	5	7	17
20–34	2,496	2.5	10	1	1	1	3	5	7	13
35–49	2,103	3.2	16	1	1	2	4	6	9	17
50–64	2,114	3.6	27	1	1	2	4	7	10	20
65+	5,088	3.7	14	1	2	3	4	7	9	17
TOTAL SINGLE DX	236	1.4	1	1	1	1	1	2	3	9
TOTAL MULTIPLE DX	12,878	3.2	15	1	1	2	4	6	9	17
TOTAL										
0–19 Years	1,175	2.3	10	1	1	1	3	4	6	17
20–34	2,567	2.5	10	1	1	2	3	5	7	13
35–49	2,152	3.1	16	1	1	2	4	6	9	17
50–64	2,127	3.6	26	1	1	2	4	7	10	20
65+	5,093	3.7	14	1	2	3	4	7	9	17
GRAND TOTAL	13,114	3.2	15	1	1	2	4	6	9	17

LOS by Diagnosis and Operation, Western Region, 45th Edition

Western Region, October 2007–September 2008 Data, by Operation

86.59: SKIN CLOSURE NEC

Type of Patients	Observed Patients	Avg. Stay	Variance	Percentiles						
				10th	25th	50th	75th	90th	95th	99th
1. SINGLE DX										
0–19 Years	98	1.3	<1	1	1	1	1	2	2	3
20–34	71	1.5	2	1	1	1	1	2	3	10
35–49	48	1.5	2	1	1	1	1	2	4	11
50–64	13	1.5	<1	1	1	1	2	2	4	4
65+	5	2.6	13	1	1	1	1	9	9	9
2. MULTIPLE DX										
0–19 Years	1,076	2.4	11	1	1	1	3	5	7	17
20–34	2,495	2.5	10	1	1	1	3	5	7	13
35–49	2,102	3.1	15	1	1	2	4	6	9	17
50–64	2,112	3.6	27	1	1	2	4	7	10	20
65+	5,087	3.7	14	1	2	3	4	7	9	17
TOTAL SINGLE DX	235	1.4	1	1	1	1	1	2	3	9
TOTAL MULTIPLE DX	12,872	3.2	15	1	1	2	4	6	9	17
TOTAL										
0–19 Years	1,174	2.3	10	1	1	1	3	4	6	17
20–34	2,566	2.5	10	1	1	1	3	5	7	13
35–49	2,150	3.1	15	1	1	2	4	6	9	17
50–64	2,125	3.6	26	1	1	2	4	7	10	20
65+	5,092	3.7	14	1	2	3	4	7	9	17
GRAND TOTAL	13,107	3.2	15	1	1	2	4	6	9	17

86.6: FREE SKIN GRAFT

Type of Patients	Observed Patients	Avg. Stay	Variance	Percentiles						
				10th	25th	50th	75th	90th	95th	99th
1. SINGLE DX										
0–19 Years	50	2.7	6	1	1	1	4	6	7	13
20–34	55	5.6	77	1	1	4	7	10	14	64
35–49	36	4.3	15	1	1	5	5	10	15	17
50–64	36	4.7	15	1	1	5	7	9	10	20
65+	12	4.2	46	1	1	1	4	6	25	25
2. MULTIPLE DX										
0–19 Years	582	12.4	195	1	3	8	16	27	36	77
20–34	696	12.6	152	2	5	9	17	27	36	84
35–49	966	14.0	189	2	5	10	19	31	42	69
50–64	1,185	12.5	169	2	4	8	16	29	43	77
65+	1,019	9.3	98	1	3	6	12	21	28	46
TOTAL SINGLE DX	189	4.1	29	1	1	3	5	8	11	20
TOTAL MULTIPLE DX	4,448	12.1	163	1	4	8	16	27	37	74
TOTAL										
0–19 Years	632	11.6	187	1	3	8	14	25	35	77
20–34	751	12.1	150	2	5	9	16	26	34	71
35–49	1,002	13.7	186	2	4	10	19	30	41	67
50–64	1,221	12.3	166	2	4	8	15	29	42	72
65+	1,031	9.3	98	1	3	6	12	21	28	46
GRAND TOTAL	4,637	11.8	160	1	4	8	15	27	36	74

86.62: HAND SKIN GRAFT NEC

Type of Patients	Observed Patients	Avg. Stay	Variance	Percentiles						
				10th	25th	50th	75th	90th	95th	99th
1. SINGLE DX										
0–19 Years	1	1.0	0	1	1	1	1	1	1	1
20–34	4	2.0	2	1	1	2	3	4	4	4
35–49	0									
50–64	1	2.0	0	2	2	2	2	2	2	2
65+	0									
2. MULTIPLE DX										
0–19 Years	33	8.3	118	1	2	5	14	15	18	63
20–34	45	8.6	46	1	3	8	13	18	22	25
35–49	75	8.2	50	2	3	5	12	18	21	32
50–64	50	9.8	107	1	3	6	14	29	32	44
65+	28	9.3	108	1	3	6	11	29	37	40
TOTAL SINGLE DX	6	1.8	1	1	1	2	2	4	4	4
TOTAL MULTIPLE DX	231	8.8	78	1	3	6	13	18	28	40
TOTAL										
0–19 Years	34	8.1	116	1	2	5	13	15	18	63
20–34	49	8.1	45	1	2	5	13	18	22	25
35–49	75	8.2	50	2	3	5	12	18	21	32
50–64	51	9.6	106	1	3	6	14	28	32	44
65+	28	9.3	108	1	3	6	11	29	37	40
GRAND TOTAL	237	8.6	77	1	2	5	13	18	28	40

86.63: FTHICK SKIN GRAFT NEC

Type of Patients	Observed Patients	Avg. Stay	Variance	Percentiles						
				10th	25th	50th	75th	90th	95th	99th
1. SINGLE DX										
0–19 Years	10	1.4	1	1	1	1	1	3	3	6
20–34	7	4.3	14	1	1	4	6	11	11	11
35–49	4	4.0	5	1	4	5	6	6	6	6
50–64	3	1.0	0	1	1	1	1	1	1	1
65+	4	1.0	0	1	1	1	1	1	1	1
2. MULTIPLE DX										
0–19 Years	40	4.6	26	1	1	2	7	13	14	21
20–34	23	7.3	86	1	2	5	7	18	21	43
35–49	37	10.6	127	2	3	7	14	22	33	58
50–64	49	7.3	28	2	4	6	8	15	17	27
65+	79	6.8	56	1	2	5	8	14	24	44
TOTAL SINGLE DX	28	2.0	4	1	1	1	1	6	6	11
TOTAL MULTIPLE DX	228	6.5	53	1	1	5	8	14	21	33
TOTAL										
0–19 Years	50	3.9	23	1	1	1	6	13	14	21
20–34	30	6.6	70	1	1	5	7	11	21	43
35–49	41	9.9	118	2	3	6	13	22	25	58
50–64	52	6.9	29	1	3	6	8	15	17	27
65+	83	6.5	55	1	2	4	8	14	22	44
GRAND TOTAL	256	5.9	49	1	1	3	7	14	21	33

LOS by Diagnosis and Operation, Western Region, 45th Edition

412

Western Region, October 2007–September 2008 Data, by Operation

86.65: HETEROGRAFT TO SKIN

Type of Patients	Observed Patients	Avg. Stay	Vari-ance	Percentiles						
				10th	25th	50th	75th	90th	95th	99th
1. SINGLE DX										
0–19 Years	0									
20–34	0									
35–49	0									
50–64	0									
65+	0									
2. MULTIPLE DX										
0–19 Years	26	17.7	135	7	10	17	20	26	43	61
20–34	21	19.8	170	10	13	17	22	32	39	64
35–49	29	16.6	65	5	11	19	21	27	30	36
50–64	20	14.8	159	2	8	14	19	43	48	48
65+	16	10.0	81	2	5	7	13	27	28	28
TOTAL SINGLE DX	0									
TOTAL MULTIPLE DX	112	16.2	125	4	9	15	21	27	39	61
TOTAL										
0–19 Years	26	17.7	135	7	10	17	20	26	43	61
20–34	21	19.8	170	10	13	17	22	32	39	64
35–49	29	16.6	65	5	11	19	21	27	30	36
50–64	20	14.8	159	2	8	14	19	43	48	48
65+	16	10.0	81	2	5	7	13	27	28	28
GRAND TOTAL	112	16.2	125	4	9	15	21	27	39	61

86.66: HOMOGRAFT TO SKIN

Type of Patients	Observed Patients	Avg. Stay	Vari-ance	Percentiles						
				10th	25th	50th	75th	90th	95th	99th
1. SINGLE DX										
0–19 Years	2	4.6	13	3	3	3	3	11	11	11
20–34	2	6.0	49	1	1	6	11	11	11	11
35–49	1	13.0	0	13	13	13	13	13	13	13
50–64	6	7.8	42	1	5	7	9	20	20	20
65+	0									
2. MULTIPLE DX										
0–19 Years	66	16.7	222	3	7	12	21	34	46	>99
20–34	61	21.1	466	4	9	13	24	59	84	>99
35–49	87	22.4	361	2	10	19	30	44	65	92
50–64	87	17.5	286	2	5	14	28	55	69	>99
65+	59	12.8	159	1	4	10	17	26	40	74
TOTAL SINGLE DX	11	6.8	29	1	3	5	11	13	20	20
TOTAL MULTIPLE DX	360	18.4	309	2	7	13	25	43	66	>99
TOTAL										
0–19 Years	68	15.9	217	3	7	11	21	34	46	>99
20–34	63	20.6	459	4	9	13	24	59	84	>99
35–49	88	22.3	358	2	10	18	30	44	65	92
50–64	93	16.9	276	2	5	11	26	53	69	>99
65+	59	12.8	159	1	4	10	17	26	40	74
GRAND TOTAL	371	17.9	303	2	7	12	24	41	65	>99

86.67: DERMAL REGENERATIVE GRFT

Type of Patients	Observed Patients	Avg. Stay	Vari-ance	Percentiles						
				10th	25th	50th	75th	90th	95th	99th
1. SINGLE DX										
0–19 Years	3	7.1	35	1	1	7	13	13	13	13
20–34	4	2.5	9	1	1	1	4	7	7	7
35–49	2	1.5	<1	1	1	2	2	2	2	2
50–64	2	3.0	8	1	1	3	5	5	5	5
65+	1	1.0	0	1	1	1	1	1	1	1
2. MULTIPLE DX										
0–19 Years	25	14.5	348	2	3	5	20	54	70	>99
20–34	30	11.3	152	2	3	5	15	33	44	45
35–49	58	8.8	105	2	3	6	11	20	43	>99
50–64	86	8.4	136	1	2	5	10	16	18	84
65+	71	8.0	39	2	4	7	11	19	22	>99
TOTAL SINGLE DX	12	3.4	15	1	1	1	7	7	13	13
TOTAL MULTIPLE DX	270	9.4	132	1	3	6	12	21	39	>99
TOTAL										
0–19 Years	28	13.8	323	1	3	5	20	54	70	>99
20–34	34	10.3	142	1	2	4	14	27	44	45
35–49	60	8.6	103	2	2	5	11	20	22	>99
50–64	88	8.3	134	1	2	5	10	16	18	84
65+	72	8.0	39	1	4	7	11	19	22	>99
GRAND TOTAL	282	9.2	129	1	2	5	12	21	35	>99

86.69: FREE SKIN GRAFT NEC

Type of Patients	Observed Patients	Avg. Stay	Vari-ance	Percentiles						
				10th	25th	50th	75th	90th	95th	99th
1. SINGLE DX										
0–19 Years	30	3.3	6	1	1	3	4	7	8	10
20–34	34	7.1	114	1	3	5	8	10	16	64
35–49	28	4.4	15	1	1	4	5	10	15	17
50–64	24	4.6	8	1	2	5	8	8	9	10
65+	7	6.4	71	1	1	4	6	25	25	25
2. MULTIPLE DX										
0–19 Years	360	14.4	218	2	6	10	18	29	36	77
20–34	499	12.4	116	2	5	9	16	27	33	55
35–49	661	14.4	184	3	5	10	19	31	42	65
50–64	877	12.9	168	3	5	8	16	30	43	72
65+	759	9.4	102	2	4	6	12	21	28	50
TOTAL SINGLE DX	123	5.0	41	1	2	4	6	9	10	25
TOTAL MULTIPLE DX	3,156	12.6	161	2	5	9	16	28	36	74
TOTAL										
0–19 Years	390	13.7	213	2	5	10	17	29	36	77
20–34	533	12.0	117	2	5	9	15	26	32	55
35–49	689	14.0	181	2	5	10	18	31	42	65
50–64	901	12.7	165	2	5	8	16	29	42	72
65+	766	9.4	102	1	3	6	12	21	28	50
GRAND TOTAL	3,279	12.3	159	2	4	8	15	28	36	72

LOS by Diagnosis and Operation, Western Region, 45th Edition

Western Region, October 2007–September 2008 Data, by Operation

86.7: PEDICLE GRAFTS OR FLAPS

Type of Patients	Observed Patients	Avg. Stay	Vari- ance	10th	25th	50th	75th	90th	95th	99th
1. SINGLE DX										
0–19 Years	33	2.1	5	1	1	1	3	4	4	14
20–34	24	1.9	3	1	1	1	2	5	5	7
35–49	22	3.3	12	1	1	2	4	7	9	15
50–64	22	2.8	11	1	1	2	4	5	6	16
65+	12	1.9	1	1	1	2	3	4	4	4
2. MULTIPLE DX										
0–19 Years	212	6.7	158	1	1	2	6	18	35	89
20–34	360	8.4	114	1	2	5	10	21	28	66
35–49	515	8.9	128	1	2	5	11	22	36	64
50–64	694	9.6	174	1	2	5	11	23	38	85
65+	788	8.3	97	1	2	5	10	20	26	59
TOTAL SINGLE DX	113	2.3	6	1	1	1	3	4	6	15
TOTAL MULTIPLE DX	2,569	8.4	135	1	2	5	10	20	32	73
TOTAL										
0–19 Years	245	6.0	139	1	1	2	5	16	32	89
20–34	384	8.0	109	1	2	4	10	20	28	66
35–49	537	8.6	124	1	2	5	10	21	34	64
50–64	716	9.4	170	1	2	5	10	23	37	84
65+	800	8.2	96	1	2	5	10	19	26	55
GRAND TOTAL	2,682	8.1	130	1	2	4	9	20	30	69

86.70: PEDICLE/FLAP GRAFT NOS

Type of Patients	Observed Patients	Avg. Stay	Vari- ance	10th	25th	50th	75th	90th	95th	99th
1. SINGLE DX										
0–19 Years	2	7.4	83	1	1	1	14	14	14	14
20–34	2	1.0	0	1	1	1	1	1	1	1
35–49	1	1.0	0	1	1	1	1	1	1	1
50–64	0									
65+	0									
2. MULTIPLE DX										
0–19 Years	11	6.6	83	1	1	2	6	26	26	26
20–34	17	12.2	224	1	2	7	13	40	54	54
35–49	23	7.3	68	1	2	4	10	19	21	32
50–64	33	7.3	77	1	2	3	12	16	24	43
65+	34	10.3	274	1	2	6	11	23	38	90
TOTAL SINGLE DX	5	3.6	33	1	1	1	1	14	14	14
TOTAL MULTIPLE DX	118	8.5	145	1	2	4	11	23	29	54
TOTAL										
0–19 Years	13	6.6	80	1	1	2	6	26	26	26
20–34	19	11.1	212	1	2	5	13	40	54	54
35–49	24	7.0	66	1	2	3	9	19	21	32
50–64	33	7.3	77	1	2	3	12	16	24	43
65+	34	10.3	274	1	2	6	11	23	38	90
GRAND TOTAL	123	8.4	142	1	2	3	11	23	29	54

86.72: PEDICLE GRAFT ADV

Type of Patients	Observed Patients	Avg. Stay	Vari- ance	10th	25th	50th	75th	90th	95th	99th
1. SINGLE DX										
0–19 Years	2	2.0	1	1	1	3	3	3	3	3
20–34	4	2.0	4	1	1	1	1	5	5	5
35–49	3	6.0	60	1	1	2	15	15	15	15
50–64	2	1.7	1	1	1	3	3	3	3	3
65+	1	4.0	0	4	4	4	4	4	4	4
2. MULTIPLE DX										
0–19 Years	18	8.6	258	1	1	1	5	51	51	51
20–34	30	6.9	134	1	2	3	8	17	21	63
35–49	33	9.4	184	2	3	4	7	39	42	54
50–64	49	10.0	345	1	2	4	6	29	67	84
65+	57	5.1	27	1	1	3	7	13	17	25
TOTAL SINGLE DX	12	2.7	10	1	1	1	3	5	15	15
TOTAL MULTIPLE DX	187	7.9	185	1	1	3	7	18	40	67
TOTAL										
0–19 Years	20	7.4	217	1	1	3	3	20	51	51
20–34	34	6.3	121	1	2	3	8	12	21	63
35–49	36	9.1	173	2	2	4	8	39	42	54
50–64	51	9.6	329	1	2	4	6	19	67	84
65+	58	5.1	26	1	1	3	7	13	17	25
GRAND TOTAL	199	7.4	172	1	1	3	6	17	39	67

86.73: ATTACH PEDICLE TO HAND

Type of Patients	Observed Patients	Avg. Stay	Vari- ance	10th	25th	50th	75th	90th	95th	99th
1. SINGLE DX										
0–19 Years	5	3.6	28	1	1	1	2	13	13	13
20–34	6	1.5	<1	1	1	2	2	2	2	2
35–49	1	4.0	0	4	4	4	4	4	4	4
50–64	1	1.0	0	1	1	1	1	1	1	1
65+	0									
2. MULTIPLE DX										
0–19 Years	13	3.1	6	1	1	2	7	7	7	7
20–34	44	2.4	2	1	1	2	3	4	5	6
35–49	67	3.5	10	1	2	3	4	6	8	17
50–64	40	3.1	7	1	1	2	4	5	7	16
65+	24	3.6	9	1	1	2	6	8	10	11
TOTAL SINGLE DX	13	2.5	11	1	1	1	2	4	13	13
TOTAL MULTIPLE DX	188	3.1	7	1	1	2	4	6	8	16
TOTAL										
0–19 Years	18	3.2	10	1	1	2	7	7	7	13
20–34	50	2.3	2	1	1	2	3	4	5	6
35–49	68	3.6	10	1	2	3	4	6	8	17
50–64	41	3.0	7	1	1	2	4	5	6	16
65+	24	3.6	9	1	1	2	6	8	10	11
GRAND TOTAL	201	3.1	7	1	1	2	4	6	8	15

LOS by Diagnosis and Operation, Western Region, 45th Edition

Western Region, October 2007–September 2008 Data, by Operation

86.74: ATTACH PEDICLE GRAFT NEC

Type of Patients	Observed Patients	Avg. Stay	Vari-ance	Percentiles						
				10th	25th	50th	75th	90th	95th	99th
1. SINGLE DX										
0–19 Years	21	2.0	2	1	1	1	3	4	4	8
20–34	10	2.2	4	1	1	1	2	4	7	7
35–49	16	2.9	6	1	1	2	4	7	9	9
50–64	18	3.0	13	1	1	2	4	6	16	16
65+	10	1.8	1	1	1	2	2	3	4	4
2. MULTIPLE DX										
0–19 Years	151	6.9	178	1	1	2	6	18	35	89
20–34	243	9.5	124	1	3	6	12	22	28	68
35–49	345	10.1	148	1	3	6	13	27	38	81
50–64	483	10.1	167	1	3	6	12	26	40	99
65+	610	8.6	98	1	2	6	11	20	27	55
TOTAL SINGLE DX	75	2.3	5	1	1	1	3	4	6	9
TOTAL MULTIPLE DX	1,832	9.0	141	1	2	5	11	22	34	81
TOTAL										
0–19 Years	172	6.2	156	1	1	2	5	15	32	89
20–34	253	9.2	122	1	3	6	12	22	28	68
35–49	361	9.8	144	1	3	6	12	25	38	81
50–64	501	9.9	163	1	3	6	11	26	38	85
65+	620	8.5	97	1	2	5	10	20	27	55
GRAND TOTAL	1,907	8.7	136	1	2	5	10	21	32	78

86.75: REV PEDICLE/FLAP GRAFT

Type of Patients	Observed Patients	Avg. Stay	Vari-ance	Percentiles						
				10th	25th	50th	75th	90th	95th	99th
1. SINGLE DX										
0–19 Years	2	1.0	0	1	1	1	1	1	1	1
20–34	2	2.0	2	1	1	3	3	3	3	3
35–49	1	2.0	0	1	2	2	2	2	2	2
50–64	1	4.0	0	4	4	4	4	4	4	4
65+	1	1.0	0	1	1	1	1	1	1	1
2. MULTIPLE DX										
0–19 Years	18	4.5	29	1	1	2	5	16	16	22
20–34	17	6.9	39	1	2	5	8	20	21	21
35–49	38	7.8	88	1	2	5	10	20	37	44
50–64	70	10.2	234	1	3	5	11	19	32	86
65+	52	8.0	53	1	3	5	11	18	29	>99
TOTAL SINGLE DX	7	1.9	1	1	1	1	3	4	4	4
TOTAL MULTIPLE DX	195	7.9	114	1	2	4	10	18	25	78
TOTAL										
0–19 Years	20	4.3	28	1	1	2	5	16	16	22
20–34	19	6.4	37	1	2	4	8	20	21	21
35–49	39	7.6	86	1	2	5	10	20	37	44
50–64	71	10.1	231	1	3	5	11	18	32	86
65+	53	7.8	53	1	3	5	11	18	29	>99
GRAND TOTAL	202	7.7	112	1	2	4	10	18	23	78

86.8: OTHER SKIN & SUBCU REP

Type of Patients	Observed Patients	Avg. Stay	Vari-ance	Percentiles						
				10th	25th	50th	75th	90th	95th	99th
1. SINGLE DX										
0–19 Years	29	1.2	<1	1	1	1	1	2	3	3
20–34	25	1.4	<1	1	1	1	2	2	3	4
35–49	45	1.3	<1	1	1	1	2	2	3	3
50–64	41	1.2	<1	1	1	1	1	2	2	3
65+	14	1.1	<1	1	1	1	1	1	2	2
2. MULTIPLE DX										
0–19 Years	103	2.2	3	1	1	1	3	5	7	8
20–34	212	2.2	10	1	1	2	3	4	5	9
35–49	517	2.3	8	1	1	2	3	4	6	13
50–64	793	2.7	23	1	1	1	3	5	8	22
65+	235	2.7	7	1	1	1	3	6	8	13
TOTAL SINGLE DX	154	1.2	<1	1	1	1	1	2	3	3
TOTAL MULTIPLE DX	1,860	2.5	14	1	1	2	3	5	7	15
TOTAL										
0–19 Years	132	2.0	3	1	1	1	2	4	6	8
20–34	237	2.1	9	1	1	2	2	4	5	9
35–49	562	2.2	8	1	1	2	3	4	5	13
50–64	834	2.7	22	1	1	1	3	5	7	18
65+	249	2.6	6	1	1	1	3	6	8	13
GRAND TOTAL	2,014	2.4	12	1	1	1	3	4	7	15

86.82: FACIAL RHYTIDECTOMY

Type of Patients	Observed Patients	Avg. Stay	Vari-ance	Percentiles						
				10th	25th	50th	75th	90th	95th	99th
1. SINGLE DX										
0–19 Years	0									
20–34	0									
35–49	3	1.0	0	1	1	1	1	1	1	1
50–64	23	1.1	<1	1	1	1	1	1	2	3
65+	10	1.0	0	1	1	1	1	1	1	1
2. MULTIPLE DX										
0–19 Years	0									
20–34	0									
35–49	18	1.2	<1	1	1	1	1	2	3	3
50–64	149	1.2	<1	1	1	1	1	2	2	3
65+	68	1.2	<1	1	1	1	1	2	2	5
TOTAL SINGLE DX	36	1.1	<1	1	1	1	1	1	2	3
TOTAL MULTIPLE DX	235	1.2	<1	1	1	1	1	2	2	3
TOTAL										
0–19 Years	0									
20–34	0									
35–49	21	1.2	<1	1	1	1	1	2	2	3
50–64	172	1.2	<1	1	1	1	1	2	2	3
65+	78	1.2	<1	1	1	1	1	2	2	5
GRAND TOTAL	271	1.2	<1	1	1	1	1	2	2	3

LOS by Diagnosis and Operation, Western Region, 45th Edition

Western Region, October 2007–September 2008 Data, by Operation

86.83: SIZE RED PLASTIC OP

Type of Patients	Observed Patients	Avg. Stay	Vari- ance	Percentiles						
				10th	25th	50th	75th	90th	95th	99th
1. SINGLE DX										
0–19 Years	0									
20–34	14	1.4	<1	1	1	1	1	2	4	4
35–49	37	1.2	<1	1	1	1	1	2	2	3
50–64	17	1.3	<1	1	1	1	1	2	3	3
65+	4	1.3	<1	1	1	1	1	2	2	2
2. MULTIPLE DX										
0–19 Years	1	8.0	0	8	8	8	8	8	8	8
20–34	144	1.7	<1	1	1	1	2	3	4	5
35–49	423	2.1	4	1	1	2	2	4	5	13
50–64	578	3.0	29	1	1	2	3	5	9	28
65+	108	3.1	9	1	1	2	4	7	9	14
TOTAL SINGLE DX	72	1.3	<1	1	1	1	1	2	2	4
TOTAL MULTIPLE DX	1,254	2.6	16	1	1	2	3	5	7	17
TOTAL										
0–19 Years	1	8.0	0	8	8	8	8	8	8	8
20–34	158	1.7	<1	1	1	1	2	3	4	5
35–49	460	2.0	4	1	1	2	2	4	5	13
50–64	595	3.0	29	1	1	2	3	5	9	28
65+	112	3.0	8	1	1	2	4	7	9	14
GRAND TOTAL	1,326	2.5	15	1	1	2	3	4	7	17

86.9: OTHER SKIN & SUBCU OPS

Type of Patients	Observed Patients	Avg. Stay	Vari- ance	Percentiles						
				10th	25th	50th	75th	90th	95th	99th
1. SINGLE DX										
0–19 Years	11	1.3	2	1	1	1	1	1	1	7
20–34	7	1.3	<1	1	1	1	2	2	2	2
35–49	14	1.5	2	1	1	1	1	4	5	5
50–64	16	1.6	1	1	1	1	1	4	5	5
65+	7	1.4	<1	1	1	1	2	3	3	3
2. MULTIPLE DX										
0–19 Years	59	2.3	3	1	1	2	3	5	5	9
20–34	37	3.1	16	1	1	1	3	7	11	22
35–49	86	2.5	7	1	1	1	3	5	8	16
50–64	125	2.2	15	1	1	1	2	4	6	11
65+	121	2.3	13	1	1	1	2	4	6	11
TOTAL SINGLE DX	55	1.4	1	1	1	1	1	2	4	7
TOTAL MULTIPLE DX	428	2.4	10	1	1	1	3	5	6	12
TOTAL										
0–19 Years	70	2.2	3	1	1	1	3	4	5	9
20–34	44	2.8	14	1	1	1	3	6	9	22
35–49	100	2.4	7	1	1	1	3	5	8	16
50–64	141	2.1	14	1	1	1	2	4	5	11
65+	128	2.2	12	1	1	1	2	4	6	11
GRAND TOTAL	483	2.3	9	1	1	1	2	4	6	11

86.89: SKIN REP & RECONST NEC

Type of Patients	Observed Patients	Avg. Stay	Vari- ance	Percentiles						
				10th	25th	50th	75th	90th	95th	99th
1. SINGLE DX										
0–19 Years	12	1.6	<1	1	1	1	2	3	3	3
20–34	10	1.4	<1	1	1	1	2	2	2	2
35–49	5	2.2	<1	1	2	2	3	3	3	3
50–64	0									
65+	0									
2. MULTIPLE DX										
0–19 Years	58	2.2	2	1	1	2	3	4	6	6
20–34	55	3.2	35	1	1	2	3	5	7	44
35–49	60	3.9	37	1	1	2	4	6	10	45
50–64	53	3.7	12	1	1	2	6	8	10	18
65+	53	3.6	7	1	2	3	4	7	10	11
TOTAL SINGLE DX	27	1.6	<1	1	1	1	2	3	3	3
TOTAL MULTIPLE DX	279	3.1	16	1	1	2	4	6	8	13
TOTAL										
0–19 Years	70	2.1	2	1	1	2	3	4	6	6
20–34	65	2.9	30	1	1	2	3	5	6	44
35–49	65	3.8	34	1	1	2	4	6	10	45
50–64	53	3.7	12	1	1	2	6	8	10	18
65+	53	3.6	7	1	2	3	4	7	10	11
GRAND TOTAL	306	3.0	15	1	1	2	3	6	7	13

86.94: INS 1 ARRAY NEURSTIM GEN

Type of Patients	Observed Patients	Avg. Stay	Vari- ance	Percentiles						
				10th	25th	50th	75th	90th	95th	99th
1. SINGLE DX										
0–19 Years	0									
20–34	3	1.0	0	1	1	1	1	1	1	1
35–49	7	1.6	2	1	1	1	4	5	5	5
50–64	8	1.9	3	1	1	1	4	5	5	5
65+	3	1.7	1	1	1	1	3	3	3	3
2. MULTIPLE DX										
0–19 Years	4	1.5	<1	1	1	1	1	3	3	3
20–34	10	2.5	2	1	1	2	4	4	5	5
35–49	31	2.2	7	1	1	1	2	3	10	13
50–64	53	1.9	2	1	1	1	2	4	5	9
65+	55	1.6	2	1	1	1	2	3	6	6
TOTAL SINGLE DX	21	1.6	2	1	1	1	1	4	5	5
TOTAL MULTIPLE DX	153	1.9	3	1	1	1	2	4	5	10
TOTAL										
0–19 Years	4	1.5	<1	1	1	1	1	3	3	3
20–34	13	2.2	2	1	1	1	3	4	5	5
35–49	38	2.1	6	1	1	1	3	4	10	13
50–64	61	1.9	2	1	1	1	2	4	5	9
65+	58	1.6	2	1	1	1	2	3	6	6
GRAND TOTAL	174	1.8	3	1	1	1	2	4	5	10

LOS by Diagnosis and Operation, Western Region, 45th Edition

Western Region, October 2007–September 2008 Data, by Operation

87.0: HEAD/NECK SFT TISS X-RAY

Type of Patients	Observed Patients	Avg. Stay	Variance	10th	25th	50th	75th	90th	95th	99th
1. SINGLE DX										
0–19 Years	313	1.9	4	1	1	1	2	3	4	7
20–34	86	1.8	2	1	1	1	2	3	4	13
35–49	67	2.0	4	1	1	2	2	3	5	14
50–64	56	2.0	5	1	1	2	2	3	4	17
65+	17	1.5	2	1	1	1	1	3	6	6
2. MULTIPLE DX										
0–19 Years	1,119	3.2	23	1	1	2	3	6	9	22
20–34	1,365	3.0	17	1	1	2	4	6	9	15
35–49	2,571	3.4	22	1	1	2	4	6	9	18
50–64	4,406	3.6	19	1	2	3	4	7	10	22
65+	10,827	3.8	13	1	2	3	5	7	9	17
TOTAL SINGLE DX	539	1.9	4	1	1	1	2	3	4	9
TOTAL MULTIPLE DX	20,288	3.6	16	1	2	3	4	7	9	18
TOTAL										
0–19 Years	1,432	2.9	19	1	1	2	3	6	8	20
20–34	1,451	3.0	16	1	1	2	3	6	9	15
35–49	2,638	3.3	21	1	1	2	4	6	9	18
50–64	4,462	3.6	19	1	1	2	4	7	10	22
65+	10,844	3.8	12	1	2	3	5	7	9	17
GRAND TOTAL	20,827	3.5	16	1	1	3	4	7	9	18

87.02: BRAIN/SKULL CONTR X-RAY

Type of Patients	Observed Patients	Avg. Stay	Variance	10th	25th	50th	75th	90th	95th	99th
1. SINGLE DX										
0–19 Years	0									
20–34	0									
35–49	1	1.0	0	1	1	1	1	1	1	1
50–64	0									
65+	0									
2. MULTIPLE DX										
0–19 Years	5	2.2	<1	2	2	2	2	3	3	3
20–34	15	4.8	8	1	3	4	7	10	10	10
35–49	7	3.0	1	2	1	3	3	5	5	5
50–64	9	4.0	9	1	1	3	7	8	8	8
65+	23	7.1	18	2	4	6	9	14	16	17
TOTAL SINGLE DX	1	1.0	0	1	1	1	1	1	1	1
TOTAL MULTIPLE DX	59	5.0	13	2	2	4	7	10	11	17
TOTAL										
0–19 Years	5	2.2	<1	2	2	2	2	3	3	3
20–34	15	4.8	8	1	3	4	7	10	10	10
35–49	8	2.8	1	1	2	3	3	5	5	5
50–64	9	4.0	9	1	1	3	7	8	8	8
65+	23	7.1	18	2	4	6	9	14	16	17
GRAND TOTAL	60	5.0	13	2	2	4	7	10	11	17

87.03: CAT SCAN HEAD

Type of Patients	Observed Patients	Avg. Stay	Variance	10th	25th	50th	75th	90th	95th	99th
1. SINGLE DX										
0–19 Years	311	1.9	4	1	1	1	2	3	4	7
20–34	86	1.8	2	1	1	1	2	3	4	13
35–49	64	2.1	4	1	1	2	2	3	5	14
50–64	56	2.0	5	1	1	2	2	3	4	17
65+	17	1.5	2	1	1	1	1	3	6	6
2. MULTIPLE DX										
0–19 Years	1,109	3.2	23	1	1	2	3	6	9	21
20–34	1,347	3.0	17	1	1	2	3	6	9	15
35–49	2,561	3.4	22	1	1	2	4	6	9	18
50–64	4,391	3.6	19	1	2	3	4	7	10	22
65+	10,788	3.8	12	1	2	3	5	7	9	17
TOTAL SINGLE DX	534	1.9	4	1	1	1	2	3	4	9
TOTAL MULTIPLE DX	20,196	3.6	16	1	2	3	4	7	9	18
TOTAL										
0–19 Years	1,420	2.9	19	1	1	2	3	6	8	20
20–34	1,433	2.9	16	1	1	2	3	6	9	15
35–49	2,625	3.3	21	1	1	2	4	6	9	18
50–64	4,447	3.5	19	1	1	2	4	7	10	22
65+	10,805	3.7	12	1	2	3	5	7	9	17
GRAND TOTAL	20,730	3.5	16	1	1	3	4	7	9	18

87.04: HEAD TOMOGRAPHY NEC

Type of Patients	Observed Patients	Avg. Stay	Variance	10th	25th	50th	75th	90th	95th	99th
1. SINGLE DX										
0–19 Years	0									
20–34	0									
35–49	1	2.0	0	2	2	2	2	2	2	2
50–64	0									
65+	0									
2. MULTIPLE DX										
0–19 Years	0									
20–34	0									
35–49	0									
50–64	1	4.0	0	4	4	4	4	4	4	4
65+	5	8.6	11	5	6	8	11	13	13	13
TOTAL SINGLE DX	1	2.0	0	2	2	2	2	2	2	2
TOTAL MULTIPLE DX	6	7.8	13	4	5	6	11	13	13	13
TOTAL										
0–19 Years	0									
20–34	0									
35–49	1	2.0	0	2	2	2	2	2	2	2
50–64	1	4.0	0	4	4	4	4	4	4	4
65+	5	8.6	11	5	6	8	11	13	13	13
GRAND TOTAL	7	7.0	15	2	4	6	11	13	13	13

LOS by Diagnosis and Operation, Western Region, 45th Edition

Western Region, October 2007–September 2008 Data, by Operation

87.1: OTHER HEAD/NECK X-RAY

Type of Patients	Observed Patients	Avg. Stay	Variance	Percentiles						
				10th	25th	50th	75th	90th	95th	99th
1. SINGLE DX										
0–19 Years	0									
20–34	1	3.0	0	3	3	3	3	3	3	3
35–49	1	1.0	0	1	1	1	1	1	1	1
50–64	0									
65+	0									
2. MULTIPLE DX										
0–19 Years	17	3.4	19	1	1	2	3	8	17	17
20–34	5	10.5	119	1	1	8	15	27	27	27
35–49	4	2.3	<1	2	2	2	3	3	3	3
50–64	2	3.0	8	1	1	5	5	5	5	5
65+	3	5.7	2	4	4	6	7	7	7	7
TOTAL SINGLE DX	2	2.0	2	1	1	1	3	3	3	3
TOTAL MULTIPLE DX	31	4.4	31	1	1	2	4	8	17	27
TOTAL										
0–19 Years	17	3.4	19	1	1	2	3	8	17	17
20–34	6	9.2	105	1	1	8	15	27	27	27
35–49	5	2.0	<1	1	2	2	2	3	3	3
50–64	2	3.0	8	1	1	5	5	5	5	5
65+	3	5.7	2	4	4	6	7	7	7	7
GRAND TOTAL	33	4.2	30	1	1	2	4	8	17	27

87.2: X-RAY OF SPINE

Type of Patients	Observed Patients	Avg. Stay	Variance	Percentiles						
				10th	25th	50th	75th	90th	95th	99th
1. SINGLE DX										
0–19 Years	2	1.0	0	1	1	1	1	1	1	1
20–34	0									
35–49	5	3.6	3	2	2	3	5	6	6	6
50–64	7	3.6	6	1	1	3	5	8	8	8
65+	3	6.0	7	4	4	5	9	9	9	9
2. MULTIPLE DX										
0–19 Years	6	4.7	18	1	1	2	10	10	10	10
20–34	32	5.5	20	1	2	4	9	11	15	18
35–49	81	4.9	18	1	2	4	6	10	13	26
50–64	109	5.2	34	1	2	4	5	10	17	26
65+	160	5.8	22	2	3	5	7	10	12	33
TOTAL SINGLE DX	17	3.7	6	1	2	3	5	8	9	9
TOTAL MULTIPLE DX	388	5.4	24	1	3	4	7	10	13	26
TOTAL										
0–19 Years	8	3.8	16	1	1	2	10	10	10	10
20–34	32	5.5	20	1	2	8	9	11	15	18
35–49	86	4.8	17	1	2	3	6	10	13	26
50–64	116	5.1	32	1	2	4	5	9	17	26
65+	163	5.8	22	2	3	5	7	10	12	33
GRAND TOTAL	405	5.3	24	1	2	4	7	10	13	26

87.21: CONTRAST MYELOGRAM

Type of Patients	Observed Patients	Avg. Stay	Variance	Percentiles						
				10th	25th	50th	75th	90th	95th	99th
1. SINGLE DX										
0–19 Years	1	1.0	0	1	1	1	1	1	1	1
20–34	0									
35–49	4	3.8	4	2	2	5	6	6	6	6
50–64	6	3.8	6	1	2	4	5	8	8	8
65+	3	6.0	7	4	4	5	9	9	9	9
2. MULTIPLE DX										
0–19 Years	5	5.2	21	1	1	4	10	10	10	10
20–34	24	5.0	16	1	2	4	9	11	11	15
35–49	65	4.9	13	1	2	4	6	10	13	16
50–64	83	6.0	41	2	3	5	7	11	19	43
65+	142	6.0	23	2	3	5	7	10	12	33
TOTAL SINGLE DX	14	4.1	6	1	2	4	5	8	9	9
TOTAL MULTIPLE DX	319	5.7	25	2	3	4	7	10	14	26
TOTAL										
0–19 Years	6	4.5	20	1	1	1	10	10	10	10
20–34	24	5.0	16	1	2	4	9	11	11	15
35–49	69	4.8	13	1	2	4	6	10	13	16
50–64	89	5.8	39	1	2	4	7	11	19	43
65+	145	6.0	23	2	3	5	7	10	12	33
GRAND TOTAL	333	5.6	25	2	3	4	7	10	14	26

87.3: THORAX SOFT TISSUE X-RAY

Type of Patients	Observed Patients	Avg. Stay	Variance	Percentiles						
				10th	25th	50th	75th	90th	95th	99th
1. SINGLE DX										
0–19 Years	7	1.3	<1	1	1	1	2	2	2	2
20–34	0									
35–49	0									
50–64	0									
65+										
2. MULTIPLE DX										
0–19 Years	87	3.0	4	1	2	2	4	6	7	11
20–34	16	4.6	15	2	2	3	6	13	14	14
35–49	26	3.6	28	1	2	2	4	5	6	29
50–64	71	3.2	5	1	2	2	4	6	7	12
65+	170	3.3	4	1	2	3	4	6	7	13
TOTAL SINGLE DX	7	1.3	<1	1	1	1	2	2	2	2
TOTAL MULTIPLE DX	370	3.3	6	1	2	3	4	6	7	13
TOTAL										
0–19 Years	94	2.9	4	1	2	2	4	6	7	11
20–34	16	4.6	15	2	2	3	6	13	14	14
35–49	26	3.6	28	1	2	2	4	5	6	29
50–64	71	3.2	5	1	2	2	4	6	7	12
65+	170	3.3	4	1	2	3	4	6	7	13
GRAND TOTAL	377	3.2	6	1	2	3	4	6	7	13

Western Region, October 2007–September 2008 Data, by Operation

87.39: THOR SOFT TISS X-RAY NEC

Type of Patients	Observed Patients	Avg. Stay	Variance	10th	25th	50th	75th	90th	95th	99th
1. SINGLE DX										
0–19 Years	7	1.3	<1	1	1	1	2	2	2	2
20–34	0									
35–49	0									
50–64	0									
65+	0									
2. MULTIPLE DX										
0–19 Years	81	2.8	3	1	2	2	3	5	7	10
20–34	15	4.4	15	2	2	3	5	13	14	14
35–49	24	2.6	2	1	2	2	3	4	5	6
50–64	65	3.2	5	1	2	2	4	7	7	12
65+	165	3.2	4	1	2	3	4	6	7	8
TOTAL SINGLE DX	7	1.3	<1	1	1	1	2	2	2	2
TOTAL MULTIPLE DX	350	3.1	4	1	2	3	4	6	7	12
TOTAL										
0–19 Years	88	2.7	3	1	2	2	3	4	7	10
20–34	15	4.4	15	2	2	3	5	13	14	14
35–49	24	2.6	2	1	2	2	3	4	5	6
50–64	65	3.2	5	1	2	2	4	7	7	12
65+	165	3.2	4	1	2	3	4	6	7	8
GRAND TOTAL	357	3.1	4	1	2	3	4	6	7	12

87.4: OTHER X-RAY OF THORAX

Type of Patients	Observed Patients	Avg. Stay	Variance	10th	25th	50th	75th	90th	95th	99th
1. SINGLE DX										
0–19 Years	77	3.2	17	1	1	2	3	6	11	24
20–34	72	3.2	31	1	1	1	3	5	13	34
35–49	69	2.2	5	1	1	1	3	5	6	14
50–64	41	2.1	2	1	1	1	3	4	6	6
65+	10	3.5	25	1	1	2	3	17	17	17
2. MULTIPLE DX										
0–19 Years	401	4.9	26	1	2	3	6	11	14	22
20–34	1,055	3.8	24	1	1	2	4	7	11	23
35–49	2,235	3.7	19	1	1	2	5	7	10	20
50–64	3,851	3.7	17	1	1	3	4	7	10	19
65+	5,468	4.1	13	2	2	3	5	8	10	18
TOTAL SINGLE DX	269	2.8	16	1	1	1	3	5	8	24
TOTAL MULTIPLE DX	13,010	3.9	16	1	2	3	5	7	10	19
TOTAL										
0–19 Years	478	4.6	25	1	2	2	3	6	11	22
20–34	1,127	3.7	25	1	1	2	4	7	11	24
35–49	2,304	3.7	19	1	1	3	5	7	10	20
50–64	3,892	3.7	17	1	1	3	4	7	9	19
65+	5,478	4.1	13	2	2	3	5	8	10	18
GRAND TOTAL	13,279	3.9	16	1	2	3	5	7	10	19

87.41: CAT SCAN THORAX

Type of Patients	Observed Patients	Avg. Stay	Variance	10th	25th	50th	75th	90th	95th	99th
1. SINGLE DX										
0–19 Years	31	3.8	29	1	1	2	3	5	18	24
20–34	45	4.0	44	1	1	2	3	8	16	34
35–49	49	2.5	6	1	1	1	3	6	7	14
50–64	23	2.3	2	1	1	2	3	4	6	6
65+	8	4.0	31	1	1	2	6	17	17	17
2. MULTIPLE DX										
0–19 Years	203	5.3	21	2	2	4	7	12	15	22
20–34	812	3.7	19	1	1	3	5	7	10	21
35–49	1,755	3.8	19	1	2	3	5	7	10	18
50–64	3,084	3.8	16	1	2	3	5	7	10	18
65+	4,820	4.2	13	1	2	3	5	8	10	18
TOTAL SINGLE DX	156	3.2	23	1	1	2	3	6	10	29
TOTAL MULTIPLE DX	10,674	4.1	16	1	2	3	5	8	10	18
TOTAL										
0–19 Years	234	5.2	22	1	2	4	7	11	15	22
20–34	857	3.7	20	1	1	3	5	7	10	23
35–49	1,804	3.8	18	1	2	3	5	7	9	18
50–64	3,107	3.8	16	1	2	3	5	7	10	17
65+	4,828	4.2	13	1	2	3	5	8	10	18
GRAND TOTAL	10,830	4.0	16	1	2	3	5	8	10	18

87.44: ROUTINE CHEST X-RAY

Type of Patients	Observed Patients	Avg. Stay	Variance	10th	25th	50th	75th	90th	95th	99th
1. SINGLE DX										
0–19 Years	34	3.3	8	1	1	2	4	6	11	12
20–34	5	2.4	2	1	1	3	3	4	4	4
35–49	7	1.7	<1	1	1	1	2	3	3	3
50–64	2	2.0	0	2	2	2	2	2	2	2
65+	1	1.0	0	1	1	1	1	1	1	1
2. MULTIPLE DX										
0–19 Years	120	4.3	18	1	2	3	6	9	12	22
20–34	53	7.1	144	1	1	2	7	18	25	75
35–49	83	6.4	53	1	2	2	8	19	24	30
50–64	104	4.9	58	1	1	2	4	10	22	43
65+	39	3.3	35	1	1	2	3	6	12	37
TOTAL SINGLE DX	49	2.9	6	1	1	2	3	6	9	12
TOTAL MULTIPLE DX	399	5.2	55	1	1	3	6	12	21	38
TOTAL										
0–19 Years	154	4.1	16	1	2	3	5	9	12	22
20–34	58	6.7	133	1	1	3	7	18	25	75
35–49	90	6.1	50	1	1	3	8	19	24	30
50–64	106	4.9	57	1	1	2	4	10	22	43
65+	40	3.2	34	1	1	2	3	5	7	37
GRAND TOTAL	448	4.9	50	1	1	2	5	12	19	37

LOS by Diagnosis and Operation, Western Region, 45th Edition

87.49: CHEST X-RAY NEC

Type of Patients	Observed Patients	Avg. Stay	Vari-ance	10th	25th	50th	75th	90th	95th	99th
1. SINGLE DX										
0–19 Years	12	1.3	<1	1	1	1	1	3	3	3
20–34	18	1.8	1	1	1	1	1	2	3	13
35–49	12	1.7	1	1	1	1	2	3	4	4
50–64	16	1.9	3	1	1	1	2	5	6	6
65+	1	2.0	0	2	2	2	2	2	2	2
2. MULTIPLE DX										
0–19 Years	62	4.0	69	1	1	2	3	5	12	61
20–34	182	2.9	8	1	1	2	3	6	8	14
35–49	390	2.8	10	1	1	2	3	5	7	17
50–64	652	2.9	13	1	1	2	3	6	8	18
65+	585	3.0	8	1	2	2	4	6	7	16
TOTAL SINGLE DX	59	1.7	3	1	1	1	2	3	5	13
TOTAL MULTIPLE DX	1,871	2.9	12	1	1	2	3	6	8	17
TOTAL										
0–19 Years	74	3.6	59	1	1	2	3	5	12	61
20–34	200	2.8	8	1	1	2	3	6	8	14
35–49	402	2.7	10	1	1	2	3	5	7	14
50–64	668	2.9	13	1	1	2	3	6	8	18
65+	586	3.0	8	1	2	2	4	6	7	16
GRAND TOTAL	1,930	2.9	12	1	1	2	3	5	8	17

87.51: PERC HEPAT CHOLANGIOGRAM

Type of Patients	Observed Patients	Avg. Stay	Vari-ance	10th	25th	50th	75th	90th	95th	99th
1. SINGLE DX										
0–19 Years	0									
20–34	1	11.0	0	11	11	11	11	11	11	11
35–49	1	5.0	0	5	5	5	5	5	5	5
50–64	0									
65+	0									
2. MULTIPLE DX										
0–19 Years	16	8.4	59	2	2	3	16	22	22	22
20–34	9	6.5	17	1	2	7	8	12	12	12
35–49	32	7.7	45	2	4	6	10	15	16	35
50–64	71	7.7	59	1	3	5	10	14	30	33
65+	118	7.1	23	2	3	6	10	14	16	21
TOTAL SINGLE DX	2	8.0	18	5	5	5	11	11	11	11
TOTAL MULTIPLE DX	246	7.5	40	2	3	6	11	16	19	32
TOTAL										
0–19 Years	16	8.4	59	2	2	3	16	22	22	22
20–34	10	6.9	17	2	2	8	11	12	12	12
35–49	33	7.6	44	2	4	6	10	15	16	35
50–64	71	7.7	59	1	3	5	10	14	30	33
65+	118	7.1-	23	2	3	6	10	14	16	21
GRAND TOTAL	248	7.5	40	2	3	6	11	16	19	32

87.5: BILIARY TRACT X-RAY

Type of Patients	Observed Patients	Avg. Stay	Vari-ance	10th	25th	50th	75th	90th	95th	99th
1. SINGLE DX										
0–19 Years	0									
20–34	8	4.6	10	1	3	3	7	11	11	11
35–49	3	3.7	5	1	1	5	5	5	5	5
50–64	1	1.0	0	1	1	1	1	1	1	1
65+	1	1.0	0	1	1	1	1	1	1	1
2. MULTIPLE DX										
0–19 Years	27	7.6	45	2	2	5	14	18	22	22
20–34	43	5.1	11	1	3	4	7	10	12	12
35–49	92	6.3	48	1	2	4	7	14	16	43
50–64	187	6.0	44	1	2	4	7	13	20	33
65+	233	6.2	23	2	3	5	9	12	14	23
TOTAL SINGLE DX	13	3.9	9	1	1	3	5	7	11	11
TOTAL MULTIPLE DX	582	6.2	35	1	2	4	8	14	16	32
TOTAL										
0–19 Years	27	7.6	45	2	2	5	14	18	22	22
20–34	51	5.0	11	1	2	4	7	10	12	12
35–49	95	6.3	47	1	3	4	7	14	16	43
50–64	188	6.0	44	1	2	4	7	13	20	33
65+	234	6.2	23	2	3	5	9	12	14	23
GRAND TOTAL	595	6.2	34	1	2	4	8	13	16	32

87.53: INTRAOP CHOLANGIOGRAM

Type of Patients	Observed Patients	Avg. Stay	Vari-ance	10th	25th	50th	75th	90th	95th	99th
1. SINGLE DX										
0–19 Years	0									
20–34	3	2.3	1	1	1	3	3	3	3	3
35–49	1	5.0	0	5	5	5	5	5	5	5
50–64	1	1.0	0	1	1	1	1	1	1	1
65+	0									
2. MULTIPLE DX										
0–19 Years	3	4.0	2	2	2	5	5	5	5	5
20–34	14	4.2	7	2	2	3	5	10	10	10
35–49	16	6.4	108	1	3	6	6	16	43	43
50–64	18	8.3	81	1	3	4	10	18	38	38
65+	39	6.8	39	2	3	5	9	11	25	34
TOTAL SINGLE DX	5	2.6	3	1	1	3	3	5	5	5
TOTAL MULTIPLE DX	90	6.4	52	2	3	4	6	11	18	43
TOTAL										
0–19 Years	3	4.0	2	2	2	5	5	5	5	5
20–34	17	3.9	7	1	2	4	5	10	10	10
35–49	17	6.3	102	1	2	4	5	16	43	43
50–64	19	7.9	80	1	3	4	10	18	38	38
65+	39	6.8	39	2	3	5	9	11	25	34
GRAND TOTAL	95	6.2	50	1	3	4	6	11	18	43

LOS by Diagnosis and Operation, Western Region, 45th Edition

Western Region, October 2007–September 2008 Data, by Operation

87.54: CHOLANGIOGRAM NEC

Type of Patients	Observed Patients	Avg. Stay	Variance	Percentiles						
				10th	25th	50th	75th	90th	95th	99th
1. SINGLE DX										
0–19 Years	0									
20–34	3	5.3	4	3	3	6	7	7	7	7
35–49	1	1.0	0	1	1	1	1	1	1	1
50–64	0									
65+	1	1.0	0	1	1	1	1	1	1	1
2. MULTIPLE DX										
0–19 Years	8	7.1	25	2	3	6	14	14	14	14
20–34	16	5.6	12	2	3	4	7	11	12	12
35–49	34	5.5	36	1	3	4	6	11	16	34
50–64	93	4.4	23	2	2	3	6	9	14	29
65+	69	4.2	8	2	2	3	6	9	9	14
TOTAL SINGLE DX	5	3.6	8	1	1	3	6	7	7	7
TOTAL MULTIPLE DX	220	4.8	20	1	2	3	6	10	14	24
TOTAL										
0–19 Years	8	7.1	25	2	3	6	14	14	14	14
20–34	19	5.5	11	1	3	5	7	11	12	12
35–49	35	5.3	36	1	3	4	6	11	16	34
50–64	93	4.4	23	2	2	3	6	9	14	29
65+	70	4.1	8	1	2	3	6	8	9	14
GRAND TOTAL	225	4.7	20	1	2	3	6	9	14	24

87.6: OTH DIGESTIVE SYST X-RAY

Type of Patients	Observed Patients	Avg. Stay	Variance	Percentiles						
				10th	25th	50th	75th	90th	95th	99th
1. SINGLE DX										
0–19 Years	67	1.7	2	1	1	1	2	4	4	9
20–34	2	2.5	<1	2	2	3	3	3	3	3
35–49	4	2.0	1	1	1	3	3	3	3	3
50–64	2	2.5	4	1	1	3	4	4	4	4
65+	3	2.3	<1	2	2	2	3	3	3	3
2. MULTIPLE DX										
0–19 Years	196	5.5	29	1	2	4	6	11	17	27
20–34	41	4.8	17	1	2	4	6	14	14	16
35–49	80	4.4	10	2	2	4	5	9	11	23
50–64	141	4.2	7	1	2	3	6	7	9	13
65+	373	5.4	14	2	3	4	7	10	13	21
TOTAL SINGLE DX	78	1.8	2	1	1	1	2	4	4	9
TOTAL MULTIPLE DX	831	5.1	18	2	3	4	6	10	13	23
TOTAL										
0–19 Years	263	4.3	24	1	1	3	5	9	13	27
20–34	43	4.7	16	1	2	4	5	14	14	16
35–49	84	4.3	10	2	2	4	5	8	9	23
50–64	143	4.2	7	1	2	3	6	7	9	13
65+	376	5.3	14	2	3	4	7	10	13	21
GRAND TOTAL	909	4.7	17	1	2	4	6	9	13	23

87.61: BARIUM SWALLOW

Type of Patients	Observed Patients	Avg. Stay	Variance	Percentiles						
				10th	25th	50th	75th	90th	95th	99th
1. SINGLE DX										
0–19 Years	2	1.0	0	1	1	1	1		1	1
20–34	0									
35–49	3	2.3	1	1	1	3	3	3	3	3
50–64	1	1.0	0	1	1	1	1	1	1	1
65+	0									
2. MULTIPLE DX										
0–19 Years	11	7.4	52	2	2	5	8	23	23	23
20–34	8	3.6	3	1	3	4	5	6	6	6
35–49	16	5.0	6	2	3	4	6	9	11	11
50–64	39	4.3	8	1	2	3	6	9	9	15
65+	163	5.7	16	2	3	5	7	10	13	23
TOTAL SINGLE DX	6	1.7	1	1	1	1	3	3	3	3
TOTAL MULTIPLE DX	237	5.4	16	2	3	4	6	10	13	23
TOTAL										
0–19 Years	13	6.7	50	1	2	5	8	23	23	23
20–34	8	3.6	3	1	3	4	5	6	6	6
35–49	19	4.6	7	2	3	4	6	9	11	11
50–64	40	4.2	8	1	2	3	6	10	9	15
65+	163	5.7	16	2	3	5	7	10	13	23
GRAND TOTAL	243	5.4	16	2	3	4	6	10	13	23

87.62: UPPER GI SERIES

Type of Patients	Observed Patients	Avg. Stay	Variance	Percentiles						
				10th	25th	50th	75th	90th	95th	99th
1. SINGLE DX										
0–19 Years	25	2.7	4	1	1	2	4	6	6	9
20–34	1	2.0	0	2	2	2	2	2	2	2
35–49	1	1.0	0	1	1	1	1	1	1	1
50–64	0									
65+	0									
2. MULTIPLE DX										
0–19 Years	144	5.1	20	1	2	4	6	10	13	19
20–34	20	3.3	4	1	2	3	5	6	7	7
35–49	28	3.5	6	1	2	3	4	6	9	12
50–64	30	4.4	9	2	2	4	5	8	11	13
65+	47	3.9	7	2	2	4	5	7	10	13
TOTAL SINGLE DX	27	2.7	4	1	1	2	4	6	6	9
TOTAL MULTIPLE DX	269	4.6	15	1	2	4	5	8	12	19
TOTAL										
0–19 Years	169	4.7	18	1	2	4	6	9	13	19
20–34	21	3.2	3	1	2	3	5	6	6	7
35–49	29	3.4	6	1	2	3	4	6	9	12
50–64	30	4.4	9	2	2	4	5	8	11	13
65+	47	3.9	7	2	2	4	5	7	10	13
GRAND TOTAL	296	4.4	14	1	2	4	5	8	11	18

LOS by Diagnosis and Operation, Western Region, 45th Edition

Western Region, October 2007–September 2008 Data, by Operation

87.69: DIGEST TRACT X-RAY NEC

Type of Patients	Observed Patients	Avg. Stay	Variance	10th	25th	50th	75th	90th	95th	99th
1. SINGLE DX										
0–19 Years	4	1.3	<1	1	1	1	2	2	2	2
20–34	0									
35–49	0									
50–64	0									
65+	0									
2. MULTIPLE DX										
0–19 Years	11	10.1	99	2	2	8	11	27	27	27
20–34	7	7.7	35	1	1	7	14	14	14	14
35–49	3	11.0	107	5	5	5	23	23	23	23
50–64	25	4.6	9	1	1	4	7	8	9	11
65+	96	6.2	17	2	3	5	8	11	14	24
TOTAL SINGLE DX	4	1.3	<1	1	1	1	2	2	2	2
TOTAL MULTIPLE DX	142	6.6	29	2	3	5	8	13	16	27
TOTAL										
0–19 Years	15	8.4	92	1	2	3	8	27	27	27
20–34	7	7.7	35	1	1	7	14	14	14	14
35–49	3	11.0	107	5	5	5	23	23	23	23
50–64	25	4.6	9	1	1	4	7	8	9	11
65+	96	6.2	17	2	3	5	8	11	14	24
GRAND TOTAL	146	6.4	29	2	3	5	8	13	16	27

87.71: CAT SCAN OF KIDNEY

Type of Patients	Observed Patients	Avg. Stay	Variance	10th	25th	50th	75th	90th	95th	99th
1. SINGLE DX										
0–19 Years	1	1.0	0	1	1	1	1	1	1	1
20–34	2	1.0	0	1	1	1	1	1	1	1
35–49	1	6.0	0	6	6	6	6	6	6	6
50–64	0									
65+	0									
2. MULTIPLE DX										
0–19 Years	4	2.9	3	1	1	3	3	6	6	6
20–34	14	2.2	1	1	2	2	2	4	5	5
35–49	24	3.8	11	1	2	3	5	10	11	13
50–64	24	3.0	5	1	2	2	3	7	7	10
65+	23	2.9	4	1	1	3	4	4	7	9
TOTAL SINGLE DX	4	2.3	6	1	1	1	6	6	6	6
TOTAL MULTIPLE DX	89	3.0	6	1	1	2	3	6	9	13
TOTAL										
0–19 Years	5	2.6	3	1	1	3	3	6	6	6
20–34	16	2.1	1	1	1	2	2	4	5	5
35–49	25	3.9	11	1	2	3	6	10	11	13
50–64	24	3.0	5	1	2	2	3	7	7	10
65+	23	2.9	4	1	1	3	4	4	7	9
GRAND TOTAL	93	3.0	6	1	1	2	3	6	9	13

87.7: X-RAY OF URINARY SYSTEM

Type of Patients	Observed Patients	Avg. Stay	Variance	10th	25th	50th	75th	90th	95th	99th
1. SINGLE DX										
0–19 Years	85	3.3	3	1	2	3	4	6	7	8
20–34	18	1.4	1	1	1	1	1	2	6	6
35–49	13	2.3	2	1	1	2	2	5	6	6
50–64	7	1.0	0	1	1	1	1	1	1	1
65+	3	1.7	1	1	1	1	3	3	3	3
2. MULTIPLE DX										
0–19 Years	1,357	4.8	21	2	2	4	6	9	11	21
20–34	271	3.2	6	1	1	2	4	7	8	13
35–49	409	3.9	19	1	2	3	5	7	11	24
50–64	475	4.3	22	1	2	3	5	9	12	20
65+	630	5.6	21	1	3	4	7	11	14	21
TOTAL SINGLE DX	126	2.8	3	1	1	2	3	5	7	8
TOTAL MULTIPLE DX	3,142	4.7	20	1	2	3	6	9	12	21
TOTAL										
0–19 Years	1,442	4.7	20	2	2	3	6	9	11	21
20–34	289	3.1	6	1	1	2	4	6	8	13
35–49	422	3.8	18	1	2	3	5	7	10	24
50–64	482	4.2	22	1	2	3	5	9	11	20
65+	633	5.5	21	1	3	4	7	11	14	21
GRAND TOTAL	3,268	4.6	20	1	2	3	6	9	12	20

87.73: IV PYELOGRAM

Type of Patients	Observed Patients	Avg. Stay	Variance	10th	25th	50th	75th	90th	95th	99th
1. SINGLE DX										
0–19 Years	0									
20–34	2	3.5	12	1	1	1	6	6	6	6
35–49	3	1.7	<1	1	1	2	2	2	2	2
50–64	1	1.0	0	1	1	1	1	1	1	1
65+	0									
2. MULTIPLE DX										
0–19 Years	8	3.9	2	2	3	3	6	6	6	6
20–34	53	2.4	2	1	2	2	3	4	5	7
35–49	46	4.0	26	2	2	3	4	6	7	36
50–64	38	3.5	5	2	2	3	4	7	9	11
65+	46	5.3	20	2	3	4	6	12	13	21
TOTAL SINGLE DX	6	2.2	4	1	1	1	2	6	6	6
TOTAL MULTIPLE DX	191	3.8	13	1	2	3	4	6	9	21
TOTAL										
0–19 Years	8	3.9	2	2	3	3	6	6	6	6
20–34	55	2.5	2	1	2	3	3	4	6	7
35–49	49	3.8	25	1	2	3	4	6	7	36
50–64	39	3.5	5	2	2	3	4	7	7	11
65+	46	5.3	20	2	3	4	6	12	13	21
GRAND TOTAL	197	3.7	13	1	2	3	4	6	9	21

LOS by Diagnosis and Operation, Western Region, 45th Edition

Western Region, October 2007–September 2008 Data, by Operation

87.74: RETROGRADE PYELOGRAM

Type of Patients	Observed Patients	Avg. Stay	Vari-ance	Percentiles 10th	25th	50th	75th	90th	95th	99th
1. SINGLE DX										
0–19 Years	0									
20–34	8	1.1	<1	1	1	1	1	2	2	2
35–49	4	1.5	<1	1	1	2	2	2	2	2
50–64	6	1.0	0	1	1	1	1	1	1	1
65+	1	1.0	0	1	1	1	1	1	1	1
2. MULTIPLE DX										
0–19 Years	37	3.0	25	1	1	2	3	5	6	43
20–34	125	3.3	8	1	1	2	4	7	8	15
35–49	193	3.7	22	1	1	2	4	7	10	28
50–64	224	4.1	14	1	2	3	5	8	12	20
65+	289	5.8	22	1	2	5	8	12	14	24
TOTAL SINGLE DX	19	1.2	<1	1	1	1	1	2	2	2
TOTAL MULTIPLE DX	868	4.3	19	1	2	3	6	9	12	20
TOTAL										
0–19 Years	37	3.0	25	1	1	2	3	5	6	43
20–34	133	3.2	8	1	1	2	4	7	8	15
35–49	197	3.7	22	1	1	2	4	7	10	28
50–64	230	4.0	14	1	1	3	5	8	12	20
65+	290	5.7	22	1	2	5	8	12	14	24
GRAND TOTAL	887	4.3	19	1	2	3	6	9	12	20

87.75: PERCUTANEOUS PYELOGRAM

Type of Patients	Observed Patients	Avg. Stay	Vari-ance	Percentiles 10th	25th	50th	75th	90th	95th	99th
1. SINGLE DX										
0–19 Years	1	1.0	0	1	1	1	1	1	1	1
20–34	0									
35–49	0									
50–64	0									
65+	0									
2. MULTIPLE DX										
0–19 Years	2	3.4	<1	3	3	3	3	5	5	5
20–34	12	2.8	4	1	2	2	4	4	8	8
35–49	33	3.7	4	1	2	4	5	6	9	10
50–64	41	5.8	14	2	3	5	8	10	11	19
65+	52	5.5	14	2	3	5	8	9	15	19
TOTAL SINGLE DX	1	1.0	0	1	1	1	1	1	1	1
TOTAL MULTIPLE DX	140	4.9	11	2	2	4	6	9	10	19
TOTAL										
0–19 Years	3	2.3	2	1	1	3	3	5	5	5
20–34	12	2.8	4	1	2	4	4	4	8	8
35–49	33	3.7	4	1	2	4	5	6	9	10
50–64	41	5.8	14	2	3	5	8	10	11	19
65+	52	5.5	14	2	3	5	8	9	15	19
GRAND TOTAL	141	4.7	12	2	2	4	6	9	10	19

87.76: RETRO CYSTOURETHROGRAM

Type of Patients	Observed Patients	Avg. Stay	Vari-ance	Percentiles 10th	25th	50th	75th	90th	95th	99th
1. SINGLE DX										
0–19 Years	70	3.4	3	2	2	3	4	6	7	9
20–34	1	2.0	0	2	2	2	2	2	2	2
35–49	0									
50–64	0									
65+	0									
2. MULTIPLE DX										
0–19 Years	1,215	4.9	21	2	3	4	6	9	11	21
20–34	22	4.5	10	1	2	3	6	8	10	13
35–49	26	4.5	30	1	2	3	5	7	13	28
50–64	23	5.5	21	1	3	4	8	12	13	19
65+	27	7.6	56	2	3	5	8	15	19	38
TOTAL SINGLE DX	71	3.4	3	2	2	3	4	6	7	9
TOTAL MULTIPLE DX	1,313	5.0	21	2	3	4	6	9	12	21
TOTAL										
0–19 Years	1,285	4.9	20	2	3	4	6	9	11	21
20–34	23	4.3	10	1	2	3	6	8	10	13
35–49	26	4.5	30	1	2	3	5	7	13	28
50–64	23	5.5	21	1	2	4	8	12	13	19
65+	27	7.6	56	2	3	5	8	15	19	38
GRAND TOTAL	1,384	4.9	21	2	3	4	6	9	11	21

87.77: CYSTOGRAM NEC

Type of Patients	Observed Patients	Avg. Stay	Vari-ance	Percentiles 10th	25th	50th	75th	90th	95th	99th
1. SINGLE DX										
0–19 Years	4	3.3	7	1	1	2	7	7	7	7
20–34	1	2.0	0	2	2	2	2	2	2	2
35–49	2	1.5	<1	1	1	2	2	2	2	2
50–64	0									
65+	1	3.0	0	3	3	3	3	3	3	3
2. MULTIPLE DX										
0–19 Years	59	5.0	26	2	3	3	5	7	17	32
20–34	20	3.3	4	1	2	3	4	6	8	8
35–49	25	5.1	7	2	3	5	7	9	11	11
50–64	47	5.5	24	1	2	4	7	12	18	22
65+	154	5.4	10	2	3	5	7	10	11	15
TOTAL SINGLE DX	8	2.6	4	1	1	2	3	7	7	7
TOTAL MULTIPLE DX	305	5.2	15	2	3	4	6	10	12	19
TOTAL										
0–19 Years	63	4.9	25	2	2	3	5	7	17	32
20–34	21	3.2	4	1	2	3	4	6	7	8
35–49	27	4.8	8	2	2	5	7	9	11	11
50–64	47	5.5	24	1	2	4	7	12	18	22
65+	155	5.4	10	2	3	5	7	10	11	15
GRAND TOTAL	313	5.1	15	2	3	4	6	10	12	19

LOS by Diagnosis and Operation, Western Region, 45th Edition

Western Region, October 2007–September 2008 Data, by Operation

87.79: URINARY SYSTEM X-RAY NEC

Type of Patients	Observed Patients	Avg. Stay	Vari-ance	Percentiles						
				10th	25th	50th	75th	90th	95th	99th
1. SINGLE DX										
0–19 Years	9	2.9	5	1	1	2	3	8	8	8
20–34	4	1.0	0	1	1	1	1	1	1	1
35–49	3	3.3	2	2	2	3	5	5	5	5
50–64	0									
65+	1	1.0	0	1	1	1	1	1	1	1
2. MULTIPLE DX										
0–19 Years	32	3.1	9	1	2	2	4	7	12	14
20–34	24	3.9	10	1	2	3	4	9	10	13
35–49	61	3.6	13	1	2	2	4	6	11	20
50–64	70	2.8	5	1	2	2	3	6	8	10
65+	23	4.8	65	1	2	3	5	6	6	41
TOTAL SINGLE DX	**17**	**2.4**	**4**	**1**	**1**	**2**	**3**	**5**	**8**	**8**
TOTAL MULTIPLE DX	**210**	**3.4**	**15**	**1**	**2**	**2**	**4**	**6**	**10**	**17**
TOTAL										
0–19 Years	41	3.1	8	1	2	2	4	7	8	14
20–34	28	3.5	9	1	1	2	4	9	10	13
35–49	64	3.6	13	1	2	2	4	6	11	20
50–64	70	2.8	5	1	2	3	3	6	8	10
65+	24	4.6	63	1	2	3	5	6	6	41
GRAND TOTAL	**227**	**3.3**	**14**	**1**	**2**	**2**	**4**	**6**	**9**	**17**

87.9: MALE GENITAL X-RAY

Type of Patients	Observed Patients	Avg. Stay	Vari-ance	Percentiles						
				10th	25th	50th	75th	90th	95th	99th
1. SINGLE DX										
0–19 Years	0									
20–34	0									
35–49	0									
50–64	0									
65+	0									
2. MULTIPLE DX										
0–19 Years	0									
20–34	0									
35–49	0									
50–64	0									
65+	0									
TOTAL SINGLE DX	**0**									
TOTAL MULTIPLE DX	**0**									
TOTAL										
0–19 Years	0									
20–34	0									
35–49	0									
50–64	0									
65+	0									
GRAND TOTAL	**0**									

87.8: FEMALE GENITAL X-RAY

Type of Patients	Observed Patients	Avg. Stay	Vari-ance	Percentiles						
				10th	25th	50th	75th	90th	95th	99th
1. SINGLE DX										
0–19 Years	0									
20–34	0									
35–49	0									
50–64	0									
65+	0									
2. MULTIPLE DX										
0–19 Years	0									
20–34	1	1.0	0	1	1	1	1	1	1	1
35–49	0									
50–64	0									
65+	0									
TOTAL SINGLE DX	**0**									
TOTAL MULTIPLE DX	**1**	**1.0**	**0**	**1**	**1**	**1**	**1**	**1**	**1**	**1**
TOTAL										
0–19 Years	0									
20–34	1	1.0	0	1	1	1	1	1	1	1
35–49	0									
50–64	0									
65+	0									
GRAND TOTAL	**1**	**1.0**	**0**	**1**	**1**	**1**	**1**	**1**	**1**	**1**

88.0: ABD SOFT TISSUE X-RAY

Type of Patients	Observed Patients	Avg. Stay	Vari-ance	Percentiles						
				10th	25th	50th	75th	90th	95th	99th
1. SINGLE DX										
0–19 Years	252	2.2	3	1	1	2	2	4	6	9
20–34	254	2.1	3	1	1	1	3	4	6	10
35–49	185	2.5	4	1	1	2	3	5	5	10
50–64	111	2.5	2	1	1	2	3	5	6	7
65+	23	2.2	1	1	1	2	3	4	4	4
2. MULTIPLE DX										
0–19 Years	726	3.7	15	1	1	2	5	8	11	21
20–34	1,892	3.1	9	1	1	2	4	6	8	15
35–49	3,097	3.4	9	1	2	3	4	6	8	15
50–64	3,781	3.7	10	1	2	3	4	7	9	15
65+	5,042	4.0	11	1	2	3	5	8	10	18
TOTAL SINGLE DX	**825**	**2.3**	**3**	**1**	**1**	**2**	**3**	**4**	**6**	**9**
TOTAL MULTIPLE DX	**14,538**	**3.7**	**11**	**1**	**2**	**3**	**4**	**7**	**9**	**17**
TOTAL										
0–19 Years	978	3.4	13	1	1	2	4	8	10	19
20–34	2,146	3.0	9	1	2	2	4	6	7	14
35–49	3,282	3.4	9	1	2	3	4	6	8	15
50–64	3,892	3.6	10	1	2	3	4	7	9	15
65+	5,065	4.0	11	1	2	3	5	8	10	18
GRAND TOTAL	**15,363**	**3.6**	**10**	**1**	**2**	**3**	**4**	**7**	**9**	**16**

LOS by Diagnosis and Operation, Western Region, 45th Edition

Western Region, October 2007–September 2008 Data, by Operation

88.01: ABDOMEN CAT SCAN

Type of Patients	Observed Patients	Avg. Stay	Vari-ance	Percentiles						
				10th	25th	50th	75th	90th	95th	99th
1. SINGLE DX										
0–19 Years	251	2.2	3	1	1	2	2	4	6	9
20–34	253	2.2	3	1	1	1	3	4	6	10
35–49	185	2.5	4	1	1	2	3	5	5	10
50–64	111	2.5	2	1	1	2	3	5	6	7
65+	23	2.2	1	1	1	2	3	4	4	4
2. MULTIPLE DX										
0–19 Years	723	3.7	15	1	1	2	4	8	11	21
20–34	1,868	3.1	9	1	1	2	4	6	8	14
35–49	3,078	3.4	9	1	2	3	4	6	8	15
50–64	3,745	3.6	10	1	2	3	4	7	9	15
65+	4,999	4.0	11	1	2	3	5	8	10	17
TOTAL SINGLE DX	823	2.3	3	1	1	2	3	4	6	9
TOTAL MULTIPLE DX	14,413	3.7	10	1	2	3	4	7	9	17
TOTAL										
0–19 Years	974	3.3	13	1	1	2	4	8	10	19
20–34	2,121	3.0	9	1	1	2	4	6	7	14
35–49	3,263	3.4	9	1	2	3	4	6	8	15
50–64	3,856	3.6	10	1	2	3	4	7	9	15
65+	5,022	4.0	11	1	2	3	5	7	10	17
GRAND TOTAL	15,236	3.6	10	1	2	3	4	7	9	16

88.1: OTHER ABDOMINAL X-RAY

Type of Patients	Observed Patients	Avg. Stay	Vari-ance	Percentiles						
				10th	25th	50th	75th	90th	95th	99th
1. SINGLE DX										
0–19 Years	3	3.0	12	1	1	1	7	7	7	7
20–34	2	2.5	<1	2	2	3	3	3	3	3
35–49	0									
50–64	1	2.0	0	2	2	2	2	2	2	2
65+	0									
2. MULTIPLE DX										
0–19 Years	13	6.2	168	1	1	2	4	5	49	49
20–34	10	5.0	12	2	2	4	9	10	10	10
35–49	14	4.1	16	1	1	2	6	9	14	14
50–64	23	3.1	6	1	1	2	4	7	8	9
65+	26	4.6	17	1	2	3	5	10	12	19
TOTAL SINGLE DX	6	2.7	5	1	1	2	3	7	7	7
TOTAL MULTIPLE DX	86	4.4	35	1	2	3	5	9	10	49
TOTAL										
0–19 Years	16	5.6	138	1	1	2	5	7	49	49
20–34	12	4.6	11	2	2	3	9	10	10	10
35–49	14	4.1	16	1	1	2	6	9	14	14
50–64	24	3.1	6	1	2	3	4	7	8	9
65+	26	4.6	17	1	2	3	5	10	12	19
GRAND TOTAL	92	4.3	33	1	2	3	5	9	10	49

88.11: PELV DYE CONTRAST X-RAY

Type of Patients	Observed Patients	Avg. Stay	Vari-ance	Percentiles						
				10th	25th	50th	75th	90th	95th	99th
1. SINGLE DX										
0–19 Years	0									
20–34	0									
35–49	0									
50–64	1	2.0	0	2	2	2	2	2	2	2
65+	0									
2. MULTIPLE DX										
0–19 Years	1	2.0	0	2	2	2	2	2	2	2
20–34	2	1.5	<1	1	1	2	2	2	2	2
35–49	4	7.0	32	1	4	4	9	14	14	14
50–64	8	2.5	2	1	1	5	3	5	5	5
65+	10	7.2	28	1	4	5	10	12	19	19
TOTAL SINGLE DX	1	2.0	0	2	2	2	2	2	2	2
TOTAL MULTIPLE DX	25	5.0	21	1	2	4	7	12	14	19
TOTAL										
0–19 Years	1	2.0	0	2	2	2	2	2	2	2
20–34	2	1.5	<1	1	1	2	2	2	2	2
35–49	4	7.0	32	1	4	4	9	14	14	14
50–64	9	2.4	2	1	1	5	3	5	5	5
65+	10	7.2	28	1	4	5	10	12	19	19
GRAND TOTAL	26	4.9	21	1	2	4	7	12	14	19

88.2: EXT & PELVIS SKEL X-RAY

Type of Patients	Observed Patients	Avg. Stay	Vari-ance	Percentiles						
				10th	25th	50th	75th	90th	95th	99th
1. SINGLE DX										
0–19 Years	13	1.1	<1	1	1	1	1	1	2	2
20–34	23	1.4	<1	1	1	1	1	3	3	4
35–49	17	2.1	5	1	1	1	2	7	8	8
50–64	11	1.3	<1	1	1	1	1	1	4	4
65+	1	1.0	0	1	1	1	1	1	1	1
2. MULTIPLE DX										
0–19 Years	46	4.0	42	1	1	2	4	6	10	38
20–34	80	3.4	22	1	1	2	3	8	11	34
35–49	108	3.4	18	1	1	2	3	8	12	23
50–64	128	3.8	42	1	1	2	3	6	15	33
65+	50	4.6	23	1	2	3	6	8	14	30
TOTAL SINGLE DX	65	1.5	2	1	1	1	1	3	4	8
TOTAL MULTIPLE DX	412	3.7	30	1	1	2	4	8	12	30
TOTAL										
0–19 Years	59	3.4	34	1	1	2	3	5	10	38
20–34	103	3.0	18	1	1	2	3	6	10	17
35–49	125	3.2	17	1	1	2	3	7	12	23
50–64	139	3.6	40	1	1	2	3	6	15	33
65+	51	4.5	23	1	2	3	6	8	14	30
GRAND TOTAL	477	3.4	26	1	1	2	3	7	12	30

LOS by Diagnosis and Operation, Western Region, 45th Edition

Western Region, October 2007–September 2008 Data, by Operation

88.3: OTHER X-RAY

Type of Patients	Observed Patients	Avg. Stay	Vari-ance	Percentiles						
				10th	25th	50th	75th	90th	95th	99th
1. SINGLE DX										
0–19 Years	118	2.3	3	1	1	2	3	4	6	8
20–34	58	1.7	<1	1	1	1	2	3	4	5
35–49	34	2.2	4	1	1	1	3	4	7	9
50–64	29	2.4	9	1	1	1	3	4	5	17
65+	5	1.6	<1	1	1	1	2	3	3	3
2. MULTIPLE DX										
0–19 Years	317	3.7	11	1	2	2	5	8	9	21
20–34	346	3.1	16	1	1	2	4	6	8	22
35–49	407	3.9	24	1	2	3	5	7	11	21
50–64	548	3.9	14	1	2	3	5	8	11	18
65+	836	4.1	22	1	2	3	5	7	10	19
TOTAL SINGLE DX	244	2.2	3	1	1	2	3	4	5	8
TOTAL MULTIPLE DX	2,454	3.8	18	1	2	3	5	7	10	21
TOTAL										
0–19 Years	435	3.3	9	1	1	2	4	7	9	14
20–34	404	2.9	14	1	1	2	3	5	8	21
35–49	441	3.8	22	1	1	3	4	7	10	21
50–64	577	3.8	14	1	1	3	5	8	11	18
65+	841	4.1	22	1	2	3	5	7	10	19
GRAND TOTAL	2,698	3.7	16	1	1	3	4	7	10	20

88.4: CONTRAST ARTERIOGRAPHY

Type of Patients	Observed Patients	Avg. Stay	Vari-ance	Percentiles						
				10th	25th	50th	75th	90th	95th	99th
1. SINGLE DX										
0–19 Years	33	2.3	3	1	1	2	3	5	6	6
20–34	35	2.7	4	1	1	2	4	6	6	8
35–49	47	3.5	9	1	1	3	4	8	10	14
50–64	50	2.3	5	1	1	1	2	4	7	14
65+	21	1.4	<1	1	1	1	2	2	2	3
2. MULTIPLE DX										
0–19 Years	184	4.7	24	1	1	3	6	10	13	24
20–34	614	4.1	17	1	2	3	5	8	10	19
35–49	1,441	4.3	23	1	2	3	6	8	11	22
50–64	2,918	4.5	18	1	2	3	6	9	12	20
65+	5,337	4.4	15	1	2	3	6	9	11	18
TOTAL SINGLE DX	186	2.5	5	1	1	2	3	6	6	11
TOTAL MULTIPLE DX	10,494	4.4	18	1	2	3	6	9	11	20
TOTAL										
0–19 Years	217	4.3	22	1	1	3	6	9	13	24
20–34	649	4.0	16	1	2	3	5	8	10	19
35–49	1,488	4.2	22	1	2	3	6	9	11	22
50–64	2,968	4.4	18	1	2	3	6	9	12	20
65+	5,358	4.4	15	1	2	3	6	9	11	18
GRAND TOTAL	10,680	4.4	17	1	2	3	6	9	11	19

88.38: CAT SCAN NEC

Type of Patients	Observed Patients	Avg. Stay	Vari-ance	Percentiles						
				10th	25th	50th	75th	90th	95th	99th
1. SINGLE DX										
0–19 Years	103	2.4	3	1	1	2	3	4	6	8
20–34	56	1.7	<1	1	1	1	2	3	4	5
35–49	32	2.3	4	1	1	2	3	4	7	9
50–64	27	2.5	10	1	1	1	3	4	5	17
65+	5	1.6	<1	1	1	1	2	3	3	3
2. MULTIPLE DX										
0–19 Years	291	3.7	11	1	2	2	5	8	9	21
20–34	329	3.1	16	1	1	2	3	6	8	22
35–49	396	3.9	24	1	2	3	5	7	11	23
50–64	519	3.9	15	1	1	3	5	8	11	18
65+	800	4.0	15	1	2	3	5	7	10	18
TOTAL SINGLE DX	223	2.3	3	1	1	2	3	4	5	9
TOTAL MULTIPLE DX	2,335	3.8	16	1	2	3	5	7	10	21
TOTAL										
0–19 Years	394	3.4	9	1	1	2	4	7	8	16
20–34	385	2.9	14	1	1	2	3	5	8	22
35–49	428	3.8	23	1	1	3	4	7	10	21
50–64	546	3.9	14	1	2	3	5	8	11	18
65+	805	4.0	15	1	2	3	5	7	10	16
GRAND TOTAL	2,558	3.6	15	1	1	3	4	7	9	20

88.41: CEREBRAL ARTERIOGRAM

Type of Patients	Observed Patients	Avg. Stay	Vari-ance	Percentiles						
				10th	25th	50th	75th	90th	95th	99th
1. SINGLE DX										
0–19 Years	16	2.5	3	1	1	2	4	6	6	6
20–34	22	2.8	4	1	1	2	4	6	6	8
35–49	31	4.2	12	1	2	2	6	9	11	14
50–64	27	2.7	8	1	1	2	3	6	8	14
65+	9	1.3	<1	1	1	1	2	2	2	2
2. MULTIPLE DX										
0–19 Years	104	4.7	27	1	1	3	6	11	13	24
20–34	267	3.8	8	1	2	3	5	8	9	14
35–49	616	4.6	26	1	2	3	6	8	11	29
50–64	1,162	4.7	23	1	2	3	6	10	12	21
65+	1,811	4.3	13	1	2	3	5	8	10	18
TOTAL SINGLE DX	105	3.0	7	1	1	2	4	6	8	14
TOTAL MULTIPLE DX	3,960	4.4	18	1	2	3	6	8	11	20
TOTAL										
0–19 Years	120	4.3	23	1	1	2	6	10	13	24
20–34	289	3.7	8	1	2	3	5	8	9	14
35–49	647	4.6	25	1	2	3	6	8	11	29
50–64	1,189	4.7	23	1	2	3	6	10	12	21
65+	1,820	4.2	13	1	2	3	5	8	10	18
GRAND TOTAL	4,065	4.4	18	1	2	3	6	8	11	20

LOS by Diagnosis and Operation, Western Region, 45th Edition

Western Region, October 2007–September 2008 Data, by Operation

88.42: CONTRAST AORTOGRAM

Type of Patients	Observed Patients	Avg. Stay	Vari-ance	Percentiles						
				10th	25th	50th	75th	90th	95th	99th
1. SINGLE DX										
0–19 Years	2	1.0	0	1	1	1	1		1	1
20–34	1	2.0	0	2	2	2	2	2	2	2
35–49	1	1.0	0	1	1	1	1	1	1	1
50–64	5	1.4	<1	1	1	1	1	3	3	3
65+	6	1.3	<1	1	1	1	2	2	2	2
2. MULTIPLE DX										
0–19 Years	6	2.4	9	1	1	1	3	10	10	10
20–34	32	5.5	15	2	3	4	8	10	14	17
35–49	84	5.5	32	1	2	4	8	11	15	36
50–64	358	4.7	19	1	2	3	6	10	13	21
65+	795	4.8	19	1	2	3	7	10	13	22
TOTAL SINGLE DX	15	1.3	<1	1	1	1	2	2	3	3
TOTAL MULTIPLE DX	1,275	4.8	20	1	2	3	7	10	13	22
TOTAL										
0–19 Years	8	2.2	7	1	1	1	3	3	10	10
20–34	33	5.4	14	2	3	4	8	10	14	17
35–49	85	5.5	32	1	2	4	8	11	15	36
50–64	363	4.7	19	1	2	3	6	10	13	21
65+	801	4.8	19	1	2	3	7	10	13	20
GRAND TOTAL	1,290	4.8	20	1	2	3	7	10	13	22

88.43: PULMONARY ARTERIOGRAM

Type of Patients	Observed Patients	Avg. Stay	Vari-ance	Percentiles						
				10th	25th	50th	75th	90th	95th	99th
1. SINGLE DX										
0–19 Years	1	2.0	0	2	2	2	2	2	2	2
20–34	4	3.8	3	2	2	4	6	6	6	6
35–49	4	2.7	2	1	1	3	3	4	4	4
50–64	4	3.5	6	2	2	3	3	7	7	7
65+	0									
2. MULTIPLE DX										
0–19 Years	15	4.3	26	1	1	2	5	13	18	18
20–34	161	3.4	10	1	1	3	4	7	8	19
35–49	390	3.4	8	1	2	3	4	7	9	12
50–64	669	3.9	9	1	2	3	5	7	10	16
65+	1,219	4.2	15	1	2	3	5	8	10	16
TOTAL SINGLE DX	13	3.2	3	2	2	3	4	6	7	7
TOTAL MULTIPLE DX	2,454	3.9	12	1	2	3	5	7	9	16
TOTAL										
0–19 Years	16	4.2	25	1	1	3	5	13	18	18
20–34	165	3.4	10	1	1	3	4	7	8	19
35–49	394	3.4	8	1	1	3	4	7	9	12
50–64	673	3.9	9	1	2	3	5	7	10	16
65+	1,219	4.2	15	1	2	3	5	8	10	16
GRAND TOTAL	2,467	3.9	12	1	2	3	5	7	9	16

88.44: THOR ARTERIOGRAM NEC

Type of Patients	Observed Patients	Avg. Stay	Vari-ance	Percentiles						
				10th	25th	50th	75th	90th	95th	99th
1. SINGLE DX										
0–19 Years	0									
20–34	0									
35–49	2	1.5	<1	1	1	2	2	2	2	2
50–64	2	1.5	<1	1	1	2	2	2	2	2
65+	1	3.0	0	3	3	3	3	3	3	3
2. MULTIPLE DX										
0–19 Years	9	4.2	10	1	2	3	7	9	9	9
20–34	51	3.8	6	1	2	3	5	7	10	11
35–49	119	3.4	29	1	1	2	4	6	8	16
50–64	199	3.6	17	1	1	2	4	7	9	24
65+	358	3.7	10	1	2	3	5	7	9	14
TOTAL SINGLE DX	5	1.8	<1	1	1	2	2	3	3	3
TOTAL MULTIPLE DX	736	3.7	14	1	2	3	5	7	9	14
TOTAL										
0–19 Years	9	4.2	10	1	2	3	7	9	9	9
20–34	51	3.8	6	1	2	3	5	7	10	11
35–49	121	3.4	29	1	1	2	4	6	7	16
50–64	201	3.6	17	1	1	2	4	7	9	14
65+	359	3.7	9	1	2	3	5	7	9	14
GRAND TOTAL	741	3.7	14	1	2	3	5	7	9	14

88.45: RENAL ARTERIOGRAM

Type of Patients	Observed Patients	Avg. Stay	Vari-ance	Percentiles						
				10th	25th	50th	75th	90th	95th	99th
1. SINGLE DX										
0–19 Years	2	4.0	8	2	2	4	6	6	6	6
20–34	1	2.0	0	2	2	2	2	2	2	2
35–49	0									
50–64	2	1.5	<1	1	1	2	2	2	2	2
65+	0									
2. MULTIPLE DX										
0–19 Years	12	5.9	6	2	6	6	9	9	9	10
20–34	9	4.8	7	1	4	5	6	10	10	10
35–49	38	4.8	25	2	3	4	5	11	13	29
50–64	55	5.1	9	1	3	4	7	9	12	16
65+	123	5.0	17	1	2	4	7	11	13	17
TOTAL SINGLE DX	5	2.6	4	1	2	2	2	6	6	6
TOTAL MULTIPLE DX	237	5.0	15	1	2	4	6	10	12	17
TOTAL										
0–19 Years	14	5.8	6	2	5	6	6	9	9	10
20–34	10	4.5	7	1	2	5	6	10	10	10
35–49	38	4.8	25	2	2	3	5	11	13	29
50–64	57	4.9	10	1	3	4	7	9	12	16
65+	123	5.0	17	1	2	4	7	11	13	17
GRAND TOTAL	242	5.0	15	1	2	4	6	10	12	17

LOS by Diagnosis and Operation, Western Region, 45th Edition

Western Region, October 2007–September 2008 Data, by Operation

88.47: ABD ARTERIOGRAM NEC

Type of Patients	Observed Patients	Avg. Stay	Variance	10th	25th	50th	75th	90th	95th	99th
1. SINGLE DX										
0–19 Years	1	1.0	0	1	1	1	1	1	1	1
20–34	0									
35–49	4	2.7	4	1	1	1	5	5	5	5
50–64	2	1.0	0	1	1	1	1	1	1	1
65+	2	1.0	0	1	1	1	1	1	1	1
2. MULTIPLE DX										
0–19 Years	12	7.0	62	1	1	6	8	16	32	32
20–34	40	6.3	30	2	2	5	8	12	22	26
35–49	53	5.2	79	1	2	4	6	8	11	65
50–64	134	4.9	17	1	2	4	6	11	13	21
65+	266	5.8	27	1	3	4	7	12	15	27
TOTAL SINGLE DX	9	1.8	2	1	1	1	1	5	5	5
TOTAL MULTIPLE DX	505	5.6	31	1	2	4	7	11	14	26
TOTAL										
0–19 Years	13	6.7	60	1	1	6	8	16	32	32
20–34	40	6.3	30	2	2	5	8	12	22	26
35–49	57	5.0	74	1	2	4	6	8	11	65
50–64	136	4.8	17	1	2	4	6	11	13	21
65+	268	5.8	27	1	3	4	7	12	15	27
GRAND TOTAL	514	5.5	31	1	2	4	7	11	14	26

88.49: CONTRAST ARTERIOGRAM NEC

Type of Patients	Observed Patients	Avg. Stay	Variance	10th	25th	50th	75th	90th	95th	99th
1. SINGLE DX										
0–19 Years	3	1.3	<1	1	1	1	2	2	2	2
20–34	5	2.2	5	1	1	1	2	6	6	6
35–49	3	1.0	0	1	1	1	1	1	1	1
50–64	3	1.0	0	1	1	1	1	1	1	1
65+	1	1.0	0	1	1	1	1	1	1	1
2. MULTIPLE DX										
0–19 Years	16	4.2	14	1	1	3	6	6	17	17
20–34	33	6.2	117	1	2	3	6	8	35	57
35–49	73	4.7	14	1	2	3	6	10	11	19
50–64	120	5.1	24	1	2	4	7	12	15	24
65+	172	4.9	17	1	2	4	7	10	14	19
TOTAL SINGLE DX	15	1.5	2	1	1	1	1	2	6	6
TOTAL MULTIPLE DX	414	5.0	26	1	2	4	6	10	14	24
TOTAL										
0–19 Years	19	3.8	13	1	1	3	6	6	6	17
20–34	38	5.7	104	1	1	3	6	8	35	57
35–49	76	4.6	14	1	2	3	5	10	11	19
50–64	123	5.0	24	1	2	4	7	12	15	24
65+	173	4.9	17	1	2	4	7	10	14	19
GRAND TOTAL	429	4.9	25	1	2	4	6	10	14	24

88.48: CONTRAST ARTERIOGRAM-LEG

Type of Patients	Observed Patients	Avg. Stay	Variance	10th	25th	50th	75th	90th	95th	99th
1. SINGLE DX										
0–19 Years	8	1.9	2	1	1	1	2	4	5	5
20–34	2	1.0	0	1	1	1	1	1	1	1
35–49	2	2.5	<1	2	2	2	3	3	3	3
50–64	5	1.4	<1	1	1	1	1	3	3	3
65+	2	1.5	<1	1	1	1	2	2	2	2
2. MULTIPLE DX										
0–19 Years	10	2.5	6	1	1	2	3	9	9	9
20–34	20	3.7	18	1	1	2	3	7	18	18
35–49	67	4.4	12	1	2	3	6	8	11	17
50–64	214	4.3	17	1	1	3	6	9	12	18
65+	588	4.5	15	1	1	3	6	10	12	19
TOTAL SINGLE DX	19	1.7	1	1	1	1	2	3	4	5
TOTAL MULTIPLE DX	899	4.4	15	1	1	3	6	10	12	18
TOTAL										
0–19 Years	18	2.2	4	1	1	1	3	4	5	9
20–34	22	3.4	17	1	1	2	3	7	11	18
35–49	69	4.4	12	1	2	3	6	8	11	17
50–64	219	4.3	17	1	1	3	6	9	12	18
65+	590	4.5	15	1	1	3	6	10	12	19
GRAND TOTAL	918	4.4	15	1	1	3	6	10	12	18

88.5: CONTRAST ANGIOCARDIOGRAM

Type of Patients	Observed Patients	Avg. Stay	Variance	10th	25th	50th	75th	90th	95th	99th
1. SINGLE DX										
0–19 Years	2	1.2	<1	1	1	1	1	2	2	2
20–34	3	2.0	<1	1	1	2	3	3	3	3
35–49	2	1.0	0	1	1	1	1	1	1	1
50–64	5	1.2	<1	1	1	1	1	2	2	2
65+	2	1.0	0	1	1	1	1	1	1	1
2. MULTIPLE DX										
0–19 Years	15	4.0	8	2	2	3	6	7	7	13
20–34	42	4.2	13	1	2	3	5	9	10	18
35–49	255	3.3	11	1	1	2	4	6	10	15
50–64	764	3.5	13	1	1	3	4	8	9	19
65+	1,269	3.9	12	1	2	3	5	8	11	17
TOTAL SINGLE DX	14	1.3	<1	1	1	1	1	2	3	3
TOTAL MULTIPLE DX	2,345	3.7	12	1	1	3	5	8	10	18
TOTAL										
0–19 Years	17	3.4	8	1	2	3	4	7	7	13
20–34	45	4.1	12	1	1	2	5	9	10	18
35–49	257	3.3	11	1	1	2	4	6	10	15
50–64	769	3.5	13	1	1	3	4	7	9	18
65+	1,271	3.9	12	1	2	3	5	8	11	17
GRAND TOTAL	2,359	3.7	12	1	1	3	5	7	10	18

LOS by Diagnosis and Operation, Western Region, 45th Edition

Western Region, October 2007–September 2008 Data, by Operation

88.51: VC ANGIOCARDIOGRAM

Type of Patients	Observed Patients	Avg. Stay	Variance	10th	25th	50th	75th	90th	95th	99th
1. SINGLE DX										
0–19 Years	0									
20–34	0									
35–49	0									
50–64	0									
65+										
2. MULTIPLE DX										
0–19 Years	1	6.0	0	6	6	6	6	6	6	6
20–34	12	4.8	12	1	2	5	9	10	10	10
35–49	18	7.3	62	1	2	5	10	15	35	35
50–64	27	8.8	93	2	3	6	11	19	30	45
65+	38	5.4	20	1	2	4	7	13	15	20
TOTAL SINGLE DX	0									
TOTAL MULTIPLE DX	96	6.7	48	1	3	5	8	14	19	45
TOTAL										
0–19 Years	1	6.0	0	6	6	6	6	6	6	6
20–34	12	4.8	12	1	2	5	9	10	10	10
35–49	18	7.3	62	1	2	5	10	15	35	35
50–64	27	8.8	93	2	3	6	11	19	30	45
65+	38	5.4	20	1	2	4	7	13	15	20
GRAND TOTAL	96	6.7	48	1	3	5	8	14	19	45

88.53: LT HEART ANGIOCARDIOGRAM

Type of Patients	Observed Patients	Avg. Stay	Variance	10th	25th	50th	75th	90th	95th	99th
1. SINGLE DX										
0–19 Years	0									
20–34	0									
35–49	0									
50–64	1	2.0	0	2	2	2	2	2	2	2
65+	0									
2. MULTIPLE DX										
0–19 Years	3	4.0	9	1	1	4	7	7	7	7
20–34	2	7.0	2	6	6	6	8	8	8	8
35–49	8	3.3	4	1	1	3	6	6	6	6
50–64	28	2.5	3	1	1	2	4	5	5	7
65+	40	4.9	19	1	2	4	6	12	13	22
TOTAL SINGLE DX	1	2.0	0	2	2	2	2	2	2	2
TOTAL MULTIPLE DX	81	3.9	12	1	2	3	5	8	11	22
TOTAL										
0–19 Years	3	4.0	9	1	1	4	7	7	7	7
20–34	2	7.0	2	6	6	6	8	8	8	8
35–49	8	3.3	4	1	1	3	6	6	6	6
50–64	29	2.5	3	1	1	2	4	5	5	7
65+	40	4.9	19	1	2	4	6	12	13	22
GRAND TOTAL	82	3.9	12	1	2	3	5	8	11	22

88.56: COR ARTERIOGRAM-2 CATH

Type of Patients	Observed Patients	Avg. Stay	Variance	10th	25th	50th	75th	90th	95th	99th
1. SINGLE DX										
0–19 Years	2	1.2	<1	1	1	1	1	2	2	2
20–34	1	3.0	0	3	3	3	3	3	3	3
35–49	2	1.0	0	1	1	1	1	1	1	1
50–64	4	1.0	0	1	1	1	1	1	1	1
65+	2	1.0	0	1	1	1	1	1	1	1
2. MULTIPLE DX										
0–19 Years	5	2.8	1	2	2	3	3	3	6	6
20–34	22	4.2	15	1	2	3	4	9	11	18
35–49	192	2.9	7	1	1	2	4	6	8	12
50–64	619	3.3	9	1	2	3	4	7	9	15
65+	1,074	3.8	11	1	2	3	5	8	10	16
TOTAL SINGLE DX	11	1.2	<1	1	1	1	1	2	3	3
TOTAL MULTIPLE DX	1,912	3.5	10	1	1	3	4	7	9	15
TOTAL										
0–19 Years	7	2.3	2	1	2	2	3	3	6	6
20–34	23	4.2	14	1	2	3	4	9	11	18
35–49	194	2.9	7	1	1	2	4	6	8	12
50–64	623	3.3	9	1	2	3	4	7	9	15
65+	1,076	3.8	11	1	2	3	5	8	10	16
GRAND TOTAL	1,923	3.5	10	1	1	3	4	7	9	15

88.57: CORONARY ARTERIOGRAM NEC

Type of Patients	Observed Patients	Avg. Stay	Variance	10th	25th	50th	75th	90th	95th	99th
1. SINGLE DX										
0–19 Years	0									
20–34	1	2.0	0	2	2	2	2	2	2	2
35–49	0									
50–64	0									
65+	0									
2. MULTIPLE DX										
0–19 Years	3	4.3	6	2	2	4	7	7	7	7
20–34	5	1.8	3	1	1	1	1	5	5	5
35–49	14	2.6	4	1	2	2	5	6	7	7
50–64	43	4.0	16	1	2	3	5	10	10	22
65+	46	5.0	23	1	2	3	6	13	14	23
TOTAL SINGLE DX	1	2.0	0	2	2	2	2	2	2	2
TOTAL MULTIPLE DX	111	4.1	17	1	2	3	5	10	13	22
TOTAL										
0–19 Years	3	4.3	6	2	2	4	7	7	7	7
20–34	6	1.8	3	1	1	1	2	5	5	5
35–49	14	2.6	4	1	2	2	4	6	7	7
50–64	43	4.0	16	1	2	3	5	10	10	22
65+	46	5.0	23	1	2	3	6	13	14	23
GRAND TOTAL	112	4.1	17	1	2	3	5	10	13	22

LOS by Diagnosis and Operation, Western Region, 45th Edition

Western Region, October 2007–September 2008 Data, by Operation

88.6: PHLEBOGRAPHY

Type of Patients	Observed Patients	Avg. Stay	Variance	10th	25th	50th	75th	90th	95th	99th
1. SINGLE DX										
0–19 Years	0									
20–34	4	4.2	13	1	1	2	5	9	9	9
35–49	2	2.0	0	2	2	2	2	2	2	2
50–64	1	2.0	0	2	2	2	2	2	2	2
65+	0									
2. MULTIPLE DX										
0–19 Years	9	7.2	32	2	2	4	14	14	14	14
20–34	38	5.3	23	1	2	5	6	9	12	28
35–49	77	4.3	7	1	2	4	6	8	10	14
50–64	107	6.7	40	1	2	4	8	14	20	30
65+	94	5.1	19	1	3	4	7	9	11	35
TOTAL SINGLE DX	7	3.3	8	1	2	2	5	9	9	9
TOTAL MULTIPLE DX	325	5.5	25	1	2	4	7	11	14	28
TOTAL										
0–19 Years	9	7.2	32	2	2	4	14	14	14	14
20–34	42	5.2	22	1	2	4	6	9	11	28
35–49	79	4.2	7	1	2	4	6	8	10	14
50–64	108	6.7	40	1	2	4	8	14	20	30
65+	94	5.1	19	1	3	4	7	9	11	35
GRAND TOTAL	332	5.5	25	1	2	4	7	11	14	28

88.67: CONTRAST PHLEBOGRAM NEC

Type of Patients	Observed Patients	Avg. Stay	Variance	10th	25th	50th	75th	90th	95th	99th
1. SINGLE DX										
0–19 Years	0									
20–34	3	2.7	4	1	1	2	5	5	5	5
35–49	2	2.0	0	2	2	2	2	2	2	2
50–64	0									
65+	0									
2. MULTIPLE DX										
0–19 Years	0									
20–34	15	5.7	48	1	2	3	6	12	28	28
35–49	42	4.5	8	2	2	4	6	8	10	14
50–64	46	6.1	25	1	2	4	9	12	13	28
65+	47	5.0	27	1	2	4	6	9	11	35
TOTAL SINGLE DX	5	2.4	2	1	2	2	2	5	5	5
TOTAL MULTIPLE DX	150	5.3	23	1	2	4	7	10	12	28
TOTAL										
0–19 Years	0									
20–34	18	5.2	41	1	2	4	6	12	28	28
35–49	44	4.4	8	2	2	4	6	8	10	14
50–64	46	6.1	25	1	2	4	9	12	13	28
65+	47	5.0	27	1	2	4	6	9	11	35
GRAND TOTAL	155	5.2	23	1	2	4	7	10	12	28

88.66: CONTRAST PHLEBOGRAM-LEG

Type of Patients	Observed Patients	Avg. Stay	Variance	10th	25th	50th	75th	90th	95th	99th
1. SINGLE DX										
0–19 Years	0									
20–34	1	9.0	0	9	9	9	9	9	9	9
35–49	0									
50–64	1	2.0	0	2	2	2	2	2	2	2
65+	0									
2. MULTIPLE DX										
0–19 Years	1	6.0	0	6	6	6	6	6	6	6
20–34	14	5.4	9	2	3	5	8	9	11	11
35–49	21	4.2	8	1	1	4	5	7	9	12
50–64	36	7.3	57	1	3	4	8	17	30	34
65+	36	5.5	12	1	3	5	7	11	13	14
TOTAL SINGLE DX	2	5.5	24	2	2	2	9	9	9	9
TOTAL MULTIPLE DX	108	5.8	27	1	3	5	7	11	13	30
TOTAL										
0–19 Years	1	6.0	0	6	6	6	6	6	6	6
20–34	15	5.7	9	2	3	5	9	9	11	11
35–49	21	4.2	8	1	1	4	5	7	9	12
50–64	37	7.2	56	1	2	4	8	17	30	34
65+	36	5.5	12	1	3	5	7	11	13	14
GRAND TOTAL	110	5.8	26	1	2	5	7	11	13	30

88.7: DIAGNOSTIC ULTRASOUND

Type of Patients	Observed Patients	Avg. Stay	Variance	10th	25th	50th	75th	90th	95th	99th
1. SINGLE DX										
0–19 Years	387	2.4	3	1	1	2	3	4	5	8
20–34	318	2.1	4	1	1	2	2	4	5	8
35–49	157	2.2	2	1	1	2	3	4	6	7
50–64	92	1.9	3	1	1	1	3	4	5	10
65+	27	1.6	<1	1	1	1	2	3	4	4
2. MULTIPLE DX										
0–19 Years	2,758	5.2	53	1	2	3	5	11	19	41
20–34	3,323	3.7	25	1	1	3	4	7	10	23
35–49	6,028	3.8	16	1	2	3	4	7	10	20
50–64	11,269	4.0	18	1	2	3	5	8	10	19
65+	25,749	4.2	12	1	2	3	5	8	10	16
TOTAL SINGLE DX	981	2.2	3	1	1	2	3	4	5	8
TOTAL MULTIPLE DX	49,127	4.1	17	1	2	3	5	8	11	19
TOTAL										
0–19 Years	3,145	4.9	47	1	2	3	5	10	17	38
20–34	3,641	3.5	23	1	1	3	4	7	9	22
35–49	6,185	3.7	16	1	2	3	4	7	10	20
50–64	11,361	3.9	18	1	2	3	5	8	10	19
65+	25,776	4.2	12	1	2	3	5	8	10	16
GRAND TOTAL	50,108	4.1	17	1	2	3	5	8	11	19

LOS by Diagnosis and Operation, Western Region, 45th Edition

Western Region, October 2007–September 2008 Data, by Operation

88.71: HEAD & NECK ULTRASOUND

Type of Patients	Observed Patients	Avg. Stay	Vari- ance	Percentiles						
				10th	25th	50th	75th	90th	95th	99th
1. SINGLE DX										
0–19 Years	14	3.3	3	1	2	3	4	7	7	7
20–34	1	1.0	0	1	1	1	1	1	1	1
35–49	4	1.5	1	1	1	1	3	3	3	3
50–64	4	1.3	<1	1	1	1	2	2	2	2
65+	3	3.0	<1	2	2	3	4	4	4	4
2. MULTIPLE DX										
0–19 Years	177	14.2	162	2	4	9	23	33	41	55
20–34	36	3.6	6	1	2	3	5	7	10	10
35–49	90	3.5	14	1	1	3	4	7	8	27
50–64	284	3.3	9	1	2	2	4	7	8	16
65+	756	3.1	5	1	2	2	4	6	7	14
TOTAL SINGLE DX	26	2.6	3	1	1	2	3	5	7	7
TOTAL MULTIPLE DX	1,343	5.0	49	1	2	3	5	10	19	38
TOTAL										
0–19 Years	191	13.5	159	2	3	9	21	32	38	55
20–34	37	3.5	6	1	2	3	4	7	10	10
35–49	94	3.4	14	1	1	3	4	6	8	27
50–64	288	3.2	8	1	2	2	4	7	8	16
65+	759	3.1	5	2	2	2	4	6	7	14
GRAND TOTAL	1,369	4.9	48	1	2	3	5	10	19	38

88.72: HEART ULTRASOUND

Type of Patients	Observed Patients	Avg. Stay	Vari- ance	Percentiles						
				10th	25th	50th	75th	90th	95th	99th
1. SINGLE DX										
0–19 Years	117	2.6	3	1	1	2	3	5	5	9
20–34	39	2.3	2	1	1	2	3	4	6	7
35–49	43	2.0	2	1	1	1	2	4	5	7
50–64	50	1.5	2	1	1	1	2	3	3	3
65+	18	1.3	<1	1	1	1	1	2	3	3
2. MULTIPLE DX										
0–19 Years	1,289	5.4	60	1	2	3	6	11	19	42
20–34	1,126	4.2	27	1	1	3	5	9	12	23
35–49	3,552	3.8	16	1	2	3	5	8	10	21
50–64	8,058	4.0	19	1	2	3	5	8	11	19
65+	21,249	4.3	12	1	2	3	5	8	10	17
TOTAL SINGLE DX	267	2.2	3	1	1	2	3	4	5	9
TOTAL MULTIPLE DX	35,274	4.2	16	1	2	3	5	8	11	19
TOTAL										
0–19 Years	1,406	5.2	55	1	2	3	5	10	18	42
20–34	1,165	4.2	26	1	1	3	5	8	12	23
35–49	3,595	3.8	16	1	1	3	5	8	10	21
50–64	8,108	4.0	19	1	2	3	5	8	11	19
65+	21,267	4.3	12	1	2	3	5	8	10	17
GRAND TOTAL	35,541	4.2	16	1	2	3	5	8	11	19

88.73: THORAX ULTRASOUND NEC

Type of Patients	Observed Patients	Avg. Stay	Vari- ance	Percentiles						
				10th	25th	50th	75th	90th	95th	99th
1. SINGLE DX										
0–19 Years	2	2.0	2	1	1	3	3	3	3	3
20–34	0									
35–49	0									
50–64	0									
65+										
2. MULTIPLE DX										
0–19 Years	3	6.3	4	4	4	7	8	8	8	8
20–34	14	3.9	17	1	1	2	4	6	17	17
35–49	20	3.9	4	2	2	3	5	7	7	8
50–64	23	3.1	5	1	2	3	4	8	8	9
65+	55	4.9	21	1	2	3	7	9	16	24
TOTAL SINGLE DX	2	2.0	2	1	1	3	3	3	3	3
TOTAL MULTIPLE DX	115	4.3	14	1	2	3	6	8	12	17
TOTAL										
0–19 Years	5	4.6	8	1	3	4	7	8	8	8
20–34	14	3.9	17	1	1	2	4	6	17	17
35–49	20	3.9	4	2	2	3	5	7	7	8
50–64	23	3.1	5	1	2	3	4	8	8	9
65+	55	4.9	21	1	2	3	7	9	16	24
GRAND TOTAL	117	4.2	14	1	2	3	6	8	12	17

88.74: DIGEST SYSTEM ULTRASOUND

Type of Patients	Observed Patients	Avg. Stay	Vari- ance	Percentiles						
				10th	25th	50th	75th	90th	95th	99th
1. SINGLE DX										
0–19 Years	5	2.0	1	1	1	2	3	3	3	3
20–34	8	1.6	<1	1	1	2	2	2	2	2
35–49	10	3.2	4	1	1	3	5	6	6	6
50–64	4	2.3	<1	1	1	3	3	3	3	3
65+	0									
2. MULTIPLE DX										
0–19 Years	18	3.2	11	1	1	2	3	10	13	13
20–34	46	2.3	2	1	1	2	3	4	5	7
35–49	68	2.9	7	1	2	3	4	5	8	16
50–64	63	3.6	8	1	2	3	4	7	10	16
65+	73	3.8	8	1	2	3	5	7	10	14
TOTAL SINGLE DX	27	2.4	2	1	1	2	3	5	6	6
TOTAL MULTIPLE DX	268	3.2	7	1	1	2	4	6	10	14
TOTAL										
0–19 Years	23	2.9	9	1	1	2	3	6	10	13
20–34	54	2.2	2	1	1	2	3	4	5	7
35–49	78	3.0	7	1	1	3	4	6	10	16
50–64	67	3.5	7	1	2	3	4	7	10	16
65+	73	3.8	8	1	2	3	5	7	10	14
GRAND TOTAL	295	3.1	7	1	1	2	4	6	8	14

431

LOS by Diagnosis and Operation, Western Region, 45th Edition

Western Region, October 2007–September 2008 Data, by Operation

88.75: URINARY SYST ULTRASOUND

Type of Patients	Observed Patients	Avg. Stay	Variance	Percentiles						
				10th	25th	50th	75th	90th	95th	99th
1. SINGLE DX										
0–19 Years	34	2.4	1	1	2	2	3	3	5	7
20–34	4	2.0	<1	1	2	2	3	3	3	3
35–49	1	1.0	0	1	1	1	1	1	1	1
50–64	0									
65+	0									
2. MULTIPLE DX										
0–19 Years	400	3.7	14	1	2	3	4	6	9	15
20–34	170	3.1	6	1	2	2	4	6	7	14
35–49	162	4.2	27	1	2	3	5	7	9	35
50–64	289	4.5	15	1	2	3	5	9	11	21
65+	652	4.5	11	2	2	4	6	8	11	17
TOTAL SINGLE DX	39	2.3	1	1	2	2	3	3	4	7
TOTAL MULTIPLE DX	1,673	4.1	14	1	2	3	5	7	10	19
TOTAL										
0–19 Years	434	3.6	13	1	2	3	4	6	9	15
20–34	174	3.1	6	1	2	2	4	6	7	14
35–49	163	4.2	27	1	2	3	5	7	9	35
50–64	289	4.5	15	1	2	3	5	9	11	21
65+	652	4.5	11	2	2	4	6	8	11	17
GRAND TOTAL	1,712	4.1	13	1	2	3	5	7	10	19

88.76: ABD & RETROPERITON US

Type of Patients	Observed Patients	Avg. Stay	Variance	Percentiles						
				10th	25th	50th	75th	90th	95th	99th
1. SINGLE DX										
0–19 Years	159	2.3	3	1	1	2	3	5	6	8
20–34	100	1.9	1	1	1	1	2	3	4	6
35–49	56	2.4	2	1	1	2	3	4	6	7
50–64	14	2.1	2	1	1	2	3	5	5	5
65+	4	1.5	<1	1	1	1	2	2	2	2
2. MULTIPLE DX										
0–19 Years	594	3.9	19	1	2	3	5	7	11	23
20–34	895	3.4	27	1	1	2	4	6	8	21
35–49	1,266	3.5	13	1	2	3	4	7	9	15
50–64	1,480	3.7	11	1	2	3	4	7	9	15
65+	1,367	4.0	9	2	2	3	5	7	9	15
TOTAL SINGLE DX	333	2.2	2	1	1	2	3	4	5	8
TOTAL MULTIPLE DX	5,602	3.7	14	1	2	3	4	7	9	17
TOTAL										
0–19 Years	753	3.5	16	1	2	2	4	7	9	19
20–34	995	3.3	24	1	1	2	4	6	8	20
35–49	1,322	3.5	13	1	2	3	4	7	9	14
50–64	1,494	3.6	11	1	2	3	4	7	9	15
65+	1,371	4.0	9	2	2	3	5	7	9	15
GRAND TOTAL	5,935	3.6	14	1	2	3	4	7	9	16

88.77: PERIPH VASC ULTRASOUND

Type of Patients	Observed Patients	Avg. Stay	Variance	Percentiles						
				10th	25th	50th	75th	90th	95th	99th
1. SINGLE DX										
0–19 Years	9	2.9	2	1	2	3	4	4	5	5
20–34	13	1.8	2	1	1	2	2	2	6	6
35–49	17	2.4	3	1	1	2	3	5	6	6
50–64	13	3.5	8	4	4	4	5	6	10	10
65+	1	4.0	0	4	4	4	4	4	4	4
2. MULTIPLE DX										
0–19 Years	38	5.8	33	2	2	3	7	11	15	28
20–34	191	3.9	13	1	2	3	5	7	9	21
35–49	512	4.1	15	1	2	3	5	8	10	20
50–64	870	4.4	24	1	2	3	6	8	11	27
65+	1,427	4.5	15	1	2	4	6	8	10	18
TOTAL SINGLE DX	53	2.6	4	1	1	2	4	5	6	10
TOTAL MULTIPLE DX	3,038	4.3	18	1	2	3	5	8	11	20
TOTAL										
0–19 Years	47	5.3	29	1	2	3	7	11	14	28
20–34	204	3.8	12	1	2	3	5	7	9	13
35–49	529	4.0	15	1	2	3	5	8	10	20
50–64	883	4.3	24	1	2	3	6	8	11	27
65+	1,428	4.5	15	1	2	4	6	8	10	18
GRAND TOTAL	3,091	4.3	18	1	2	3	5	8	10	20

88.78: GRAVID UTERUS ULTRASOUND

Type of Patients	Observed Patients	Avg. Stay	Variance	Percentiles						
				10th	25th	50th	75th	90th	95th	99th
1. SINGLE DX										
0–19 Years	17	1.7	<1	1	1	1	2	3	3	3
20–34	129	2.3	7	1	1	2	2	4	7	19
35–49	13	1.8	<1	1	1	1	3	3	3	3
50–64	1	1.0	0	1	1	1	1	1	1	1
65+	0									
2. MULTIPLE DX										
0–19 Years	123	2.9	16	1	1	2	3	5	6	27
20–34	729	3.4	26	1	1	2	3	6	9	27
35–49	194	4.4	55	1	1	2	4	8	12	44
50–64	11	9.1	305	1	2	2	4	23	58	58
65+	0									
TOTAL SINGLE DX	160	2.2	6	1	1	2	2	4	6	19
TOTAL MULTIPLE DX	1,057	3.5	33	1	1	2	3	6	10	36
TOTAL										
0–19 Years	140	2.7	14	1	1	2	3	4	5	27
20–34	858	3.2	23	1	1	2	3	6	9	26
35–49	207	4.2	52	1	1	2	4	7	12	44
50–64	12	8.5	283	1	2	2	4	23	58	58
65+	0									
GRAND TOTAL	1,217	3.4	30	1	1	2	3	6	9	33

Western Region, October 2007–September 2008 Data, by Operation

88.79: ULTRASOUND NEC

Type of Patients	Observed Patients	Avg. Stay	Vari-ance	Percentiles						
				10th	25th	50th	75th	90th	95th	99th
1. SINGLE DX										
0–19 Years	30	1.7	<1	1	1	2	2	3	3	5
20–34	24	1.7	<1	1	1	1	2	3	3	4
35–49	13	2.1	2	1	1	1	3	3	6	6
50–64	6	1.5	0	1	1	2	1	4	4	4
65+	1	2.0	0	2	2	2	2	2	2	2
2. MULTIPLE DX										
0–19 Years	116	3.0	5	1	2	2	4	5	6	15
20–34	116	3.6	35	1	1	2	4	7	8	19
35–49	164	3.1	8	1	1	2	4	6	7	17
50–64	191	3.7	15	1	2	3	4	6	10	25
65+	170	3.7	10	1	2	3	5	7	8	18
TOTAL SINGLE DX	74	1.8	1	1	1	1	2	3	4	6
TOTAL MULTIPLE DX	757	3.4	14	1	2	2	4	6	8	17
TOTAL										
0–19 Years	146	2.8	5	1	1	2	3	4	6	15
20–34	140	3.3	29	1	1	2	3	6	8	19
35–49	177	3.0	7	1	1	2	4	6	7	17
50–64	197	3.7	15	1	2	3	4	6	10	25
65+	171	3.6	10	2	2	3	5	7	8	18
GRAND TOTAL	831	3.3	13	1	1	2	4	6	8	17

88.9: OTHER DIAGNOSTIC IMAGING

Type of Patients	Observed Patients	Avg. Stay	Vari-ance	Percentiles						
				10th	25th	50th	75th	90th	95th	99th
1. SINGLE DX										
0–19 Years	409	2.7	4	1	1	2	3	5	7	11
20–34	97	2.8	4	1	1	2	4	5	6	14
35–49	83	3.2	32	1	1	2	3	5	7	51
50–64	41	3.6	32	1	1	2	4	7	8	36
65+	18	2.4	5	1	1	2	2	6	9	9
2. MULTIPLE DX										
0–19 Years	2,003	5.0	34	1	2	3	6	11	14	32
20–34	1,081	4.0	18	1	2	3	5	8	11	22
35–49	2,197	4.3	27	1	2	3	5	8	12	26
50–64	3,807	4.5	30	1	2	3	5	9	13	27
65+	5,531	4.2	17	1	2	3	5	8	10	19
TOTAL SINGLE DX	648	2.7	7	1	1	2	3	5	7	11
TOTAL MULTIPLE DX	14,619	4.5	26	1	2	3	5	9	12	25
TOTAL										
0–19 Years	2,412	4.6	30	1	2	3	5	10	13	30
20–34	1,178	3.9	17	1	2	3	5	8	10	21
35–49	2,280	4.3	27	1	2	3	5	8	12	26
50–64	3,848	4.5	30	1	2	3	5	9	13	27
65+	5,549	4.2	17	1	2	3	5	8	10	19
GRAND TOTAL	15,267	4.4	25	1	2	3	5	9	12	25

88.8: THERMOGRAPHY

Type of Patients	Observed Patients	Avg. Stay	Vari-ance	Percentiles						
				10th	25th	50th	75th	90th	95th	99th
1. SINGLE DX										
0–19 Years	0									
20–34	0									
35–49	0									
50–64	0									
65+	0									
2. MULTIPLE DX										
0–19 Years	0									
20–34	0									
35–49	0									
50–64	0									
65+	0									
TOTAL SINGLE DX	0									
TOTAL MULTIPLE DX	0									
TOTAL										
0–19 Years	0									
20–34	0									
35–49	0									
50–64	0									
65+	0									
GRAND TOTAL	0									

88.91: BRAIN & BRAIN STEM MRI

Type of Patients	Observed Patients	Avg. Stay	Vari-ance	Percentiles						
				10th	25th	50th	75th	90th	95th	99th
1. SINGLE DX										
0–19 Years	319	2.6	3	1	1	2	3	5	6	9
20–34	43	2.4	2	1	1	2	4	5	5	6
35–49	43	3.7	59	1	1	2	4	5	7	51
50–64	23	3.1	53	1	1	2	2	3	7	36
65+	11	1.7	<1	1	1	2	2	2	4	4
2. MULTIPLE DX										
0–19 Years	1,508	5.0	34	1	2	3	6	11	14	32
20–34	591	3.7	16	1	2	2	4	7	10	21
35–49	1,262	3.9	26	1	2	3	5	7	10	23
50–64	2,364	4.3	36	1	2	3	5	8	12	32
65+	3,901	4.0	17	1	2	3	5	7	9	19
TOTAL SINGLE DX	439	2.6	8	1	1	2	3	5	6	9
TOTAL MULTIPLE DX	9,626	4.3	27	1	2	3	5	8	12	26
TOTAL										
0–19 Years	1,827	4.6	30	1	2	3	5	10	13	32
20–34	634	3.6	15	1	2	3	4	7	9	20
35–49	1,305	3.9	27	1	2	3	4	7	10	23
50–64	2,387	4.3	37	1	2	3	5	8	12	32
65+	3,912	4.0	17	1	2	3	5	7	9	19
GRAND TOTAL	10,065	4.2	26	1	2	3	5	8	12	25

LOS by Diagnosis and Operation, Western Region, 45th Edition

Western Region, October 2007–September 2008 Data, by Operation

88.93: SPINAL CANAL MRI

Type of Patients	Observed Patients	Avg. Stay	Vari-ance	10th	25th	50th	75th	90th	95th	99th
1. SINGLE DX										
0–19 Years	21	3.2	10	1	1	2	3	9	9	15
20–34	27	3.1	8	1	1	2	4	7	8	14
35–49	22	2.2	2	1	1	2	3	4	4	6
50–64	5	3.4	8	1	2	2	4	8	8	8
65+	3	5.3	16	1	1	6	6	9	9	9
2. MULTIPLE DX										
0–19 Years	176	5.1	39	1	2	3	5	10	15	28
20–34	208	4.2	29	1	2	3	5	9	13	25
35–49	390	4.7	35	1	2	3	5	9	13	36
50–64	536	4.9	24	1	2	3	5	10	14	25
65+	704	4.8	16	2	2	4	6	9	12	19
TOTAL SINGLE DX	78	3.0	8	1	1	2	4	7	9	15
TOTAL MULTIPLE DX	2,014	4.8	27	1	2	3	6	9	13	25
TOTAL										
0–19 Years	197	4.9	37	1	2	3	5	9	15	28
20–34	235	4.1	27	1	1	3	4	9	13	25
35–49	412	4.6	33	1	2	3	5	9	13	31
50–64	541	4.9	24	1	2	3	5	10	14	25
65+	707	4.8	16	2	2	4	6	9	12	19
GRAND TOTAL	2,092	4.7	26	1	2	3	6	9	13	25

88.95: PELVIS/PROS/BLADDER MRI

Type of Patients	Observed Patients	Avg. Stay	Vari-ance	10th	25th	50th	75th	90th	95th	99th
1. SINGLE DX										
0–19 Years	2	1.8	<1			2	2	2	2	2
20–34	0									
35–49	0									
50–64	1	1.0	0	1	1	1	1	1	1	1
65+	1									
2. MULTIPLE DX										
0–19 Years	27	5.1	33	1	2	3	6	11	11	32
20–34	19	4.9	13	1	2	4	7	11	14	14
35–49	31	6.9	78	1	2	4	10	15	45	>99
50–64	36	6.2	17	2	3	5	7	12	14	22
65+	50	4.9	19	2	2	4	5	10	12	25
TOTAL SINGLE DX	3	1.7	<1	1	1	2	2	2	2	2
TOTAL MULTIPLE DX	163	5.5	32	1	2	4	7	11	15	45
TOTAL										
0–19 Years	29	4.8	31	1	2	3	6	11	11	32
20–34	19	4.9	13	1	2	4	7	11	14	14
35–49	31	6.9	78	1	2	4	10	15	45	>99
50–64	36	6.2	17	3	3	5	7	12	14	22
65+	51	4.9	19	2	2	4	5	10	12	25
GRAND TOTAL	166	5.4	31	1	2	4	6	11	14	32

88.94: MUSCULOSKELETAL MRI

Type of Patients	Observed Patients	Avg. Stay	Vari-ance	10th	25th	50th	75th	90th	95th	99th
1. SINGLE DX										
0–19 Years	39	3.2	8	1	1	2	4	5	12	12
20–34	4	3.5	3	2	2	3	6	6	6	6
35–49	8	3.4	8	1	2	2	7	8	8	8
50–64	2	3.0	0	1	1	1	5	5	5	5
65+	1	2.0		2	2	2	2	2	2	2
2. MULTIPLE DX										
0–19 Years	147	4.9	16	1	2	4	6	9	13	21
20–34	95	4.7	12	1	2	4	6	9	10	23
35–49	260	5.5	25	2	3	4	7	11	13	29
50–64	401	5.5	20	2	3	4	7	11	13	17
65+	283	5.5	17	2	3	4	6	12	14	25
TOTAL SINGLE DX	54	3.2	8	1	1	2	4	7	10	12
TOTAL MULTIPLE DX	1,186	5.3	19	2	3	4	7	10	13	23
TOTAL										
0–19 Years	186	4.5	15	1	2	3	5	9	12	18
20–34	99	4.6	12	1	2	3	6	9	10	23
35–49	268	5.5	24	2	3	4	7	11	13	29
50–64	403	5.5	20	2	3	4	7	11	13	17
65+	284	5.4	17	2	3	4	6	12	14	25
GRAND TOTAL	1,240	5.2	18	2	2	4	6	10	13	22

88.97: MRI SITE NEC & NOS

Type of Patients	Observed Patients	Avg. Stay	Vari-ance	10th	25th	50th	75th	90th	95th	99th
1. SINGLE DX										
0–19 Years	24	2.8	7	1	1	2	4	5	11	11
20–34	22	3.3	4	2	2	3	5	6	6	9
35–49	10	3.1	5	1	1	3	3	5	8	8
50–64	11	5.0	5	3	3	4	7	7	9	9
65+	2	2.5	4	1	1	4	4	4	4	4
2. MULTIPLE DX										
0–19 Years	132	6.0	37	1	2	4	8	11	18	31
20–34	155	4.1	10	1	2	3	5	8	12	15
35–49	245	4.4	17	1	2	3	5	8	11	23
50–64	429	4.1	11	1	2	3	5	8	10	16
65+	567	4.2	12	2	2	3	5	8	9	20
TOTAL SINGLE DX	69	3.2	6	1	2	2	4	6	9	11
TOTAL MULTIPLE DX	1,528	4.5	16	1	2	3	5	9	11	23
TOTAL										
0–19 Years	156	5.4	33	1	2	3	7	11	16	31
20–34	177	4.0	10	1	2	3	5	8	11	15
35–49	255	4.3	16	1	2	3	5	8	11	23
50–64	440	4.1	10	1	2	3	6	8	10	16
65+	569	4.2	12	2	2	3	5	8	9	20
GRAND TOTAL	1,597	4.4	16	1	2	3	5	8	11	23

LOS by Diagnosis and Operation, Western Region, 45th Edition

Western Region, October 2007–September 2008 Data, by Operation

89.0: DX INTERVIEW/CONSUL/EXAM

Type of Patients	Observed Patients	Avg. Stay	Variance	10th	25th	50th	75th	90th	95th	99th
1. SINGLE DX										
0–19 Years	43	2.3	<1	1	2	2	3	3	4	4
20–34	1	2.0	0	2	2	2	2	2	2	2
35–49	1	2.0	0	2	2	2	2	2	2	2
50–64	0									
65+	0									
2. MULTIPLE DX										
0–19 Years	305	3.4	8	1	2	3	4	6	9	16
20–34	213	8.9	44	3	4	7	11	20	24	29
35–49	248	9.1	54	3	5	7	11	17	23	42
50–64	153	11.3	118	3	5	9	14	22	27	54
65+	24	6.8	24	2	4	6	7	13	18	21
TOTAL SINGLE DX	45	2.2	<1	1	2	2	3	3	4	4
TOTAL MULTIPLE DX	943	7.5	55	2	3	5	9	15	22	34
TOTAL										
0–19 Years	348	3.2	7	1	2	3	3	5	9	16
20–34	214	8.8	44	3	4	7	11	20	24	29
35–49	249	9.1	54	3	5	7	11	17	23	42
50–64	153	11.3	118	3	5	9	14	22	27	54
65+	24	6.8	24	2	4	6	7	13	18	21
GRAND TOTAL	988	7.3	54	2	3	5	9	15	22	34

89.03: COMPR INTERVIEW/EVAL

Type of Patients	Observed Patients	Avg. Stay	Variance	10th	25th	50th	75th	90th	95th	99th
1. SINGLE DX										
0–19 Years	0									
20–34	0									
35–49	0									
50–64	0									
65+	0									
2. MULTIPLE DX										
0–19 Years	0									
20–34	1	2.0	0	2	2	2	2	2	2	2
35–49	0									
50–64	0									
65+	0									
TOTAL SINGLE DX	0									
TOTAL MULTIPLE DX	1	2.0	0	2	2	2	2	2	2	2
TOTAL										
0–19 Years	0									
20–34	1	2.0	0	2	2	2	2	2	2	2
35–49	0									
50–64	0									
65+	0									
GRAND TOTAL	1	2.0	0	2	2	2	2	2	2	2

89.06: LIMITED CONSULTATION

Type of Patients	Observed Patients	Avg. Stay	Variance	10th	25th	50th	75th	90th	95th	99th
1. SINGLE DX										
0–19 Years	0									
20–34	0									
35–49	0									
50–64	0									
65+	0									
2. MULTIPLE DX										
0–19 Years	57	6.4	16	3	4	5	8	12	15	22
20–34	167	8.8	45	3	4	6	11	20	25	29
35–49	177	9.1	56	3	5	7	10	18	22	43
50–64	113	11.6	134	3	5	9	14	22	27	54
65+	9	8.5	31	4	5	6	10	21	21	21
TOTAL SINGLE DX	0									
TOTAL MULTIPLE DX	523	9.2	67	3	4	7	11	19	24	42
TOTAL										
0–19 Years	57	6.4	16	3	4	5	8	12	15	22
20–34	167	8.8	45	3	4	6	11	20	25	29
35–49	177	9.1	56	3	5	7	10	18	22	43
50–64	113	11.6	134	3	5	9	14	22	27	54
65+	9	8.5	31	4	5	6	10	21	21	21
GRAND TOTAL	523	9.2	67	3	4	7	11	19	24	42

89.1: NERVOUS SYSTEM EXAMS

Type of Patients	Observed Patients	Avg. Stay	Variance	10th	25th	50th	75th	90th	95th	99th
1. SINGLE DX										
0–19 Years	1,133	1.9	2	1	1	2	2	3	4	7
20–34	203	3.9	6	1	2	3	5	7	8	13
35–49	95	4.1	5	2	3	4	5	7	8	15
50–64	60	3.8	3	1	3	3	4	6	7	7
65+	9	3.1	1	1	3	3	4	5	5	5
2. MULTIPLE DX										
0–19 Years	2,795	2.5	12	1	1	2	3	5	6	14
20–34	732	3.8	10	1	2	3	4	7	8	16
35–49	920	4.3	15	1	2	3	5	8	10	21
50–64	994	4.7	24	1	2	3	5	9	13	26
65+	1,666	4.7	16	2	2	4	6	9	12	22
TOTAL SINGLE DX	1,500	2.3	3	1	1	2	3	4	6	8
TOTAL MULTIPLE DX	7,107	3.5	15	1	1	2	4	7	9	19
TOTAL										
0–19 Years	3,928	2.4	9	1	1	2	3	4	6	12
20–34	935	3.9	9	1	2	3	5	7	8	14
35–49	1,015	4.3	14	1	2	3	5	8	10	20
50–64	1,054	4.7	23	1	2	4	5	9	12	26
65+	1,675	4.7	16	2	2	4	6	9	12	22
GRAND TOTAL	8,607	3.3	13	1	1	2	4	6	8	17

LOS by Diagnosis and Operation, Western Region, 45th Edition

Western Region, October 2007–September 2008 Data, by Operation

89.14: ELECTROENCEPHALOGRAM

Type of Patients	Observed Patients	Avg. Stay	Vari-ance	Percentiles						
				10th	25th	50th	75th	90th	95th	99th
1. SINGLE DX										
0–19 Years	171	2.3	3	1	1	2	3	4	6	11
20–34	22	2.1	2	1	1	2	3	4	5	5
35–49	14	2.7	2	1	2	2	4	4	6	6
50–64	6	2.7	1	1	2	3	4	4	4	4
65+	1	1.0	0	1	1	1	1	1	1	1
2. MULTIPLE DX										
0–19 Years	484	3.6	20	1	1	2	4	7	10	22
20–34	258	3.9	20	1	2	3	4	8	10	23
35–49	440	4.4	26	1	2	3	5	9	14	26
50–64	643	4.9	31	1	2	3	6	10	16	28
65+	1,503	4.8	17	2	2	4	6	9	12	24
TOTAL SINGLE DX	214	2.3	3	1	1	2	3	4	6	11
TOTAL MULTIPLE DX	3,328	4.4	22	1	2	3	5	9	12	24
TOTAL										
0–19 Years	655	3.2	16	1	1	2	3	7	9	20
20–34	280	3.8	18	1	2	3	4	7	10	23
35–49	454	4.3	25	1	2	3	5	8	13	26
50–64	649	4.9	31	1	2	3	5	10	16	28
65+	1,504	4.8	17	2	2	4	6	9	12	24
GRAND TOTAL	3,542	4.3	21	1	2	3	5	9	12	24

89.17: POLYSOMNOGRAM

Type of Patients	Observed Patients	Avg. Stay	Vari-ance	Percentiles						
				10th	25th	50th	75th	90th	95th	99th
1. SINGLE DX										
0–19 Years	3	1.8	<1	1	2	2	2	2	2	2
20–34	0									
35–49	0									
50–64	0									
65+	0									
2. MULTIPLE DX										
0–19 Years	24	8.6	238	1	2	3	7	13	59	59
20–34	0									
35–49	1	4.0	0	4	4	4	4	4	4	4
50–64	2	5.5	40	1	1	6	10	10	10	10
65+	1	2.0	0	2	2	2	2	2	2	2
TOTAL SINGLE DX	3	1.8	<1	1	2	2	2	2	2	2
TOTAL MULTIPLE DX	28	8.3	223	1	2	3	7	13	59	59
TOTAL										
0–19 Years	27	7.9	217	1	2	3	6	13	59	59
20–34	0									
35–49	1	4.0	0	4	4	4	4	4	4	4
50–64	2	5.5	40	1	1	6	10	10	10	10
65+	1	2.0	0	2	2	2	2	2	2	2
GRAND TOTAL	31	7.7	205	1	2	3	6	13	59	59

89.15: NEURO FUNCTION TEST NEC

Type of Patients	Observed Patients	Avg. Stay	Vari-ance	Percentiles						
				10th	25th	50th	75th	90th	95th	99th
1. SINGLE DX										
0–19 Years	538	1.3	<1	1	1	1	1	2	2	3
20–34	2	1.5	<1	1	1	1	2	2	2	2
35–49	1	1.0	0	1	1	1	1	1	1	1
50–64	0									
65+	0									
2. MULTIPLE DX										
0–19 Years	1,320	1.5	8	1	1	1	2	2	3	5
20–34	1	2.0	0	2	2	2	2	2	2	2
35–49	1	3.0	0	3	3	3	3	3	3	3
50–64	1	2.0	0	2	2	2	2	2	2	2
65+	13	6.8	16	3	4	5	8	14	15	15
TOTAL SINGLE DX	541	1.3	<1	1	1	1	1	2	2	3
TOTAL MULTIPLE DX	1,336	1.5	8	1	1	1	2	2	3	5
TOTAL										
0–19 Years	1,858	1.4	6	1	1	1	2	2	2	4
20–34	3	1.7	<1	1	1	1	2	3	3	3
35–49	2	2.0	2	1	1	2	2	3	3	3
50–64	1	2.0	0	2	2	2	2	2	2	2
65+	13	6.8	16	3	4	5	8	14	15	15
GRAND TOTAL	1,877	1.4	6	1	1	1	2	2	3	5

89.19: VIDEO/TELEMETRIC EEG MON

Type of Patients	Observed Patients	Avg. Stay	Vari-ance	Percentiles						
				10th	25th	50th	75th	90th	95th	99th
1. SINGLE DX										
0–19 Years	420	2.2	2	1	1	2	3	4	5	7
20–34	179	4.2	6	2	3	4	5	7	8	14
35–49	80	4.4	5	2	3	4	5	8	8	15
50–64	53	3.9	3	2	3	4	5	6	7	7
65+	8	3.4	<1	2	3	3	4	5	5	5
2. MULTIPLE DX										
0–19 Years	945	2.8	5	1	1	2	3	5	6	12
20–34	468	3.8	5	2	2	3	5	7	8	11
35–49	475	4.2	6	2	3	4	5	7	8	13
50–64	343	4.4	9	2	3	4	5	8	9	14
65+	146	4.0	9	1	2	3	5	8	9	16
TOTAL SINGLE DX	740	2.7	4	1	1	2	3	5	7	9
TOTAL MULTIPLE DX	2,377	3.3	6	1	2	3	4	6	7	12
TOTAL										
0–19 Years	1,365	2.6	4	1	1	2	3	5	6	11
20–34	647	3.9	5	2	3	4	5	7	8	13
35–49	555	4.3	6	2	3	4	5	7	8	13
50–64	396	4.3	8	2	3	4	5	7	8	14
65+	154	3.9	8	1	2	3	5	8	9	16
GRAND TOTAL	3,117	3.2	6	1	2	3	4	6	7	12

LOS by Diagnosis and Operation, Western Region, 45th Edition

Western Region, October 2007–September 2008 Data, by Operation

89.2: GU SYSTEM-EXAMINATION

Type of Patients	Observed Patients	Avg. Stay	Vari-ance	Percentiles						
				10th	25th	50th	75th	90th	95th	99th
1. SINGLE DX										
0–19 Years	4	1.4	<1	1	1	1	1	2	4	4
20–34	0									
35–49	1	1.0	0	1	1	1	1	1	1	1
50–64	1	1.0	0	1	1	1	1	1	1	1
65+	0									
2. MULTIPLE DX										
0–19 Years	22	2.6	8	1	1	2	3	4	5	19
20–34	23	3.3	13	1	1	2	3	6	9	17
35–49	25	5.3	31	1	2	4	5	12	13	26
50–64	25	5.4	63	1	1	3	4	9	27	34
65+	61	6.1	30	1	3	5	8	11	12	32
TOTAL SINGLE DX	6	1.3	<1	1	1	1	1	2	4	4
TOTAL MULTIPLE DX	156	4.7	29	1	2	3	6	9	13	32
TOTAL										
0–19 Years	26	2.4	7	1	1	2	3	4	5	19
20–34	23	3.3	13	1	1	2	3	6	9	17
35–49	26	5.1	30	1	2	4	5	12	13	26
50–64	26	5.2	62	1	1	3	4	9	27	34
65+	61	6.1	30	1	3	5	8	11	12	32
GRAND TOTAL	162	4.5	28	1	1	3	5	9	12	32

89.29: GU SYSTEM EXAMS NEC

Type of Patients	Observed Patients	Avg. Stay	Vari-ance	Percentiles						
				10th	25th	50th	75th	90th	95th	99th
1. SINGLE DX										
0–19 Years	0									
20–34	0									
35–49	1	1.0	0	1	1	1	1	1	1	1
50–64	0									
65+	0									
2. MULTIPLE DX										
0–19 Years	1	1.0	0	1	1	1	1	1	1	1
20–34	2	2.0	2	1	1	1	3	3	3	3
35–49	5	3.0	2	1	1	4	4	4	4	4
50–64	6	3.5	9	1	1	3	4	9	9	9
65+	42	5.5	8	2	3	5	8	9	11	12
TOTAL SINGLE DX	1	1.0	0	1	1	1	1	1	1	1
TOTAL MULTIPLE DX	55	4.7	9	1	2	4	6	9	11	12
TOTAL										
0–19 Years	1	1.0	0	1	1	1	1	1	1	1
20–34	2	2.0	2	1	1	1	3	3	3	3
35–49	5	2.6	2	1	1	3	4	4	4	4
50–64	6	3.5	9	1	1	3	4	9	9	9
65+	42	5.5	8	2	3	5	8	9	11	12
GRAND TOTAL	56	4.6	9	1	2	4	6	9	11	12

89.22: CYSTOMETROGRAM

Type of Patients	Observed Patients	Avg. Stay	Vari-ance	Percentiles						
				10th	25th	50th	75th	90th	95th	99th
1. SINGLE DX										
0–19 Years	0									
20–34	0									
35–49	0									
50–64	0									
65+	0									
2. MULTIPLE DX										
0–19 Years	2	1.0	0	1	1	1	1	1	1	1
20–34	1	9.0	0	9	9	9	9	9	9	9
35–49	4	12.8	86	5	5	12	26	26	26	26
50–64	5	14.7	220	1	4	7	27	34	34	34
65+	5	12.3	134	3	6	8	12	32	32	32
TOTAL SINGLE DX	0									
TOTAL MULTIPLE DX	17	11.6	123	1	4	8	12	32	34	34
TOTAL										
0–19 Years	2	1.0	0	1	1	1	1	1	1	1
20–34	1	9.0	0	9	9	9	9	9	9	9
35–49	4	12.8	86	5	5	12	26	26	26	26
50–64	5	14.7	220	1	4	7	27	34	34	34
65+	5	12.3	134	3	6	8	12	32	32	32
GRAND TOTAL	17	11.6	123	1	4	8	12	32	34	34

89.3: OTHER EXAMINATIONS

Type of Patients	Observed Patients	Avg. Stay	Vari-ance	Percentiles						
				10th	25th	50th	75th	90th	95th	99th
1. SINGLE DX										
0–19 Years	110	3.0	5	1	1	2	4	5	7	12
20–34	2	5.5	4	4	4	4	7	7	7	7
35–49	1	1.0	0	1	1	1	1	1	1	1
50–64	1	5.0	0	5	5	5	5	5	5	5
65+	1	1.0	0	1	1	1	1	1	1	1
2. MULTIPLE DX										
0–19 Years	576	6.9	54	1	2	5	9	16	21	38
20–34	39	5.6	38	1	2	3	7	14	22	28
35–49	37	3.8	12	1	2	2	5	9	17	>99
50–64	78	4.8	12	1	2	4	6	9	11	20
65+	107	5.6	19	1	2	4	7	12	14	20
TOTAL SINGLE DX	115	3.0	5	1	1	2	4	5	7	12
TOTAL MULTIPLE DX	837	6.5	46	1	2	4	8	14	20	38
TOTAL										
0–19 Years	686	6.3	48	1	2	4	8	14	20	38
20–34	41	5.6	36	1	2	4	7	11	20	28
35–49	38	3.7	12	1	1	2	5	9	17	>99
50–64	79	4.8	12	1	2	4	6	9	11	20
65+	108	5.6	19	1	2	4	7	12	14	20
GRAND TOTAL	952	6.0	42	1	2	4	7	13	20	35

LOS by Diagnosis and Operation, Western Region, 45th Edition

Western Region, October 2007–September 2008 Data, by Operation

89.37: VITAL CAPACITY

Type of Patients	Observed Patients	Avg. Stay	Variance	10th	25th	50th	75th	90th	95th	99th
1. SINGLE DX										
0–19 Years	4	4.8	3	3	4	5	7	7	7	7
20–34	0									
35–49	0									
50–64	1	5.0	0	5	5	5	5	5	5	5
65+	0									
2. MULTIPLE DX										
0–19 Years	33	6.6	33	2	3	4	8	20	21	21
20–34	6	10.4	98	1	2	10	14	28	28	28
35–49	10	2.8	5	1	1	2	5	8	>99	>99
50–64	33	3.9	5	2	2	3	5	6	8	11
65+	35	6.1	19	2	3	5	7	13	14	20
TOTAL SINGLE DX	5	4.8	2	3	4	5	5	7	7	7
TOTAL MULTIPLE DX	117	5.7	25	2	2	4	7	14	20	28
TOTAL										
0–19 Years	37	6.4	30	2	3	4	8	15	21	21
20–34	6	10.4	98	1	2	10	14	28	28	28
35–49	10	2.8	5	1	1	2	5	8	>99	>99
50–64	34	3.9	5	2	2	3	5	6	8	11
65+	35	6.1	19	2	3	5	7	13	14	20
GRAND TOTAL	122	5.7	24	2	3	4	7	13	20	28

89.38: RESPIRATORY MEASURE NEC

Type of Patients	Observed Patients	Avg. Stay	Variance	10th	25th	50th	75th	90th	95th	99th
1. SINGLE DX										
0–19 Years	51	2.6	3	1	1	2	4	5	5	7
20–34	0									
35–49	0									
50–64	0									
65+										
2. MULTIPLE DX										
0–19 Years	240	9.6	84	1	3	7	13	21	28	44
20–34	4	3.0	<1	2	2	3	3	4	4	4
35–49	3	3.0	3	3	2	3	5	5	5	5
50–64	8	6.1	16	3	3	6	7	15	15	15
65+	14	2.6	2	1	2	3	3	5	5	5
TOTAL SINGLE DX	51	2.6	3	1	1	2	4	5	5	7
TOTAL MULTIPLE DX	269	9.0	79	1	3	6	12	20	27	44
TOTAL										
0–19 Years	291	8.3	76	1	2	5	11	20	27	43
20–34	4	3.0	<1	2	2	3	3	4	4	4
35–49	3	3.0	3	2	2	2	5	5	5	5
50–64	8	6.1	16	3	3	6	7	15	15	15
65+	14	2.6	2	1	2	3	3	5	5	5
GRAND TOTAL	320	7.9	72	1	2	5	11	19	26	43

89.39: NONOPERATIVE EXAMS NEC

Type of Patients	Observed Patients	Avg. Stay	Variance	10th	25th	50th	75th	90th	95th	99th
1. SINGLE DX										
0–19 Years	55	3.1	7	1	1	3	4	6	12	12
20–34	2	5.5	4	4	4	4	7	7	7	7
35–49	1	1.0	0	1	1	1	1	1	1	1
50–64	0									
65+	0									
2. MULTIPLE DX										
0–19 Years	288	5.4	34	1	2	4	7	10	17	35
20–34	19	5.0	21	1	2	4	6	11	20	20
35–49	12	5.4	25	1	1	4	7	12	17	17
50–64	26	5.2	12	1	2	4	8	10	11	14
65+	42	6.1	24	1	2	5	8	13	16	21
TOTAL SINGLE DX	58	3.2	7	1	1	3	4	7	12	12
TOTAL MULTIPLE DX	387	5.4	31	1	2	4	7	11	17	32
TOTAL										
0–19 Years	343	5.1	31	1	2	3	6	10	16	32
20–34	21	5.0	19	1	3	4	6	10	11	20
35–49	13	5.1	24	1	1	4	7	12	17	17
50–64	26	5.2	12	1	3	4	8	10	11	14
65+	42	6.1	24	1	2	5	8	13	16	21
GRAND TOTAL	445	5.2	29	1	2	4	6	10	16	32

89.4: CARD STRESS/DEVICE CHECK

Type of Patients	Observed Patients	Avg. Stay	Variance	10th	25th	50th	75th	90th	95th	99th
1. SINGLE DX										
0–19 Years	1	3.0	0	3	3	3	3	3	3	3
20–34	19	1.2	<1	1	1	1	1	2	4	4
35–49	67	1.3	<1	1	1	1	1	2	3	3
50–64	79	1.2	<1	1	1	1	1	2	2	3
65+	6	1.3	<1	1	1	1	2	2	2	2
2. MULTIPLE DX										
0–19 Years	19	2.3	4	1	1	1	3	6	6	7
20–34	244	2.2	6	1	1	1	2	4	5	8
35–49	2,409	2.0	3	1	1	1	2	4	5	8
50–64	5,446	2.1	4	1	1	1	2	4	5	9
65+	7,110	2.8	6	1	1	2	3	5	7	13
TOTAL SINGLE DX	172	1.2	<1	1	1	1	1	2	3	3
TOTAL MULTIPLE DX	15,228	2.4	5	1	1	2	3	5	6	11
TOTAL										
0–19 Years	20	2.3	4	1	1	1	3	6	6	7
20–34	263	2.1	5	1	1	1	2	4	5	8
35–49	2,476	1.9	3	1	1	1	2	4	5	8
50–64	5,525	2.1	3	1	1	1	2	4	5	9
65+	7,116	2.8	6	1	1	2	3	5	7	13
GRAND TOTAL	15,400	2.4	5	1	1	2	3	5	6	11

Western Region, October 2007–September 2008 Data, by Operation

89.41: TREADMILL STRESS TEST

Type of Patients	Observed Patients	Avg. Stay	Variance	10th	25th	50th	75th	90th	95th	99th
1. SINGLE DX										
0–19 Years	1	3.0	0	3	3	3	3	3	3	3
20–34	11	1.4	<1	1	1	1	1	3	4	4
35–49	41	1.1	<1	1	1	1	1	3	2	3
50–64	42	1.1	<1	1	1	1	1	1	1	2
65+	3	1.3	<1	1	1	1	2	2	2	2
2. MULTIPLE DX										
0–19 Years	7	1.2	<1	1	1	1	1	2	2	2
20–34	102	1.6	1	1	1	1	2	3	3	6
35–49	1,031	1.6	2	1	1	1	2	3	4	7
50–64	1,954	1.5	2	1	1	1	2	3	3	6
65+	1,250	2.1	3	1	1	1	2	4	5	10
TOTAL SINGLE DX	98	1.2	<1	1	1	1	1	2	2	3
TOTAL MULTIPLE DX	4,344	1.7	2	1	1	1	2	3	4	8
TOTAL										
0–19 Years	8	1.6	<1	1	1	1	2	3	3	3
20–34	113	1.6	1	1	1	1	2	3	3	6
35–49	1,072	1.6	2	1	1	1	2	3	4	7
50–64	1,996	1.5	2	1	1	1	2	3	3	6
65+	1,253	2.1	3	1	1	1	2	4	5	10
GRAND TOTAL	4,442	1.7	2	1	1	1	2	3	4	7

89.44: CV STRESS TEST NEC

Type of Patients	Observed Patients	Avg. Stay	Variance	10th	25th	50th	75th	90th	95th	99th
1. SINGLE DX										
0–19 Years	0									
20–34	8	1.0	<1	1	1	1	1	1	1	1
35–49	26	1.5	<1	1	1	1	2	3	3	3
50–64	37	1.3	<1	1	1	1	1	2	3	3
65+	3	1.3	<1	1	1	1	2	2	2	2
2. MULTIPLE DX										
0–19 Years	5	1.6	<1	1	1	1	2	3	3	3
20–34	102	2.6	11	1	1	2	3	5	5	8
35–49	1,230	2.1	3	1	1	2	3	4	5	8
50–64	3,018	2.3	4	1	1	2	3	4	5	9
65+	4,343	2.7	5	1	1	2	3	5	7	11
TOTAL SINGLE DX	74	1.3	<1	1	1	1	2	2	3	3
TOTAL MULTIPLE DX	8,698	2.5	4	1	1	2	3	5	6	10
TOTAL										
0–19 Years	5	1.6	<1	1	1	1	2	3	3	3
20–34	110	2.5	10	1	1	2	3	5	5	8
35–49	1,256	2.1	3	1	1	2	3	4	5	8
50–64	3,055	2.3	4	1	1	2	3	4	5	9
65+	4,346	2.7	5	1	1	2	3	5	7	11
GRAND TOTAL	8,772	2.5	4	1	1	2	3	5	6	10

89.45: PACEMAKER RATE CHECK

Type of Patients	Observed Patients	Avg. Stay	Variance	10th	25th	50th	75th	90th	95th	99th
1. SINGLE DX										
0–19 Years	0	0								
20–34	0	0								
35–49	0	0								
50–64	0	0								
65+	0									
2. MULTIPLE DX										
0–19 Years	5	2.2	5	1	1	1	1	7	7	7
20–34	17	2.6	5	1	1	2	3	8	8	8
35–49	31	2.7	3	1	1	2	4	5	6	6
50–64	101	3.4	7	1	1	3	4	6	9	13
65+	847	3.8	10	1	2	3	5	7	9	17
TOTAL SINGLE DX	0									
TOTAL MULTIPLE DX	1,001	3.7	10	1	2	3	5	7	9	17
TOTAL										
0–19 Years	5	2.2	5	1	1	1	1	7	7	7
20–34	17	2.6	5	1	1	2	3	8	8	8
35–49	31	2.7	3	1	1	2	4	5	6	6
50–64	101	3.4	7	1	1	3	4	6	9	13
65+	847	3.8	10	1	2	3	5	7	9	17
GRAND TOTAL	1,001	3.7	10	1	2	3	5	7	9	17

89.49: AICD CHECK

Type of Patients	Observed Patients	Avg. Stay	Variance	10th	25th	50th	75th	90th	95th	99th
1. SINGLE DX										
0–19 Years	0	0								
20–34	0	0								
35–49	0	0								
50–64	0	0								
65+	0									
2. MULTIPLE DX										
0–19 Years	1	1.0	0	1	1	1	1	1	1	1
20–34	22	2.5	3	1	1	2	3	4	4	8
35–49	114	3.4	10	1	2	2	4	7	10	16
50–64	366	3.1	9	1	1	2	4	6	8	14
65+	649	3.6	11	1	2	3	4	7	10	17
TOTAL SINGLE DX	0									
TOTAL MULTIPLE DX	1,152	3.4	10	1	1	2	4	7	9	16
TOTAL										
0–19 Years	1	1.0	0	1	1	1	1	1	1	1
20–34	22	2.5	3	1	1	2	3	4	4	8
35–49	114	3.4	10	1	2	2	4	7	10	16
50–64	366	3.1	9	1	1	2	4	6	8	14
65+	649	3.6	11	1	2	3	4	7	10	17
GRAND TOTAL	1,152	3.4	10	1	1	2	4	7	9	16

LOS by Diagnosis and Operation, Western Region, 45th Edition

Western Region, October 2007–September 2008 Data, by Operation

89.5: OTHER CARDIAC FUNCT TEST

Type of Patients	Observed Patients	Avg. Stay	Vari-ance	Percentiles						
				10th	25th	50th	75th	90th	95th	99th
1. SINGLE DX										
0–19 Years	15	1.4	1	1	1	1	1	2	5	5
20–34	37	1.8	2	1	1	1	2	2	5	6
35–49	55	1.8	3	1	1	1	2	4	4	11
50–64	36	1.7	3	1	1	1	2	3	4	11
65+	7	2.8	8	1	1	2	4	9	9	9
2. MULTIPLE DX										
0–19 Years	140	3.3	7	1	1	2	4	7	9	14
20–34	481	3.4	24	1	1	2	3	6	11	28
35–49	1,254	2.7	13	1	1	2	3	5	7	20
50–64	1,971	2.6	9	1	1	2	3	5	7	14
65+	2,041	3.2	8	1	1	2	4	6	8	14
TOTAL SINGLE DX	150	1.8	3	1	1	1	2	4	5	11
TOTAL MULTIPLE DX	5,887	2.9	11	1	1	2	3	6	8	16
TOTAL										
0–19 Years	155	3.0	7	1	1	2	4	6	8	14
20–34	518	3.3	23	1	1	2	3	6	11	26
35–49	1,309	2.7	13	1	1	2	3	5	7	20
50–64	2,007	2.6	9	1	1	2	3	5	7	14
65+	2,048	3.2	8	1	1	2	4	6	8	14
GRAND TOTAL	6,037	2.9	11	1	1	2	3	6	8	16

89.52: ELECTROCARDIOGRAM

Type of Patients	Observed Patients	Avg. Stay	Vari-ance	Percentiles						
				10th	25th	50th	75th	90th	95th	99th
1. SINGLE DX										
0–19 Years	4	1.0	0	1	1	1	1	1	1	1
20–34	23	1.7	7	1	1	1	2	4	4	5
35–49	37	1.9	3	1	1	1	2	4	5	11
50–64	27	1.6	4	1	1	1	1	3	3	11
65+	7	2.8	8	1	1	2	4	9	9	9
2. MULTIPLE DX										
0–19 Years	61	3.4	7	1	2	2	4	7	11	12
20–34	233	3.5	30	1	1	2	3	7	12	32
35–49	711	2.5	9	1	1	2	3	5	7	16
50–64	1,156	2.3	6	1	1	2	3	5	7	12
65+	738	2.6	7	1	1	2	3	5	8	13
TOTAL SINGLE DX	98	1.8	3	1	1	1	2	4	4	11
TOTAL MULTIPLE DX	2,899	2.5	9	1	1	2	3	5	7	16
TOTAL										
0–19 Years	65	3.1	7	1	1	2	4	7	9	12
20–34	256	3.3	27	1	1	2	3	6	12	32
35–49	748	2.5	8	1	1	1	3	5	7	16
50–64	1,183	2.3	6	1	1	2	3	5	7	12
65+	745	2.6	7	1	1	2	3	5	8	13
GRAND TOTAL	2,997	2.5	9	1	1	2	3	5	7	16

89.50: AMBULATORY CARD MONITOR

Type of Patients	Observed Patients	Avg. Stay	Vari-ance	Percentiles						
				10th	25th	50th	75th	90th	95th	99th
1. SINGLE DX										
0–19 Years	3	3.2	4	1	1	2	5	5	5	5
20–34	2	1.5	<1	1	1	2	2	2	2	2
35–49	1	3.0	0	3	3	3	3	3	3	3
50–64	0									
65+	0									
2. MULTIPLE DX										
0–19 Years	5	6.8	8	2	5	7	8	10	10	10
20–34	4	13.1	386	3	3	3	4	43	43	43
35–49	9	3.4	4	2	2	3	4	7	7	7
50–64	13	3.4	3	2	2	3	4	6	7	7
65+	47	4.3	23	1	2	3	4	7	16	25
TOTAL SINGLE DX	6	2.7	3	1	1	2	5	5	5	5
TOTAL MULTIPLE DX	78	4.7	34	1	2	3	5	8	10	43
TOTAL										
0–19 Years	8	5.6	9	2	2	5	8	10	10	10
20–34	6	9.2	267	1	2	3	4	43	43	43
35–49	10	3.2	4	1	2	3	4	7	7	7
50–64	13	3.4	3	2	2	3	4	6	7	7
65+	47	4.3	23	1	2	3	4	7	16	25
GRAND TOTAL	84	4.5	32	1	2	3	5	8	10	43

89.54: ECG MONITORING

Type of Patients	Observed Patients	Avg. Stay	Vari-ance	Percentiles						
				10th	25th	50th	75th	90th	95th	99th
1. SINGLE DX										
0–19 Years	5	1.0	0	1	1	1	1	1	1	1
20–34	12	2.1	3	1	1	1	3	5	6	6
35–49	16	1.5	<1	1	1	1	2	2	4	4
50–64	8	2.0	1	1	1	2	3	4	4	4
65+	0									
2. MULTIPLE DX										
0–19 Years	56	2.4	4	1	1	2	3	5	6	14
20–34	207	3.1	14	1	1	2	3	6	9	22
35–49	477	3.1	21	1	1	2	3	5	8	23
50–64	696	3.1	15	1	1	2	3	6	8	16
65+	1,013	3.5	7	1	2	3	4	6	9	14
TOTAL SINGLE DX	41	1.7	1	1	1	1	2	3	4	6
TOTAL MULTIPLE DX	2,449	3.2	13	1	1	2	4	6	8	17
TOTAL										
0–19 Years	61	2.3	4	1	1	2	3	5	5	14
20–34	219	3.1	13	1	1	2	3	6	9	22
35–49	493	3.0	20	1	1	2	3	5	7	23
50–64	704	3.0	15	1	1	2	3	6	8	16
65+	1,013	3.5	7	1	2	3	4	6	9	14
GRAND TOTAL	2,490	3.2	12	1	1	2	4	6	8	17

Western Region, October 2007–September 2008 Data, by Operation

89.59: NONOP CARD/VASC EXAM NEC

Type of Patients	Observed Patients	Avg. Stay	Variance	10th	25th	50th	75th	90th	95th	99th
1. SINGLE DX										
0–19 Years	3	1.0	0	1	1	1	1	1	1	1
20–34	0									
35–49	1	2.0	0	2	2	2	2	2	2	2
50–64	1	2.0	0	2	2	2	2	2	2	2
65+	0									
2. MULTIPLE DX										
0–19 Years	14	4.5	11	1	2	4	6	8	15	15
20–34	37	3.1	10	1	1	2	4	6	7	19
35–49	57	3.1	7	1	1	2	4	8	9	12
50–64	106	3.4	5	1	2	3	4	7	8	9
65+	243	3.6	7	1	2	3	5	7	8	11
TOTAL SINGLE DX	5	1.3	<1	1	1	1	1	2	2	2
TOTAL MULTIPLE DX	457	3.5	7	1	2	3	5	7	8	12
TOTAL										
0–19 Years	17	3.6	10	1	1	3	6	6	8	15
20–34	37	3.1	10	1	1	2	4	6	7	19
35–49	58	3.1	7	1	1	2	4	8	9	12
50–64	107	3.4	5	1	2	3	4	7	8	9
65+	243	3.6	7	1	2	3	5	7	8	11
GRAND TOTAL	462	3.5	7	1	2	3	4	7	8	12

89.6: CIRCULATORY MONITORING

Type of Patients	Observed Patients	Avg. Stay	Variance	10th	25th	50th	75th	90th	95th	99th
1. SINGLE DX										
0–19 Years	30	2.4	1	1	2	2	3	4	4	5
20–34	4	2.5	9	1	1	1	7	7	7	7
35–49	4	2.0	<1	1	2	2	3	3	3	3
50–64	7	1.9	3	1	1	2	3	6	6	6
65+	1	2.0	0	2	2	2	2	2	2	2
2. MULTIPLE DX										
0–19 Years	618	6.5	118	1	2	3	5	14	23	54
20–34	221	4.4	26	1	2	3	5	9	12	21
35–49	456	5.3	23	1	2	4	7	10	14	25
50–64	845	5.9	29	2	3	4	8	12	15	24
65+	1,694	5.9	22	2	3	5	7	11	15	24
TOTAL SINGLE DX	46	2.3	2	1	1	2	3	4	5	7
TOTAL MULTIPLE DX	3,834	5.9	41	2	3	4	7	12	15	29
TOTAL										
0–19 Years	648	6.3	113	1	2	3	5	14	22	53
20–34	225	4.3	26	1	2	3	5	9	12	21
35–49	460	5.3	23	1	2	4	7	10	14	25
50–64	852	5.9	29	2	3	4	8	12	15	24
65+	1,695	5.9	22	2	3	5	7	11	15	24
GRAND TOTAL	3,880	5.8	41	2	3	4	7	11	15	29

89.61: ART PRESSURE MONITORING

Type of Patients	Observed Patients	Avg. Stay	Variance	10th	25th	50th	75th	90th	95th	99th
1. SINGLE DX										
0–19 Years	0									
20–34	0									
35–49	0									
50–64	0									
65+	0									
2. MULTIPLE DX										
0–19 Years	15	24.3	655	4	9	14	40	84	84	84
20–34	13	4.2	4	2	3	4	5	6	9	9
35–49	21	5.7	20	1	3	4	7	9	14	19
50–64	47	7.2	27	3	3	6	9	13	19	25
65+	86	7.1	26	2	4	6	9	13	15	36
TOTAL SINGLE DX	0									
TOTAL MULTIPLE DX	182	10.1	190	2	4	6	10	17	36	84
TOTAL										
0–19 Years	15	24.3	655	4	9	14	40	84	84	84
20–34	13	4.2	4	2	3	4	5	6	9	9
35–49	21	5.7	20	1	3	4	7	9	14	19
50–64	47	7.2	27	3	3	6	9	13	19	25
65+	86	7.1	26	2	4	6	9	13	15	36
GRAND TOTAL	182	10.1	190	2	4	6	10	17	36	84

89.62: CVP MONITORING

Type of Patients	Observed Patients	Avg. Stay	Variance	10th	25th	50th	75th	90th	95th	99th
1. SINGLE DX										
0–19 Years	0									
20–34	0									
35–49	0									
50–64	2	1.0	0	1	1	1	1	1	1	1
65+	0									
2. MULTIPLE DX										
0–19 Years	12	17.1	302	4	4	5	26	53	53	53
20–34	18	4.9	10	2	2	5	6	11	13	13
35–49	48	6.3	16	2	4	5	8	13	15	16
50–64	80	6.6	26	2	4	5	9	13	18	24
65+	124	7.8	21	3	4	7	10	15	18	20
TOTAL SINGLE DX	2	1.0	0	1	1	1	1	1	1	1
TOTAL MULTIPLE DX	282	8.0	58	2	4	6	10	15	20	53
TOTAL										
0–19 Years	12	17.1	302	4	4	5	26	53	53	53
20–34	18	4.9	10	2	2	5	6	11	13	13
35–49	48	6.3	16	2	4	5	8	13	15	16
50–64	82	6.5	26	3	3	5	9	13	17	24
65+	124	7.8	21	3	4	7	10	15	18	20
GRAND TOTAL	284	8.0	58	2	4	6	10	15	19	53

LOS by Diagnosis and Operation, Western Region, 45th Edition

Western Region, October 2007–September 2008 Data, by Operation

89.64: PA WEDGE MONITORING

Type of Patients	Observed Patients	Avg. Stay	Variance	10th	25th	50th	75th	90th	95th	99th
1. SINGLE DX										
0–19 Years	0									
20–34	1	1.0	0	1	1	1	1	1	1	1
35–49	0									
50–64	1	1.0	0	1	1	1	1	1	1	1
65+	0									
2. MULTIPLE DX										
0–19 Years	1	5.0	0	5	5	5	5	5	5	5
20–34	19	11.6	173	1	3	10	13	23	59	59
35–49	44	7.2	46	2	3	5	10	12	15	38
50–64	108	8.5	56	1	4	7	11	15	18	29
65+	143	9.2	43	3	5	8	12	16	24	32
TOTAL SINGLE DX	2	1.0	0	1	1	1	1	1	1	1
TOTAL MULTIPLE DX	315	8.8	56	2	4	7	12	15	23	38
TOTAL										
0–19 Years	1	5.0	0	5	5	5	5	5	5	5
20–34	20	11.1	170	1	3	9	13	23	59	59
35–49	44	7.2	46	2	3	5	10	12	15	38
50–64	109	8.5	56	1	4	7	11	15	18	29
65+	143	9.2	43	3	5	8	12	16	24	32
GRAND TOTAL	317	8.8	56	2	4	7	12	15	23	38

89.65: ARTERIAL BLD GAS MEASURE

Type of Patients	Observed Patients	Avg. Stay	Variance	10th	25th	50th	75th	90th	95th	99th
1. SINGLE DX										
0–19 Years	26	2.5	1	1	2	2	3	4	4	5
20–34	2	4.0	18	1	1	4	7	7	7	7
35–49	3	2.0	<1	1	1	2	3	3	3	3
50–64	4	2.5	6	1	1	2	6	6	6	6
65+	1	2.0	0	2	2	2	2	2	2	2
2. MULTIPLE DX										
0–19 Years	555	4.8	51	1	2	3	4	8	16	36
20–34	140	3.2	7	1	2	2	4	6	8	15
35–49	244	4.4	13	2	2	3	5	9	12	19
50–64	436	4.9	22	2	2	4	6	9	12	18
65+	1,034	5.2	17	2	3	4	6	10	12	22
TOTAL SINGLE DX	36	2.5	2	1	2	2	3	4	5	7
TOTAL MULTIPLE DX	2,409	4.9	25	1	2	4	6	9	12	24
TOTAL										
0–19 Years	581	4.7	49	1	2	3	4	8	15	34
20–34	142	3.2	7	1	2	3	4	6	8	15
35–49	247	4.4	13	1	2	3	5	9	12	19
50–64	440	4.9	22	2	2	4	6	9	12	18
65+	1,035	5.2	17	2	3	4	6	10	12	22
GRAND TOTAL	2,445	4.8	25	1	2	3	6	9	12	24

89.68: CARDIAC OUTPUT MON NEC

Type of Patients	Observed Patients	Avg. Stay	Variance	10th	25th	50th	75th	90th	95th	99th
1. SINGLE DX										
0–19 Years	0									
20–34	1	1.0	0	1	1	1	1	1	1	1
35–49	1	2.0	0	2	2	2	2	2	2	2
50–64	0									
65+	0									
2. MULTIPLE DX										
0–19 Years	4	8.0	26	1	3	12	12	12	12	12
20–34	26	5.2	7	2	3	5	7	9	10	12
35–49	93	6.3	39	2	3	5	7	11	22	42
50–64	159	6.5	28	1	3	5	9	13	16	24
65+	273	5.8	18	2	3	4	7	12	15	20
TOTAL SINGLE DX	2	1.5	<1	1	1	2	2	2	2	2
TOTAL MULTIPLE DX	555	6.1	24	2	3	5	8	12	15	24
TOTAL										
0–19 Years	4	8.0	26	1	3	12	12	12	12	12
20–34	27	5.1	8	2	3	5	7	9	10	12
35–49	94	6.3	39	2	3	5	7	11	22	42
50–64	159	6.5	28	1	3	5	9	13	16	24
65+	273	5.8	18	2	3	4	7	12	15	20
GRAND TOTAL	557	6.1	24	2	3	5	8	12	15	24

89.7: GENERAL PHYSICAL EXAM

Type of Patients	Observed Patients	Avg. Stay	Variance	10th	25th	50th	75th	90th	95th	99th
1. SINGLE DX										
0–19 Years	1	1.0	0	1	1	1	1	1	1	1
20–34	0									
35–49	0									
50–64	0									
65+										
2. MULTIPLE DX										
0–19 Years	1	1.0	0	1	1	1	1	1	1	1
20–34	5	3.4	6	1	1	3	6	6	6	6
35–49	4	4.8	6	1	3	5	8	8	8	8
50–64	2	7.0	31	3	4	7	11	11	11	11
65+	2	4.0	18	1	1	4	7	7	7	7
TOTAL SINGLE DX	1	1.0	0	1	1	1	1	1	1	1
TOTAL MULTIPLE DX	14	4.2	10	1	1	4	6	8	11	11
TOTAL										
0–19 Years	2	1.0	0	1	1	1	1	1	1	1
20–34	5	3.4	6	1	1	3	6	6	6	6
35–49	4	4.8	6	2	4	5	8	8	8	8
50–64	2	7.0	31	3	3	7	11	11	11	11
65+	2	4.0	18	1	1	4	7	7	7	7
GRAND TOTAL	15	3.5	9	1	1	2	6	8	11	11

LOS by Diagnosis and Operation, Western Region, 45th Edition

89.8: AUTOPSY

Type of Patients	Observed Patients	Avg. Stay	Variance	10th	25th	50th	75th	90th	95th	99th
1. SINGLE DX										
0–19 Years	0									
20–34	0									
35–49	0									
50–64	0									
65+	0									
2. MULTIPLE DX										
0–19 Years	0									
20–34	0									
35–49	0									
50–64	0									
65+	0									
TOTAL SINGLE DX	0									
TOTAL MULTIPLE DX	0									
TOTAL										
0–19 Years	0									
20–34	0									
35–49	0									
50–64	0									
65+	0									
GRAND TOTAL	0									

90.1: MICRO EXAM-ENDOCRINE

Type of Patients	Observed Patients	Avg. Stay	Variance	10th	25th	50th	75th	90th	95th	99th
1. SINGLE DX										
0–19 Years	0									
20–34	0									
35–49	0									
50–64	0									
65+	0									
2. MULTIPLE DX										
0–19 Years	0									
20–34	0									
35–49	0									
50–64	0									
65+	0									
TOTAL SINGLE DX	0									
TOTAL MULTIPLE DX	0									
TOTAL										
0–19 Years	0									
20–34	0									
35–49	0									
50–64	0									
65+	0									
GRAND TOTAL	0									

90.0: MICRO EXAM-NERVOUS SYST

Type of Patients	Observed Patients	Avg. Stay	Variance	10th	25th	50th	75th	90th	95th	99th
1. SINGLE DX										
0–19 Years	0									
20–34	0									
35–49	0									
50–64	0									
65+	0									
2. MULTIPLE DX										
0–19 Years	1	6.0	0	6	6	6	6	6	6	6
20–34	0									
35–49	0									
50–64	0									
65+	0									
TOTAL SINGLE DX	0									
TOTAL MULTIPLE DX	1	6.0	0	6	6	6	6	6	6	6
TOTAL										
0–19 Years	1	6.0	0	6	6	6	6	6	6	6
20–34	0									
35–49	0									
50–64	0									
65+	0									
GRAND TOTAL	1	6.0	0	6	6	6	6	6	6	6

90.2: MICRO EXAM-EYE

Type of Patients	Observed Patients	Avg. Stay	Variance	10th	25th	50th	75th	90th	95th	99th
1. SINGLE DX										
0–19 Years	0									
20–34	0									
35–49	0									
50–64	0									
65+	0									
2. MULTIPLE DX										
0–19 Years	1	3.0	0	3	3	3	3	3	3	3
20–34	0									
35–49	0									
50–64	2	9.0	18	6	6	9	12	12	12	12
65+	0									
TOTAL SINGLE DX	0									
TOTAL MULTIPLE DX	3	7.0	21	3	3	6	12	12	12	12
TOTAL										
0–19 Years	1	3.0	0	3	3	3	3	3	3	3
20–34	0									
35–49	0									
50–64	2	9.0	18	6	6	9	12	12	12	12
65+	0									
GRAND TOTAL	3	7.0	21	3	3	6	12	12	12	12

LOS by Diagnosis and Operation, Western Region, 45th Edition

Western Region, October 2007–September 2008 Data, by Operation

90.3: MICRO EXAM-ENT/LARYNX

Type of Patients	Observed Patients	Avg. Stay	Vari-ance	10th	25th	50th	75th	90th	95th	99th
1. SINGLE DX										
0–19 Years	0									
20–34	0									
35–49	0									
50–64	0									
65+	0									
2. MULTIPLE DX										
0–19 Years	0									
20–34	0									
35–49	0									
50–64	1	2.0	0	2	2	2	2	2	2	2
65+	0									
TOTAL SINGLE DX	0									
TOTAL MULTIPLE DX	1	2.0	0	2	2	2	2	2	2	2
TOTAL										
0–19 Years	0									
20–34	0									
35–49	0									
50–64	1	2.0	0	2	2	2	2	2	2	2
65+	0									
GRAND TOTAL	1	2.0	0	2	2	2	2	2	2	2

90.4: MICRO EXAM-LOWER RESP

Type of Patients	Observed Patients	Avg. Stay	Vari-ance	10th	25th	50th	75th	90th	95th	99th
1. SINGLE DX										
0–19 Years	0									
20–34	0									
35–49	0									
50–64	0									
65+	0									
2. MULTIPLE DX										
0–19 Years	1	2.0	0	2	2	2	2	2	2	2
20–34	0									
35–49	0									
50–64	0									
65+	4	5.5	9	4	4	4	10	10	10	10
TOTAL SINGLE DX	0									
TOTAL MULTIPLE DX	5	4.8	9	2	4	4	4	10	10	10
TOTAL										
0–19 Years	1	2.0	0	2	2	2	2	2	2	2
20–34	0									
35–49	0									
50–64	0									
65+	4	5.5	9	4	4	4	10	10	10	10
GRAND TOTAL	5	4.8	9	2	4	4	4	10	10	10

90.5: MICRO EXAM-BLOOD

Type of Patients	Observed Patients	Avg. Stay	Vari-ance	10th	25th	50th	75th	90th	95th	99th
1. SINGLE DX										
0–19 Years	6	3.0	4	1	2	3	3	7	7	7
20–34	0									
35–49	0									
50–64	0									
65+	0									
2. MULTIPLE DX										
0–19 Years	691	4.2	38	1	2	2	4	9	15	30
20–34	4	3.0	<1	2	2	3	3	4	4	4
35–49	8	6.8	38	1	3	4	13	18	18	18
50–64	7	5.0	21	2	2	3	5	15	15	15
65+	14	3.4	5	1	2	3	3	7	8	8
TOTAL SINGLE DX	6	3.0	4	1	2	3	3	7	7	7
TOTAL MULTIPLE DX	724	4.2	37	1	2	2	4	9	15	27
TOTAL										
0–19 Years	697	4.2	38	1	2	2	4	9	15	30
20–34	4	3.0	<1	2	2	3	3	4	4	4
35–49	8	6.8	38	1	3	4	13	18	18	18
50–64	7	5.0	21	2	2	3	5	15	15	15
65+	14	3.4	5	1	2	3	3	7	8	8
GRAND TOTAL	730	4.2	37	1	2	2	4	9	15	27

90.52: CULTURE-BLOOD

Type of Patients	Observed Patients	Avg. Stay	Vari-ance	10th	25th	50th	75th	90th	95th	99th
1. SINGLE DX										
0–19 Years	5	2.2	<1	1	2	2	3	3	3	3
20–34	0									
35–49	0									
50–64	0									
65+	0									
2. MULTIPLE DX										
0–19 Years	675	4.2	39	1	2	2	4	9	15	30
20–34	0									
35–49	0									
50–64	0									
65+	1	7.0	0	7	7	7	7	7	7	7
TOTAL SINGLE DX	5	2.2	<1	1	2	2	3	3	3	3
TOTAL MULTIPLE DX	676	4.3	39	1	2	2	4	9	15	30
TOTAL										
0–19 Years	680	4.2	38	1	2	2	4	9	15	30
20–34	0									
35–49	0									
50–64	0									
65+	1	7.0	0	7	7	7	7	7	7	7
GRAND TOTAL	681	4.2	38	1	2	2	4	9	15	30

444

LOS by Diagnosis and Operation, Western Region, 45th Edition

Western Region, October 2007–September 2008 Data, by Operation

90.6: MICRO EXAM-SPLEEN/MARROW

Type of Patients	Observed Patients	Avg. Stay	Vari-ance	10th	25th	50th	75th	90th	95th	99th
1. SINGLE DX										
0–19 Years	0									
20–34	0									
35–49	0									
50–64	0									
65+	0									
2. MULTIPLE DX										
0–19 Years	0									
20–34	0									
35–49	0									
50–64	0									
65+	0									
TOTAL SINGLE DX	0									
TOTAL MULTIPLE DX	0									
TOTAL										
0–19 Years	0									
20–34	0									
35–49	0									
50–64	0									
65+	0									
GRAND TOTAL	0									

90.7: MICRO EXAM-LYMPH SYSTEM

Type of Patients	Observed Patients	Avg. Stay	Vari-ance	10th	25th	50th	75th	90th	95th	99th
1. SINGLE DX										
0–19 Years	0									
20–34	0									
35–49	0									
50–64	0									
65+	0									
2. MULTIPLE DX										
0–19 Years	0									
20–34	1	2.0	0	2	2	2	2	2	2	2
35–49	0									
50–64	0									
65+	0									
TOTAL SINGLE DX	0									
TOTAL MULTIPLE DX	1	2.0	0	2	2	2	2	2	2	2
TOTAL										
0–19 Years	0									
20–34	1	2.0	0	2	2	2	2	2	2	2
35–49	0									
50–64	0									
65+	0									
GRAND TOTAL	1	2.0	0	2	2	2	2	2	2	2

90.8: MICRO EXAM-UPPER GI

Type of Patients	Observed Patients	Avg. Stay	Vari-ance	10th	25th	50th	75th	90th	95th	99th
1. SINGLE DX										
0–19 Years	0									
20–34	0									
35–49	0									
50–64	0									
65+	0									
2. MULTIPLE DX										
0–19 Years	1	4.0	0	4	4	4	4	4	4	4
20–34	0									
35–49	0									
50–64	0									
65+	1	2.0	0	2	2	2	2	2	2	2
TOTAL SINGLE DX	0									
TOTAL MULTIPLE DX	2	3.0	2	2	2	3	4	4	4	4
TOTAL										
0–19 Years	1	4.0	0	4	4	4	4	4	4	4
20–34	0									
35–49	0									
50–64	0									
65+	1	2.0	0	2	2	2	2	2	2	2
GRAND TOTAL	2	3.0	2	2	2	3	4	4	4	4

90.9: MICRO EXAM-LOWER GI

Type of Patients	Observed Patients	Avg. Stay	Vari-ance	10th	25th	50th	75th	90th	95th	99th
1. SINGLE DX										
0–19 Years	0									
20–34	0									
35–49	0									
50–64	0									
65+	0									
2. MULTIPLE DX										
0–19 Years	1	4.0	0	4	4	4	4	4	4	4
20–34	0									
35–49	0									
50–64	1	6.0	0	6	6	6	6	6	6	6
65+	1	1.0	0	1	1	1	1	1	1	1
TOTAL SINGLE DX	0									
TOTAL MULTIPLE DX	3	3.7	6	1	1	4	6	6	6	6
TOTAL										
0–19 Years	1	4.0	0	4	4	4	4	4	4	4
20–34	0									
35–49	0									
50–64	1	6.0	0	6	6	6	6	6	6	6
65+	1	1.0	0	1	1	1	1	1	1	1
GRAND TOTAL	3	3.7	6	1	1	4	6	6	6	6

LOS by Diagnosis and Operation, Western Region, 45th Edition

Western Region, October 2007–September 2008 Data, by Operation

91.0: MICRO EXAM-BIL/PANCREAS

Type of Patients	Observed Patients	Avg. Stay	Vari-ance	Percentiles						
				10th	25th	50th	75th	90th	95th	99th
1. SINGLE DX										
0–19 Years	0									
20–34	0									
35–49	0									
50–64	0									
65+	0									
2. MULTIPLE DX										
0–19 Years	0									
20–34	0									
35–49	0									
50–64	0									
65+	0									
TOTAL SINGLE DX	0									
TOTAL MULTIPLE DX	0									
TOTAL										
0–19 Years	0									
20–34	0									
35–49	0									
50–64	0									
65+	0									
GRAND TOTAL	0									

91.1: MICRO EXAM-PERITONEUM

Type of Patients	Observed Patients	Avg. Stay	Vari-ance	Percentiles						
				10th	25th	50th	75th	90th	95th	99th
1. SINGLE DX										
0–19 Years	0									
20–34	0									
35–49	0									
50–64	0									
65+	0									
2. MULTIPLE DX										
0–19 Years	0									
20–34	0									
35–49	0									
50–64	0									
65+	0									
TOTAL SINGLE DX	0									
TOTAL MULTIPLE DX	0									
TOTAL										
0–19 Years	0									
20–34	0									
35–49	0									
50–64	0									
65+	0									
GRAND TOTAL	0									

91.2: MICRO EXAM-UPPER URINARY

Type of Patients	Observed Patients	Avg. Stay	Vari-ance	Percentiles						
				10th	25th	50th	75th	90th	95th	99th
1. SINGLE DX										
0–19 Years	0									
20–34	0									
35–49	0									
50–64	0									
65+	0									
2. MULTIPLE DX										
0–19 Years	0									
20–34	0									
35–49	0									
50–64	0									
65+	0									
TOTAL SINGLE DX	0									
TOTAL MULTIPLE DX	0									
TOTAL										
0–19 Years	0									
20–34	0									
35–49	0									
50–64	0									
65+	0									
GRAND TOTAL	0									

91.3: MICRO EXAM-LOWER URINARY

Type of Patients	Observed Patients	Avg. Stay	Vari-ance	Percentiles						
				10th	25th	50th	75th	90th	95th	99th
1. SINGLE DX										
0–19 Years	0									
20–34	0									
35–49	0									
50–64	0									
65+										
2. MULTIPLE DX										
0–19 Years	81	2.5	14	1	1	2	2	4	6	32
20–34	27	3.3	12	1	1	2	4	7	13	15
35–49	15	4.3	21	1	1	3	6	10	18	18
50–64	9	9.8	62	3	5	7	11	23	23	23
65+	0									
TOTAL SINGLE DX	0									
TOTAL MULTIPLE DX	132	3.4	21	1	1	2	3	7	12	23
TOTAL										
0–19 Years	81	2.5	14	1	1	2	2	4	6	32
20–34	27	3.3	12	1	1	2	4	7	13	15
35–49	15	4.3	21	1	1	3	6	10	18	18
50–64	9	9.8	62	3	5	7	11	23	23	23
65+	0									
GRAND TOTAL	132	3.4	21	1	1	2	3	7	12	23

LOS by Diagnosis and Operation, Western Region, 45th Edition

Western Region, October 2007–September 2008 Data, by Operation

91.4: MICRO EXAM-FEMALE GENIT

Type of Patients	Observed Patients	Avg. Stay	Variance	Percentiles						
				10th	25th	50th	75th	90th	95th	99th
1. SINGLE DX										
0–19 Years	0									
20–34	0									
35–49	0									
50–64	0									
65+	0									
2. MULTIPLE DX										
0–19 Years	1	5.0	0	5	5	5	5	5	5	5
20–34	2	4.0	18	1	1	1	7	7	7	7
35–49	1	4.0	0	4	4	4	4	4	4	4
50–64	3	2.0	3	1	1	1	4	4	4	4
65+	1	7.0	0	7	7	7	7	7	7	7
TOTAL SINGLE DX	0									
TOTAL MULTIPLE DX	8	3.7	6	1	1	4	5	7	7	7
TOTAL										
0–19 Years	1	5.0	0	5	5	5	5	5	5	5
20–34	2	4.0	18	1	1	1	7	7	7	7
35–49	1	4.0	0	4	4	4	4	4	4	4
50–64	3	2.0	3	1	1	1	4	4	4	4
65+	1	7.0	0	7	7	7	7	7	7	7
GRAND TOTAL	8	3.7	6	1	1	4	5	7	7	7

91.5: MICRO EXAM-MS/JT FLUID

Type of Patients	Observed Patients	Avg. Stay	Variance	Percentiles						
				10th	25th	50th	75th	90th	95th	99th
1. SINGLE DX										
0–19 Years	0									
20–34	0									
35–49	0									
50–64	0									
65+	0									
2. MULTIPLE DX										
0–19 Years	0									
20–34	0									
35–49	0									
50–64	0									
65+	0									
TOTAL SINGLE DX	0									
TOTAL MULTIPLE DX	0									
TOTAL										
0–19 Years	0									
20–34	0									
35–49	0									
50–64	0									
65+	0									
GRAND TOTAL	0									

91.6: MICRO EXAM-INTEGUMENT

Type of Patients	Observed Patients	Avg. Stay	Variance	Percentiles						
				10th	25th	50th	75th	90th	95th	99th
1. SINGLE DX										
0–19 Years	0									
20–34	0									
35–49	0									
50–64	0									
65+	0									
2. MULTIPLE DX										
0–19 Years	5	2.8	<1	2	2	3	3	4	4	4
20–34	0									
35–49	1	3.0	0	3	3	3	3	3	3	3
50–64	3	6.7	40	3	3	3	14	14	14	14
65+	13	4.9	6	2	3	4	7	8	9	9
TOTAL SINGLE DX	0									
TOTAL MULTIPLE DX	22	4.6	9	2	3	3	6	8	9	14
TOTAL										
0–19 Years	5	2.8	<1	2	2	3	3	4	4	4
20–34	0									
35–49	1	3.0	0	3	3	3	3	3	3	3
50–64	3	6.7	40	3	3	3	14	14	14	14
65+	13	4.9	6	2	3	4	7	8	9	9
GRAND TOTAL	22	4.6	9	2	3	3	6	8	9	14

91.7: MICRO EXAM-OP WOUND

Type of Patients	Observed Patients	Avg. Stay	Variance	Percentiles						
				10th	25th	50th	75th	90th	95th	99th
1. SINGLE DX										
0–19 Years	0									
20–34	0									
35–49	0									
50–64	0									
65+	0									
2. MULTIPLE DX										
0–19 Years	0									
20–34	0									
35–49	0									
50–64	1	6.0	0	6	6	6	6	6	6	6
65+	0									
TOTAL SINGLE DX	0									
TOTAL MULTIPLE DX	1	6.0	0	6	6	6	6	6	6	6
TOTAL										
0–19 Years	0									
20–34	0									
35–49	0									
50–64	1	6.0	0	6	6	6	6	6	6	6
65+	0									
GRAND TOTAL	1	6.0	0	6	6	6	6	6	6	6

LOS by Diagnosis and Operation, Western Region, 45th Edition

Western Region, October 2007–September 2008 Data, by Operation

91.8: MICRO EXAM NEC

Type of Patients	Observed Patients	Avg. Stay	Vari-ance	10th	25th	50th	75th	90th	95th	99th
1. SINGLE DX										
0–19 Years	1	4.0	0	4	4	4	4	4	4	4
20–34	0									
35–49	0									
50–64	0									
65+	0									
2. MULTIPLE DX										
0–19 Years	0									
20–34	0									
35–49	0									
50–64	1	3.0	0	3	3	3	3	3	3	3
65+	1	5.0	0	5	5	5	5	5	5	5
TOTAL SINGLE DX	1	4.0	0	4	4	4	4	4	4	4
TOTAL MULTIPLE DX	2	4.0	2	3	3	5	5	5	5	5
TOTAL										
0–19 Years	1	4.0	0	4	4	4	4	4	4	4
20–34	0									
35–49	0									
50–64	1	3.0	0	3	3	3	3	3	3	3
65+	1	5.0	0	5	5	5	5	5	5	5
GRAND TOTAL	3	4.0	1	3	3	4	5	5	5	5

92.0: ISOTOPE SCAN & FUNCTION

Type of Patients	Observed Patients	Avg. Stay	Vari-ance	10th	25th	50th	75th	90th	95th	99th
1. SINGLE DX										
0–19 Years	9	1.4	<1	1	1	1	2	2	2	2
20–34	15	1.8	<1	1	1	2	2	3	3	3
35–49	18	2.2	2	1	1	2	3	4	7	7
50–64	14	1.8	<1	1	1	2	3	3	4	4
65+	3	2.7	<1	2	2	3	3	3	3	3
2. MULTIPLE DX										
0–19 Years	43	6.2	38	1	2	3	9	16	17	33
20–34	155	3.1	4	1	2	3	4	6	8	10
35–49	648	2.8	6	1	1	2	3	5	8	14
50–64	1,465	2.7	8	1	1	2	3	5	7	13
65+	2,155	3.2	8	2	2	2	4	6	8	14
TOTAL SINGLE DX	59	1.9	1	1	1	2	2	3	4	7
TOTAL MULTIPLE DX	4,466	3.0	8	1	1	2	4	6	8	14
TOTAL										
0–19 Years	52	5.6	36	1	2	3	7	16	17	33
20–34	170	3.0	4	1	2	3	4	5	7	10
35–49	666	2.8	6	1	1	2	3	5	7	14
50–64	1,479	2.7	8	1	1	2	3	5	7	13
65+	2,158	3.2	8	2	2	2	4	6	8	14
GRAND TOTAL	4,525	3.0	8	1	1	2	4	6	8	14

91.9: MICRO EXAM NOS

Type of Patients	Observed Patients	Avg. Stay	Vari-ance	10th	25th	50th	75th	90th	95th	99th
1. SINGLE DX										
0–19 Years	0									
20–34	0									
35–49	0									
50–64	0									
65+	0									
2. MULTIPLE DX										
0–19 Years	0									
20–34	1	29.0	0	29	29	29	29	29	29	29
35–49	0									
50–64	0									
65+	0									
TOTAL SINGLE DX	0									
TOTAL MULTIPLE DX	1	29.0	0	29	29	29	29	29	29	29
TOTAL										
0–19 Years	0									
20–34	1	29.0	0	29	29	29	29	29	29	29
35–49	0									
50–64	0									
65+	0									
GRAND TOTAL	1	29.0	0	29	29	29	29	29	29	29

92.02: LIVER SCAN/ISOTOPE FUNCT

Type of Patients	Observed Patients	Avg. Stay	Vari-ance	10th	25th	50th	75th	90th	95th	99th
1. SINGLE DX										
0–19 Years	4	1.3	<1	1	1	1	2	2	2	2
20–34	10	1.8	<1	1	1	2	2	3	3	3
35–49	6	3.0	4	1	2	3	3	7	7	7
50–64	4	2.5	2	1	2	3	3	4	4	4
65+	2	2.5	<1	2	2	3	3	3	3	3
2. MULTIPLE DX										
0–19 Years	9	3.4	26	1	1	2	3	6	19	19
20–34	81	3.0	3	1	2	3	4	5	6	9
35–49	104	3.8	7	1	2	3	5	7	9	14
50–64	115	3.9	6	2	2	3	5	6	9	13
65+	246	4.6	11	2	2	4	6	9	11	15
TOTAL SINGLE DX	26	2.2	2	1	1	2	3	3	4	7
TOTAL MULTIPLE DX	555	4.1	8	1	2	3	5	8	10	15
TOTAL										
0–19 Years	13	2.9	20	1	1	1	3	6	19	19
20–34	91	2.9	3	1	2	3	4	5	6	9
35–49	110	3.7	7	1	2	3	5	7	9	14
50–64	119	3.9	6	1	2	3	5	6	9	13
65+	248	4.6	11	2	2	4	6	9	11	15
GRAND TOTAL	581	4.0	8	1	2	3	5	8	10	15

LOS by Diagnosis and Operation, Western Region, 45th Edition

Western Region, October 2007–September 2008 Data, by Operation

92.03: RENAL SCAN/ISOTOPE STUDY

Type of Patients	Observed Patients	Avg. Stay	Vari-ance	Percentiles						
				10th	25th	50th	75th	90th	95th	99th
1. SINGLE DX										
0–19 Years	0									
20–34	0									
35–49	0									
50–64	0									
65+	0									
2. MULTIPLE DX										
0–19 Years	13	5.7	19	1	3	3	7	16	16	16
20–34	3	5.7	4	4	4	5	8	8	8	8
35–49	12	6.7	28	2	3	4	10	13	19	19
50–64	21	6.5	40	2	3	5	7	11	16	30
65+	33	5.4	15	2	3	4	6	10	15	17
TOTAL SINGLE DX	0									
TOTAL MULTIPLE DX	82	5.9	23	2	3	4	7	13	16	30
TOTAL										
0–19 Years	13	5.7	19	1	3	3	7	16	16	16
20–34	3	5.7	4	4	4	5	8	8	8	8
35–49	12	6.7	28	2	3	4	10	13	19	19
50–64	21	6.5	40	2	3	5	7	11	16	30
65+	33	5.4	15	2	3	4	6	10	15	17
GRAND TOTAL	82	5.9	23	2	3	4	7	13	16	30

92.04: GI SCAN & ISOTOPE STUDY

Type of Patients	Observed Patients	Avg. Stay	Vari-ance	Percentiles						
				10th	25th	50th	75th	90th	95th	99th
1. SINGLE DX										
0–19 Years	4	1.5	<1	1	1	1	2	2	2	2
20–34	3	1.7	1	1	1	1	3	3	3	3
35–49	2	2.5	4	1	1	3	4	4	4	4
50–64	0									
65+	0									
2. MULTIPLE DX										
0–19 Years	19	7.8	58	2	3	5	12	17	17	33
20–34	20	3.9	8	1	2	3	5	9	10	10
35–49	33	5.3	10	2	3	5	7	9	12	15
50–64	50	4.3	7	1	3	4	5	9	11	13
65+	58	4.1	5	2	2	4	5	7	8	11
TOTAL SINGLE DX	9	1.8	1	1	1	1	2	4	4	4
TOTAL MULTIPLE DX	180	4.8	14	2	2	4	6	9	12	17
TOTAL										
0–19 Years	23	6.9	54	1	2	3	9	17	17	33
20–34	23	3.6	7	1	1	3	5	9	9	10
35–49	35	5.1	10	2	3	4	7	9	12	15
50–64	50	4.3	7	1	3	4	5	9	11	13
65+	58	4.1	5	2	2	4	5	7	8	11
GRAND TOTAL	189	4.6	14	2	2	4	5	9	11	17

92.05: CV SCAN/ISOTOPE STUDY

Type of Patients	Observed Patients	Avg. Stay	Vari-ance	Percentiles						
				10th	25th	50th	75th	90th	95th	99th
1. SINGLE DX										
0–19 Years	1	2.0	0	2	2	2	2	2	2	2
20–34	1	2.0	0	2	2	2	2	2	2	2
35–49	7	1.6	<1	1	1	1	3	3	3	3
50–64	8	1.4	<1	1	1	1	3	3	3	3
65+	1	3.0	0	3	3	3	3	3	3	3
2. MULTIPLE DX										
0–19 Years	1	3.0	0	3	3	3	3	3	3	3
20–34	41	2.8	6	1	1	2	3	6	8	10
35–49	487	2.3	4	1	1	2	3	4	6	11
50–64	1,260	2.4	6	1	1	2	3	5	6	10
65+	1,799	2.9	6	1	1	2	3	6	8	12
TOTAL SINGLE DX	18	1.6	<1	1	1	1	2	3	3	3
TOTAL MULTIPLE DX	3,588	2.6	6	1	1	2	3	5	7	11
TOTAL										
0–19 Years	2	2.5	<1	2	2	3	3	3	3	3
20–34	42	2.7	6	1	1	2	3	6	8	10
35–49	494	2.3	4	1	1	2	3	4	6	11
50–64	1,268	2.4	6	1	1	2	3	5	6	10
65+	1,800	2.9	6	1	1	2	3	6	8	12
GRAND TOTAL	3,606	2.6	6	1	1	2	3	5	7	11

92.1: OTHER RADIOISOTOPE SCAN

Type of Patients	Observed Patients	Avg. Stay	Vari-ance	Percentiles						
				10th	25th	50th	75th	90th	95th	99th
1. SINGLE DX										
0–19 Years	9	3.2	2	1	2	3	5	5	5	5
20–34	6	4.3	2	3	3	3	6	6	6	6
35–49	3	6.3	55	2	2	2	15	15	15	15
50–64	3	3.7	8	2	2	2	7	7	7	7
65+	1	1.0	0	1	1	1	1	1	1	1
2. MULTIPLE DX										
0–19 Years	95	4.6	24	1	2	3	6	9	11	17
20–34	111	4.3	19	1	2	3	5	9	10	22
35–49	223	4.3	20	1	2	3	5	8	10	28
50–64	463	4.6	26	1	2	3	6	9	11	19
65+	1,243	4.8	13	2	2	4	6	9	11	18
TOTAL SINGLE DX	22	3.6	6	1	2	3	5	6	7	15
TOTAL MULTIPLE DX	2,135	4.7	17	1	2	4	6	9	11	19
TOTAL										
0–19 Years	104	4.4	21	1	2	3	5	9	11	17
20–34	117	4.3	18	1	2	3	6	9	10	22
35–49	226	4.3	21	1	2	3	5	8	11	28
50–64	466	4.6	26	1	2	3	6	9	11	19
65+	1,244	4.8	13	2	2	4	6	9	11	18
GRAND TOTAL	2,157	4.7	17	1	2	4	6	9	11	19

LOS by Diagnosis and Operation, Western Region, 45th Edition

Western Region, October 2007–September 2008 Data, by Operation

92.14: BONE SCAN

Type of Patients	Observed Patients	Avg. Stay	Vari-ance	Percentiles						
				10th	25th	50th	75th	90th	95th	99th
1. SINGLE DX										
0–19 Years	6	2.7	3	1	1	3	5	5	5	5
20–34	4	5.0	2	3	3	5	6	6	6	6
35–49	1	15.0	0	15	15	15	15	15	15	15
50–64	0									
65+	0									
2. MULTIPLE DX										
0–19 Years	48	5.3	37	1	2	4	8	10	11	49
20–34	19	5.2	12	1	2	5	8	10	14	14
35–49	53	6.0	35	2	3	5	6	11	17	39
50–64	102	6.1	17	2	3	5	7	11	14	20
65+	266	5.6	14	2	3	5	7	10	13	19
TOTAL SINGLE DX	11	3.8	10	1	1	3	5	6	6	15
TOTAL MULTIPLE DX	488	5.7	20	2	3	5	7	10	13	20
TOTAL										
0–19 Years	54	4.9	32	1	2	4	6	9	11	49
20–34	23	5.1	10	1	3	5	6	9	10	14
35–49	54	6.2	35	2	3	5	6	12	17	39
50–64	102	6.1	17	2	3	5	7	11	14	20
65+	266	5.6	14	2	3	5	7	10	13	19
GRAND TOTAL	499	5.6	20	2	3	5	7	10	13	20

92.18: TOTAL BODY SCAN

Type of Patients	Observed Patients	Avg. Stay	Vari-ance	Percentiles						
				10th	25th	50th	75th	90th	95th	99th
1. SINGLE DX										
0–19 Years	1	5.0	0	5	5	5	5	5	5	5
20–34	0									
35–49	1	2.0	0	2	2	2	2	2	2	2
50–64	0									
65+	0									
2. MULTIPLE DX										
0–19 Years	14	5.9	21	1	2	7	7	16	17	17
20–34	5	5.8	10	2	3	7	8	9	9	9
35–49	9	6.6	66	2	3	4	5	28	28	28
50–64	27	5.4	11	1	4	5	7	9	9	18
65+	68	5.7	14	2	3	5	7	10	14	22
TOTAL SINGLE DX	2	4.4	2	2	5	5	5	5	5	5
TOTAL MULTIPLE DX	123	5.7	17	2	3	5	7	9	15	22
TOTAL										
0–19 Years	15	5.7	17	2	3	5	7	9	16	17
20–34	5	5.8	10	2	3	7	8	9	9	9
35–49	10	6.1	61	2	3	4	5	28	28	28
50–64	27	5.4	11	1	4	5	7	9	9	18
65+	68	5.7	14	2	3	5	7	10	14	22
GRAND TOTAL	125	5.7	17	2	3	5	7	9	15	22

92.15: PULMONARY SCAN

Type of Patients	Observed Patients	Avg. Stay	Vari-ance	Percentiles						
				10th	25th	50th	75th	90th	95th	99th
1. SINGLE DX										
0–19 Years	0									
20–34	0									
35–49	1	2.0	0	2	2	2	2	2	2	2
50–64	1	2.0	0	2	2	2	2	2	2	2
65+	1	1.0	0	1	1	1	1	1	1	1
2. MULTIPLE DX										
0–19 Years	6	3.6	2	1	3	4	4	5	5	5
20–34	80	3.9	19	1	1	2	5	7	10	29
35–49	154	3.5	12	1	2	3	4	7	9	15
50–64	311	4.1	30	1	2	3	5	7	9	16
65+	877	4.5	12	1	2	4	6	8	11	18
TOTAL SINGLE DX	3	1.7	<1	1	1	2	2	2	2	2
TOTAL MULTIPLE DX	1,428	4.2	16	1	2	3	5	8	10	18
TOTAL										
0–19 Years	6	3.6	2	1	3	4	4	5	5	5
20–34	80	3.9	19	1	1	2	5	7	10	29
35–49	155	3.5	12	1	2	3	4	7	9	15
50–64	312	4.1	30	1	2	3	5	7	9	16
65+	878	4.5	12	1	2	4	6	8	11	18
GRAND TOTAL	1,431	4.2	16	1	2	3	5	8	10	18

92.19: SCAN OF SITE NEC

Type of Patients	Observed Patients	Avg. Stay	Vari-ance	Percentiles						
				10th	25th	50th	75th	90th	95th	99th
1. SINGLE DX										
0–19 Years	0									
20–34	1	3.0	0	3	3	3	3	3	3	3
35–49	0									
50–64	0									
65+	0									
2. MULTIPLE DX										
0–19 Years	14	3.4	2	2	3	3	4	6	6	6
20–34	0									
35–49	3	7.3	20	3	3	7	12	12	12	12
50–64	8	6.5	15	1	4	4	9	13	13	13
65+	7	3.9	3	2	2	4	6	6	6	6
TOTAL SINGLE DX	1	3.0	0	3	3	3	3	3	3	3
TOTAL MULTIPLE DX	32	4.6	8	2	3	4	6	9	12	13
TOTAL										
0–19 Years	14	3.4	2	2	3	3	4	6	6	6
20–34	1	3.0	0	3	3	3	3	3	3	3
35–49	3	7.3	20	3	3	7	12	12	12	12
50–64	8	6.5	15	1	4	4	9	13	13	13
65+	7	3.9	3	2	2	4	6	6	6	6
GRAND TOTAL	33	4.6	8	2	3	4	6	9	12	13

LOS by Diagnosis and Operation, Western Region, 45th Edition

92.2: THER RADIOLOGY & NU MED

Type of Patients	Observed Patients	Avg. Stay	Vari-ance	Percentiles						
				10th	25th	50th	75th	90th	95th	99th
1. SINGLE DX										
0–19 Years	10	2.1	2	1	1	2	2	5	5	5
20–34	115	1.8	<1	1	1	2	2	3	3	4
35–49	167	1.8	<1	1	1	2	2	3	3	3
50–64	149	1.9	<1	1	1	2	2	3	3	5
65+	89	1.7	<1	1	1	2	2	3	3	7
2. MULTIPLE DX										
0–19 Years	84	8.0	155	1	2	4	7	16	30	62
20–34	304	3.9	40	1	2	2	4	6	10	33
35–49	796	4.5	32	1	2	3	5	10	15	32
50–64	1,536	5.6	34	1	2	3	7	13	17	29
65+	1,872	5.9	31	1	2	4	7	13	16	30
TOTAL SINGLE DX	530	1.8	<1	1	1	2	2	3	3	5
TOTAL MULTIPLE DX	4,592	5.5	38	1	2	3	7	12	16	32
TOTAL										
0–19 Years	94	7.6	148	1	2	4	7	16	29	62
20–34	419	3.4	30	1	2	2	3	6	9	29
35–49	963	4.0	27	1	2	3	4	8	12	32
50–64	1,685	5.2	32	1	2	3	6	13	16	28
65+	1,961	5.7	31	1	2	4	7	12	16	29
GRAND TOTAL	5,122	5.1	35	1	2	3	6	11	16	30

92.24: PHOTON TELERADIOTHERAPY

Type of Patients	Observed Patients	Avg. Stay	Vari-ance	Percentiles						
				10th	25th	50th	75th	90th	95th	99th
1. SINGLE DX										
0–19 Years	0									
20–34	0									
35–49	0									
50–64	0									
65+	0									
2. MULTIPLE DX										
0–19 Years	13	6.6	22	1	4	4	11	12	16	16
20–34	11	4.3	8	2	2	3	8	8	10	10
35–49	54	7.4	62	2	3	5	8	16	25	43
50–64	174	8.6	54	2	3	6	13	20	26	33
65+	279	7.3	31	2	4	6	10	14	17	30
TOTAL SINGLE DX	0									
TOTAL MULTIPLE DX	531	7.6	41	2	4	5	10	16	21	33
TOTAL										
0–19 Years	13	6.6	22	1	4	4	11	12	16	16
20–34	11	4.3	8	2	2	3	8	8	10	10
35–49	54	7.4	62	2	3	5	8	16	25	43
50–64	174	8.6	54	2	3	6	13	20	26	33
65+	279	7.3	31	2	4	6	10	14	17	30
GRAND TOTAL	531	7.6	41	2	4	5	10	16	21	33

92.27: RADIOACTIVE ELEMENT IMPL

Type of Patients	Observed Patients	Avg. Stay	Vari-ance	Percentiles						
				10th	25th	50th	75th	90th	95th	99th
1. SINGLE DX										
0–19 Years	0									
20–34	14	1.6	1	1	1	1	2	3	5	5
35–49	48	1.8	<1	1	1	2	2	3	3	3
50–64	56	1.8	<1	1	1	2	2	3	4	5
65+	51	1.4	<1	1	1	1	2	2	3	3
2. MULTIPLE DX										
0–19 Years	0									
20–34	18	5.3	167	1	2	2	3	5	57	57
35–49	100	2.7	8	1	2	2	3	4	7	10
50–64	210	2.6	16	1	1	2	3	4	7	14
65+	308	2.7	17	1	1	2	2	5	8	24
TOTAL SINGLE DX	169	1.7	<1	1	1	1	2	3	3	5
TOTAL MULTIPLE DX	636	2.8	19	1	1	2	3	4	8	25
TOTAL										
0–19 Years	0									
20–34	32	3.7	96	1	1	2	2	4	5	57
35–49	148	2.4	6	1	1	2	3	4	6	10
50–64	266	2.5	13	1	1	2	2	4	6	14
65+	359	2.5	15	1	1	2	2	4	7	24
GRAND TOTAL	805	2.5	16	1	1	2	2	4	6	24

92.28: ISOTOPE INJECT/INSTILL

Type of Patients	Observed Patients	Avg. Stay	Vari-ance	Percentiles						
				10th	25th	50th	75th	90th	95th	99th
1. SINGLE DX										
0–19 Years	1	1.0	0	1	1	1	1	1	1	1
20–34	30	1.9	<1	1	2	2	2	2	3	4
35–49	34	1.9	<1	1	2	2	2	3	3	3
50–64	19	1.8	<1	1	2	2	2	3	3	3
65+	7	1.9	<1	1	2	2	2	2	2	2
2. MULTIPLE DX										
0–19 Years	13	14.1	554	1	1	2	7	62	62	62
20–34	41	2.4	3	1	2	2	2	3	5	9
35–49	70	2.5	4	1	1	2	3	4	6	15
50–64	78	2.8	8	1	1	2	3	5	10	18
65+	74	3.3	31	2	2	2	3	5	9	43
TOTAL SINGLE DX	91	1.9	<1	1	2	2	2	3	3	4
TOTAL MULTIPLE DX	276	3.7	63	1	2	2	3	5	9	62
TOTAL										
0–19 Years	14	13.5	537	1	1	2	7	62	62	62
20–34	71	2.2	2	1	2	2	2	3	4	9
35–49	104	2.3	3	1	1	2	2	3	4	9
50–64	97	2.6	7	1	1	2	3	4	9	18
65+	81	3.2	28	1	2	2	3	4	8	43
GRAND TOTAL	367	3.3	48	1	2	2	3	4	8	62

LOS by Diagnosis and Operation, Western Region, 45th Edition

Western Region, October 2007–September 2008 Data, by Operation

92.29: RADIOTHERAPEUTIC PX NEC

Type of Patients	Observed Patients	Avg. Stay	Vari-ance	Percentiles						
				10th	25th	50th	75th	90th	95th	99th
1. SINGLE DX										
0–19 Years	9	2.2	2	1	1	2	2	5	5	5
20–34	70	1.8	<1	1	1	2	2	3	3	3
35–49	85	1.8	<1	1	1	2	2	3	3	3
50–64	73	2.0	<1	1	2	2	2	3	3	5
65+	31	2.0	1	1	1	2	2	3	3	7
2. MULTIPLE DX										
0–19 Years	47	5.9	65	1	2	3	5	12	29	43
20–34	225	4.1	38	1	2	2	4	6	13	33
35–49	545	4.8	35	1	2	3	5	10	15	35
50–64	1,006	5.8	32	2	2	4	7	13	17	28
65+	1,149	6.4	31	2	3	5	8	13	17	30
TOTAL SINGLE DX	268	1.9	<1	1	1	2	2	3	3	5
TOTAL MULTIPLE DX	2,972	5.7	34	2	2	4	7	13	17	31
TOTAL										
0–19 Years	56	5.5	59	1	2	2	5	12	29	43
20–34	295	3.5	30	1	2	2	3	6	9	33
35–49	630	4.4	32	1	2	3	5	10	14	32
50–64	1,079	5.5	31	1	2	3	7	13	16	28
65+	1,180	6.3	30	2	3	5	8	13	17	30
GRAND TOTAL	3,240	5.4	32	1	2	3	6	12	16	30

92.32: MULTI-SOURCE PHOTON SURG

Type of Patients	Observed Patients	Avg. Stay	Vari-ance	Percentiles						
				10th	25th	50th	75th	90th	95th	99th
1. SINGLE DX										
0–19 Years	0									
20–34	0									
35–49	0									
50–64	2	1.0	0	1	1	1	1	1	1	1
65+	1	1.0	0	1	1	1	1	1	1	1
2. MULTIPLE DX										
0–19 Years	0									
20–34	3	2.3	5	1	1	1	5	5	5	5
35–49	14	1.4	1	1	1	1	1	4	4	4
50–64	41	2.2	7	1	1	1	1	6	10	10
65+	86	1.5	5	1	1	1	1	1	3	18
TOTAL SINGLE DX	3	1.0	0	1	1	1	1	1	1	1
TOTAL MULTIPLE DX	144	1.7	5	1	1	1	1	3	6	10
TOTAL										
0–19 Years	0									
20–34	3	2.3	5	1	1	1	5	5	5	5
35–49	14	1.4	1	1	1	1	1	4	4	4
50–64	43	2.1	7	1	1	1	1	6	10	10
65+	87	1.5	5	1	1	1	1	1	3	18
GRAND TOTAL	147	1.7	5	1	1	1	1	3	6	10

92.3: STEREOTACTIC RADIOSURG

Type of Patients	Observed Patients	Avg. Stay	Vari-ance	Percentiles						
				10th	25th	50th	75th	90th	95th	99th
1. SINGLE DX										
0–19 Years	1	2.0	0	2	2	2	2	2	2	2
20–34	1	2.0	0	2	2	2	2	2	2	2
35–49	0									
50–64	4	1.0	0	1	1	1	1	1	1	1
65+	2	1.0	0	1	1	1	1	1	1	1
2. MULTIPLE DX										
0–19 Years	4	4.4	7	3	3	3	8	8	8	8
20–34	4	26.3	>999	1	1	1	5	99	99	99
35–49	24	4.0	33	1	1	1	5	10	14	26
50–64	60	3.2	9	1	1	1	5	9	10	10
65+	102	2.0	9	1	1	1	1	4	9	17
TOTAL SINGLE DX	8	1.5	<1	1	1	1	2	2	2	2
TOTAL MULTIPLE DX	194	3.2	57	1	1	1	3	8	10	18
TOTAL										
0–19 Years	5	3.8	6	2	2	3	3	8	8	8
20–34	5	21.5	>999	1	1	1	5	99	99	99
35–49	24	4.0	33	1	1	1	4	10	14	26
50–64	64	3.1	9	1	1	1	4	9	10	10
65+	104	2.0	9	1	1	1	1	4	9	17
GRAND TOTAL	202	3.1	54	1	1	1	3	8	10	18

92.4: INTRA-OP RADIATION PX

Type of Patients	Observed Patients	Avg. Stay	Vari-ance	Percentiles						
				10th	25th	50th	75th	90th	95th	99th
1. SINGLE DX										
0–19 Years	0									
20–34	0									
35–49	0									
50–64	0									
65+	0									
2. MULTIPLE DX										
0–19 Years	0									
20–34	0									
35–49	1	14.0	0	14	14	14	14	14	14	14
50–64	0									
65+	0									
TOTAL SINGLE DX	0									
TOTAL MULTIPLE DX	1	14.0	0	14	14	14	14	14	14	14
TOTAL										
0–19 Years	0									
20–34	0									
35–49	1	14.0	0	14	14	14	14	14	14	14
50–64	0									
65+	0									
GRAND TOTAL	1	14.0	0	14	14	14	14	14	14	14

LOS by Diagnosis and Operation, Western Region, 45th Edition

Western Region, October 2007–September 2008 Data, by Operation

93.0: DXTIC PHYSICAL TX

Type of Patients	Observed Patients	Avg. Stay	Vari-ance	Percentiles						
				10th	25th	50th	75th	90th	95th	99th
1. SINGLE DX										
0–19 Years	5	2.0	1	1	1	2	3	3	3	3
20–34	6	2.2	4	1	1	3	3	6	6	6
35–49	2	2.5	5	1	1	3	4	4	4	4
50–64	2	3.0	8	1	1	3	5	5	5	5
65+	1	1.0	0	1	1	1	1	1	1	1
2. MULTIPLE DX										
0–19 Years	44	10.8	103	2	2	7	15	27	31	37
20–34	28	7.7	70	2	2	4	9	21	27	29
35–49	74	8.0	114	1	3	5	8	16	25	81
50–64	165	10.5	211	2	3	5	12	22	37	76
65+	441	7.3	46	2	3	5	9	17	22	32
TOTAL SINGLE DX	16	2.1	2	1	1	1	3	4	5	6
TOTAL MULTIPLE DX	752	8.4	96	2	3	5	10	21	26	45
TOTAL										
0–19 Years	49	9.9	100	1	2	6	14	27	31	37
20–34	34	6.7	63	1	2	3	7	21	27	29
35–49	76	7.8	111	1	3	5	8	16	25	81
50–64	167	10.4	209	2	3	5	12	22	37	76
65+	442	7.2	46	2	3	4	9	17	22	32
GRAND TOTAL	768	8.3	94	2	3	5	10	20	26	45

93.08: ELECTROMYOGRAPHY

Type of Patients	Observed Patients	Avg. Stay	Vari-ance	Percentiles						
				10th	25th	50th	75th	90th	95th	99th
1. SINGLE DX										
0–19 Years	0									
20–34	2	6.0	0	6	6	6	6	6	6	6
35–49	2	2.5	5	1	1	3	4	4	4	4
50–64	0									
65+	0									
2. MULTIPLE DX										
0–19 Years	6	2.9	2	1	1	3	4	5	5	5
20–34	5	3.2	5	1	2	3	3	7	7	7
35–49	6	7.0	31	1	3	5	11	16	16	16
50–64	13	9.2	44	2	6	7	11	19	25	25
65+	21	8.9	60	4	5	6	8	21	24	31
TOTAL SINGLE DX	3	3.7	6	1	1	4	6	6	6	6
TOTAL MULTIPLE DX	51	7.4	44	2	3	6	9	16	24	31
TOTAL										
0–19 Years	6	2.9	2	1	1	3	4	5	5	5
20–34	6	3.7	5	1	2	3	6	7	7	7
35–49	8	5.9	27	1	1	4	6	16	16	16
50–64	13	9.2	44	2	6	7	11	19	25	25
65+	21	8.9	60	4	5	6	8	21	24	31
GRAND TOTAL	54	7.2	42	1	3	5	8	16	24	31

93.01: FUNCTIONAL PT EVALUATION

Type of Patients	Observed Patients	Avg. Stay	Vari-ance	Percentiles						
				10th	25th	50th	75th	90th	95th	99th
1. SINGLE DX										
0–19 Years	5	2.0	1	1	1	2	3	3	3	3
20–34	3	1.0	0	1	1	1	1	1	1	1
35–49	0									
50–64	1	5.0	0	5	5	5	5	5	5	5
65+	1	1.0	0	1	1	1	1	1	1	1
2. MULTIPLE DX										
0–19 Years	33	11.9	106	2	3	8	21	27	31	37
20–34	21	9.3	83	1	3	5	15	21	27	29
35–49	63	8.3	130	2	3	5	8	16	25	81
50–64	140	11.4	237	2	3	6	14	24	48	76
65+	414	7.2	46	2	3	4	9	16	22	32
TOTAL SINGLE DX	10	1.9	2	1	1	1	3	3	5	5
TOTAL MULTIPLE DX	671	8.7	101	2	3	5	11	21	27	48
TOTAL										
0–19 Years	38	10.8	104	1	2	7	15	27	31	37
20–34	24	8.2	80	1	3	5	15	21	27	29
35–49	63	8.3	130	1	3	5	9	17	25	81
50–64	141	11.3	236	2	3	6	14	24	48	76
65+	415	7.2	46	2	3	4	9	16	22	32
GRAND TOTAL	681	8.6	100	2	3	5	11	21	27	48

93.1: PT EXERCISES

Type of Patients	Observed Patients	Avg. Stay	Vari-ance	Percentiles						
				10th	25th	50th	75th	90th	95th	99th
1. SINGLE DX										
0–19 Years	3	2.7	<1	1	3	3	3	3	3	3
20–34	2	3.0	0	3	3	3	3	3	3	3
35–49	2	1.0	0	1	1	1	1	1	1	1
50–64	1	3.0	0	3	3	3	3	3	3	3
65+	1	2.0	0	2	2	2	2	2	2	2
2. MULTIPLE DX										
0–19 Years	7	3.1	16	1	1	2	2	8	15	15
20–34	8	7.1	139	2	3	3	4	36	36	36
35–49	37	3.0	40	1	1	2	3	4	4	40
50–64	90	2.5	20	1	1	2	3	4	6	42
65+	73	3.1	8	1	1	2	3	8	11	14
TOTAL SINGLE DX	9	2.4	<1	1	2	3	3	3	3	3
TOTAL MULTIPLE DX	215	3.0	23	1	1	2	3	4	8	36
TOTAL										
0–19 Years	10	3.0	11	1	1	2	3	8	15	15
20–34	10	6.2	111	2	3	3	3	36	36	36
35–49	39	2.9	38	1	1	2	3	4	4	40
50–64	91	2.5	20	1	1	2	3	4	6	42
65+	74	3.1	8	1	1	2	3	8	11	14
GRAND TOTAL	224	3.0	22	1	1	2	3	4	8	36

LOS by Diagnosis and Operation, Western Region, 45th Edition

Western Region, October 2007–September 2008 Data, by Operation

93.16: JOINT MOBILIZATION NEC

Type of Patients	Observed Patients	Avg. Stay	Vari-ance	Percentiles						
				10th	25th	50th	75th	90th	95th	99th
1. SINGLE DX										
0–19 Years	3	2.7	<1	1	3	3	3	3	3	3
20–34	1	3.0	0	3	3	3	3	3	3	3
35–49	2	1.0	0	1	1	1	1	1	1	1
50–64	1	3.0	0	3	3	3	3	3	3	3
65+	1	2.0	0	2	2	2	2	2	2	2
2. MULTIPLE DX										
0–19 Years	6	3.2	17	1	1	2	2	8	15	15
20–34	7	7.5	160	2	2	3	3	36	36	36
35–49	35	3.0	42	1	1	2	3	3	4	40
50–64	88	2.0	2	1	1	2	3	4	4	8
65+	64	2.3	2	1	1	2	3	3	4	9
TOTAL SINGLE DX	8	2.4	<1	1	1	3	3	3	3	3
TOTAL MULTIPLE DX	200	2.5	15	1	1	2	3	3	5	15
TOTAL										
0–19 Years	9	3.1	11	1	1	2	3	8	15	15
20–34	8	6.9	140	2	3	3	3	36	36	36
35–49	37	2.9	40	1	1	2	3	3	4	40
50–64	89	2.0	2	1	1	2	3	4	4	8
65+	65	2.3	2	1	1	2	3	3	4	9
GRAND TOTAL	208	2.5	14	1	1	2	3	3	5	15

93.22: AMB & GAIT TRAINING

Type of Patients	Observed Patients	Avg. Stay	Vari-ance	Percentiles						
				10th	25th	50th	75th	90th	95th	99th
1. SINGLE DX										
0–19 Years	0									
20–34	0									
35–49	0									
50–64	0									
65+	0									
2. MULTIPLE DX										
0–19 Years	3	11.1	86	2	2	8	23	23	23	23
20–34	0									
35–49	1	9.0	0	9	9	9	9	9	9	9
50–64	6	3.8	2	2	3	4	4	6	6	6
65+	21	6.4	12	3	4	5	9	12	13	13
TOTAL SINGLE DX	0									
TOTAL MULTIPLE DX	31	7.5	38	2	3	5	9	23	23	23
TOTAL										
0–19 Years	3	11.1	86	2	2	8	23	23	23	23
20–34	0									
35–49	1	9.0	0	9	9	9	9	9	9	9
50–64	6	3.8	2	2	3	4	4	6	6	6
65+	21	6.4	12	3	4	5	9	12	13	13
GRAND TOTAL	31	7.5	38	2	3	5	9	23	23	23

93.2: OTH PT MS MANIPULATION

Type of Patients	Observed Patients	Avg. Stay	Vari-ance	Percentiles						
				10th	25th	50th	75th	90th	95th	99th
1. SINGLE DX										
0–19 Years	4	2.5	1	2	2	2	4	4	4	4
20–34	7	2.4	5	1	1	1	3	7	7	7
35–49	1	3.0	0	3	3	3	3	3	3	3
50–64	4	2.0	2	1	1	1	2	4	4	4
65+	2	2.0	2	1	1	3	3	3	3	3
2. MULTIPLE DX										
0–19 Years	38	5.3	33	2	2	3	7	9	23	23
20–34	17	3.5	24	1	1	2	3	9	21	21
35–49	47	3.3	41	1	1	2	3	4	7	45
50–64	120	2.5	9	1	1	2	3	5	6	14
65+	133	3.0	7	1	1	2	4	6	9	13
TOTAL SINGLE DX	18	2.3	2	1	1	2	3	4	7	7
TOTAL MULTIPLE DX	355	3.2	17	1	1	2	3	7	9	23
TOTAL										
0–19 Years	42	5.1	32	2	2	3	4	9	23	23
20–34	24	3.2	18	1	1	2	3	7	9	21
35–49	48	3.3	40	1	1	2	3	4	7	45
50–64	124	2.5	9	1	1	2	3	4	6	14
65+	135	3.0	7	1	1	2	4	6	9	13
GRAND TOTAL	373	3.2	16	1	1	2	3	6	9	23

93.26: MANUAL RUPT JOINT ADHES

Type of Patients	Observed Patients	Avg. Stay	Vari-ance	Percentiles						
				10th	25th	50th	75th	90th	95th	99th
1. SINGLE DX										
0–19 Years	2	2.0	0	2	2	2	2	2	2	2
20–34	6	2.4	6	1	1	1	3	7	7	7
35–49	1	3.0	0	3	3	3	3	3	3	3
50–64	2	1.0	0	1	1	1	1	1	1	1
65+	2	2.0	2	1	1	2	3	3	3	3
2. MULTIPLE DX										
0–19 Years	1	3.0	0	3	3	3	3	3	3	3
20–34	7	2.6	<1	1	2	3	3	4	4	4
35–49	28	2.1	1	1	1	2	3	4	5	5
50–64	85	1.9	2	1	1	1	2	3	5	7
65+	77	1.8	1	1	1	1	2	3	4	6
TOTAL SINGLE DX	13	2.1	3	1	1	1	3	3	7	7
TOTAL MULTIPLE DX	198	1.9	1	1	1	2	2	3	4	6
TOTAL										
0–19 Years	3	2.3	<1	2	2	2	3	3	3	3
20–34	13	2.5	3	1	1	2	3	4	7	7
35–49	29	2.1	1	1	1	2	3	4	4	5
50–64	87	1.9	2	1	1	1	2	3	5	7
65+	79	1.8	1	1	1	1	2	3	4	6
GRAND TOTAL	211	1.9	2	1	1	2	3	3	4	6

Western Region, October 2007–September 2008 Data, by Operation

93.3: OTHER PT THERAPEUTIC PX

Type of Patients	Observed Patients	Avg. Stay	Vari-ance	Percentiles						
				10th	25th	50th	75th	90th	95th	99th
1. SINGLE DX										
0–19 Years	15	3.3	4	1	1	3	5	6	6	11
20–34	2	2.0	2	1	1	3	3	3	3	3
35–49	2	2.5	<1	2	2	3	3	3	3	3
50–64	5	2.4	2	1	2	2	2	5	5	5
65+	3	3.3	6	1	1	3	6	6	6	6
2. MULTIPLE DX										
0–19 Years	176	11.3	142	2	4	7	14	27	38	61
20–34	152	12.7	118	2	5	9	18	26	36	51
35–49	320	12.4	115	3	5	9	17	26	33	56
50–64	1,061	13.1	123	3	5	10	17	28	35	65
65+	3,967	9.9	58	3	4	8	14	20	24	32
TOTAL SINGLE DX	27	3.2	4	1	1	3	5	6	6	11
TOTAL MULTIPLE DX	5,676	10.8	82	3	4	8	15	22	27	47
TOTAL										
0–19 Years	191	10.6	135	2	3	6	13	24	36	55
20–34	154	12.6	118	2	5	9	18	26	36	51
35–49	322	12.3	115	3	5	9	17	25	32	56
50–64	1,066	13.0	123	3	5	10	17	28	35	65
65+	3,970	9.9	58	3	4	8	14	20	24	32
GRAND TOTAL	5,703	10.7	82	2	4	8	15	21	27	47

93.38: COMBINED PT NOS

Type of Patients	Observed Patients	Avg. Stay	Vari-ance	Percentiles						
				10th	25th	50th	75th	90th	95th	99th
1. SINGLE DX										
0–19 Years	0									
20–34	0									
35–49	0									
50–64	0									
65+	0									
2. MULTIPLE DX										
0–19 Years	13	11.1	70	1	6	7	20	24	24	29
20–34	7	10.8	116	2	4	8	13	34	34	34
35–49	32	13.3	79	4	5	11	20	22	32	35
50–64	131	12.0	67	4	5	11	16	22	26	42
65+	421	12.2	77	4	6	10	17	22	27	33
TOTAL SINGLE DX	0									
TOTAL MULTIPLE DX	604	12.2	75	4	6	10	17	22	27	36
TOTAL										
0–19 Years	13	11.1	70	1	6	7	20	24	24	29
20–34	7	10.8	116	2	4	8	13	34	34	34
35–49	32	13.3	79	4	5	11	20	22	32	35
50–64	131	12.0	67	4	5	11	16	22	26	42
65+	421	12.2	77	4	6	10	17	22	27	33
GRAND TOTAL	604	12.2	75	4	6	10	17	22	27	36

93.39: PHYSICAL THERAPY NEC

Type of Patients	Observed Patients	Avg. Stay	Vari-ance	Percentiles						
				10th	25th	50th	75th	90th	95th	99th
1. SINGLE DX										
0–19 Years	14	3.2	3	1	1	3	5	6	6	6
20–34	1	1.0	0	1	1	1	1	1	1	1
35–49	2	2.5	<1	2	2	3	3	3	3	3
50–64	4	2.5	3	1	1	2	5	5	5	5
65+	3	3.3	6	1	1	3	6	6	6	6
2. MULTIPLE DX										
0–19 Years	130	11.9	156	2	4	7	15	27	40	63
20–34	127	14.1	122	3	6	12	19	27	36	51
35–49	269	12.8	122	3	5	9	17	27	34	57
50–64	908	13.4	131	3	5	10	17	28	36	66
65+	3,531	9.6	55	2	4	8	14	19	23	32
TOTAL SINGLE DX	24	3.1	3	1	1	3	5	6	6	6
TOTAL MULTIPLE DX	4,965	10.7	84	3	4	8	15	21	27	49
TOTAL										
0–19 Years	144	11.0	147	2	3	6	14	27	38	61
20–34	128	14.0	122	2	6	11	19	27	36	51
35–49	271	12.8	122	3	5	9	17	26	34	57
50–64	912	13.3	131	3	5	10	17	28	36	66
65+	3,534	9.6	55	2	4	8	14	19	23	32
GRAND TOTAL	4,989	10.6	83	2	4	8	14	21	27	49

93.4: SKELETAL & OTH TRACTION

Type of Patients	Observed Patients	Avg. Stay	Vari-ance	Percentiles						
				10th	25th	50th	75th	90th	95th	99th
1. SINGLE DX										
0–19 Years	1	3.0	0	3	3	3	3	3	3	3
20–34	0									
35–49	2	3.0	8	1	1	3	5	5	5	5
50–64	0									
65+	0									
2. MULTIPLE DX										
0–19 Years	8	5.5	14	1	3	5	10	10	10	10
20–34	14	3.1	1	2	2	3	4	5	5	5
35–49	14	8.1	57	2	4	5	12	26	>99	>99
50–64	21	7.7	31	2	4	6	12	18	23	>99
65+	70	7.8	84	1	3	6	8	16	22	54
TOTAL SINGLE DX	3	3.0	4	1	1	3	5	5	5	5
TOTAL MULTIPLE DX	127	7.1	60	2	3	5	9	17	23	>99
TOTAL										
0–19 Years	9	5.3	13	1	3	5	10	10	10	10
20–34	14	3.1	1	2	2	3	4	5	5	5
35–49	16	7.4	53	2	4	5	10	26	>99	>99
50–64	21	7.7	31	2	4	6	12	18	23	>99
65+	70	7.8	84	1	3	6	8	16	22	54
GRAND TOTAL	130	7.0	59	2	3	5	8	16	23	>99

LOS by Diagnosis and Operation, Western Region, 45th Edition

Western Region, October 2007–September 2008 Data, by Operation

93.5: OTH IMMOB/PRESS/WND ATTN

Type of Patients	Observed Patients	Avg. Stay	Variance	10th	25th	50th	75th	90th	95th	99th
1. SINGLE DX										
0–19 Years	210	1.3	1	1	1	1	2	2	3	4
20–34	65	2.3	18	1	1	1	2	4	6	33
35–49	39	2.1	4	1	1	1	2	4	7	10
50–64	19	1.5	<1	1	1	1	2	3	3	3
65+	5	2.0	1	1	1	2	3	3	3	3
2. MULTIPLE DX										
0–19 Years	675	3.1	18	1	1	2	3	7	9	18
20–34	611	3.6	36	1	1	2	4	7	11	20
35–49	695	4.3	27	1	2	3	5	8	12	26
50–64	1,003	4.6	25	1	2	3	6	10	13	28
65+	2,354	4.4	14	1	2	3	5	8	11	22
TOTAL SINGLE DX	338	1.6	4	1	1	1	2	2	3	7
TOTAL MULTIPLE DX	5,338	4.1	21	1	2	3	5	8	11	22
TOTAL										
0–19 Years	885	2.7	14	1	1	2	3	6	8	17
20–34	676	3.5	35	1	1	2	4	7	10	21
35–49	734	4.2	26	1	2	3	5	8	11	25
50–64	1,022	4.6	25	1	2	3	5	9	13	28
65+	2,359	4.4	14	1	2	3	5	8	11	22
GRAND TOTAL	5,676	3.9	20	1	1	3	5	8	11	21

93.52: NECK SUPPORT APPLICATION

Type of Patients	Observed Patients	Avg. Stay	Variance	10th	25th	50th	75th	90th	95th	99th
1. SINGLE DX										
0–19 Years	1	2.0	0	2	2	2	2	2	2	2
20–34	0									
35–49	1	1.0	0	1	1	1	1	1	1	1
50–64	0									
65+	1	2.0	0	2	2	2	2	2	2	2
2. MULTIPLE DX										
0–19 Years	5	3.8	3	1	3	5	5	5	5	5
20–34	16	2.4	5	1	1	2	2	4	10	10
35–49	19	2.4	2	1	2	2	4	4	6	6
50–64	17	3.5	3	1	2	3	5	6	6	6
65+	35	4.7	10	1	2	4	6	11	11	11
TOTAL SINGLE DX	3	1.7	<1	1	1	2	2	2	2	2
TOTAL MULTIPLE DX	92	3.6	7	1	2	3	5	7	10	11
TOTAL										
0–19 Years	6	3.5	3	1	2	5	5	5	5	5
20–34	16	2.4	5	1	1	2	2	4	10	10
35–49	20	2.4	2	1	1	2	4	4	6	6
50–64	17	3.5	3	1	2	3	5	6	6	6
65+	36	4.6	10	1	2	4	6	11	11	11
GRAND TOTAL	95	3.5	7	1	2	3	5	7	10	11

93.53: CAST APPLICATION NEC

Type of Patients	Observed Patients	Avg. Stay	Variance	10th	25th	50th	75th	90th	95th	99th
1. SINGLE DX										
0–19 Years	85	1.3	2	1	1	1	1	2	2	7
20–34	12	2.0	8	1	1	1	1	2	11	11
35–49	9	1.9	2	1	1	1	2	4	4	4
50–64	5	1.8	<1	1	1	2	2	3	3	3
65+	1	1.0	0	1	1	1	1	1	1	1
2. MULTIPLE DX										
0–19 Years	135	3.0	20	1	1	2	3	6	8	20
20–34	51	3.1	13	1	1	2	3	6	16	17
35–49	54	4.3	24	1	2	3	6	8	10	34
50–64	121	4.9	20	1	2	4	6	10	13	26
65+	262	4.4	13	2	2	3	5	8	10	23
TOTAL SINGLE DX	112	1.4	2	1	1	1	1	2	2	11
TOTAL MULTIPLE DX	623	3.9	18	1	2	3	5	8	10	21
TOTAL										
0–19 Years	220	2.3	13	1	1	2	2	5	7	20
20–34	63	2.9	13	1	1	2	3	6	11	17
35–49	63	4.0	22	1	1	3	5	7	9	34
50–64	126	4.8	20	1	2	4	6	10	13	26
65+	263	4.4	13	2	2	3	5	8	10	23
GRAND TOTAL	735	3.4	15	1	1	2	4	7	9	20

93.54: APPLICATION OF SPLINT

Type of Patients	Observed Patients	Avg. Stay	Variance	10th	25th	50th	75th	90th	95th	99th
1. SINGLE DX										
0–19 Years	75	1.5	<1	1	1	1	2	3	3	4
20–34	35	1.7	<1	1	1	1	2	3	3	5
35–49	20	1.5	<1	1	1	1	2	2	4	4
50–64	5	1.6	<1	1	1	2	2	3	3	3
65+	0									
2. MULTIPLE DX										
0–19 Years	192	2.3	6	1	1	2	3	4	6	12
20–34	287	3.1	55	1	1	2	3	5	7	45
35–49	295	3.8	31	1	2	2	4	7	11	37
50–64	444	3.9	19	1	2	3	5	7	10	27
65+	1,202	3.8	9	1	2	3	5	7	9	15
TOTAL SINGLE DX	135	1.5	<1	1	1	1	2	3	3	4
TOTAL MULTIPLE DX	2,420	3.6	19	1	2	3	4	7	9	19
TOTAL										
0–19 Years	267	2.1	5	1	1	2	3	4	5	6
20–34	322	2.9	49	1	1	2	3	4	6	17
35–49	315	3.6	29	1	1	2	4	7	10	33
50–64	449	3.9	19	1	2	3	5	7	10	27
65+	1,202	3.8	9	1	2	3	5	7	9	15
GRAND TOTAL	2,555	3.5	18	1	1	3	4	6	9	18

Western Region, October 2007–September 2008 Data, by Operation

93.56: PRESSURE DRESSING APPL

Type of Patients	Observed Patients	Avg. Stay	Vari-ance	Percentiles						
				10th	25th	50th	75th	90th	95th	99th
1. SINGLE DX										
0–19 Years	0									
20–34	0									
35–49	0									
50–64	1	1.0	0	1	1	1	1	1	1	1
65+	0									
2. MULTIPLE DX										
0–19 Years	8	5.5	31	1	1	2	13	13	13	13
20–34	10	6.8	22	2	2	6	10	13	14	14
35–49	18	5.9	7	2	3	6	7	10	11	11
50–64	43	7.0	78	1	2	4	7	13	31	37
65+	82	6.6	36	2	3	4	7	14	22	30
TOTAL SINGLE DX	1	1.0	0	1	1	1	1	1	1	1
TOTAL MULTIPLE DX	161	6.5	42	1	3	5	8	13	22	35
TOTAL										
0–19 Years	8	5.5	31	1	1	2	13	13	13	13
20–34	10	6.8	22	2	2	6	10	13	14	14
35–49	18	5.9	7	2	3	6	7	10	11	11
50–64	44	6.9	77	1	2	4	7	13	31	37
65+	82	6.6	36	2	3	4	7	14	22	30
GRAND TOTAL	162	6.5	42	1	3	5	8	13	22	35

93.57: APPL WOUND DRESSING NEC

Type of Patients	Observed Patients	Avg. Stay	Vari-ance	Percentiles						
				10th	25th	50th	75th	90th	95th	99th
1. SINGLE DX										
0–19 Years	8	1.2	<1	1	1	1	1	1	2	3
20–34	3	2.0	3	1	1	1	4	4	4	4
35–49	2	1.5	<1	1	1	1	2	2	2	2
50–64	1	1.0	0	1	1	1	1	1	1	1
65+	2	3.0	0	3	3	3	3	3	3	3
2. MULTIPLE DX										
0–19 Years	245	3.4	24	1	1	2	4	7	9	15
20–34	163	4.4	27	1	2	3	5	9	16	28
35–49	180	4.6	14	1	2	3	6	9	13	18
50–64	188	4.9	18	1	2	3	7	11	14	21
65+	254	6.1	23	2	3	4	8	13	17	22
TOTAL SINGLE DX	16	1.4	<1	1	1	1	1	3	3	4
TOTAL MULTIPLE DX	1,030	4.5	23	1	2	3	6	10	13	21
TOTAL										
0–19 Years	253	3.3	23	1	1	2	4	7	9	13
20–34	166	4.4	27	1	1	3	5	9	16	28
35–49	182	4.5	14	1	2	3	6	9	13	18
50–64	189	4.9	18	1	2	3	7	11	14	21
65+	256	6.1	23	2	3	4	8	13	17	22
GRAND TOTAL	1,046	4.5	22	1	1	3	6	10	13	21

93.59: IMMOB/PRESS/WND ATTN NEC

Type of Patients	Observed Patients	Avg. Stay	Vari-ance	Percentiles						
				10th	25th	50th	75th	90th	95th	99th
1. SINGLE DX										
0–19 Years	7	1.6	<1	1	1	1	2	3	3	3
20–34	12	5.0	83	1	1	1	4	7	33	33
35–49	7	4.3	13	1	1	2	7	10	10	10
50–64	7	1.3	<1	1	1	1	2	2	2	2
65+	1	1.0	0	1	1	1	1	1	1	1
2. MULTIPLE DX										
0–19 Years	68	4.4	19	1	2	3	5	12	17	18
20–34	79	3.9	10	1	2	3	5	9	11	15
35–49	124	5.0	44	1	2	3	6	9	13	26
50–64	188	5.4	36	1	3	4	7	12	18	39
65+	516	4.7	18	1	3	4	6	9	11	22
TOTAL SINGLE DX	34	3.2	32	1	1	1	3	7	10	33
TOTAL MULTIPLE DX	975	4.8	24	1	2	3	6	9	13	23
TOTAL										
0–19 Years	75	4.2	18	1	2	2	5	10	14	17
20–34	91	4.0	19	1	1	3	5	8	11	33
35–49	131	4.9	42	1	2	3	6	9	13	26
50–64	195	5.3	35	1	2	3	6	12	18	39
65+	517	4.7	18	1	3	4	6	9	11	22
GRAND TOTAL	1,009	4.7	24	1	2	3	6	9	13	26

93.6: OSTEOPATHIC MANIPULATION

Type of Patients	Observed Patients	Avg. Stay	Vari-ance	Percentiles						
				10th	25th	50th	75th	90th	95th	99th
1. SINGLE DX										
0–19 Years	0									
20–34	0									
35–49	0									
50–64	1	2.0	0	2	2	2	2	2	2	2
65+	0									
2. MULTIPLE DX										
0–19 Years	0									
20–34	10	2.2	2	1	1	2	3	4	4	4
35–49	15	2.5	3	1	1	2	3	4	8	8
50–64	19	2.5	2	1	2	2	3	5	6	6
65+	27	3.8	6	2	2	3	5	6	9	12
TOTAL SINGLE DX	1	2.0	0	2	2	2	2	2	2	2
TOTAL MULTIPLE DX	71	2.9	4	1	2	2	3	5	6	12
TOTAL										
0–19 Years	0									
20–34	10	2.2	2	1	1	2	3	4	4	4
35–49	15	2.5	3	1	1	2	3	4	8	8
50–64	20	2.5	2	1	2	2	3	5	5	6
65+	27	3.8	6	2	2	3	5	6	9	12
GRAND TOTAL	72	2.9	4	1	2	2	3	5	6	12

LOS by Diagnosis and Operation, Western Region, 45th Edition

Western Region, October 2007–September 2008 Data, by Operation

93.67: OMT NEC

Type of Patients	Observed Patients	Avg. Stay	Variance	10th	25th	50th	75th	90th	95th	99th
1. SINGLE DX										
0–19 Years	0									
20–34	0									
35–49	0									
50–64	0									
65+	0									
2. MULTIPLE DX										
0–19 Years	0									
20–34	9	2.3	2	1	1	2	3	4	4	4
35–49	14	2.6	3	1	2	2	3	4	8	8
50–64	16	2.5	3	1	1	2	3	5	6	6
65+	22	3.9	6	2	2	3	5	6	9	12
TOTAL SINGLE DX	0									
TOTAL MULTIPLE DX	61	3.0	4	1	2	2	3	5	6	12
TOTAL										
0–19 Years	0									
20–34	9	2.3	2	1	1	2	3	4	4	4
35–49	14	2.6	3	1	2	2	3	4	8	8
50–64	16	2.5	3	1	1	2	3	5	6	6
65+	22	3.9	6	2	2	3	5	6	9	12
GRAND TOTAL	61	3.0	4	1	2	2	3	5	6	12

93.75: SPEECH THERAPY NEC

Type of Patients	Observed Patients	Avg. Stay	Variance	10th	25th	50th	75th	90th	95th	99th
1. SINGLE DX										
0–19 Years	1	1.0	0							1
20–34	0									
35–49	0									
50–64	0									
65+	0									
2. MULTIPLE DX										
0–19 Years	19	11.3	338	1	1	2	8	52	52	52
20–34	20	6.1	400	1	1	1	2	5	5	91
35–49	16	4.3	91	1	1	2	3	4	40	40
50–64	39	9.4	191	1	2	4	9	35	47	62
65+	186	6.0	34	1	3	4	7	12	19	34
TOTAL SINGLE DX	1	1.0	0	1	1	1	1	1	1	1
TOTAL MULTIPLE DX	280	6.8	111	1	2	4	7	13	23	52
TOTAL										
0–19 Years	20	10.9	329	1	1	2	8	52	52	52
20–34	20	6.1	400	1	1	1	2	5	5	91
35–49	16	4.3	91	1	1	2	3	4	40	40
50–64	39	9.4	191	1	2	4	9	35	47	62
65+	186	6.0	34	1	3	4	7	12	19	34
GRAND TOTAL	281	6.8	111	1	2	4	7	13	23	52

93.7: SPEECH/READ/BLIND REHAB

Type of Patients	Observed Patients	Avg. Stay	Variance	10th	25th	50th	75th	90th	95th	99th
1. SINGLE DX										
0–19 Years	1	1.0	0	1	1	1	1	1	1	1
20–34	0									
35–49	0									
50–64	0									
65+	0									
2. MULTIPLE DX										
0–19 Years	20	11.5	325	1	1	5	8	52	52	52
20–34	20	6.1	400	1	1	1	2	5	5	91
35–49	17	6.0	137	1	1	2	3	34	40	40
50–64	39	9.4	191	1	2	4	9	35	47	62
65+	186	6.0	34	1	3	4	7	12	19	34
TOTAL SINGLE DX	1	1.0	0	1	1	1	1	1	1	1
TOTAL MULTIPLE DX	282	7.0	113	1	2	4	7	15	30	52
TOTAL										
0–19 Years	21	11.1	317	1	1	2	8	52	52	52
20–34	20	6.1	400	1	1	1	2	5	5	91
35–49	17	6.0	137	1	1	2	3	34	40	40
50–64	39	9.4	191	1	2	4	9	35	47	62
65+	186	6.0	34	1	3	4	7	12	19	34
GRAND TOTAL	283	6.9	113	1	2	4	7	15	30	52

93.8: OTHER REHAB THERAPY

Type of Patients	Observed Patients	Avg. Stay	Variance	10th	25th	50th	75th	90th	95th	99th
1. SINGLE DX										
0–19 Years	22	4.8	10	2	2	5	6	8	11	16
20–34	183	8.3	70	2	3	6	10	17	24	45
35–49	128	7.0	40	2	3	6	9	15	20	29
50–64	100	9.4	96	2	3	6	10	21	34	47
65+	3	14.7	154	6	6	9	29	29	29	29
2. MULTIPLE DX										
0–19 Years	145	9.5	126	2	3	6	11	22	28	56
20–34	619	11.2	166	2	4	7	14	26	35	74
35–49	636	10.3	130	3	4	8	12	23	34	62
50–64	641	12.2	143	3	4	8	16	27	36	64
65+	557	12.4	70	3	6	11	17	24	27	44
TOTAL SINGLE DX	436	8.0	65	2	3	5	9	17	23	42
TOTAL MULTIPLE DX	2,598	11.2	129	2	4	7	15	25	33	61
TOTAL										
0–19 Years	167	9.1	119	2	3	6	11	21	28	56
20–34	802	10.6	146	2	4	6	13	24	34	69
35–49	764	9.7	116	2	4	6	12	21	31	60
50–64	741	11.8	137	3	4	8	15	26	36	61
65+	560	12.4	70	3	6	11	17	24	27	44
GRAND TOTAL	3,034	10.8	122	2	4	7	14	23	32	57

LOS by Diagnosis and Operation, Western Region, 45th Edition

Western Region, October 2007–September 2008 Data, by Operation

93.81: RECREATIONAL THERAPY

Type of Patients	Observed Patients	Avg. Stay	Variance	10th	25th	50th	75th	90th	95th	99th
1. SINGLE DX										
0–19 Years	0									
20–34	25	6.2	35	2	2	4	7	18	18	24
35–49	10	4.1	3	2	3	3	5	6	7	7
50–64	6	4.5	7	2	2	5	5	9	9	9
65+	0									
2. MULTIPLE DX										
0–19 Years	0									
20–34	17	7.5	18	4	4	7	9	15	17	17
35–49	39	6.1	30	4	3	4	7	14	20	29
50–64	64	11.5	60	4	5	10	17	23	27	32
65+	137	13.7	56	6	8	12	17	26	28	36
TOTAL SINGLE DX	41	5.4	23	2	2	4	6	10	18	24
TOTAL MULTIPLE DX	257	11.6	58	4	6	10	15	22	27	35
TOTAL										
0–19 Years	0									
20–34	42	6.7	28	2	4	5	9	15	18	24
35–49	49	5.7	25	2	3	4	6	14	14	29
50–64	70	10.9	59	3	5	9	15	23	27	32
65+	137	13.7	56	6	8	12	17	26	28	36
GRAND TOTAL	298	10.8	58	3	5	9	15	21	26	35

93.83: OCCUPATIONAL THERAPY

Type of Patients	Observed Patients	Avg. Stay	Variance	10th	25th	50th	75th	90th	95th	99th
1. SINGLE DX										
0–19 Years	22	4.8	10	2	2	5	6	8	11	16
20–34	158	8.6	75	2	3	6	10	17	27	45
35–49	118	7.3	43	2	3	5	11	17	21	29
50–64	94	9.7	101	2	3	6	11	21	34	48
65+	3	14.7	154	6	6	9	29	29	29	29
2. MULTIPLE DX										
0–19 Years	143	9.4	125	2	3	6	11	21	28	56
20–34	600	11.3	170	2	4	7	14	26	35	75
35–49	589	10.5	136	2	4	6	13	25	37	62
50–64	551	12.0	153	3	4	8	15	27	38	66
65+	388	11.4	72	3	5	9	16	23	27	44
TOTAL SINGLE DX	395	8.2	68	2	3	6	10	17	27	42
TOTAL MULTIPLE DX	2,271	11.0	137	2	4	7	14	24	34	64
TOTAL										
0–19 Years	165	9.1	118	2	3	6	10	21	28	56
20–34	758	10.7	151	2	4	7	13	24	34	69
35–49	707	9.9	122	2	3	6	12	22	34	60
50–64	645	11.6	146	2	4	9	15	26	37	64
65+	391	11.4	72	3	5	9	16	23	27	44
GRAND TOTAL	2,666	10.6	128	2	4	7	13	23	33	61

93.89: REHABILITATION NEC

Type of Patients	Observed Patients	Avg. Stay	Variance	10th	25th	50th	75th	90th	95th	99th
1. SINGLE DX										
0–19 Years	0									
20–34	0									
35–49	0									
50–64	0									
65+	0									
2. MULTIPLE DX										
0–19 Years	2	24.0	12	22	22	22	28	28	28	28
20–34	2	24.6	261	13	13	36	36	36	36	36
35–49	8	14.3	66	1	8	13	16	28	28	28
50–64	26	18.0	104	6	12	17	23	34	35	44
65+	32	18.2	54	8	11	19	26	28	28	29
TOTAL SINGLE DX	0									
TOTAL MULTIPLE DX	70	18.1	76	7	12	18	25	28	34	44
TOTAL										
0–19 Years	2	24.0	12	22	22	22	28	28	28	28
20–34	2	24.6	261	13	13	36	36	36	36	36
35–49	8	14.3	66	1	8	13	16	28	28	28
50–64	26	18.0	104	6	12	17	23	34	35	44
65+	32	18.2	54	8	11	19	26	28	28	29
GRAND TOTAL	70	18.1	76	7	12	18	25	28	34	44

93.9: RESPIRATORY THERAPY

Type of Patients	Observed Patients	Avg. Stay	Variance	10th	25th	50th	75th	90th	95th	99th
1. SINGLE DX										
0–19 Years	1,675	2.4	2	1	2	2	3	4	4	7
20–34	29	1.6	<1	1	1	1	2	3	3	4
35–49	21	2.0	2	1	1	1	2	4	5	6
50–64	24	2.2	2	1	1	2	2	4	5	7
65+	10	3.2	11	1	1	2	4	4	12	12
2. MULTIPLE DX										
0–19 Years	9,948	9.3	153	2	2	4	10	24	36	62
20–34	766	5.0	30	1	2	3	6	10	14	29
35–49	2,493	4.9	31	2	2	4	6	9	12	26
50–64	6,357	5.3	25	2	2	4	6	10	14	24
65+	13,159	5.9	21	2	3	5	7	11	14	22
TOTAL SINGLE DX	1,759	2.4	2	1	2	2	3	4	4	7
TOTAL MULTIPLE DX	32,723	6.8	68	2	3	4	8	13	21	45
TOTAL										
0–19 Years	11,623	8.4	138	1	2	4	9	22	34	59
20–34	795	4.9	29	1	2	3	6	10	14	28
35–49	2,514	4.9	31	1	2	3	6	9	12	24
50–64	6,381	5.3	25	1	2	4	6	10	14	24
65+	13,169	5.9	21	2	3	5	7	11	14	22
GRAND TOTAL	34,482	6.6	66	2	2	4	7	13	20	44

LOS by Diagnosis and Operation, Western Region, 45th Edition

Western Region, October 2007–September 2008 Data, by Operation

93.90: CPAP

Type of Patients	Observed Patients	Avg. Stay	Vari-ance	Percentiles						
				10th	25th	50th	75th	90th	95th	99th
1. SINGLE DX										
0–19 Years	104	2.6	4	1	2	2	2	4	7	7
20–34	6	2.0	2	1	1	1	3	4	4	4
35–49	2	1.0	0	1	1	1	1	1	1	1
50–64	5	1.6	<1	1	1	2	2	2	2	2
65+	4	5.7	17	3	3	4	4	12	12	12
2. MULTIPLE DX										
0–19 Years	5,563	12.9	214	2	3	7	17	33	44	68
20–34	447	6.0	40	1	2	4	8	13	16	38
35–49	1,729	5.5	37	1	2	4	7	10	14	30
50–64	4,738	5.8	25	2	3	4	7	11	14	25
65+	10,065	6.3	23	3	3	5	8	12	15	23
TOTAL SINGLE DX	121	2.6	4	1	1	2	2	4	7	12
TOTAL MULTIPLE DX	22,542	7.9	85	2	3	5	9	16	25	51
TOTAL										
0–19 Years	5,667	12.7	212	2	3	7	16	33	44	68
20–34	453	6.0	39	1	2	4	7	13	16	38
35–49	1,731	5.5	37	1	2	4	7	10	14	30
50–64	4,743	5.8	25	2	3	4	7	11	14	25
65+	10,069	6.3	23	2	3	5	8	12	15	23
GRAND TOTAL	22,663	7.9	84	2	3	5	9	16	25	51

93.91: IPPB

Type of Patients	Observed Patients	Avg. Stay	Vari-ance	Percentiles						
				10th	25th	50th	75th	90th	95th	99th
1. SINGLE DX										
0–19 Years	45	1.7	<1	1	1	2	2	2	3	3
20–34	0									
35–49	1	1.0	0	1	1	1	1	1	1	1
50–64	0									
65+	0									
2. MULTIPLE DX										
0–19 Years	202	2.8	8	1	1	2	3	5	9	13
20–34	4	6.0	3	4	5	6	8	8	8	8
35–49	7	4.7	4	2	2	4	6	7	7	7
50–64	18	9.8	380	2	3	4	7	14	87	87
65+	53	7.3	24	2	3	6	10	15	18	21
TOTAL SINGLE DX	46	1.7	<1	1	1	2	2	2	3	3
TOTAL MULTIPLE DX	284	4.1	38	1	2	2	5	9	12	21
TOTAL										
0–19 Years	247	2.6	7	1	1	2	3	4	8	13
20–34	8	6.0	3	4	5	6	8	8	8	8
35–49	8	4.3	5	1	2	6	6	7	7	7
50–64	18	9.8	380	2	3	4	7	14	87	87
65+	53	7.3	24	2	3	6	10	15	18	21
GRAND TOTAL	330	3.8	33	1	1	2	4	9	11	19

93.93: NONMECH RESUSCITATION

Type of Patients	Observed Patients	Avg. Stay	Vari-ance	Percentiles						
				10th	25th	50th	75th	90th	95th	99th
1. SINGLE DX										
0–19 Years	16	2.4	<1	1	2	2	3	3	4	4
20–34	0									
35–49	0									
50–64	0									
65+										
2. MULTIPLE DX										
0–19 Years	328	3.3	11	1	2	3	3	5	9	19
20–34	4	1.5	<1	1	1	2	2	2	2	2
35–49	4	2.3	2	1	2	2	2	4	4	4
50–64	8	4.6	10	1	2	5	6	11	11	11
65+	7	4.2	10	1	2	4	6	10	10	10
TOTAL SINGLE DX	16	2.4	<1	1	2	2	3	3	4	4
TOTAL MULTIPLE DX	349	3.4	11	1	2	3	3	6	9	19
TOTAL										
0–19 Years	344	3.3	11	1	2	3	3	5	9	19
20–34	2	1.5	<1	1	1	2	2	2	2	2
35–49	4	2.3	2	1	2	2	2	4	4	4
50–64	8	4.6	10	1	2	5	6	11	11	11
65+	7	4.2	10	1	2	4	6	10	10	10
GRAND TOTAL	365	3.3	11	1	2	3	3	5	9	19

93.94: NEBULIZER THERAPY

Type of Patients	Observed Patients	Avg. Stay	Vari-ance	Percentiles						
				10th	25th	50th	75th	90th	95th	99th
1. SINGLE DX										
0–19 Years	289	2.2	2	1	1	2	3	4	5	7
20–34	12	1.7	<1	1	1	1	2	3	3	3
35–49	7	2.2	3	1	1	1	4	5	5	5
50–64	13	2.6	4	1	1	2	4	5	7	7
65+	4	1.5	<1	1	1	1	2	2	2	2
2. MULTIPLE DX										
0–19 Years	673	2.7	5	1	1	2	3	5	7	11
20–34	140	3.4	15	1	1	2	4	6	11	22
35–49	372	3.5	19	1	2	3	4	7	9	15
50–64	806	3.9	25	1	2	3	4	6	8	19
65+	1,855	4.7	13	2	3	4	6	8	11	18
TOTAL SINGLE DX	325	2.1	2	1	1	2	3	4	5	7
TOTAL MULTIPLE DX	3,846	4.0	15	1	2	3	5	7	9	18
TOTAL										
0–19 Years	962	2.6	4	1	1	2	3	5	6	10
20–34	152	3.3	15	1	1	3	4	5	8	22
35–49	379	3.5	19	1	2	3	4	7	9	15
50–64	819	3.8	24	2	2	3	4	6	8	19
65+	1,859	4.7	13	2	3	4	6	8	11	18
GRAND TOTAL	4,171	3.8	14	1	2	3	5	7	9	17

LOS by Diagnosis and Operation, Western Region, 45th Edition

Western Region, October 2007–September 2008 Data, by Operation

93.95: HYPERBARIC OXYGENATION

Type of Patients	Observed Patients	Avg. Stay	Vari-ance	Percentiles						
				10th	25th	50th	75th	90th	95th	99th
1. SINGLE DX										
0–19 Years	2	2.5	<1	2	2	2	3	3	3	3
20–34	1	1.0	0	1	1	1	1	1	1	1
35–49	0									
50–64	1	1.0	0	1	1	1	1	1	1	1
65+	0									
2. MULTIPLE DX										
0–19 Years	3	6.9	13	3	3	5	10	10	10	10
20–34	5	1.4	<1	1	1	1	2	2	2	2
35–49	10	5.2	80	1	1	2	4	30	30	30
50–64	20	6.8	53	1	2	4	12	17	30	30
65+	15	7.8	47	1	3	6	9	19	26	26
TOTAL SINGLE DX	4	1.8	<1	1	1	2	2	3	3	3
TOTAL MULTIPLE DX	53	6.3	49	1	2	3	8	13	26	30
TOTAL										
0–19 Years	5	5.4	13	2	3	3	10	10	10	10
20–34	6	1.3	<1	1	1	1	2	2	2	2
35–49	10	5.2	80	1	1	2	4	30	30	30
50–64	21	6.5	52	1	2	3	9	13	17	30
65+	15	7.8	47	1	3	6	9	19	26	26
GRAND TOTAL	57	6.0	47	1	1	3	7	13	26	30

93.99: RESPIRATORY THERAPY NEC

Type of Patients	Observed Patients	Avg. Stay	Vari-ance	Percentiles						
				10th	25th	50th	75th	90th	95th	99th
1. SINGLE DX										
0–19 Years	67	1.9	2	1	1	1	2	4	5	7
20–34	1	1.0	0	1	1	1	1	1	1	1
35–49	1	2.0	0	2	2	2	2	2	2	2
50–64	0									
65+	0									
2. MULTIPLE DX										
0–19 Years	273	6.0	37	1	2	4	8	14	17	29
20–34	52	3.3	14	1	1	2	3	8	12	21
35–49	97	3.1	11	1	1	2	3	6	11	19
50–64	138	2.9	11	1	1	2	3	6	9	28
65+	42	2.7	5	1	1	2	3	6	8	10
TOTAL SINGLE DX	69	1.9	2	1	1	1	2	4	5	7
TOTAL MULTIPLE DX	602	4.4	25	1	1	3	5	10	15	25
TOTAL										
0–19 Years	340	5.2	32	1	2	3	7	13	16	29
20–34	53	3.2	14	1	1	2	3	8	12	21
35–49	98	3.1	11	1	1	2	3	6	11	19
50–64	138	2.9	11	1	1	2	3	6	9	28
65+	42	2.7	5	1	1	2	3	6	8	10
GRAND TOTAL	671	4.1	23	1	1	2	4	10	14	25

93.96: OXYGEN ENRICHMENT NEC

Type of Patients	Observed Patients	Avg. Stay	Vari-ance	Percentiles						
				10th	25th	50th	75th	90th	95th	99th
1. SINGLE DX										
0–19 Years	1,152	2.6	1	1	2	3	3	4	4	6
20–34	9	1.5	<1	1	1	1	1	3	3	3
35–49	6	2.2	3	1	1	2	3	5	6	6
50–64	5	1.8	2	1	1	1	2	4	4	4
65+	2	1.5	<1	1	1	2	2	2	2	2
2. MULTIPLE DX										
0–19 Years	2,905	4.9	37	2	2	3	5	9	14	33
20–34	116	3.6	7	1	2	3	4	7	8	15
35–49	274	3.5	11	1	2	3	4	7	8	20
50–64	629	3.9	10	1	2	3	5	7	10	15
65+	1,122	4.7	12	2	2	4	6	9	11	19
TOTAL SINGLE DX	1,178	2.5	1	1	2	3	3	4	4	6
TOTAL MULTIPLE DX	5,046	4.6	26	1	2	3	5	9	12	28
TOTAL										
0–19 Years	4,057	4.2	28	1	2	3	4	8	11	30
20–34	125	3.5	7	1	2	3	4	7	8	15
35–49	284	3.4	11	1	1	2	4	6	8	20
50–64	634	3.9	10	1	2	3	5	7	10	15
65+	1,124	4.7	12	2	2	4	6	9	11	19
GRAND TOTAL	6,224	4.2	22	1	2	3	5	8	11	24

94.0: PSYCH EVAL & TESTING

Type of Patients	Observed Patients	Avg. Stay	Vari-ance	Percentiles						
				10th	25th	50th	75th	90th	95th	99th
1. SINGLE DX										
0–19 Years	1	5.0	0	5	5	5	5	5	5	5
20–34	1	2.0	0	2	2	2	2	2	2	2
35–49	0									
50–64	0									
65+	0									
2. MULTIPLE DX										
0–19 Years	8	8.7	20	4	6	8	9	19	19	19
20–34	19	5.9	36	2	2	3	7	14	25	25
35–49	9	4.3	13	2	2	3	6	13	13	13
50–64	2	1.5	<1	1	1	2	2	2	2	2
65+	1	12.0	0	12	12	12	12	12	12	12
TOTAL SINGLE DX	2	3.5	4	2	2	2	5	5	5	5
TOTAL MULTIPLE DX	39	6.0	28	2	2	4	8	13	19	25
TOTAL										
0–19 Years	9	8.3	19	4	6	8	9	19	19	19
20–34	20	5.7	35	2	2	3	7	14	25	25
35–49	9	4.3	13	2	2	3	6	13	13	13
50–64	2	1.5	<1	1	1	2	2	2	2	2
65+	1	12.0	0	12	12	12	12	12	12	12
GRAND TOTAL	41	5.9	27	2	2	4	8	13	14	25

Western Region, October 2007–September 2008 Data, by Operation

94.1: PSYCH EVAL/CONSULT

Type of Patients	Observed Patients	Avg. Stay	Variance	Percentiles						
				10th	25th	50th	75th	90th	95th	99th
1. SINGLE DX										
0–19 Years	1	9.0	0	9	9	9	9	9	9	9
20–34	0									
35–49	0									
50–64	0									
65+	0									
2. MULTIPLE DX										
0–19 Years	66	6.3	23	1	3	5	8	13	17	24
20–34	421	6.4	22	2	3	5	8	13	15	21
35–49	457	7.1	36	2	4	6	9	14	19	28
50–64	220	7.8	68	2	3	5	9	15	20	47
65+	40	8.1	36	2	4	7	11	19	22	25
TOTAL SINGLE DX	1	9.0	0	9	9	9	9	9	9	9
TOTAL MULTIPLE DX	1,204	7.0	37	2	3	5	9	14	17	28
TOTAL										
0–19 Years	67	6.3	23	1	3	5	9	13	17	24
20–34	421	6.4	22	2	3	5	8	13	15	21
35–49	457	7.1	36	2	4	6	9	14	19	28
50–64	220	7.8	68	2	3	5	9	15	20	47
65+	40	8.1	36	2	4	7	11	19	22	25
GRAND TOTAL	1,205	7.0	37	2	3	5	9	14	17	28

94.11: PSYCH MENTAL STATUS

Type of Patients	Observed Patients	Avg. Stay	Variance	Percentiles						
				10th	25th	50th	75th	90th	95th	99th
1. SINGLE DX										
0–19 Years	1	9.0	0	9	9	9	9	9	9	9
20–34	0									
35–49	0									
50–64	0									
65+	0									
2. MULTIPLE DX										
0–19 Years	63	6.4	23	1	3	5	9	13	17	24
20–34	419	6.4	22	2	3	5	8	13	15	21
35–49	453	7.1	36	2	4	6	9	14	19	28
50–64	219	7.8	68	2	3	5	9	15	20	47
65+	40	8.1	36	2	4	7	11	19	22	25
TOTAL SINGLE DX	1	9.0	0	9	9	9	9	9	9	9
TOTAL MULTIPLE DX	1,194	7.0	37	2	3	5	9	14	17	28
TOTAL										
0–19 Years	64	6.5	23	1	3	5	9	13	17	24
20–34	419	6.4	22	2	3	5	8	13	15	21
35–49	453	7.1	36	2	4	6	9	14	19	28
50–64	219	7.8	68	2	3	5	9	15	20	47
65+	40	8.1	36	2	4	7	11	19	22	25
GRAND TOTAL	1,195	7.0	37	2	3	5	9	14	17	28

94.19: PSYCH INTERVIEW/EVAL NEC

Type of Patients	Observed Patients	Avg. Stay	Variance	Percentiles						
				10th	25th	50th	75th	90th	95th	99th
1. SINGLE DX										
0–19 Years	0									
20–34	0									
35–49	0									
50–64	0									
65+										
2. MULTIPLE DX										
0–19 Years	3	3.3	6	1	1	3	6	6	6	6
20–34	2	4.0	0	4	4	4	4	4	4	4
35–49	2	1.0	0	1	1	1	1	1	1	1
50–64	1	14.0	0	14	14	14	14	14	14	14
65+	0									
TOTAL SINGLE DX	0									
TOTAL MULTIPLE DX	8	4.3	19	1	1	3	6	14	14	14
TOTAL										
0–19 Years	3	3.3	6	1	1	3	6	6	6	6
20–34	2	4.0	0	4	4	4	4	4	4	4
35–49	2	1.0	0	1	1	1	1	1	1	1
50–64	1	14.0	0	14	14	14	14	14	14	14
65+	0									
GRAND TOTAL	8	4.3	19	1	1	3	6	14	14	14

94.2: PSYCH SOMATOTHERAPY

Type of Patients	Observed Patients	Avg. Stay	Variance	Percentiles						
				10th	25th	50th	75th	90th	95th	99th
1. SINGLE DX										
0–19 Years	57	11.3	100	3	5	7	14	29	33	47
20–34	116	17.5	394	2	6	10	20	48	69	90
35–49	77	14.7	212	3	4	10	19	36	57	>99
50–64	60	19.5	409	3	5	13	26	54	67	88
65+	6	22.3	323	2	4	28	33	49	49	49
2. MULTIPLE DX										
0–19 Years	290	9.3	69	2	3	7	12	20	28	45
20–34	855	8.3	98	2	3	5	9	18	32	54
35–49	1,146	9.4	105	2	3	6	11	21	31	55
50–64	1,021	12.2	168	2	4	8	15	29	43	78
65+	651	16.5	177	4	7	13	22	35	43	74
TOTAL SINGLE DX	316	16.2	303	2	5	10	20	43	60	88
TOTAL MULTIPLE DX	3,963	11.0	137	2	3	7	14	26	37	65
TOTAL										
0–19 Years	347	9.6	74	3	4	7	12	21	29	45
20–34	971	9.4	141	2	3	6	10	21	37	72
35–49	1,223	9.7	114	3	3	6	11	23	32	57
50–64	1,081	12.6	183	2	4	8	15	31	44	87
65+	657	16.6	179	4	7	13	22	35	43	74
GRAND TOTAL	4,279	11.4	151	2	4	7	14	27	38	71

LOS by Diagnosis and Operation, Western Region, 45th Edition

Western Region, October 2007–September 2008 Data, by Operation

94.22: LITHIUM THERAPY

Type of Patients	Observed Patients	Avg. Stay	Variance	Percentiles						
				10th	25th	50th	75th	90th	95th	99th
1. SINGLE DX										
0–19 Years	0									
20–34	0									
35–49	1	13.0	0	13	13	13	13	13	13	13
50–64	0									
65+	0									
2. MULTIPLE DX										
0–19 Years	4	6.0	28	3	3	4	4	14	14	14
20–34	14	5.0	13	3	3	4	5	12	13	13
35–49	11	6.5	26	2	3	5	13	13	15	15
50–64	11	6.2	31	1	2	4	7	17	17	17
65+	2	9.0	2	8	8	8	10	10	10	10
TOTAL SINGLE DX	1	13.0	0	13	13	13	13	13	13	13
TOTAL MULTIPLE DX	42	6.0	21	2	3	4	8	13	15	17
TOTAL										
0–19 Years	4	6.0	28	3	3	4	4	14	14	14
20–34	14	5.0	13	3	3	4	5	12	13	13
35–49	12	7.1	28	1	2	5	13	13	15	15
50–64	11	6.2	31	2	3	4	7	17	17	17
65+	2	9.0	2	8	8	8	10	10	10	10
GRAND TOTAL	43	6.2	22	2	3	4	9	13	15	17

94.23: NEUROLEPTIC THERAPY

Type of Patients	Observed Patients	Avg. Stay	Variance	Percentiles						
				10th	25th	50th	75th	90th	95th	99th
1. SINGLE DX										
0–19 Years	0									
20–34	1	5.0	0	5	5	5	5	5	5	5
35–49	0									
50–64	0									
65+	0									
2. MULTIPLE DX										
0–19 Years	0									
20–34	3	5.3	10	3	3	4	9	9	9	9
35–49	10	10.9	31	4	8	8	16	21	21	21
50–64	42	11.9	42	4	7	12	16	21	22	28
65+	137	14.2	84	5	7	12	18	27	33	41
TOTAL SINGLE DX	1	5.0	0	5	5	5	5	5	5	5
TOTAL MULTIPLE DX	192	13.4	73	5	7	12	17	25	30	41
TOTAL										
0–19 Years	0									
20–34	4	5.2	7	3	4	5	5	9	9	9
35–49	10	10.9	31	4	8	8	16	21	21	21
50–64	42	11.9	42	4	7	12	16	21	22	28
65+	137	14.2	84	5	7	12	18	27	33	41
GRAND TOTAL	193	13.3	73	5	7	12	17	25	30	41

94.25: PSYCH DRUG THERAPY NEC

Type of Patients	Observed Patients	Avg. Stay	Variance	Percentiles						
				10th	25th	50th	75th	90th	95th	99th
1. SINGLE DX										
0–19 Years	56	11.5	101	3	5	7	14	29	33	47
20–34	111	17.6	409	2	5	10	20	48	69	90
35–49	71	14.6	213	2	4	10	20	35	57	>99
50–64	48	21.8	468	3	6	14	33	55	67	88
65+	4	22.0	521	2	3	19	41	49	49	49
2. MULTIPLE DX										
0–19 Years	282	9.3	69	2	3	7	12	20	27	45
20–34	776	7.8	89	2	3	5	9	15	26	52
35–49	892	7.7	79	2	3	5	9	15	23	52
50–64	720	10.4	155	2	3	7	12	23	43	78
65+	255	12.4	106	3	6	10	15	23	29	46
TOTAL SINGLE DX	290	16.4	319	2	5	10	20	43	61	90
TOTAL MULTIPLE DX	2,925	8.9	104	2	3	6	10	19	29	61
TOTAL										
0–19 Years	338	9.6	75	3	4	7	12	21	29	45
20–34	887	9.0	139	2	3	5	10	20	36	72
35–49	963	8.2	92	2	3	5	9	17	27	57
50–64	768	11.1	181	2	3	7	12	25	45	87
65+	259	12.5	112	3	6	10	15	24	31	49
GRAND TOTAL	3,215	9.6	128	2	3	6	11	20	34	69

94.27: ELECTROSHOCK THERAPY NEC

Type of Patients	Observed Patients	Avg. Stay	Variance	Percentiles						
				10th	25th	50th	75th	90th	95th	99th
1. SINGLE DX										
0–19 Years	1	3.0	0	3	3	3	3	3	3	3
20–34	3	17.4	91	7	7	19	26	26	26	26
35–49	5	16.6	311	1	4	10	16	47	47	47
50–64	12	10.0	73	1	4	8	20	28	27	27
65+	2	23.0	49	18	18	28	28	28	28	28
2. MULTIPLE DX										
0–19 Years	3	16.3	141	8	8	11	30	30	30	30
20–34	62	15.8	174	4	6	12	22	38	49	>99
35–49	233	16.1	158	4	8	13	23	32	44	58
50–64	248	17.8	191	4	8	14	24	36	45	91
65+	257	22.0	250	3	10	20	30	44	53	81
TOTAL SINGLE DX	23	13.3	128	2	4	10	20	27	28	47
TOTAL MULTIPLE DX	803	18.5	204	3	8	15	26	39	49	80
TOTAL										
0–19 Years	4	13.0	138	3	8	10	30	30	30	30
20–34	65	15.9	169	4	6	12	22	38	49	>99
35–49	238	16.2	160	3	8	12	23	32	45	58
50–64	260	17.5	188	4	8	14	24	35	45	91
65+	259	22.0	248	3	11	20	30	43	53	81
GRAND TOTAL	826	18.4	203	3	8	15	26	38	49	80

LOS by Diagnosis and Operation, Western Region, 45th Edition

Western Region, October 2007–September 2008 Data, by Operation

94.3: INDIVIDUAL PSYCHOTHERAPY

Type of Patients	Observed Patients	Avg. Stay	Vari- ance	Percentiles						
				10th	25th	50th	75th	90th	95th	99th
1. SINGLE DX										
0–19 Years	8	4.0	9	1	1		7	8	8	8
20–34	70	3.7	6	1	1	3	5	8	9	11
35–49	24	4.1	11	1	2	3	5	7	8	17
50–64	14	6.1	6	3	5	7	8	9	10	10
65+	2	11.0	49	6	6	11	16	16	16	16
2. MULTIPLE DX										
0–19 Years	161	6.0	41	2	3	4	6	12	18	40
20–34	796	5.1	22	2	3	4	6	8	12	24
35–49	773	5.9	27	2	3	5	7	12	16	25
50–64	764	7.2	37	3	3	5	8	16	21	30
65+	203	10.1	43	4	5	8	14	19	22	29
TOTAL SINGLE DX	118	4.2	9	1	2	4	6	8	9	16
TOTAL MULTIPLE DX	2,697	6.4	32	2	3	5	7	14	18	28
TOTAL										
0–19 Years	169	5.9	39	2	3	4	6	11	18	40
20–34	866	5.0	21	2	3	4	6	8	11	24
35–49	797	5.9	27	2	3	5	7	12	16	24
50–64	778	7.2	37	2	3	5	8	16	21	30
65+	205	10.1	43	4	5	8	14	19	22	29
GRAND TOTAL	2,815	6.3	32	2	3	5	7	13	18	28

94.37: EXPL VERBAL PSYCHTX

Type of Patients	Observed Patients	Avg. Stay	Vari- ance	Percentiles						
				10th	25th	50th	75th	90th	95th	99th
1. SINGLE DX										
0–19 Years	0									
20–34	0									
35–49	0									
50–64	0									
65+	0									
2. MULTIPLE DX										
0–19 Years	0									
20–34	0									
35–49	0									
50–64	0									
65+	0									
TOTAL SINGLE DX	0									
TOTAL MULTIPLE DX	0									
TOTAL										
0–19 Years	0									
20–34	0									
35–49	0									
50–64	0									
65+	0									
GRAND TOTAL	0									

94.38: SUPP VERBAL PSYCHTX

Type of Patients	Observed Patients	Avg. Stay	Vari- ance	Percentiles						
				10th	25th	50th	75th	90th	95th	99th
1. SINGLE DX										
0–19 Years	0									
20–34	0									
35–49	0									
50–64	0									
65+	0									
2. MULTIPLE DX										
0–19 Years	0									
20–34	1	7.0	0	7	7	7	7	7	7	7
35–49	2	23.0	18	20	20	26	26	26	26	26
50–64	0									
65+	0									
TOTAL SINGLE DX	0									
TOTAL MULTIPLE DX	3	17.7	94	7	7	20	26	26	26	26
TOTAL										
0–19 Years	0									
20–34	1	7.0	0	7	7	7	7	7	7	7
35–49	0									
50–64	2	23.0	18	20	20	26	26	26	26	26
65+	0									
GRAND TOTAL	3	17.7	94	7	7	20	26	26	26	26

94.39: INDIVIDUAL PSYCHTX NEC

Type of Patients	Observed Patients	Avg. Stay	Vari- ance	Percentiles						
				10th	25th	50th	75th	90th	95th	99th
1. SINGLE DX										
0–19 Years	7	4.0	10	1	1	2	7	8	8	8
20–34	69	3.6	6	1	1	3	5	8	8	11
35–49	22	4.3	12	2	2	3	5	7	8	17
50–64	14	6.1	6	3	5	7	8	9	10	10
65+	2	11.0	49	6	6	11	16	16	16	16
2. MULTIPLE DX										
0–19 Years	120	5.2	15	2	3	4	6	10	14	19
20–34	744	5.0	22	2	3	4	6	8	11	25
35–49	727	5.6	23	2	3	4	7	11	15	24
50–64	745	7.2	37	2	4	5	8	16	21	30
65+	194	10.3	44	4	5	9	14	19	23	36
TOTAL SINGLE DX	114	4.2	9	1	2	4	6	8	9	16
TOTAL MULTIPLE DX	2,530	6.2	30	2	3	5	7	13	18	27
TOTAL										
0–19 Years	127	5.2	15	2	3	4	6	10	14	19
20–34	813	4.9	21	2	3	4	6	8	11	21
35–49	749	5.6	22	2	3	4	7	11	15	24
50–64	759	7.2	37	2	4	5	8	16	21	30
65+	196	10.3	44	4	5	9	14	19	23	36
GRAND TOTAL	2,644	6.1	29	2	3	5	7	13	17	27

LOS by Diagnosis and Operation, Western Region, 45th Edition

Western Region, October 2007–September 2008 Data, by Operation

94.4: OTH PSYCHTX/COUNSELLING

Type of Patients	Observed Patients	Avg. Stay	Variance	Percentiles						
				10th	25th	50th	75th	90th	95th	99th
1. SINGLE DX										
0–19 Years	9	3.8	4	1	2	4	5	7	7	7
20–34	28	4.7	9	2	3	4	6	8	12	14
35–49	27	6.3	15	3	3	5	8	12	13	17
50–64	14	11.5	63	3	5	12	14	27	28	28
65+	0									
2. MULTIPLE DX										
0–19 Years	156	5.8	40	2	3	4	6	10	14	39
20–34	700	6.3	40	2	3	5	7	12	17	32
35–49	869	6.9	28	2	3	5	9	13	17	25
50–64	793	8.8	40	3	4	7	12	17	22	30
65+	314	11.9	41	4	7	11	15	20	24	29
TOTAL SINGLE DX	78	6.4	26	2	3	5	8	13	14	28
TOTAL MULTIPLE DX	2,832	7.8	39	2	4	6	10	15	20	29
TOTAL										
0–19 Years	165	5.7	38	2	3	4	6	10	13	39
20–34	728	6.2	39	2	3	5	7	12	17	30
35–49	896	6.9	27	2	3	5	9	13	17	25
50–64	807	8.8	40	3	4	7	12	17	22	29
65+	314	11.9	41	4	7	11	15	20	24	29
GRAND TOTAL	2,910	7.7	39	2	4	6	10	15	20	28

94.44: GROUP THERAPY NEC

Type of Patients	Observed Patients	Avg. Stay	Variance	Percentiles						
				10th	25th	50th	75th	90th	95th	99th
1. SINGLE DX										
0–19 Years	9	3.8	4	1	2	4	5	7	7	7
20–34	28	4.7	9	2	3	4	6	8	12	14
35–49	27	6.3	15	3	3	5	8	12	13	17
50–64	14	11.5	63	3	5	12	14	27	28	28
65+	0									
2. MULTIPLE DX										
0–19 Years	147	5.8	41	2	3	4	6	10	13	39
20–34	699	6.3	40	2	3	5	7	12	17	32
35–49	868	6.9	27	2	3	5	9	13	17	25
50–64	793	8.8	40	3	4	7	12	17	22	30
65+	313	12.0	41	5	7	11	15	20	24	29
TOTAL SINGLE DX	78	6.4	26	2	3	5	8	13	14	28
TOTAL MULTIPLE DX	2,820	7.8	39	2	4	6	10	15	20	29
TOTAL										
0–19 Years	156	5.7	39	2	3	4	6	10	13	39
20–34	727	6.2	39	2	3	5	7	12	17	30
35–49	895	6.9	27	2	3	5	9	13	17	25
50–64	807	8.8	40	3	4	7	12	17	22	29
65+	313	12.0	41	5	7	11	15	20	24	29
GRAND TOTAL	2,898	7.7	39	2	4	6	10	15	20	29

94.49: COUNSELLING NEC

Type of Patients	Observed Patients	Avg. Stay	Variance	Percentiles						
				10th	25th	50th	75th	90th	95th	99th
1. SINGLE DX										
0–19 Years	0									
20–34	0									
35–49	0									
50–64	0									
65+	0									
2. MULTIPLE DX										
0–19 Years	0									
20–34	1	2.0	0	2	2	2	2	2	2	2
35–49	1	24.0	0	24	24	24	24	24	24	24
50–64	0									
65+	0									
TOTAL SINGLE DX	0									
TOTAL MULTIPLE DX	2	13.1	239	2	2	24	24	24	24	24
TOTAL										
0–19 Years	0									
20–34	1	2.0	0	2	2	2	2	2	2	2
35–49	1	24.0	0	24	24	24	24	24	24	24
50–64	0									
65+	0									
GRAND TOTAL	2	13.1	239	2	2	24	24	24	24	24

94.5: REFERRAL PSYCH REHAB

Type of Patients	Observed Patients	Avg. Stay	Variance	Percentiles						
				10th	25th	50th	75th	90th	95th	99th
1. SINGLE DX										
0–19 Years	0									
20–34	0									
35–49	0									
50–64	0									
65+	0									
2. MULTIPLE DX										
0–19 Years	0									
20–34	0									
35–49	0									
50–64	1	6.0	0	6	6	6	6	6	6	6
65+	0									
TOTAL SINGLE DX	0									
TOTAL MULTIPLE DX	1	6.0	0	6	6	6	6	6	6	6
TOTAL										
0–19 Years	0									
20–34	0									
35–49	0									
50–64	1	6.0	0	6	6	6	6	6	6	6
65+	0									
GRAND TOTAL	1	6.0	0	6	6	6	6	6	6	6

LOS by Diagnosis and Operation, Western Region, 45th Edition

Western Region, October 2007–September 2008 Data, by Operation

94.6: ALCOHOL/DRUG REHAB/DETOX

Type of Patients	Observed Patients	Avg. Stay	Variance	Percentiles						
				10th	25th	50th	75th	90th	95th	99th
1. SINGLE DX										
0–19 Years	15	9.2	112	1	2	4	18	30	32	32
20–34	98	14.9	400	2	2	5	27	31	61	90
35–49	121	8.6	144	2	2	4	10	29	30	62
50–64	54	5.8	50	2	3	4	5	14	30	30
65+	9	16.1	208	4	4	6	30	37	37	37
2. MULTIPLE DX										
0–19 Years	553	11.2	167	2	3	5	14	41	42	42
20–34	4,698	6.2	52	1	2	4	7	14	22	31
35–49	9,213	5.4	30	2	2	4	6	11	15	30
50–64	7,480	5.8	35	2	3	4	7	11	15	30
65+	1,573	6.2	31	2	3	5	7	12	16	30
TOTAL SINGLE DX	297	10.4	222	1	2	4	14	30	34	90
TOTAL MULTIPLE DX	23,517	5.9	40	2	3	4	7	12	17	30
TOTAL										
0–19 Years	568	11.1	166	2	3	5	14	40	42	42
20–34	4,796	6.4	60	1	2	4	7	14	24	32
35–49	9,334	5.4	31	2	2	4	6	11	15	30
50–64	7,534	5.8	35	2	3	4	7	11	15	30
65+	1,582	6.3	33	2	3	5	7	12	16	30
GRAND TOTAL	23,814	5.9	42	2	3	4	7	12	17	31

94.61: ALCOHOL REHABILITATION

Type of Patients	Observed Patients	Avg. Stay	Variance	Percentiles						
				10th	25th	50th	75th	90th	95th	99th
1. SINGLE DX										
0–19 Years	1	32.0	0	32	32	32	32	32	32	32
20–34	15	37.5	679	14	18	30	59	90	90	90
35–49	17	25.1	317	7	13	28	30	62	>99	>99
50–64	2	9.5	39	5	5	14	14	14	14	14
65+	2	27.5	82	21	21	28	34	34	34	34
2. MULTIPLE DX										
0–19 Years	5	8.2	38	1	2	11	13	14	14	14
20–34	104	17.2	174	7	10	13	28	30	30	58
35–49	262	12.5	96	4	9	11	14	28	29	30
50–64	186	13.4	126	5	9	11	14	21	30	60
65+	50	12.6	48	4	9	13	14	21	30	33
TOTAL SINGLE DX	37	29.6	466	9	14	28	32	67	90	>99
TOTAL MULTIPLE DX	607	13.6	117	4	9	11	14	29	30	60
TOTAL										
0–19 Years	6	12.2	125	1	2	13	14	32	32	32
20–34	119	19.8	278	7	10	14	28	30	58	90
35–49	279	13.3	117	4	9	11	14	29	30	87
50–64	188	13.3	125	5	9	11	14	21	30	60
65+	52	13.2	56	4	10	13	14	21	30	34
GRAND TOTAL	644	14.5	150	5	9	11	14	29	30	87

94.62: ALCOHOL DETOXIFICATION

Type of Patients	Observed Patients	Avg. Stay	Variance	Percentiles						
				10th	25th	50th	75th	90th	95th	99th
1. SINGLE DX										
0–19 Years	2	2.5	4	1	1	1	4	4	4	4
20–34	22	3.4	2	1	2	4	4	5	6	6
35–49	61	3.0	3	1	1	3	4	5	5	9
50–64	34	3.7	1	2	3	4	4	5	6	6
65+	5	4.4	<1	4	4	4	4	6	6	6
2. MULTIPLE DX										
0–19 Years	61	3.4	14	1	1	2	4	7	7	21
20–34	1,767	3.6	11	1	2	3	4	6	8	17
35–49	5,756	4.2	14	1	2	3	5	7	10	19
50–64	4,798	4.8	25	2	3	4	6	9	12	24
65+	1,135	5.3	22	2	3	4	6	10	12	25
TOTAL SINGLE DX	124	3.3	2	1	2	3	4	5	6	7
TOTAL MULTIPLE DX	13,517	4.4	18	1	2	3	5	8	11	21
TOTAL										
0–19 Years	63	3.4	14	1	1	2	4	7	7	21
20–34	1,789	3.6	11	1	2	3	4	6	8	17
35–49	5,817	4.1	13	1	2	3	5	7	10	19
50–64	4,832	4.8	25	1	2	4	5	9	12	23
65+	1,140	5.3	22	2	3	4	6	10	12	25
GRAND TOTAL	13,641	4.4	18	1	2	3	5	8	11	21

94.63: ALCOHOL REHAB/DETOX

Type of Patients	Observed Patients	Avg. Stay	Variance	Percentiles						
				10th	25th	50th	75th	90th	95th	99th
1. SINGLE DX										
0–19 Years	1	12.0	0	12	12	12	12	12	12	12
20–34	8	26.3	296	4	14	29	31	61	61	61
35–49	14	17.1	213	3	5	14	26	30	55	55
50–64	6	12.4	189	1	4	5	30	30	30	30
65+	1	30.0	0	30	30	30	30	30	30	30
2. MULTIPLE DX										
0–19 Years	12	15.0	81	7	9	12	22	30	30	30
20–34	172	12.5	87	3	5	11	17	29	30	39
35–49	487	10.4	74	4	5	7	14	24	30	33
50–64	508	10.5	73	4	5	7	14	21	30	33
65+	143	11.5	72	4	5	8	15	21	30	41
TOTAL SINGLE DX	30	18.9	231	4	5	14	30	31	55	61
TOTAL MULTIPLE DX	1,322	10.9	75	3	5	8	14	22	30	34
TOTAL										
0–19 Years	13	14.8	75	7	9	12	21	30	30	30
20–34	180	13.2	103	3	5	12	17	30	30	58
35–49	501	10.5	78	3	5	7	14	24	30	35
50–64	514	10.5	74	4	5	7	14	21	30	33
65+	144	11.6	74	4	5	8	15	21	30	41
GRAND TOTAL	1,352	11.0	80	3	5	8	14	24	30	34

Western Region, October 2007–September 2008 Data, by Operation

94.64: DRUG REHABILITATION

Type of Patients	Observed Patients	Avg. Stay	Variance	Percentiles						
				10th	25th	50th	75th	90th	95th	99th
1. SINGLE DX										
0–19 Years	1	19.0	0	19	19	19	19	19	19	19
20–34	13	27.4	625	5	8	18	31	56	88	88
35–49	5	14.2	38	4	14	15	18	20	20	20
50–64	3	15.3	95	4	4	21	21	21	21	21
65+	0									
2. MULTIPLE DX										
0–19 Years	17	12.0	85	2	6	8	18	30	30	30
20–34	117	12.2	110	2	6	8	15	27	30	50
35–49	102	9.9	85	3	5	7	13	19	28	55
50–64	53	9.1	42	2	5	7	14	15	21	30
65+	4	5.8	8	4	4	5	5	10	10	10
TOTAL SINGLE DX	22	22.4	413	4	8	18	30	53	56	88
TOTAL MULTIPLE DX	293	10.7	87	2	5	7	14	22	30	55
TOTAL										
0–19 Years	18	12.4	82	2	6	8	19	30	30	30
20–34	130	13.7	178	2	6	8	19	30	35	60
35–49	107	10.1	83	3	5	7	14	19	28	55
50–64	56	9.4	45	2	5	7	14	20	21	30
65+	4	5.8	8	4	4	5	5	10	10	10
GRAND TOTAL	315	11.5	118	2	5	8	14	24	30	56

94.65: DRUG DETOXIFICATION

Type of Patients	Observed Patients	Avg. Stay	Variance	Percentiles						
				10th	25th	50th	75th	90th	95th	99th
1. SINGLE DX										
0–19 Years	7	3.0	1	1	2	3	4	4	4	4
20–34	33	2.8	3	1	1	2	4	5	6	7
35–49	18	3.0	8	1	1	2	3	10	10	10
50–64	7	1.9	<1	1	1	2	3	3	3	3
65+	0									
2. MULTIPLE DX										
0–19 Years	226	4.5	28	1	2	3	5	7	9	28
20–34	1,541	4.7	19	2	3	4	5	8	10	27
35–49	1,304	4.7	12	2	3	4	6	8	10	19
50–64	958	4.9	12	2	3	4	6	8	10	20
65+	151	5.7	15	2	3	5	7	10	14	18
TOTAL SINGLE DX	65	2.8	4	1	1	2	4	5	6	10
TOTAL MULTIPLE DX	4,180	4.8	16	2	3	4	6	8	10	23
TOTAL										
0–19 Years	233	4.4	27	1	2	3	5	7	9	28
20–34	1,574	4.6	19	2	3	4	5	8	10	27
35–49	1,322	4.7	12	2	3	4	6	8	10	19
50–64	965	4.9	12	2	3	4	6	8	10	20
65+	151	5.7	15	2	3	5	7	10	14	18
GRAND TOTAL	4,245	4.7	15	2	3	4	6	8	10	22

94.66: DRUG REHAB/DETOX

Type of Patients	Observed Patients	Avg. Stay	Variance	Percentiles						
				10th	25th	50th	75th	90th	95th	99th
1. SINGLE DX										
0–19 Years	2	24.0	72	18	18	24	30	30	30	30
20–34	7	23.8	90	4	19	29	30	30	30	30
35–49	6	12.5	112	4	5	9	21	30	30	30
50–64	2	17.0	332	4	4	17	30	30	30	30
65+	1	37.0	0	37	37	37	37	37	37	37
2. MULTIPLE DX										
0–19 Years	50	11.3	59	4	5	11	14	21	28	37
20–34	348	13.3	116	5	6	10	17	29	30	45
35–49	304	9.4	42	4	5	7	13	18	23	30
50–64	310	8.9	38	3	5	7	10	16	22	30
65+	29	8.6	29	4	5	7	10	15	15	30
TOTAL SINGLE DX	18	20.0	135	4	6	25	30	30	37	37
TOTAL MULTIPLE DX	1,041	10.6	70	4	5	8	14	21	29	35
TOTAL										
0–19 Years	52	11.8	64	4	5	12	15	21	30	37
20–34	355	13.5	117	5	6	11	17	29	30	45
35–49	310	9.4	44	4	5	7	13	19	24	30
50–64	312	8.9	39	3	5	7	10	16	22	30
65+	30	9.5	55	4	5	7	10	15	30	37
GRAND TOTAL	1,059	10.7	72	4	5	8	14	22	30	35

94.67: ALC/DRUG REHABILITATION

Type of Patients	Observed Patients	Avg. Stay	Variance	Percentiles						
				10th	25th	50th	75th	90th	95th	99th
1. SINGLE DX										
0–19 Years	0									
20–34	0									
35–49	0									
50–64	0									
65+										
2. MULTIPLE DX										
0–19 Years	81	36.1	111	21	32	42	42	42	42	42
20–34	102	17.0	90	5	9	14	28	29	30	30
35–49	93	15.8	123	3	8	14	21	30	30	61
50–64	36	15.1	68	5	10	14	19	27	30	42
65+	2	6.5	25	3	3	7	10	10	10	10
TOTAL SINGLE DX	0									
TOTAL MULTIPLE DX	314	21.3	178	4	11	19	30	42	42	42
TOTAL										
0–19 Years	81	36.1	111	21	32	42	42	42	42	42
20–34	102	17.0	90	5	9	14	28	29	30	30
35–49	93	15.8	123	3	8	14	21	30	30	61
50–64	36	15.1	68	5	10	14	19	27	30	42
65+	2	6.5	25	3	3	7	10	10	10	10
GRAND TOTAL	314	21.3	178	4	11	19	30	42	42	42

LOS by Diagnosis and Operation, Western Region, 45th Edition

Western Region, October 2007–September 2008 Data, by Operation

94.68: ALC/DRUG DETOXIFICATION

Type of Patients	Observed Patients	Avg. Stay	Variance	Percentiles						
				10th	25th	50th	75th	90th	95th	99th
1. SINGLE DX										
0–19 Years	0									
20–34	0									
35–49	0									
50–64	0									
65+	0									
2. MULTIPLE DX										
0–19 Years	41	5.1	19	1	3	4	6	8	13	21
20–34	386	4.7	18	1	2	4	6	8	11	28
35–49	622	4.7	17	2	3	4	5	8	11	23
50–64	402	4.8	10	2	3	4	6	8	10	17
65+	32	5.2	11	2	3	4	7	9	13	15
TOTAL SINGLE DX	0									
TOTAL MULTIPLE DX	1,483	4.7	15	2	3	4	6	8	11	21
TOTAL										
0–19 Years	41	5.1	19	1	3	4	6	8	13	21
20–34	386	4.7	18	1	2	4	6	8	11	28
35–49	622	4.7	17	2	3	4	5	8	11	23
50–64	402	4.8	10	2	3	4	6	8	10	17
65+	32	5.2	11	2	3	4	7	9	13	15
GRAND TOTAL	1,483	4.7	15	2	3	4	6	8	11	21

94.69: ALC/DRUG REHAB/DETOX

Type of Patients	Observed Patients	Avg. Stay	Variance	Percentiles						
				10th	25th	50th	75th	90th	95th	99th
1. SINGLE DX										
0–19 Years	1	1.0	0	1	1	1	1	1	1	1
20–34	0									
35–49	0									
50–64	0									
65+										
2. MULTIPLE DX										
0–19 Years	60	13.9	68	3	7	12	20	29	30	31
20–34	161	13.5	97	4	6	10	18	30	31	40
35–49	283	9.9	60	4	5	7	12	21	30	36
50–64	229	9.1	50	4	5	7	11	16	25	30
65+	27	8.0	21	4	5	7	8	14	18	24
TOTAL SINGLE DX	1	1.0	0	1	1	1	1	1	1	1
TOTAL MULTIPLE DX	760	10.7	67	4	5	8	14	23	30	37
TOTAL										
0–19 Years	61	13.6	70	3	7	12	20	27	30	31
20–34	161	13.5	97	4	6	10	18	30	31	40
35–49	283	9.9	60	3	5	7	12	21	30	36
50–64	229	9.1	50	4	5	7	11	16	25	30
65+	27	8.0	21	4	5	7	8	14	18	24
GRAND TOTAL	761	10.7	67	4	5	8	14	23	30	37

95.0: GEN/SUBJECTIVE EYE EXAM

Type of Patients	Observed Patients	Avg. Stay	Variance	Percentiles						
				10th	25th	50th	75th	90th	95th	99th
1. SINGLE DX										
0–19 Years	12	1.2	<1	1	1	1	1	2	2	2
20–34	0	1.0	0	1	1	1	1	1	1	1
35–49	0									
50–64	0									
65+										
2. MULTIPLE DX										
0–19 Years	61	4.4	98	1	1	2	4	6	19	55
20–34	4	2.0	2	1	1	1	3	5	5	5
35–49	4	2.5	<1	2	2	2	3	3	3	3
50–64	4	3.1	14	1	2	1	5	11	11	11
65+	4	1.0	0	1	1	1	1	1	1	1
TOTAL SINGLE DX	13	1.2	<1	1	1	1	1	2	2	2
TOTAL MULTIPLE DX	77	4.1	87	1	1	2	4	6	11	55
TOTAL										
0–19 Years	73	3.9	83	1	1	1	3	6	9	55
20–34	5	1.9	2	1	1	1	2	5	5	5
35–49	4	2.5	<1	2	2	2	3	3	3	3
50–64	4	3.1	14	1	2	1	5	11	11	11
65+	4	1.0	0	1	1	1	1	1	1	1
GRAND TOTAL	90	3.7	74	1	1	1	3	6	9	44

95.1: FORM & STRUCT EYE EXAM

Type of Patients	Observed Patients	Avg. Stay	Variance	Percentiles						
				10th	25th	50th	75th	90th	95th	99th
1. SINGLE DX										
0–19 Years	0									
20–34	0									
35–49	0									
50–64	0									
65+										
2. MULTIPLE DX										
0–19 Years	3	1.2	<1	1	1	1	1	2	2	2
20–34	5	3.0	4	1	2	2	4	6	6	6
35–49	1	5.0	0	5	5	5	5	5	5	5
50–64	2	5.0	2	4	4	6	6	6	6	6
65+	2	2.5	5	1	1	3	4	4	4	4
TOTAL SINGLE DX	0									
TOTAL MULTIPLE DX	13	2.8	4	1	1	2	4	6	6	6
TOTAL										
0–19 Years	3	1.2	<1	1	1	1	1	2	2	2
20–34	5	3.0	4	1	2	2	4	6	6	6
35–49	1	5.0	0	5	5	5	5	5	5	5
50–64	2	5.0	2	4	4	6	6	6	6	6
65+	2	2.5	5	1	1	3	4	4	4	4
GRAND TOTAL	13	2.8	4	1	1	2	4	6	6	6

LOS by Diagnosis and Operation, Western Region, 45th Edition

Western Region, October 2007–September 2008 Data, by Operation

95.2: OBJECTIVE FUNCT EYE TEST

Type of Patients	Observed Patients	Avg. Stay	Vari-ance	10th	25th	50th	75th	90th	95th	99th
1. SINGLE DX										
0–19 Years	0									
20–34	0									
35–49	0									
50–64	0									
65+	0									
2. MULTIPLE DX										
0–19 Years	2	5.7	<1	5	5	6	6	6	6	6
20–34	1	10.0	0	10	10	10	10	10	10	10
35–49	1	11.0	0	11	11	11	11	11	11	11
50–64	3	3.0	7	1	1	2	6	6	6	6
65+	0									
TOTAL SINGLE DX	0									
TOTAL MULTIPLE DX	7	5.9	12	1	2	6	10	11	11	11
TOTAL										
0–19 Years	2	5.7	<1	5	5	6	6	6	6	6
20–34	1	10.0	0	10	10	10	10	10	10	10
35–49	1	11.0	0	11	11	11	11	11	11	11
50–64	3	3.0	7	1	1	2	6	6	6	6
65+	0									
GRAND TOTAL	7	5.9	12	1	2	6	10	11	11	11

95.3: SPECIAL VISION SERVICES

Type of Patients	Observed Patients	Avg. Stay	Vari-ance	10th	25th	50th	75th	90th	95th	99th
1. SINGLE DX										
0–19 Years	0									
20–34	0									
35–49	0									
50–64	0									
65+	0									
2. MULTIPLE DX										
0–19 Years	0									
20–34	1	12.0	0	12	12	12	12	12	12	12
35–49	0									
50–64	0									
65+	0									
TOTAL SINGLE DX	0									
TOTAL MULTIPLE DX	1	12.0	0	12	12	12	12	12	12	12
TOTAL										
0–19 Years	0									
20–34	1	12.0	0	12	12	12	12	12	12	12
35–49	0									
50–64	0									
65+	0									
GRAND TOTAL	1	12.0	0	12	12	12	12	12	12	12

95.4: NONOP HEARING PROCEDURE

Type of Patients	Observed Patients	Avg. Stay	Vari-ance	10th	25th	50th	75th	90th	95th	99th
1. SINGLE DX										
0–19 Years	8,587	1.8	<1	1	1	2	2	3	3	4
20–34	0									
35–49	0									
50–64	0									
65+	0									
2. MULTIPLE DX										
0–19 Years	23,606	2.5	7	1	2	2	3	4	4	11
20–34	1	2.0	0	1	2	2	2	2	2	2
35–49	2	2.5	5	1	1	3	4	4	4	4
50–64	2	7.5	83	1	1	1	14	14	14	14
65+	0									
TOTAL SINGLE DX	8,587	1.8	<1	1	1	2	2	3	3	4
TOTAL MULTIPLE DX	23,611	2.5	7	1	2	2	3	4	4	11
TOTAL										
0–19 Years	32,193	2.3	5	1	1	2	3	4	4	9
20–34	1	2.0	0	2	2	2	2	2	2	2
35–49	2	2.5	5	1	1	3	4	4	4	4
50–64	2	7.5	83	1	1	1	14	14	14	14
65+	0									
GRAND TOTAL	32,198	2.3	5	1	1	2	3	4	4	9

95.41: AUDIOMETRY

Type of Patients	Observed Patients	Avg. Stay	Vari-ance	10th	25th	50th	75th	90th	95th	99th
1. SINGLE DX										
0–19 Years	1,651	1.9	<1	1	1	2	2	3	3	4
20–34	0									
35–49	0									
50–64	0									
65+	0									
2. MULTIPLE DX										
0–19 Years	6,355	2.5	9	1	2	2	3	4	4	14
20–34	1	2.0	0	2	2	2	2	2	2	2
35–49	1	4.0	0	4	4	4	4	4	4	4
50–64	1	14.0	0	14	14	14	14	14	14	14
65+	0									
TOTAL SINGLE DX	1,651	1.9	<1	1	1	2	2	3	3	4
TOTAL MULTIPLE DX	6,358	2.5	9	1	2	2	3	4	4	14
TOTAL										
0–19 Years	8,006	2.4	7	1	1	2	3	4	4	11
20–34	1	2.0	0	2	2	2	2	2	2	2
35–49	1	4.0	0	4	4	4	4	4	4	4
50–64	1	14.0	0	14	14	14	14	14	14	14
65+	0									
GRAND TOTAL	8,009	2.4	7	1	1	2	3	4	4	11

LOS by Diagnosis and Operation, Western Region, 45th Edition

Western Region, October 2007–September 2008 Data, by Operation

95.42: CLINICAL HEARING TEST

Type of Patients	Observed Patients	Avg. Stay	Variance	Percentiles						
				10th	25th	50th	75th	90th	95th	99th
1. SINGLE DX										
0–19 Years	15	1.5	<1	1	1	1	2	2	3	3
20–34	0									
35–49	0									
50–64	0									
65+	0									
2. MULTIPLE DX										
0–19 Years	213	2.1	1	1	1	2	2	3	4	6
20–34	0									
35–49	0									
50–64	0									
65+	0									
TOTAL SINGLE DX	15	1.5	<1	1	1	1	2	2	3	3
TOTAL MULTIPLE DX	213	2.1	1	1	1	2	2	3	4	6
TOTAL										
0–19 Years	228	2.0	1	1	1	2	2	3	3	6
20–34	0									
35–49	0									
50–64	0									
65+	0									
GRAND TOTAL	228	2.0	1	1	1	2	2	3	3	6

95.43: AUDIOLOGICAL EVALUATION

Type of Patients	Observed Patients	Avg. Stay	Variance	Percentiles						
				10th	25th	50th	75th	90th	95th	99th
1. SINGLE DX										
0–19 Years	764	1.7	<1	1	1	2	2	3	3	4
20–34	0									
35–49	0									
50–64	0									
65+	0									
2. MULTIPLE DX										
0–19 Years	1,211	2.5	12	1	1	2	2	4	7	17
20–34	0									
35–49	0									
50–64	1	1.0	0	1	1	1	1	1	1	1
65+	0									
TOTAL SINGLE DX	764	1.7	<1	1	1	2	2	3	3	4
TOTAL MULTIPLE DX	1,212	2.5	12	1	1	2	2	4	7	17
TOTAL										
0–19 Years	1,975	2.2	8	1	1	2	2	3	5	12
20–34	0									
35–49	0									
50–64	1	1.0	0	1	1	1	1	1	1	1
65+	0									
GRAND TOTAL	1,976	2.2	8	1	1	2	2	3	5	12

95.46: AUDITORY & VEST TEST NEC

Type of Patients	Observed Patients	Avg. Stay	Variance	Percentiles						
				10th	25th	50th	75th	90th	95th	99th
1. SINGLE DX										
0–19 Years	1,528	2.2	<1	1	2	2	2	3	3	4
20–34	0									
35–49	0									
50–64	0									
65+	0									
2. MULTIPLE DX										
0–19 Years	5,912	2.5	2	2	2	2	3	4	4	5
20–34	0									
35–49	0									
50–64	0									
65+	0									
TOTAL SINGLE DX	1,528	2.2	<1	1	2	2	2	3	3	4
TOTAL MULTIPLE DX	5,912	2.5	2	2	2	2	3	4	4	5
TOTAL										
0–19 Years	7,440	2.5	1	2	2	2	3	4	4	5
20–34	0									
35–49	0									
50–64	0									
65+	0									
GRAND TOTAL	7,440	2.5	1	2	2	2	3	4	4	5

95.47: HEARING EXAMINATION NOS

Type of Patients	Observed Patients	Avg. Stay	Variance	Percentiles						
				10th	25th	50th	75th	90th	95th	99th
1. SINGLE DX										
0–19 Years	4,620	1.7	<1	1	1	2	2	3	3	4
20–34	0									
35–49	0									
50–64	0									
65+	0									
2. MULTIPLE DX										
0–19 Years	9,892	2.4	8	1	1	2	3	4	4	12
20–34	0									
35–49	0									
50–64	0									
65+	0									
TOTAL SINGLE DX	4,620	1.7	<1	1	1	2	2	3	3	4
TOTAL MULTIPLE DX	9,892	2.4	8	1	1	2	3	4	4	12
TOTAL										
0–19 Years	14,512	2.2	5	1	1	2	2	3	4	10
20–34	0									
35–49	0									
50–64	0									
65+	0									
GRAND TOTAL	14,512	2.2	5	1	1	2	2	3	4	10

LOS by Diagnosis and Operation, Western Region, 45th Edition

Western Region, October 2007–September 2008 Data, by Operation

95.49: NONOP HEARING PX NEC

Type of Patients	Observed Patients	Avg. Stay	Variance	Percentiles						
				10th	25th	50th	75th	90th	95th	99th
1. SINGLE DX										
0–19 Years	9	1.7	<1	1	1	2	2	2	2	2
20–34	0									
35–49	0									
50–64	0									
65+	0									
2. MULTIPLE DX										
0–19 Years	23	2.2	1	1	2	2	2	4	4	5
20–34	0									
35–49	1	1.0	0	1	1	1	1	1	1	1
50–64	0									
65+	0									
TOTAL SINGLE DX	9	1.7	<1	1	1	2	2	2	2	2
TOTAL MULTIPLE DX	24	2.2	1	1	2	2	2	4	4	5
TOTAL										
0–19 Years	32	2.1	<1	1	1	2	2	4	4	5
20–34	0									
35–49	1	1.0	0	1	1	1	1	1	1	1
50–64	0									
65+	0									
GRAND TOTAL	33	2.0	<1	1	1	2	2	4	4	5

96.0: NONOP GI & RESP INTUB

Type of Patients	Observed Patients	Avg. Stay	Variance	Percentiles						
				10th	25th	50th	75th	90th	95th	99th
1. SINGLE DX										
0–19 Years	96	2.2	3	1	1	2	3	4	5	7
20–34	49	2.8	6	1	1	2	3	5	7	16
35–49	38	2.8	2	1	2	2	4	4	5	6
50–64	41	2.7	3	1	2	3	3	5	5	9
65+	19	3.4	4	1	2	3	4	6	10	10
2. MULTIPLE DX										
0–19 Years	5,926	15.7	448	1	2	6	22	54	74	>99
20–34	1,786	5.3	55	1	2	3	6	12	17	42
35–49	2,854	6.4	58	1	2	4	8	14	20	36
50–64	4,206	7.5	66	2	3	5	9	17	23	46
65+	5,422	7.6	48	2	3	5	10	16	21	32
TOTAL SINGLE DX	243	2.5	4	1	1	2	3	5	6	10
TOTAL MULTIPLE DX	20,194	9.8	196	1	2	5	11	24	43	86
TOTAL										
0–19 Years	6,022	15.5	444	1	2	5	21	53	73	>99
20–34	1,835	5.3	54	1	2	3	6	11	17	41
35–49	2,892	6.4	57	1	2	4	8	14	20	36
50–64	4,247	7.4	66	2	3	5	9	16	23	46
65+	5,441	7.6	48	2	3	5	10	16	21	32
GRAND TOTAL	20,437	9.7	194	1	2	5	10	23	43	86

96.04: INSERT ENDOTRACHEAL TUBE

Type of Patients	Observed Patients	Avg. Stay	Variance	Percentiles						
				10th	25th	50th	75th	90th	95th	99th
1. SINGLE DX										
0–19 Years	49	2.6	4	1	1	2	3	4	5	13
20–34	16	3.1	17	1	1	1	4	8	16	16
35–49	3	2.4	2	1	1	2	4	4	4	4
50–64	5	1.2	<1	1	1	1	1	2	2	2
65+	0									
2. MULTIPLE DX										
0–19 Years	4,735	18.6	509	1	3	8	30	59	80	>99
20–34	1,377	5.7	63	1	2	3	9	13	18	42
35–49	2,001	7.4	73	1	2	5	9	17	23	45
50–64	2,481	9.7	90	2	4	7	12	21	27	55
65+	2,505	10.6	66	3	5	9	14	21	25	39
TOTAL SINGLE DX	73	2.6	6	1	1	2	3	5	6	16
TOTAL MULTIPLE DX	13,099	12.5	266	2	3	7	15	34	54	97
TOTAL										
0–19 Years	4,784	18.4	506	1	3	8	30	59	79	>99
20–34	1,393	5.7	62	1	2	3	6	13	18	42
35–49	2,004	7.4	73	1	2	5	9	17	23	43
50–64	2,486	9.7	90	2	4	7	12	20	27	55
65+	2,505	10.6	66	3	5	9	14	21	25	39
GRAND TOTAL	13,172	12.5	265	1	3	7	15	34	54	97

96.05: RESP TRACT INTUB NEC

Type of Patients	Observed Patients	Avg. Stay	Variance	Percentiles						
				10th	25th	50th	75th	90th	95th	99th
1. SINGLE DX										
0–19 Years	15	2.1	2	1	1	2	2	5	6	6
20–34	0									
35–49	1	3.0	0	3	3	3	3	3	3	3
50–64	0									
65+	0									
2. MULTIPLE DX										
0–19 Years	714	3.8	35	1	2	2	3	7	12	25
20–34	16	8.0	194	1	3	4	8	11	64	64
35–49	34	6.2	28	1	3	6	9	17	17	18
50–64	67	7.6	34	1	3	6	11	14	19	29
65+	135	10.1	68	3	5	8	13	18	22	38
TOTAL SINGLE DX	16	2.1	2	1	1	2	3	5	6	6
TOTAL MULTIPLE DX	966	5.1	48	1	2	3	5	12	16	29
TOTAL										
0–19 Years	729	3.7	34	1	2	2	3	6	12	25
20–34	16	8.0	194	1	3	4	8	11	64	64
35–49	35	6.1	27	1	2	4	9	17	17	18
50–64	67	7.6	34	1	3	6	11	14	19	29
65+	135	10.1	68	3	5	8	13	18	22	38
GRAND TOTAL	982	5.1	47	1	2	3	5	12	16	29

LOS by Diagnosis and Operation, Western Region, 45th Edition

Western Region, October 2007–September 2008 Data, by Operation

96.07: INSERT GASTRIC TUBE NEC

Type of Patients	Observed Patients	Avg. Stay	Vari-ance	Percentiles						
				10th	25th	50th	75th	90th	95th	99th
1. SINGLE DX										
0–19 Years	32	1.7	2	1	1	1	2	3	4	7
20–34	32	2.6	1	2	2	2	3	3	5	6
35–49	33	2.8	2	1	2	3	4	4	5	6
50–64	33	2.7	2	1	2	2	3	4	5	9
65+	18	3.4	5	1	2	3	4	6	10	10
2. MULTIPLE DX										
0–19 Years	430	4.1	28	1	2	3	4	8	12	25
20–34	368	3.6	10	1	2	3	4	7	10	15
35–49	782	4.0	13	1	2	3	5	7	10	16
50–64	1,567	4.1	14	1	2	3	5	7	10	21
65+	2,588	4.7	13	2	2	4	6	9	12	18
TOTAL SINGLE DX	148	2.5	2	1	1	2	3	4	5	9
TOTAL MULTIPLE DX	5,735	4.3	14	1	2	3	5	8	11	18
TOTAL										
0–19 Years	462	3.9	26	1	2	3	4	8	12	25
20–34	400	3.5	9	1	2	3	4	6	9	15
35–49	815	4.0	13	1	2	3	5	7	10	15
50–64	1,600	4.1	14	1	2	3	5	7	10	20
65+	2,606	4.7	13	2	2	4	6	9	11	18
GRAND TOTAL	5,883	4.3	14	1	2	3	5	8	11	18

96.08: INSERT INTESTINAL TUBE

Type of Patients	Observed Patients	Avg. Stay	Vari-ance	Percentiles						
				10th	25th	50th	75th	90th	95th	99th
1. SINGLE DX										
0–19 Years	0									
20–34	1	1.0	0	1	1	1	1	1	1	1
35–49	1	2.0	0	2	2	2	2	2	2	2
50–64	3	5.0	4	3	3	5	7	7	7	7
65+	1	3.0	0	3	3	3	3	3	3	3
2. MULTIPLE DX										
0–19 Years	16	17.1	336	2	4	9	22	59	59	59
20–34	23	8.3	146	2	2	4	7	16	44	46
35–49	33	5.5	25	1	2	4	7	14	15	21
50–64	77	5.1	22	1	2	4	6	11	14	31
65+	140	6.9	36	2	3	5	8	15	19	34
TOTAL SINGLE DX	6	3.5	5	1	2	3	5	7	7	7
TOTAL MULTIPLE DX	289	7.6	85	2	3	5	8	16	22	59
TOTAL										
0–19 Years	16	17.1	336	2	4	9	22	59	59	59
20–34	24	8.0	142	2	2	4	6	16	44	46
35–49	34	5.4	24	1	2	3	7	14	15	21
50–64	80	5.1	21	1	2	4	7	10	13	31
65+	141	6.8	36	2	3	5	8	13	19	34
GRAND TOTAL	295	7.5	84	2	3	5	8	15	22	59

96.09: INSERT RECTAL TUBE

Type of Patients	Observed Patients	Avg. Stay	Vari-ance	Percentiles						
				10th	25th	50th	75th	90th	95th	99th
1. SINGLE DX										
0–19 Years	0									
20–34	0									
35–49	0									
50–64	0									
65+	0									
2. MULTIPLE DX										
0–19 Years	3	14.8	378	2	2	5	37	37	37	37
20–34	1	4.0	0	4	4	4	4	4	4	4
35–49	3	7.0	75	1	1	3	17	17	17	17
50–64	6	6.2	51	3	4	5	7	20	20	20
65+	45	6.6	15	3	4	6	8	11	15	19
TOTAL SINGLE DX	0									
TOTAL MULTIPLE DX	58	6.9	36	1	4	6	8	15	19	37
TOTAL										
0–19 Years	3	14.8	378	2	2	5	37	37	37	37
20–34	1	4.0	0	4	4	4	4	4	4	4
35–49	3	7.0	75	1	1	5	17	17	17	17
50–64	6	6.2	51	3	4	6	8	20	20	20
65+	45	6.6	15	3	4	6	8	11	15	19
GRAND TOTAL	58	6.9	36	1	4	6	8	15	19	37

96.1: OTHER NONOP INSERTION

Type of Patients	Observed Patients	Avg. Stay	Vari-ance	Percentiles						
				10th	25th	50th	75th	90th	95th	99th
1. SINGLE DX										
0–19 Years	0									
20–34	0									
35–49	0									
50–64	0									
65+	0									
2. MULTIPLE DX										
0–19 Years	3	3.8	12	1	1	5	8	8	8	8
20–34	7	2.5	2	1	1	2	4	4	4	4
35–49	10	3.3	2	2	2	3	3	5	7	7
50–64	7	2.0	1	1	1	2	3	4	4	4
65+	16	6.2	21	2	3	5	7	11	20	20
TOTAL SINGLE DX	0									
TOTAL MULTIPLE DX	43	4.0	12	1	2	3	5	8	10	20
TOTAL										
0–19 Years	3	3.8	12	1	1	5	8	8	8	8
20–34	7	2.5	2	1	1	2	4	4	4	4
35–49	10	3.3	2	2	2	3	3	5	7	7
50–64	7	2.0	1	1	1	2	3	4	4	4
65+	16	6.2	21	2	3	5	7	11	20	20
GRAND TOTAL	43	4.0	12	1	2	3	5	8	10	20

LOS by Diagnosis and Operation, Western Region, 45th Edition

Western Region, October 2007–September 2008 Data, by Operation

96.2: NONOP DILATION & MANIP

Type of Patients	Observed Patients	Avg. Stay	Vari-ance	Percentiles						
				10th	25th	50th	75th	90th	95th	99th
1. SINGLE DX										
0–19 Years	83	1.5	<1	1	1	1	2	3	3	5
20–34	5	1.8	<1	1	1	2	2	3	3	3
35–49	6	1.0	0	1	1	1	1	1	1	1
50–64	10	1.2	<1	1	1	1	1	2	2	2
65+	4	1.3	<1	1	1	1	1	2	2	2
2. MULTIPLE DX										
0–19 Years	88	2.6	9	1	1	2	3	5	7	14
20–34	23	3.8	13	1	1	3	5	6	11	16
35–49	64	3.4	24	1	1	2	4	6	12	34
50–64	119	2.9	8	1	1	2	4	6	9	13
65+	240	3.5	13	1	1	2	4	7	10	21
TOTAL SINGLE DX	**108**	**1.5**	**<1**	**1**	**1**	**1**	**2**	**3**	**3**	**5**
TOTAL MULTIPLE DX	**534**	**3.1**	**12**	**1**	**1**	**2**	**4**	**6**	**10**	**19**
TOTAL										
0–19 Years	171	2.0	5	1	1	1	2	4	5	11
20–34	28	3.4	11	1	1	2	4	6	11	16
35–49	70	3.2	22	1	1	2	4	6	12	34
50–64	129	2.7	8	1	1	2	3	6	8	13
65+	244	3.4	13	1	1	2	4	7	10	21
GRAND TOTAL	**642**	**2.7**	**10**	**1**	**1**	**2**	**3**	**5**	**7**	**17**

96.27: MANUAL REDUCTION HERNIA

Type of Patients	Observed Patients	Avg. Stay	Vari-ance	Percentiles						
				10th	25th	50th	75th	90th	95th	99th
1. SINGLE DX										
0–19 Years	5	1.0	0	1	1	1	1	1	1	1
20–34	2	1.5	<1	1	1	1	2	2	2	2
35–49	3	1.0	0	1	1	1	1	1	1	1
50–64	5	1.0	0	1	1	1	1	1	1	1
65+	2	1.0	0	1	1	1	1	1	1	1
2. MULTIPLE DX										
0–19 Years	20	3.6	40	1	1	2	3	5	10	32
20–34	3	1.7	1	1	1	1	3	3	3	3
35–49	33	2.2	6	1	1	1	2	4	5	14
50–64	75	2.6	5	1	1	2	4	6	8	12
65+	155	3.0	9	1	1	2	4	6	9	20
TOTAL SINGLE DX	**17**	**1.1**	**<1**	**1**	**1**	**1**	**1**	**1**	**1**	**2**
TOTAL MULTIPLE DX	**286**	**2.9**	**10**	**1**	**1**	**2**	**4**	**5**	**8**	**20**
TOTAL										
0–19 Years	25	3.0	31	1	1	1	3	4	10	32
20–34	5	1.6	<1	1	1	1	2	3	3	3
35–49	36	2.1	6	1	1	1	2	4	5	14
50–64	80	2.5	5	1	1	2	3	5	7	12
65+	157	3.0	9	1	1	2	4	6	9	20
GRAND TOTAL	**303**	**2.8**	**10**	**1**	**1**	**2**	**3**	**5**	**8**	**14**

96.29: ALIMENTARY INTUSS RED

Type of Patients	Observed Patients	Avg. Stay	Vari-ance	Percentiles						
				10th	25th	50th	75th	90th	95th	99th
1. SINGLE DX										
0–19 Years	76	1.5	<1	1	1	1	2	3	3	4
20–34	0									
35–49	0									
50–64	0									
65+	0									
2. MULTIPLE DX										
0–19 Years	38	1.8	1	1	1	1	2	3	4	5
20–34	1									
35–49	1	1.0	0	1	1	1	1	1	1	1
50–64	0									
65+	0									
TOTAL SINGLE DX	**76**	**1.5**	**<1**	**1**	**1**	**1**	**2**	**3**	**3**	**4**
TOTAL MULTIPLE DX	**39**	**1.8**	**1**	**1**	**1**	**1**	**2**	**3**	**4**	**5**
TOTAL										
0–19 Years	114	1.6	<1	1	1	1	2	3	4	4
20–34	0									
35–49	1	1.0	0	1	1	1	1	1	1	1
50–64	0									
65+	0									
GRAND TOTAL	**115**	**1.6**	**<1**	**1**	**1**	**1**	**2**	**3**	**4**	**4**

96.3: NONOP GI IRRIG/INSTILL

Type of Patients	Observed Patients	Avg. Stay	Vari-ance	Percentiles						
				10th	25th	50th	75th	90th	95th	99th
1. SINGLE DX										
0–19 Years	121	1.7	<1	1	1	1	2	3	3	4
20–34	3	1.7	<1	1	1	2	2	2	3	2
35–49	3	3.3	4	1	1	4	5	5	5	5
50–64	3	2.3	2	1	1	2	4	4	4	4
65+	1	2.0	0	2	2	2	2	2	2	2
2. MULTIPLE DX										
0–19 Years	1,021	6.3	71	1	2	3	7	16	22	41
20–34	134	2.8	17	1	1	2	3	5	7	11
35–49	105	3.0	9	1	1	2	4	6	8	14
50–64	121	3.8	13	1	2	3	4	8	11	16
65+	395	4.7	13	1	2	4	6	9	12	19
TOTAL SINGLE DX	**131**	**1.8**	**<1**	**1**	**1**	**1**	**2**	**3**	**3**	**5**
TOTAL MULTIPLE DX	**1,776**	**5.4**	**50**	**1**	**2**	**3**	**6**	**13**	**18**	**37**
TOTAL										
0–19 Years	1,142	5.7	64	1	2	3	6	14	20	41
20–34	137	2.7	17	1	1	2	3	5	7	11
35–49	108	3.0	9	1	1	2	4	6	8	14
50–64	124	3.8	13	1	2	3	4	8	11	16
65+	396	4.7	13	1	2	4	6	9	12	19
GRAND TOTAL	**1,907**	**5.1**	**47**	**1**	**2**	**3**	**6**	**12**	**17**	**36**

LOS by Diagnosis and Operation, Western Region, 45th Edition

Western Region, October 2007–September 2008 Data, by Operation

96.33: GASTRIC LAVAGE

Type of Patients	Observed Patients	Avg. Stay	Vari-ance	Percentiles						
				10th	25th	50th	75th	90th	95th	99th
1. SINGLE DX										
0–19 Years	86	2.1	<1	1	1	2	3	3	4	5
20–34	2	2.0	0	2	2	2	2	2	2	2
35–49	2	4.5	<1	4	4	5	5	5	5	5
50–64	1	4.0	0	4	4	4	4	4	4	4
65+	0									
2. MULTIPLE DX										
0–19 Years	579	2.6	6	1	1	2	3	4	5	9
20–34	96	2.6	22	1	1	2	3	4	6	45
35–49	69	2.8	5	1	1	2	4	6	8	11
50–64	56	3.8	15	1	2	3	4	7	10	25
65+	60	5.0	16	1	2	4	6	11	13	18
TOTAL SINGLE DX	91	2.2	1	1	1	2	3	3	4	5
TOTAL MULTIPLE DX	860	2.8	9	1	1	2	3	5	7	13
TOTAL										
0–19 Years	665	2.5	5	1	1	2	3	4	5	9
20–34	98	2.6	21	1	1	2	3	4	6	45
35–49	71	2.8	5	1	1	2	4	5	8	11
50–64	57	3.8	15	1	2	3	4	7	10	25
65+	60	5.0	16	1	2	4	6	11	13	18
GRAND TOTAL	951	2.8	9	1	1	2	3	4	7	13

96.35: GASTRIC GAVAGE

Type of Patients	Observed Patients	Avg. Stay	Vari-ance	Percentiles						
				10th	25th	50th	75th	90th	95th	99th
1. SINGLE DX										
0–19 Years	2	1.5	<1	1	1	2	2	2	2	2
20–34	0									
35–49	0									
50–64	0									
65+	0									
2. MULTIPLE DX										
0–19 Years	343	13.3	112	3	6	11	17	25	34	54
20–34	2	1.0	0	1	1	1	1	1	1	1
35–49	6	4.2	25	1	1	3	4	14	14	14
50–64	1	3.0	0	3	3	3	3	3	3	3
65+	0									
TOTAL SINGLE DX	2	1.5	<1	1	1	2	2	2	2	2
TOTAL MULTIPLE DX	352	13.1	112	3	6	11	17	24	34	54
TOTAL										
0–19 Years	345	13.2	113	3	6	11	17	24	34	54
20–34	2	1.0	0	1	1	1	1	1	1	1
35–49	6	4.2	25	1	1	3	4	14	14	14
50–64	1	3.0	0	3	3	3	3	3	3	3
65+	0									
GRAND TOTAL	354	13.0	113	3	6	11	17	24	34	54

96.38: IMPACTED FECES REMOVAL

Type of Patients	Observed Patients	Avg. Stay	Vari-ance	Percentiles						
				10th	25th	50th	75th	90th	95th	99th
1. SINGLE DX										
0–19 Years	18	1.3	<1	1	1	1	2	2	3	3
20–34	1	1.0	0	1	1	1	1	1	1	1
35–49	0									
50–64	2	1.5	<1	1	1	2	2	2	2	2
65+	1	2.0	0	2	2	2	2	2	2	2
2. MULTIPLE DX										
0–19 Years	76	3.2	13	1	1	2	4	6	8	26
20–34	25	3.7	7	1	1	3	6	7	8	9
35–49	24	3.3	19	1	2	2	4	6	6	22
50–64	48	3.4	8	1	2	3	4	9	10	13
65+	304	4.7	13	2	2	4	6	9	11	19
TOTAL SINGLE DX	22	1.4	<1	1	1	1	2	2	3	3
TOTAL MULTIPLE DX	477	4.1	13	1	2	3	5	8	11	20
TOTAL										
0–19 Years	94	2.9	11	1	1	2	3	5	6	17
20–34	26	3.6	7	1	1	2	6	7	8	9
35–49	24	3.3	19	1	2	3	4	6	6	22
50–64	50	3.4	8	1	2	3	4	6	10	13
65+	305	4.7	13	1	2	4	6	9	11	19
GRAND TOTAL	499	3.9	13	1	2	3	5	8	10	19

96.4: DIGEST/GU IRRIG/INSTILL

Type of Patients	Observed Patients	Avg. Stay	Vari-ance	Percentiles						
				10th	25th	50th	75th	90th	95th	99th
1. SINGLE DX										
0–19 Years	103	1.6	<1	1	1	1	2	3	3	4
20–34	612	1.5	<1	1	1	1	2	2	3	4
35–49	103	1.3	<1	1	1	1	2	2	3	3
50–64	11	1.6	<1	1	1	1	2	3	3	3
65+	4	2.0	<1			2	3	3	3	3
2. MULTIPLE DX										
0–19 Years	191	2.2	1	1	1	2	3	4	4	6
20–34	1,195	2.1	2	1	1	2	3	3	4	8
35–49	328	1.9	2	1	1	2	2	3	4	7
50–64	124	3.2	11	1	1	2	3	7	9	16
65+	418	3.8	11	1	2	3	5	7	11	15
TOTAL SINGLE DX	833	1.5	<1	1	1	1	2	2	3	4
TOTAL MULTIPLE DX	2,256	2.4	5	1	1	2	3	4	6	12
TOTAL										
0–19 Years	294	2.0	1	1	1	2	3	3	4	6
20–34	1,807	1.9	2	1	1	1	2	3	3	6
35–49	431	1.7	2	1	1	2	2	3	3	6
50–64	135	3.1	10	1	1	2	3	7	9	16
65+	422	3.7	11	1	2	3	5	7	11	15
GRAND TOTAL	3,089	2.2	4	1	1	2	3	4	5	11

LOS by Diagnosis and Operation, Western Region, 45th Edition

Western Region, October 2007–September 2008 Data, by Operation

96.48: INDWELL CATH IRRIG NEC

Type of Patients	Observed Patients	Avg. Stay	Variance	Percentiles						
				10th	25th	50th	75th	90th	95th	99th
1. SINGLE DX										
0–19 Years	1	7.0	0	7	7	7	7	7	7	7
20–34	0									
35–49	0									
50–64	2	1.5	<1	1	1	2	2	2	2	2
65+	2	2.0	0	2	2	2	2	2	2	2
2. MULTIPLE DX										
0–19 Years	0									
20–34	5	3.6	8	1	2	2	5	8	8	8
35–49	7	4.8	30	1	1	1	11	14	14	14
50–64	68	3.4	14	1	2	2	3	8	10	24
65+	224	3.6	11	1	2	3	4	7	9	18
TOTAL SINGLE DX	5	2.8	6	1	2	2	2	7	7	7
TOTAL MULTIPLE DX	304	3.6	12	1	2	3	4	7	10	18
TOTAL										
0–19 Years	1	7.0	0	7	7	7	7	7	7	7
20–34	5	3.6	8	1	2	2	5	8	8	8
35–49	7	4.8	30	1	1	1	11	14	14	14
50–64	70	3.4	14	1	1	2	3	7	10	24
65+	226	3.6	11	1	2	3	4	7	9	18
GRAND TOTAL	309	3.6	12	1	2	3	4	7	10	18

96.5: OTHER NONOP IRRIG/CLEAN

Type of Patients	Observed Patients	Avg. Stay	Variance	Percentiles						
				10th	25th	50th	75th	90th	95th	99th
1. SINGLE DX										
0–19 Years	4	2.0	<1	1	1	2	2	3	3	3
20–34	3	1.0	0	1	1	1	1	1	1	1
35–49	2	3.5	12	1	1	1	6	6	6	6
50–64	3	2.7	8	1	1	1	3	6	6	6
65+	1	3.0	0	3	3	3	3	3	3	3
2. MULTIPLE DX										
0–19 Years	97	4.9	35	1	2	3	7	14	30	>99
20–34	55	5.6	31	1	2	4	7	11	20	28
35–49	109	6.0	30	2	2	4	7	14	18	25
50–64	126	7.8	57	1	3	5	10	18	24	32
65+	410	8.4	54	2	4	7	11	16	21	30
TOTAL SINGLE DX	13	2.2	3	1	1	1	3	6	6	6
TOTAL MULTIPLE DX	797	7.2	48	1	3	5	10	15	21	33
TOTAL										
0–19 Years	101	4.8	35	1	2	3	7	14	25	>99
20–34	58	5.4	31	1	2	4	7	11	20	28
35–49	111	6.0	30	2	2	4	7	13	18	25
50–64	129	7.6	56	1	3	5	10	18	24	32
65+	411	8.3	54	2	4	7	11	16	21	30
GRAND TOTAL	810	7.1	48	1	3	5	10	15	21	33

96.49: GU INSTILLATION NEC

Type of Patients	Observed Patients	Avg. Stay	Variance	Percentiles						
				10th	25th	50th	75th	90th	95th	99th
1. SINGLE DX										
0–19 Years	102	1.5	<1	1	1	1	2	3	3	3
20–34	611	1.5	<1	1	1	1	2	2	3	4
35–49	103	1.3	<1	1	1	1	2	2	3	3
50–64	9	1.7	<1	1	1	1	2	3	3	3
65+	2	2.0	2	1	1	2	3	3	3	3
2. MULTIPLE DX										
0–19 Years	184	2.2	1	1	1	2	3	4	4	6
20–34	1,185	2.0	2	1	1	2	3	3	4	6
35–49	319	1.8	2	1	1	1	2	3	4	6
50–64	46	2.6	5	1	1	2	3	4	7	14
65+	169	3.8	11	1	1	3	5	8	11	15
TOTAL SINGLE DX	827	1.5	<1	1	1	1	2	2	3	4
TOTAL MULTIPLE DX	1,903	2.2	3	1	1	2	3	4	5	9
TOTAL										
0–19 Years	286	2.0	1	1	1	2	2	3	4	6
20–34	1,796	1.8	1	1	1	2	2	3	3	5
35–49	422	1.7	1	1	1	1	2	3	4	6
50–64	55	2.4	5	1	1	2	3	4	7	14
65+	171	3.8	11	1	1	3	5	8	11	15
GRAND TOTAL	2,730	2.0	2	1	1	2	2	3	4	8

96.52: IRRIGATION OF EAR

Type of Patients	Observed Patients	Avg. Stay	Variance	Percentiles						
				10th	25th	50th	75th	90th	95th	99th
1. SINGLE DX										
0–19 Years	1	3.0	0	3	3	3	3	3	3	3
20–34	0									
35–49	0									
50–64	0									
65+	0									
2. MULTIPLE DX										
0–19 Years	28	3.1	6	1	2	2	4	7	7	10
20–34	4	3.3	5	1	3	4	6	6	6	6
35–49	7	7.9	124	2	1	4	6	33	33	33
50–64	11	4.0	28	1	1	1	6	11	17	17
65+	51	4.7	23	1	2	3	6	12	18	20
TOTAL SINGLE DX	1	3.0	0	3	3	3	3	3	3	3
TOTAL MULTIPLE DX	101	4.2	22	1	2	3	5	9	14	20
TOTAL										
0–19 Years	29	3.1	5	1	2	2	4	7	7	10
20–34	5	3.3	5	1	2	4	6	6	6	6
35–49	7	7.9	124	2	3	4	6	33	33	33
50–64	11	4.0	28	1	1	1	6	11	17	17
65+	51	4.7	23	1	2	3	6	12	18	20
GRAND TOTAL	102	4.2	22	1	2	3	5	9	14	20

LOS by Diagnosis and Operation, Western Region, 45th Edition

Western Region, October 2007–September 2008 Data, by Operation

96.56: BRONCH/TRACH LAVAGE NEC

Type of Patients	Observed Patients	Avg. Stay	Vari-ance	Percentiles						
				10th	25th	50th	75th	90th	95th	99th
1. SINGLE DX										
0–19 Years	0									
20–34	0									
35–49	0									
50–64	0									
65+	0									
2. MULTIPLE DX										
0–19 Years	16	13.9	74	5	9	14	30	>99	>99	>99
20–34	19	8.9	53	2	4	7	11	24	28	28
35–49	48	8.6	33	2	4	7	11	18	22	25
50–64	64	9.9	50	3	5	8	12	20	25	32
65+	298	9.7	61	3	5	8	13	18	22	34
TOTAL SINGLE DX	0									
TOTAL MULTIPLE DX	445	9.8	58	3	5	8	13	20	25	92
TOTAL										
0–19 Years	16	13.9	74	5	9	14	30	>99	>99	>99
20–34	19	8.9	53	2	4	7	11	24	28	28
35–49	48	8.6	33	2	4	7	11	18	22	25
50–64	64	9.9	50	3	5	8	12	20	25	32
65+	298	9.7	61	3	5	8	13	18	22	34
GRAND TOTAL	445	9.8	58	3	5	8	13	20	25	92

96.59: WOUND IRRIGATION NEC

Type of Patients	Observed Patients	Avg. Stay	Vari-ance	Percentiles						
				10th	25th	50th	75th	90th	95th	99th
1. SINGLE DX										
0–19 Years	3	1.7	<1	1	1	2	2	2	2	2
20–34	3	1.0	0	1	1	1	1	1	1	1
35–49	2	3.5	12	1	1	1	6	6	6	6
50–64	3	2.7	8	1	1	1	6	6	6	6
65+	1	3.0	0	3	3	3	3	3	3	3
2. MULTIPLE DX										
0–19 Years	33	2.5	3	1	1	2	3	5	5	10
20–34	30	3.9	14	1	1	3	5	7	8	20
35–49	44	3.6	6	1	2	3	5	7	9	10
50–64	33	3.6	6	1	1	3	4	7	9	10
65+	30	3.9	9	1	2	3	5	8	10	12
TOTAL SINGLE DX	12	2.2	4	1	1	1	3	6	6	6
TOTAL MULTIPLE DX	170	3.5	7	1	2	3	4	7	9	12
TOTAL										
0–19 Years	36	2.5	3	1	1	2	3	5	5	10
20–34	33	3.6	14	1	1	3	4	7	8	20
35–49	46	3.6	6	1	2	3	5	7	9	10
50–64	36	3.6	6	1	1	3	4	7	9	10
65+	31	3.8	8	1	2	3	5	8	10	12
GRAND TOTAL	182	3.4	7	1	1	3	4	7	9	12

96.6: ENTERAL NUTRITION

Type of Patients	Observed Patients	Avg. Stay	Vari-ance	Percentiles						
				10th	25th	50th	75th	90th	95th	99th
1. SINGLE DX										
0–19 Years	8	4.2	5	3	3	3	5	9	10	10
20–34	3	2.3	<1	3	2	2	3	3	3	3
35–49	2	6.0	18	3	3	6	9	9	9	9
50–64	1	3.0	0	3	3	3	3	3	3	3
65+	0									
2. MULTIPLE DX										
0–19 Years	1,385	7.1	57	1	3	5	9	16	20	35
20–34	161	8.3	68	2	3	5	10	19	24	53
35–49	207	8.0	64	2	3	6	10	17	27	52
50–64	494	8.5	57	2	4	7	10	16	23	41
65+	1,631	7.9	41	3	4	6	10	15	19	32
TOTAL SINGLE DX	14	4.0	5	2	3	3	5	9	9	10
TOTAL MULTIPLE DX	3,878	7.5	54	2	3	5	9	16	21	35
TOTAL										
0–19 Years	1,393	7.1	57	1	3	5	9	16	20	35
20–34	164	8.2	67	2	3	5	10	19	24	53
35–49	209	8.0	64	2	3	6	10	17	27	52
50–64	495	8.5	57	2	4	7	10	16	23	41
65+	1,631	7.9	41	3	4	6	10	15	19	32
GRAND TOTAL	3,892	7.5	53	2	3	5	9	16	21	35

96.7: CONT MECH VENT NEC

Type of Patients	Observed Patients	Avg. Stay	Vari-ance	Percentiles						
				10th	25th	50th	75th	90th	95th	99th
1. SINGLE DX										
0–19 Years	60	3.1	4	1	1	3	4	6	7	11
20–34	17	3.2	7	1	1	2	3	8	8	8
35–49	10	2.5	6	1	1	2	5	7	7	7
50–64	4	6.7	47	1	1	2	8	16	16	16
65+	5	7.8	49	2	3	3	15	16	16	16
2. MULTIPLE DX										
0–19 Years	6,400	17.0	379	2	4	10	22	49	68	>99
20–34	3,648	6.7	72	1	2	4	8	15	22	39
35–49	6,311	8.9	79	3	5	6	12	19	25	44
50–64	10,821	10.9	86	3	5	8	14	21	28	50
65+	16,535	11.0	68	4	6	9	14	21	26	42
TOTAL SINGLE DX	96	3.3	8	1	1	3	4	7	8	16
TOTAL MULTIPLE DX	43,715	11.6	149	2	4	8	14	24	35	75
TOTAL										
0–19 Years	6,460	16.9	377	2	4	10	22	49	68	>99
20–34	3,665	6.7	71	1	2	4	8	15	22	39
35–49	6,321	8.9	79	3	5	6	12	19	25	44
50–64	10,825	10.9	86	3	5	8	14	21	28	50
65+	16,540	11.0	68	4	6	9	14	21	26	42
GRAND TOTAL	43,811	11.6	148	2	4	8	14	24	35	75

LOS by Diagnosis and Operation, Western Region, 45th Edition

96.71: CONT MECH VENT-<96 HOURS

Type of Patients	Observed Patients	Avg. Stay	Vari-ance	Percentiles						
				10th	25th	50th	75th	90th	95th	99th
1. SINGLE DX										
0–19 Years	56	2.8	3	1	1	2	4	5	6	8
20–34	17	3.2	7	1	1	2	3	8	8	8
35–49	10	2.5	6	1	1	1	5	8	7	7
50–64	4	6.7	47	1	1	2	8	16	16	16
65+	4	5.7	38	2	2	3	3	15	15	15
2. MULTIPLE DX										
0–19 Years	4,457	13.0	289	1	3	6	15	38	54	80
20–34	2,859	4.3	23	1	2	3	5	9	11	24
35–49	4,298	5.7	31	1	2	4	7	11	15	28
50–64	6,584	7.4	39	2	4	6	9	14	17	31
65+	9,786	8.1	33	3	4	7	10	15	18	29
TOTAL SINGLE DX	91	3.0	6	1	1	2	4	6	7	15
TOTAL MULTIPLE DX	27,984	8.3	96	2	3	6	10	16	24	57
TOTAL										
0–19 Years	4,513	12.8	287	1	3	6	14	38	54	80
20–34	2,876	4.3	23	1	2	3	5	9	11	24
35–49	4,308	5.7	31	1	2	4	7	11	15	27
50–64	6,588	7.4	39	2	4	6	9	14	17	31
65+	9,790	8.1	33	3	4	7	10	15	18	29
GRAND TOTAL	28,075	8.3	96	2	3	6	10	16	24	57

96.72: CONT MECH VENT->95 HOURS

Type of Patients	Observed Patients	Avg. Stay	Vari-ance	Percentiles						
				10th	25th	50th	75th	90th	95th	99th
1. SINGLE DX										
0–19 Years	4	7.1	4	4	7	7	7	11	11	11
20–34	0									
35–49	0									
50–64	0									
65+	1	16.0	0	16	16	16	16	16	16	16
2. MULTIPLE DX										
0–19 Years	1,929	24.7	459	7	11	17	34	68	88	>99
20–34	780	15.4	150	5	8	12	18	28	37	84
35–49	2,006	15.9	111	6	9	13	19	28	35	62
50–64	4,218	16.3	111	7	10	14	20	29	36	62
65+	6,711	15.3	88	6	9	13	19	26	32	51
TOTAL SINGLE DX	5	8.2	13	4	7	7	7	16	16	16
TOTAL MULTIPLE DX	15,644	17.5	187	6	9	14	21	32	48	95
TOTAL										
0–19 Years	1,933	24.6	458	7	11	17	34	68	88	>99
20–34	780	15.4	150	5	8	12	18	28	37	84
35–49	2,006	15.9	111	6	9	13	19	28	35	62
50–64	4,218	16.3	111	7	10	14	20	29	36	62
65+	6,712	15.3	88	6	9	13	19	26	32	51
GRAND TOTAL	15,649	17.5	187	6	9	14	21	32	48	95

97.0: GI APPLIANCE REPLACEMENT

Type of Patients	Observed Patients	Avg. Stay	Vari-ance	Percentiles						
				10th	25th	50th	75th	90th	95th	99th
1. SINGLE DX										
0–19 Years	3	1.0	0	1	1	1	1	1	1	1
20–34	1	4.0	0	4	4	4	4	4	4	4
35–49	4	1.5	<1	1	1	1	2	2	2	2
50–64	6	1.3	<1	1	1	2	2	2	2	2
65+	1	2.0	0	2	2	2	2	2	2	2
2. MULTIPLE DX										
0–19 Years	310	7.3	103	1	2	3	9	17	22	53
20–34	142	6.3	58	1	2	4	8	13	19	46
35–49	248	6.8	64	2	2	5	8	13	17	50
50–64	505	5.5	29	1	2	4	7	11	16	30
65+	1,328	6.2	34	2	3	5	8	12	16	30
TOTAL SINGLE DX	15	1.5	<1	1	1	1	2	2	4	4
TOTAL MULTIPLE DX	2,533	6.4	52	1	2	4	8	13	18	42
TOTAL										
0–19 Years	313	7.3	102	1	2	3	9	17	22	53
20–34	143	6.3	58	1	2	4	8	13	19	46
35–49	252	6.7	64	2	2	5	8	13	17	50
50–64	511	5.5	29	1	2	4	7	10	16	30
65+	1,329	6.2	33	2	3	5	8	12	16	30
GRAND TOTAL	2,548	6.4	52	1	2	4	8	13	18	42

97.02: REPL GASTROSTOMY TUBE

Type of Patients	Observed Patients	Avg. Stay	Vari-ance	Percentiles						
				10th	25th	50th	75th	90th	95th	99th
1. SINGLE DX										
0–19 Years	2	1.0	0	1	1	1	1	1	1	1
20–34	0									
35–49	0									
50–64	1	1.0	0	1	1	1	1	1	1	1
65+	0									
2. MULTIPLE DX										
0–19 Years	224	7.5	101	1	2	4	9	18	21	45
20–34	84	7.3	71	1	2	4	9	17	21	57
35–49	148	7.1	54	2	3	5	8	14	18	37
50–64	268	6.0	32	1	3	4	8	11	17	31
65+	971	6.5	34	2	3	5	8	12	17	30
TOTAL SINGLE DX	3	1.0	0	1	1	1	1	1	1	1
TOTAL MULTIPLE DX	1,695	6.7	53	1	3	5	8	14	19	40
TOTAL										
0–19 Years	226	7.5	101	1	2	4	9	18	21	45
20–34	84	7.3	71	1	2	4	9	17	21	57
35–49	148	7.1	54	2	3	5	9	14	18	37
50–64	269	6.0	32	1	3	4	8	11	17	31
65+	971	6.5	34	2	3	5	8	12	17	30
GRAND TOTAL	1,698	6.7	53	1	3	5	8	14	19	40

LOS by Diagnosis and Operation, Western Region, 45th Edition

Western Region, October 2007–September 2008 Data, by Operation

97.03: REPL SMALL INTEST TUBE

Type of Patients	Observed Patients	Avg. Stay	Vari-ance	Percentiles						
				10th	25th	50th	75th	90th	95th	99th
1. SINGLE DX										
0–19 Years	1	1.0	0	1	1	1	1	1	1	1
20–34	0									
35–49	0									
50–64	1	1.0	0	1	1	1	1	1	1	1
65+	0									
2. MULTIPLE DX										
0–19 Years	59	7.9	132	1	1	3	9	16	25	61
20–34	24	5.3	78	1	2	4	6	6	7	46
35–49	39	6.3	21	1	3	5	7	11	15	23
50–64	61	5.6	34	1	2	4	7	11	18	31
65+	112	6.6	49	2	3	5	8	13	18	44
TOTAL SINGLE DX	2	1.0	0	1	1	1	1	1	1	1
TOTAL MULTIPLE DX	295	6.8	77	1	2	4	8	15	22	53
TOTAL										
0–19 Years	60	7.8	131	1	1	3	9	16	25	61
20–34	24	5.3	78	1	2	4	6	6	7	46
35–49	39	6.3	21	1	3	5	9	11	15	23
50–64	62	5.6	34	1	2	4	7	11	18	31
65+	112	6.6	49	2	3	5	8	13	18	44
GRAND TOTAL	297	6.8	77	1	2	4	8	15	22	53

97.1: REPL MS APPLIANCE

Type of Patients	Observed Patients	Avg. Stay	Vari-ance	Percentiles						
				10th	25th	50th	75th	90th	95th	99th
1. SINGLE DX										
0–19 Years	4	7.1	182	1	1	1	1	31	31	31
20–34	2	2.5	<1	2	2	3	3	3	3	3
35–49	0									
50–64	1	4.0	0	4	4	4	4	4	4	4
65+	0									
2. MULTIPLE DX										
0–19 Years	16	3.6	10	1	1	1	7	9	9	9
20–34	8	4.4	42	1	1	2	3	20	20	20
35–49	20	4.1	9	1	3	4	5	11	12	12
50–64	17	5.3	56	1	2	4	5	9	33	33
65+	28	4.6	7	2	3	4	5	8	10	14
TOTAL SINGLE DX	7	5.6	108	1	1	2	4	31	31	31
TOTAL MULTIPLE DX	89	4.3	18	1	1	3	5	9	10	20
TOTAL										
0–19 Years	20	4.0	28	1	1	1	7	9	9	31
20–34	10	4.0	33	1	1	2	3	20	20	20
35–49	20	4.1	9	1	3	4	5	11	12	12
50–64	18	5.2	52	1	2	4	5	9	33	33
65+	28	4.6	7	2	3	4	5	8	10	14
GRAND TOTAL	96	4.4	23	1	1	3	5	9	11	31

97.05: REPL PANC/BILIARY STENT

Type of Patients	Observed Patients	Avg. Stay	Vari-ance	Percentiles						
				10th	25th	50th	75th	90th	95th	99th
1. SINGLE DX										
0–19 Years	0									
20–34	1	4.0	0	4	4	4	4	4	4	4
35–49	4	1.5	<1	1	1	1	2	2	2	2
50–64	4	1.5	<1	1	1	1	2	2	2	2
65+	1	2.0	0	2	2	2	2	2	2	2
2. MULTIPLE DX										
0–19 Years	15	4.4	27	1	1	2	4	15	15	15
20–34	33	4.4	6	2	2	4	6	8	10	10
35–49	59	6.7	122	1	2	4	6	11	50	57
50–64	170	4.7	22	1	2	4	5	9	13	30
65+	228	4.9	22	1	2	3	6	9	14	26
TOTAL SINGLE DX	10	1.8	<1	1	1	2	2	4	4	4
TOTAL MULTIPLE DX	505	5.0	33	1	2	4	6	9	14	31
TOTAL										
0–19 Years	15	4.4	27	1	1	2	4	15	15	15
20–34	34	4.4	6	2	2	4	6	8	10	10
35–49	63	6.3	116	1	2	3	6	9	17	57
50–64	174	4.7	22	1	2	4	5	9	13	30
65+	229	4.9	22	1	2	3	6	9	14	26
GRAND TOTAL	515	4.9	32	1	2	3	6	9	14	31

97.2: OTHER NONOP REPLACEMENT

Type of Patients	Observed Patients	Avg. Stay	Vari-ance	Percentiles						
				10th	25th	50th	75th	90th	95th	99th
1. SINGLE DX										
0–19 Years	1	3.0	0	3	3	3	3	3	3	3
20–34	0									
35–49	1	6.0	0	6	6	6	6	6	6	6
50–64	0									
65+	3	3.3	<1	3	3	3	4	4	4	4
2. MULTIPLE DX										
0–19 Years	41	15.4	325	1	2	9	24	53	53	79
20–34	18	10.1	287	1	2	5	9	25	73	73
35–49	63	5.9	57	1	2	4	6	11	16	37
50–64	121	6.8	99	1	2	4	8	15	19	36
65+	127	7.4	48	2	3	5	10	16	22	30
TOTAL SINGLE DX	5	3.7	1	3	3	3	4	6	6	6
TOTAL MULTIPLE DX	370	8.4	130	1	2	5	9	19	28	56
TOTAL										
0–19 Years	42	15.1	320	1	2	8	19	53	53	79
20–34	18	10.1	287	1	2	5	9	25	73	73
35–49	64	5.9	56	1	1	5	6	11	16	37
50–64	121	6.8	99	1	2	4	8	15	19	36
65+	130	7.3	48	2	3	5	10	16	22	30
GRAND TOTAL	375	8.3	128	1	2	5	9	19	28	56

LOS by Diagnosis and Operation, Western Region, 45th Edition

Western Region, October 2007–September 2008 Data, by Operation

97.23: REPL TRACH TUBE

Type of Patients	Observed Patients	Avg. Stay	Variance	10th	25th	50th	75th	90th	95th	99th
1. SINGLE DX										
0–19 Years	0									
20–34	0									
35–49	0									
50–64	0									
65+	1	3.0	0	3	3	3	3	3	3	3
2. MULTIPLE DX										
0–19 Years	41	15.4	325	1	2	9	24	53	53	79
20–34	11	14.9	420	3	3	8	19	25	73	73
35–49	53	6.1	64	1	1	4	6	11	33	37
50–64	87	7.0	126	1	2	4	7	18	20	92
65+	90	7.3	48	2	3	6	8	15	21	42
TOTAL SINGLE DX	1	3.0	0	3	3	3	3	3	3	3
TOTAL MULTIPLE DX	282	9.0	155	1	2	5	10	20	30	56
TOTAL										
0–19 Years	41	15.4	325	1	2	9	24	53	53	79
20–34	11	14.9	420	3	3	8	19	25	73	73
35–49	53	6.1	64	1	1	4	6	11	33	37
50–64	87	7.0	126	1	2	4	7	18	20	92
65+	91	7.2	48	2	3	6	8	15	21	42
GRAND TOTAL	283	9.0	155	1	2	5	9	20	30	56

97.3: RMVL THER DEV-HEAD/NECK

Type of Patients	Observed Patients	Avg. Stay	Variance	10th	25th	50th	75th	90th	95th	99th
1. SINGLE DX										
0–19 Years	7	2.2	1	1	1	3	3	3	4	4
20–34	1	2.0	0	2	2	2	2	2	2	2
35–49	2	1.5	<1	1	1	1	2	2	2	2
50–64	0									
65+	0									
2. MULTIPLE DX										
0–19 Years	45	1.7	2	1	1	1	2	2	3	10
20–34	19	7.2	56	1	2	4	12	22	24	24
35–49	25	7.6	121	2	2	7	7	17	31	51
50–64	28	7.5	79	1	1	3	11	18	19	42
65+	50	5.2	20	2	2	3	8	12	13	22
TOTAL SINGLE DX	10	2.1	1	1	1	2	3	3	4	4
TOTAL MULTIPLE DX	167	4.4	40	1	2	2	5	11	16	31
TOTAL										
0–19 Years	52	1.8	2	1	1	1	2	3	4	10
20–34	20	7.0	55	1	2	4	12	22	24	24
35–49	27	7.2	114	1	2	3	7	17	31	51
50–64	28	7.5	79	1	1	3	11	18	19	42
65+	50	5.2	20	2	2	3	8	12	13	22
GRAND TOTAL	177	4.3	37	1	1	2	4	11	16	31

97.37: RMVL TRACHEOSTOMY TUBE

Type of Patients	Observed Patients	Avg. Stay	Variance	10th	25th	50th	75th	90th	95th	99th
1. SINGLE DX										
0–19 Years	1	1.0	0	1	1	1	1	1	1	1
20–34	1	2.0	0	2	2	2	2	2	2	2
35–49	1	1.0	0	1	1	1	1	1	1	1
50–64	0									
65+	0									
2. MULTIPLE DX										
0–19 Years	30	1.6	2	1	1	1	2	2	5	10
20–34	5	6.9	77	1	1	4	6	22	22	22
35–49	11	8.4	76	2	2	6	10	17	31	31
50–64	15	10.8	118	1	2	11	16	19	42	42
65+	13	4.7	17	1	2	4	6	12	13	13
TOTAL SINGLE DX	3	1.3	<1	1	1	1	2	2	2	2
TOTAL MULTIPLE DX	74	4.0	39	1	1	2	4	11	17	31
TOTAL										
0–19 Years	31	1.6	2	1	1	1	2	2	5	10
20–34	6	6.1	66	1	1	4	6	22	22	22
35–49	12	7.8	73	2	2	5	10	17	31	31
50–64	15	10.8	118	1	2	11	16	19	42	42
65+	13	4.7	17	1	2	4	6	12	13	13
GRAND TOTAL	77	4.0	38	1	1	2	4	11	17	31

97.4: RMVL THOR THER DEVICE

Type of Patients	Observed Patients	Avg. Stay	Variance	10th	25th	50th	75th	90th	95th	99th
1. SINGLE DX										
0–19 Years	0									
20–34	1	2.0	0	2	2	2	2	2	2	2
35–49	1	1.0	0	1	1	1	1	1	1	1
50–64	0									
65+	0									
2. MULTIPLE DX										
0–19 Years	65	10.0	82	3	5	8	13	17	28	54
20–34	52	4.7	8	2	3	4	6	8	10	15
35–49	96	6.5	25	2	3	5	9	12	14	32
50–64	133	6.0	19	2	3	5	7	11	13	23
65+	133	6.2	21	2	3	5	7	13	16	23
TOTAL SINGLE DX	2	1.5	<1	1	1	1	2	2	2	2
TOTAL MULTIPLE DX	479	7.1	41	2	3	5	9	14	17	32
TOTAL										
0–19 Years	65	10.0	82	3	5	8	13	17	28	54
20–34	53	4.7	8	2	3	4	6	8	10	15
35–49	97	6.4	25	1	3	5	9	12	14	32
50–64	133	6.0	19	2	3	5	7	11	13	23
65+	133	6.2	21	2	3	5	7	13	16	23
GRAND TOTAL	481	7.1	41	2	3	5	9	14	17	32

LOS by Diagnosis and Operation, Western Region, 45th Edition

Western Region, October 2007–September 2008 Data, by Operation

97.49: RMVL DEV FROM THORAX NEC

Type of Patients	Observed Patients	Avg. Stay	Vari-ance	10th	25th	50th	75th	90th	95th	99th
1. SINGLE DX										
0–19 Years	0									
20–34	0									
35–49	0									
50–64	0									
65+	0									
2. MULTIPLE DX										
0–19 Years	61	10.2	84	3	5	8	14	17	28	54
20–34	47	5.0	8	2	3	4	6	9	10	15
35–49	87	6.2	20	2	3	5	9	12	14	26
50–64	124	6.1	20	2	3	5	8	11	13	23
65+	105	6.3	23	2	3	5	7	14	17	23
TOTAL SINGLE DX	0									
TOTAL MULTIPLE DX	424	7.3	43	2	3	6	9	14	17	29
TOTAL										
0–19 Years	61	10.2	84	3	5	8	14	17	28	54
20–34	47	5.0	8	2	3	4	6	9	10	15
35–49	87	6.2	20	2	3	5	9	12	14	26
50–64	124	6.1	20	2	3	5	8	11	13	23
65+	105	6.3	23	2	3	5	7	14	17	23
GRAND TOTAL	424	7.3	43	2	3	6	9	14	17	29

97.51: RMVL GASTROSTOMY TUBE

Type of Patients	Observed Patients	Avg. Stay	Vari-ance	10th	25th	50th	75th	90th	95th	99th
1. SINGLE DX										
0–19 Years	0									
20–34	1	1.0	0	1	1	1	1	1	1	1
35–49	0									
50–64	0									
65+	0									
2. MULTIPLE DX										
0–19 Years	18	6.5	143	1	1	2	7	14	37	53
20–34	21	12.8	163	2	6	9	17	29	39	55
35–49	40	13.3	146	3	4	9	21	34	39	49
50–64	92	11.9	259	2	3	6	13	33	46	>99
65+	128	8.3	65	2	3	6	10	17	26	34
TOTAL SINGLE DX	1	1.0	0	1	1	1	1	1	1	1
TOTAL MULTIPLE DX	299	10.0	151	1	3	6	11	26	35	56
TOTAL										
0–19 Years	18	6.5	143	1	1	2	7	14	37	53
20–34	22	12.3	162	1	6	9	14	29	39	55
35–49	40	13.3	146	3	4	9	21	34	39	49
50–64	92	11.9	259	2	3	6	13	33	46	>99
65+	128	8.3	65	2	3	6	10	17	26	34
GRAND TOTAL	300	10.0	151	1	3	6	11	26	35	56

97.5: NONOP RMVL GI THER DEV

Type of Patients	Observed Patients	Avg. Stay	Vari-ance	10th	25th	50th	75th	90th	95th	99th
1. SINGLE DX										
0–19 Years	0									
20–34	4	3.3	7	1	1	3	7	7	7	7
35–49	0									
50–64	1	2.0	0	2	2	2	2	2	2	2
65+	0									
2. MULTIPLE DX										
0–19 Years	29	5.3	93	1	1	2	5	10	25	53
20–34	46	8.1	106	1	2	4	9	18	29	55
35–49	69	10.3	132	1	2	5	14	29	35	49
50–64	171	9.0	193	1	2	5	9	21	39	99
65+	185	7.3	51	2	3	6	9	14	19	34
TOTAL SINGLE DX	5	3.0	6	1	2	2	3	7	7	7
TOTAL MULTIPLE DX	500	8.0	118	1	2	4	9	18	31	55
TOTAL										
0–19 Years	29	5.3	93	1	1	2	5	10	25	53
20–34	50	7.7	100	1	2	4	9	18	29	55
35–49	69	10.3	132	2	3	5	14	29	35	49
50–64	172	8.9	193	1	2	5	9	21	39	99
65+	185	7.3	51	2	3	6	9	14	19	34
GRAND TOTAL	505	8.0	117	1	2	4	9	18	31	55

97.55: RMVL BILIARY/LIVER TUBE

Type of Patients	Observed Patients	Avg. Stay	Vari-ance	10th	25th	50th	75th	90th	95th	99th
1. SINGLE DX										
0–19 Years	0									
20–34	2	2.5	<1	2	2	3	3	3	3	3
35–49	0									
50–64	0									
65+	0									
2. MULTIPLE DX										
0–19 Years	5	1.2	<1	1	1	1	1	2	2	2
20–34	20	3.0	3	2	2	3	3	5	7	7
35–49	19	6.4	109	1	1	3	6	13	48	48
50–64	59	3.9	16	1	1	2	5	10	15	20
65+	46	4.9	12	1	2	4	7	10	12	13
TOTAL SINGLE DX	2	2.5	<1	2	2	3	3	3	3	3
TOTAL MULTIPLE DX	149	4.3	25	1	2	3	6	9	13	20
TOTAL										
0–19 Years	5	1.2	<1	1	1	3	1	2	2	2
20–34	22	3.0	2	2	2	3	3	5	6	7
35–49	19	6.4	109	1	1	3	6	13	48	48
50–64	59	3.9	16	1	1	2	5	10	15	20
65+	46	4.9	12	1	2	4	7	10	12	13
GRAND TOTAL	151	4.3	25	1	2	3	6	9	13	20

LOS by Diagnosis and Operation, Western Region, 45th Edition

Western Region, October 2007–September 2008 Data, by Operation

97.6: NONOP RMVL URIN THER DEV

Type of Patients	Observed Patients	Avg. Stay	Variance	10th	25th	50th	75th	90th	95th	99th
1. SINGLE DX										
0–19 Years	1	2.0	0	2	2	2	2	2	2	2
20–34	2	1.0	0	1	1	1	1	1	1	1
35–49	4	2.3	<1	1	2	3	3	3	3	3
50–64	2	2.0	2	1	1	1	3	3	3	3
65+	2	1.3	<1	1	1	1	2	2	2	2
2. MULTIPLE DX										
0–19 Years	35	3.4	9	1	2	3	4	6	6	25
20–34	103	4.5	63	1	2	3	4	8	9	18
35–49	108	4.0	10	1	2	3	5	9	11	13
50–64	148	5.8	28	1	2	5	7	11	16	27
65+	152	5.8	27	1	2	4	8	11	16	26
TOTAL SINGLE DX	11	1.8	<1	1	1	2	2	3	3	3
TOTAL MULTIPLE DX	546	4.9	29	1	2	4	6	10	13	26
TOTAL										
0–19 Years	36	3.4	9	1	2	3	4	6	6	25
20–34	105	4.5	62	1	2	3	4	8	9	18
35–49	112	4.0	10	1	2	3	5	8	11	13
50–64	150	5.8	28	1	2	4	7	11	16	27
65+	154	5.7	26	1	2	4	8	11	16	26
GRAND TOTAL	557	4.9	28	1	2	3	6	9	13	26

97.7: RMVL THER DEV GENIT SYST

Type of Patients	Observed Patients	Avg. Stay	Variance	10th	25th	50th	75th	90th	95th	99th
1. SINGLE DX										
0–19 Years	2	1.7	1	1	1	1	3	3	3	3
20–34	9	2.0	1	1	1	2	3	4	4	4
35–49	4	3.3	11	1	1	3	8	8	8	8
50–64	1	1.0	0	1	1	1	1	1	1	1
65+	0									
2. MULTIPLE DX										
0–19 Years	10	2.3	1	1	2	2	3	4	4	4
20–34	98	2.5	3	1	1	2	3	4	6	9
35–49	33	4.3	9	2	3	3	5	7	11	15
50–64	10	3.0	3	1	2	3	4	6	6	6
65+	18	5.5	22	1	2	3	7	13	18	18
TOTAL SINGLE DX	16	2.2	3	1	1	1	3	4	8	8
TOTAL MULTIPLE DX	169	3.2	7	1	2	3	4	6	8	15
TOTAL										
0–19 Years	12	2.2	1	1	1	2	3	4	4	4
20–34	107	2.5	2	1	1	2	3	4	5	8
35–49	37	4.2	9	1	3	3	5	8	11	15
50–64	11	2.8	3	1	2	3	4	5	6	6
65+	18	5.5	22	1	2	3	7	13	18	18
GRAND TOTAL	185	3.1	6	1	1	3	4	6	8	15

97.62: RMVL URETERAL DRAIN

Type of Patients	Observed Patients	Avg. Stay	Variance	10th	25th	50th	75th	90th	95th	99th
1. SINGLE DX										
0–19 Years	1	2.0	0	2	2	2	2	2	2	2
20–34	2	1.0	0	1	1	1	1	1	1	1
35–49	4	2.3	<1	1	2	3	3	3	3	3
50–64	2	2.0	2	1	1	1	3	3	3	3
65+	0									
2. MULTIPLE DX										
0–19 Years	28	3.3	3	1	2	3	4	6	6	9
20–34	91	3.2	4	1	2	2	4	6	8	9
35–49	93	4.0	10	1	2	3	5	8	11	16
50–64	107	6.0	30	1	3	5	7	11	16	27
65+	104	5.9	23	1	2	4	8	11	16	23
TOTAL SINGLE DX	9	1.9	<1	1	1	2	3	3	3	3
TOTAL MULTIPLE DX	423	4.6	17	1	2	3	6	9	11	26
TOTAL										
0–19 Years	29	3.3	3	1	2	3	4	6	6	9
20–34	93	3.1	4	1	2	2	4	6	8	9
35–49	97	3.9	9	1	2	3	5	8	11	16
50–64	109	5.9	30	1	3	5	7	11	16	27
65+	104	5.9	23	1	2	5	8	11	12	23
GRAND TOTAL	432	4.6	17	1	2	3	6	9	11	26

97.71: REMOVAL IUD

Type of Patients	Observed Patients	Avg. Stay	Variance	10th	25th	50th	75th	90th	95th	99th
1. SINGLE DX										
0–19 Years	2	1.7	1	1	1	1	3	3	3	3
20–34	8	2.1	1	1	1	2	3	4	4	4
35–49	4	3.3	11	1	1	3	8	8	8	8
50–64	1	1.0	0	1	1	1	1	1	1	1
65+	0									
2. MULTIPLE DX										
0–19 Years	10	2.3	1	1	2	2	3	4	4	4
20–34	96	2.5	3	1	1	2	3	4	6	9
35–49	32	4.4	9	2	3	3	5	7	11	15
50–64	8	3.1	3	1	2	3	5	6	6	6
65+	0									
TOTAL SINGLE DX	15	2.3	3	1	1	2	3	4	8	8
TOTAL MULTIPLE DX	146	3.0	4	1	2	3	4	5	7	11
TOTAL										
0–19 Years	12	2.2	1	1	1	2	3	4	4	4
20–34	104	2.5	2	1	1	2	3	4	5	8
35–49	36	4.3	9	1	3	3	5	8	11	15
50–64	9	2.9	3	1	2	3	3	6	6	6
65+	0									
GRAND TOTAL	161	2.9	4	1	1	2	3	5	7	11

LOS by Diagnosis and Operation, Western Region, 45th Edition

Western Region, October 2007–September 2008 Data, by Operation

97.8: OTH NONOP RMVL THER DEV

Type of Patients	Observed Patients	Avg. Stay	Vari-ance	Percentiles						
				10th	25th	50th	75th	90th	95th	99th
1. SINGLE DX										
0–19 Years	1	4.0	0	4	4	4	4	4	4	4
20–34	1	3.0	0	3	3	3	3	3	3	3
35–49	3	2.3	2	1	1	2	3	4	4	4
50–64	2	1.5	<1	1	1	2	2	2	2	2
65+	0									
2. MULTIPLE DX										
0–19 Years	29	7.1	63	1	2	3	9	14	31	31
20–34	28	5.4	22	1	2	4	8	15	16	16
35–49	50	4.2	10	1	2	3	6	9	11	14
50–64	62	6.3	40	2	2	4	7	18	21	30
65+	75	5.3	21	1	3	4	6	10	15	25
TOTAL SINGLE DX	7	2.4	2	1	1	2	4	4	4	4
TOTAL MULTIPLE DX	244	5.7	33	1	2	4	7	14	18	31
TOTAL										
0–19 Years	30	7.0	62	1	2	3	9	14	31	31
20–34	29	5.3	22	1	2	3	8	15	16	16
35–49	53	4.1	10	1	2	3	6	7	11	14
50–64	64	6.1	39	2	2	4	7	18	21	30
65+	75	5.3	21	1	3	4	6	10	15	25
GRAND TOTAL	251	5.6	32	1	2	3	7	14	18	31

97.89: RMVL THERAPEUTIC DEV NEC

Type of Patients	Observed Patients	Avg. Stay	Vari-ance	Percentiles						
				10th	25th	50th	75th	90th	95th	99th
1. SINGLE DX										
0–19 Years	1	4.0	0	4	4	4	4	4	4	4
20–34	0									
35–49	1	1.0	0	1	1	1	1	1	1	1
50–64	0									
65+	0									
2. MULTIPLE DX										
0–19 Years	9	6.6	23	3	3	5	14	14	14	14
20–34	11	4.1	17	1	1	3	4	8	15	15
35–49	25	3.9	7	1	2	3	6	7	9	10
50–64	23	5.0	25	2	2	3	6	11	14	22
65+	31	4.7	19	2	3	3	5	8	10	25
TOTAL SINGLE DX	2	2.5	4	1	1	1	4	4	4	4
TOTAL MULTIPLE DX	99	4.8	18	1	2	3	6	10	14	22
TOTAL										
0–19 Years	10	6.5	22	3	3	5	14	14	14	14
20–34	11	4.1	17	1	1	3	4	8	15	15
35–49	26	3.8	7	1	2	3	6	7	9	10
50–64	23	5.0	25	2	2	3	6	11	14	22
65+	31	4.7	19	2	3	3	5	8	10	25
GRAND TOTAL	101	4.7	18	1	2	3	6	10	14	22

98.0: RMVL INTRALUM GI FB

Type of Patients	Observed Patients	Avg. Stay	Vari-ance	Percentiles						
				10th	25th	50th	75th	90th	95th	99th
1. SINGLE DX										
0–19 Years	161	1.1	<1	1	1	1	1	1	2	2
20–34	14	1.0	0	1	1	1	1	1	1	1
35–49	18	1.3	<1	1	1	1	1	2	3	3
50–64	13	1.1	<1	1	1	1	1	1	2	2
65+	0									
2. MULTIPLE DX										
0–19 Years	92	2.1	6	1	1	1	2	6	7	13
20–34	36	2.6	9	1	1	1	3	5	9	16
35–49	81	2.7	14	1	1	1	3	6	9	20
50–64	71	2.1	3	1	1	2	3	4	6	9
65+	129	3.4	14	1	1	2	4	9	11	17
TOTAL SINGLE DX	206	1.1	<1	1	1	1	1	1	2	2
TOTAL MULTIPLE DX	409	2.5	9	1	1	1	3	6	9	16
TOTAL										
0–19 Years	253	1.4	2	1	1	1	1	2	3	9
20–34	50	2.2	7	1	1	1	2	5	6	16
35–49	99	2.4	11	1	1	1	2	6	9	20
50–64	84	1.9	3	1	1	2	2	4	5	9
65+	129	3.4	14	1	1	2	4	9	11	17
GRAND TOTAL	615	1.9	6	1	1	1	2	3	6	13

98.02: RMVL INTRALUM ESOPH FB

Type of Patients	Observed Patients	Avg. Stay	Vari-ance	Percentiles						
				10th	25th	50th	75th	90th	95th	99th
1. SINGLE DX										
0–19 Years	153	1.1	<1	1	1	1	1	1	2	2
20–34	1	1.0	0	1	1	1	1	1	1	1
35–49	4	1.8	<1	1	1	2	2	3	3	3
50–64	1	1.0	0	1	1	1	1	1	1	1
65+	0									
2. MULTIPLE DX										
0–19 Years	85	2.0	6	1	1	1	2	6	7	13
20–34	12	2.9	18	1	1	1	3	4	16	16
35–49	31	3.1	21	1	1	1	2	7	17	20
50–64	46	1.9	2	1	1	1	2	4	5	8
65+	114	3.3	13	1	1	2	4	9	11	17
TOTAL SINGLE DX	159	1.1	<1	1	1	1	1	1	2	2
TOTAL MULTIPLE DX	288	2.5	9	1	1	1	2	6	9	16
TOTAL										
0–19 Years	238	1.4	2	1	1	1	1	2	3	9
20–34	13	2.8	17	1	1	1	3	4	16	16
35–49	35	3.0	19	1	1	1	3	7	17	20
50–64	47	1.9	2	1	1	1	2	4	5	8
65+	114	3.3	13	1	1	2	4	9	11	17
GRAND TOTAL	447	1.8	5	1	1	1	1	3	6	13

LOS by Diagnosis and Operation, Western Region, 45th Edition

Western Region, October 2007–September 2008 Data, by Operation

98.1: RMVL INTRALUM FB NEC

Type of Patients	Observed Patients	Avg. Stay	Variance	10th	25th	50th	75th	90th	95th	99th
1. SINGLE DX										
0–19 Years	63	1.2	<1	1	1	1	1	2	2	2
20–34	4	1.3	<1	1	1	1	2	2	2	2
35–49	4	1.3	<1	1	1	1	1	2	2	2
50–64	2	1.0	0	1	1	1	1	1	1	1
65+	0									
2. MULTIPLE DX										
0–19 Years	85	2.2	3	1	1	2	3	4	5	8
20–34	31	2.2	3	1	1	2	3	4	9	>99
35–49	39	5.6	118	1	1	2	5	9	46	53
50–64	34	3.0	25	1	1	1	4	5	11	28
65+	62	4.1	11	1	1	3	5	9	10	15
TOTAL SINGLE DX	73	1.2	<1	1	1	1	1	2	2	2
TOTAL MULTIPLE DX	251	3.0	21	1	1	2	3	6	9	28
TOTAL										
0–19 Years	148	1.7	2	1	1	1	2	3	4	8
20–34	35	2.1	2	1	1	2	3	4	9	>99
35–49	43	5.2	108	1	1	2	5	7	18	53
50–64	36	2.9	23	1	1	1	3	5	11	28
65+	62	4.1	11	1	1	3	5	9	10	15
GRAND TOTAL	324	2.5	15	1	1	1	3	5	8	18

98.2: RMVL OTH FB W/O INC

Type of Patients	Observed Patients	Avg. Stay	Variance	10th	25th	50th	75th	90th	95th	99th
1. SINGLE DX										
0–19 Years	10	1.4	2	1	1	1	1	2	7	7
20–34	9	1.2	<1	1	1	1	1	2	2	2
35–49	4	1.0	0	1	1	1	1	1	1	1
50–64	0									
65+	0									
2. MULTIPLE DX										
0–19 Years	33	4.0	53	1	1	2	4	8	8	45
20–34	46	2.7	8	1	1	2	3	5	7	16
35–49	27	2.7	6	1	1	2	4	7	8	8
50–64	25	8.0	137	1	1	3	8	21	41	44
65+	31	3.2	5	1	1	3	5	6	6	10
TOTAL SINGLE DX	23	1.3	1	1	1	1	1	2	2	7
TOTAL MULTIPLE DX	162	3.9	39	1	1	2	4	8	10	44
TOTAL										
0–19 Years	43	3.1	37	1	1	2	2	7	8	45
20–34	55	2.4	7	1	1	1	3	5	7	16
35–49	31	2.5	6	1	1	1	4	7	8	8
50–64	25	8.0	137	1	1	3	8	21	41	44
65+	31	3.2	5	1	1	3	5	6	6	10
GRAND TOTAL	185	3.5	33	1	1	2	4	7	9	44

98.15: RMVL INTRALUM TRACH FB

Type of Patients	Observed Patients	Avg. Stay	Variance	10th	25th	50th	75th	90th	95th	99th
1. SINGLE DX										
0–19 Years	34	1.2	<1	1	1	1	1	2	2	2
20–34	0									
35–49	0									
50–64	1	1.0	0	1	1	1	1	1	1	1
65+	0									
2. MULTIPLE DX										
0–19 Years	44	2.3	3	1	1	2	3	4	5	8
20–34	3	2.5	<1	1	2	3	3	3	3	3
35–49	5	5.2	8	2	3	5	7	9	9	9
50–64	9	2.1	2	1	1	1	4	4	4	4
65+	20	4.7	15	1	1	4	9	10	12	12
TOTAL SINGLE DX	35	1.2	<1	1	1	1	1	2	2	2
TOTAL MULTIPLE DX	81	2.7	5	1	1	2	3	5	8	10
TOTAL										
0–19 Years	78	1.8	2	1	1	1	2	4	4	8
20–34	3	2.5	<1	1	2	3	3	3	3	3
35–49	5	5.2	8	2	3	5	7	9	9	9
50–64	10	2.0	2	1	1	1	4	4	4	4
65+	20	4.7	15	1	1	4	9	10	12	12
GRAND TOTAL	116	2.1	4	1	1	1	3	4	8	9

98.5: ESWL

Type of Patients	Observed Patients	Avg. Stay	Variance	10th	25th	50th	75th	90th	95th	99th
1. SINGLE DX										
0–19 Years	2	1.5	<1	1	1	2	2	2	2	2
20–34	22	1.9	<1	1	1	2	2	3	4	4
35–49	20	1.6	<1	1	1	1	2	3	3	3
50–64	18	1.5	<1	1	1	1	2	3	4	4
65+	4	2.3	2	1	2	2	4	4	4	4
2. MULTIPLE DX										
0–19 Years	22	2.2	3	1	1	2	2	5	6	7
20–34	143	2.7	8	1	1	2	3	5	6	15
35–49	264	2.9	6	1	1	2	4	6	7	12
50–64	257	2.9	16	1	1	2	4	5	7	14
65+	229	3.7	11	1	2	3	5	8	11	14
TOTAL SINGLE DX	66	1.7	<1	1	1	1	2	3	4	4
TOTAL MULTIPLE DX	915	3.1	10	1	1	2	4	6	8	14
TOTAL										
0–19 Years	24	2.2	3	1	1	2	2	5	6	7
20–34	165	2.6	7	1	1	2	3	5	6	15
35–49	284	2.9	6	1	1	2	3	6	7	12
50–64	275	2.8	15	1	2	3	3	5	6	14
65+	233	3.7	11	1	2	3	5	8	11	14
GRAND TOTAL	981	3.0	10	1	1	2	4	6	8	14

LOS by Diagnosis and Operation, Western Region, 45th Edition

Western Region, October 2007–September 2008 Data, by Operation

98.51: RENAL/URETER/BLAD ESWL

Type of Patients	Observed Patients	Avg. Stay	Variance	10th	25th	50th	75th	90th	95th	99th
1. SINGLE DX										
0–19 Years	2	1.5	<1	1	1	2	2	2	2	2
20–34	22	1.9	<1	1	1	2	2	3	4	4
35–49	20	1.6	<1	1	1	1	2	2	3	3
50–64	18	1.5	<1	1	1	1	2	3	4	4
65+	4	2.3	2	1	2	2	4	4	4	4
2. MULTIPLE DX										
0–19 Years	21	2.2	3	1	1	2	3	5	6	7
20–34	143	2.7	8	1	1	2	3	5	6	15
35–49	261	3.0	6	1	1	2	4	6	7	12
50–64	250	2.9	16	1	1	2	4	5	6	11
65+	228	3.7	11	2	2	3	5	8	11	14
TOTAL SINGLE DX	66	1.7	<1	1	1	1	2	3	4	4
TOTAL MULTIPLE DX	903	3.1	10	1	1	2	4	6	8	14
TOTAL										
0–19 Years	23	2.2	3	1	1	2	2	5	6	7
20–34	165	2.6	7	1	1	2	3	5	6	15
35–49	281	2.9	6	1	1	2	3	6	7	12
50–64	268	2.8	15	1	1	2	3	5	6	11
65+	232	3.7	10	1	2	3	5	8	11	14
GRAND TOTAL	969	3.0	10	1	1	2	4	6	8	14

99.0: BLOOD TRANSFUSION

Type of Patients	Observed Patients	Avg. Stay	Variance	10th	25th	50th	75th	90th	95th	99th
1. SINGLE DX										
0–19 Years	245	2.6	5	1	1	2	3	5	7	11
20–34	140	2.8	6	1	1	2	4	5	8	11
35–49	130	2.1	5	1	1	1	2	4	7	12
50–64	86	1.7	2	1	1	1	2	4	5	8
65+	149	1.3	<1	1	1	1	1	2	3	6
2. MULTIPLE DX										
0–19 Years	3,543	5.6	48	1	2	4	7	12	16	37
20–34	4,772	4.6	27	1	2	3	6	9	13	27
35–49	10,469	4.4	23	1	2	3	5	9	12	23
50–64	18,906	5.0	25	1	2	4	6	10	13	25
65+	61,290	5.0	18	1	2	4	6	10	13	21
TOTAL SINGLE DX	750	2.3	4	1	1	1	3	5	7	11
TOTAL MULTIPLE DX	98,980	5.0	23	1	2	4	6	10	13	23
TOTAL										
0–19 Years	3,788	5.5	46	1	2	4	7	11	15	36
20–34	4,912	4.6	27	1	2	3	6	9	13	27
35–49	10,599	4.3	23	1	2	3	5	9	12	23
50–64	18,992	5.0	25	1	2	4	6	10	13	25
65+	61,439	5.0	18	1	2	4	6	10	13	21
GRAND TOTAL	99,730	5.0	22	1	2	4	6	10	13	23

99.01: EXCHANGE TRANSFUSION

Type of Patients	Observed Patients	Avg. Stay	Variance	10th	25th	50th	75th	90th	95th	99th
1. SINGLE DX										
0–19 Years	2	2.6	<1	1	3	3	3	3	3	3
20–34	2	3.0	0	3	3	3	3	3	3	3
35–49	0									
50–64	4	1.0	0	1	1	1	1	1	1	1
65+	0									
2. MULTIPLE DX										
0–19 Years	54	6.4	16	2	3	6	8	12	14	21
20–34	23	6.4	24	3	3	3	9	14	15	19
35–49	10	5.7	12	2	3	5	6	10	13	13
50–64	10	7.3	33	1	2	7	9	17	17	17
65+	4	7.5	35	2	6	6	16	16	16	16
TOTAL SINGLE DX	8	2.1	1	1	1	3	3	3	3	3
TOTAL MULTIPLE DX	97	6.5	18	2	3	6	9	13	16	19
TOTAL										
0–19 Years	56	6.2	16	2	3	5	8	12	14	21
20–34	25	6.2	23	3	3	3	9	14	15	19
35–49	10	5.7	12	2	3	5	6	10	13	13
50–64	10	4.8	29	1	1	1	8	9	17	17
65+	4	7.5	35	2	6	6	16	16	16	16
GRAND TOTAL	105	6.1	18	2	3	5	8	13	15	19

99.03: WHOLE BLOOD TRANSFUS NEC

Type of Patients	Observed Patients	Avg. Stay	Variance	10th	25th	50th	75th	90th	95th	99th
1. SINGLE DX										
0–19 Years	0									
20–34	0									
35–49	0									
50–64	1	1.0	0	1	1	1	1	1	1	1
65+	1	1.0	0	1	1	1	1	1	1	1
2. MULTIPLE DX										
0–19 Years	6	5.2	3	3	3	6	7	7	>99	>99
20–34	8	2.8	4	1	2	2	3	7	7	7
35–49	15	3.7	7	1	2	3	4	8	11	11
50–64	23	4.0	9	1	2	3	6	6	7	15
65+	70	5.0	20	1	3	4	6	9	10	27
TOTAL SINGLE DX	2	1.0	0	1	1	1	1	1	1	1
TOTAL MULTIPLE DX	122	4.6	14	1	2	4	6	8	10	27
TOTAL										
0–19 Years	6	5.2	3	3	3	6	7	7	>99	>99
20–34	8	2.8	4	1	2	2	3	7	7	7
35–49	15	3.7	7	1	2	3	4	8	11	11
50–64	24	3.8	9	1	1	3	5	6	7	15
65+	71	5.0	20	1	2	4	6	9	10	27
GRAND TOTAL	124	4.5	14	1	2	4	6	8	10	27

LOS by Diagnosis and Operation, Western Region, 45th Edition

Western Region, October 2007–September 2008 Data, by Operation

99.04: PACKED CELL TRANSFUSION

Type of Patients	Observed Patients	Avg. Stay	Variance	10th	25th	50th	75th	90th	95th	99th
1. SINGLE DX										
0–19 Years	204	2.6	5	1	1	2	3	5	7	11
20–34	125	2.8	6	1	1	2	4	6	8	11
35–49	115	2.0	4	1	1	1	2	4	6	12
50–64	67	1.9	3	1	1	1	2	4	6	8
65+	140	1.2	<1	1	1	1	1	2	2	4
2. MULTIPLE DX										
0–19 Years	2,847	5.6	49	1	2	4	7	11	16	38
20–34	4,264	4.6	27	1	2	3	6	9	13	27
35–49	9,327	4.2	22	1	2	3	5	9	12	22
50–64	16,726	5.0	24	1	2	4	6	10	13	25
65+	55,380	5.0	18	1	2	4	6	10	13	21
TOTAL SINGLE DX	651	2.3	4	1	1	1	3	5	7	11
TOTAL MULTIPLE DX	88,544	4.9	22	1	2	4	6	10	13	23
TOTAL										
0–19 Years	3,051	5.4	47	1	2	3	6	11	15	38
20–34	4,389	4.5	27	1	2	3	6	9	13	27
35–49	9,442	4.2	22	1	2	3	5	9	12	22
50–64	16,793	5.0	24	1	2	4	6	10	13	24
65+	55,520	5.0	18	1	2	4	6	10	13	21
GRAND TOTAL	89,195	4.9	22	1	2	4	6	10	13	23

99.05: PLATELET TRANSFUSION

Type of Patients	Observed Patients	Avg. Stay	Variance	10th	25th	50th	75th	90th	95th	99th
1. SINGLE DX										
0–19 Years	26	2.2	6	1	1	1	2	5	6	13
20–34	7	2.0	<1	1	1	2	3	3	3	3
35–49	10	2.8	4	1	1	3	4	4	7	7
50–64	9	1.2	<1	1	1	1	1	3	3	3
65+	2	1.0	0	1	1	1	1	1	1	1
2. MULTIPLE DX										
0–19 Years	491	6.2	49	1	2	4	8	13	17	34
20–34	268	5.7	33	2	2	4	7	11	14	37
35–49	537	5.7	31	1	2	4	7	12	17	30
50–64	895	5.8	33	1	2	4	7	12	15	29
65+	1,609	5.4	20	1	2	4	7	11	13	24
TOTAL SINGLE DX	54	2.1	4	1	1	1	2	4	6	13
TOTAL MULTIPLE DX	3,800	5.7	32	1	2	4	7	11	15	28
TOTAL										
0–19 Years	517	6.1	49	1	2	4	8	13	16	34
20–34	275	5.6	33	2	2	4	7	11	14	37
35–49	547	5.6	31	1	2	4	7	12	16	30
50–64	904	5.7	33	1	2	4	7	12	15	28
65+	1,611	5.4	20	1	2	4	7	11	13	24
GRAND TOTAL	3,854	5.7	32	1	2	4	7	11	15	28

99.06: COAG FACTOR TRANSFUSION

Type of Patients	Observed Patients	Avg. Stay	Variance	10th	25th	50th	75th	90th	95th	99th
1. SINGLE DX										
0–19 Years	10	2.6	4	1	2	2	3	3	9	9
20–34	0									
35–49	0									
50–64	1	1.0	0	1	1	1	1	1	1	1
65+	0									
2. MULTIPLE DX										
0–19 Years	53	4.0	9	1	2	3	6	7	10	13
20–34	35	4.9	23	1	2	3	6	10	18	18
35–49	20	3.9	7	1	1	3	5	9	9	11
50–64	15	5.3	47	1	2	3	6	13	27	27
65+	22	5.2	20	1	2	4	8	10	12	19
TOTAL SINGLE DX	11	2.5	4	1	1	2	3	3	9	9
TOTAL MULTIPLE DX	145	4.3	15	1	2	3	6	10	11	18
TOTAL										
0–19 Years	63	3.7	9	1	2	3	6	7	10	13
20–34	35	4.9	23	1	2	3	6	10	18	18
35–49	20	3.9	7	1	1	3	5	7	9	11
50–64	16	5.1	45	1	2	2	6	13	27	27
65+	22	5.2	20	1	2	4	8	10	12	19
GRAND TOTAL	156	4.2	14	1	2	3	6	9	10	18

99.07: SERUM TRANSFUSION NEC

Type of Patients	Observed Patients	Avg. Stay	Variance	10th	25th	50th	75th	90th	95th	99th
1. SINGLE DX										
0–19 Years	3	2.0	3	1	1	1	3	5	5	5
20–34	5	2.0	<1	1	2	2	5	3	3	3
35–49	4	2.8	4	1	1	2	5	5	5	5
50–64	4	2.0	2	1	1	2	4	4	4	4
65+	6	2.9	8	1	1	1	6	7	7	7
2. MULTIPLE DX										
0–19 Years	76	5.8	41	1	2	4	7	12	15	33
20–34	157	4.3	11	1	2	3	5	9	12	15
35–49	541	5.4	33	1	2	4	6	11	15	27
50–64	1,196	5.2	31	1	2	4	7	11	14	28
65+	4,100	5.1	17	1	2	4	7	10	13	20
TOTAL SINGLE DX	22	2.3	3	1	1	1	3	5	6	7
TOTAL MULTIPLE DX	6,070	5.1	22	1	2	4	7	10	13	22
TOTAL										
0–19 Years	79	5.6	40	1	2	4	6	11	14	33
20–34	162	4.2	11	1	2	3	5	9	12	15
35–49	545	5.4	33	1	2	4	7	11	15	27
50–64	1,200	5.2	31	1	2	4	6	11	14	28
65+	4,106	5.1	17	1	2	4	7	10	13	24
GRAND TOTAL	6,092	5.1	22	1	2	4	7	10	13	22

LOS by Diagnosis and Operation, Western Region, 45th Edition

485

Western Region, October 2007–September 2008 Data, by Operation

99.09: TRANSFUSION NEC

Type of Patients	Observed Patients	Avg. Stay	Vari-ance	Percentiles						
				10th	25th	50th	75th	90th	95th	99th
1. SINGLE DX										
0–19 Years	0									
20–34	1	1.0	0	1	1	1	1	1	1	1
35–49	1	11.0	0	11	11	11	11	11	11	11
50–64	0									
65+	0									
2. MULTIPLE DX										
0–19 Years	12	6.1	9	1	6	6	7	7	7	17
20–34	16	4.1	18	1	1	4	4	11	19	19
35–49	17	5.1	30	1	1	3	7	14	20	20
50–64	29	7.4	113	1	2	4	8	13	35	51
65+	85	6.1	30	2	3	5	7	10	13	41
TOTAL SINGLE DX	2	6.0	50	1	1	1	11	11	11	11
TOTAL MULTIPLE DX	159	6.0	39	1	3	5	7	11	14	41
TOTAL										
0–19 Years	12	6.1	9	1	6	6	7	7	7	17
20–34	17	4.0	18	1	1	4	4	5	19	19
35–49	18	5.5	30	1	1	4	8	14	20	20
50–64	29	7.4	113	1	2	4	8	13	35	51
65+	85	6.1	30	2	3	5	7	10	13	41
GRAND TOTAL	161	6.0	39	1	3	5	7	11	14	41

99.10: INJECT THROMBOLYTIC

Type of Patients	Observed Patients	Avg. Stay	Vari-ance	Percentiles						
				10th	25th	50th	75th	90th	95th	99th
1. SINGLE DX										
0–19 Years	7	1.4	<1	1	1	1	2	3	3	3
20–34	3	2.3	2	1	1	2	4	4	4	4
35–49	9	2.4	2	1	1	2	3	5	5	5
50–64	6	3.3	9	1	2	2	4	9	9	9
65+	1	4.0	0	4	4	4	4	4	4	4
2. MULTIPLE DX										
0–19 Years	45	5.5	28	1	1	4	8	12	18	22
20–34	98	7.0	47	2	3	5	8	17	18	35
35–49	280	5.4	19	2	3	4	7	11	14	22
50–64	688	6.3	51	2	3	4	7	11	16	41
65+	1,577	6.3	28	2	3	5	8	11	16	26
TOTAL SINGLE DX	26	2.4	3	1	1	2	3	4	5	9
TOTAL MULTIPLE DX	2,688	6.2	33	2	3	5	7	11	16	31
TOTAL										
0–19 Years	52	5.2	27	1	1	4	7	12	18	22
20–34	101	6.8	46	2	3	5	8	16	18	35
35–49	289	5.3	19	1	3	4	7	11	14	22
50–64	694	6.2	51	2	3	4	7	11	16	41
65+	1,578	6.3	28	2	3	5	8	11	16	26
GRAND TOTAL	2,714	6.2	33	2	3	5	7	11	16	31

99.11: INJECT RH IMMUNE GLOB

Type of Patients	Observed Patients	Avg. Stay	Vari-ance	Percentiles						
				10th	25th	50th	75th	90th	95th	99th
1. SINGLE DX										
0–19 Years	11	2.9	4	1	1	2	5	6	6	6
20–34	27	1.6	<1	1	1	1	2	3	3	4
35–49	3	2.3	2	1	1	2	4	4	4	4
50–64	0									
65+	0									
2. MULTIPLE DX										
0–19 Years	94	3.0	22	1	1	2	3	4	7	35
20–34	186	3.2	37	1	1	2	3	5	9	37
35–49	40	7.2	187	1	2	3	5	23	44	58
50–64	9	3.9	12	1	1	3	5	11	11	11
65+	4	6.2	12	2	2	5	10	10	10	10
TOTAL SINGLE DX	41	2.0	2	1	1	2	2	4	5	6
TOTAL MULTIPLE DX	333	3.7	51	1	1	2	3	7	10	44
TOTAL										
0–19 Years	105	2.9	20	1	1	2	3	5	7	30
20–34	213	3.0	33	1	1	2	3	5	9	32
35–49	43	6.9	176	1	2	2	3	23	44	58
50–64	9	3.9	12	2	1	3	5	11	11	11
65+	4	6.2	12	2	2	5	10	10	10	10
GRAND TOTAL	374	3.5	45	1	1	2	3	6	10	44

99.1: INJECT/INFUSE THER SUBST

Type of Patients	Observed Patients	Avg. Stay	Vari-ance	Percentiles						
				10th	25th	50th	75th	90th	95th	99th
1. SINGLE DX										
0–19 Years	307	2.4	3	1	1	2	3	4	6	9
20–34	76	2.3	3	1	1	2	3	4	7	10
35–49	46	2.6	3	1	1	2	3	5	6	7
50–64	25	3.1	15	1	1	2	4	7	9	19
65+	13	1.8	2	1	1	1	2	4	5	5
2. MULTIPLE DX										
0–19 Years	6,394	10.9	136	2	3	7	15	26	35	56
20–34	1,133	6.0	42	1	2	4	7	13	17	34
35–49	1,713	6.6	40	1	3	5	8	14	19	29
50–64	3,046	6.5	42	1	3	5	8	13	18	31
65+	5,099	7.0	36	2	3	5	9	14	18	30
TOTAL SINGLE DX	467	2.5	3	1	1	2	3	5	6	9
TOTAL MULTIPLE DX	17,385	8.5	86	2	3	6	11	19	26	47
TOTAL										
0–19 Years	6,701	10.4	133	1	3	6	14	25	34	54
20–34	1,209	5.8	40	1	2	4	7	13	17	34
35–49	1,759	6.5	39	1	2	4	8	14	19	29
50–64	3,071	6.5	41	1	3	5	8	13	18	31
65+	5,112	7.0	36	2	3	5	9	14	18	29
GRAND TOTAL	17,852	8.3	85	2	3	5	10	19	26	47

LOS by Diagnosis and Operation, Western Region, 45th Edition

Western Region, October 2007–September 2008 Data, by Operation

99.14: INJECT/INFUSE GAMMA GLOB

Type of Patients	Observed Patients	Avg. Stay	Variance	10th	25th	50th	75th	90th	95th	99th
1. SINGLE DX										
0–19 Years	261	2.3	2	1	1	2	3	4	6	8
20–34	16	1.9	2	1	1	1	3	3	7	7
35–49	11	2.3	3	1	1	2	3	4	7	7
50–64	12	1.4	<1	1	1	1	1	2	4	4
65+	9	1.3	<1	1	1	1	2	2	2	2
2. MULTIPLE DX										
0–19 Years	1,522	3.3	17	1	1	2	3	6	10	25
20–34	132	4.0	10	1	2	3	5	7	10	17
35–49	160	4.1	10	1	2	3	5	8	9	12
50–64	291	3.7	15	1	2	3	5	8	11	20
65+	224	5.6	19	2	2	4	7	12	14	21
TOTAL SINGLE DX	309	2.3	2	1	1	2	3	4	5	8
TOTAL MULTIPLE DX	2,329	3.6	17	1	1	2	4	7	11	23
TOTAL										
0–19 Years	1,783	3.1	15	1	1	2	3	6	9	23
20–34	148	3.8	9	1	2	3	5	7	9	17
35–49	171	3.9	9	1	2	3	5	8	9	12
50–64	303	3.6	14	1	1	2	5	8	10	18
65+	233	5.5	19	2	2	4	7	12	14	21
GRAND TOTAL	2,638	3.4	15	1	1	2	4	7	10	20

99.15: PARENTERAL NUTRITION

Type of Patients	Observed Patients	Avg. Stay	Variance	10th	25th	50th	75th	90th	95th	99th
1. SINGLE DX										
0–19 Years	10	5.6	6	4	4	6	6	9	9	11
20–34	11	3.9	10	1	1	3	7	8	10	10
35–49	8	3.3	4	1	1	6	6	6	6	6
50–64	4	9.0	45	4	6	7	7	19	19	19
65+	1	5.0	0	5	5	5	5	5	5	5
2. MULTIPLE DX										
0–19 Years	4,542	14.0	152	3	6	10	18	30	39	63
20–34	444	8.8	43	3	4	7	11	17	22	37
35–49	748	9.4	48	3	5	7	12	19	22	35
50–64	1,328	8.9	48	3	4	7	11	17	21	30
65+	1,883	9.7	50	3	5	8	12	18	22	35
TOTAL SINGLE DX	34	5.1	11	1	3	4	6	9	10	19
TOTAL MULTIPLE DX	8,945	12.0	114	3	5	9	15	25	33	54
TOTAL										
0–19 Years	4,552	13.9	152	3	6	10	18	30	39	63
20–34	455	8.7	43	3	4	7	11	17	22	37
35–49	756	9.3	48	3	5	8	12	19	22	35
50–64	1,332	8.9	48	3	4	7	11	17	21	30
65+	1,884	9.7	50	3	5	8	12	18	22	35
GRAND TOTAL	8,979	12.0	114	3	5	9	15	24	33	54

99.17: INJECT INSULIN

Type of Patients	Observed Patients	Avg. Stay	Variance	10th	25th	50th	75th	90th	95th	99th
1. SINGLE DX										
0–19 Years	11	2.2	1	1	1	2	3	4	4	4
20–34	6	3.6	4	1	3	3	5	7	7	7
35–49	5	2.6	2	1	2	2	3	5	5	5
50–64	0									
65+	1	1.0	0	1	1	1	1	1	1	1
2. MULTIPLE DX										
0–19 Years	100	3.6	8	1	2	3	5	7	9	9
20–34	138	2.8	5	1	1	2	3	5	6	13
35–49	209	3.5	8	1	2	3	4	6	9	16
50–64	246	3.0	5	1	2	3	4	6	9	12
65+	467	4.1	12	1	2	3	5	8	10	16
TOTAL SINGLE DX	23	2.6	2	1	1	2	3	5	5	7
TOTAL MULTIPLE DX	1,160	3.6	9	1	2	3	4	7	9	13
TOTAL										
0–19 Years	111	3.5	8	1	2	3	5	7	8	9
20–34	144	2.9	5	1	1	2	3	5	7	13
35–49	214	3.5	8	1	2	3	4	6	9	16
50–64	246	3.0	5	1	2	3	4	6	9	12
65+	468	4.1	12	2	2	3	5	8	10	16
GRAND TOTAL	1,183	3.6	9	1	2	3	4	7	9	13

99.18: INJECT ELECTROLYTES

Type of Patients	Observed Patients	Avg. Stay	Variance	10th	25th	50th	75th	90th	95th	99th
1. SINGLE DX										
0–19 Years	5	1.2	<1	1	1	1	1	2	2	2
20–34	2	2.0	2	1	1	3	3	3	3	3
35–49	0									
50–64	0									
65+	0									
2. MULTIPLE DX										
0–19 Years	43	4.0	36	1	1	2	4	12	13	34
20–34	17	3.0	6	1	2	2	3	6	11	11
35–49	28	3.8	29	1	2	2	3	8	15	27
50–64	48	3.2	5	1	2	2	5	6	8	8
65+	101	3.8	10	1	2	3	5	8	10	13
TOTAL SINGLE DX	7	1.4	<1	1	1	1	2	3	3	3
TOTAL MULTIPLE DX	237	3.7	15	1	1	2	5	8	11	19
TOTAL										
0–19 Years	48	3.7	33	1	1	2	3	12	13	34
20–34	19	2.9	6	1	1	2	3	6	11	11
35–49	28	3.8	29	1	2	2	3	8	15	27
50–64	48	3.2	5	1	2	2	5	6	8	8
65+	101	3.8	10	1	2	3	5	8	10	13
GRAND TOTAL	244	3.6	15	1	1	2	4	8	11	19

LOS by Diagnosis and Operation, Western Region, 45th Edition

Western Region, October 2007–September 2008 Data, by Operation

99.19: INJECT ANTICOAGULANT

Type of Patients	Observed Patients	Avg. Stay	Vari-ance	Percentiles						
				10th	25th	50th	75th	90th	95th	99th
1. SINGLE DX										
0–19 Years	0									
20–34	8	2.3	1	1	1	3	3	4	4	4
35–49	8	3.1	3	1	1	3	5	6	6	6
50–64	2	2.0	2	1	1	1	3	3	3	3
65+	0									
2. MULTIPLE DX										
0–19 Years	35	3.9	11	1	2	3	4	9	12	19
20–34	109	5.2	71	1	2	4	6	9	11	24
35–49	228	3.9	17	1	2	3	5	7	9	19
50–64	401	4.2	15	1	2	3	6	8	10	17
65+	829	4.5	15	1	2	4	6	8	11	16
TOTAL SINGLE DX	18	2.7	2	1	1	3	3	5	6	6
TOTAL MULTIPLE DX	1,602	4.4	19	1	2	3	5	8	10	18
TOTAL										
0–19 Years	35	3.9	11	1	2	3	4	9	12	19
20–34	117	5.0	67	1	2	4	6	8	11	24
35–49	236	3.9	17	1	2	3	5	7	9	19
50–64	403	4.2	15	1	2	3	6	8	10	17
65+	829	4.5	15	1	2	4	6	8	11	16
GRAND TOTAL	1,620	4.4	19	1	2	3	5	8	10	18

99.2: OTH INJECT THER SUBST

Type of Patients	Observed Patients	Avg. Stay	Vari-ance	Percentiles						
				10th	25th	50th	75th	90th	95th	99th
1. SINGLE DX										
0–19 Years	1,835	1.9	4	1	1	1	2	3	4	8
20–34	562	2.5	9	1	1	2	3	4	6	16
35–49	195	2.6	16	1	1	2	3	5	8	28
50–64	134	2.2	6	1	1	1	2	4	5	11
65+	30	2.1	3	1	1	1	3	5	5	7
2. MULTIPLE DX										
0–19 Years	11,887	5.8	78	1	2	3	5	11	23	50
20–34	5,672	5.1	44	1	2	3	5	9	18	35
35–49	7,359	4.7	32	1	2	3	5	8	15	31
50–64	11,568	4.9	38	1	2	3	6	9	16	33
65+	12,061	4.9	30	1	2	3	6	9	14	30
TOTAL SINGLE DX	2,756	2.1	6	1	1	1	2	3	5	10
TOTAL MULTIPLE DX	48,547	5.2	52	1	2	3	5	9	18	39
TOTAL										
0–19 Years	13,722	5.5	73	1	2	3	5	10	21	48
20–34	6,234	4.9	41	1	2	3	5	9	17	34
35–49	7,554	4.6	32	1	2	3	5	8	15	31
50–64	11,702	4.9	38	1	2	3	6	9	16	33
65+	12,091	4.9	30	1	2	3	6	9	14	30
GRAND TOTAL	51,303	5.1	50	1	2	3	5	9	17	38

99.20: INJECT PLATELET INHIB

Type of Patients	Observed Patients	Avg. Stay	Vari-ance	Percentiles						
				10th	25th	50th	75th	90th	95th	99th
1. SINGLE DX										
0–19 Years	1	2.0	0	2	2	2	2	2	2	2
20–34	0									
35–49	1	7.0	0	7	7	7	7	7	7	7
50–64	0									
65+	0									
2. MULTIPLE DX										
0–19 Years	1	4.0	0	4	4	4	4	4	4	4
20–34	4	3.0	<1	2	2	3	4	4	4	4
35–49	35	2.5	4	1	1	1	4	5	7	8
50–64	100	2.9	4	1	1	3	4	6	7	9
65+	252	4.4	12	2	2	3	5	8	11	18
TOTAL SINGLE DX	2	4.5	12	2	2	7	7	7	7	7
TOTAL MULTIPLE DX	392	3.8	10	1	2	3	5	7	10	17
TOTAL										
0–19 Years	2	3.0	2	2	2	2	4	4	4	4
20–34	4	3.0	<1	2	2	3	4	4	4	4
35–49	36	2.6	4	1	1	2	4	5	7	8
50–64	100	2.9	4	1	1	3	4	6	7	9
65+	252	4.4	12	2	2	3	5	8	11	18
GRAND TOTAL	394	3.8	10	1	2	3	5	7	10	17

99.21: INJECT ANTIBIOTIC

Type of Patients	Observed Patients	Avg. Stay	Vari-ance	Percentiles						
				10th	25th	50th	75th	90th	95th	99th
1. SINGLE DX										
0–19 Years	182	2.6	3	1	2	2	3	4	7	9
20–34	57	2.3	2	1	1	2	3	4	6	8
35–49	37	2.5	5	1	1	2	3	5	6	13
50–64	28	2.5	2	1	1	2	3	4	6	11
65+	4	3.3	4	1	1	2	5	5	5	7
2. MULTIPLE DX										
0–19 Years	1,718	4.9	30	1	2	3	6	10	14	27
20–34	898	3.7	22	1	2	2	4	7	10	20
35–49	1,141	3.8	14	1	2	3	5	7	9	21
50–64	1,749	4.1	14	1	2	3	5	8	11	18
65+	3,762	4.5	15	1	2	3	5	8	11	19
TOTAL SINGLE DX	308	2.5	3	1	1	2	3	4	6	9
TOTAL MULTIPLE DX	9,268	4.3	19	1	2	3	5	8	11	21
TOTAL										
0–19 Years	1,900	4.7	28	1	2	3	5	10	14	25
20–34	955	3.6	21	1	2	3	4	7	10	20
35–49	1,178	3.7	13	1	2	3	4	7	9	21
50–64	1,777	4.1	14	1	2	3	5	8	10	18
65+	3,766	4.5	15	1	2	3	5	8	11	19
GRAND TOTAL	9,576	4.3	18	1	2	3	5	8	11	21

LOS by Diagnosis and Operation, Western Region. 45th Edition

Western Region, October 2007–September 2008 Data, by Operation

99.22: INJECT ANTI-INFECT NEC

Type of Patients	Observed Patients	Avg. Stay	Vari- ance	Percentiles						
				10th	25th	50th	75th	90th	95th	99th
1. SINGLE DX										
0–19 Years	1	3.0	0	3	3	3	3	3	3	3
20–34	1	1.0	0	1	1	1	1	1	1	1
35–49	2	1.0	0	1	1	1	1	1	1	1
50–64	0									
65+	0									
2. MULTIPLE DX										
0–19 Years	25	8.0	185	2	4	4	7	18	24	79
20–34	9	4.2	15	1	2	2	5	12	12	12
35–49	16	3.9	15	1	2	3	5	6	17	17
50–64	12	4.9	11	2	2	4	5	9	12	12
65+	16	4.6	15	2	2	3	7	8	17	17
TOTAL SINGLE DX	4	1.5	1	1	1	1	3	3	3	3
TOTAL MULTIPLE DX	78	5.8	82	2	2	4	6	12	17	79
TOTAL										
0–19 Years	26	7.9	181	2	4	4	7	18	24	79
20–34	10	3.9	14	1	1	2	5	9	12	12
35–49	18	3.6	14	1	2	3	5	6	17	17
50–64	12	4.9	11	2	2	4	7	9	12	12
65+	16	4.6	15	2	2	3	7	8	17	17
GRAND TOTAL	82	5.6	79	1	2	4	6	9	17	79

99.23: INJECT STEROID

Type of Patients	Observed Patients	Avg. Stay	Vari- ance	Percentiles						
				10th	25th	50th	75th	90th	95th	99th
1. SINGLE DX										
0–19 Years	27	1.7	<1	1	1	1	2	3	4	4
20–34	15	3.7	21	1	1	2	4	10	18	18
35–49	2	12.9	240	2	2	2	24	24	24	24
50–64	2	2.0	0	2	2	2	2	2	2	2
65+	0									
2. MULTIPLE DX										
0–19 Years	93	3.0	6	1	1	2	3	8	9	11
20–34	101	3.5	14	1	2	2	4	6	10	19
35–49	107	3.8	19	1	2	3	5	7	8	22
50–64	184	3.7	18	1	2	3	4	7	9	17
65+	369	4.3	16	1	2	3	5	8	11	22
TOTAL SINGLE DX	46	2.8	18	1	1	2	2	4	10	24
TOTAL MULTIPLE DX	854	3.9	15	1	2	3	5	7	10	21
TOTAL										
0–19 Years	120	2.7	5	1	1	2	3	5	9	11
20–34	116	3.5	15	1	2	2	4	6	13	19
35–49	109	4.0	22	1	2	3	5	7	9	24
50–64	186	3.7	18	1	2	3	4	7	9	17
65+	369	4.3	16	1	2	3	5	8	11	22
GRAND TOTAL	900	3.8	16	1	2	3	5	7	10	21

99.25: INJECT CA CHEMO AGENT

Type of Patients	Observed Patients	Avg. Stay	Vari- ance	Percentiles						
				10th	25th	50th	75th	90th	95th	99th
1. SINGLE DX										
0–19 Years	58	3.7	11	1	1	3	5	7	10	20
20–34	32	2.6	3	1	1	2	4	4	6	9
35–49	10	2.8	4	1	1	2	5	5	6	6
50–64	26	2.4	3	1	1	2	4	5	5	5
65+	8	2.6	5	1	1	3	4	7	7	7
2. MULTIPLE DX										
0–19 Years	7,461	5.1	46	1	2	4	5	8	17	36
20–34	3,051	6.1	54	1	3	4	6	12	22	36
35–49	4,255	5.6	43	1	2	4	5	10	20	34
50–64	7,493	5.6	50	1	2	4	5	11	21	37
65+	5,098	5.7	51	1	2	4	6	11	20	36
TOTAL SINGLE DX	134	3.1	7	1	1	2	5	6	7	11
TOTAL MULTIPLE DX	27,358	5.4	48	1	2	4	5	10	20	36
TOTAL										
0–19 Years	7,519	5.1	46	1	2	4	5	8	17	36
20–34	3,083	6.0	53	1	3	4	6	12	22	36
35–49	4,265	5.6	43	1	2	4	5	10	20	34
50–64	7,519	5.6	50	1	2	4	5	11	21	37
65+	5,106	5.7	51	1	2	4	6	11	20	36
GRAND TOTAL	27,492	5.4	48	1	2	4	5	10	20	36

99.26: INJECT TRANQUILIZER

Type of Patients	Observed Patients	Avg. Stay	Vari- ance	Percentiles						
				10th	25th	50th	75th	90th	95th	99th
1. SINGLE DX										
0–19 Years	0									
20–34	0									
35–49	0									
50–64	0									
65+	0									
2. MULTIPLE DX										
0–19 Years	0									
20–34	1	1.0	0	1	1	1	1	1	1	1
35–49	2	1.5	<1	1	1	2	2	2	2	2
50–64	1	1.0	0	1	1	1	1	1	1	1
65+	2	4.0	18	1	1	4	7	7	7	7
TOTAL SINGLE DX	0									
TOTAL MULTIPLE DX	6	2.2	6	1	1	1	2	7	7	7
TOTAL										
0–19 Years	0									
20–34	1	1.0	0	1	1	1	1	1	1	1
35–49	2	1.5	<1	1	1	2	2	2	2	2
50–64	1	1.0	0	1	1	1	1	1	1	1
65+	2	4.0	18	1	1	4	7	7	7	7
GRAND TOTAL	6	2.2	6	1	1	1	2	7	7	7

LOS by Diagnosis and Operation, Western Region, 45th Edition

Western Region, October 2007–September 2008 Data, by Operation

99.28: INJECT BRM/ANTINEO AGENT

Type of Patients	Observed Patients	Avg. Stay	Vari-ance	Percentiles						
				10th	25th	50th	75th	90th	95th	99th
1. SINGLE DX										
0–19 Years	4	1.6	2	1	1	1	1	5	5	5
20–34	3	1.7	<1	1	1	1	2	2	2	2
35–49	5	2.4	3	1	1	2	3	5	5	5
50–64	3	1.7	1	1	1	1	3	3	3	3
65+	3	2.0	3	1	1	1	4	4	4	4
2. MULTIPLE DX										
0–19 Years	83	3.2	16	1	1	2	4	5	7	27
20–34	63	4.6	16	1	2	4	5	6	8	23
35–49	149	4.3	7	1	3	4	5	6	8	18
50–64	219	5.5	23	2	4	5	7	9	17	24
65+	255	4.9	25	1	2	4	6	8	12	31
TOTAL SINGLE DX	18	1.9	2	1	1	1	2	4	5	5
TOTAL MULTIPLE DX	769	4.5	19	1	2	4	5	7	11	24
TOTAL										
0–19 Years	87	3.2	16	1	1	1	4	5	7	20
20–34	66	4.4	16	1	2	4	5	6	8	23
35–49	154	4.2	7	1	2	4	5	6	8	18
50–64	222	5.5	22	2	3	4	5	8	16	24
65+	258	4.9	25	1	2	4	6	8	12	31
GRAND TOTAL	787	4.5	19	1	2	4	5	7	11	23

99.29: INJECT/INFUSE NEC

Type of Patients	Observed Patients	Avg. Stay	Vari-ance	Percentiles						
				10th	25th	50th	75th	90th	95th	99th
1. SINGLE DX										
0–19 Years	1,559	1.7	4	1	1	1	2	3	3	5
20–34	445	2.5	9	1	1	2	3	4	6	16
35–49	138	2.5	18	1	1	1	2	4	8	28
50–64	75	2.0	8	1	1	1	2	3	8	21
65+	15	1.6	1	1	1	1	2	4	4	4
2. MULTIPLE DX										
0–19 Years	2,502	10.9	297	1	1	3	12	36	53	85
20–34	1,540	4.1	36	1	1	2	4	8	13	34
35–49	1,652	3.2	17	1	1	2	4	6	9	24
50–64	1,808	3.2	12	1	1	2	4	7	10	18
65+	2,303	3.6	12	2	2	3	5	7	9	17
TOTAL SINGLE DX	2,232	1.9	6	1	1	1	2	3	4	10
TOTAL MULTIPLE DX	9,805	5.5	106	1	1	2	5	11	23	63
TOTAL										
0–19 Years	4,061	7.5	209	1	1	2	5	24	43	78
20–34	1,985	3.7	31	1	1	2	4	7	12	32
35–49	1,790	3.1	17	1	1	2	3	6	9	24
50–64	1,883	3.2	12	1	1	2	4	7	10	18
65+	2,318	3.6	12	2	2	3	5	7	9	17
GRAND TOTAL	12,037	4.9	90	1	1	2	4	9	19	57

99.3: PROPHYL VACC-BACT DIS

Type of Patients	Observed Patients	Avg. Stay	Vari-ance	Percentiles						
				10th	25th	50th	75th	90th	95th	99th
1. SINGLE DX										
0–19 Years	2	1.0	0	1	1	1	1	1	1	1
20–34	3	1.0	0	1	1	1	1	1	1	1
35–49	3	3.0	7	1	1	2	6	6	6	6
50–64	0									
65+	0									
2. MULTIPLE DX										
0–19 Years	45	9.4	304	1	1	3	10	17	44	82
20–34	78	2.9	16	1	1	2	3	6	11	29
35–49	63	3.0	13	1	1	2	3	6	8	25
50–64	76	3.6	15	1	1	3	4	7	10	28
65+	92	3.8	9	1	2	3	5	8	10	16
TOTAL SINGLE DX	8	1.8	3	1	1	1	1	6	6	6
TOTAL MULTIPLE DX	354	4.4	68	1	1	2	4	9	13	44
TOTAL										
0–19 Years	47	9.2	297	1	1	3	10	17	44	82
20–34	81	2.9	15	1	1	2	3	6	8	29
35–49	66	3.0	12	1	1	3	3	6	8	25
50–64	76	3.6	15	1	2	3	4	7	10	28
65+	92	3.8	9	1	2	3	5	8	10	16
GRAND TOTAL	362	4.4	66	1	1	2	4	9	13	44

99.36: DIPHTHERIA TOXOID ADMIN

Type of Patients	Observed Patients	Avg. Stay	Vari-ance	Percentiles						
				10th	25th	50th	75th	90th	95th	99th
1. SINGLE DX										
0–19 Years	0									
20–34	1	1.0	0	1	1	1	1	1	1	1
35–49	0									
50–64	0									
65+	0									
2. MULTIPLE DX										
0–19 Years	9	4.4	36	1	2	2	4	20	20	20
20–34	46	2.8	19	1	1	1	3	6	8	29
35–49	45	2.6	6	1	1	3	3	6	8	11
50–64	46	3.2	6	1	1	3	4	7	7	13
65+	58	3.5	7	1	1	3	5	9	10	10
TOTAL SINGLE DX	1	1.0	0	1	1	1	1	1	1	1
TOTAL MULTIPLE DX	204	3.1	11	1	1	2	4	6	9	13
TOTAL										
0–19 Years	9	4.4	36	1	1	2	4	20	20	20
20–34	47	2.7	19	1	1	2	3	6	8	29
35–49	45	2.6	6	1	1	2	3	6	8	11
50–64	46	3.2	6	1	1	3	4	7	7	13
65+	58	3.5	7	1	1	3	5	9	10	10
GRAND TOTAL	205	3.1	10	1	1	2	4	6	9	13

LOS by Diagnosis and Operation, Western Region, 45th Edition

Western Region, October 2007–September 2008 Data, by Operation

99.38: TETANUS TOXOID ADMIN

Type of Patients	Observed Patients	Avg. Stay	Vari-ance	10th	25th	50th	75th	90th	95th	99th
1. SINGLE DX										
0–19 Years	2	1.0	0	1	1	1	1	1	1	1
20–34	2	1.0	0	1	1	1	1	1	1	1
35–49	1	2.0	0	2	2	2	2	2	2	2
50–64	0									
65+	0									
2. MULTIPLE DX										
0–19 Years	4	23.6	>999	2	2	2	82	82	82	82
20–34	24	3.5	15	1	1	2	4	11	13	14
35–49	16	4.0	33	1	2	3	4	6	25	25
50–64	22	5.1	37	1	2	3	4	10	14	28
65+	27	4.0	9	1	2	3	5	8	12	13
TOTAL SINGLE DX	5	1.2	<1	1	1	1	1	2	2	2
TOTAL MULTIPLE DX	93	5.0	86	1	2	3	4	10	14	82
TOTAL										
0–19 Years	6	16.1	>999	1	1	2	6	82	82	82
20–34	26	3.3	14	1	2	2	3	11	13	14
35–49	17	3.9	31	1	2	3	4	6	25	25
50–64	22	5.1	37	1	2	3	4	10	14	28
65+	27	4.0	9	1	2	3	5	8	12	13
GRAND TOTAL	98	4.8	83	1	2	3	4	10	14	82

99.4: VIRAL IMMUNIZATION

Type of Patients	Observed Patients	Avg. Stay	Vari-ance	10th	25th	50th	75th	90th	95th	99th
1. SINGLE DX										
0–19 Years	1	1.0	0	1	1	1	1	1	1	1
20–34	5	2.2	<1	1	2	2	3	3	3	3
35–49	1	1.0	0	1	1	1	1	1	1	1
50–64	0									
65+	0									
2. MULTIPLE DX										
0–19 Years	19	2.5	<1	1	2	2	3	4	4	4
20–34	38	1.9	<1	1	1	2	2	3	3	6
35–49	6	1.9	<1	1	2	2	2	3	3	3
50–64	5	2.8	3	1	2	2	4	5	5	5
65+	4	6.8	17	2	2	6	12	12	12	12
TOTAL SINGLE DX	7	1.9	<1	1	1	2	3	3	3	3
TOTAL MULTIPLE DX	72	2.4	3	1	1	2	3	4	6	12
TOTAL										
0–19 Years	20	2.4	<1	1	2	2	3	4	4	4
20–34	43	1.9	<1	1	1	2	2	3	3	6
35–49	7	1.9	<1	1	1	2	2	3	3	3
50–64	5	2.8	3	1	2	2	4	5	5	5
65+	4	6.8	17	2	2	6	12	12	12	12
GRAND TOTAL	79	2.3	3	1	1	2	3	4	5	12

99.5: OTHER IMMUNIZATION

Type of Patients	Observed Patients	Avg. Stay	Vari-ance	10th	25th	50th	75th	90th	95th	99th
1. SINGLE DX										
0–19 Years	3,589	1.8	<1	1	1	2	2	3	3	4
20–34	11	3.0	8	1	1	2	3	4	11	11
35–49	2	2.0	0	2	2	2	2	2	2	2
50–64	4	2.0	2	1	1	2	4	4	4	4
65+	2	1.0	0	1	1	1	1	1	1	1
2. MULTIPLE DX										
0–19 Years	195,857	2.3	6	1	1	2	3	3	4	11
20–34	604	3.2	8	1	2	2	4	6	8	12
35–49	1,569	3.8	16	1	2	3	4	7	9	21
50–64	2,993	3.9	17	1	2	3	5	7	10	17
65+	6,798	4.3	12	1	2	3	5	8	10	18
TOTAL SINGLE DX	3,608	1.8	<1	1	1	2	2	3	3	4
TOTAL MULTIPLE DX	207,821	2.4	6	1	1	2	3	4	4	12
TOTAL										
0–19 Years	199,446	2.3	5	1	1	2	3	3	4	11
20–34	615	3.2	8	1	2	2	4	6	8	12
35–49	1,571	3.8	16	1	2	3	4	7	9	21
50–64	2,997	3.9	17	1	2	3	5	7	10	17
65+	6,800	4.3	12	1	2	3	5	8	10	18
GRAND TOTAL	211,429	2.4	6	1	1	2	3	4	4	12

99.52: INFLUENZA VACCINATION

Type of Patients	Observed Patients	Avg. Stay	Vari-ance	10th	25th	50th	75th	90th	95th	99th
1. SINGLE DX										
0–19 Years	18	1.9	<1	1	1	2	3	3	3	3
20–34	6	4.0	13	1	2	3	4	11	11	11
35–49	1	2.0	0	2	2	2	2	2	2	2
50–64	1	2.0	0	2	2	2	2	2	2	2
65+	2	1.0	0	1	1	1	1	1	1	1
2. MULTIPLE DX										
0–19 Years	275	2.7	9	1	1	2	3	5	7	12
20–34	315	3.1	11	1	2	3	3	5	7	13
35–49	690	3.7	17	1	2	3	4	7	9	25
50–64	1,273	4.0	17	1	2	3	5	7	9	20
65+	2,134	4.2	15	2	2	3	5	7	10	17
TOTAL SINGLE DX	28	2.2	3	1	1	2	3	3	4	11
TOTAL MULTIPLE DX	4,687	3.9	15	1	2	3	5	7	9	18
TOTAL										
0–19 Years	293	2.6	9	1	1	2	3	5	6	12
20–34	321	3.1	11	1	2	3	3	5	7	13
35–49	691	3.7	17	1	2	3	4	7	9	25
50–64	1,274	4.0	17	1	2	3	5	7	9	20
65+	2,136	4.2	15	2	2	3	5	7	10	17
GRAND TOTAL	4,715	3.9	15	2	2	3	5	7	9	18

LOS by Diagnosis and Operation, Western Region, 45th Edition

Western Region, October 2007–September 2008 Data, by Operation

99.55: VACCINATION NEC

Type of Patients	Observed Patients	Avg. Stay	Variance	Percentiles						
				10th	25th	50th	75th	90th	95th	99th
1. SINGLE DX										
0–19 Years	3,458	1.8	<1	1	1	2	2	3	3	4
20–34	5	1.8	<1	1	1	2	2	3	3	3
35–49	0									
50–64	3	2.0	3	1	1	1	4	4	4	4
65+	0									
2. MULTIPLE DX										
0–19 Years	195,346	2.3	5	1	1	2	3	3	4	11
20–34	284	3.2	5	1	2	3	4	6	8	12
35–49	869	3.8	15	1	2	3	5	7	9	21
50–64	1,700	3.9	17	1	2	3	5	7	10	15
65+	4,641	4.3	11	1	2	3	5	8	10	18
TOTAL SINGLE DX	3,466	1.8	<1	1	1	2	2	3	3	4
TOTAL MULTIPLE DX	202,840	2.3	6	1	1	2	3	4	4	12
TOTAL										
0–19 Years	198,804	2.3	5	1	1	2	3	3	4	11
20–34	289	3.2	5	1	2	3	4	6	8	12
35–49	869	3.8	15	1	2	3	5	7	9	21
50–64	1,703	3.9	17	1	2	3	5	7	10	15
65+	4,641	4.3	11	1	2	3	5	8	10	18
GRAND TOTAL	206,306	2.3	6	1	1	2	3	4	4	11

99.59: VACC/INOCULATION NEC

Type of Patients	Observed Patients	Avg. Stay	Variance	Percentiles						
				10th	25th	50th	75th	90th	95th	99th
1. SINGLE DX										
0–19 Years	113	1.9	<1	1	1	2	2	3	3	4
20–34	0									
35–49	0									
50–64	0									
65+	0									
2. MULTIPLE DX										
0–19 Years	196	3.5	29	1	2	2	3	4	11	28
20–34	3	4.7	22	1	1	3	10	10	10	10
35–49	5	4.0	11	2	2	3	3	10	10	10
50–64	11	3.9	3	2	2	3	4	4	7	7
65+	13	2.9	2	1	2	3	4	5	5	5
TOTAL SINGLE DX	113	1.9	<1	1	1	2	2	3	3	4
TOTAL MULTIPLE DX	228	3.5	27	1	2	2	3	5	10	28
TOTAL										
0–19 Years	309	3.0	21	1	1	2	3	4	7	28
20–34	5	4.7	22	1	1	3	10	10	10	10
35–49	5	4.0	11	2	2	3	3	10	10	10
50–64	11	3.0	3	2	2	3	4	4	7	7
65+	13	2.9	2	1	2	3	4	5	5	5
GRAND TOTAL	341	3.0	20	1	2	2	3	4	7	28

99.6: CARD RHYTHM CONVERSION

Type of Patients	Observed Patients	Avg. Stay	Variance	Percentiles						
				10th	25th	50th	75th	90th	95th	99th
1. SINGLE DX										
0–19 Years	11	3.2	8	1	1	2	3	9	9	9
20–34	17	2.1	2	1	1	2	3	7	>99	>99
35–49	29	1.4	<1	1	1	1	2	3	3	3
50–64	44	1.7	2	1	1	1	2	3	3	10
65+	28	1.5	<1	1	1	1	2	3	3	3
2. MULTIPLE DX										
0–19 Years	205	5.6	95	1	2	3	6	10	16	62
20–34	192	3.1	17	1	1	2	4	6	7	45
35–49	657	3.3	15	1	1	2	4	7	9	19
50–64	2,008	3.6	15	1	1	3	4	7	10	19
65+	4,603	4.2	16	2	2	3	5	8	11	19
TOTAL SINGLE DX	129	1.9	3	1	1	2	2	3	7	10
TOTAL MULTIPLE DX	7,665	4.0	19	1	2	3	5	8	11	20
TOTAL										
0–19 Years	216	5.4	90	1	2	3	6	10	15	62
20–34	209	3.0	16	1	1	2	4	6	7	45
35–49	686	3.2	15	1	1	2	4	7	9	19
50–64	2,052	3.5	15	1	1	2	4	7	10	19
65+	4,631	4.2	16	2	2	3	5	8	11	19
GRAND TOTAL	7,794	4.0	19	1	2	3	5	8	11	20

99.60: CPR NOS

Type of Patients	Observed Patients	Avg. Stay	Variance	Percentiles						
				10th	25th	50th	75th	90th	95th	99th
1. SINGLE DX										
0–19 Years	3	2.7	<1	2	2	3	3	3	3	3
20–34	0									
35–49	0									
50–64	0									
65+	0									
2. MULTIPLE DX										
0–19 Years	99	8.3	220	2	2	4	7	16	40	78
20–34	22	6.1	31	1	2	4	8	15	22	>99
35–49	41	7.9	100	2	3	6	8	17	24	55
50–64	117	9.0	72	2	3	6	12	20	29	37
65+	204	8.6	65	2	4	7	11	16	23	53
TOTAL SINGLE DX	3	2.7	<1	2	2	3	>99	>99	>99	>99
TOTAL MULTIPLE DX	483	8.5	103	2	3	5	10	18	28	62
TOTAL										
0–19 Years	102	8.1	215	2	2	4	7	16	40	78
20–34	22	6.1	31	1	2	4	5	22	>99	>99
35–49	41	7.9	100	1	2	6	8	17	24	55
50–64	117	9.0	72	2	3	6	12	20	29	37
65+	204	8.6	65	2	4	7	11	16	23	53
GRAND TOTAL	486	8.4	103	2	3	5	10	18	28	72

99.61: ATRIAL CARDIOVERSION

Type of Patients	Observed Patients	Avg. Stay	Vari-ance	Percentiles						
				10th	25th	50th	75th	90th	95th	99th
1. SINGLE DX										
0–19 Years	2	1.7	<1	1	1	2	2	2	2	2
20–34	6	1.8	<1	1	1	1	3	3	3	3
35–49	9	1.4	<1	1	1	1	3	3	3	3
50–64	20	1.8	<1	1	1	1	3	3	4	4
65+	14	1.5	<1	1	1	1	2	3	3	3
2. MULTIPLE DX										
0–19 Years	35	4.0	16	1	1	3	4	12	15	15
20–34	57	2.4	2	1	1	2	4	4	5	6
35–49	251	2.8	6	1	1	2	4	6	8	13
50–64	731	3.3	11	1	1	2	4	6	8	14
65+	1,678	4.1	12	1	2	3	5	8	10	16
TOTAL SINGLE DX	51	1.7	<1	1	1	1	2	3	3	4
TOTAL MULTIPLE DX	2,752	3.7	11	1	2	3	5	7	10	15
TOTAL										
0–19 Years	37	3.9	15	1	1	3	4	12	15	15
20–34	63	2.4	2	1	1	2	3	4	5	6
35–49	260	2.8	6	1	1	2	3	6	7	13
50–64	751	3.2	11	1	1	2	4	6	8	14
65+	1,692	4.0	12	1	2	3	5	8	10	16
GRAND TOTAL	2,803	3.7	11	1	2	3	5	7	10	15

99.62: HEART COUNTERSHOCK NEC

Type of Patients	Observed Patients	Avg. Stay	Vari-ance	Percentiles						
				10th	25th	50th	75th	90th	95th	99th
1. SINGLE DX										
0–19 Years	3	6.0	15	1	1	9	9	9	9	9
20–34	11	2.2	3	1	1	2	2	4	7	7
35–49	17	1.5	<1	1	1	1	1	3	3	3
50–64	21	1.7	4	1	1	1	1	2	3	10
65+	12	1.3	<1	1	1	1	1	2	3	3
2. MULTIPLE DX										
0–19 Years	46	4.2	23	2	2	3	5	8	10	33
20–34	86	2.8	23	1	1	2	3	4	5	45
35–49	310	3.2	10	1	1	2	4	8	9	15
50–64	966	3.3	9	1	1	2	4	7	9	14
65+	2,217	4.1	14	1	2	3	5	8	11	18
TOTAL SINGLE DX	64	2.1	5	1	1	1	2	4	9	10
TOTAL MULTIPLE DX	3,625	3.8	13	1	2	3	5	8	10	18
TOTAL										
0–19 Years	49	4.3	23	2	2	3	5	9	10	24
20–34	97	2.8	21	1	1	2	3	4	5	45
35–49	327	3.2	9	1	1	2	4	7	9	15
50–64	987	3.2	9	1	1	2	4	7	9	14
65+	2,229	4.1	14	1	2	3	5	8	11	18
GRAND TOTAL	3,689	3.8	13	1	1	3	5	8	10	17

99.69: CARDIAC RHYTHM CONV NEC

Type of Patients	Observed Patients	Avg. Stay	Vari-ance	Percentiles						
				10th	25th	50th	75th	90th	95th	99th
1. SINGLE DX										
0–19 Years	3	1.8	1	1	1	1	3	3	3	3
20–34	0									
35–49	3	1.0	0	1	1	1	1	1	1	1
50–64	3	1.0	0	1	1	1	1	1	1	1
65+	2	2.0	0	2	2	2	2	2	2	2
2. MULTIPLE DX										
0–19 Years	14	2.8	7	1	1	2	2	8	10	10
20–34	27	3.2	13	1	1	2	4	7	7	20
35–49	54	2.4	5	1	1	2	3	3	7	13
50–64	193	3.0	9	1	1	2	3	6	9	17
65+	499	3.5	11	1	2	3	5	7	9	13
TOTAL SINGLE DX	11	1.6	<1	1	1	1	2	3	3	3
TOTAL MULTIPLE DX	787	3.3	10	1	1	2	4	7	9	14
TOTAL										
0–19 Years	17	2.5	6	1	1	2	3	6	8	10
20–34	27	3.2	13	1	1	2	4	7	7	20
35–49	57	2.3	5	1	1	2	3	3	7	13
50–64	196	2.9	8	1	1	2	3	6	10	17
65+	501	3.5	11	2	2	3	5	7	9	13
GRAND TOTAL	798	3.2	10	1	1	2	4	6	9	14

99.7: THER APHERESIS/ADMIN NEC

Type of Patients	Observed Patients	Avg. Stay	Vari-ance	Percentiles						
				10th	25th	50th	75th	90th	95th	99th
1. SINGLE DX										
0–19 Years	11	1.3	1	1	1	1	1	3	5	5
20–34	8	7.3	26	1	5	7	12	17	17	17
35–49	34	3.5	9	1	1	5	7	7	7	7
50–64	34	1.8	3	1	1	1	1	4	6	8
65+	3	2.0	3	1	1	1	4	4	4	4
2. MULTIPLE DX										
0–19 Years	100	8.2	126	1	2	4	9	20	26	67
20–34	126	9.7	61	2	4	7	14	20	26	31
35–49	207	8.5	71	2	3	6	11	19	24	43
50–64	399	6.8	47	1	2	5	9	15	20	35
65+	331	7.2	49	1	3	5	8	15	24	36
TOTAL SINGLE DX	60	2.4	8	1	1	1	3	6	7	17
TOTAL MULTIPLE DX	1,163	7.7	65	1	3	5	10	17	24	39
TOTAL										
0–19 Years	111	7.5	118	1	1	4	8	20	24	67
20–34	134	9.6	59	1	4	7	13	20	26	31
35–49	211	8.4	71	1	3	6	11	19	24	43
50–64	433	6.4	45	1	2	4	9	14	19	30
65+	334	7.1	49	1	3	5	8	15	24	36
GRAND TOTAL	1,223	7.4	64	1	2	5	9	17	24	39

LOS by Diagnosis and Operation, Western Region, 45th Edition

Western Region, October 2007–September 2008 Data, by Operation

99.71: THER PLASMAPHERESIS

Type of Patients	Observed Patients	Avg. Stay	Vari- ance	10th	25th	50th	75th	90th	95th	99th
1. SINGLE DX										
0–19 Years	4	1.6	2	1	1	1	1	5	5	5
20–34	6	6.7	9	3	5	7	7	12	12	12
35–49	3	4.3	9	1	1	7	7	7	7	7
50–64	30	1.7	3	1	1	1	1	4	6	8
65+	1	1.0	0	1	1	1	1	1	1	1
2. MULTIPLE DX										
0–19 Years	47	7.7	66	1	1	5	12	22	28	28
20–34	89	10.6	69	1	5	8	15	24	28	43
35–49	127	10.0	96	2	4	7	12	22	27	43
50–64	230	7.4	58	1	2	5	10	17	22	39
65+	141	9.1	66	2	4	7	10	20	26	39
TOTAL SINGLE DX	44	2.5	7	1	1	1	4	7	7	12
TOTAL MULTIPLE DX	634	8.7	70	1	3	6	11	20	26	42
TOTAL										
0–19 Years	51	7.2	63	1	1	4	11	22	28	28
20–34	95	10.4	66	1	5	7	14	24	28	43
35–49	130	9.8	94	2	4	7	12	22	27	43
50–64	260	6.7	55	1	1	5	9	16	21	39
65+	142	9.0	66	2	4	7	10	20	26	39
GRAND TOTAL	678	8.3	69	1	3	6	11	19	26	42

99.79: THER APHERESIS NEC

Type of Patients	Observed Patients	Avg. Stay	Vari- ance	10th	25th	50th	75th	90th	95th	99th
1. SINGLE DX										
0–19 Years	5	1.2	<1	1	1	1	1	3	3	3
20–34	0									
35–49	0									
50–64	1	4.0	0	4	4	4	4	4	4	4
65+	0									
2. MULTIPLE DX										
0–19 Years	25	5.3	23	1	2	4	6	13	20	20
20–34	5	6.8	7	4	6	6	7	11	11	11
35–49	15	6.4	25	1	3	5	9	12	20	20
50–64	23	6.1	17	2	3	5	10	12	12	14
65+	14	10.1	86	2	4	7	12	24	31	31
TOTAL SINGLE DX	6	1.5	1	1	1	1	1	4	4	4
TOTAL MULTIPLE DX	82	6.2	30	1	3	4	7	13	20	24
TOTAL										
0–19 Years	30	4.8	22	1	2	4	6	13	20	20
20–34	5	6.8	7	4	6	6	7	11	11	11
35–49	15	6.4	25	1	3	5	9	12	20	20
50–64	24	6.0	16	2	3	4	10	12	12	14
65+	14	10.1	86	2	4	7	12	24	31	31
GRAND TOTAL	88	5.8	29	1	2	4	7	12	20	24

99.74: THER PLATELETPHERESIS

Type of Patients	Observed Patients	Avg. Stay	Vari- ance	10th	25th	50th	75th	90th	95th	99th
1. SINGLE DX										
0–19 Years	2	1.0	0	1	1	1	1	1	1	1
20–34	2	9.0	125	1	1	17	17	17	17	17
35–49	1	1.0	0	1	1	1	1	1	1	1
50–64	2	2.5	<1	2	2	3	3	3	3	3
65+	2	2.5	4	1	1	4	4	4	4	4
2. MULTIPLE DX										
0–19 Years	20	19.1	562	2	3	8	24	67	67	67
20–34	26	6.7	33	2	3	5	8	18	20	21
35–49	50	6.0	27	2	3	4	7	12	18	24
50–64	104	5.8	35	1	2	4	7	13	18	28
65+	138	5.4	25	1	2	4	7	10	15	29
TOTAL SINGLE DX	9	3.5	27	1	1	1	3	17	17	17
TOTAL MULTIPLE DX	338	6.6	75	1	2	4	7	13	19	67
TOTAL										
0–19 Years	22	17.7	540	1	3	8	21	67	67	67
20–34	28	6.9	35	1	3	5	9	18	20	21
35–49	51	5.9	27	1	3	4	7	12	18	24
50–64	106	5.7	34	1	2	4	7	13	18	28
65+	140	5.3	25	1	2	4	7	10	14	29
GRAND TOTAL	347	6.5	74	1	2	4	7	14	19	67

99.8: MISC PHYSICAL PROCEDURES

Type of Patients	Observed Patients	Avg. Stay	Vari- ance	10th	25th	50th	75th	90th	95th	99th
1. SINGLE DX										
0–19 Years	6,207	1.6	<1	1	1	1	2	2	3	4
20–34	0									
35–49	1	1.0	0	1	1	1	1	1	1	1
50–64	0									
65+	1	4.0	0	4	4	4	4	4	4	4
2. MULTIPLE DX										
0–19 Years	26,234	5.7	47	2	2	4	5	13	19	36
20–34	20	4.0	24	1	2	2	3	7	21	21
35–49	28	4.5	39	1	2	3	4	32	>99	>99
50–64	31	2.6	2	1	2	2	3	5	6	7
65+	48	7.4	39	3	4	5	9	14	18	36
TOTAL SINGLE DX	6,209	1.6	<1	1	1	1	2	2	3	4
TOTAL MULTIPLE DX	26,361	5.7	47	2	2	4	5	13	19	36
TOTAL										
0–19 Years	32,441	4.8	40	1	2	3	5	10	17	33
20–34	20	4.0	24	1	2	2	3	7	21	21
35–49	29	4.4	38	1	2	3	4	14	>99	>99
50–64	31	2.6	2	1	2	2	3	5	6	7
65+	49	7.3	38	3	4	5	8	14	18	36
GRAND TOTAL	32,570	4.8	40	1	2	3	5	10	17	33

Western Region, October 2007–September 2008 Data, by Operation

99.82: UV LIGHT THERAPY

Type of Patients	Observed Patients	Avg. Stay	Vari-ance	Percentiles						
				10th	25th	50th	75th	90th	95th	99th
1. SINGLE DX										
0–19 Years	367	1.6	<1	1	1	1	2	2	3	4
20–34	0									
35–49	0									
50–64	0									
65+	0									
2. MULTIPLE DX										
0–19 Years	1,314	5.1	35	2	2	3	5	11	18	30
20–34	0									
35–49	0									
50–64	0									
65+	0									
TOTAL SINGLE DX	367	1.6	<1	1	1	1	2	2	3	4
TOTAL MULTIPLE DX	1,314	5.1	35	2	2	3	5	11	18	30
TOTAL										
0–19 Years	1,681	4.3	29	1	2	3	4	8	15	28
20–34	0									
35–49	0									
50–64	0									
65+	0									
GRAND TOTAL	1,681	4.3	29	1	2	3	4	8	15	28

99.83: PHOTOTHERAPY NEC

Type of Patients	Observed Patients	Avg. Stay	Vari-ance	Percentiles						
				10th	25th	50th	75th	90th	95th	99th
1. SINGLE DX										
0–19 Years	5,838	1.6	<1	1	1	1	2	2	3	4
20–34	0									
35–49	0									
50–64	0									
65+	0									
2. MULTIPLE DX										
0–19 Years	24,902	5.7	48	2	2	4	5	13	20	37
20–34	0									
35–49	0									
50–64	0									
65+	2	5.0	8	3	3	7	7	7	7	7
TOTAL SINGLE DX	5,838	1.6	<1	1	1	1	2	2	3	4
TOTAL MULTIPLE DX	24,904	5.7	48	2	2	4	5	13	20	37
TOTAL										
0–19 Years	30,740	4.9	41	1	2	3	5	10	17	33
20–34	0									
35–49	0									
50–64	0									
65+	2	5.0	8	3	3	7	7	7	7	7
GRAND TOTAL	30,742	4.9	41	1	2	3	5	10	17	33

99.84: ISOLATION

Type of Patients	Observed Patients	Avg. Stay	Vari-ance	Percentiles						
				10th	25th	50th	75th	90th	95th	99th
1. SINGLE DX										
0–19 Years	1	2.0	0	2	2	2	2	2	2	2
20–34	0									
35–49	1	1.0	0	1	1	1	1	1	1	1
50–64	0									
65+	1	4.0	0	4	4	4	4	4	4	4
2. MULTIPLE DX										
0–19 Years	9	5.3	17	1	1	6	7	10	10	15
20–34	12	4.3	32	1	1	2	4	7	21	21
35–49	14	2.6	3	1	1	3	4	7	>99	>99
50–64	19	2.8	3	1	1	2	4	6	7	7
65+	45	7.4	40	3	4	5	8	14	18	36
TOTAL SINGLE DX	3	2.3	2	1	1	2	4	4	4	4
TOTAL MULTIPLE DX	99	5.3	27	1	2	4	7	10	15	36
TOTAL										
0–19 Years	10	5.2	17	1	1	6	7	10	10	15
20–34	12	4.3	32	1	1	2	4	7	21	21
35–49	15	2.5	3	1	1	3	4	7	>99	>99
50–64	19	2.8	3	1	1	2	4	6	7	7
65+	46	7.3	39	3	4	5	8	14	18	36
GRAND TOTAL	102	5.2	26	1	2	4	7	10	15	36

99.88: THER PHOTOPHERESIS

Type of Patients	Observed Patients	Avg. Stay	Vari-ance	Percentiles						
				10th	25th	50th	75th	90th	95th	99th
1. SINGLE DX										
0–19 Years	1	1.0	0	1	1	1	1	1	1	1
20–34	0									
35–49	0									
50–64	0									
65+	0									
2. MULTIPLE DX										
0–19 Years	7	2.8	2	1	2	3	4	5	5	5
20–34	8	3.5	15	2	2	2	2	13	13	13
35–49	14	6.4	70	2	2	3	11	32	>99	>99
50–64	12	2.3	<1	2	2	2	2	2	5	5
65+	0									
TOTAL SINGLE DX	1	1.0	0	1	1	1	1	1	1	1
TOTAL MULTIPLE DX	41	4.0	28	2	2	2	4	11	14	>99
TOTAL										
0–19 Years	8	2.6	2	1	2	2	3	5	5	5
20–34	8	3.5	15	2	2	2	2	13	13	13
35–49	14	6.4	70	2	2	3	11	32	>99	>99
50–64	12	2.3	<1	2	2	2	2	2	5	5
65+	0									
GRAND TOTAL	42	3.9	28	2	2	2	4	11	14	>99

LOS by Diagnosis and Operation, Western Region, 45th Edition

Western Region, October 2007–September 2008 Data, by Operation

99.9: OTHER MISC PROCEDURES

Type of Patients	Observed Patients	Avg. Stay	Vari-ance	Percentiles						
				10th	25th	50th	75th	90th	95th	99th
1. SINGLE DX										
0–19 Years	8	2.7	2	1	2	2	3	6	6	6
20–34	4	3.5	2	2	2	3	4	5	5	5
35–49	0									
50–64	0									
65+	1	2.0	0	2	2	2	2	2	2	2
2. MULTIPLE DX										
0–19 Years	129	3.5	6	1	2	3	4	6	8	14
20–34	33	4.5	41	1	2	3	5	7	9	40
35–49	47	3.5	5	1	2	3	4	7	7	12
50–64	66	4.6	10	1	2	4	7	9	11	13
65+	486	4.6	16	2	3	4	6	8	10	17
TOTAL SINGLE DX	**13**	**2.7**	**2**	**1**	**2**	**2**	**3**	**6**	**6**	**6**
TOTAL MULTIPLE DX	**761**	**4.1**	**12**	**1**	**2**	**3**	**5**	**8**	**9**	**14**
TOTAL										
0–19 Years	137	3.5	6	1	2	3	4	6	8	14
20–34	37	4.4	37	1	2	3	5	7	7	40
35–49	47	3.5	5	1	2	3	4	7	7	12
50–64	66	4.6	10	1	2	4	7	9	11	13
65+	487	4.6	16	2	3	4	6	8	10	17
GRAND TOTAL	**774**	**4.0**	**12**	**1**	**2**	**3**	**5**	**7**	**9**	**14**

99.99: MISC PROCEDURES NEC

Type of Patients	Observed Patients	Avg. Stay	Vari-ance	Percentiles						
				10th	25th	50th	75th	90th	95th	99th
1. SINGLE DX										
0–19 Years	7	2.7	2	1	2	2	3	6	6	6
20–34	3	3.0	<1	2	2	3	4	4	4	4
35–49	0									
50–64	0									
65+	1	2.0	0	2	2	2	2	2	2	2
2. MULTIPLE DX										
0–19 Years	123	3.5	5	2	2	3	4	6	8	13
20–34	28	4.7	47	1	2	3	5	7	9	40
35–49	45	3.5	6	1	2	3	4	7	7	12
50–64	61	4.5	10	2	2	4	7	8	11	13
65+	474	4.6	16	2	3	4	6	8	10	17
TOTAL SINGLE DX	**11**	**2.7**	**2**	**1**	**2**	**2**	**3**	**6**	**6**	**6**
TOTAL MULTIPLE DX	**731**	**4.0**	**12**	**1**	**2**	**3**	**5**	**7**	**9**	**14**
TOTAL										
0–19 Years	130	3.4	5	1	2	3	4	6	8	13
20–34	31	4.6	43	1	2	3	5	7	9	40
35–49	45	3.5	6	1	2	3	4	7	7	12
50–64	61	4.5	10	2	2	4	7	8	11	13
65+	475	4.6	16	2	3	4	6	8	10	17
GRAND TOTAL	**742**	**4.0**	**12**	**1**	**2**	**3**	**5**	**7**	**9**	**14**

LOS by Diagnosis and Operation, Western Region, 45th Edition

APPENDIX A
Hospital Characteristics
Short-Term, General, Nonfederal Hospitals[1]

HOSPITAL CATEGORY	U.S. TOTAL
Bed Size	
6–24 Beds	1,064
25–49	1,576
50–99	1,386
100–199	1,393
200–299	701
300–399	392
400–499	181
500+	264
Unknown	70
Total	**7,027**
Region and Census Division	
Northeast	**970**
New England	304
Middle Atlantic	666
North Central	**1,912**
East North Central	1,055
West North Central	858
South	**2,830**
South Atlantic	1,071
East South Central	571
West South Central	1,186
West	**1,315**
Mountain	526
Pacific	789
Location	
Urban	4,678
Rural	2,346
Teaching Intensity	
High/Medium	409
Low	6,521

---

[1] For a definition of short-term, general, and nonfederal hospitals, see "Description of the Database."

APPENDIX B
States Included in Each Region

Northeast

Connecticut
Maine
Massachusetts
New Hampshire
New Jersey
New York
Pennsylvania
Rhode Island
Vermont

North Central

Illinois
Indiana
Iowa
Kansas
Michigan
Minnesota
Missouri
Nebraska
North Dakota
Ohio
South Dakota
Wisconsin

South

Alabama
Arkansas
Delaware
District of Columbia
Florida
Georgia
Kentucky
Louisiana
Maryland
Mississippi
North Carolina
Oklahoma
South Carolina
Tennessee
Texas
Virginia
West Virginia

West

Alaska
Arizona
California
Colorado
Hawaii
Idaho
Montana
Nevada
New Mexico
Oregon
Utah
Washington
Wyoming

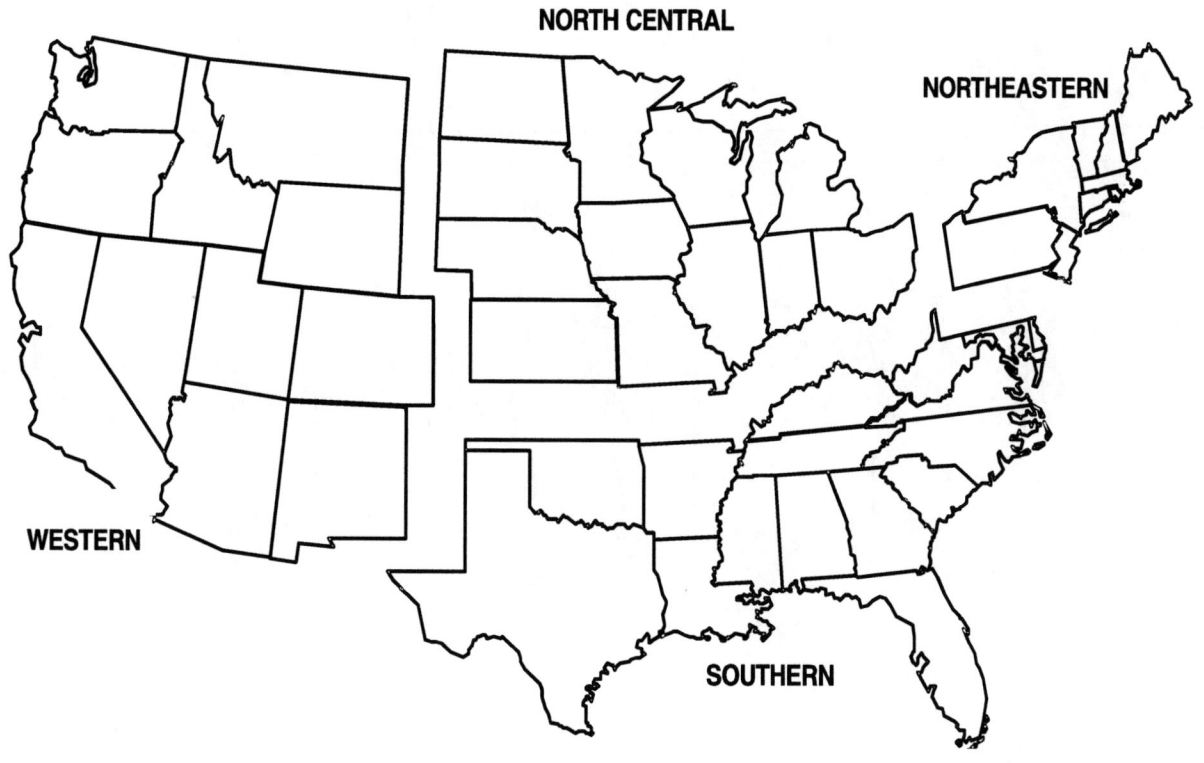

NORTH CENTRAL

NORTHEASTERN

WESTERN

SOUTHERN

APPENDIX C
Operative Status of Procedure Codes

The following table lists every ICD-9-CM procedure code included in this book, its description, and its CMS-defined operative status (*i.e.,* operative or non-operative). Operative procedures are those classified by CMS as "operating room" procedures. CMS physician panels classify every ICD-9-CM procedure code according to whether the procedure would, in most hospitals, be performed in the operating room. For codes that contain both operative and non-operative detail codes, the notation "Mixed," followed by the number of each type, will appear in the "Operative Status" column. For example, a chapter code containing three operative and two non-operative detail codes will be identified as "Mixed (3, 2)."

Code	Description	Operative Status	Code	Description	Operative Status
00.0	Therapeutic ultrasound	Non-Operative	01.51	Exc cereb meningeal les	Operative
00.1	Pharmaceuticals	Non-Operative	01.53	Brain lobectomy	Operative
00.13	Inject nesiritide	Non-Operative	01.59	Exc/destr brain les NEC	Operative
00.14	Inject oxazol antibio	Non-Operative	01.6	Excision of skull lesion	Operative
00.15	High-dose interleukin-2	Non-Operative	02.0	Cranioplasty	Operative
00.17	Infuse vasopressor agent	Non-Operative	02.01	Opening cranial suture	Operative
00.2	Intravascular imaging	Non-Operative	02.02	Elevation skull fx frag	Operative
00.3	Computer assisted surg	Non-Operative	02.03	Cran bone flap formation	Operative
00.4	Adjunct vasc syst px	Non-Operative	02.04	Bone graft to skull	Operative
00.5	Oth cardiovascular px	Mixed (7, 1)	02.05	Skull plate insertion	Operative
00.50	Impl CRT-P total system	Operative	02.06	Cranial osteoplasty NEC	Operative
00.51	Impl CRT-D total system	Operative	02.1	Cerebral meninges repair	Operative
00.52	Impl lead cor ven system	Operative	02.12	REP cerebral mening NEC	Operative
00.54	Impl CRT-D generator	Operative	02.2	Ventriculostomy	Operative
00.6	Blood vessel px	Mixed (3, 3)	02.3	Extracranial vent shunt	Operative
00.61	PERC ather precereb vess	Operative	02.34	Vent shunt to abd cavity	Operative
00.62	PERC ather IC vessel	Operative	02.39	Ops to estab vent drain	Operative
00.66	PTCA/atherectomy	Operative	02.4	Vent shunt rev/rmvl	Mixed (2, 1)
00.7	Other hip px	Mixed (4, 4)	02.42	Repl ventricular shunt	Operative
00.70	Rev hip repl-both COMP	Operative	02.43	Rmvl ventricular shunt	Operative
00.71	Rev hip repl-acetab COMP	Operative	02.9	Skull & brain ops NEC	Mixed (5, 2)
00.72	Rev hip repl-FEM COMP	Operative	02.93	Impl/repl IC neurstim ld	Operative
00.73	Rev hip repl-liner/head	Operative	02.94	Insert/repl skull tongs	Operative
00.8	Other knee & hip px	Operative	03.0	Spinal canal exploration	Operative
00.80	Rev knee repl-total	Operative	03.02	Reopen laminectomy site	Operative
00.81	Rev knee repl-tib COMP	Operative	03.09	Spinal canal expl NEC	Operative
00.82	Rev knee repl-FEM COMP	Operative	03.1	Intraspin nerve root div	Operative
00.83	Rev knee repl-PAT COMP	Operative	03.2	Chordotomy	Operative
00.84	Rev knee repl-tib insert	Operative	03.3	Dxtic px on spinal canal	Mixed (2, 1)
00.85	Hip resurfacing-total	Operative	03.31	Spinal tap	Non-Operative
00.86	Hip resurfacing-FEM head	Operative	03.32	Spinal cord/meninges Bx	Operative
00.9	Px & intervention NEC	Non-Operative	03.4	Exc spinal cord lesion	Operative
01.0	Cranial puncture	Non-Operative	03.5	Spinal cord plastic ops	Operative
01.02	Ventriculopunct via cath	Non-Operative	03.51	Spinal meningocele REP	Operative
01.1	Dxtic px on skull/brain	Mixed (5, 5)	03.53	Vertebral fx repair	Operative
01.10	IC pressure monitoring	Non-Operative	03.59	Spinal struct repair NEC	Operative
01.13	Closed brain biopsy	Non-Operative	03.6	Spinal cord adhesiolysis	Operative
01.14	Open biopsy of brain	Operative	03.7	Spinal thecal shunt	Operative
01.2	Craniotomy & craniectomy	Mixed (6, 2)	03.71	Subarach-periton shunt	Operative
01.23	Reopen craniotomy site	Operative	03.8	Destr inject-spine canal	Non-Operative
01.24	Craniotomy NEC	Operative	03.9	Spinal cord ops NEC	Mixed (5, 5)
01.25	Craniectomy NEC	Operative	03.90	Insert spinal canal cath	Non-Operative
01.3	Inc brain/cereb meninges	Operative	03.91	Inject anes-spinal canal	Non-Operative
01.31	Inc cerebral meninges	Operative	03.92	Inject spinal canal NEC	Non-Operative
01.39	Brain incision NEC	Operative	03.93	Impl/repl sp neurstim ld	Operative
01.4	Thalamus/globus pall ops	Operative	03.94	Rmvl sp neurostim lead	Operative
01.5	Exc/destr brain/meninges	Operative	03.95	Spinal blood patch	Non-Operative

Code	Description	Operative Status	Code	Description	Operative Status
03.97	Rev spinal thecal shunt	Operative	08.09	Other eyelid incision	Non-Operative
04.0	Periph nerve inc/div/exc	Operative	08.1	Dxtic px on eyelid	Mixed (1, 1)
04.01	Exc acoustic neuroma	Operative	08.2	Exc/destr eyelid lesion	Operative
04.07	Periph/cran nerv exc NEC	Operative	08.3	Ptosis/lid retract REP	Operative
04.1	Dxtic px periph nerv	Mixed (2, 1)	08.4	Entropion/ectropion REP	Operative
04.2	Destr periph/cran nerves	Non-Operative	08.5	Oth adjust lid position	Operative
04.3	Cran/periph nerve suture	Operative	08.6	Eyelid reconst w graft	Operative
04.4	Periph nerv adhesiolysis	Operative	08.7	Other eyelid reconst	Operative
04.41	Decomp trigeminal root	Operative	08.8	Other repair of eyelid	Non-Operative
04.42	Cranial nerve decomp NEC	Operative	08.81	Linear REP eyelid lac	Non-Operative
04.43	Carpal tunnel release	Operative	08.9	Other eyelid operations	Operative
04.49	Periph nerv ADHESIO NEC	Operative	09.0	Lacrimal gland incision	Operative
04.5	Cran or periph nerv grft	Operative	09.1	Lacrimal system dxtic px	Operative
04.6	Periph nerves transpos	Operative	09.2	Lacrimal gland les exc	Operative
04.7	Other periph neuroplasty	Operative	09.3	Other lacrimal gland ops	Operative
04.8	Peripheral nerve inject	Non-Operative	09.4	Lacrimal passage manip	Operative
04.81	Anes inject periph nerve	Non-Operative	09.5	Inc lacrimal sac/passg	Operative
04.9	Oth periph nerve ops	Operative	09.6	Lacrimal sac/passage exc	Operative
04.92	Impl periph neurostim ld	Operative	09.7	Canaliculus/punctum REP	Operative
05.0	Sympath nerve division	Operative	09.8	NL fistulization	Operative
05.1	Sympath nerve dxtic px	Operative	09.9	Oth lacrimal syst ops	Operative
05.2	Sympathectomy	Operative	10.0	Inc/rmvl FB-conjunctiva	Operative
05.3	Sympath nerve injection	Non-Operative	10.1	Conjunctiva incision NEC	Operative
05.31	Anes inject sympath nerv	Non-Operative	10.2	Conjunctiva dxtic px	Operative
05.8	Oth sympath nerve ops	Operative	10.3	Exc/destr conjunct les	Operative
05.9	Other nervous system ops	Operative	10.4	Conjunctivoplasty	Operative
06.0	Thyroid field incision	Mixed (2, 1)	10.5	Conjunct/lid ADHESIO	Operative
06.09	Inc thyroid field NEC	Operative	10.6	Repair conjunct lac	Operative
06.1	Thyroid/parathy dxtic px	Mixed (3, 1)	10.9	Other conjunctival ops	Operative
06.11	Closed thyroid biopsy	Non-Operative	11.0	Magnet removal cornea FB	Operative
06.2	Unilat thyroid lobectomy	Operative	11.1	Corneal incision	Operative
06.3	Other part thyroidectomy	Operative	11.2	Dxtic px on cornea	Operative
06.31	Excision thyroid lesion	Operative	11.3	Excision of pterygium	Operative
06.39	Part thyroidectomy NEC	Operative	11.4	Exc/destr corneal lesion	Operative
06.4	Complete thyroidectomy	Operative	11.5	Corneal repair	Operative
06.5	Substernal thyroidectomy	Operative	11.51	Suture of corneal lac	Operative
06.51	Part substern thyroidect	Operative	11.6	Corneal transplant	Operative
06.52	Tot substern thyroidect	Operative	11.7	Other cornea reconst	Operative
06.6	Lingual thyroid excision	Operative	11.9	Other corneal operations	Operative
06.7	Thyroglossal duct exc	Operative	12.0	Rmvl inOc FB ant segment	Operative
06.8	Parathyroidectomy	Operative	12.1	Iridotomy/smp iridectomy	Operative
06.81	Total parathyroidectomy	Operative	12.2	Anterior SEG dxtic px	Operative
06.89	Other parathyroidectomy	Operative	12.3	Iridoplasty/coreoplasty	Operative
06.9	Thyroid/parathy ops NEC	Operative	12.4	Destr iris/cil body les	Operative
07.0	Adrenal field expl	Operative	12.5	InOc circulat facilitat	Operative
07.1	Oth endocrine dxtic px	Mixed (7, 1)	12.6	Scleral fistulization	Operative
07.11	Clsd adrenal gland Bx	Non-Operative	12.7	Elevat inOc press relief	Operative
07.2	Partial adrenalectomy	Operative	12.8	Operations on sclera	Operative
07.22	Unilateral adrenalectomy	Operative	12.9	Oth anterior segment ops	Operative
07.3	Bilateral adrenalectomy	Operative	13.0	Removal FB from lens	Operative
07.4	Other adrenal operations	Operative	13.1	Intracap lens extraction	Operative
07.5	Pineal gland operations	Operative	13.2	Lin extracaps lens extr	Operative
07.6	Hypophysectomy	Operative	13.3	Simp asp lens extraction	Operative
07.61	Exc pit les-transfrontal	Operative	13.4	Frag-asp extracaps lens	Operative
07.62	Exc pit les-transsphen	Operative	13.5	Oth extracaps lens extr	Operative
07.65	Tot exc pit-transsphen	Operative	13.6	Oth cataract extraction	Operative
07.7	Other hypophysis ops	Operative	13.7	Insert prosthetic lens	Operative
07.8	Thymectomy	Operative	13.8	Implanted lens removal	Operative
07.82	Tot excision thymus NEC	Operative	13.9	Other operations on lens	Operative
07.9	Other thymus operations	Operative	14.0	Rmvl of post segment FB	Operative
08.0	Eyelid incision	Non-Operative	14.1	Dxtic px posterior SEG	Operative

Code	Description	Operative Status	Code	Description	Operative Status
14.2	Retina-choroid les destr	Mixed (5, 3)	21.0	Control of epistaxis	Mixed (5, 4)
14.3	Repair of retinal tear	Mixed (3, 3)	21.01	Ant NAS pack for epistx	Non-Operative
14.4	REP retina detach/buckle	Operative	21.02	Post NAS pack for epistx	Non-Operative
14.49	Scleral buckling NEC	Operative	21.03	Caut to cntrl epistaxis	Non-Operative
14.5	Oth repair retina detach	Operative	21.09	Epistaxis control NEC	Operative
14.6	Rmvl prosth mat post SEG	Operative	21.1	Nose incision	Non-Operative
14.7	Operations on vitreous	Operative	21.2	Nasal diagnostic px	Non-Operative
14.74	Mech vitrectomy NEC	Operative	21.21	Rhinoscopy	Non-Operative
14.9	Other post segment ops	Operative	21.3	Nasal lesion destr/exc	Non-Operative
15.0	ExOc musc-tend dxtic px	Operative	21.4	Resection of nose	Operative
15.1	1 ExOc musc ops w detach	Operative	21.5	Submuc NAS septum resect	Operative
15.2	Oth ops on 1 ExOc muscle	Operative	21.6	Turbinectomy	Operative
15.3	Temp detach >1 ExOc musc	Operative	21.7	Nasal fracture reduction	Mixed (1, 1)
15.4	Oth ops on >1 ExOc musc	Operative	21.71	Clsd reduction nasal fx	Non-Operative
15.5	ExOc musc transposition	Operative	21.72	Open reduction nasal fx	Operative
15.6	Rev ExOc muscle surgery	Operative	21.8	Nasal REP & plastic ops	Mixed (8, 1)
15.7	ExOc muscle injury REP	Operative	21.81	Nasal laceration suture	Non-Operative
15.9	Oth ExOc musc-tend ops	Operative	21.88	Septoplasty NEC	Operative
16.0	Orbitotomy	Operative	21.89	Nasal repair NEC	Operative
16.09	Orbitotomy NEC	Operative	21.9	Other nasal operations	Mixed (1, 1)
16.1	Rmvl penetr FB eye NOS	Operative	22.0	Nasal sinus asp & lavage	Non-Operative
16.2	Orbit & eyeball dxtic px	Mixed (3, 1)	22.1	Nasal sinus dxtic px	Mixed (1, 2)
16.3	Evisceration of eyeball	Operative	22.19	Nasal sinus dxtic px NEC	Non-Operative
16.4	Enucleation of eyeball	Operative	22.2	Intranasal antrotomy	Non-Operative
16.5	Exenteration of orbit	Operative	22.3	Ext maxillary antrotomy	Operative
16.6	2nd px post rmvl eyeball	Operative	22.4	Front sinusot & sinusect	Operative
16.7	Ocular/orbital impl rmvl	Operative	22.5	Other nasal sinusotomy	Operative
16.8	Eyeball/orbit inj repair	Operative	22.6	Other nasal sinusectomy	Operative
16.82	Repair eyeball rupture	Operative	22.62	Exc max sinus lesion NEC	Operative
16.9	Other eye & orbit ops	Mixed (4, 1)	22.63	Ethmoidectomy	Operative
18.0	External ear incision	Non-Operative	22.7	Nasal sinus repair	Operative
18.09	External ear inc NEC	Non-Operative	22.9	Other nasal sinus ops	Operative
18.1	External ear dxtic px	Non-Operative	23.0	Forceps tooth extraction	Non-Operative
18.2	Exc/destr ext ear lesion	Mixed (1, 1)	23.09	Tooth extraction NEC	Non-Operative
18.29	Destr ext ear les NEC	Non-Operative	23.1	Surg removal of tooth	Non-Operative
18.3	Other external ear exc	Operative	23.19	Surg tooth extract NEC	Non-Operative
18.4	Suture ext ear lac	Non-Operative	23.2	Tooth restor by filling	Non-Operative
18.5	Correction prominent ear	Operative	23.3	Tooth restor by inlay	Non-Operative
18.6	Ext audit canal reconst	Operative	23.4	Other dental restoration	Non-Operative
18.7	Oth plastic REP ext ear	Operative	23.5	Tooth implantation	Non-Operative
18.79	Plastic REP ext ear NEC	Operative	23.6	Prosthetic dental impl	Non-Operative
18.9	Other ext ear operations	Operative	23.7	Root canal Tx & apicoect	Non-Operative
19.0	Stapes mobilization	Operative	24.0	Gum or alveolar incision	Non-Operative
19.1	Stapedectomy	Operative	24.1	Tooth & gum dxtic px	Non-Operative
19.2	Stapedectomy revision	Operative	24.2	Gingivoplasty	Operative
19.3	Ossicular chain ops NEC	Operative	24.3	Other operations on gums	Non-Operative
19.4	Myringoplasty	Operative	24.4	Exc of dental les of jaw	Operative
19.5	Other tympanoplasty	Operative	24.5	Alveoloplasty	Operative
19.6	Tympanoplasty revision	Operative	24.6	Exposure of tooth	Non-Operative
19.9	Middle ear repair NEC	Operative	24.7	Appl orthodont appliance	Non-Operative
20.0	Myringotomy	Mixed (1, 1)	24.8	Other orthodontic op	Non-Operative
20.01	Myringotomy w intubation	Operative	24.9	Other dental operation	Non-Operative
20.1	Tympanostomy tube rmvl	Non-Operative	25.0	Dxtic px on tongue	Mixed (1, 2)
20.2	Mastoid & mid ear inc	Operative	25.1	Exc/destr tongue les	Operative
20.3	Mid & inner ear dxtic px	Mixed (2, 1)	25.2	Partial glossectomy	Operative
20.4	Mastoidectomy	Operative	25.3	Complete glossectomy	Operative
20.5	Oth middle ear excision	Operative	25.4	Radical glossectomy	Operative
20.6	Fenestration inner ear	Operative	25.5	Repair of tongue	Mixed (1, 1)
20.7	Inc/exc/destr inner ear	Operative	25.9	Other tongue operations	Mixed (2, 3)
20.8	Eustachian tube ops	Non-Operative	25.91	Lingual frenotomy	Non-Operative
20.9	Other ME & IE ops	Mixed (8, 1)	25.92	Lingual frenectomy	Non-Operative

Code	Description	Operative Status	Code	Description	Operative Status
26.0	Inc salivary gland/duct	Non-Operative	31.69	Other laryngeal repair	Operative
26.1	Salivary gland dxtic px	Mixed (1, 2)	31.7	Repair of trachea	Operative
26.2	Exc of SG lesion	Operative	31.73	Trach fistula close NEC	Operative
26.29	Salivary les exc NEC	Operative	31.74	Revision of tracheostomy	Operative
26.3	Sialoadenectomy	Operative	31.9	Other larynx/trachea ops	Mixed (4, 3)
26.30	Sialoadenectomy NOS	Operative	31.99	Tracheal operation NEC	Operative
26.31	Partial sialoadenectomy	Operative	32.0	Loc exc/destr bronch les	Mixed (1, 1)
26.32	Complete sialoadenectomy	Operative	32.1	Bronchial excision NEC	Operative
26.4	SG & duct repair	Operative	32.2	Loc exc/destr lung les	Mixed (8, 1)
26.9	Oth salivary operations	Mixed (1, 1)	32.20	Thorscpy exc lung les	Operative
27.0	Drain face & mouth floor	Operative	32.29	Loc exc lung les NEC	Operative
27.1	Incision of palate	Operative	32.3	SEG resection lung	Operative
27.2	Oral cavity dxtic px	Mixed (2, 3)	32.30	Thorscpy SEG lung resect	Operative
27.3	Exc bony palate les/tiss	Operative	32.39	SEG resect lung NEC&NOS	Operative
27.4	Other excision of mouth	Mixed (3, 1)	32.4	Lung lobectomy	Operative
27.49	Excision of mouth NEC	Operative	32.41	Thorscpy lung lobectomy	Operative
27.5	Mouth plastic repair	Mixed (6, 2)	32.49	Lung lobectomy NEC	Operative
27.51	Suture of lip laceration	Non-Operative	32.5	Pneumonectomy	Operative
27.54	Repair of cleft lip	Operative	32.59	Pneumonectomy NEC & NOS	Operative
27.59	Mouth repair NEC	Operative	32.6	RAD dissect thor struct	Operative
27.6	Palatoplasty	Mixed (4, 1)	32.9	Lung excision NEC	Operative
27.62	Cleft palate correction	Operative	33.0	Bronchus incision	Operative
27.63	Rev cleft palate repair	Operative	33.1	Lung incision	Operative
27.69	Other plastic REP palate	Operative	33.2	Bronchial/lung dxtic px	Mixed (5, 5)
27.7	Operations on uvula	Operative	33.20	Thoracoscopic lung Bx	Operative
27.9	Oth ops on mouth & face	Mixed (2, 1)	33.21	Bronchoscopy thru stoma	Non-Operative
27.92	Mouth struct inc NOS	Operative	33.22	Fiber-optic bronchoscopy	Non-Operative
28.0	Tonsil/peritonsillar I&D	Operative	33.23	Bronchoscopy NEC	Non-Operative
28.1	Tonsil&adenoid dxtic px	Operative	33.24	Closed bronchus biopsy	Non-Operative
28.2	Tonsillectomy	Operative	33.26	Closed lung biopsy	Non-Operative
28.3	T&A	Operative	33.27	Endoscopic lung biopsy	Operative
28.4	Excision of tonsil tag	Operative	33.28	Open biopsy of lung	Operative
28.5	Excision lingual tonsil	Operative	33.3	Surg collapse of lung	Mixed (2, 3)
28.6	Adenoidectomy	Operative	33.39	Surg collaps of lung NEC	Operative
28.7	Hemor control post T&A	Operative	33.4	Lung & bronchus repair	Operative
28.9	Other tonsil/adenoid ops	Operative	33.5	Lung transplantation	Operative
29.0	Pharyngotomy	Operative	33.52	Bilat lung transplant	Operative
29.1	Pharyngeal dxtic px	Non-Operative	33.6	Heart-lung transplant	Operative
29.11	Pharyngoscopy	Non-Operative	33.7	Endo ins/repl/rmv resp	Non-Operative
29.2	Exc branchial cleft cyst	Operative	33.9	Other bronchial lung ops	Mixed (4, 1)
29.3	Exc/destr pharyngeal les	Operative	33.93	Puncture of lung	Operative
29.32	PHAR diverticulectomy	Operative	34.0	Inc chest wall & pleura	Mixed (3, 4)
29.4	Plastic op on pharynx	Operative	34.01	Chest wall incision	Non-Operative
29.5	Other pharyngeal repair	Operative	34.02	Exploratory thoracotomy	Operative
29.9	Other pharyngeal ops	Mixed (2, 1)	34.03	Reopen thoracotomy site	Operative
30.0	Exc/destr les larynx	Operative	34.04	Insert intercostal cath	Non-Operative
30.09	Exc/destr larynx les NEC	Operative	34.06	Thorscpy pleural drain	Operative
30.1	Hemilaryngectomy	Operative	34.09	Pleural incision NEC	Non-Operative
30.2	Partial laryngectomy NEC	Operative	34.1	Mediastinum incision	Operative
30.3	Complete laryngectomy	Operative	34.2	Thorax dxtic procedures	Mixed (7, 3)
30.4	Radical laryngectomy	Operative	34.20	Thoracoscopic pleural Bx	Operative
31.0	Larynx injection	Non-Operative	34.21	Transpleura thoracoscopy	Operative
31.1	Temporary tracheostomy	Non-Operative	34.22	Mediastinoscopy	Operative
31.2	Permanent tracheostomy	Operative	34.23	Chest wall biopsy	Non-Operative
31.29	Other perm tracheostomy	Operative	34.24	Pleural biopsy NEC	Non-Operative
31.3	Inc larynx/trachea NEC	Operative	34.25	Closed mediastinal Bx	Non-Operative
31.4	Larynx/trachea dxtic px	Mixed (1, 6)	34.26	Open mediastinal biopsy	Operative
31.42	Laryngoscopy/tracheoscpy	Non-Operative	34.3	Destr mediastinum les	Operative
31.43	Closed larynx biopsy	Non-Operative	34.4	Exc/destr chest wall les	Operative
31.5	Loc exc/destr larynx les	Operative	34.5	Pleurectomy	Operative
31.6	Repair of larynx	Operative	34.51	Decortication of lung	Operative

Code	Description	Operative Status	Code	Description	Operative Status
34.52	Thorscpy decort lung	Operative	37.22	Left heart cardiac cath	Non-Operative
34.59	Pleural excision NEC	Operative	37.23	Rt/left heart card cath	Non-Operative
34.6	Pleural scarification	Operative	37.25	Cardiac biopsy	Non-Operative
34.7	Repair of chest wall	Mixed (3, 2)	37.26	Cath based invas EPS	Non-Operative
34.74	Pectus deformity repair	Operative	37.3	Pericardiect/exc hrt les	Operative
34.79	Chest wall repair NEC	Operative	37.31	Pericardiectomy	Operative
34.8	Operations on diaphragm	Operative	37.33	Heart les exc NEC-open	Operative
34.82	Suture diaphragm lac	Operative	37.34	Heart les exc appr NEC	Operative
34.9	Other ops on thorax	Mixed (2, 2)	37.4	REP heart & pericardium	Operative
34.91	Thoracentesis	Non-Operative	37.5	Heart replacement px	Operative
34.92	Inject into thor cavit	Non-Operative	37.51	Heart transplantation	Operative
35.0	Closed heart valvotomy	Operative	37.6	Impl circulatory & HAS	Operative
35.1	Open heart valvuloplasty	Operative	37.61	Pulsation balloon impl	Operative
35.11	Opn aortic valvuloplasty	Operative	37.66	Insert implantable HAS	Operative
35.12	Opn mitral valvuloplasty	Operative	37.7	Card lead px/pocket rev	Mixed (5, 5)
35.14	Opn tricusp valvuloplast	Operative	37.71	Insert TV lead-ventricle	Non-Operative
35.2	Heart valve replacement	Operative	37.72	Insert TV lead-ATR&vent	Non-Operative
35.21	Repl aortic valve-tissue	Operative	37.73	Insert TV lead-atrium	Non-Operative
35.22	Repl aortic valve NEC	Operative	37.74	Insert epicardial lead	Operative
35.23	Repl mitral valve w tiss	Operative	37.75	Revision cardiac lead	Operative
35.24	Repl mitral valve NEC	Operative	37.76	Repl transvenous lead	Operative
35.25	Repl pulmon valve w tiss	Operative	37.77	Removal cardiac lead	Operative
35.3	Tiss adj to hrt valv ops	Operative	37.78	Insert temp TV pacer	Non-Operative
35.33	Annuloplasty	Operative	37.79	Rev cardiac dev pocket	Operative
35.4	Septal defect production	Mixed (1, 1)	37.8	Cardiac pacemaker dev op	Mixed (5, 3)
35.5	Prosth REP heart septa	Operative	37.80	Insert pacemaker dev NOS	Operative
35.52	Prosth REP ASD clsd tech	Operative	37.81	Insert single chamb dev	Non-Operative
35.53	Open prosth REP VSD	Operative	37.82	Insert rate-respon dev	Non-Operative
35.6	Tiss grft REP hrt septa	Operative	37.83	Insert dual-chamber dev	Non-Operative
35.61	Repair ASD w tiss graft	Operative	37.85	Repl w 1-chamber device	Operative
35.62	Repair VSD w tiss graft	Operative	37.86	Repl w rate-respon dev	Operative
35.63	Repair ECD w tiss graft	Operative	37.87	Repl w dual-chamb device	Operative
35.7	Heart septa repair NEC	Operative	37.89	Rev/rmvl pacemaker dev	Operative
35.71	Repair ASD NEC & NOS	Operative	37.9	Hrt/pericardium ops NEC	Mixed (7, 3)
35.8	Tot REP cong card anom	Operative	37.94	Impl/repl AICD tot syst	Operative
35.81	Tot REP tetralogy Fallot	Operative	37.97	Replace AICD lead only	Operative
35.9	Valves & septa ops NEC	Operative	37.98	Repl AICD generator only	Operative
35.92	Creat conduit rt vent-PA	Operative	38.0	Incision of vessel	Operative
35.94	Creat conduit atrium-PA	Operative	38.03	Upper limb vessel inc	Operative
35.96	PERC valvuloplasty	Operative	38.06	Abdominal art incision	Operative
36.0	Rmvl cor art obstr/stent	Mixed (2, 3)	38.08	Lower limb artery inc	Operative
36.06	Non-drug-elut cor stent	Non-Operative	38.1	Endarterectomy	Operative
36.07	Drug-eluting cor stent	Non-Operative	38.12	Head/nk endarterect NEC	Operative
36.1	Hrt revasc bypass anast	Operative	38.16	Abdominal endarterectomy	Operative
36.11	Cor bypass-1 cor art	Operative	38.18	Lower limb endarterect	Operative
36.12	Cor bypass-2 cor art	Operative	38.2	Dxtic blood vessels px	Mixed (2, 1)
36.13	Cor bypass-3 cor art	Operative	38.21	Blood vessel biopsy	Operative
36.14	Cor bypass-4+ cor art	Operative	38.3	Vessel resect w anast	Operative
36.15	1 int mam-cor art bypass	Operative	38.34	Aorta resection w anast	Operative
36.16	2 int mam-cor art bypass	Operative	38.4	Vessel resect w repl	Operative
36.2	Arterial implant revasc	Operative	38.44	Abd aorta resect w repl	Operative
36.3	Other heart revasc	Operative	38.45	Thor vess resect w repl	Operative
36.31	Open transmyo revasc	Operative	38.48	Leg artery resect w repl	Operative
36.9	Other heart vessel ops	Operative	38.5	Lig&strip varicose veins	Operative
36.99	Heart vessel ops NEC	Operative	38.59	Lower limb VV lig&strip	Operative
37.0	Pericardiocentesis	Non-Operative	38.6	Other vessel excision	Operative
37.1	Cardiotomy & pericardiot	Operative	38.63	Up limb vessel exc NEC	Operative
37.12	Pericardiotomy	Operative	38.7	Interruption vena cava	Operative
37.2	Dxtic px hrt/pericardium	Mixed (1, 9)	38.8	Other surg vessel occl	Operative
37.20	NIPS	Non-Operative	38.82	Occl head/neck vess NEC	Operative
37.21	Rt heart cardiac cath	Non-Operative	38.83	Occl upper limb vess NEC	Operative

Code	Description	Operative Status	Code	Description	Operative Status
38.85	Occl thoracic vess NEC	Operative	40.5	Oth RAD node dissection	Operative
38.86	Surg occl abd artery NEC	Operative	40.51	RAD exc axillary nodes	Operative
38.9	Puncture of vessel	Non-Operative	40.52	RAD exc periaortic nodes	Operative
38.91	Arterial catheterization	Non-Operative	40.53	RAD exc iliac lymph node	Operative
38.92	Umbilical vein cath	Non-Operative	40.59	RAD exc lymph node NEC	Operative
38.93	Venous catheter NEC	Non-Operative	40.6	Thoracic duct operations	Operative
38.94	Venous cutdown	Non-Operative	40.9	Lymphatic struct ops NEC	Operative
38.95	Venous cath for RD	Non-Operative	41.0	Bone marrow transplant	Operative
38.98	Arterial puncture NEC	Non-Operative	41.03	Allo marrow transpl NEC	Operative
38.99	Venous puncture NEC	Non-Operative	41.04	Autlog stem cell transpl	Operative
39.0	Systemic to PA shunt	Operative	41.05	Allo stem cell transpl	Operative
39.1	Intra-abd venous shunt	Operative	41.1	Puncture of spleen	Non-Operative
39.2	Other shunt/vasc bypass	Operative	41.2	Splenotomy	Operative
39.21	Caval-PA anastomosis	Operative	41.3	Marrow & spleen dxtic px	Mixed (1, 4)
39.22	Aorta-scl-carotid bypass	Operative	41.31	Bone marrow biopsy	Non-Operative
39.25	Aorta-iliac-femoral byp	Operative	41.4	Exc/destr splenic tissue	Operative
39.26	Intra-abd vasc shunt NEC	Operative	41.5	Total splenectomy	Operative
39.27	Arteriovenostomy for RD	Operative	41.9	Oth spleen & marrow ops	Mixed (4, 3)
39.28	EC-IC vascular bypass	Operative	42.0	Esophagotomy	Operative
39.29	Vasc shunt & bypass NEC	Operative	42.1	Esophagostomy	Operative
39.3	Suture of vessel	Operative	42.2	Esophageal dxtic px	Mixed (2, 4)
39.31	Suture of artery	Operative	42.23	Esophagoscopy NEC	Non-Operative
39.32	Suture of vein	Operative	42.24	Closed esophageal biopsy	Non-Operative
39.4	Vascular px revision	Operative	42.3	Exc/destr esoph les/tiss	Mixed (3, 1)
39.42	Rev AV shunt for RD	Operative	42.33	Endo exc/destr esoph les	Non-Operative
39.43	Rmvl AV shunt for RD	Operative	42.4	Excision of esophagus	Operative
39.49	Vascular px revision NEC	Operative	42.41	Partial esophagectomy	Operative
39.5	Other vessel repair	Operative	42.42	Total esophagectomy	Operative
39.50	PTA/atherect oth vessel	Operative	42.5	Intrathor esoph anast	Operative
39.51	Clipping of aneurysm	Operative	42.6	Antesternal esoph anast	Operative
39.52	Aneurysm repair NEC	Operative	42.7	Esophagomyotomy	Operative
39.53	AV fistula repair	Operative	42.8	Other esophageal repair	Mixed (7, 1)
39.56	REP vess w tiss patch	Operative	42.81	Insert perm tube esoph	Non-Operative
39.57	REP vess w synth patch	Operative	42.9	Other esophageal ops	Mixed (1, 2)
39.59	Repair of vessel NEC	Operative	42.92	Esophageal dilation	Non-Operative
39.6	Open heart auxiliary px	Mixed (1, 5)	43.0	Gastrotomy	Operative
39.7	Endovascular vessel REP	Operative	43.1	Gastrostomy	Non-Operative
39.71	Endovascular graft-AAA	Operative	43.11	PEG	Non-Operative
39.72	Endov REP HN vessel	Operative	43.19	Gastrostomy NEC	Non-Operative
39.73	Endov graft thor aorta	Operative	43.3	Pyloromyotomy	Operative
39.74	Endov rmvl HN vess obstr	Operative	43.4	Loc exc gastric les	Mixed (2, 1)
39.79	Endov REP vessels NEC	Operative	43.41	Endo exc gastric les	Non-Operative
39.8	Vascular body operations	Operative	43.42	Loc gastric les exc NEC	Operative
39.9	Other vessel operations	Mixed (6, 4)	43.5	Proximal gastrectomy	Operative
39.90	Non-drug periph stent	Non-Operative	43.6	Distal gastrectomy	Operative
39.93	Insert vess-vess cannula	Operative	43.7	Part gastrectomy w anast	Operative
39.95	Hemodialysis	Non-Operative	43.8	Oth partial gastrectomy	Operative
39.98	Hemorrhage control NOS	Operative	43.89	Partial gastrectomy NEC	Operative
39.99	Vessel operation NEC	Operative	43.9	Total gastrectomy	Operative
40.0	Inc lymphatic structure	Operative	43.99	Total gastrectomy NEC	Operative
40.1	Lymphatic dxtic px	Operative	44.0	Vagotomy	Operative
40.11	Lymphatic struct biopsy	Operative	44.1	Gastric dxtic px	Mixed (2, 4)
40.2	Smp exc lymphatic struct	Operative	44.13	Gastroscopy NEC	Non-Operative
40.21	Exc deep cervical node	Operative	44.14	Closed gastric biopsy	Non-Operative
40.23	Exc axillary lymph node	Operative	44.2	Pyloroplasty	Mixed (2, 1)
40.24	Exc inguinal lymph node	Operative	44.22	Endo dilation pylorus	Non-Operative
40.29	Smp exc lymphatic NEC	Operative	44.29	Other pyloroplasty	Operative
40.3	Regional lymph node exc	Operative	44.3	Gastroenterostomy	Operative
40.4	RAD exc cerv lymph node	Operative	44.31	High gastric bypass	Operative
40.41	Unilat RAD neck dissect	Operative	44.32	PERC gastrojejunostomy	Operative
40.42	Bilat RAD neck dissect	Operative	44.38	Lapscp gastroenterostomy	Operative

Code	Description	Operative Status	Code	Description	Operative Status
44.39	Gastroenterostomy NEC	Operative	46.11	Temporary colostomy	Operative
44.4	Cntrl peptic ulcer hemor	Mixed (3, 3)	46.13	Permanent colostomy	Operative
44.41	Sut gastric ulcer site	Operative	46.2	Ileostomy	Mixed (4, 1)
44.42	Sut duodenal ulcer site	Operative	46.20	Ileostomy NOS	Operative
44.43	Endo cntrl gastric bleed	Non-Operative	46.23	Permanent ileostomy NEC	Operative
44.5	Revision gastric anast	Operative	46.3	Other enterostomy	Non-Operative
44.6	Other gastric repair	Mixed (8, 1)	46.32	PEJ	Non-Operative
44.61	Suture gastric lac	Operative	46.39	Enterostomy NEC	Non-Operative
44.63	Close stom fistula NEC	Operative	46.4	Intestinal stoma rev	Operative
44.66	Creat EG sphinct compet	Operative	46.41	Sm intest stoma revision	Operative
44.67	Lapscp px EGS compet	Operative	46.42	Pericolostomy hernia REP	Operative
44.68	Lapscp gastroplasty	Operative	46.43	Lg intest stoma rev NEC	Operative
44.69	Gastric repair NEC	Operative	46.5	Intestinal stoma closure	Operative
44.9	Other stomach operations	Mixed (7, 2)	46.51	Sm intest stoma closure	Operative
44.95	Lapscp gastric rest px	Operative	46.52	Lg intest stoma closure	Operative
44.96	Lapscp rev gast rest px	Operative	46.6	Fixation of intestine	Operative
44.97	Lapscp rmv gast rest dev	Operative	46.7	Other intestinal repair	Operative
44.99	Gastric operation NEC	Operative	46.71	Duodenal lac suture	Operative
45.0	Enterotomy	Operative	46.73	Small intest suture NEC	Operative
45.02	Sm intest incision NEC	Operative	46.74	Closure SmB fistula NEC	Operative
45.1	Small intest dxtic px	Mixed (2, 5)	46.75	Large intestine suture	Operative
45.12	Endo S-intest thru stoma	Non-Operative	46.79	Repair of intestine NEC	Operative
45.13	Sm intest endoscopy NEC	Non-Operative	46.8	Bowel dilation & manip	Mixed (3, 1)
45.14	Closed small intest Bx	Non-Operative	46.81	Intra-abd S-intest manip	Operative
45.16	EGD w closed biopsy	Non-Operative	46.82	Intra-abd L-intest manip	Operative
45.2	Lg intestine dxtic px	Mixed (2, 7)	46.85	Dilation of intestine	Non-Operative
45.22	Endo L-intest thru stoma	Non-Operative	46.9	Other intestinal ops	Mixed (6, 2)
45.23	Colonoscopy	Non-Operative	46.93	Revision sm intest anast	Operative
45.24	Flexible sigmoidoscopy	Non-Operative	47.0	Appendectomy	Operative
45.25	Closed lg intest biopsy	Non-Operative	47.01	Lapscp appendectomy	Operative
45.3	Loc exc/destr SmB les	Mixed (4, 1)	47.09	Other appendectomy	Operative
45.30	Endo exc/destr duod les	Non-Operative	47.1	Incidental appendectomy	Operative
45.31	Loc exc duod les NEC	Operative	47.11	Lapscp incidental APPY	Operative
45.33	Loc exc S-intest les NEC	Operative	47.2	Drain appendiceal absc	Operative
45.4	Loc destr lg intest les	Mixed (2, 2)	47.9	Other appendiceal ops	Operative
45.41	Exc lg intest lesion	Operative	48.0	Proctotomy	Operative
45.42	Endo colon polypectomy	Non-Operative	48.1	Proctostomy	Operative
45.43	Endo destr colon les NEC	Non-Operative	48.2	Rectal/perirect dxtic px	Mixed (2, 5)
45.5	Intestinal SEG isolation	Operative	48.23	Rig proctosigmoidoscopy	Non-Operative
45.6	Sm intest excision NEC	Operative	48.24	Closed rectal biopsy	Non-Operative
45.61	Mult SEG S-intest resect	Operative	48.3	Loc destr rectal lesion	Mixed (1, 5)
45.62	Part S-intest resect NEC	Operative	48.35	Loc exc rectal les/tiss	Operative
45.7	Part lg intest excision	Operative	48.36	Endo rectal polypectomy	Non-Operative
45.71	Mult SEG L-intest resect	Operative	48.4	Pull-thru rect resection	Operative
45.72	Cecectomy	Operative	48.49	Pull-thru rect resect	Operative
45.73	Right hemicolectomy	Operative	48.5	Abd-perineal rect resect	Operative
45.74	Transverse colon resect	Operative	48.6	Other rectal resection	Operative
45.75	Left hemicolectomy	Operative	48.62	Ant rect resect w colost	Operative
45.76	Sigmoidectomy	Operative	48.63	Anterior rect resect NEC	Operative
45.79	Part lg intest exc NEC	Operative	48.69	Rectal resection NEC	Operative
45.8	Tot intra-abd colectomy	Operative	48.7	Repair of rectum	Operative
45.9	Intestinal anastomosis	Operative	48.75	Abdominal proctopexy	Operative
45.91	Sm-to-sm intest anast	Operative	48.76	Proctopexy NEC	Operative
45.93	Sm-lg intest anast NEC	Operative	48.8	Perirect tiss inc/exc	Operative
45.94	Lg-to-lg intest anast	Operative	48.81	Perirectal incision	Operative
45.95	Anastomosis to anus	Operative	48.9	Oth rectal/perirect op	Operative
46.0	Intest exteriorization	Operative	49.0	Perianal tiss inc/exc	Mixed (3, 1)
46.01	S-intest exteriorization	Operative	49.01	Inc perianal abscess	Operative
46.03	L-intest exteriorization	Operative	49.1	Inc/exc of anal fistula	Operative
46.1	Colostomy	Mixed (3, 1)	49.11	Anal fistulotomy	Operative
46.10	Colostomy NOS	Operative	49.12	Anal fistulectomy	Operative

Code	Description	Operative Status	Code	Description	Operative Status
49.2	Anal & perianal dxtic px	Non-Operative	52.1	Pancreatic dxtic px	Mixed (2, 3)
49.21	Anoscopy	Non-Operative	52.11	Pancreas aspiration Bx	Non-Operative
49.3	Loc destr anal les NEC	Mixed (1, 1)	52.2	Panc/panc duct les destr	Mixed (1, 1)
49.39	Oth loc destr anal les	Operative	52.22	Panc duct les destr NEC	Operative
49.4	Hemorrhoid procedures	Mixed (4, 4)	52.3	Pancreatic cyst marsup	Operative
49.45	Hemorrhoid ligation	Operative	52.4	Int drain panc cyst	Operative
49.46	Exc of hemorrhoids	Operative	52.5	Partial pancreatectomy	Operative
49.5	Anal sphincter division	Operative	52.52	Distal pancreatectomy	Operative
49.6	Excision of anus	Operative	52.59	Part pancreatectomy NEC	Operative
49.7	Repair of anus	Operative	52.6	Total pancreatectomy	Operative
49.73	Closure of anal fistula	Operative	52.7	RAD panc/duodenectomy	Operative
49.79	Anal sphincter REP NEC	Operative	52.8	Transplant of pancreas	Mixed (4, 3)
49.9	Oth operations on anus	Operative	52.9	Other ops on pancreas	Mixed (4, 4)
50.0	Hepatotomy	Operative	52.93	Endo insert panc stent	Non-Operative
50.1	Hepatic dxtic px	Mixed (3, 2)	52.96	Pancreatic anastomosis	Operative
50.11	Closed liver biopsy	Non-Operative	53.0	Unilat IH repair	Operative
50.12	Open biopsy of liver	Operative	53.00	Unilat IH repair NOS	Operative
50.13	Transjugular liver Bx	Non-Operative	53.01	Unilat REP direct IH	Operative
50.14	Laparoscopic liver Bx	Operative	53.02	Unilat REP indirect IH	Operative
50.2	Loc exc/destr liver les	Operative	53.03	Unilat REP DIR IH/graft	Operative
50.22	Partial hepatectomy	Operative	53.04	Unilat indirect IH/graft	Operative
50.23	Open ablat liver lesion	Operative	53.05	Unilat REP IH/graft NOS	Operative
50.24	PERC ablat liver lesion	Operative	53.1	Bilat IH repair	Operative
50.25	Lapscp ablat liver les	Operative	53.10	Bilat IH repair NOS	Operative
50.29	Hepatic lesion destr NEC	Operative	53.12	Bilat indirect IH repair	Operative
50.3	Hepatic lobectomy	Operative	53.14	Bilat direct IH REP-grft	Operative
50.4	Total hepatectomy	Operative	53.15	Bilat indirect IH-graft	Operative
50.5	Liver transplant	Operative	53.16	Direct/indirect IH-graft	Operative
50.59	Liver transplant NEC	Operative	53.17	Bilat IH REP-graft NOS	Operative
50.6	Repair of liver	Operative	53.2	Unilat FH repair	Operative
50.61	Closure of liver lac	Operative	53.21	Unilat FH REP w graft	Operative
50.9	Other liver operations	Non-Operative	53.29	Unilat FH REP NEC	Operative
50.91	PERC liver aspiration	Non-Operative	53.3	Bilat FH repair	Operative
50.94	Hepatic injection NEC	Non-Operative	53.4	Umbilical hernia repair	Operative
51.0	GB inc & cholecystostomy	Mixed (3, 1)	53.41	UH REP-graft/prosth	Operative
51.01	PERC aspiration of GB	Non-Operative	53.49	Umb hernia repair NEC	Operative
51.03	Cholecystostomy NEC	Operative	53.5	REP oth abd wall hernia	Operative
51.04	Cholecystotomy NEC	Operative	53.51	Incisional hernia repair	Operative
51.1	Biliary tract dxtic px	Mixed (2, 5)	53.59	Abd wall hernia REP NEC	Operative
51.10	ERCP	Non-Operative	53.6	REP oth abd hernia-graft	Operative
51.14	Clsd BD/sphinct Oddi Bx	Non-Operative	53.61	Inc hern REP-grft/prosth	Operative
51.2	Cholecystectomy	Operative	53.69	Hern NEC REP-grft/prosth	Operative
51.22	Cholecystectomy NOS	Operative	53.7	Abd REP-diaph hernia	Operative
51.23	Lapscp cholecystectomy	Operative	53.8	Repair DH thor appr	Operative
51.3	Biliary tract anast	Operative	53.80	Repair DH thor appr NOS	Operative
51.36	Choledochoenterostomy	Operative	53.9	Other hernia repair	Operative
51.37	Hepatic duct-GI anast	Operative	54.0	Abdominal wall incision	Operative
51.4	Inc bile duct obstr	Operative	54.1	Laparotomy	Operative
51.43	Insert CBD-hep tube	Operative	54.11	Exploratory laparotomy	Operative
51.5	Other bile duct incision	Operative	54.12	Reopen recent LAP site	Operative
51.6	Loc exc BD & S of O les	Mixed (4, 1)	54.19	Laparotomy NEC	Operative
51.7	Repair of bile ducts	Operative	54.2	Abd region dxtic px	Mixed (4, 2)
51.8	Sphincter of Oddi op NEC	Mixed (4, 5)	54.21	Laparoscopy	Operative
51.84	Endo ampulla & BD dilat	Non-Operative	54.22	Abd wall or umbilicus Bx	Operative
51.85	Endo sphinctot/papillot	Non-Operative	54.23	Peritoneal biopsy	Operative
51.87	Endo insert BD stent	Non-Operative	54.24	Clsd intra-abd mass Bx	Non-Operative
51.88	Endo rmvl biliary stone	Non-Operative	54.3	Exc/destr abd wall les	Operative
51.9	Other biliary tract ops	Mixed (6, 2)	54.4	Exc/destr periton tiss	Operative
51.98	PERC op on bil tract NEC	Non-Operative	54.5	Peritoneal adhesiolysis	Operative
52.0	Pancreatotomy	Operative	54.51	Lapscp periton ADHESIO	Operative
52.01	Drain panc cyst by cath	Operative	54.59	Periton adhesiolysis NEC	Operative

Code	Description	Operative Status	Code	Description	Operative Status
54.6	Abd wall/periton suture	Operative	57.4	TU exc/destr bladder les	Operative
54.61	Reclose postop disrupt	Operative	57.49	TU destr bladder les NEC	Operative
54.63	Abd wall suture NEC	Operative	57.5	Bladder les destr NEC	Operative
54.7	Oth abd wall periton REP	Operative	57.59	Oth bladder lesion destr	Operative
54.71	Repair of gastroschisis	Operative	57.6	Partial cystectomy	Operative
54.72	Abdomen wall repair NEC	Operative	57.7	Total cystectomy	Operative
54.9	Other abd region ops	Mixed (4, 5)	57.71	Radical cystectomy	Operative
54.91	PERC abd drainage	Non-Operative	57.79	Total cystectomy NEC	Operative
54.92	Rmvl FB periton cavity	Operative	57.8	Oth urin bladder repair	Operative
54.93	Create cutaneoperit fist	Operative	57.81	Suture bladder lac	Operative
54.95	Peritoneal incision	Operative	57.83	Enterovesical fist REP	Operative
54.98	Peritoneal dialysis	Non-Operative	57.84	REP oth fistula bladder	Operative
55.0	Nephrotomy & nephrostomy	Operative	57.87	Urinary bladder reconst	Operative
55.01	Nephrotomy	Operative	57.89	Bladder repair NEC	Operative
55.02	Nephrostomy	Operative	57.9	Other bladder operations	Mixed (6, 3)
55.03	PERC nephrostomy s frag	Operative	57.91	Bladder sphincterotomy	Operative
55.04	PERC nephrostomy w frag	Operative	57.93	Control bladder hemor	Operative
55.1	Pyelotomy & pyelostomy	Operative	57.94	Insert indwell urin cath	Non-Operative
55.11	Pyelotomy	Operative	57.95	Repl indwell urin cath	Non-Operative
55.2	Renal diagnostic px	Mixed (2, 3)	58.0	Urethrotomy	Operative
55.23	Closed renal biopsy	Non-Operative	58.1	Urethral meatotomy	Operative
55.3	Loc exc/destr renal les	Operative	58.2	Urethral diagnostic px	Non-Operative
55.33	PERC ablat renal lesion	Operative	58.3	Exc/destr urethral les	Non-Operative
55.34	Lapscp ablat renal les	Operative	58.31	Endo urethral les destr	Non-Operative
55.39	Loc destr renal les NEC	Operative	58.4	Repair of urethra	Operative
55.4	Partial nephrectomy	Operative	58.45	Hypospad/epispadias REP	Operative
55.5	Complete nephrectomy	Operative	58.46	Urethral reconst NEC	Operative
55.51	Nephroureterectomy	Operative	58.49	Urethral repair NEC	Operative
55.53	Rejected kid nephrectomy	Operative	58.5	Urethral stricture rel	Operative
55.54	Bilateral nephrectomy	Operative	58.6	Urethral dilation	Non-Operative
55.6	Kidney transplant	Operative	58.9	Other urethral ops	Operative
55.69	Kidney transplant NEC	Operative	58.93	Implantation of AUS	Operative
55.7	Nephropexy	Operative	58.99	Periurethral ops NEC	Operative
55.8	Other kidney repair	Operative	59.0	Retroperiton dissection	Operative
55.87	Correction of UPJ	Operative	59.02	Perirenal ADHESIO NEC	Operative
55.9	Other renal operations	Mixed (4, 5)	59.1	Perivesical incision	Operative
55.92	PERC renal aspiration	Non-Operative	59.2	Perirenal dxtic px	Operative
55.93	Repl nephrostomy tube	Non-Operative	59.3	Urethroves junct plicat	Operative
56.0	TU rmvl ureteral obstr	Operative	59.4	Suprapubic sling op	Operative
56.1	Ureteral meatotomy	Operative	59.5	Retropubic urethral susp	Operative
56.2	Ureterotomy	Operative	59.6	Paraurethral suspension	Operative
56.3	Ureteral diagnostic px	Mixed (2, 4)	59.7	Oth urinary incont REP	Mixed (2, 1)
56.31	Ureteroscopy	Non-Operative	59.79	Urin incont repair NEC	Operative
56.4	Ureterectomy	Operative	59.8	Ureteral catheterization	Non-Operative
56.41	Partial ureterectomy	Operative	59.9	Other urinary system ops	Mixed (2, 4)
56.5	Cutan uretero-ileostomy	Operative	59.94	Repl cystostomy tube	Non-Operative
56.51	Form cutan ileoureterost	Operative	60.0	Incision of prostate	Operative
56.6	Ext urin diversion NEC	Operative	60.1	Pros/sem vesicl dxtic px	Mixed (5, 2)
56.7	Other ureteral anast	Operative	60.11	Clsd prostatic Bx	Non-Operative
56.74	Ureteroneocystostomy	Operative	60.2	TU prostatectomy	Operative
56.8	Repair of ureter	Operative	60.21	TULIP procedure	Operative
56.9	Other ureteral operation	Mixed (5, 1)	60.29	TU prostatectomy NEC	Operative
57.0	TU bladder clearance	Non-Operative	60.3	Suprapubic prostatectomy	Operative
57.1	Cystotomy & cystostomy	Mixed (3, 2)	60.4	Retropubic prostatectomy	Operative
57.17	Percutaneous cystostomy	Non-Operative	60.5	Radical prostatectomy	Operative
57.18	S/P cystostomy NEC	Operative	60.6	Other prostatectomy	Operative
57.19	Cystotomy NEC	Operative	60.62	Perineal prostatectomy	Operative
57.2	Vesicostomy	Operative	60.69	Prostatectomy NEC	Operative
57.3	Bladder diagnostic px	Mixed (3, 2)	60.7	Seminal vesicle ops	Mixed (3, 1)
57.32	Cystoscopy NEC	Non-Operative	60.8	Periprostatic inc or exc	Operative
57.33	Closed bladder biopsy	Operative	60.9	Other prostatic ops	Mixed (6, 2)

Code	Description	Operative Status	Code	Description	Operative Status
60.94	Cntrl postop pros hemor	Operative	65.9	Other ovarian operations	Operative
61.0	Scrotum & tunica vag I&D	Non-Operative	65.91	Aspiration of ovary	Operative
61.1	Scrotum/tunica dxtic px	Non-Operative	66.0	Salpingostomy/salpingot	Operative
61.2	Excision of hydrocele	Operative	66.02	Salpingostomy	Operative
61.3	Scrotal les exc/destr	Non-Operative	66.1	Fallopian tube dxtic px	Operative
61.4	Scrotum & tunica vag REP	Mixed (2, 1)	66.2	Bilat endo occl FALL	Operative
61.9	Oth scrot/tunica vag ops	Mixed (2, 1)	66.22	Bilat endo lig/div FALL	Operative
62.0	Incision of testis	Operative	66.29	Bilat endo occl FALL NEC	Operative
62.1	Testes dxtic px	Mixed (2, 1)	66.3	Oth bilat FALL destr/exc	Operative
62.2	Testicular les exc/destr	Operative	66.32	Bilat FALL lig & div NEC	Operative
62.3	Unilateral orchiectomy	Operative	66.39	Bilat FALL destr NEC	Operative
62.4	Bilateral orchiectomy	Operative	66.4	Tot unilat salpingectomy	Operative
62.41	Rmvl both testes	Operative	66.5	Tot bilat salpingectomy	Operative
62.5	Orchiopexy	Operative	66.51	Rmvl both FALL tubes	Operative
62.6	Testes repair	Operative	66.6	Other salpingectomy	Operative
62.7	Insert testicular prosth	Operative	66.61	Exc/destr FALL les	Operative
62.9	Other testicular ops	Mixed (1, 2)	66.62	Rmvl FALL & tubal preg	Operative
63.0	Spermatic cord dxtic px	Mixed (1, 1)	66.69	Partial FALL rmvl NEC	Operative
63.1	Exc spermatic varicocele	Operative	66.7	Repair of fallopian tube	Operative
63.2	Exc epididymis cyst	Operative	66.79	FALL tube repair NEC	Operative
63.3	Exc sperm cord les NEC	Operative	66.8	FALL tube insufflation	Non-Operative
63.4	Epididymectomy	Operative	66.9	Other fallopian tube ops	Mixed (7, 1)
63.5	Sperm cord/epid repair	Mixed (3, 1)	67.0	Cervical canal dilation	Non-Operative
63.6	Vasotomy	Non-Operative	67.1	Cervical diagnostic px	Operative
63.7	Vasectomy & vas def lig	Non-Operative	67.12	Cervical biopsy NEC	Operative
63.8	Vas def & epid repair	Mixed (5, 1)	67.2	Conization of cervix	Operative
63.9	Oth sperm cord/epid ops	Mixed (5, 1)	67.3	Exc/destr cerv les NEC	Operative
64.0	Circumcision	Non-Operative	67.4	Amputation of cervix	Operative
64.1	Penile diagnostic px	Mixed (1, 1)	67.5	Int cervical os repair	Operative
64.2	Loc exc/destr penile les	Operative	67.59	Int cervical os REP NEC	Operative
64.3	Amputation of penis	Operative	67.6	Other repair of cervix	Operative
64.4	Penile REP/plastic ops	Operative	68.0	Hysterotomy	Operative
64.49	Penile repair NEC	Operative	68.1	Uter/adnexa dxtic px	Mixed (5, 2)
64.5	Sex transformation NEC	Operative	68.16	Closed uterine biopsy	Operative
64.9	Other male genital ops	Mixed (7, 2)	68.2	Uterine les exc/destr	Operative
64.92	Penile incision	Operative	68.23	Endometrial ablation	Operative
64.96	Rmvl int penile prosth	Operative	68.29	Uter les exc/destr NEC	Operative
64.97	Insert or repl IPP	Operative	68.3	Subtot abd hysterectomy	Operative
64.98	Penile operation NEC	Operative	68.31	LSH	Operative
65.0	Oophorotomy	Operative	68.39	Subtot abd hyst NEC&NOS	Operative
65.01	Lapscp oophorotomy	Operative	68.4	Total abd hysterectomy	Operative
65.1	Dxtic px on ovaries	Operative	68.41	TLH	Operative
65.2	Loc exc/destr ovary les	Operative	68.49	TAH NEC & NOS	Operative
65.25	Lapscp ov les exc NEC	Operative	68.5	Vaginal hysterectomy	Operative
65.29	Loc exc/destr ov les NEC	Operative	68.51	LAVH	Operative
65.3	Unilateral oophorectomy	Operative	68.59	Vag hyst NEC & NOS	Operative
65.31	Lapscp unilat oophorect	Operative	68.6	Radical abd hysterectomy	Operative
65.39	Unilat oophorectomy NEC	Operative	68.61	TLRH	Operative
65.4	Unilateral S-O	Operative	68.69	Rad abd hyst NEC & NOS	Operative
65.41	Lapscp unilateral S-O	Operative	68.7	Radical vag hysterectomy	Operative
65.49	Unilateral S-O NEC	Operative	68.79	Rad vag hyst NEC & NOS	Operative
65.5	Bilateral oophorectomy	Operative	68.8	Pelvic evisceration	Operative
65.51	Rmvl both ovaries NEC	Operative	68.9	Hysterectomy NEC & NOS	Operative
65.6	Bilat salpingo-oophorect	Operative	69.0	Uterine D&C	Operative
65.61	Rmvl both ov & FALL NEC	Operative	69.01	D&C for term of preg	Operative
65.62	Rmvl rem ov & FALL NEC	Operative	69.02	D&C post del or AB	Operative
65.63	Lapscp rmvl both ov/FALL	Operative	69.09	D&C NEC	Operative
65.7	Repair of ovary	Operative	69.1	Exc/destr uter/supp les	Operative
65.8	Tubo-ovarian ADHESIO	Operative	69.19	Exc uter/supp struct NEC	Operative
65.81	Lapscp ADHESIO ov/FALL	Operative	69.2	Uterine supp struct REP	Operative
65.89	ADHESIO ov/FALL tube NEC	Operative	69.3	Paracerv uterine denerv	Operative

Code	Description	Operative Status
69.4	Uterine repair	Operative
69.5	Asp curettage uterus	Mixed (2, 1)
69.51	Asp curettage-preg term	Operative
69.52	Asp curette post del/AB	Operative
69.59	Asp curettage uterus NEC	Non-Operative
69.6	Menstrual extraction	Non-Operative
69.7	Insertion of IUD	Non-Operative
69.9	Other ops uterus/adnexa	Mixed (4, 5)
69.96	Rmvl cervical cerclage	Non-Operative
70.0	Culdocentesis	Non-Operative
70.1	Inc vagina & cul-de-sac	Mixed (3, 1)
70.12	Culdotomy	Operative
70.14	Vaginotomy NEC	Operative
70.2	Vag/cul-de-sac dxtic px	Mixed (3, 2)
70.24	Vaginal biopsy	Operative
70.3	Loc exc/destr vag/cul	Operative
70.33	Exc/destr vaginal lesion	Operative
70.4	Vaginal obliteration	Operative
70.5	Cystocele/rectocele REP	Operative
70.50	REP cystocele/rectocele	Operative
70.51	Cystocele repair	Operative
70.52	Rectocele repair	Operative
70.53	Cyst&rect REP-gft/prosth	Operative
70.54	Cystocele REP-gft/prosth	Operative
70.55	Rectocele REP-gft/prosth	Operative
70.6	Vaginal constr/reconst	Operative
70.7	Other vaginal repair	Operative
70.71	Suture vagina laceration	Operative
70.73	REP rectovaginal fistula	Operative
70.77	Vaginal susp & fixation	Operative
70.78	Vag susp/fix-grft/prosth	Operative
70.79	Vaginal repair NEC	Operative
70.8	Vaginal vault oblit	Operative
70.9	Oth vag & cul-de-sac ops	Mixed (3, 2)
70.92	Cul-de-sac operation NEC	Operative
70.93	Cul op NEC-graft/prosth	Operative
71.0	Inc vulva & perineum	Operative
71.09	Inc vulva/perineum NEC	Operative
71.1	Vulvar diagnostic px	Operative
71.11	Vulvar biopsy	Operative
71.2	Bartholin's gland ops	Mixed (4, 1)
71.22	Inc Bartholin's gland	Operative
71.3	Loc vulvar/peri exc NEC	Operative
71.4	Operations on clitoris	Operative
71.5	Radical vulvectomy	Operative
71.6	Other vulvectomy	Operative
71.61	Unilateral vulvectomy	Operative
71.7	Vulvar & perineal repair	Operative
71.71	Suture vulvar/peri lac	Operative
71.79	Vulvar/perineum REP NEC	Operative
71.8	Vulvar operations NEC	Operative
71.9	Female genital ops NEC	Operative
72.0	Low forceps operation	Non-Operative
72.1	Low forceps w episiotomy	Non-Operative
72.2	Mid forceps operation	Non-Operative
72.21	Mid forceps w episiotomy	Non-Operative
72.3	High forceps operation	Non-Operative
72.4	Forceps ROT fetal head	Non-Operative
72.5	Breech extraction	Non-Operative
72.54	Tot breech extract NEC	Non-Operative
72.6	Forceps-aftercoming head	Non-Operative
72.7	Vacuum extraction del	Non-Operative
72.71	VED w episiotomy	Non-Operative
72.79	Vacuum extract del NEC	Non-Operative
72.8	Instrumental del NEC	Non-Operative
72.9	Instrumental del NOS	Non-Operative
73.0	Artificial rupt membrane	Non-Operative
73.01	Induction labor by AROM	Non-Operative
73.09	Artif rupt membranes NEC	Non-Operative
73.1	Surg induction labor NEC	Non-Operative
73.2	Int/comb version/extract	Non-Operative
73.3	Failed forceps	Non-Operative
73.4	Medical induction labor	Non-Operative
73.5	Manually assisted del	Non-Operative
73.51	Manual ROT fetal head	Non-Operative
73.59	Manual assisted del NEC	Non-Operative
73.6	Episiotomy	Non-Operative
73.8	Fetal ops-facilitate del	Non-Operative
73.9	Oth ops assisting del	Mixed (2, 3)
74.0	Classical CD	Operative
74.1	Low cervical CD	Operative
74.2	Extraperitoneal CD	Operative
74.3	Rmvl extratubal preg	Operative
74.4	Cesarean section NEC	Operative
74.9	Cesarean section NOS	Operative
74.99	Other CD type NOS	Operative
75.0	Intra-amnio inject-AB	Non-Operative
75.1	Diagnostic amniocentesis	Non-Operative
75.2	Intrauterine transfusion	Non-Operative
75.3	IU ops fetus & amnio NEC	Mixed (1, 7)
75.32	Fetal EKG	Non-Operative
75.34	Fetal monitoring NEC	Non-Operative
75.35	Dxtic px fetus/amnio NEC	Non-Operative
75.37	Amnioinfusion	Non-Operative
75.4	Man rmvl of ret placenta	Non-Operative
75.5	REP current OB lac uter	Operative
75.51	REP current OB lac cerv	Operative
75.6	REP oth current OB lac	Mixed (1, 2)
75.61	REP OB lac blad/urethra	Operative
75.62	REP OB lac rectum/anus	Non-Operative
75.69	REP current OB lac NEC	Non-Operative
75.7	PP manual expl uterus	Non-Operative
75.8	OB tamponade uterus/vag	Non-Operative
75.9	Other obstetrical ops	Mixed (2, 3)
76.0	Facial bone incision	Operative
76.1	Dxtic px facial bone/jt	Operative
76.2	Exc/destr fac bone les	Operative
76.3	Partial facial ostectomy	Operative
76.31	Partial mandibulectomy	Operative
76.39	Part facial ostect NEC	Operative
76.4	Facial bone exc/reconst	Operative
76.5	TMJ arthroplasty	Operative
76.6	Other facial bone repair	Operative
76.62	Open osty mand ramus	Operative
76.64	Mand orthognathic op NEC	Operative
76.65	SEG osteoplasty maxilla	Operative
76.66	Tot osteoplasty maxilla	Operative
76.7	Reduction of facial fx	Mixed (6, 4)
76.72	Open red malar/ZMC fx	Operative
76.74	Open red maxillary fx	Operative
76.75	Clsd red mandibular fx	Non-Operative
76.76	Open red mandibular fx	Operative

Code	Description	Operative Status	Code	Description	Operative Status
76.79	Open red facial fx NEC	Operative	78.63	Rmvl impl dev rad/ulna	Operative
76.9	Oth ops facial bone/jt	Mixed (5, 3)	78.65	Rmvl impl dev femur	Operative
76.91	Bone graft to face bone	Operative	78.67	Rmvl impl dev tib & fib	Operative
76.97	Rmvl int fix face bone	Operative	78.68	Rmvl impl dev MT/tarsal	Operative
77.0	Sequestrectomy	Operative	78.69	Rmvl impl dev site NEC	Operative
77.1	Bone inc NEC w/o div	Operative	78.7	Osteoclasis	Operative
77.2	Wedge osteotomy	Operative	78.8	Other bone diagnostic px	Operative
77.25	Femoral wedge osteotomy	Operative	78.9	Insert bone growth stim	Operative
77.27	Tib & fib wedge osty	Operative	79.0	Clsd fx red w/o int fix	Non-Operative
77.3	Other division of bone	Operative	79.01	Clsd fx red humerus	Non-Operative
77.35	Femoral division NEC	Operative	79.02	Clsd fx red radius/ulna	Non-Operative
77.37	Tibia/fibula div NEC	Operative	79.05	Clsd fx red femur	Non-Operative
77.4	Biopsy of bone	Operative	79.06	Clsd fx red tibia/fibula	Non-Operative
77.41	Chest cage bone biopsy	Operative	79.09	Closed fx reduction NEC	Non-Operative
77.42	Humerus biopsy	Operative	79.1	Clsd fx red w int fix	Operative
77.45	Femoral biopsy	Operative	79.11	CRIF humerus	Operative
77.47	Tibia & fibula biopsy	Operative	79.12	CRIF radius/ulna	Operative
77.48	Metatarsal/tarsal biopsy	Operative	79.13	CRIF MC/carpals	Operative
77.49	Bone biopsy NEC	Operative	79.14	CRIF finger	Operative
77.5	Toe deformity exc/REP	Operative	79.15	CRIF femur	Operative
77.6	Loc exc bone lesion	Operative	79.16	CRIF tibia & fibula	Operative
77.61	Exc chest cage bone les	Operative	79.17	CRIF metatarsal/tarsal	Operative
77.62	Loc exc humerus lesion	Operative	79.2	Open fracture reduction	Operative
77.63	Loc exc radius/ulna les	Operative	79.22	Open red radius/ulna fx	Operative
77.65	Local exc femur lesion	Operative	79.26	Open red tibia/fib fx	Operative
77.67	Loc exc tibia/fibula les	Operative	79.3	Op fx reduction int fix	Operative
77.68	Local exc MT/tarsal les	Operative	79.31	ORIF humerus	Operative
77.69	Loc exc bone lesion NEC	Operative	79.32	ORIF radius/ulna	Operative
77.7	Exc bone for graft	Operative	79.33	ORIF carpals/metacarpals	Operative
77.77	Exc tib/fib for graft	Operative	79.34	ORIF finger	Operative
77.79	Exc bone for graft NEC	Operative	79.35	ORIF femur	Operative
77.8	Other partial ostectomy	Operative	79.36	ORIF tibia & fibula	Operative
77.81	Chest cage ostectomy NEC	Operative	79.37	ORIF metatarsal/tarsal	Operative
77.85	Part ostectomy femur	Operative	79.38	ORIF toe	Operative
77.86	Partial patellectomy	Operative	79.39	ORIF bone NEC X facial	Operative
77.87	Part ostectomy tib/fib	Operative	79.4	CR sep epiphysis	Operative
77.88	Part ostectomy MT/tarsal	Operative	79.5	Open red sep epiphysis	Operative
77.89	Partial ostectomy NEC	Operative	79.56	Op red sep epiph tib/fib	Operative
77.9	Total ostectomy	Operative	79.6	Open fx site debridement	Operative
77.91	Tot chest cage ostectomy	Operative	79.61	Debride open fx humerus	Operative
78.0	Bone graft	Operative	79.62	Debride open fx rad/ulna	Operative
78.05	Bone graft to femur	Operative	79.64	Debride open fx finger	Operative
78.07	Bone graft tibia/fibula	Operative	79.65	Debride open femur fx	Operative
78.1	Appl ext fixator device	Operative	79.66	Debride opn fx tibia/fib	Operative
78.13	Appl ext fix rad/ulna	Operative	79.67	Debride opn fx MT/tarsal	Operative
78.15	Appl ext fix dev femur	Operative	79.7	Closed red dislocation	Non-Operative
78.17	Appl ext fix dev tib/fib	Operative	79.71	Clsd red shoulder disloc	Non-Operative
78.2	Limb shortening px	Operative	79.72	Clsd red elbow disloc	Non-Operative
78.25	Limb short px femur	Operative	79.74	Clsd red hand/finger DIS	Non-Operative
78.3	Limb lengthening px	Operative	79.75	Clsd red hip disloc	Non-Operative
78.35	Limb length px femur	Operative	79.76	Clsd red knee disloc	Non-Operative
78.4	Other bone repair	Operative	79.8	Open red dislocation	Operative
78.45	Femoral repair NEC	Operative	79.85	Open red hip disloc	Operative
78.47	Tibia/fibula repair NEC	Operative	79.87	Open red ankle disloc	Operative
78.5	Int fix w/o fx reduction	Operative	79.9	Bone injury op NOS	Operative
78.52	Int fix w/o red humerus	Operative	80.0	Arthrotomy rmvl prosth	Operative
78.55	Int fix w/o red femur	Operative	80.05	Rmvl prosth hip inc	Operative
78.57	Int fix w/o red tib/fib	Operative	80.06	Rmvl prosth knee inc	Operative
78.59	Int fix w/o fx red NEC	Operative	80.1	Other arthrotomy	Operative
78.6	Rmvl impl dev from bone	Operative	80.11	Arthrotomy NEC shoulder	Operative
78.62	Rmvl impl dev humerus	Operative	80.12	Arthrotomy NEC elbow	Operative

Code	Description	Operative Status	Code	Description	Operative Status
0.13	Arthrotomy NEC wrist	Operative	81.53	Hip repl revision NOS	Operative
0.14	Arthrotomy NEC hand/fing	Operative	81.54	Total knee replacement	Operative
0.15	Arthrotomy NEC hip	Operative	81.55	Knee repl revision NOS	Operative
0.16	Arthrotomy NEC knee	Operative	81.56	Total ankle replacement	Operative
0.17	Arthrotomy NEC ankle	Operative	81.6	Oth spinal procedures	Mixed (2, 3)
0.2	Arthroscopy	Operative	81.65	Vertebroplasty	Operative
0.21	Shoulder arthroscopy	Operative	81.66	Kyphoplasty	Operative
0.26	Knee arthroscopy	Operative	81.7	Hand/finger arthroplasty	Operative
0.3	Biopsy joint structure	Non-Operative	81.8	Should/elb arthroplasty	Operative
0.36	Knee joint biopsy	Non-Operative	81.80	Total shoulder repl	Operative
0.39	Joint biopsy NEC	Non-Operative	81.81	Partial shoulder repl	Operative
0.4	Jt capsule/LIG/cart div	Operative	81.82	Recur should disloc REP	Operative
0.46	Knee structure division	Operative	81.83	Should arthroplasty NEC	Operative
0.5	IV disc exc/destruction	Mixed (3, 1)	81.84	Total elbow replacement	Operative
0.50	IV disc exc/destr NOS	Operative	81.85	Elbow arthroplasty NEC	Operative
0.51	IV disc excision	Operative	81.9	Other joint structure op	Mixed (7, 2)
0.6	Exc knee semilunar cart	Operative	81.91	Arthrocentesis	Non-Operative
0.7	Synovectomy	Operative	81.92	Injection into joint	Non-Operative
0.76	Knee synovectomy	Operative	81.97	Rev joint repl UE	Operative
0.8	Oth exc/destr joint les	Operative	82.0	Inc hand soft tissue	Mixed (4, 1)
0.81	Exc/destr should les NEC	Operative	82.01	Expl tendon sheath hand	Operative
0.82	Exc/destr elbow les NEC	Operative	82.09	Inc soft tissue hand NEC	Operative
0.84	Exc/destr hand les NEC	Operative	82.1	Div hand musc/tend/fasc	Operative
0.85	Exc/destr hip lesion NEC	Operative	82.2	Exc les hand soft tissue	Operative
0.86	Exc/destr knee les NEC	Operative	82.29	Exc les sft tiss hnd NEC	Operative
0.87	Exc/destr ankle les NEC	Operative	82.3	Oth exc hand soft tissue	Operative
0.88	Exc/destr ft jt les NEC	Operative	82.33	Hand tenonectomy NEC	Operative
0.9	Other joint excision	Operative	82.4	Suture hand soft tissue	Operative
0.99	Excision of joint NEC	Operative	82.44	Sut flexor tend hand NEC	Operative
31.0	Spinal fusion	Operative	82.45	Suture hand tendon NEC	Operative
31.00	Spinal fusion NOS	Operative	82.5	Hand musc/tend transpl	Operative
31.01	Atlas-axis spinal fusion	Operative	82.6	Reconstruction of thumb	Operative
31.02	Ant cervical fusion NEC	Operative	82.7	Plastic op hnd grft/impl	Operative
31.03	Post cervical fusion NEC	Operative	82.8	Other plastic ops hand	Operative
31.04	Anterior dorsal fusion	Operative	82.9	Oth hand soft tissue ops	Mixed (2, 5)
31.05	Posterior dorsal fusion	Operative	83.0	Inc musc/tend/fasc/bursa	Operative
31.06	Anterior lumbar fusion	Operative	83.02	Myotomy	Operative
31.07	Lat trans lumbar fusion	Operative	83.03	Bursotomy	Operative
31.08	Posterior lumbar fusion	Operative	83.09	Soft tissue incision NEC	Operative
31.1	Foot & ankle arthrodesis	Operative	83.1	Musc/tend/fasc division	Operative
31.11	Ankle fusion	Operative	83.12	Adductor tenotomy of hip	Operative
31.12	Triple arthrodesis	Operative	83.13	Tenotomy NEC	Operative
31.13	Subtalar fusion	Operative	83.14	Fasciotomy	Operative
31.2	Arthrodesis of oth joint	Operative	83.2	Soft tissue dxtic px	Operative
31.22	Arthrodesis of knee	Operative	83.21	Soft tissue biopsy	Operative
31.3	Spinal refusion	Operative	83.3	Exc lesion soft tissue	Operative
31.32	Ant cerv refusion NEC	Operative	83.32	Exc muscle lesion	Operative
31.33	Post cerv refusion NEC	Operative	83.39	Exc les soft tissue NEC	Operative
31.35	Post dorsal refusion	Operative	83.4	Other exc musc/tend/fasc	Operative
31.36	Ant lumbar refusion	Operative	83.42	Tenonectomy NEC	Operative
31.37	Lat trans lumb refusion	Operative	83.44	Fasciectomy NEC	Operative
31.38	Post lumbar refusion	Operative	83.45	Myectomy NEC	Operative
31.4	Other low limb joint REP	Operative	83.49	Soft tissue exc NEC	Operative
31.40	Hip repair NEC	Operative	83.5	Bursectomy	Operative
31.44	Patellar stabilization	Operative	83.6	Suture musc/tendon/fasc	Operative
31.45	Cruciate LIG repair NEC	Operative	83.61	Tendon sheath suture	Operative
31.47	Repair of knee NEC	Operative	83.63	Rotator cuff repair	Operative
31.49	Repair of ankle NEC	Operative	83.64	Suture of tendon NEC	Operative
31.5	Joint repl lower EXT	Operative	83.65	Muscle/fasc suture NEC	Operative
31.51	Total hip replacement	Operative	83.7	Muscle/tendon reconst	Operative
31.52	Partial hip replacement	Operative	83.72	Tendon recession	Operative

Code	Description	Operative Status	Code	Description	Operative Status
83.75	Tendon transf/transpl	Operative	86.04	Skin & subcu I&D NEC	Non-Operative
83.8	Musc/tend/fasc op NEC	Operative	86.05	Inc w rmvl FB/dev skin	Non-Operative
83.81	Tendon graft	Operative	86.06	Insertion infusion pump	Operative
83.82	Muscle or fascia graft	Operative	86.07	VAD insertion	Non-Operative
83.85	Change in m/t length NEC	Operative	86.09	Skin/subcu incision NEC	Non-Operative
83.86	Quadricepsplasty	Operative	86.1	Skin & subcu dxtic px	Non-Operative
83.88	Plastic ops tendon NEC	Operative	86.11	Skin & subcu biopsy	Non-Operative
83.9	Other conn tissue ops	Mixed (4, 5)	86.2	Exc/destr skin lesion	Mixed (3, 5)
83.94	Aspiration of bursa	Non-Operative	86.21	Excision pilonidal cyst	Operative
83.95	Soft tissue asp NEC	Non-Operative	86.22	Exc debride WND/infect	Operative
83.96	Injection into bursa	Non-Operative	86.23	Nail removal	Non-Operative
84.0	Amputation of upper limb	Operative	86.26	Lig dermal appendage	Non-Operative
84.01	Finger amputation	Operative	86.27	Debridement of nail	Non-Operative
84.02	Thumb amputation	Operative	86.28	Nonexc debridement wound	Non-Operative
84.1	Amputation of lower limb	Operative	86.3	Loc exc/destr skin NEC	Non-Operative
84.11	Toe amputation	Operative	86.4	RAD excision skin lesion	Operative
84.12	Amputation through foot	Operative	86.5	Skin/subcu suture/close	Non-Operative
84.15	BK amputation NEC	Operative	86.59	Skin closure NEC	Non-Operative
84.17	Above knee amputation	Operative	86.6	Free skin graft	Mixed (8, 1)
84.2	Extremity reattachment	Operative	86.62	Hand skin graft NEC	Operative
84.3	Amputation stump rev	Operative	86.63	Fthick skin graft NEC	Operative
84.4	Impl or fit prosth limb	Mixed (3, 6)	86.65	Heterograft to skin	Operative
84.5	Impl oth MS dev & subst	Mixed (1, 7)	86.66	Homograft to skin	Operative
84.6	Spinal disc replacement	Operative	86.67	Dermal regenerative grft	Operative
84.62	Insert tot C IVD prosth	Operative	86.69	Free skin graft NEC	Operative
84.65	Insert tot LS IVD prosth	Operative	86.7	Pedicle grafts or flaps	Operative
84.7	Adjunct code ext fix dev	Non-Operative	86.70	Pedicle/flap graft NOS	Operative
84.8	Insert/repl/rev spin dev	Operative	86.72	Pedicle graft adv	Operative
84.80	Ins/repl intsp proc dev	Operative	86.73	Attach pedicle to hand	Operative
84.9	Other musculoskeletal op	Operative	86.74	Attach pedicle graft NEC	Operative
85.0	Mastotomy	Non-Operative	86.75	Rev pedicle/flap graft	Operative
85.1	Breast diagnostic px	Mixed (1, 2)	86.8	Other skin & subcu REP	Operative
85.11	PERC breast biopsy	Non-Operative	86.82	Facial rhytidectomy	Operative
85.12	Open biopsy of breast	Operative	86.83	Size red plastic op	Operative
85.2	Exc/destr breast tissue	Operative	86.89	Skin REP & reconst NEC	Operative
85.21	Local exc breast lesion	Operative	86.9	Other skin & subcu ops	Mixed (7, 2)
85.23	Subtotal mastectomy	Operative	86.94	Ins 1 array neurstim gen	Operative
85.3	Red mammoplasty/ectomy	Operative	87.0	Head/neck sft tiss x-ray	Non-Operative
85.32	Bilat red mammoplasty	Operative	87.02	Brain/skull contr x-ray	Non-Operative
85.34	Uni subcu mammectomy NEC	Operative	87.03	CAT scan head	Non-Operative
85.36	Bilat subcu mammect NEC	Operative	87.04	Head tomography NEC	Non-Operative
85.4	Mastectomy	Operative	87.1	Other head/neck x-ray	Non-Operative
85.41	Unilat simple mastectomy	Operative	87.2	X-ray of spine	Non-Operative
85.42	Bilat simple mastectomy	Operative	87.21	Contrast myelogram	Non-Operative
85.43	Unilat exten simple MAST	Operative	87.3	Thorax soft tissue x-ray	Non-Operative
85.44	Bilat exten simple MAST	Operative	87.39	Thor soft tiss x-ray NEC	Non-Operative
85.45	Unilat RAD mastectomy	Operative	87.4	Other x-ray of thorax	Non-Operative
85.5	Augmentation mammoplasty	Mixed (3, 2)	87.41	CAT scan thorax	Non-Operative
85.6	Mastopexy	Operative	87.44	Routine chest x-ray	Non-Operative
85.7	Total breast reconst	Operative	87.49	Chest x-ray NEC	Non-Operative
85.8	Other breast repair	Mixed (7, 1)	87.5	Biliary tract x-ray	Mixed (1, 4)
85.84	Breast pedicle graft	Operative	87.51	PERC hepat cholangiogram	Non-Operative
85.85	Breast muscle flap graft	Operative	87.53	Intraop cholangiogram	Operative
85.89	Mammoplasty NEC	Operative	87.54	Cholangiogram NEC	Non-Operative
85.9	Other breast operations	Mixed (5, 2)	87.6	Oth digestive syst x-ray	Non-Operative
85.91	Aspiration of breast	Non-Operative	87.61	Barium swallow	Non-Operative
85.94	Breast implant removal	Operative	87.62	Upper GI series	Non-Operative
85.96	Rmvl brst tiss expander	Operative	87.69	Digest tract x-ray NEC	Non-Operative
86.0	Incision skin & subcu	Mixed (1, 7)	87.7	X-ray of urinary system	Non-Operative
86.01	Aspiration skin & subcu	Non-Operative	87.71	CAT scan of kidney	Non-Operative
86.03	Incision pilonidal sinus	Non-Operative	87.73	IV pyelogram	Non-Operative

Code	Description	Operative Status	Code	Description	Operative Status
7.74	Retrograde pyelogram	Non-Operative	89.38	Respiratory measure NEC	Non-Operative
7.75	Percutaneous pyelogram	Non-Operative	89.39	Nonoperative exams NEC	Non-Operative
7.76	Retro cystourethrogram	Non-Operative	89.4	Card stress/device check	Non-Operative
7.77	Cystogram NEC	Non-Operative	89.41	Treadmill stress test	Non-Operative
7.79	Urinary system x-ray NEC	Non-Operative	89.44	CV stress test NEC	Non-Operative
7.8	Female genital x-ray	Non-Operative	89.45	Pacemaker rate check	Non-Operative
7.9	Male genital x-ray	Non-Operative	89.49	AICD check	Non-Operative
8.0	Abd soft tissue x-ray	Non-Operative	89.5	Other cardiac funct test	Non-Operative
8.01	Abdomen CAT scan	Non-Operative	89.50	Ambulatory card monitor	Non-Operative
8.1	Other abdominal x-ray	Non-Operative	89.52	Electrocardiogram	Non-Operative
8.11	Pelv dye contrast x-ray	Non-Operative	89.54	ECG monitoring	Non-Operative
8.2	EXT & pelvis skel x-ray	Non-Operative	89.59	Nonop card/vasc exam NEC	Non-Operative
8.3	Other x-ray	Non-Operative	89.6	Circulatory monitoring	Non-Operative
8.38	CAT scan NEC	Non-Operative	89.61	Art pressure monitoring	Non-Operative
8.4	Contrast arteriography	Non-Operative	89.62	CVP monitoring	Non-Operative
8.41	Cerebral arteriogram	Non-Operative	89.64	PA wedge monitoring	Non-Operative
8.42	Contrast aortogram	Non-Operative	89.65	Arterial bld gas measure	Non-Operative
8.43	Pulmonary arteriogram	Non-Operative	89.68	Cardiac output MON NEC	Non-Operative
8.44	Thor arteriogram NEC	Non-Operative	89.7	General physical exam	Non-Operative
8.45	Renal arteriogram	Non-Operative	89.8	Autopsy	Non-Operative
8.47	Abd arteriogram NEC	Non-Operative	90.0	Micro exam-nervous syst	Non-Operative
8.48	Contrast arteriogram-leg	Non-Operative	90.1	Micro exam-endocrine	Non-Operative
8.49	Contrast arteriogram NEC	Non-Operative	90.2	Micro exam-eye	Non-Operative
8.5	Contrast angiocardiogram	Non-Operative	90.3	Micro exam-ENT/larynx	Non-Operative
8.51	VC angiocardiogram	Non-Operative	90.4	Micro exam-lower resp	Non-Operative
8.53	Lt heart angiocardiogram	Non-Operative	90.5	Micro exam-blood	Non-Operative
8.56	Cor arteriogram-2 cath	Non-Operative	90.52	Culture-blood	Non-Operative
8.57	Coronary arteriogram NEC	Non-Operative	90.6	Micro exam-spleen/marrow	Non-Operative
8.6	Phlebography	Non-Operative	90.7	Micro exam-lymph system	Non-Operative
8.66	Contrast phlebogram-leg	Non-Operative	90.8	Micro exam-upper GI	Non-Operative
8.67	Contrast phlebogram NEC	Non-Operative	90.9	Micro exam-lower GI	Non-Operative
8.7	Diagnostic ultrasound	Non-Operative	91.0	Micro exam-bil/pancreas	Non-Operative
8.71	Head & neck ultrasound	Non-Operative	91.1	Micro exam-peritoneum	Non-Operative
8.72	Heart ultrasound	Non-Operative	91.2	Micro exam-upper urinary	Non-Operative
8.73	Thorax ultrasound NEC	Non-Operative	91.3	Micro exam-lower urinary	Non-Operative
8.74	Digest system ultrasound	Non-Operative	91.4	Micro exam-female genit	Non-Operative
8.75	Urinary syst ultrasound	Non-Operative	91.5	Micro exam-MS/jt fluid	Non-Operative
8.76	Abd & retroperiton US	Non-Operative	91.6	Micro exam-integument	Non-Operative
8.77	Periph vasc ultrasound	Non-Operative	91.7	Micro exam-op wound	Non-Operative
8.78	Gravid uterus ultrasound	Non-Operative	91.8	Micro exam NEC	Non-Operative
8.79	Ultrasound NEC	Non-Operative	91.9	Micro exam NOS	Non-Operative
8.8	Thermography	Non-Operative	92.0	Isotope scan & function	Non-Operative
8.9	Other diagnostic imaging	Non-Operative	92.02	Liver scan/isotope funct	Non-Operative
8.91	Brain & brain stem MRI	Non-Operative	92.03	Renal scan/isotope study	Non-Operative
8.93	Spinal canal MRI	Non-Operative	92.04	GI scan & isotope study	Non-Operative
8.94	Musculoskeletal MRI	Non-Operative	92.05	CV scan/isotope study	Non-Operative
8.95	Pelvis/pros/bladder MRI	Non-Operative	92.1	Other radioisotope scan	Non-Operative
8.97	MRI site NEC & NOS	Non-Operative	92.14	Bone scan	Non-Operative
9.0	Dx interview/consul/exam	Non-Operative	92.15	Pulmonary scan	Non-Operative
9.03	Compr interview/eval	Non-Operative	92.18	Total body scan	Non-Operative
9.06	Limited consultation	Non-Operative	92.19	Scan of site NEC	Non-Operative
9.1	Nervous system exams	Non-Operative	92.2	Ther radiology & nu med	Mixed (1, 9)
9.14	Electroencephalogram	Non-Operative	92.24	Photon teleradiotherapy	Non-Operative
9.15	Neuro function test NEC	Non-Operative	92.27	Radioactive element impl	Operative
9.17	Polysomnogram	Non-Operative	92.28	Isotope inject/instill	Non-Operative
9.19	Video/telemetric EEG MON	Non-Operative	92.29	Radiotherapeutic px NEC	Non-Operative
9.2	GU system-examination	Non-Operative	92.3	Stereotactic radiosurg	Non-Operative
9.22	Cystometrogram	Non-Operative	92.32	Multi-source photon surg	Non-Operative
9.29	GU system exams NEC	Non-Operative	92.4	Intra-op radiation px	Non-Operative
9.3	Other examinations	Non-Operative	93.0	Dxtic physical Tx	Non-Operative
9.37	Vital capacity	Non-Operative	93.01	Functional PT evaluation	Non-Operative

Code	Description	Operative Status	Code	Description	Operative Status
93.08	Electromyography	Non-Operative	95.1	Form & struct eye exam	Non-Operative
93.1	PT exercises	Non-Operative	95.2	Objective funct eye test	Non-Operative
93.16	Joint mobilization NEC	Non-Operative	95.3	Special vision services	Non-Operative
93.2	Oth PT MS manipulation	Non-Operative	95.4	Nonop hearing procedure	Non-Operative
93.22	Amb & gait training	Non-Operative	95.41	Audiometry	Non-Operative
93.26	Manual rupt joint adhes	Non-Operative	95.42	Clinical hearing test	Non-Operative
93.3	Other PT therapeutic px	Non-Operative	95.43	Audiological evaluation	Non-Operative
93.38	Combined PT NOS	Non-Operative	95.46	Auditory & vest test NEC	Non-Operative
93.39	Physical therapy NEC	Non-Operative	95.47	Hearing examination NOS	Non-Operative
93.4	Skeletal & oth traction	Non-Operative	95.49	Nonop hearing px NEC	Non-Operative
93.5	Oth immob/press/WND attn	Non-Operative	96.0	Nonop GI & resp intub	Non-Operative
93.52	Neck support application	Non-Operative	96.04	Insert endotracheal tube	Non-Operative
93.53	Cast application NEC	Non-Operative	96.05	Resp tract intub NEC	Non-Operative
93.54	Application of splint	Non-Operative	96.07	Insert gastric tube NEC	Non-Operative
93.56	Pressure dressing appl	Non-Operative	96.08	Insert intestinal tube	Non-Operative
93.57	Appl wound dressing NEC	Non-Operative	96.09	Insert rectal tube	Non-Operative
93.59	Immob/press/WND attn NEC	Non-Operative	96.1	Other nonop insertion	Non-Operative
93.6	Osteopathic manipulation	Non-Operative	96.2	Nonop dilation & manip	Non-Operative
93.67	OMT NEC	Non-Operative	96.27	Manual reduction hernia	Non-Operative
93.7	Speech/read/blind rehab	Non-Operative	96.29	Alimentary intuss red	Non-Operative
93.75	Speech therapy NEC	Non-Operative	96.3	Nonop GI irrig/instill	Non-Operative
93.8	Other rehab therapy	Non-Operative	96.33	Gastric lavage	Non-Operative
93.81	Recreational therapy	Non-Operative	96.35	Gastric gavage	Non-Operative
93.83	Occupational therapy	Non-Operative	96.38	Impacted feces removal	Non-Operative
93.89	Rehabilitation NEC	Non-Operative	96.4	Digest/GU irrig/instill	Non-Operative
93.9	Respiratory therapy	Non-Operative	96.48	Indwell cath irrig NEC	Non-Operative
93.90	CPAP	Non-Operative	96.49	GU instillation NEC	Non-Operative
93.91	IPPB	Non-Operative	96.5	Other nonop irrig/clean	Non-Operative
93.93	Nonmech resuscitation	Non-Operative	96.52	Irrigation of ear	Non-Operative
93.94	Nebulizer therapy	Non-Operative	96.56	Bronch/trach lavage NEC	Non-Operative
93.95	Hyperbaric oxygenation	Non-Operative	96.59	Wound irrigation NEC	Non-Operative
93.96	Oxygen enrichment NEC	Non-Operative	96.6	Enteral nutrition	Non-Operative
93.99	Respiratory therapy NEC	Non-Operative	96.7	Cont mech vent NEC	Non-Operative
94.0	Psych eval & testing	Non-Operative	96.71	Cont mech vent-<96 hours	Non-Operative
94.1	Psych eval/consult	Non-Operative	96.72	Cont mech vent->95 hours	Non-Operative
94.11	Psych mental status	Non-Operative	97.0	GI appliance replacement	Non-Operative
94.19	Psych interview/eval NEC	Non-Operative	97.02	Repl gastrostomy tube	Non-Operative
94.2	Psych somatotherapy	Non-Operative	97.03	Repl small intest tube	Non-Operative
94.22	Lithium therapy	Non-Operative	97.05	Repl panc/biliary stent	Non-Operative
94.23	Neuroleptic therapy	Non-Operative	97.1	Repl MS appliance	Non-Operative
94.25	Psych drug therapy NEC	Non-Operative	97.2	Other nonop replacement	Non-Operative
94.27	Electroshock therapy NEC	Non-Operative	97.23	Repl TRACH tube	Non-Operative
94.3	Individual psychotherapy	Non-Operative	97.3	Rmvl ther dev-head/neck	Non-Operative
94.37	Expl verbal psychTx	Non-Operative	97.37	Rmvl tracheostomy tube	Non-Operative
94.38	Supp verbal psychTx	Non-Operative	97.4	Rmvl thor ther device	Non-Operative
94.39	Individual psychTx NEC	Non-Operative	97.49	Rmvl dev from thorax NEC	Non-Operative
94.4	Oth psychTx/counselling	Non-Operative	97.5	Nonop rmvl GI ther dev	Non-Operative
94.44	Group therapy NEC	Non-Operative	97.51	Rmvl gastrostomy tube	Non-Operative
94.49	Counselling NEC	Non-Operative	97.55	Rmvl biliary/liver tube	Non-Operative
94.5	Referral psych rehab	Non-Operative	97.6	Nonop rmvl urin ther dev	Non-Operative
94.6	Alcohol/drug rehab/detox	Non-Operative	97.62	Rmvl ureteral drain	Non-Operative
94.61	Alcohol rehabilitation	Non-Operative	97.7	Rmvl ther dev genit syst	Non-Operative
94.62	Alcohol detoxification	Non-Operative	97.71	Removal IUD	Non-Operative
94.63	Alcohol rehab/detox	Non-Operative	97.8	Oth nonop rmvl ther dev	Non-Operative
94.64	Drug rehabilitation	Non-Operative	97.89	Rmvl therapeutic dev NEC	Non-Operative
94.65	Drug detoxification	Non-Operative	98.0	Rmvl intralum GI FB	Non-Operative
94.66	Drug rehab/detox	Non-Operative	98.02	Rmvl intralum esoph FB	Non-Operative
94.67	ALC/drug rehabilitation	Non-Operative	98.1	Rmvl intralum FB NEC	Non-Operative
94.68	ALC/drug detoxification	Non-Operative	98.15	Rmvl intralum trach FB	Non-Operative
94.69	ALC/drug rehab/detox	Non-Operative	98.2	Rmvl oth FB w/o inc	Non-Operative
95.0	Gen/subjective eye exam	Mixed (1, 7)	98.5	ESWL	Non-Operative

Code	Description	Operative Status	Code	Description	Operative Status
8.51	Renal/ureter/blad ESWL	Non-Operative	99.29	Inject/infuse NEC	Non-Operative
9.0	Blood transfusion	Non-Operative	99.3	Prophyl vacc-bact dis	Non-Operative
9.01	Exchange transfusion	Non-Operative	99.36	Diphtheria toxoid admin	Non-Operative
9.03	Whole blood transfus NEC	Non-Operative	99.38	Tetanus toxoid admin	Non-Operative
9.04	Packed cell transfusion	Non-Operative	99.4	Viral immunization	Non-Operative
9.05	Platelet transfusion	Non-Operative	99.5	Other immunization	Non-Operative
9.06	Coag factor transfusion	Non-Operative	99.52	Influenza vaccination	Non-Operative
9.07	Serum transfusion NEC	Non-Operative	99.55	Vaccination NEC	Non-Operative
9.09	Transfusion NEC	Non-Operative	99.59	Vacc/inoculation NEC	Non-Operative
9.1	Inject/infuse ther subst	Non-Operative	99.6	Card rhythm conversion	Non-Operative
9.10	Inject thrombolytic	Non-Operative	99.60	CPR NOS	Non-Operative
9.11	Inject Rh immune glob	Non-Operative	99.61	Atrial cardioversion	Non-Operative
9.14	Inject/infuse gamma glob	Non-Operative	99.62	Heart countershock NEC	Non-Operative
9.15	Parenteral nutrition	Non-Operative	99.69	Cardiac rhythm conv NEC	Non-Operative
9.17	Inject insulin	Non-Operative	99.7	Ther apheresis/admin NEC	Non-Operative
9.18	Inject electrolytes	Non-Operative	99.71	Ther plasmapheresis	Non-Operative
9.19	Inject anticoagulant	Non-Operative	99.74	Ther plateletpheresis	Non-Operative
9.2	Oth inject ther subst	Non-Operative	99.79	Ther apheresis NEC	Non-Operative
9.20	Inject platelet inhib	Non-Operative	99.8	Misc physical procedures	Non-Operative
9.21	Inject antibiotic	Non-Operative	99.82	UV light therapy	Non-Operative
9.22	Inject anti-infect NEC	Non-Operative	99.83	Phototherapy NEC	Non-Operative
9.23	Inject steroid	Non-Operative	99.84	Isolation	Non-Operative
9.25	Inject CA chemo agent	Non-Operative	99.88	Ther photopheresis	Non-Operative
9.26	Inject tranquilizer	Non-Operative	99.9	Other misc procedures	Non-Operative
9.28	Inject BRM/antineo agent	Non-Operative	99.99	Misc procedures NEC	Non-Operative

GLOSSARY

Average Length of Stay Calculated from the admission and discharge dates by counting the day of admission as the first day; the day of discharge is not included. The average is figured by adding the lengths of stay for each patient and then dividing by the total number of patients. Patients discharged on the day of admission are counted as staying one day in the calculation of average length of stay. Patients with stays over 99 days (>99) are excluded from this calculation.

Distribution Percentiles A length of stay percentile for a stratified group of patients is determined by arranging the individual patient stays from low to high. Counting up from the lowest stay to the point where one-half of the patients have been counted yields the value of the 50th percentile. Counting one-tenth of the total patients gives the 10th percentile, and so on. The 10th, 25th, 50th, 75th, 90th, 95th, and 99th percentiles of stay are displayed in days. If, for example, the 10th percentile for a group of patients is four, then 10 percent of the patients stayed four days or less. The 50th percentile is the median. Any percentile with a value of 100 days or more is listed as >99. Patients who were hospitalized more than 99 days (>99) are not included in the total patients, average stay, and variance categories. The percentiles, however, do include these patients.

Multiple Diagnoses Patients Patients are classified in the multiple diagnoses category if they had at least one valid secondary diagnosis in addition to the principal one. The following codes are not considered valid secondary diagnoses for purposes of this classification

1. Manifestation codes (conditions that evolved from underlying diseases [etiology] and are in italics in ICD-9-CM, Volume 1)

2. Codes V27.0-V27.9 (outcome of delivery)

3. E Codes (external causes of injury and poisoning)

Observed Patients The number of patients in the stratified group as reported in our projected inpatient database. Patients with stays longer than 99 days (>99) are not included. This data element does not use the projection factor.

Operated Patients In the diagnosis tables, operated patients are those who had at least one procedure that is classified by CMS as an operating room procedure. CMS physician panels classify every ICD-9-CM procedure code according to whether the procedure would in most hospitals be performed in the operating room. This classification system differs slightly from that used in Length of Stay publications published previous to 1995, in which patients were categorized as operated if any of their procedures were labeled as Uniform Hospital Discharge Data Set (UHDDS) Class 1. Appendix C contains a list of procedure codes included in this book and their CMS-defined operative status.

Variance A measure of the spread of the data around the average, the variance shows how much individual patient lengths of stay from the average. The smallest variance is zero, indicating that all lengths of stay are equal. In tables in which there is a large variance and the patient group size is relatively small, the average stay may appear high. This sometimes occurs when one or two patients with long hospitalizations fall into the group.

ALPHABETIC INDEX

This index provides an alphabetical listing by descriptive title for all chapter ICD-9-CM diagnoses and procedures codes included in the book. For ease of use, titles are grouped into major classification chapters (i.e., *Diseases of the Circulatory System*). These classification chapters are listed for your reference below.

ICD-9-CM Classification Chapters

Procedure Chapters

Procedure Codes

Procedure Codes

Procedure Codes

Procedure Codes

Procedure Codes

Code	Description	Page	Code	Description	Pag
64.0	Circumcision	277	65.0	Oophorotomy	28
63.4	Epididymectomy	275	71.4	Operations on clitoris	31
63.2	Exc epididymis cyst	275	66.3	Oth bilat FALL destr/exc	28
63.3	Exc sperm cord les NEC	275	70.9	Oth vag & cul-de-sac ops	30
63.1	Exc spermatic varicocele	275	66.9	Other fallopian tube ops	29
61.2	Excision of hydrocele	271	69.9	Other ops uterus/adnexa	30
60.0	Incision of prostate	266	65.9	Other ovarian operations	28
62.0	Incision of testis	272	67.6	Other repair of cervix	29
62.7	Insert testicular prosth	274	66.6	Other salpingectomy	28
64.2	Loc exc/destr penile les	277	70.7	Other vaginal repair	30
62.5	Orchiopexy	273	71.6	Other vulvectomy	31
61.9	Oth scrot/tunica vag ops	272	69.3	Paracerv uterine denerv	30
63.9	Oth sperm cord/epid ops	277	68.8	Pelvic evisceration	29
64.9	Other male genital ops	279	68.6	Radical abd hysterectomy	29
60.6	Other prostatectomy	269	68.7	Radical vag hysterectomy	29
60.9	Other prostatic ops	270	71.5	Radical vulvectomy	31
62.9	Other testicular ops	274	66.7	Repair of fallopian tube	29
64.4	Penile REP/plastic ops	278	65.7	Repair of ovary	28
64.1	Penile diagnostic px	277	66.0	Salpingostomy/salpingot	28
60.8	Periprostatic inc or exc	270	68.3	Subtot abd hysterectomy	29
60.1	Pros/sem vesicl dxtic px	267	66.5	Tot bilat salpingectomy	28
60.5	Radical prostatectomy	268	66.4	Tot unilat salpingectomy	28
60.4	Retropubic prostatectomy	268	68.4	Total abd hysterectomy	29
61.3	Scrotal les exc/destr	271	65.8	Tubo-ovarian ADHESIO	28
61.0	Scrotum & tunica vag I&D	270	65.4	Unilateral S-O	28
61.4	Scrotum & tunica vag REP	271	65.3	Unilateral oophorectomy	28
61.1	Scrotum/tunica dxtic px	271	68.1	Uter/adnexa dxtic px	29
60.7	Seminal vesicle ops	269	69.0	Uterine D&C	29
64.5	Sex transformation NEC	278	68.2	Uterine les exc/destr	29
63.5	Sperm cord/epid repair	276	69.4	Uterine repair	30
63.0	Spermatic cord dxtic px	274	69.2	Uterine supp struct REP	30
60.3	Suprapubic prostatectomy	268	70.2	Vag/cul-de-sac dxtic px	30
60.2	TU prostatectomy	267	70.6	Vaginal constr/reconst	30
62.1	Testes dxtic px	272	68.5	Vaginal hysterectomy	29
62.6	Testes repair	274	70.4	Vaginal obliteration	30
62.2	Testicular les exc/destr	272	70.8	Vaginal vault oblit	30
62.3	Unilateral orchiectomy	273	71.7	Vulvar & perineal repair	31
63.8	Vas def & epid repair	276	71.1	Vulvar diagnostic px	31
63.7	Vasectomy & vas def lig	276	71.8	Vulvar operations NEC	31
63.6	Vasotomy	276			

OPERATIONS ON THE FEMALE GENITAL ORGANS (65-71)

Code	Description	Page
67.4	Amputation of cervix	292
69.5	Asp curettage uterus	301
71.2	Bartholin's gland ops	311
66.2	Bilat endo occl FALL	287
65.6	Bilat salpingo-oophorect	283
65.5	Bilateral oophorectomy	283
67.0	Cervical canal dilation	291
67.1	Cervical diagnostic px	291
67.2	Conization of cervix	292
70.0	Culdocentesis	303
70.5	Cystocele/rectocele REP	305
65.1	Dxtic px on ovaries	280
67.3	Exc/destr cerv les NEC	292
69.1	Exc/destr uter/supp les	300
66.8	FALL tube insufflation	290
66.1	Fallopian tube dxtic px	286
71.9	Female genital ops NEC	313
68.9	Hysterectomy NEC & NOS	298
68.0	Hysterotomy	293
70.1	Inc vagina & cul-de-sac	303
71.0	Inc vulva & perineum	310
69.7	Insertion of IUD	302
67.5	Int cervical os repair	292
65.2	Loc exc/destr ovary les	281
70.3	Loc exc/destr vag/cul	304
71.3	Loc vulvar/peri exc NEC	311
69.6	Menstrual extraction	302

OBSTETRICAL PROCEDURES (72-75)

Code	Description	Pag
73.0	Artificial rupt membrane	3
72.5	Breech extraction	3
74.4	Cesarean section NEC	32
74.9	Cesarean section NOS	32
74.0	Classical CD	32
75.1	Diagnostic amniocentesis	32
73.6	Episiotomy	32
74.2	Extraperitoneal CD	32
73.3	Failed forceps	3
73.8	Fetal ops-facilitate del	3
72.4	Forceps ROT fetal head	3
72.6	Forceps-aftercoming head	3
72.3	High forceps operation	3
75.3	IU ops fetus & amnio NEC	32
72.8	Instrumental del NEC	3
72.9	Instrumental del NOS	3
73.2	Int/comb version/extract	3
75.0	Intra-amnio inject-AB	3
75.2	Intrauterine transfusion	32
74.1	Low cervical CD	32
72.0	Low forceps operation	3
72.1	Low forceps w episiotomy	3
75.4	Man rmvl of ret placenta	32
73.5	Manually assisted del	3
73.4	Medical induction labor	3
72.2	Mid forceps operation	3
75.8	OB tamponade uterus/vag	3
73.9	Oth ops assisting del	32

Procedure Codes